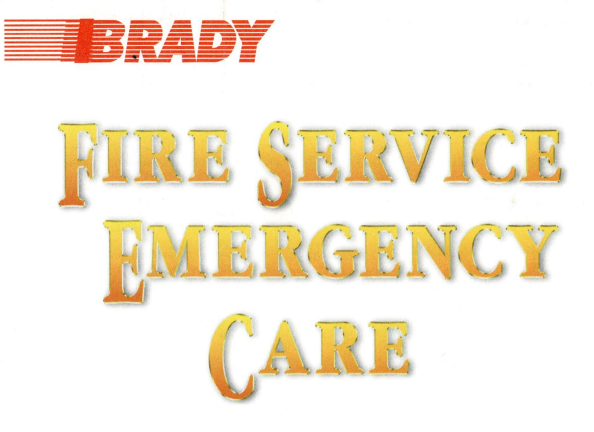

FIRE SERVICE EMERGENCY CARE

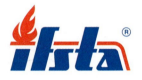

Edward T. Dickinson, M.D., NREMT-P, FACEP

Validated by: The International Fire Service Training Association

IFSTA Senior Editor: Michael A. Wieder

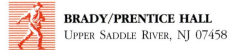

BRADY/PRENTICE HALL
UPPER SADDLE RIVER, NJ 07458

Library of Congress Cataloging-in-Publication Data

Dickinson, Edward T.
    Fire service emergency care / Edward T. Dickinson ; validated by
the International Fire Service Training Association, IFSTA senior
editor, Michael A. Wieder.
        p.   cm.
    Includes bibliographical references and index.
    ISBN 0-8359-5279-7 (case). — ISBN 0-8359-5133-2 (pbk).
    1. Emergency medicine.   2. Emergency medical technicians.
I. Wieder, Michael A.   II. International Fire Service Training
Association.   III. Title.
RC86.7.D55   1998
616.02′5—dc21   98-25811
                                                              CIP

PUBLISHER: Susan Katz
MANAGING DEVELOPMENT EDITOR: Lois Berlowitz
DEVELOPMENT EDITOR: Dan Zinkus
DIRECTOR OF MANUFACTURING AND PRODUCTION: Bruce Johnson
MANAGING PRODUCTION EDITOR: Patrick Walsh
PRODUCTION EDITOR: Julie Boddorf
SENIOR PRODUCTION MANAGER: Ilene Sanford
MARKETING MANAGER: Tiffany Price
MARKETING COORDINATOR: Cindy Frederick
EDITORIAL ASSISTANT: Carol Sobel
MANAGING PHOTOGRAPHY EDITOR: Michal Heron
PHOTOGRAPHERS: Stephen Bell, Michael Gallitelli, Don Hall
    Productions, Michal Heron, Richard Logan, Mark
    Longwood
COVER PHOTOGRAPHY: top left, Mark C. Ide; top right, Mark C.
    Ide; bottom, Craig Jackson, In The Dark Photography
COVER DESIGN: Bruce Kenselaar
INTERIOR DESIGN: Sue Walrath
COMPOSITION: The Clarinda Company
PRINTING AND BINDING: Von Hoffman Press

Printed in the United States of America

10 9 8 7 6 5 4 3 2 1

ISBN 08359-5279-7
ISBN 08359-5133-2[pbk]

PRENTICE-HALL INTERNATIONAL (UK) LIMITED, *London*
PRENTICE-HALL OF AUSTRALIA PTY. LIMITED, *Sydney*
PRENTICE-HALL CANADA, INC., *Toronto*
PRENTICE-HALL HISPANOAMERICANA, S.A., *Mexico*
PRENTICE-HALL OF INDIA PRIVATE LIMITED, *New Delhi*
PRENTICE-HALL OF JAPAN, INC., *Tokyo*
SIMON & SCHUSTER ASIA PTE LTD., *Singapore*
EDITORA PRENTICE-HALL DO BRASIL, LTDA., *Rio de Janeiro*

NOTICE ON CARE PROCEDURES

It is the intent of the author and publisher that this textbook be used as part of a formal EMT-Basic education program taught by qualified instructors and supervised by a licensed physician. The procedures described in this textbook are based upon consultation with EMT and medical authorities. The author and publisher have taken care to make certain that these procedures reflect currently accepted clinical practice; however, they cannot be considered absolute recommendations.

The material in this textbook contains the most current information available at the time of publication. However, federal, state, and local guidelines concerning clinical practices, including without limitation, those governing infection control and universal precautions, change rapidly. The reader should note, therefore, that the new regulations may require changes in some procedures.

It is the responsibility of the reader to familiarize himself or herself with the policies and procedures set by federal, state, and local agencies as well as the institution or agency where the reader is employed. The authors and the publisher of this textbook and the supplements written to accompany it disclaim any liability, loss, or risk resulting directly or indirectly from the suggested procedures and theory, from any undetected errors, or from the reader's misunderstanding of the text. It is the reader's responsibility to stay informed of any new changes or recommendations made by any federal, state, and local agency as well as by his or her employing institution or agency.

NOTICE ON GENDER USAGE

The English language has historically given preference to the male gender. Among many words, the pronouns "he" and "his" are commonly used to describe both genders. Society evolves faster than language, and the male pronouns still predominate in our speech. Thus, in many instances, male pronouns may be used in this book to describe both males and females solely for the purpose of brevity. This is not intended to offend any readers of the female gender.

NOTICE RE "ON SCENE"

The names used and situations depicted in "On Scene" scenarios throughout the text are fictitious.

*To Debbie, Stephen, and Alex for their
endless love and patience throughout
this and many other projects.*

and

*To the firefighters of the Tri-Village Fire Company
and the Hamilton Fire Department
for their comradery and for instilling in me a
love and dedication to the fire service.*

E.T.D.

Brief Contents

PART 1   **ESSENTIALS**   **1**
Chapter 1   Introduction to Emergency Medical Care   3
Chapter 2   The Well-being of the EMT-Basic   19
Chapter 3   Infection Control and Body Substance Isolation   35
Chapter 4   Medical/Legal Issues   51
Chapter 5   Anatomy and Physiology   67
Chapter 6   Airway Management   95
Chapter 7   Patient Assessment   141
             SECTION I: An Overview   142
             SECTION II: Scene Size-up   145
             SECTION III: Initial Assessment   163
             SECTION IV: SAMPLE History and Vital Signs   176
             SECTION V: Focused History and Physical Examination/
                 Detailed Physical Examination—Medical Patients   187
             SECTION VI: Focused History and Physical Examination/
                 Detailed Physical Examination—Trauma Patients   197
             SECTION VII: The Ongoing Assessment   217
Chapter 8   Communication and Documentation   225
Chapter 9   Transition of Prehospital Care   253
Chapter 10   Lifting and Moving Patients   261

PART 2   **MEDICAL AND TRAUMA EMERGENCIES**   **285**
Chapter 11   General Pharmacology   287
Chapter 12   Respiratory Emergencies   301
Chapter 13   Cardiac Emergencies   319
Chapter 14   Altered Mental Status Emergencies—Diabetes and Other Causes   347
Chapter 15   Poisonings and Allergic Reactions   363
Chapter 16   Environmental Emergencies   385
Chapter 17   Obstetrics and Gynecology   411
Chapter 18   Behavioral Emergencies   443
Chapter 19   Bleeding and Shock   457
Chapter 20   Soft Tissue Injuries   481
Chapter 21   Musculoskeletal Injuries   517
Chapter 22   Injuries to the Head and Spine   547
Chapter 23   Infants and Children   593
Chapter 24   Geriatrics   631

PART 3   **OPERATIONS**   **645**
Chapter 25   Emergency Vehicle Operations   647
Chapter 26   Gaining Access and Basics of Extrication   671
Chapter 27   Emergency Incident Rehabilitation   699
Chapter 28   EMS Special Operations   715

ADVANCED AIRWAY ELECTIVE   **755**
Chapter 29   Advanced Airway Management   757

APPENDICES
Appendix A   ALS-Assist Skills   797
Appendix B   Basic Cardiac Life Support Review   805
Appendix C   National Registry EMT-B Practical Examinations   833
Glossary   **845**
Index   **855**

Detailed Contents

PART 1   ESSENTIALS   1

Introduction to Emergency Medical Care   3

OBJECTIVES	4
ON SCENE	4
The Fire Service and Emergency Medical Care	5
Overview of the EMS System	6
Elements of the EMS System	8
Public Information and Education	8
Communications Systems	8
Human Resources and Training	9
Medical Direction	10
Evaluation	11
Facilities and Trauma Systems	12
Roles and Responsibilities of the EMT	14
Professionalism	14
CHAPTER REVIEW	16
At a Glance	17

The Well-being of the EMT-Basic   19

OBJECTIVES	20
ON SCENE	20
Emotional Aspects of Emergency Care	21
Death and Dying	21
Other Stressful Situations	22
Stress Management	24
Family and Friends' Responses	24
Comprehensive Critical Incident Stress Management	25
Personal Safety and the EMT	26
Scene Safety	26
Violence	30
CHAPTER REVIEW	32
At a Glance	33

Infection Control and Body Substance Isolation   35

OBJECTIVES	36
ON SCENE	36

Infectious Diseases and Body Substance Isolation	38
Basic Safety Precautions	38
Handwashing	38
Personal Protective Equipment	38
Protection from Airborne Pathogens	41
Monitoring Personal Health	43
Cleaning and Disinfection of Equipment	43
Infection Control and the Law	45
Bloodborne Pathogens	45
Tuberculosis Guidelines	46
The Ryan White Act	47
CHAPTER REVIEW	49
At a Glance	50

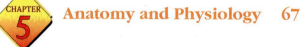

Medical/Legal Issues   51

OBJECTIVES	52
ON SCENE	52
Laws and Ethics	53
Scope of Practice	54
Consent	54
Advance Directives	55
Refusal of Care/Abandonment	55
Negligence	58
Assault/Battery	59
Minors and Special Risk Patients	60
Confidentiality	60
Potential Organ Donors	61
Special Reporting Situations	61
Suspected Crime Scenes	63
Minimizing Liability	63
CHAPTER REVIEW	64
At a Glance	65

Anatomy and Physiology   67

OBJECTIVES	68
ON SCENE	68

Human Anatomy Basics   68
   Anatomical Terms   69
   Body Positioning   72
Anatomy and Physiology of Body Systems   73
   Musculoskeletal System   73
   Respiratory System   77
   Circulatory System   81
   Nervous System   87
   Endocrine System   88
   Gastrointestinal System   88
   Genitourinary System   88
   The Skin   89
CHAPTER REVIEW   92
At a Glance   93

Airway Management 95

OBJECTIVES   96
ON SCENE   97
The Importance of Airway Management   98
Respiration   99
   Adequate and Inadequate Breathing   99
   Assessment of Respiratory Failure
   and Arrest   99
Opening the Airway   102
   Head-Tilt, Chin-Lift Maneuver   102
   Jaw-Thrust Maneuver   104
Techniques of Artificial Ventilation   105
   Mouth-to-Mask Ventilation   106
   The Bag-Valve Mask   107
   The Flow-Restricted, Oxygen-Powered
   Ventilation Device   112
Airway Adjuncts   112
   Rules for Using Airway Adjuncts   113
   Oropharyngeal Airways   113
   Nasopharyngeal Airways   117
Suction and Suction Devices   118
   Mounted Suction Systems   118
   Portable Suction Units   118
   Tubing, Tips, and Catheters   119
   Techniques of Suctioning   120
Oxygen Therapy   121
   The Importance of Supplemental Oxygen 121
   Hypoxia   124
   Pulse Oximetry   124
   Hazards of Oxygen Therapy   126
   Oxygen Therapy Equipment   127
   Administering Oxygen   130

Special Considerations   135
CHAPTER REVIEW   138
At a Glance   139

Patient Assessment 141

SECTION I: An Overview   142
Scene Size-up   142
Initial Assessment   143
Focused History and Physical Examination   143
Detailed Physical Examination   144
Ongoing Assessment   144
SECTION II: Scene Size-up   145
OBJECTIVES   145
Dispatch Information   146
Scene Safety   146
   Body Substance Isolation (BSI)   147
   Personal Safety of the EMT   147
   Patient Safety   150
   Bystander Safety   152
Scene Assessment   152
   Nature of Illness   152
   Mechanism of Injury   153
Determining the Number of Patients   162
SECTION III: Initial Assessment   163
OBJECTIVES   163
Steps of Initial Assessment   164
Forming a General Impression   165
Assessment of Mental Status   168
Assessment of Airway Status   170
Assessment of Breathing Status   171
   Assessment of Breathing—Responsive
   Patient   171
   Assessment of Breathing—Unresponsive
   Patient   171
Assessment of Circulation Status   172
   Assessment of the Pulse   172
   Assessment for External Bleeding   172
   Assessment of the Skin   172
Initial Assessment of Infants and Children   173
Identification of Priority Patients   175
SECTION IV: SAMPLE History and
   Vital Signs   176
OBJECTIVES   176
The SAMPLE History   177

Signs and Symptoms 178
Allergies 178
Medications 178
Pertinent Past Medical History 179
Last Oral Intake 179
Events Leading Up to the Illness
or Injury 180
Vital Signs 180
Pulse 180
Respirations 182
Blood Pressure 183
Skin 185
Pupils 186

SECTION V: Focused History and
Physical Exam/Detailed Physical
Exam—Medical Patients 187
OBJECTIVES 188
Approaches to the Focused History
and Physical Exam 188
The Unresponsive Medical Patient 189
ON SCENE 189
The Rapid Physical Examination—
Unresponsive Patient 189
Determining Baseline Vital Signs 192
Positioning the Patient 192
Obtain a SAMPLE History 193
The Detailed Physical Examination—
Unresponsive Medical Patient 194
The Responsive Medical Patient 194
ON SCENE 194
History of the Present Illness—OPQRST 195
Completing the SAMPLE History 195
The Focused Physical Examination—
Responsive Medical Patient 196
Assessing Baseline Vital Signs 196
Providing Emergency Care 196
The Detailed Physical Examination—
Responsive Medical Patient 196

SECTION VI: Focused History and
Physical Examination/Detailed Physical
Examination—Trauma Patients 197
OBJECTIVES 197
Reconsidering the Mechanism of Injury 198
Trauma Patient—Significant Mechanism
of Injury 199
ON SCENE 199
Priorities with the Trauma Patient with
Significant Mechanism of Injury 200
Continuing Spinal Stabilization 200

Requesting ALS Support 200
Reconsidering the Transport Decision 200
Reassessing Mental Status 201
Performing the Rapid Trauma
Assessment 201
Assessing Baseline Vital Signs 201
Obtaining the SAMPLE History 204
Detailed Physical Examination—Trauma
Patient with a Significant Mechanism
of Injury 210
Trauma Patient—No Significant Mechanism
of Injury 210
ON SCENE 216
Priorities with the Trauma Patient—
No Significant Mechanism of Injury 216
The Focused Physical Examination 216
Vital Signs and SAMPLE History 217
Detailed Physical Examination—Trauma
Patient with No Significant Mechanism
of Injury 217
SECTION VII: The Ongoing Assessment 217
OBJECTIVES 217
Steps of the Ongoing Assessment 218
Trending of Assessment Components 218
When to Perform the Ongoing Assessment 219
The Ongoing Assessment in Practice 219
Unresponsive Medical Patient 219
Responsive Medical Patient 220
Trauma Patient with Significant
Mechanism of Injury 221
Trauma Patient with No Significant
Mechanism of Injury 221
CHAPTER REVIEW 221
At a Glance 223

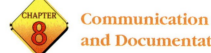

**Communication
and Documentation** 225

OBJECTIVES 226
ON SCENE 227
Interpersonal Communication 228
General Guidelines 229
Communications Systems 232
Communications System Components 232
System Maintenance 234
Radio Communications Basics 234
General Rules 234

Communication and Dispatch 235
Communication with Medical Direction 236
Communications En Route to the
    Hospital/Receiving Facility 237
Communications After Arrival at
    the Hospital/Receiving Facility 237
Documentation 237
Reasons for Documentation 238
The Prehospital Care Report 239
Legal Issues 246
Falsification 248
Correcting Errors 248
Special Situations 249
CHAPTER REVIEW 250
At a Glance 252

CHAPTER 9 Transition of Prehospital Care 253

OBJECTIVES 254
ON SCENE 254
Transition of Care 255
Tiered EMS Systems 255
Transition of Care Procedures 256
Special Circumstances in Transition of Care 258
Bystander Care 258
Aviation Crews 259
CHAPTER REVIEW 260
At a Glance 260

CHAPTER 10 Lifting and Moving Patients 261

OBJECTIVES 262
ON SCENE 262
Planning for Lifting and Moving 263
Body Mechanics and Lifting and Moving 263
The Power Lift and Power Grip 263
Special Lifting and Carrying
    Considerations 265
Patient Safety Considerations 268
Types of Patient Moves 268
Patient-Carrying Equipment 276
Wheeled Ambulance Stretcher 276
Portable Ambulance Stretcher 277
Stair Chair 279
Scoop Stretcher 280

Spine Boards 280
Basket Stretcher 281
Flexible Stretcher 281
Positioning of Patients 282
CHAPTER REVIEW 283
At a Glance 284

PART 2   MEDICAL AND TRAUMA EMERGENCIES   285

CHAPTER 11 General Pharmacology 287

OBJECTIVES 288
ON SCENE 288
Essentials of Pharmacology 289
Medications 289
Medication Names 289
Routes of Administration 290
Forms of Medication 290
Prescription Labeling 290
Understanding Medications 291
Administration of Medications 292
Medications Administered by EMTs 293
Medications the EMT May Assist
    in Administering 293
Medications Carried on the EMS Unit 295
Commonly Encountered Medications 296
CHAPTER REVIEW 299
At a Glance 300

CHAPTER 12 Respiratory Emergencies 301

OBJECTIVES 302
ON SCENE 302
Anatomy and Physiology of the
    Respiratory System 303
Adequate and Inadequate Breathing 304
Adequate Breathing 305
Inadequate Breathing 305
Adequate and Inadequate Artificial
    Ventilation 305
Respiratory Distress 306
Assessment of the Patient in
    Respiratory Distress 307
Hypoxic Drive 310

The Prescribed Inhaler   310
The Home Nebulizer   311
Infants and Children with Respiratory
    Complaints   311
Smoke Inhalation   315
CHAPTER REVIEW   317
At a Glance   318

Cardiac Emergencies   319

OBJECTIVES   320
ON SCENE   322
Anatomy and Physiology of the
    Cardiovascular System   322
Cardiac Compromise   324
    Assessment of the Cardiac
        Compromise Patient   324
    Nitroglycerin   327
Cardiac Arrest   328
Defibrillation   332
Defibrillators   333
    Internal Defibrillators   333
    External Defibrillators   333
Automated External Defibrillators (AEDs)   333
    Fully Automated AEDs   333
    Semi-Automated AEDs   333
    Advantages of AEDs   334
    When and When Not to Use the AED   335
    Safety Concerns with AEDs   335
    CPR and AEDs   336
    Assessment of the Cardiac Arrest
        Patient   337
    Key Ideas in AED   339
    Post-Resuscitation Care   339
    Recurring Cardiac Arrest   342
    Single Rescuer Use of the AED   342
    Using a Fully Automated AED   343
    AED Maintenance   343
    AED Training and Quality Assurance   343
CHAPTER REVIEW   345
At a Glance   346

Altered Mental Status Emergencies—Diabetes and Other Causes   347

OBJECTIVES   348

ON SCENE   348
Altered Mental Status   349
    Assessment of the Patient with Altered
        Mental Status—No History of Diabetes 349
Diabetes and Altered Mental Status   351
    Physiology of Diabetes   351
    Assessment of the Altered Mental Status
        Patient with History of Diabetes   352
Seizures   356
    Assessment of the Seizure Patient   356
Cerebrovascular Accidents   358
CHAPTER REVIEW   360
At a Glance   361

Poisonings and Allergic Reactions   363

OBJECTIVES   364
ON SCENE   365
Poisoning   365
    Routes of Exposure   367
    Assessment of the Poisoning Patient   368
    Assessment and Management
        Techniques   368
Allergic Reactions   376
    Assessment of the Patient with an
        Allergic Reaction   377
CHAPTER REVIEW   382
At a Glance   383

Environmental Emergencies   385

OBJECTIVES   386
ON SCENE   386
Temperature Regulation and the Body   387
Cold-Related Emergencies   388
    Generalized Hypothermia   389
    Assessment of the Hypothermic Patient   390
    Local Cold Injuries   393
Heat-Related Emergencies   395
    Heat Cramps   396
    Heat Exhaustion   396
    Heat Stroke   397
Water-Related Emergencies   398
    Special Water-Related Emergencies   400
Bites and Stings   403
    Insect Stings   403

Spider Bites 404
Scorpion Stings 405
Snake Bites 405
CHAPTER REVIEW 407
At a Glance 408

CHAPTER 17 Obstetrics and Gynecology 411

OBJECTIVES 412
ON SCENE 412
Anatomy and Physiology of Pregnancy 413
Normal Childbirth 417
The Role of the EMT 417
Equipment and Supplies 417
Evaluating the Mother 418
Delivery Procedures 419
Assessment and Care of the Newborn 423
Ongoing Care of the Mother 427
Childbirth Complications 429
Prolapsed Umbilical Cord 429
Breech Presentation 430
Limb Presentation 431
Multiple Births 431
Premature Birth 432
Meconium 433
Emergencies in Pregnancy 434
Spontaneous Abortion (Miscarriage) 434
Seizures During Pregnancy 435
Vaginal Bleeding Late in Pregnancy 435
Trauma During Pregnancy 436
Gynecological Emergencies 437
Vaginal Bleeding 437
Trauma to External Genitalia 437
Sexual Assault 438
CHAPTER REVIEW 439
At a Glance 440

CHAPTER 18 Behavioral Emergencies 443

OBJECTIVES 444
ON SCENE 444
Behavioral Emergencies 445
Behavioral Changes 445
Situational Stress Reactions 446
Psychiatric Emergencies 446
Assessment of Behavioral Emergency
Patients 447

Special Considerations 448
Suicide 448
Hostile or Aggressive Patients 449
Reasonable Force and Restraint 450
Documenting Behavioral Emergencies 452
Medical/Legal Considerations 453
CHAPTER REVIEW 454
At a Glance 455

CHAPTER 19 Bleeding and Shock 457

OBJECTIVES 458
ON SCENE 458
The Circulatory System 459
The Heart 459
The Blood Vessels 461
The Blood 461
Bleeding 461
Body Substance Isolation 462
External Bleeding 462
Types of Bleeding 462
Control of Bleeding 464
Devices Used in Controlling Bleeding 465
Special Situations 468
Internal Bleeding 469
Mechanisms of Injury Associated
with Internal Bleeding 469
Signs and Symptoms Associated
with Internal Bleeding 470
Shock (Hypoperfusion) 471
CHAPTER REVIEW 478
At a Glance 479

CHAPTER 20 Soft Tissue Injuries 481

OBJECTIVES 482
ON SCENE 483
Skin Functions and Structures 484
Soft Tissue Injuries 485
Closed Soft Tissue Injuries 485
Assessment of Closed Soft Tissue
Injuries 486
Open Soft Tissue Injuries 487
Assessment of Open Soft Tissue
Injuries 489
Dressings and Bandages 490

Emergency Care Considerations
  for Specific Injuries   494
Burns   502
  Classification of Burns   503
  Burn Severity   506
  Assessment of the Patient with Burns   507
  Special Considerations with Infants
    and Children   510
  Chemical and Electrical Burns   510
CHAPTER REVIEW   514
At a Glance   515

CHAPTER 21 Musculoskeletal Injuries — 517

OBJECTIVES   518
ON SCENE   518
Anatomy and Physiology of the
  Musculoskeletal System   519
  Bones of the Pelvis and Extremities   519
  Connective Tissue, Joints, and Muscles   521
Trauma and the Musculoskeletal System   521
  Mechanisms of Musculoskeletal Injury   523
  Types of Musculoskeletal Injuries   524
  Open and Closed Musculoskeletal
    Injuries   524
  Assessment of Musculoskeletal Injuries   526
Splinting   527
  Types of Splints   527
  General Guidelines for Splinting   528
  Realigning Injured Extremities   531
  Splinting Long Bone Injuries   532
  Special Techniques for Long Bone
    Injuries   532
CHAPTER REVIEW   545
At a Glance   546

CHAPTER 22 Injuries to the Head and Spine — 547

OBJECTIVES   548
ON SCENE   548
Anatomy of the Skull, Spine, and
  Central Nervous System   550
  The Skull   550
  The Spine   550
  The Central Nervous System   551
Spinal Injuries   552
  Mechanisms of Injury   552

Assessment of Spinal Injury Patients   553
Immobilization and Spinal Injuries   557
Injuries to the Head   580
  Scalp and Facial Injuries   581
  Skull Injuries   581
  Brain Injuries   581
  Assessment of Head Injuries   583
Helmet Removal   585
CHAPTER REVIEW   589
At a Glance   590

CHAPTER 23 Infants and Children — 593

OBJECTIVES   594
ON SCENE   594
Introduction to Pediatric Emergency Care   595
Anatomy and Physiology Considerations   595
Developmental Considerations   598
Management of the Pediatric Airway
  and Breathing   598
  Airway Skills   601
  Supplemental Oxygen Therapy   606
  Artificial Ventilation   607
Assessment of the Pediatric Patient   608
  Initial Assessment   608
  History and Physical Examination   611
Common Medical Problems in Infants
  and Children   611
  Airway Obstruction   611
  Respiratory Emergencies   613
  Seizures   614
  Altered Mental Status   615
  Fever   615
  Poisonings   616
  Shock (Hypoperfusion)   616
  Near Drowning   617
  Sudden Infant Death Syndrome   618
Trauma in Infants and Children   618
  Trauma Considerations by Mechanism
    of Injury   618
  Trauma Considerations by Body
    Region   619
Child Abuse and Neglect   622
  Approaches to Suspected Abuse
    or Neglect Situations   623
Infants and Children with Special Needs   624
  Tracheostomy Tubes   625

Home Ventilators   626
Central Intravenous Lines   626
Gastric Feeding Tubes and
    Gastrostomy Tubes   626
Shunts   627
Additional Considerations   627
Advance Directives   627
The Family   627
The EMT's Response to Pediatric
    Patients   628
CHAPTER REVIEW   629
At a Glance   630

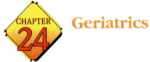

Geriatrics   **631**

OBJECTIVES   632
ON SCENE   632
Anatomy and Physiology in Aging   633
Approaches to the Geriatric Patient   634
Scene Size-up   635
Assessment of the Geriatric Patient   635
Geriatric Trauma Emergencies   636
Medical Emergencies   639
CHAPTER REVIEW   642
At a Glance   643

PART 3   OPERATIONS   645

Emergency Vehicle Operations   **647**

OBJECTIVES   648
ON SCENE   648
Phases of an Emergency Response   649
Preparing for the Call   649
Dispatch and Response   651
En Route to the Scene   655
At the Scene   658
En Route to the Receiving Facility   661
At the Receiving Facility   662
Returning to Service   662
Air Medical Transport   665
Requesting Air Medical Support   665
Selecting a Landing Zone   665
Ground Safety Procedures   666
Transition of Care   666

CHAPTER REVIEW   668
At a Glance   669

Gaining Access and Basics of Extrication   **671**

OBJECTIVES   672
ON SCENE   672
Vehicle Rescue   674
Preparing for the Rescue   674
Sizing-up the Scene   674
Recognizing and Managing Hazards   675
Stabilizing a Vehicle   685
Access   686
Simple vs. Complex Access   686
Initial and Rapid Trauma Assessment   692
Extrication   693
Normal vs. Rapid Extrication   693
Partial vs. Full Extrication   694
Transport, Detailed Physical Exam,
    and Ongoing Assessment   695
Terminating the Rescue   695
CHAPTER REVIEW   696
At a Glance   697

Emergency Incident Rehabilitation   **699**

OBJECTIVES   700
ON SCENE   700
Emergency Incident Rehabilitation   701
Stress- and Heat-Related Emergencies   701
Mechanisms of Heat Loss   702
Heat Cramps   703
Heat Exhaustion   703
Heat Stroke   703
The Rehab Sector/Group   704
Functions in the Rehab Sector/Group   704
Staffing of the Rehab Sector/Group   704
Design and Location of the Rehab
    Sector/Group   705
Criteria for Entering the Rehab
    Sector/Group   707
Accountability in the Rehab
    Sector/Group   707
Entry and Triage   708
Medical Evaluation/Treatment Area   709
Hydration and Nourishment in the
    Rehab Sector/Group   710

CHAPTER REVIEW   712
At a Glance   713

CHAPTER 28 — EMS Special Operations   715

OBJECTIVES   716
On Scene   716
Rescue Situation Hazards   718
  Water-Related Hazards   718
  Ice Rescue   723
  Confined Spaces and Hazardous
    Atmospheres   724
  Trench Collapses   727
  Rough Terrain Evacuation   728
  Helicopters in Rescue Operations   729
Hazardous Materials   732
  Training for Hazardous Materials
    Emergencies   732
  The Role of EMTs at Hazmat Incidents   733
Multiple-Casualty Incidents   742
  The Incident Management System   742
  Psychological Considerations   752
CHAPTER REVIEW   753
At a Glance   754

ADVANCED AIRWAY ELECTIVE   755

CHAPTER 29 — Advanced Airway Management   757

OBJECTIVES   758
On Scene   759
Respiratory Anatomy and Physiology   760
  Anatomy   760
  Physiology   760
  Pediatric Airway and Anatomy   762

Mangement of the Airway   763
  Suctioning the Airway   763
  Orotracheal Intubation   763
  Nasogastric Intubation of Infants
    and Children   781
  Orotracheal and Endotracheal
    Suctioning   781
Additional Advanced Airway Techniques   783
  Automatic Transport Ventilators   783
  Esophageal and Multilumen Airways   786
CHAPTER REVIEW   794
At a Glance   794

APPENDICES

APPENDIX A — ALS-Assist Skills   797

Assisting with Endotracheal Intubation   797
Applying ECG/Defibrillator Electrodes   800
Using a Pulse Oximeter   801
Assisting in IV Therapy   802

APPENDIX B — Basic Cardiac Life Support Review   805

Before Beginning Resuscitation: First Steps   805
Rescue Breathing   809
CPR   812
Clearing Airway Obstructions   826

APPENDIX C — National Registry EMT-B Practical Examinations   833

Glossary   **845**
Index   **855**

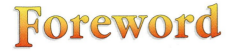

Foreword

The fire service has always had an important role in EMS and, likewise, EMS is extremely important to the fire service. In 1975, the International Association of Fire Chiefs endorsed, by resolution, emergency medical care as a legitimate role of the fire service. Sixteen years later, the IAFC and the International Association of Fire Fighters adopted a joint resolution reaffirming prehospital emergency care as a major service provided by the fire service.

From very humble beginnings as an add-on service, EMS has evolved into a critical component within an overwhelming majority of fire departments. In spite of this well-established role, there have been no textbooks produced with a fire service background and orientation. Training for fire-based EMTs has been provided by adopting texts designed for ambulance service personnel—until now. In the book you are holding, Dr. Edward T. Dickinson has provided an outstanding text, written with a fire service outlook.

While EMS is essentially the same regardless of who provides it, there are nuances and issues unique to the fire service. A text like this one that offers a fire service perspective for firefighter-EMTs is long overdue. This book is a joint venture between Brady Publishing and the International Fire Service Training Association (IFSTA). You will find it very easy to read and understand. It contains basic information that every EMT trainee needs, and it offers added coverage particularly relevant for fire service personnel on topics such as emergency incident rehabilitation and the Incident Management System. Unique features titled Company Officer's Notes and Transition of Care appear throughout the text, highlighting areas of special concern to firefighter-EMTs. In addition, the real-world scenarios that open each chapter were clearly written by someone who has been in the field.

At last, there is a book specifically designed to address fire service training of Emergency Medical Technicians. It will mean better prepared and more competent firefighter-EMTs, which will mean better service and care for the people who call 9-1-1.

Chief Richard A. Marinucci
President
International Association of Fire Chiefs

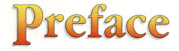
Preface

You are about to begin training to become an Emergency Medical Technician-Basic in the fire service. This textbook, which will provide much of the information you will use as an EMT, is unique. *Fire Service Emergency Care* is the product of an unprecedented joint venture by Brady Publishing and the International Fire Service Training Association (IFSTA), two leading producers of fire service training materials. It is the first textbook written specifically for EMTs who are members of the fire service.

Fire Service Emergency Care is based on and complies with the guidelines established for the training of EMTs set by the U.S. Department of Transportation (DOT). The book, however, organizes and presents its content with an awareness of the particular situations in which firefighter-EMTs work. The book's author, Dr. Edward T. Dickinson, is a board-certified emergency physician and a former firefighter-EMT/Paramedic. He presents the EMT course content in a way that recognizes the distinct needs and requirements of members of the fire service. Using it will enable you to confront the special situations that firefighter-EMTs face.

Although this book uses the DOT curriculum as a foundation, materials in it are at times rearranged or amplified on to enhance your understanding or to take into account the needs of fire service members. In addition, the physicians and instructors who have designed your course have done so to meet the specific needs of your community. They may suggest following different steps in carrying out emergency procedures from those described in the DOT curriculum and in this textbook.

Such variations in procedures are common. There are cases where more than one procedure works. Your EMS system may have tested one of the procedures and found it effective and easy to teach. Your system, therefore, may have decided to follow that procedure rather than an alternative described in the DOT curriculum and this book. In such cases, your instructors will train you to use the methods employed in your EMS system. In cases where many common variations of a procedure may be used, this book will remind you to "follow local protocols."

Emergency medicine is a constantly changing field. New technologies and new research will lead to changes in they types of procedures EMTs are allowed to perform and in the methods by which they carry out emergency care procedures. The content of this book and of your EMT course will not mark the end of your training. You must continue to stay up-to-date with changes in emergency medicine. Your instructor will tell you how continuing education programs for EMTs are presented in your area. The instructor can also suggest books, prehospital emergency care journals, videos, and state- or locally-produced newsletters that can help you stay current.

THE 1994 EMT-BASIC CURRICULUM

In 1994, the U.S. DOT released a revision of the EMT-Basic National Standard Curriculum. This curriculum made significant changes in what EMTs learn and what care they can provide. The content and approaches of the U.S. DOT curriculum provide the basis for this textbook.

The intent of the curriculum is for students to follow a particular sequence in learning the knowledge and skills of an EMT. After completing the CPR prerequisite, students cover some essentials of EMS—foundation materials that they need to know in order to understand later topics. Airway management, for example, is one of these essentials that is taught early on because evaluation and maintenance of the airway is so vital to patient care.

Following airway management, students learn the assessment skills that they will use with any type of patient, medical or trauma. The curriculum, and the textbook, then go on to teach the assessment and care of specific types of medical and trauma emergencies. This section of the textbook ends with chapters devoted to the special needs of infants, children, and elderly patients in medical and trauma emergencies.

After medical and trauma emergencies, the curriculum and book deal with operations. These are the nonmedical situations, such as ambulance and rescue operations and multiple-casualty and hazardous materials incidents that are still essential parts essential elements of EMS.

The last chapter in the textbook deals with advanced airway management, including the skills of orotracheal and nasogastric intubation. The U.S. DOT curriculum describes these skills as elective. They may or may not be taught in your jurisdiction.

INTERVENTIONS

The basics of emergency treatment provided by EMTs have traditionally included provision of oxygen, spinal immobilization, and splinting. With the 1994 curriculum, EMTs were allowed to perform additional treatments with the approval of medical direction. For example, EMTs can now administer or assist in administering several medications either carried on the emergency vehicle or prescribed to patients. These medications include oral glucose, activated charcoal, epinephrine auto-injectors, metered dose inhalers, and nitroglycerin. EMTs can also perform an additional procedure, automated defibrillation. (As noted above, advanced airway procedures are an elective that may be taught in certain jurisdictions.)

FEATURES OF THE TEXTBOOK

The following features of Fire Service Emergency Care are intended to make teaching and studying of the EMT-Basic course easier.

Objectives Knowledge and Understanding Objectives and Skills Objectives from the 1994 EMT-Basic National Standard Curriculum are listed at the start of each chapter. Every objective is covered in this textbook. Page references appearing after the Knowledge and Understanding Objectives are to textbook pages on which the objectives are discussed. Students should be able to master these objectives by reading the text. Mastery of the Skills Objectives, however, requires hands-on practice obtained by working with an instructor. For this reason, no page references appear after the Skill Objectives, although the skills are discussed in the text.

On Scene Each chapter opens with a scenario in which firefighter-EMTs encounter a real-life situation in which a patient is suffering from a medical or trauma emergency. These case studies are intended to convey a sense of what providing emergency care in the field is like. They will also give students a way of tying the textbook discussion of a topic to its application in the real world.

Special Fire Service Chapters *Fire Service Emergency Care* covers all topics discussed in the U.S. DOT curriculum. However, it goes beyond the curriculum in some cases to present information that is particularly relevant to the needs of firefighter-EMTs. Two chapters of the book are especially targeted to those needs. Chapter 9 deals with Transition of Prehospital Care. Firefighter-EMTs often provide emergency medical services as part of a tiered response system. This chapter describes policies and procedures to ensure that information about a patient is properly passed along among responders in such systems in order to assure optimal patient care. Chapter 27 deals with Emergency Incident Rehabilitation. Because of the nature of their duties, firefighters are often exposed to the possibility of heat- and stress-related emergencies. Firefighter-EMTs often have the responsibility of providing rehabilitation to firefighters to prevent such emergencies and of caring for firefighters when the emergencies do develop. This chapter describes how to set up a Rehabilitation Sector/Group area and suggests procedures by which firefighters can be admitted to and discharged from the area.

Updated Information The U.S. DOT curriculum appeared in 1994. However, refinements and changes in emergency medicine procedures and practices have continued since then. This textbook provides the latest information available in several areas. For example, it discusses management of stroke based on the 1997 National Institutes of Health guidelines for EMT-Basics. Recognizing the growing use of pulse oximeters in EMS system, it gives step-by-step instructions for using the devices. The book also gives new information about home nebulizers and advanced airway management. Whenever such information is provided, it is always with the reminder that the use of the devices and procedures are matters of local protocol and policy.

Skill Summaries Information on skills that EMTs must master are summarized in step-by-step form through groupings of photos and art. These summaries serve as handy reminders/references for skills procedures learned in the classroom.

Medications Information about medications that EMTs are authorized to administer or assist in administering is given special highlighted treatment in the text. These features contain all the basic information students need for working with these medications including indications and contraindications for administration, dosage, side effects, and step-by-step procedures. The actual authority to use any of the medications discussed in the text must be granted locally by medical direction.

Company Officer's Notes These features appear from time to time throughout the textbook to highlight safety and patient care considerations for the personnel in charge at emergency scenes.

Transition of Care Because proper transition of care from one emergency provider to another is so crucial to patients' well-being, in addition to Chapter 9 on that topic, Transition of Care notes stressing key points and procedures have been provided throughout the text.

Pediatric and Geriatric Concerns In general, procedures for assessing and treating infants, children, and the elderly are the same as for other patients. However, issues related to anatomy and physiology can sometimes affect assessment or care for these groups. The U.S. DOT curriculum calls for a special module on assessment and care of infants and children. This material is covered in Chapter 23 of the textbook. The curriculum does not call for a separate section on the elderly. However, geriatric patients represent a large and growing segment of EMS clients. For this reason, the author has discussed special concerns with geriatric patients in Chapter 24. In addition, whenever issues involving the care of infants, children, and the elderly with specific illnesses or injuries, Pediatric Notes and Geriatric Notes have been provided at appropriate places in the text.

Chapter Review Chapter Review pages contain three elements. A Summary recaps the main ideas in the chapter. Reviewing Key Concepts asks students questions that test their understanding of significant information in the chapter. Resources to Learn More presents suggested book or journal articles that can enhance student understanding of subjects discussed in the chapter.

At a Glance Chapters conclude with diagrams, flow charts, or algorithms that provide students with an easy-to-scan summary of key ideas or procedures discussed within the chapter.

ALS-Assist Skills Firefighter-EMTs must frequently work in conjunction with EMTs who have more advanced levels of training. Although they themselves cannot perform the procedures, EMTs may be able to assist advanced EMTs in carrying out certain advanced life support (ALS) skills. Appendix A discusses some of the ways EMTs can help with these ALS skills.

Basic Cardiac Life Support Review Basic life support is a prerequisite to the EMT-Basic course. Appendix B reviews these skills, including CPR and procedures for dealing with foreign body airway obstruction.

National Registry Skill Sheets The practical skill sheets used at the EMT-Basic level by the National Registry of Emergency Medical Technicians are included in Appendix C as a tool to aid students in practicing their practical skills. The skill sheets also provide a tool that the instructor can use in making a formal evaluation of students' performance. The skill sheets contain the instructions that are provided to candidates before practical testing. Studying this material should allay students' fears and uncertainties about criteria that will be tested in the practical examination.

Supporting Materials Several ancillary materials are available as aids to instruction. These include a Student Workbook and an Instructor's Resource Manual. A testing package and a slide program are also available.

SUGGESTIONS FOR IMPROVEMENTS

Some of the best ideas for better training and education methods come from students and instructors who use educational materials in their classes. Any student, practicing EMT, or EMS instructor who has suggestions for improving this textbook, the supporting materials that accompany it, or EMT-Basic training and education should write to the author at:

Brady Marketing Department
c/o Tiffany Price
Brady/Prentice Hall
One Lake Street
Upper Saddle River, NJ 07458

You can also reach Dr. Dickinson through the Internet at:

eddickin@mail.med.upenn.edu

Visit the Brady Web Site at:

http://www.bradybooks.com

Acknowledgments

CONTRIBUTING WRITERS

Deepest appreciation to the following people who contributed chapters to this book:

Chip Beaudet
Executive Director
Mountain Lakes EMS Program
Queensbury, NY

Dr. Lawrence C. Brilliant, M.D., FACEP
Director, Department of Emergency Medicine
Episcopal Hospital
Philadelphia, PA

Daniel Limmer, EMT-P
Paramedic, Colonie EMS Department
Training Officer, Colonie Police Department
Colonie, NY

Jonathan Politis, B.A., NREMT-P
Director, Colonie EMS Department
Colonie, NY

Marc Rabdau
Assistant Chief
Eagle Fire Protection District
Eagle, ID

Andrew Stern, NREMT-P, MPA, M.A.
Senior Paramedic, Colonie EMS Department
Colonie, NY

Lawrence E. Tan, NREMT-P
Emergency Services Assistant Manager/
Commander, Emergency Services Operations
New Castle County, DE

IFSTA VALIDATING COMMITTEE

Acknowledgment and special thanks are extended to the members of the IFSTA validating committee who contributed their time, wisdom, and knowledge to a thorough review of the manuscript for this book.

IFSTA/Fire Protection Publications Staff Liaison
Michael A. Wieder
Fire Protection Publications

Oklahoma State University
Stillwater, OK

Gary Alvey
Marin County Fire Department
Healdsburg, CA

Dr. Jess Andrews, Ed.D.
Program Coordinator
Fire Service Training
Oklahoma State University
Stillwater, OK

Deborah Ayers
EMS Division Chief
Medic 7
Edmonds, WA

Douglas K. Cline, Captain-Paramedic
Chapel Hill Fire Department
Chapel Hill, NC

Eric Heckerson
Mesa Fire Department
EMS Division
Mesa, AZ

Mark Rabdau,
Assistant Chief
Eagle Fire Protection District
Eagle, ID

Jacqueline (Jackie) White
EMS Training Program Manager
Phoenix Fire Department
Phoenix, AZ

REVIEWERS

Our thanks to the many people involved in EMS for their feedback and suggestions:

Bubba Bell, EMT-P
Cleveland, MS

Samuel Bennett, EMT-B
Training and Safety Officer
Pimlico Volunteer Fire Department
Pimlico, SC

Kevin Bersche
EMS Coordinator
Farmington Hills Fire Rescue
Farmington Hills, MI

Scott Blackburn, NREMT-P
Emergency Response Training, Inc.
Baton Rouge, LA

Ken Bouvier, NREMT-I
Hazardous Materials Specialist
New Orleans, LA

Charles P. Butler
Arkansas Fire Academy
Camden, AR

Patricia A. Ciara, Assistant Deputy Chief
Paramedic
EMS/CME Supervisor
Chicago Fire Department
Chicago, IL

Stephan D. Cox
Maryland Fire & Rescue
University of Maryland
College Park, MD

Capt. Robert B. Gilliland, REMT-P
Company Officer/Paramedic
Mobile Fire Rescue Department
Mobile, AL

John Gunyon, EMT-I
Gateway Technical College
Elkhorn, WI

Rick Hilinski, BA, EMT-P
Assistant Director, Medic Program
CCAC Public Safety Institute
Pittsburgh, PA

Rusty Hollingsworth, NREMT-P
Paramedic Instructor
Beaufort County EMS
Beaufort, SC

Jack L. Johnson, C.F.I.
Master Class Instructor
Training Officer
Young America Fire Department
Galveston, IN

Linda Johnson
BCS Coordinator
Thomas Jefferson EMS Council
Charlottesville, VA

Lois Justry
Instructor Coordinator
Fire Department of New York EMS

Leo G. Kelly, Firefighter-EMT-B
Fire Service Instructor II
Emergency Medical Services Instructor
Commission on Fire Prevention and Control
Connecticut Fire Academy

Lt. John S. Kovach
Garland Fire Department
Garland, TX

Andy Lamarca
Director of Development
Mobile Life Support Service
Mobile, AL

Bill Landers, EMT-P Instructor
Atlanta Fire Department & EMS
Atlanta, TX

John A. Lewin, EMT-P, CFF III
EMS Instructor
Auburn Emergency Squad
Auburn, IL

Sgt. D. M. Magnino, EMT-P
Program Director
California Highway Patrol Emergency Medical
Services

Robert Marnatti
EMMCO East, Inc.
Kersey, PA

William D. McClincy
Regional EMS Training Coordinator
Meadville, PA

Robert McMahon, RN
Fire and EMS Coordinator
Putnam County, NY, Bureau of EMS

David Bruce Milligan, Jr.
Training Officer
Logan County Fire Department
Logan, Utah

Stephen J. Nardozzi
Assistant Professor & Director, EMS Studies
Westchester Community College
Valhalla, NY

Walter Nelson, EMT-D
NYS Regional Faculty Member

Chester H. Penn, NREMT-P
Paramedic Instructor
Horry-Georgetown Technical College
Myrtle Beach, SC

Fitzgerald J. Peterson, Firefighter EMT-P
Salt Lake County Fire Department
Salt Lake City, UT

Mark Register, BS, NREMT-P
Islandton, SC

Theodore J. Roberts, Firefighter EMT-P
Columbus Division of Fire
Columbus, OH

Robert Rose
Center for Emergency Care Training
Broad Channel Volunteer Fire Department
Spring Creek Volunteer Ambulance
New York State

Frank C. Schaper
Deputy Chief
St. Louis Fire Department
St. Louis, MO

Brent Smith, Firefighter, NREMT-P
Jacksonville Fire Department
Jacksonville, TX

Eva Aileen Sowinski, NREMT-B, BSN, RN
Emergency Services Training Administrator
Delaware State Fire School
Dover, DE

Patricia A. Strizak, EMT-P
Emergency Care Institute, NYU Downtown
Hospital
New York, NY

Pat Trevathan, MS
Kentucky Tech Fire/Rescue Training
West Kentucky State Training Institute
Paducah, KY

Alfred G. Tucker
Rural/Metro Ambulance
Employee Development
Northwest Florida/Alabama

Phyllis R. Vinson, BS, REMT-P
EMS Manager
Mobile County EMS
Mobile, AL

PHOTO CREDITS

Photo sources not otherwise credited include the following:

Robert J Bennett: 7-14, 7-20, 7-21B
John Callan, Shout Pictures: 20-10B, 24-03
Mary E. Dickinson, xxiv
Harvey Eisner CO 16, 25-4, 27-3, cover
David Handschuh: 7-6, 15-6, CO 23, CO ALS
Michal Heron: 28-07B, 28-08
Ronald Jeffers, Fire Service Publications, IFSTA: 27-10B
Kobal Collection NBC/TV: 1-1
Mark C Ide: 9-3, CO 19, CO 22, CO 25, CO 27, CO 29
In The Dark Photography: T. Mack: CO 2, 28-27
In The Dark Photography: Craig Jackson: CO 3, CO 6, CO 7, 7-1, 7-4, 7-26, 8-1, CO 9, CO 10, CO 15, 15-10, 15-11, CO 20, CO 26, 26-15, 27-2, 27-6A, 27-6C, CO BLS
Breck P. Kent: 16-15
Richard M. Levitan, MD © Airway Cam Technologies, Inc.: 29-14, 29-27, 29-28, 29-29, 29-30, 29-31, 29-32
Howard M Paul, Emergency! Stock: 2-3, 9-4, 25-07, 27-1, CO 28, 28-09
Photo Researchers: Joseph T. Collins, 16-14; Tom McHugh, 16-18; Suzanne L. Collins, Joseph T. Collins, 16-19
Sarasota County Fire Department: 7-2A
Sygma, Allen Tannenbaum: 7-24
Michael A. Wieder, Fire Protection Publications, IFSTA: CO 1, 25-12, 27-6B

PHOTO ACKNOWLEDGMENTS

The publisher wishes to express appreciation for the contribution to this book by the author, Edward T. Dickinson, M.D., of many fine photos of trauma injuries and medical conditions.

Companies We wish to thank the following companies for their cooperation in providing us with photos:

Laerdal Medical 13-10
Nellcor, Puritan, Bennett, Inc. 29-33 a & b

Organizations We wish to thank the following organizations for their assistance in creating the photo program for this book:

Carrollton Fire Department, Carrollton TX: EMS Coordinator Captain John Barnard

Fire Protection Publications, IFSTA: Michael A. Wieder

City of Plano Fire Department, Plano TX: Fire Chief Bill Peterson; EMS Coordinator Ken Klein; Monique Cardwell, Public Education

McKinney Fire Department, McKinney, TX: Assistant Chief Frank Roma

Westmere Fire Department, Guilderland, NY: Chief David Szary

While acknowledging the valuable assistance and professionalism contributed by all of the organizations participating in this project, the publisher wishes to make special mention of the extraordinary commitment of many weeks of personnel services and equipment provided by the Sarasota County Fire Department, Sarasota Florida. Our appreciation to

Sarasota County Government, County Administrator James L Ley

Sarasota County Fire Department, Fire Chief John Albritton; Deputy Fire Chief Julius Halas, Division Chief Brian Gorsky, Lt. Paul Dezzi

Sarasota County Sheriff's Department: Sheriff Geoffrey Monge

Technical Advisors Thanks to the following people for providing technical support during the photo shoots:

Richard Beebe, Paramedic Program Consultant, Bassett Health Care, Cooperstown, NY.
Lt. Paul Dezzi, Debbie Peace, Sarasota County Fire Department.
Michael A. Wieder, Fire Protection Publications, IFSTA

Among the fire fighters who worked tirelessly with us were:

Jerry Alston, Rob Bennett, Gary Collins, Jay Del Castillo, John Elwood, Greg Garrison, Kevin Moore, Leigh Paul, Debbie Peace, Mike Regnier, Susan Shyne, Vincent Thomas.

About the Author

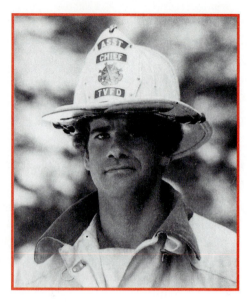

EDWARD T. DICKINSON, M.D., NREMT-P, FACEP, is currently Assistant Professor and Director of EMS Field Operations in the Department of Emergency Medicine, University of Pennsylvania School of Medicine in Philadelphia. He has also served as the Medical Director for the Town of Colonie, NY, EMS Department and the New York State Police LifeGuard Air Rescue Helicopter program. He is a residency-trained, board-certified emergency medicine physician who is a Fellow of the American College of Emergency Physicians. Dr. Dickinson holds certifications as an instructor in Pediatric Advanced Life Support (PALS), Advanced Trauma Life Support (ATLS), and Advanced Cardiac Life Support (ACLS). He has served as chairman of the EMS Education Committee of the National Association of EMS Physicians.

He began his career in EMS in 1979 as a firefighter-EMT in upstate New York. As a volunteer firefighter, he served as a company officer, assistant chief, and training officer. In 1985, he was the first volunteer firefighter in the country ever to receive the top award for heroism from the *Firehouse Magazine* Heroism and Community Awards program in recognition of his rescue of two elderly women trapped in a house fire.

Dr. Dickinson has remained active in EMS for the past 19 years. He frequently rides with EMS units on the streets and has maintained his certification as a National Registry EMT-Paramedic. He is active in pre-hospital research and has served as medical editor for numerous Brady EMT-B and First Responder texts.

PART

1

ESSENTIALS

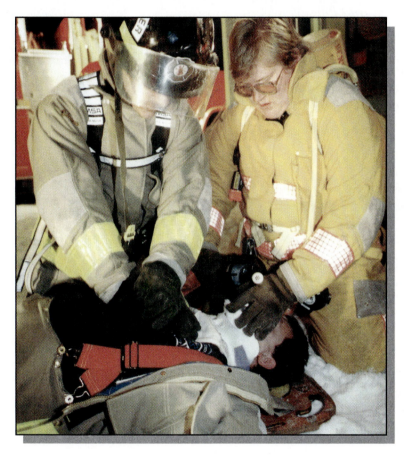

*A*s an EMT-Basic, you will be responsible for the assessment and emergency medical care of a wide variety of ill and injured patients. Before you can provide care to any patient, however, you must have a firm grasp of some basic information that you will use whenever you are on a call.

    For example, you must have a clear understanding of the overall Emergency Medical Services (EMS) system and your role in it. You must know how to assure your own well being—both physical and psychological—so that you can provide the best possible patient care. ▶

In order to provide patient care, you will have to know the basic structures and functions of the human body. Building on this information, you will learn approaches to follow whenever you assess patients. Proper procedures for communication and documentation will aid you in your assessment and in passing on information that is vital to your patient's continuing care.

These subjects and others are discussed in the chapters of Part 1.

Chapter 1   *Introduction to Emergency Medical Care*
Chapter 2   *The Well-Being of the EMT-Basic*
Chapter 3   *Infection Control and Body Substance Isolation*
Chapter 4   *Medical/Legal Issues*
Chapter 5   *Anatomy and Physiology*
Chapter 6   *Airway Management*
Chapter 7   *Patient Assessment*
Chapter 8   *Communication and Documentation*
Chapter 9   *Transition of Prehospital Care*
Chapter 10   *Lifting and Moving Patients*

Introduction to Emergency Medical Care

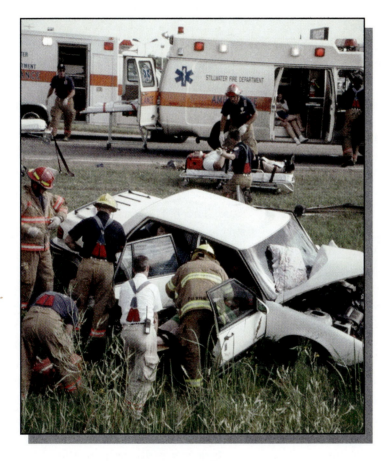

*A*s a firefighter, you are already a part of a proud tradition. Members of the fire service have always stood at the ready to save lives and to protect property. As an Emergency Medical Technician-Basic (EMT), your abilities to serve within this tradition will be enhanced. You will receive training that will enable you to assess patients and provide emergency medical care in the challenging out-of-hospital environment. You will still be a firefighter, but you will also become a competent and valuable part of the Emergency Medical Services (EMS) system.

At the completion of this chapter, the EMT-Basic student should be able to meet the following objectives:

Knowledge and Understanding

1. Define Emergency Medical Services (EMS) systems. (p. 5)
2. Differentiate the roles and responsibilities of the EMT-Basic from other prehospital care providers. (pp. 9–10, 13)
3. Describe the EMT-Basic's roles and responsibilities related to personal safety. (p. 14)
4. Discuss the roles and responsibilities of the EMT toward the safety of the crew, the patient, and bystanders. (p. 14)

5. Define quality improvement and discuss the EMT-Basic's role in the process. (pp. 11–12)
6. Define medical direction and discuss the EMT-Basic's role in the process. (pp. 10–11)
7. State the specific statutes and regulations in your state regarding the EMS system. (pp. 6, 8–11, 14–15)
8. Assess areas of personal attitude and conduct of the EMT-Basic. (pp. 14–15)
9. Characterize the various methods used to access the EMS system in your community. (pp. 8–9)

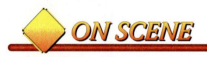

ON SCENE

Jack Brighton is practicing his swing on the community golf course when he suddenly collapses. Two golfers see him fall. Larry Kradlik and Stephanie Brown both work for a large local textile firm, and both have attended a CPR day that the firm sponsored.

Larry and Stephanie rush to Jack's side. Noting the absence of pulse and respirations, they begin CPR on him. Meanwhile, another pair of golfers come over to offer help. Stephanie directs them to call 9-1-1 for assistance. One of the golfers has a cellular phone in his bag and makes the call.

An Emergency Medical Dispatcher at the communications center takes the call. He quickly obtains information about Jack's condition and the care being provided from the caller. Then he dispatches the nearest fire department first response unit and the municipal paramedic ambulance to the golf course.

Two minutes after the golfer placed the call to 9-1-1, a Midway Fire Department unit arrives on the scene. Mark Menzies and Tom Houghton are the firefighter EMTs assigned to the unit. They grab the unit's jump kit and automated external defibrillator (AED) and rush to Jack's side. Quickly verifying that Jack has no pulse

and is not breathing, they apply the defibrillator pads and turn on the machine. It advises the crew to deliver a shock to the patient. After the first shock, the AED gives a "Check pulse" message. The EMTs reassess the patient and find a strong carotid pulse. Jack, however, is still not breathing.

Mark and Tom begin to ventilate the patient with a bag-valve-mask device and high concentration oxygen. Just as they do, the paramedic ambulance arrives. The paramedics insert an endotracheal tube to secure Jack's airway. They also start an IV and administer medications through it to stabilize Jack's heart rate. Meanwhile, Mark and Tom, at the paramedics' direction, continue to provide ventilations through the endotracheal tube.

Jack is rapidly prepared for transport in the paramedic ambulance to the local hospital. Because his condition is considered critical, the paramedics request that Mark and Tom ride along in the ambulance. Their help may be needed if Jack suffers another cardiac arrest. En route to the hospital, the paramedics contact the base station physician. She directs the paramedics to administer additional medications to the patient.

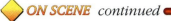

Upon arrival at the hospital, the EMTs and the paramedics provide information about Jack's condition and the treatment he has received to the emergency department physician and nurse. They then transfer Jack's care to the emergency department staff, complete their paperwork, and prepare to return to service.

Three weeks later, Jack Brighton is discharged from the hospital after open-heart surgery to correct the blockages in his coronary arteries that almost killed him. A year later, he will be back out on the golf course, trying once again to improve his game.

Jack Brighton survived only because he suffered cardiac arrest in a town with a well-developed Emergency Medical Services system. Not one person, but an entire network came together to provide him with the care he needed to return to his life and his family.

Firefighter EMTs played an important part in the system that saved Jack's life. Firefighter EMTs today can provide patients in the field with a level of care undreamed of not too long ago. To gain a better appreciation of the role of the firefighter EMT, you should understand how the system of which they are a part has developed.

THE FIRE SERVICE AND EMERGENCY MEDICAL CARE

The modern **Emergency Medical Services (EMS) system** provides patients with emergency prehospital care and transport to medical facilities. But long before the current EMS system took shape, the American fire service had been performing rescues and rendering first aid to the sick and injured. Until a few decades ago, firefighters, funeral directors, and members of volunteer rescue squads were the chief providers of emergency care to patients in the field. These providers worked to the best of their abilities, usually with training only in basic first-aid procedures and sometimes without any formal training at all. Their main goal was to transport patients to hospitals where actual care would be given.

Wartime experiences—in World Wars I and II, but especially in Korea and Vietnam—helped change ideas about emergency care. It became increasingly clear that emergency medical care provided to trauma patients in the field and during transport greatly increased patients' chances of survival and full recovery. Efforts soon began to apply these lessons learned on the battlefields to civilian life.

The EMS system we know today is the result of the hard work of many individual EMS pioneers. Not all their contributions can be cited here. However, some key events during the 1960s and early 1970s should be noted. These events laid the groundwork on which today's EMS system has been built.

- *1966*—The National Academy of Sciences, National Research Council publishes *Accidental Death and Disability: The Neglected Disease of Modern Society*. This document, known as "The White Paper," detailed the shortcomings of emergency medical care in the United States. It also made recommendations for improving emergency care, both in hospitals and in the field.

- *1966*—Congress passes the National Highway Safety Act. It charges the U.S. Department of Transportation (DOT) with developing standards that will help the states upgrade their prehospital emergency care.

- *1967*—Dr. J. Frank Pantridge describes mobile intensive care units in Northern Ireland. A report in the medical journal *Lancet* indicates that advanced life support measures can be used successfully with patients who suffer cardiac arrests in ambulances.

- *1971*—The American Academy of Orthopedic Surgeons publishes the first edition of *Emergency Care and Transportation of the Sick and Injured*. It is the first widely distributed textbook for Emergency Medical Technicians.

- *1973*—Congress passes the Emergency Medical Services Systems Act. Its goal is to provide funding and other resources for the development of comprehensive EMS systems across the country. The act included provisions covering training, equipment, and communications systems in emergency care.

- *1977*—The "Star of Life" symbol is adopted. The National Highway Traffic Safety Administration approves its use only by EMS personnel and on emergency vehicles that meet standards set by the U.S. DOT.

A different type of development turned firefighters into role models as highly trained providers of prehospital emergency medical care. This was the broadcast of the television show *Emergency!* that premiered in 1971 (Figure 1-1). On it each week, the viewing public saw firefighter EMTs and paramedics who were part of

Los Angeles County's well-defined EMS system save the lives of the seriously ill and injured. Many Americans then looked to their own communities and their own fire departments for similar levels of service and involvement in EMS and pressed for such levels if they were lacking.

Today, EMS has become a vital part of the fire service. The fire service is the largest provider of emergency medical care in the country. In some fire departments, EMS calls account for as much as 80 percent of the department's call volume. As an EMT, you will be an essential provider of emergency medical care as part of this highly evolved EMS system.

OVERVIEW OF THE EMS SYSTEM

It has been said that there are actually two "*S*"s in EMS. The first *S* stands for *services*. The second *S* stands for *system*. Although EMTs are a crucial part of the EMS system, there are many other health care providers and many other elements at work to assure that the system functions properly (Figure 1-2A-G).

The National Highway Traffic Safety Administration (NHTSA) has a Technical Assistance Program that sets standards for EMS systems across the country. The program defines 12 different parts of an EMS system and details how the system should perform in each of the 12 areas. A

Figure 1-1 The television show *Emergency!* helped raise public awareness of the fire department's role in EMS.

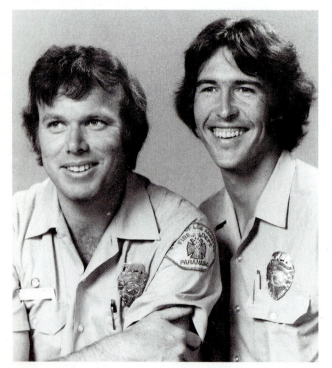

Figure 1-2A Members of the public should be able to access the EMS system easily.

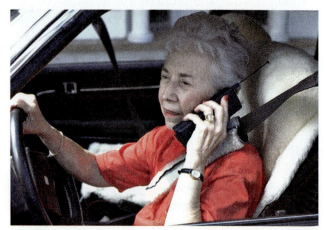

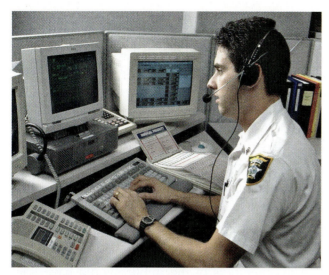

Figure 1-2B An Emergency Medical Dispatcher (EMD) directs appropriate resources to the emergency scene.

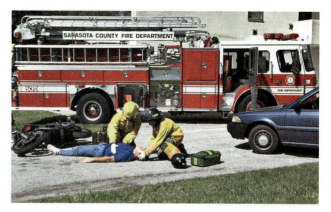

Figure 1-2C Firefighter EMTs are often the first members of the EMS system to arrive on the scene.

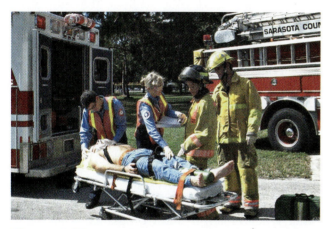

Figure 1-2D Firefighter EMTs often transfer care of the patient to other members of the EMS system.

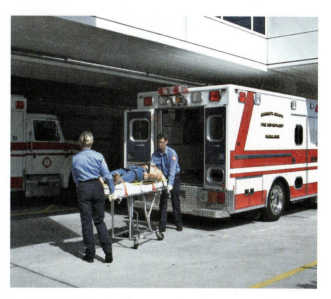

Figure 1-2E A safe, smooth trip to a receiving facility is an important part of good patient care.

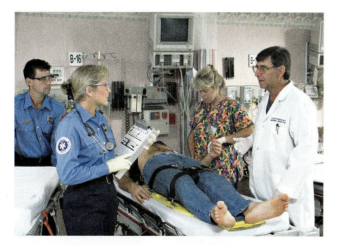

Figure 1-2F Proper transfer of patient care to emergency department personnel includes providing oral and written reports.

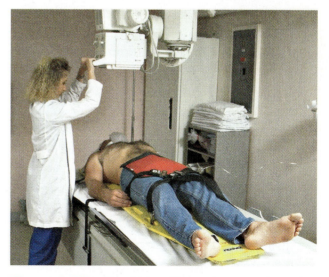

Figure 1-2G Hospital staff members continue the care of the patient.

brief description of the Technical Assistance Program standards is given below:

◆ *Regulations and policies.* Each state should have laws, policies, and procedures to govern its EMS system. A lead EMS agency should provide leadership to local jurisdictions.

◆ *Resource management.* There should be centralized control of resources available to EMS systems in a state. This is meant to ensure that all jurisdictions and all patients have equal access to an acceptable level of emergency medical care.

◆ *Human resources and training.* A standardized EMS curriculum should be taught by qualified instructors, and all personnel who transport patients in the prehospital setting should be adequately trained.

◆ *Transportation.* States should ensure that safe, reliable ground or air transportation is available for emergency patients.

◆ *Facilities.* Seriously ill or injured patients should be transported in a timely manner to an appropriate medical facility.

◆ *Communications.* A communications system must be in place that allows the public access to the EMS system. The communications system permits appropriate resources to be directed to the scene of an emergency by linking dispatchers, emergency medical care providers, and medical facilities.

◆ *Public information and education.* EMS personnel should take part in efforts to inform citizens about how they can prevent accidents and injuries and how they can access the EMS system when it is needed.

◆ *Medical direction.* Each EMS system should have a physician who serves as its medical director. The medical director delegates medical practice to non-physician caregivers, such as EMTs. The medical director oversees all aspects of patient care.

◆ *Trauma systems.* Each state should have a system for caring for trauma patients. It should include a specialized trauma center (or centers), rehabilitation programs, and guidelines for assigning patients and transporting them to the trauma center(s).

◆ *Evaluation.* Each state should have a program for continually monitoring and upgrading the quality of care in its EMS system.

ELEMENTS OF THE EMS SYSTEM

To gain a better idea of how EMS systems operate, take a closer look at parts described in the NHTSA's Technical Assistance Program.

Public Information and Education

Ideally, members of the public should have contact with their local EMS system before they ever need it. This is because the system's public information programs should be reaching out to them, providing them with information that may keep them from needing prehospital emergency care. Such programs should teach about *injury prevention*. For example, they might stress the use of seat belts in cars and precautions to be taken in cars with airbags. School programs might highlight for children the importance of wearing helmets when bike riding and wearing helmets and other protective gear when skateboarding.

Education won't prevent all emergencies, however. That is why EMS systems should offer other types of information programs. Some campaigns, for example, might inform the public about how to access EMS in case of an emergency. The system might also make more formal educational opportunities available. It might offer CPR courses or training for future First Responders or Emergency Medical Technicians.

Communications Systems

As noted above, the EMS system has the obligation of providing a system of communications. This system should allow citizens who need emergency services access to it. The system must also permit appropriate resources to be directed where they are needed.

Access to the system for citizens can be broken down into 9-1-1 and non-9-1-1 systems. A call to 9-1-1, also known as the *universal number,* connects the caller with a central communications center. A dispatcher at the center takes information about the emergency and quickly dispatches appropriate fire, police, and EMS personnel based on that information. In some areas, "enhanced" 9-1-1 (E 9-1-1) systems can automatically identify the caller's phone number and the location from which the call is coming.

In areas without a 9-1-1 system, callers may have to dial a seven-digit (or longer) phone number to reach a dispatch center. In some municipalities, callers can access emergency resources directly by using call or pull boxes.

Once a caller has contacted the EMS system, the system must have the resources to direct appropriate aid to him. It should have properly trained dispatchers who can evaluate the caller's information and dispatch the resources that are needed to the scene. The dispatchers may also be able to provide patient care instructions for callers to follow until responders reach the scene. There should be pagers or station alert systems to rapidly notify the appropriate units of the dispatch. Additionally, there must be a radio (or cellular or wireless phone) system. This system must provide two-way communications between the dispatcher and EMS units in the field. That system must also permit two-way communications between the field units and the medical facility for providing updates on the patient's status and for obtaining medical direction.

Human Resources and Training

An EMS system works because of the people in it. An EMS system may use emergency care providers with several different levels of training.

Emergency Medical Dispatcher

The EMS dispatcher receives calls from the public about emergencies and directs appropriate personnel and resources to the scene. The **Emergency Medical Dispatcher** (EMD) is specially trained to obtain essential medical information from callers. With this information and the assistance of a flip-card or computer system, an EMD can determine the urgency, or priority, of the patient's need for emergency medical assistance. Knowing the patient's priority, the EMD can then dispatch the units at the appropriate level of vehicle response (such as a red-lights-and-siren

response versus a quiet response) and the appropriate level of medical response (basic life support versus advanced life support).

First Responder

A **Certified First Responder (CFR)** is trained to provide emergency medical care until the arrival of EMTs or paramedics. Police officers, firefighters, industrial health officers, and other professionals likely to be first on the scene of emergencies are frequently trained to deliver this level of care. CFRs can perform a general patient assessment. They are also trained to provide basic emergency medical care such as bleeding control, spinal stabilization, and CPR. In some areas, they may also be allowed to administer oxygen. An increasing number of CFRs are also being trained in the use of automated external defibrillators (AEDs).

Emergency Medical Technician-Basic

The **Emergency Medical Technician-Basic (EMT-B)** is the foundation upon which modern EMS systems are built. That level of certification is the most widely obtained among prehospital care providers. As an EMT, you will be taught how to assess and provide emergency medical care for a wide variety of illnesses and injuries. **Basic life support** (BLS) skills—including CPR, oxygen administration, spinal immobilization, emergency childbirth assistance, splinting, and hemorrhage control—have long been the mainstay of the care provided by EMTs.

The adoption of the U.S. Department of Transportation 1994 EMT-Basic National Standard Curriculum brought with it changes in the EMT's job description. Some skills that had previously been considered **advanced life support** (ALS) and reserved for advanced EMTs became part of the EMT-Basic's responsibilities. Among these were using automated external defibrillators (AEDs) and assisting patients with administration of prescription medications (including epinephrine auto-injectors, nitroglycerin, and inhaled asthma medications). Definitive control of a patient's airway through endotracheal intubation is now also an *optional* EMT skill that may be taught in your local jurisdiction if approved by medical direction.

Emergency Medical Technician-Intermediate

The **EMT-Intermediate (EMT-I)** has completed training as an EMT and gone on to be certified in the use of certain ALS skills. EMT-Is are considered "advanced EMTs." They are trained to administer intravenous (IV) fluids. They can also perform advanced airway management through endotracheal intubation or use of an alternative advanced airway device. Depending on their hours of training and the state and jurisdiction in which they work, EMT-Is may be allowed to administer certain emergency IV medications much as paramedics do. A variety of terms in addition to EMT-I are used for personnel with this level of training; the terms include "cardiac technician," "critical care technician," and "AEMT-3."

Emergency Medical Technician-Paramedic

The **Emergency Medical Technician-Paramedic (EMT-P)** is the most extensively trained prehospital care provider. EMT-Ps not only complete classroom and lab teaching but also serve extensive hospital rotations and must usually complete field internships. EMT-Ps have advanced assessment skills, can interpret electrocardiograms (EKGs), administer a wide variety of medications, and perform endotracheal intubations. Many also have training in some emergency procedures such as surgical airway management.

Certification and Licensing

EMTs are certified, and in some cases licensed, by individual states. In order to be certified, an EMT or advanced EMT must pass both written examinations and tests demonstrating practical mastery of certain skills. Certified EMTs at all levels are usually required to recertify every few years. Recertification is based upon either completion of a certain number of hours of continuing education courses, successful completion of a formal recertification course, or reexamination.

In some jurisdictions, prehospital providers must receive credentials granted by regional EMS oversight agencies in order to work in specific regions. This is especially common at the ad-vanced EMT levels. This practice assures that the advanced EMTs have knowledge of and are willing to comply with local patient care protocols.

The National Registry of Emergency Medical Technicians (NREMT) provides testing and certification on a national level for Certified First Responders, EMT-Bs, EMT-Is, and EMT-Ps (Figure 1-3). Many states use the National Registry examination and certification system as the sole basis of their own state certifications. NREMT certification is desirable even if it is not required in your state. Obtaining it makes certification easier if you move to another state. Also, NREMT certification indicates that you have exhibited additional professionalism by obtaining a nationally recognized certification.

Medical Direction

Certification as an EMT is not a license to practice medicine. In modern EMS systems, physicians provide **medical direction** for the systems (Figure 1-4). This means that a physician (or physicians) must be responsible for the clinical and patient care aspects of each EMS system's operations. The care rendered by EMTs within a system is considered an extension of the medical director's authority and license as a physician.

Physicians participate at many levels in EMS systems. Regional boards of physicians may set policies and patient care guidelines. Medical

Figure 1-3 The NREMT-Basic patch indicates the wearer has successfully completed demanding practical and written examinations.

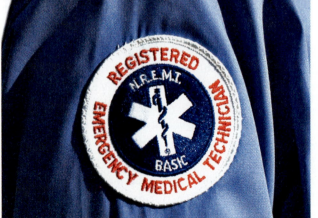

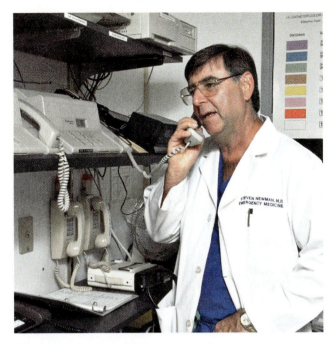

Figure 1-4 The EMS medical director can provide on-line guidance on patient care to EMS personnel in the field.

directors may provide dedicated input to an agency's EMS service. Also, on-duty emergency department physicians may provide medical direction and feedback to EMTs at the hospital.

Medical direction—sometimes called *medical control* or *medical oversight*—can take different forms. **On-line medical direction** occurs when a physician gives direct orders to a prehospital care provider either by radio or telephone. For example, an EMT might call in by radio to the emergency department physician requesting permission to administer activated charcoal to a patient who has ingested a poison. The physician may approve or disapprove the request. This is an example of on-line medical direction.

Off-line medical direction refers to medical policies, procedures, and practices that a system physician has set up in advance of a call. These policies, procedures, and practices can be followed in certain situations without speaking to a physician. For example, an EMT can assist a patient with chest pain in taking his prescribed nitroglycerin without speaking to a physician if the EMT's agency has a predetermined physician-approved protocol calling for such administration. **Protocols** are lists of steps or actions to be performed in certain situations. Other terms for protocols are **standing orders** or **treatment guidelines.**

As an EMT you are likely to interact with the physician(s) responsible for your department's medical direction in several ways:

◆ *By delivering on-scene patient care as the physician observes.* It is essential that physicians responsible for the quality of patient care in an EMS system get into the streets to see firsthand the care being provided (Figure 1-5).

◆ *By receiving on-line medical direction in certain cases.*

◆ *By participating in the department's evaluation program.* The medical director is responsible for reviewing all aspects of the department's patient care. An EMT may work with the physician as part of a quality improvement committee or may receive feedback on his patient care directly from the medical director.

Evaluation

As noted above, every EMS system must have in place a system to monitor the quality of the care it provides to its patients. In prehospital care, this evaluation system is usually referred to as **quality improvement (QI).** Other common terms for

Figure 1-5 The medical director should get out into the field to observe firsthand the quality of care the EMS system is providing.

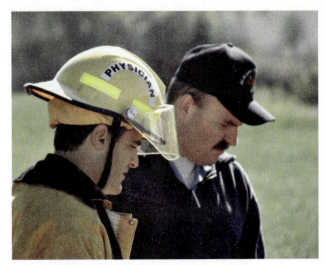

such systems are quality assessment (QA), continuous quality improvement (CQI), and total quality management (TQM). The federal Department of Transportation's EMT-B curriculum defines QI as follows: "A system of internal and external reviews and audits of all aspects of an EMS system so as to identify those aspects needing improvement to assure that the public receives the highest quality prehospital care" (Figure 1-6).

The QI system thus has two goals. One is to find problems or weaknesses within the system. The other is to bring about changes in those problem areas that will *improve the quality* of the system.

As an EMT, you have a professional obligation to participate actively in your department's QI program. You may do this by:

- Providing clear and accurate documentation of patient care
- Participating in run reviews and audits
- Serving on QI committees
- Gathering feedback from patients, hospital staff, and other prehospital providers about the quality of care rendered
- Being receptive to constructive feedback from the QI system
- Maintaining personal knowledge and skills to assure that quality care is delivered at all times
- Participating in continuing education programs

Figure 1-6 The quality improvement (QI) committee is part of a process aimed at ensuring that the EMS system is providing the best possible patient care.

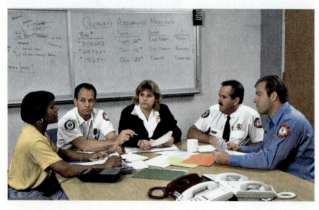

- Carrying out preventive maintenance on medical devices and other equipment to assure their proper functioning during emergency care situations

COMPANY OFFICER'S NOTES

As a company officer, you will be in a unique position to observe the quality of care provided by your crew. You may play numerous roles in the provision of QI. For example, you might provide direct feedback to the crew after a call or you might identify calls that should be referred to the system's QI committee.

Facilities and Trauma Systems

The goal of the EMS system is to minimize the patient's risk of death (mortality) and permanent disability (morbidity). To this end, the prehospital EMS system is part of a larger health care system that is designed to provide comprehensive patient care.

The component of the health care system that you as an EMT will interact with most often is the hospital emergency department. The decision about the hospital to which you will transport a patient is usually based upon the patient's request. When there is more than one hospital in an area, patients tend to go to the one with which their doctor or their health care plan is affiliated.

Special Facilities

In some cases, your local EMS system may have protocols directing that patients with certain injuries or illnesses be transported to specified receiving facilities. As part of the larger health care system, special medical centers have been developed. These centers have special equipment and medical personnel with extensive training in caring for patients with certain problems. Such centers are more common in larger metropolitan areas. Examples of specialty centers include the following:

- *Trauma centers.* At these centers, surgery teams are available 24 hours a day. The centers are equipped to handle injuries that are beyond the capabilities of standard hospital emergency departments.

- *Burn centers.* These specialize in caring for seriously burned patients. They usually also provide long-term care and rehabilitation.

- *Poison control centers.* They treat victims of poisoning. Also, they usually can provide guidance for EMS personnel in the field who are confronted with poisoning cases.

- *Spine and head injury centers.* These injuries can have serious long-term consequences. Personnel at such centers have extensive training in the delicate surgery often required in these cases. These centers usually also provide long-term care and rehabilitation.

- *Pediatric centers.* The anatomical and physiological differences in infants and children as opposed to adults often mean they respond differently to illness and injury. Medical personnel at these specialized centers are fully alert to these differences and their implications for patient care.

- *Hyperbaric centers.* These centers have special facilities for creating environments of high atmospheric pressure. Such environments are useful in treating patients suffering from smoke inhalation, carbon monoxide poisoning, and certain other illnesses.

Health Care Professionals

In addition to the prehospital workers described earlier, as an EMT you will be working with a variety of health care professionals in the hospitals and specialty centers to which you transport patients. Among these professionals will be the following:

Nurses. Your most frequent contacts will probably be with emergency department (ED) nurses. A standard practice is for each patient arriving in the ED to have a nurse assigned to him. You will usually give your oral reports on the patient's condition as well as any patient-related paperwork to this nurse.

EDs in busier areas will often have a *triage nurse.* The triage nurse screens all incoming patients, both walk-ins and ambulance patients. This nurse determines how urgent their problems are and assigns patients to specific beds based on the patients' needs for evaluation and further treatment.

Many EDs will also a have a *charge nurse* on duty for each shift. The charge nurse, along with the attending ED physician, is responsible for the smooth running of the department.

You may also encounter *nurse practitioners* (NPs) working in the emergency department. NPs are registered nurses who have received advanced education and are trained in physical diagnosis and treatment. In most states, nurse practitioners can prescribe medications and order tests for patients.

Physicians. Most emergency departments are staffed at all times by physicians. Individual states and hospitals determine the qualifications a physician must possess to staff an ED. In general, these physicians have obtained additional certification in advanced cardiac and trauma life support. Some ED physicians are specially trained and board certified as specialists in emergency medicine. You may also interact with other physician specialists in the ED, including trauma surgeons and pediatric specialists.

Physician Assistants. *Physician assistants* (PAs) are widely used in emergency departments as "physician extenders." PAs are trained to work under the direct or indirect supervision of physicians. They evaluate and treat patients and are authorized by their supervising physician to perform procedures such as suturing and more advanced procedures. In most states, PAs are allowed to prescribe medications. In some rural areas, the emergency department may be staffed only by a PA who has a physician available for on-line consultation.

Other Health Care Professionals. Other professionals and members of the health care team you may encounter in the ED include:

- Respiratory therapists
- Lab technicians
- Nursing assistants

- Radiology technicians
- Emergency room technicians

Public Safety Officers. Public safety officers, such as members of the local police department or sheriff's office, are not traditionally considered to be part of the EMS system. However, law enforcement officers and EMS personnel often work very closely together. EMTs and police officers interact extensively at motor vehicle crash scenes, crime scenes, and calls involving behavioral emergencies. Although the EMT has a responsibility to assess and assure scene safety, it is, in fact, police officers who most commonly assure the safety of both EMTs and patients at scenes such as these.

In some EMS systems, police officers may act as first responders. They are often trained to control bleeding, initiate CPR, and, in some areas, use automated external defibrillators (AEDs).

ROLES AND RESPONSIBILITIES OF THE EMT

As a trained firefighter, you already have a number of well-defined roles and responsibilities. As an EMT, those duties and responsibilities will expand greatly.

Your ultimate responsibility as an EMT will be to provide excellent patient care. To fulfill this responsibility, there are a number of different duties you must perform. These will be described at greater length throughout the rest of this book, but they are briefly summarized below:

- *Assuring personal safety.* Remember that you cannot carry out your responsibilities of caring for a patient if you yourself are injured.
- *Assuring the safety of the patient, of other firefighters and emergency care providers, and of bystanders at all times.*
- *Performing patient assessments in order to determine what care is necessary.*
- *Lifting and moving patients in a fashion that is safe for the patient and minimizes the risk of related injuries to yourself and the crew.*

- *Providing for the safe transport of the patient or the smooth transition of patient care to those who will transport him.*
- *Providing complete, accurate, and appropriate documentation of your patient as required by your department.*
- *Respecting the patient as another human at all times.*
- *Acting as a patient advocate.* This means that you must at all times speak up for the patient's rights and needs and do what you can to assure his well being. Remember that you must be sensitive to the patient's psychological as well as physical needs.

Professionalism

The EMT is a relatively new member of the health care team. After a relatively short training period (as compared to those required for many other health professionals), you will be empowered to make potential life-or-death decisions on the behalf of another human being who has been injured or become ill. This is a huge responsibility, and it should not be taken lightly.

When on duty, you must at all times conduct yourself in a professional manner that conveys to the patient, the public, and fellow firefighters that you take your responsibility seriously. Professionalism has nothing to do with salary or financial reimbursement. It has everything to do with accepting the responsibility of providing the best possible patient care. As a professional you will be expected to do the following (Figure 1-7):

- *Dress in a way that projects a positive professional image.*
- *Maintain as neat and clean an appearance as possible given the circumstances in which you are providing care.*
- *Maintain an up-to-date knowledge of current standards of emergency care and be aware of changes in medical treatment as they emerge.* You can do this by taking formal continuing education or refresher courses. You should also read articles and medical studies in journals dealing with the provision of prehospital care. Among these publications are the *Jour-*

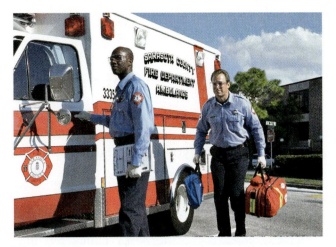

Figure 1-7 EMTs who maintain a professional appearance inspire confidence in their patients.

nal of Emergency Medical Services (JEMS); Emergency—The Journal of Emergency Services; Prehospital Emergency Care; and Annals of Emergency Medicine.

◆ *Maintain up-to-date knowledge of local, state, and national issues affecting EMS.* Be aware of financial issues, aspects of managed care programs, legislation, and, in some cases, labor-related issues that can impact on the way prehospital care is delivered in your jurisdiction.

◆ *Actively participate in your EMS system's quality improvement program.*

◆ *Be willing to participate in research studies.* When you do, report data honestly and without personal bias.

◆ *Always make the patient's medical and psychological needs your priority without endangering yourself.*

The chapter continues with *Chapter Review* on page 16.

Chapter Review

SUMMARY

As an EMT, you will be part of a comprehensive health care system designed to provide the best possible patient care. It is important that you become familiar with the many aspects of the EMS system in which you work. Knowing as much as you can about that system will help you to better understand your roles and responsibilities as an EMT.

REVIEWING KEY CONCEPTS

1. Explain the purpose of the Emergency Medical Service system.

2. List the basic methods by which a citizen can access the EMS system. Explain some of the advantages and disadvantages of these methods.

3. Describe the three standard levels of emergency medical technician certification.

4. Explain the difference between on-line and off-line medical direction.

5. Define QI and explain its purpose.

6. List the types of special facilities that may be part of an EMS system. Name some of the special facilities in your area.

RESOURCES TO LEARN MORE

Books

Bledsoe, Bryan E., Porter, Robert S., Shade, Bruce R. *Paramedic Emergency Care, Third Edition.* Upper Saddle River, NJ: Brady/Prentice Hall, 1992.

Karren, K.J., Hafen, B.Q., Limmer, D., Dickinson, E.T. *First Responder: A Skills Approach, Fifth Edition.* Upper Saddle River, NJ: Brady/Prentice Hall, 1998.

Paris, P.M., Roth, R.N., and Verdile, V.P., eds. *Prehospital Medicine: The Art of On-line Medical Command.* St. Louis: Mosby, 1996.

Steele, Susi. *Emergency Dispatching: A Medical Communicator's Guide.* Upper Saddle River, NJ: Brady/Prentice Hall, 1992.

Organizations

National Registry of EMTs. 6610 Busch Blvd., P.O. Box 29233, Columbus, OH 43229-0233. Telephone: 614-888-4484.

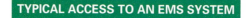

TYPICAL ACCESS TO AN EMS SYSTEM

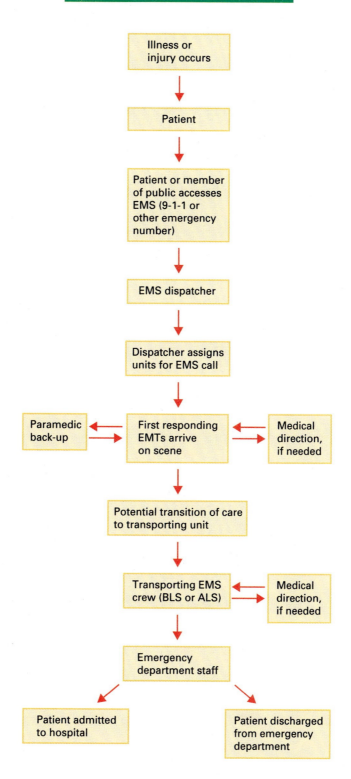

The Well-Being of the EMT-Basic

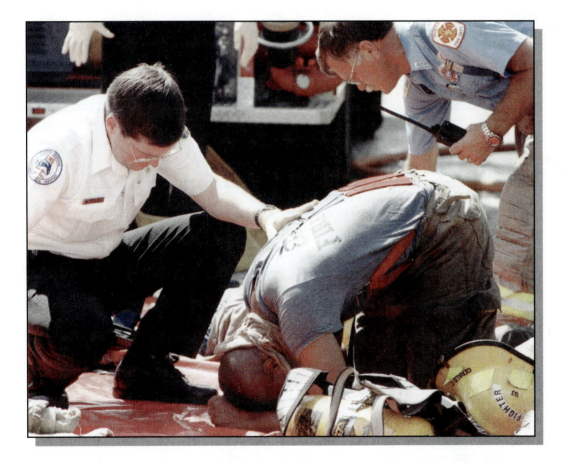

*A*s a firefighter, you have probably experienced difficult and
stressful situations. The loss of life in a fire, the injury of a
colleague, the emotional anguish of people devastated by the loss
of livelihood and property—these are all examples of stressful situations
that a firefighter confronts in the course of his or her job. As an EMT,
you will most likely face additional hazards and stress. One of the most
important skills you can learn as an EMT is how to minimize the risks of
falling victim to the physical and emotional hazards that EMS providers
commonly encounter.

At the completion of this chapter, the EMT-Basic student should be able to meet the following objectives:

Knowledge and Understanding

1. List possible emotional reactions that the EMT-Basic may experience when faced with trauma, illness, death, and dying. (pp. 20–23)

2. Discuss the possible reactions that a family member may exhibit when confronted with death and dying. (pp. 20–21)

3. State the steps in the EMT-Basic's approach to the family confronted with death and dying. (p. 21)

4. State the possible reactions that the family of the EMT-Basic may exhibit due to involvement with EMS. (pp. 24–25)

5. Recognize the signs and symptoms of critical incident stress. (pp. 23–24, 25)

6. State the possible steps that the EMT-Basic may take to help reduce/alleviate stress. (pp. 23–26)

7. Explain the need to determine scene safety. (p. 26)

8. List the personal protective equipment necessary for each of the following situations: (pp. 26–31)
   —Hazardous materials
   —Rescue operations
   —Violent scenes
   —Crime scenes

9. Explain the rationale for serving as an advocate for the use of appropriate protective equipment. (p. 26)

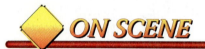

ON SCENE

DISPATCH: *KED 629, MADISON COUNTY FIRE CONTROL TO HAMILTON FIRE, HAMILTON RESCUE. RESPOND FOR A REPORTED SNOWMOBILE ACCIDENT, WEST LAKE ROAD AT SANDS LANE. TIME OUT IS 1312.*

You have just completed your EMT course. It is a cold November day and a light snow has been falling all day. You drive to the station and respond on board the department's rescue unit. As you are en route, your assistant chief arrives on the scene and radios you a scene size-up. He advises you will have as patients two children who were riding a snowmobile and were struck by an automobile while crossing the road. The chief states that one child is in cardiac arrest and the other is in respiratory arrest.

Your unit arrives on scene 2 minutes later. As you come off the back of the rescue truck, you see two bodies. The first is in the center of the road near the car involved. The second is lying by the side of the road about 25 yards (23 meters) away. A 3-foot-wide streak of blood stretches from the wrecked snowmobile down the snow-covered road to the body.

The senior rescue officer, who is a paramedic, quickly assesses the patient lying farther away and returns, confirming the cardiac arrest. Because on-scene resources are limited and the child near the car still has a pulse, he decides to not initiate any treatment on the patient in cardiac arrest.

You immediately move to the head of the child near the car and begin to provide ventilations with a pocket mask while another firefighter stabilizes the patient's neck. As you work, you notice that the child's left leg is almost completely severed at the hip.

After about a minute of ventilations, the paramedic reports a loss of pulses. He begins chest compressions and you continue ventilations as the child is rapidly secured to a spine board and moved to the rescue unit.

The ride to the hospital takes less than 4 minutes. During that time, you continue to ventilate the patient while another EMT suctions the bloody airway almost constantly. At the community hospital, the emergency department physician and the surgeon make their best efforts to revive the child. But they never regain a pulse. The child is pronounced dead 16 minutes after arrival at the emergency department.

As you begin to restock supplies and clean your equipment, the parents of both children arrive at the emergency department. The physicians take the parents into the family room. Suddenly, you hear screams. The door to the room

flies open. One mother bursts through it, shouting back at the doctors, "No! You're lying! You're lying! Josh is at school. He's okay. I know it. Oh God, take me instead and bring him back! Oh God!" Her husband comes up to her and she collapses into his arms. Clinging to each other, the couple begins to sob. The emergency department is silent as you and your crew leave to return to quarters.

That night you call your parents back home just to see how they are doing.

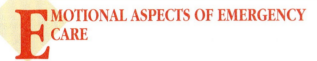

EMOTIONAL ASPECTS OF EMERGENCY CARE

Situations in which emergency medical care is provided are by their nature stressful. Patients experiencing sudden illness or injury wonder if they are going to live or die. Family members see loved ones who, just moments before had been well and healthy, suffer agonizing pain from injuries received in an accident; or they see dear friends dying after years of debilitating illness. Situations like these can produce a wide range of emotions—fear, anger, sorrow, anxiety. As an EMT, you must always be aware of the emotions your patients and their families are experiencing. Respect those emotions. At the same time, realize that you, too, are human and that caring for patients will produce emotional responses in you as well.

When your emotions are aroused, you are experiencing a form of **stress.** Sometimes stress can be positive, helping you to work effectively under pressure. At other times, though, stresses can cause negative changes. You will learn later in this chapter about ways of dealing with stress to avoid its negative effects. But first, you should be familiar with situations that can produce high levels of stress.

Death and Dying

At some time in your career, you will respond to a call involving a dead or dying patient. Perhaps the patient will be dead when you arrive on the scene. Perhaps the patient will be conscious and speak to you before his death. An inescapable reality of emergency medical care is that sometimes, despite your best possible care, your patient will die. Although all people eventually die, death is almost always a very troubling event. As an EMT, you must be aware of the ways in which patients and their families—and you yourself—are likely to react to death and dying.

Almost 20 years ago, Dr. Elisabeth Kübler-Ross described the emotional stages that dying patients went through as they tried to come to terms with their own mortality. Her studies were based on observations over time of patients with terminal illnesses. Nevertheless, many of her observations are still relevant to critically injured or ill patients and their families in emergencies.

Kübler-Ross described how patients and their loved ones pass through different stages of emotions as they try to "deal" with death. The stages in this process include the following:

◆ *Denial ("Not me.")* The patient refuses to accept that he is dying. This is often the first defense mechanism.

- *Anger ("Why me?")* This stage develops as the patient realizes his lack of control in the situation. In this stage, he and his family may lash out, verbally or even physically, at the EMT and other EMS personnel. You should recognize such anger as an outgrowth of frustration and not take it personally. However, you should never allow yourself to be physically assaulted. Try to understand what the patient and his family are feeling. Employ good listening and communication skills.

- *Bargaining ("Okay, but first let me . . .")* In this stage, the patient tries to reach some sort of deal or agreement that, in his mind, will postpone death.

- *Depression ("Okay, but I haven't . . .")* The patient may become sad, silent, despairing about things he didn't do and now will not have time to do.

- *Acceptance ("Okay, I'm not afraid.")* In this stage, the patient accepts the fact of his death, although this does not mean he is happy about dying. Often, the patient reaches this stage before his family does. Thus, the family may be the ones who will need your support most at this point.

These stages are not tidy categories. Although patients are often said to "proceed" from denial through the other stages to final acceptance, this is not always the case. Sometimes patients and families experience more than one stage at the same time. Sometimes they may not experience a stage at all.

Because of the usual suddenness of deaths that you will encounter as an EMT, few patients or their families will go through all the stages as described. However, many patients and families will experience one or more of the stages in attempting to come to terms with death. For example, the child's mother in this chapter's On Scene exhibited denial ("No! You're lying!"), anger (her shouting at the doctors), bargaining ("Oh God, take me instead"), and depression (her collapsing into her husband's arms to cry) in her response to the shock of her child's death.

When you are called to the scene of a dying or dead patient, you may be able to provide only limited medical care. Remember, though, that the patient and his family will need emotional support at this difficult time. People's responses to death and dying can differ widely. Many religious, cultural, social, and medical factors shape those responses. This means there is no single set of rules to follow when you deal with dying patients and their family members.

The key to your behavior at these times is to be alert to the needs of the patient (and family). Respect his dignity. Talk directly to him, if possible. Ask if there is anything the patient needs. (Giving him some sense of control at this critical time is important.) Listen carefully when the patient speaks to you. Respond to his needs in any way you reasonably can. If the patient expresses a desire for privacy, do not intrude any more than your duties demand.

Other general guidelines that may help you in managing these most difficult situations include the following:

- Be prepared for a wide range of responses to death from the patient and the family. Be aware that family members may express anger, rage, or despair.

- Listen with sympathy and concern to what the patient and the family are saying.

- Do not falsely reassure the patient. You can be honest without being blunt or brutal.

- Do not offer medical opinions that are beyond your expertise and training.

- Use a gentle voice.

- Make good eye contact when speaking with the patient and family.

- Let the patient know that everything that can be done is being done.

- Do not be afraid of touching the patient to offer comfort and reassurance, if such touching seems appropriate.

- Comfort the family.

Other Stressful Situations

Dealing with the dead or dying patient is one of the most stressful and emotionally taxing situations that you will face as an EMT. However, firefighter EMTs have to cope with many other difficult situations. Some of those most likely to produce high levels of stress are described below.

Remember that in these situations, you, other EMS personnel, patients, family members, and bystanders are all likely to be deeply affected by stress. People involved in events like these may respond in unpredictable ways.

Multiple-Casualty Incidents

A **multiple-casualty incident** (MCI) is any single call that involves three or more patients. MCIs are stressful for many reasons. They not only involve multiple patients, but they also are usually prolonged operations that result in physical as well as psychological fatigue.

Infants and Children

No matter how seasoned you become as an EMT, calls involving seriously ill or injured infants or children tend to affect you more deeply than calls involving adults. Stress can be heightened when the child involved is the same age as one of your own children or a child you know well. Stress levels can rise even higher because of the frustration of knowing that so many of the childhood injuries EMTs treat could be prevented with adequate supervision by parents or caregivers.

Severe Injuries

A badly damaged human body can be difficult to observe. An awareness that the damage means intense pain and a possible life of disability for the patient makes such a call even more stressful for the observer. Calls for amputations, eviscerations, blindings, and deep wounds can all produce high levels of stress.

Abuse and Neglect

Firefighter EMTs may witness the effects of abuse and neglect on children, elders, and spouses. The abuse and neglect can be physical, psychological, or both. EMTs often feel deep anger and frustration in these situations.

Death or Injury of a Coworker

As EMTs, we often forget our own vulnerability to injury and even to death. When a coworker is injured or killed on the job, it is deeply troubling. We mourn the loss of the person. But we are also shaken because that loss reminds us how fragile our own lives are.

In addition to these high-stress calls, other job-related factors can cause stress. These factors might include long working hours, fear of making errors, and boredom between calls. Add to all these the normal stresses of daily life—like difficulties in personal finances and in personal relationships—and it's clear that an EMT's stress levels can be very high indeed.

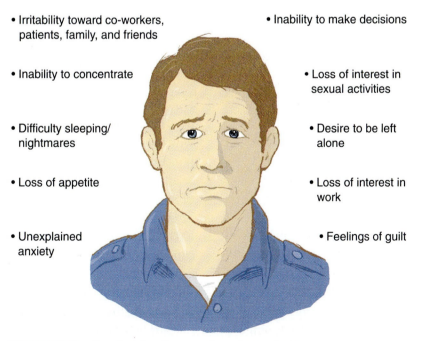

- Irritability toward co-workers, patients, family, and friends
- Inability to concentrate
- Difficulty sleeping/ nightmares
- Loss of appetite
- Unexplained anxiety
- Inability to make decisions
- Loss of interest in sexual activities
- Desire to be left alone
- Loss of interest in work
- Feelings of guilt

Figure 2-1   Be alert for the warning signs of stress.

A person under too much stress for too long will experience some form of stress reaction. The reaction might take the form of **burnout**—a state of exhaustion or irritability that decreases effectiveness on the job. If unrelieved, the high stress levels can have even more serious long-term psychological and physical complications.

Stress Management

To manage stress effectively, you must first learn how to recognize its signs in yourself and in others (Figure 2-1). Some of the most common warning signs and symptoms of stress include the following:

- Irritability with family, friends, and coworkers
- Inability to concentrate
- Difficulty sleeping or nightmares
- Loss of appetite
- Loss of sexual desire
- Anxiety
- Indecisiveness
- Guilt
- Isolation
- Loss of interest in work

If you recognize several of these symptoms in yourself, then you should act to reduce your level of stress. The key to counteracting stress is to strike a good balance between work, family, recreation, and personal health interests in your life. Specific steps to reduce stress include:

- *Increasing your exercise.* Aerobic exercises such as walking, running, or using gym equipment such as stationary bicycles and treadmills may markedly reduce your level of stress.
- *Modifying your diet.* Eat more healthy, balanced meals. Reduce the consumption of sugar, caffeine, and alcoholic beverages. Avoid fatty foods. Increase your intake of carbohydrates.
- *Using relaxation, meditation, and visual imagery techniques.* Some individuals find enrolling in programs or classes that use these techniques to be very helpful.
- *Altering your work schedule.* If you can identify specific factors relating to scheduling that increase your stress, then request a change if

possible. Being relocated to a less busy unit or scheduling larger blocks of time to spend off-duty with friends and family may be helpful.

The effects of stress can be serious. If your own attempts to control stress don't work, seek professional help. Health insurance policies or employee assistance programs may cover the costs of such care. Remember that using professional care is not a sign of weakness; it's a way to make yourself a more effective and efficient firefighter EMT.

COMPANY OFFICER'S NOTES

Always be on the lookout for signs and symptoms of stress in your crew. Watch for both signs of acute stress reaction to an immediate situation and signs of chronic stress.

A firefighter who is overwhelmed by stress in a particular situation may pose an immediate hazard to himself and to other firefighters. In such a situation, immediately reassign the firefighter to another sector if possible; when the call is over, refer him for CISD.

Some personnel will show or complain of the signs and symptoms of stress increasingly over time. It is extremely important that you reach out to such personnel. Offer to talk with them about their problems or complaints. If it seems more appropriate, suggest resources for counseling. Be sure to convey the message that there is no weakness or shame attached in seeking help for problems with stress.

Family and Friends' Responses

For many firefighters, their fellow firefighters are like a second family. The intense conditions in which firefighters often work and their common bond of duty solidify these relationships. These relationships can be a source of strength in times of stress.

Family and friends who are not firefighters or EMTs can offer support as well. However, they can often be additional sources of stress for firefighter EMTs.

There are a variety of reasons why this is so. Family and friends often do not fully understand or cannot relate to many of the factors that affect your life as a fire service EMT. At times when you want to share details about your job or a particularly troubling call, you may find that your friends and family appear uninterested or "grossed out" by what you tell them.

Family and friends also experience stress related to your work. They may worry about the dangers you face on the job. They may also feel frustration about the uncertainties that come with emergency work. For example, they may resent the fact that you are constantly "on call," making activities difficult to plan or "ruining" the ones that do take place when your pager goes off.

Reducing stress growing out of relations with family and friends requires give and take on both sides. This give-and-take begins with communicating. Each side has to be willing to share its concerns and hear those of the other side. You have to make clear that there are things you'd like to talk about. Family and friends should be willing to recognize your need to talk. Work out ground rules for communicating. Express your needs, but listen to and respect the wishes of a family member who says to you, "I'd really like to hear what happened, but could you wait till after I'm finished eating?"

There are practical steps you can take to improve these relationships. Set aside specific times to spend with family members and friends. As far as possible, don't let anything interrupt these appointments when you set them. Involve family and friends in things you are doing off the job; for example, invite them to take part in your exercise program if appropriate.

Remember, you will always have to cope with sources of stress as an EMT. The odds are good, however, that you can reduce or eliminate stress arising from relationships with family and friends. A positive attitude, a willingness to communicate, and an openness to the ideas and feelings of others can get you on the way to this goal.

Comprehensive Critical Incident Stress Management

In a section above, you read about incidents highly likely to cause stress in emergency workers. Sometimes these incidents are so large or they create such strong emotional responses that their impact is almost overwhelming. For example, a school bus plunges through a guardrail into a ravine, killing eight young children. Or an airplane crashes into a cornfield killing 176 passengers and crew members. Events like these are called **critical incidents.** Such an incident can produce an extreme stress reaction, one so powerful that it can interfere with an emergency worker's ability to function, either during the incident or after it. This intense reaction leaves the worker at increased risk of developing long-term emotional and psychological difficulties, including *post-traumatic stress syndrome.*

To counteract this risk, systems of comprehensive critical incident stress management have been developed. The cornerstone of most of these programs is the process called **critical incident stress debriefing** (CISD).

CISD is a specially organized, open discussion that takes place after a serious and emotionally taxing event. Its purpose is to provide a forum in which emergency workers can release their stress (Figure 2-2). What constitutes a "critical incident" requiring CISD should be determined by the needs of the emergency personnel who were on the scene. For example, in a big city, a motor vehicle crash in which two teenagers are killed may not be perceived as a major incident. In a small rural village, such a crash might emotionally devastate the entire community.

Usually a line officer or chief officer will initiate the CISD process after a critical incident. But

Figure 2-2 The critical incident stress debriefing helps emergency workers deal with the stress brought on by an event that had an especially strong emotional impact.

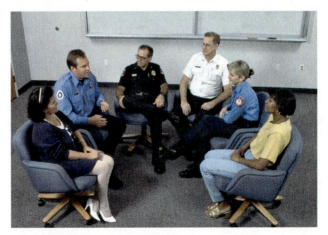

you or any emergency worker who was at the scene can request a CISD.

At a CISD, a group of specially trained peer counselors and mental health professionals sits down with the emergency workers involved in the incident. All personnel (including those in command of the incident) are encouraged, but should not be forced, to attend. The debriefing should be held within 24 to 72 hours of the incident. At the meeting, an open, confidential discussion of the responders' feelings, fears, and reactions should take place.

CISD is not an investigation or an interrogation, nor is it a tactical debriefing. It should be a non-threatening meeting in which emergency workers can openly express their emotions. The trained professionals who take part can offer concrete suggestions for ways of overcoming the stress related to the incident.

CISD is not an absolute cure for the stress related to a major incident. However, holding a CISD soon after the incident can accelerate the normal recovery process. It can also reduce or eliminate some stress reactions entirely.

A **defusing session** is a shorter form of the CISD. It is usually held within a few hours of the critical incident. The personnel who were involved in the incident are usually the only participants. The defusing session gives participants a chance to vent their emotions about the incident. It also can help them get ready for the kind of discussion that will take place in the CISD.

In addition to CISD, a comprehensive critical incident stress management program should include the following components:

◆ Pre-incident education about stress and stress reactions

◆ On-scene peer support of emergency personnel

◆ One-on-one support as needed

◆ Disaster support services

◆ Follow-up support services as needed

◆ Spouse and family support

◆ Community outreach programs

◆ Other health and wellness programs based on local needs and resources.

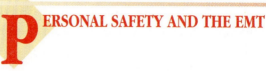

PERSONAL SAFETY AND THE EMT

Up to this point, the chapter has focused on the psychological hazards of your duties as an EMT and how to deal with them. However, there will be many calls on which your physical well being may be at risk. These calls involve exposure to hazardous materials, on-scene violence, and behavioral emergencies. In addition, you must always be alert to protect yourself from diseases that may be carried in the blood and other body fluids of patients. The risks and precautions relating to infectious diseases will be discussed in depth in Chapter 3, "Infection Control and Body Substance Isolation."

Scene Safety

There is one key fact to keep in mind whenever you are dispatched on a call. It is that if you are killed or injured at the scene, you will not be able to provide the patient with emergency medical care. Your safety, then, should be your first priority on any call.

To protect your safety, you must learn to recognize hazards and potential hazards at any scene to which you are dispatched. In Chapter 7, "Patient Assessment," you will learn how to perform a proper **scene size-up.** On every call you make, a scene size-up will be your first step in the process of evaluating and treating a patient. In the scene size-up, you examine the scene to detect any possible hazards to yourself, your crew, your patient, and any bystanders. If you discover a hazard, you must take steps to control it before proceeding with patient care. You may control the hazard yourself, if you are properly trained and equipped, or you can summon appropriate personnel to the scene.

Hazardous Materials

As a firefighter, you have probably received at least some specialized training about hazardous materials (hazmat). Most firefighters are at least

Table 2-1

Levels of Hazmat Training

LEVEL	TASKS	HOURS OF TRAINING
First Responder Awareness	Recognize a hazmat emergency; notify proper agencies	No minimum
First Responder Operations	Protect people, property, and environment at hazmat incident; remain safe distance from material; keep incident from spreading	8 minimum
Hazardous Materials Technician	Plug, patch, or stop release of hazmat	24 hours minimum
Hazardous Materials Specialist	Provide command and support activities at hazmat incident	48 minimum

trained to the First Responder Awareness level. Indeed, you may have already obtained advance training to a level such as Hazardous Materials Technician. (See Table 2-1 for the various levels of hazmat training.) Whatever the level of your previous training, the importance of personal safety when dealing with hazardous materials cannot be overemphasized (Figure 2-3). It will be discussed here briefly and in greater depth in Chapter 28, "EMS Special Operations."

Hazardous materials come in many forms. Some are toxic gases. Others are corrosive liquids. Still others are poisonous powders. No matter what their form, hazardous materials are by definition a threat to your well being. Their effects may be short term, such as a burn received through contact with a corrosive. Or the effects can be long term, such as the irreversible liver disease associated with exposure to carbon tetrachloride.

Hazardous materials can be found almost anywhere in our society. They are made or used in industrial plants, carried down streets and highways by tanker trucks, and stored in barns on farms. They can be found in most kitchens and garages.

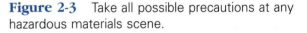

Figure 2-3 Take all possible precautions at any hazardous materials scene.

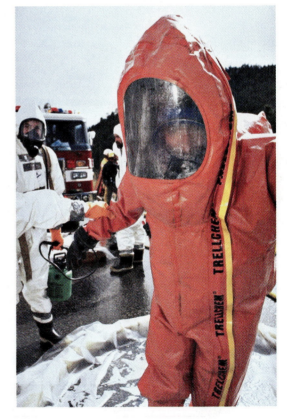

Sometimes your dispatch information will tell you that hazardous materials are present at a scene. At other times, you will have to determine their presence. There are certain scenes at which you should be especially alert for hazardous materials. Suspect hazardous materials on calls involving tanker trucks or railroad cars. Assume all calls for leaks, spills, or odd odors involve hazardous materials until proven otherwise. Finally, evaluate carefully all medical calls to industrial or residential settings where multiple patients have the same signs or symptoms. Few causes other than hazardous materials can make a number of patients at the same location suddenly ill all at the same time.

Whenever you suspect or determine the presence of hazardous material at a scene, keep a safe distance away, preferably uphill and upwind of the material. Try to identify the material involved. Use binoculars to locate any placards identifying hazardous materials on trucks, buildings, and storage containers (Figure 2-4). Check for the colors and numbers shown on the plac-

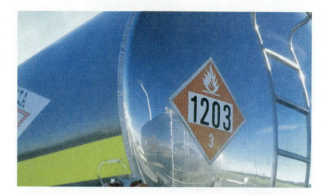

Figure 2-4 Be alert for warning placards that may indicate the presence of a hazardous material at an emergency scene.

ards in the *North American Emergency Response Handbook* (Figure 2-5). This book, which should be on every emergency vehicle, is a copublication of the United States, Canadian, and Mexican governments (Figure 2-6). It lists the chemical names of hazardous materials as identified by the numbers and colors on the placards. The book also outlines the effects of a hazardous material

Figure 2-5 Examples of hazardous materials warning placards.

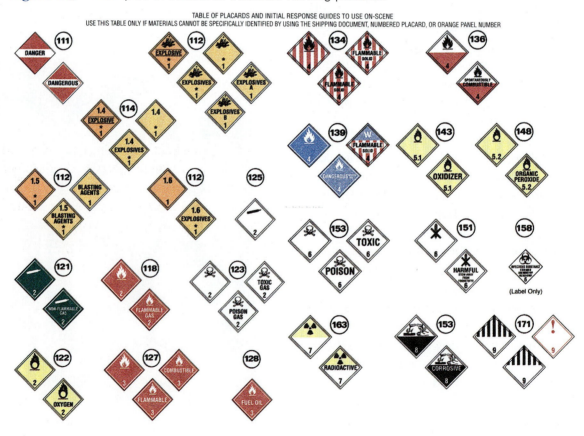

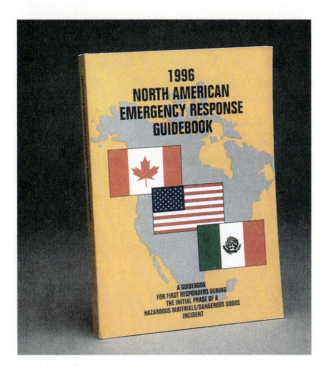

Figure 2-6 A copy of the *North American Emergency Response Guidebook* should be on board any emergency vehicle that may be dispatched to a hazardous materials incident.

on a patient as well as the steps necessary for decontamination.

If you determine that a hazardous material is involved, secure the scene from a distance, making sure that no one enters. Call for a hazmat team, providing as much information as you can about the material and the circumstances of the incident.

The officer in charge of hazmat operations will determine the level of personal protective gear that should be worn at the scene. Often, hazmat encapsulating suits and self-contained breathing apparatus (SCBA) are required.

To assure your personal safety during a hazmat incident, carefully follow the directions of the hazmat team members. In particular, pay careful attention to staging instructions. Be careful not to come in contact with contaminated patients unless you are wearing proper protective clothing and SCBA when necessary or until patient decontamination has taken place.

As an EMT, your main role at a hazmat incident will be to provide emergency medical care once the scene is made safe. You should treat

patients only after the hazmat team has provided basic decontamination. (Your role will probably be greater if you are assigned to the hazmat team.) In addition, you may be assigned to provide medical monitoring and care as part of emergency incident rehabilitation of firefighters involved in hazmat operations (see Chapter 27, "Emergency Incident Rehabilitation").

Rescue Situations

Emergency rescues are some of the most dramatic situations you will encounter in the fire service. These scenes are also among the most hazardous to an EMT's personal safety. At any rescue scene, identify specific dangers from fire, explosion, electricity, hazardous materials, or other sources during the scene size-up. Be aware that in some rescue situations such as those involving confined spaces and swift water, the conditions that injured and trapped the patient pose the same risks for you. When possible, act to remove or reduce the threats you discover. If you are properly trained and equipped, take action yourself. Otherwise, summon trained personnel who have the needed resources.

As a firefighter, you may normally be capable of controlling and monitoring many of the dangers at a rescue scene. When you are acting as an EMT, however, the situation changes somewhat. Your focus will be on evaluation and care of the patient. The best way of assuring scene safety while you carry out your medical tasks is to request that adequate numbers of appropriately trained personnel with specialized equipment be sent to the scene. Far too many firefighter injuries and deaths during rescue operations result from rushing into a scene without properly sizing it up and from failing to request adequate resources to control the scene.

There are some simple but important steps that you can follow to assure personal safety at rescue scenes. They include the following:

◆ *"Dress for the occasion."* Always use personal protective gear appropriate for the conditions (Figure 2-7). For example, always wear turnout gear, a helmet, eye protection, and puncture-resistant leather gloves at motor

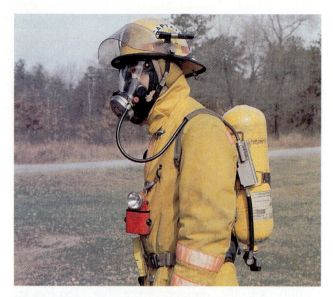

Figure 2-7 Some emergency scenes will require the use of self-contained breathing apparatus (SCBA).

vehicle extrication scenes (Figure 2-8). If your call involves water hazards, then wear a personal flotation device (PFD).

◆ *Establish the Incident Management System (IMS).* The Incident Management System provides a management framework for large-scale incidents. It is especially helpful at complex rescue scenes. Under IMS, a specific Safety Sector is set up to monitor on-scene hazards. In addition, the individual who assumes the role of Command has overall charge of the incident and can assure that adequate resources are committed to the scene. You will learn more about IMS in Chapter 28, "EMS Special Operations."

◆ *Have a rescue plan.* Form a strategy that includes safety considerations before beginning any rescue attempts. Rushing in to "rescue" a patient without a sound plan puts both patient and rescue personnel at risk.

◆ *Monitor the scene for changing conditions.* Many rescue scenes are dynamic. A scene that was initially safe can suddenly become unsafe. For example, a hostile crowd may begin to gather at the scene of a shooting. Or the level of water in a ditch where you're extricating a patient may begin to rise because of a thunderstorm in the nearby hills. Always

keep an eye out for obvious and subtle signs that conditions on the scene are changing. Be aware that the changes may require you to summon additional resources or to pull back from the scene.

◆ *Summon adequate resources to accomplish the rescue safely.* This can never be stressed too highly. Get the personnel and equipment to the scene that you need to perform the rescue safely! If your department does not have the necessary personnel or equipment, don't hesitate to request assistance or mutual aid from neighboring jurisdictions that have resources that will make the scene less hazardous.

Violence

Unfortunately, violence and its aftereffects are all too common in the prehospital environment. In your job, you may be called to the scenes of

Figure 2-8 Full protective gear includes eye protection, helmet, turnout gear, and gloves.

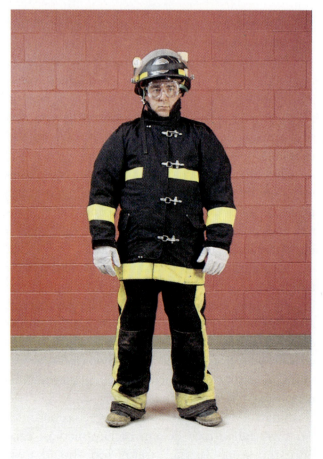

shootings, stabbings, assaults, incidents of domestic violence, and behavioral emergencies. The factors that led to the initial violence at a scene may still be present when you arrive. The violence that had been directed at your patient can easily be turned against you. Always be alert to the possibility of danger on calls where injuries were the result of violence.

In well-run EMS systems, the dispatcher will ask questions of the person who called 9-1-1 to help determine the potential for violence. If a violent or potentially violent scene is identified, law enforcement units should be dispatched to the scene immediately. It is the job of law enforcement personnel to secure the scene and make it safe before EMS units move in.

If your unit arrives on a scene that has not yet been secured, then you should **stage,** or wait, a safe distance from the scene. Contact dispatch to assure that law enforcement units have been notified. Then wait until they arrive and make the scene safe. If you see guns or hear shots, make sure that you are staged out of the range of gunfire. Remember, you can be of no assistance to a patient if you yourself are wounded or killed.

Once the scene is secure, your focus should be caring for the injured patient, family members, or suspect. It is not your job to decide who is to blame for an incident. It is your job and responsibility to provide emergency medical care to anyone on the scene who requires it or requests it.

The police officers who initially secured the scene will generally stay with fire department units to assure continued security. You should, however, remain alert to the possibility that violence may break out again at the scene while you are there. Loud voices, slamming doors, or breaking glass should warn you that the scene may once again be turning violent. If you judge that conditions are becoming unsafe and police have left the scene or cannot contain the situation, retreat from the scene. Stage a safe distance away until the police have secured the scene.

If gunfire occurs, move behind a dense structure such as your vehicle's engine block or behind a concrete or brick wall (Figure 2-9). Being inside the ambulance or behind its door does not provide adequate protection from gunfire.

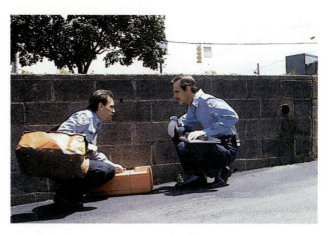

Figure 2-9 If gunfire breaks out at an emergency scene, take cover behind a solid, dense object like a concrete wall or your vehicle's engine block.

Remember, too, that violence can erupt inside the emergency vehicle. In one case, a gang member entered the back of an ambulance and shot a wounded member of a rival gang who was under the care of EMTs. Whenever a call involves violence, be prepared for the possibility that the violence will continue after your arrival. There is no such thing as being "safely inside the ambulance" on such calls.

Steps to help assure your personal safety at scenes that involve violence or the potential for violence include the following:

◆ *Immediately request the dispatch of law enforcement personnel to any scene involving violence or the potential for violence.*

◆ *Never enter a scene until it has been secured by law enforcement personnel.*

◆ *Always carry a portable two-way radio so that you can request additional assistance at any time.*

◆ *Be alert to the sounds of potential violence such as shouting, objects being thrown, or doors slamming.*

◆ *Retreat from any scene at which you believe that violence poses a threat to your safety.*

◆ *Depending upon the area in which you work and your department's policies, you may be required to wear or want to consider the use of body armor—a "bullet-proof vest"—for protection from gunfire.*

Chapter Review

As an EMT, you will face risks of both emotional stress and physical injury. Remember to keep your own well being as a priority on the job. To do this, learn how to recognize signs of stress in yourself and how you can reduce the negative effects of that stress. In addition, always remember to survey a scene carefully before you enter it. Only enter a scene after taking all appropriate steps to assure your personal safety and reduce the risk of injury.

REVIEWING KEY CONCEPTS

1. List and describe the stages that people may pass through as they try to deal with death and dying.

2. Describe things an EMT can do to help patients and family members deal with the emotions stirred up by a death.

3. List some of the job-related situations likely to cause high levels of stress in EMTs.

4. Describe some of the warning signs for high levels of stress. Explain some of the actions that an EMT might take to reduce stress levels.

5. Describe what a CISD is and how it works.

6. List some of the basic steps you should follow if you suspect the presence of hazardous materials at an emergency scene.

7. List the basic steps for assuring personal safety at a rescue scene.

8. List steps you can take to help assure personal safety at scenes that may involve violence.

RESOURCES TO LEARN MORE

EMS Safety: Techniques and Applications. Washington, D.C.: Federal Emergency Management Agency. U.S. Fire Administration, FA-144. April 1994.

Kübler-Ross, Elisabeth, M.D. *On Death and Dying.* New York: Collier Books/Macmillan, 1969.

THE CISD PROCESS

CRITICAL INCIDENT OCCURS
Produces strong emotional response in emergency workers

↓

NEED FOR CISD RECOGNIZED
Usually the company officer arranges for CISD, but any emergency worker involved in incident can request one

↓

CISD SCHEDULED
Usually held within 24 to 72 hours of incident

↓

THE CISD
Participants include those involved in incident, trained peer counselors, mental health professionals; process involves the following seven stages

↓

PHASE 1: INTRODUCTION
Sets goals for the CISD. Assures confidentiality.

↓

PHASE 2: FACTS
Sets out details of what occurred at the incident

↓

PHASE 3: FEELINGS
Encourages participants to explore feelings the incident raised in them

↓

PHASE 4: SYMPTOMS
Encourages participants to note any physical reactions the incident may have caused in them

↓

PHASE 5: TEACHING
Allows professionals to help participants sort through feelings; provides opportunity to reinforce that extreme reactions are normal in such situations

↓

PHASE 6: RE-ENTRY
Offers suggestions for coping after the CISD; may include an action plan with goals and activities to reduce stress

↓

PHASE 7: FOLLOW-UP
Explores how participants are coping months or weeks later

Infection Control and Body Substance Isolation

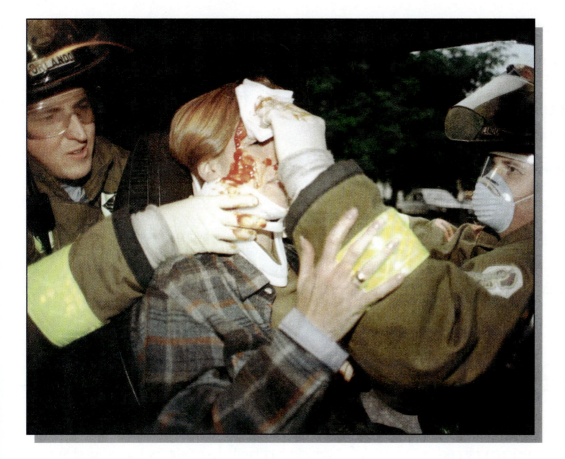

W hen working with the ill and injured, firefighter EMTs are potentially at risk from diseases transmitted either by contact with body fluids, such as blood, or by contact with airborne particles. Usually such risks are minimal. However, EMTs on the job are likely to encounter a variety of patients suffering from a wide range of illnesses under many different conditions. With all these unknowns and variables, the possibility of contracting an infectious disease is real. Therefore, EMTs—and other EMS providers—must always take *precautions in order to reduce the possibility of an occupational exposure to a disease.*

Remember that an EMT who has experienced an occupational exposure to a disease is not the only person at risk from the exposure. The EMT might expose family and co-workers to the disease. In addition, the EMT might unknowingly infect other patients he contacts.

For these reasons, it is important for you as an EMT to always use the appropriate precautions when providing care to patients and when handling equipment and materials that have been in contact with patients. These precautions are in your best interests. They are also considered the correct standard of care that should be followed by all emergency medical personnel.

OBJECTIVES

At the completion of this chapter, the EMT-Basic student should be able to meet the following objectives:

Knowledge and Understanding

1. Explain the need to determine scene safety. (pp. 37, 38)
2. Discuss the importance of body substance isolation (BSI). (pp. 38–42, 43, 45)
3. Describe the steps an EMT-Basic should take for personal protection from airborne and bloodborne pathogens. (pp. 45–48)

Skills

1. Given a scenario with potential infectious exposure, the EMT-Basic will use appropriate personal protective equipment. At the completion of the scenario, the EMT-Basic will properly remove and discard the protective garments.
2. Given the above scenario, the EMT-Basic will complete disinfection/cleaning and all reporting documentation.

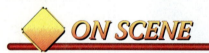 **ON SCENE**

DISPATCH: *SQUAD 5, RESCUE 10, ENGINE 7, AND BATTALION 3—RESPOND TO THE REPORT OF A SINGLE VEHICLE ROLLOVER ON INTERSTATE 90 EASTBOUND NEAR EXIT 5. AMBULANCE HAS BEEN DISPATCHED. TIME OUT IS 2315.*

You are an EMT assigned to Rescue 10, which is the first unit to reach the scene. Based on the dispatch information, you have put on full turn-out gear including latex gloves under work gloves. Upon arrival, you determine that there is only one patient, who is still inside the vehicle. Extrication will be required, but because the vehicle has landed upright and on a level surface, you estimate that it will not take long. A quick survey of the patient reveals a male in his early 20s, unconscious, breathing, with blood visible on the face, shirt, and pants.

While you size-up the scene, the other dispatched units arrive. The paramedics from Squad 5 continue to assess the patient and provide some care. They also advise the Incident Commander that rapid extrication is needed. When

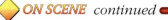

he approves, you aid them in performing it. The patient needs rapid transportation to the trauma center, and the paramedics ask you to ride along to assist.

Before getting into the ambulance you remove your turnout gear and work gloves, leaving your latex gloves on. A quick look at the patient immobilized on the stretcher reveals no signs of broken glass, so you start to remove the patient's clothing to permit a detailed physical examination. After cutting the patient's shirt, you reach to remove it. As you do, a piece of glass that went unnoticed in the patient's pocket tears through your glove and cuts your hand. You immediately cease your care of the patient and cover your wound with sterile gauze.

From the blood present on the patient's shirt, you conclude that there was probably blood on the piece of glass as well. The run time to the hospital is less than 15 minutes, and when you arrive you notify your captain about the exposure. He instructs you to remain at the hospital to have the wound cared for and to immediately begin the post-exposure management procedures.

Luckily, one of the fire department's EMS physicians works at the trauma center where you have taken the patient. She is available and takes charge of initiating the exposure control plan for your agency. With your permission, blood sam-

ples are drawn. Then you and the physician discuss the risks of your exposure.

The two major concerns are hepatitis B and HIV. Your medical file shows that you have been immunized for hepatitis B and are not at risk for that disease. The doctor tells you that the risk of your contracting HIV is extremely remote. The patient would need to have been HIV positive. Even if he had been, there would be less than a 0.3 percent, or 3 in 1,000, chance of becoming infected. She also tells you that there are drugs that you can consider taking that may reduce the risk of contracting the disease, but points out that these medications can have side effects. After she answers your questions, you decide to take the medications just in case the patient is infected.

You start the medications immediately and are informed that you will receive follow-up testing for HIV for the next year. You also receive counseling on how to change certain aspects of your life until you are sure that you have not been infected through this occupational exposure. As the months go by, all your blood tests are negative for HIV. You are obviously relieved that you were not infected. Nevertheless, taking the medications, coping with the anxiety, and modifying your personal life have made for a very stressful year.

EMTs frequently encounter unexpected elements during an emergency medical response. Extrication problems, poor lighting, violent behavior, confusion at the scene, the presence of hazardous materials, rapid changes in the environment, and exposure to infectious diseases are just some of these elements that can impact on safety. Although no scene can ever be made completely safe, there are a number of things that an EMT can do to lessen the risks that are associated with the job. This chapter focuses on things the EMT

can do to minimize the risk of experiencing occupational exposure to infectious diseases. (Other chapters highlighting personal safety measures for the EMT to follow include: Chapter 2, "The Wellbeing of the EMT-Basic"; Chapter 7, "Patient Assessment"; Chapter 10, "Lifting and Moving Patients"; Chapter 25, "Emergency Vehicle Operations"; Chapter 26, "Gaining Access and Basics of Extrication"; Chapter 27, "Emergency Incident Rehabilitation"; and Chapter 28, "EMS Special Operations.")

INFECTIOUS DISEASES AND BODY SUBSTANCE ISOLATION

Infectious diseases are those that spread from person to person. They are caused by **pathogens.** These microorganisms include bacteria and viruses. Pathogens can be spread in a number of ways. They can be carried in blood or other body fluids. Airborne pathogens can be carried in the tiny droplets that are sprayed when a person coughs or sneezes. Pathogens in blood or body fluids can enter another person's body through breaks in the skin, such as cuts and sores and chapped hands, or through mucous membranes, such as those in the eyes, nose, or mouth. Airborne pathogens are inhaled.

The diseases spread by pathogens can produce effects ranging from mild discomfort to death. Yet often a person carrying pathogens for a disease will show no outward signs of illness. Therefore, EMTs should consider *all blood and all body fluids to be infectious.* This means that EMTs must take proper precautions to protect themselves—and their patients—from possible contamination with blood or other body fluids.

The federal government has developed guidelines aimed at preventing the spread of disease through contact with blood and body fluids. These safeguards involve a form of infection control known as **body substance isolation (BSI).** BSI precautions are required by law to be part of the policies and procedures of the fire department or agency for which you provide emergency care. In addition, you as an EMT share the responsibility of preventing the spread of infection by following BSI precautions.

Basic Safety Precautions

Following BSI guidelines is vital, and those guidelines will be discussed below. However, you should remember that there are other basic steps you can take to decrease the risks of contracting an infectious disease. For example, constant assessment and reassessment of the patient and of the scene will help alert you to potential hazards. You should, for instance, look before placing your hands when rolling a patient over. Carefully check for uncontrolled bleeding, especially spurting blood, and sharp objects. Also keep in mind that just because you observe something doesn't mean that other emergency personnel at the scene have observed it too. Make sure that you let everyone around the patient know about any potential hazards.

Handwashing

Handwashing is a simple measure that can be of great help in guarding against the spread of disease. *In fact, probably the most important infection control practice for the EMT is handwashing.* As soon as possible after every patient contact, after gloves are removed, or after a decontamination procedure has been completed, you should thoroughly wash your hands (Figure 3-1).

Remove any rings or jewelry from your hands and arms. Then use plain soap and water. Lather your hands front and back vigorously up to 2 or 3 inches (50 to 76 mm) above the wrist for no less than 10 seconds. Be sure to lather and rub between the fingers and to pay attention to creases and cracks at the knuckles. Scrub under and around the fingernails with a brush. Rinse your hands under running water, holding your hands downward so that the water drains off the fingertips. Dry your hands using a paper towel.

Plain soap works perfectly well for handwashing. At those times when soap is not available, you might use anti-microbial handwashing solution or an alcohol-based foam or towelette.

Personal Protective Equipment

BSI precautions involve the use of **personal protective equipment (PPE).** This equipment includes barriers such as gloves, masks, goggles, and—when appropriate—gowns for protection against an exposure. The various types of PPE are discussed in detail below.

Gloves

Gloves should be used on all calls where there is any possibility of exposure to blood or other body fluids (Figure 3-2). They are an important safeguard against occupational exposure and should be worn whenever there is direct patient

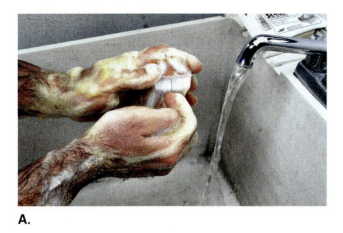

A.

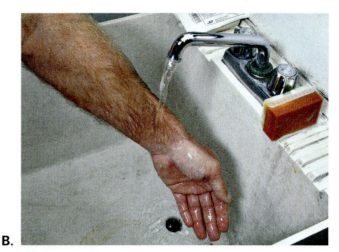

B.

Figure 3-1 Proper handwashing technique. **A.** Lather up well and be sure to scrub under the nails with a brush. **B.** When rinsing, hold hands pointing downward so that soap and water run off away from the body.

contact. Put your gloves on *before* contacting the patient so that you do not get distracted and forget to do so.

Vinyl or latex gloves specifically recommended for patient care settings are the type most commonly used by emergency care providers. They are an effective barrier against contamination from blood or other body fluids. If the gloves become grossly contaminated during a call, change them if you can do so safely.

About 10 percent of health care workers are allergic to latex in some degree. Those who either suspect or know they have an allergy to latex should discuss the situation with either their physician or agency infection control officer who can suggest appropriate gloves made of other materials.

Figure 3-2 Among the gloves that EMTs may use on the job are those made of (left to right) latex, leather, and vinyl.

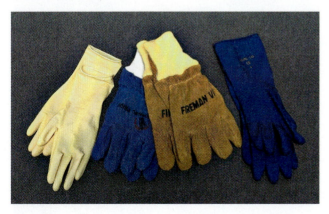

Vinyl or latex gloves will not provide protection against sharp objects. Nor will they hold up during tasks like cleaning soiled equipment or the ambulance. When performing decontamination tasks, such as cleaning up blood, a more durable glove that is specifically suited for this type of task should be used. In cases such as extrications where jagged metal and broken glass might be encountered, vinyl or latex gloves should be worn under heavier work gloves. Remember, though, that most work gloves do not provide moisture barriers. Therefore, body substance isolation is still needed if a risk of exposure exists.

Rips and tears in vinyl or latex gloves do occur. For this reason, extra gloves should be readily available. When a tear occurs and there has been no contamination, remove the torn gloves as soon as possible, wash your hands thoroughly, and put on new gloves. If there is a possibility that an occupational exposure has taken place, follow your agency's exposure control plan.

Never reuse latex or vinyl gloves. Remove them properly to avoid contaminating your hands with substances on the outside of the gloves (Figure 3-3). Once they are removed, be sure to dispose of them properly. After you remove the gloves, remember to wash your hands.

Eye Protection

When blood or other body fluids could come in contact with the eyes, eye protection should be

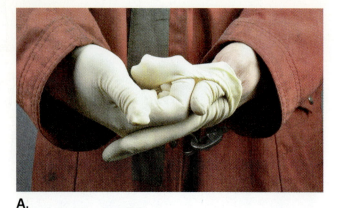

A.

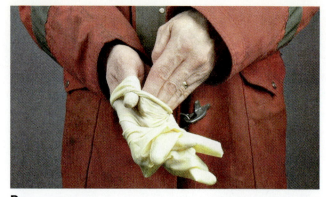

B.

Figure 3-3   Technique for removing gloves. **A.** Hook the gloved fingers of one hand under the cuff of the other glove and pull that glove off, not letting the gloved fingers come in contact with bare skin. **B.** Slide the fingers of the ungloved hand under the cuff of the remaining glove and push the glove off, being careful not to touch the glove's exterior.

worn (Figure 3-4). In these cases, wear goggles or glasses with side protectors designed to prevent such contact. Even if you normally wear glasses, they should be modified with clip-on side protectors to prevent splashing or spraying from the side. Alternatively, you might use goggles specifically designed to be worn over eyeglasses.

Protection for the eyes goes beyond the use of eyewear. You should remember not to touch or rub your eyes until after your gloves have been removed and you have properly washed and dried your hands.

Masks

There are masks designed to prevent blood and body fluids from coming into contact with the EMT's mouth and nose. These masks are usually

Figure 3-4   Proper eyewear can provide protection from splashing, splattering, or spraying fluids.

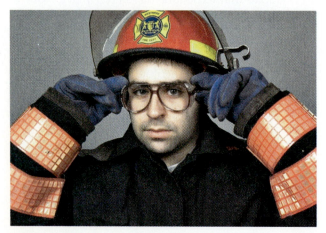

disposable and have elastic bands to hold them in place (Figure 3-5). These surgical-style masks are intended for a single use. Note that these masks *do not* provide protection from some airborne pathogens, such as those that cause tuberculosis.

Figure 3-5   A surgical-type mask can keep spraying or spattering blood or body fluids from entering the nose or mouth.

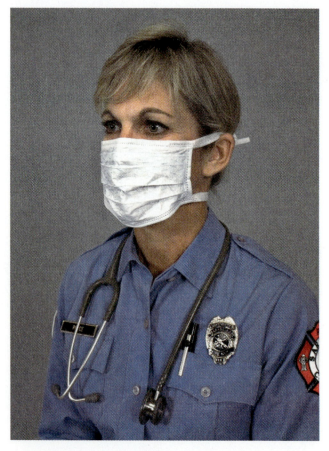

(Masks for protection from airborne particles will be discussed later in this chapter.) Some masks have eye shields attached.

Gowns

Single-use, disposable gowns provide a barrier to blood and other body fluids. They should be worn whenever the possibility of heavy bleeding and contamination of clothing exists. Such cases include major trauma with spurting (arterial) bleeding and childbirth. For other times when a gown should be used, refer to Table 3-1.

Protection from Airborne Pathogens

Pulmonary tuberculosis (TB) is an airborne infectious disease. It can be spread easily by droplets produced during coughing or sneezing and can

COMPANY OFFICER'S NOTES

The use of the proper BSI under the appropriate situations is important to the health and welfare of the EMT. With in-service training and appropriate feedback, the company officer can provide constant reminders of the importance of using BSI. The company officer should never hesitate to remind EMTs to put on gloves and other personal protective equipment when necessary. Without these barriers, the likelihood of an occupational exposure increases dramatically. Remember that such exposure can ultimately lead to devastating consequences for the exposed firefighter, potential anxiety and fear among other EMTs in the agency, and significant costs for the department/agency. All EMTs must understand that BSI is mandatory!

Table 3-1

When and Which Types of Personal Protective Equipment to Use

Activity	Gloves	Eyewear	Mask	Gown
Uncontrolled bleeding	Yes	Yes	Yes	Yes
Controlled bleeding	Yes	No	No	No
Childbirth	Yes	Yes	Yes	Yes
Endotracheal intubation	Yes	Yes	Yes	No
Oral/nasal suctioning, manually cleaning airway	Yes	Yes	Yes	Yes
Handling and cleaning possibly contaminated instruments	Yes	Yes	Yes	Yes
Measuring blood pressure	No*	No	No	No
Giving an injection	Yes	No	No	No
Measuring temperature	Yes	No	No	No
Cleaning patient compartment after a medical call	Yes	No**	No**	No**

*Unless the patient's arm is contaminated with blood or body fluids or unless required by department policy.

**Unless heavily contaminated by blood or body fluids or unless required by department policy.

present a significant risk to EMTs. In the past 10 years, multi-drug resistant TB (MDR-TB) has become prevalent in some urban areas. This type of TB does not respond well to the usual treatment for TB and, even though it is not common, it has serious consequences for anyone who contracts it.

Patients with active TB may present with a variety of signs and symptoms. However, they may also not even know that they have TB. Therefore, you should consider the possibility of TB when you encounter any patient complaining of fever, weight loss, night sweats, or who has had a persistent cough. TB is not uncommon and certain groups of patients are considered high risk (Table 3-2).

When the EMT is caring for patients who may have TB, the standard surgical mask does not provide adequate protection. Instead, an N-95 or a high-efficiency particulate air (HEPA) respirator approved by the National Institute for Occupational Safety and Health (NIOSH) should be worn during the entire call (Figure 3-6).

Also consider placing a standard surgical mask on the patient to cut down on the release of droplets into the air from coughing. Do this only if the patient's airway is not compromised and the patient has no trouble breathing. If you do place a surgical mask on the patient, monitor the patient's airway and breathing carefully (Figure 3-7).

All emergency care providers, as part of their routine physicals, should be evaluated for TB.

Usually a simple skin test (sometimes called a Mantoux or PPD) is performed. The test determines whether the provider has been exposed to TB. The department's infection control officer or physician should determine, after evaluating the potential risks to providers, how often testing should be done. Testing for TB exposure is usu-

Figure 3-6 NIOSH-approved respirators.
A. A high-efficiency particulate air (HEPA) respirator.
B. An N-95 respirator.

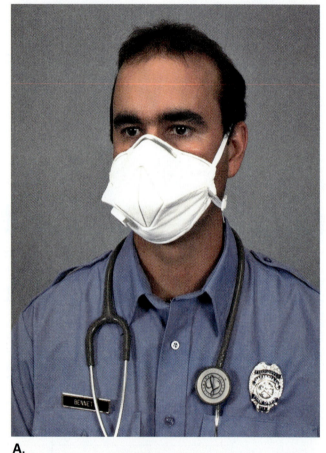

A.

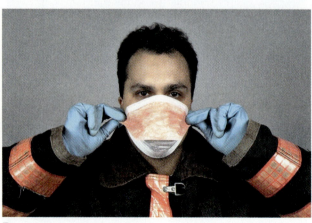

B.

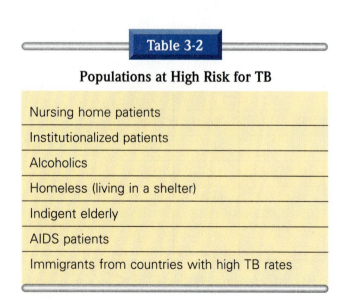

Table 3-2
Populations at High Risk for TB
Nursing home patients
Institutionalized patients
Alcoholics
Homeless (living in a shelter)
Indigent elderly
AIDS patients
Immigrants from countries with high TB rates

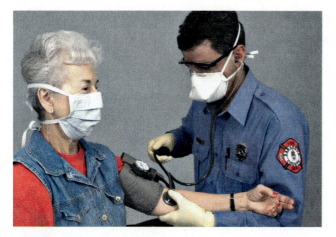

Figure 3-7 With a suspected tuberculosis patient, you may place a surgical-type mask on the patient while you wear a NIOSH-approved respirator. Monitor the patient's airway and breathing carefully.

ally done on a yearly basis or more often if there has been a possible occupational exposure.

MONITORING PERSONAL HEALTH

All EMTs should have a periodic physical examination, usually once a year. A physical should not only establish the EMT's fitness to work but also update his or her immunization and screening records. This information should include, at a minimum, the current immunization status or results of screening tests for these infectious diseases:

- Hepatitis B
- Tetanus/diphtheria
- Measles
- Mumps
- Rubella (German measles)
- Chicken pox
- Polio
- Tuberculosis (TB)
- Influenza immunization

These records will also assist in identifying an EMT's risk in the event of an occupational exposure. Without proper immunizations, an EMT can

be at needless risk of contracting a disease that may put not only himself but also co-workers and patients at risk for infection. Therefore, it is important for every EMT to know his own health status. For more information about common infectious diseases, refer to Table 3-3.

CLEANING AND DISINFECTION OF EQUIPMENT

Any personal protective equipment designed for a single use should be properly disposed of after that use. The same is true of medical devices designed for a single use that have become contaminated with blood or other body fluids during a call. Such materials, other than needles or sharp objects, should be deposited in a red bag or container marked with a biohazard seal (Figure 3-8A). Needles and other sharp objects should be placed in a puncture-proof container, sometimes called a "sharps" container that is designated for biohazard waste disposal (Figure 3-8B). Once material is placed in an appropriate container it should be disposed of following your department's procedures for biohazardous waste.

Non-disposable equipment used during a call and surfaces that may have come into contact with a patient's blood or body fluids must receive cleaning, disinfection, or sterilization. These items may include patient stretchers, the patient compartment of the ambulance, backboards, cervical collars, respiratory-assist and inhalation-therapy equipment, and laryngoscope blades. **Cleaning** refers to the washing of an object with soap and

Table 3-3

Infectious Diseases

Disease	Method of Transmission	Incubation Period*
AIDS (acquired immune deficiency syndrome)/HIV infection	AIDS- or HIV-infected blood via intravenous drug use, unprotected sexual intercourse, blood transfusions, accidental needle sticks; infected mothers may pass HIV on to their unborn children	Several months or years
Chickenpox (varicella)	Airborne droplets, contact with open sores	14 to 21 days
German measles (rubella)	Airborne droplets; infected mothers may pass the disease to their unborn children	14 to 21 days
Hepatitis	Contact with blood, stools, body fluids, or contaminated objects	Weeks to months, depending on type
Meningitis (bacterial)	Oral and nasal secretions	2 to 10 days
Mononucleosis	Respiratory secretions, airborne droplets	30 to 50 days
Mumps	Droplets of saliva or objects contaminated by saliva	12 to 26 days
Staphylococcal skin infections	Contact with infected wounds or sores or contaminated objects	Several days
Tuberculosis	Respiratory secretions, airborne droplets, contact with contaminated objects	4 to 12 weeks
Whooping cough (pertussis)	Respiratory secretions, airborne droplets	10 to 16 days

*The time between exposure to an infectious disease and the appearance of signs and symptoms.

B.

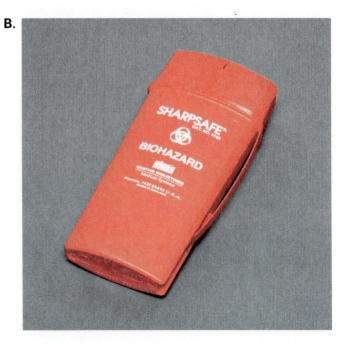

Figure 3-8 Dispose of biohazardous wastes properly. **A.** A "red bag." **B.** A portable "sharps" container.

A.

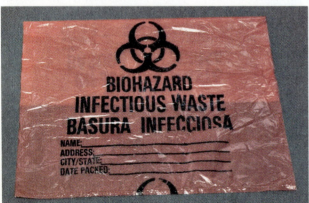

water. **Disinfection** includes cleaning, but also involves use of a disinfectant to kill many of the microorganisms that may be on the object. **Sterilization** is the use of chemical or physical methods to kill all microorganisms on an object.

Clean all work areas, such as the patient stretcher, equipment, and the patient compartment of an ambulance, after every patient encounter. Wash areas down with approved soaps or disinfectants and throw away single-use cleaning supplies in a proper biohazard container.

Generally, you should disinfect items that come into direct contact with the intact skin of a patient. These include things like backboards, splints, cervical collars, and so forth. An alternative to a commercial disinfectant is bleach solution diluted in water. Recommended concentrations are 1 part bleach to 100 parts water or 1 part bleach to 10 parts water depending on how much organic material is on an item.

Items that are inserted into the patient's body —laryngoscope blades, for example—should be sterilized by heat, steam, or radiation. There are also EPA-approved solutions for sterilization.

If equipment has become contaminated and requires extensive cleaning, it should be bagged and removed to a specific area designated for this purpose. Remember, also, that cleaning of contaminated material should never be done in or around food preparation areas.

Disposable work gloves worn during cleaning and decontamination should be discarded when done (Figure 3-9). If clothing has become contaminated, it should be bagged and washed in accordance with department or agency procedures. The person whose clothing was contaminated should take a shower before dressing again. If an occupational exposure is suspected, follow the department or agency's management procedures immediately and completely.

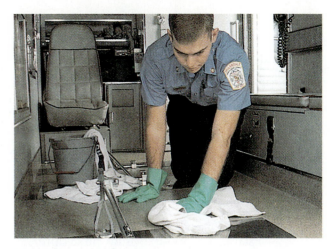

Figure 3-9 Follow your department's protocols concerning appropriate personal protective equipment when cleaning equipment after a call.

ing the health of emergency response personnel. Every fire department or EMS agency should have a comprehensive, detailed knowledge of what these standards require and a process for ensuring that the department or EMS agency is in full compliance with them.

Bloodborne Pathogens

The federal government established standards (Title 29 Code of Federal Regulation 1910.1030) in 1991 under the authority of the Occupational Safety and Health Administration (OSHA) regarding the exposure of emergency care workers to bloodborne pathogens. These standards, in part, require every emergency response agency to establish an **exposure control plan** for its employees. This plan is intended to cover employees who are potentially at risk from exposure to bloodborne pathogens. The plan must set guidelines to help minimize the chance of an exposure occurring. In addition, the plan must also contain the specific procedures to follow in the event of an exposure. The following summary, adapted from recommendations developed by the National Association of EMS Physicians, gives an overview of the OSHA standards on bloodborne pathogens. (For the specific regulations, contact the U.S. Department of Labor.)

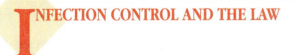

INFECTION CONTROL AND THE LAW

In recent years, the federal government has enacted a number of measures aimed at protect-

- All services shall develop a comprehensive written infection control plan for all EMS providers. The plan should:

    —Establish a list, by job title, of employees who might be at risk from an exposure

    —Create a regular infection control training program

    —Provide agency standards for dealing with all aspects of risk to bloodborne pathogens

    —Establish a post-exposure procedure.

- Administrative controls should be initiated that provide specific information about ways to prevent occupational exposure to all at-risk employees. Such information should include:

    —The use of body substance isolation

    —The appropriate methods for handling hazardous wastes

    —Procedures to follow for decontaminating equipment.

- Periodically this information should be reviewed and modified in accordance with any new scientific evidence.

- Equipment (engineering) controls should be used whenever available. Safety devices for prehospital care have largely focused on the use of needles for intravenous (IV) and medication administration. All providers should evaluate, in consultation with their infection control officer or medical director, any new device that might help to minimize the risk of exposure and, if the device is found to be effective, make the device a standard part of the agency's equipment and start using it routinely.

- Body substance isolation (BSI) precautions and personnel protective equipment (PPE) should be routinely used by all emergency responders. These protection barriers should be immediately available and used in accordance with agency policy (See Table 3-1).

- Work practice controls should be established and followed. These should provide guidelines for the handling of infectious waste and contaminated items such as work clothes, medical equipment, and emergency vehicles. These controls are intended to keep the work environment hygienically safe and to prevent cross-contamination. One important aspect of this recommendation is to ensure that food preparation and eating areas cannot come into contact with infectious materials.

- All emergency medical response agencies should have an aggressive vaccination program. Even though members can decline to receive them, vaccinations, specifically for hepatitis B (HBV), are strongly encouraged. Everyone who can potentially come into contact with body fluids and infectious materials should be vaccinated.

- In the event of an occupational exposure, there must be a plan in place for the employee to follow. This plan must provide for rapid assessment, counseling, and any necessary treatment, including post-exposure prophylaxis. It is imperative that all post-exposure medical information, both about the employee and the source patient, be handled confidentially.

Tuberculosis Guidelines

Guidelines issued in the *Morbidity and Mortality Weekly Report* from the Centers for Disease Control in 1994 established guidelines for the prevention of tuberculosis (TB) in health care facilities. A brief summary of those guidelines and others that relate to emergency medical services follows below:

- A surgical mask should be placed over the mouth and nose, if possible, of any patient suspected of active TB.

- EMS personnel should wear respiratory protection—an N-95 or HEPA respirator—when transporting a suspected TB patient.

- If feasible, the windows of the transporting vehicle should be kept open and the ventilation system should be set on the non-recirculating cycle.

- Personnel should be included in regular purified protein derivative (PPD) tuberculin testing. The frequency of this testing should be determined after the risk to TB has been evaluated.

- The agency should perform a risk assessment study and develop a TB infection control plan. The plan should contain post-exposure follow-up procedures, including counseling.

- The agency should provide for fit testing of respiratory protection devices, such as an N-95 or HEPA respirator, for all personnel who may be required to use this type of respiratory protection device.

The Ryan White Act

In 1994 a federal regulation known as Subtitle B of the Ryan White Comprehensive AIDS Resources Emergency (CARE) act regarding emergency response employees took effect. (This legislation is usually referred to as the Ryan White CARE Act.) The act required that emergency response personnel be allowed to request access to certain information about bloodborne or airborne infectious diseases to which they may have been exposed on the job. Before this regulation became law, emergency responders in many areas of the country could not get information about the medical history of patients they had cared for, even if they suspected that contact with those patients had exposed them to infectious diseases.

Occupational exposure to human immunodeficiency virus (HIV) is probably the most significant concern among emergency medical personnel. However, the Ryan White CARE Act also allows medical personnel to request information to determine if they have been exposed to other serious and potentially life-threatening viruses and diseases (see Table 3-4).

The Ryan White CARE Act specifically deals with the notification of the **emergency response employee (ERE)** about a possible exposure sustained in the line of duty (Figure 3-10). Specifically, an ERE is considered to be a firefighter, law enforcement officer, emergency medical technician, or other professional emergency responder, either paid or volunteer. The procedure for notification starts when, for example, a fire department EMT believes that in providing care to a patient he may have been exposed to a bloodborne disease through accidental contact with the patient's blood. The EMT notifies the person who has been appointed by the department as the **designated officer (DO).** The DO then submits a written request to the hospital asking if a risk from contact with the patient exists.

Risk is determined by examination of the patient's medical record, including laboratory tests, for information identifying an infectious disease. The law does not require the patient to submit to testing for HIV or other bloodborne diseases. The hospital has 48 hours to respond to the DO's request. In the event that the hospital initially believes the source patient does not have an infec-

Table 3-4

Infectious Diseases Covered Under the Ryan White CARE Act

Pathogens Carried by Body Fluids	Airborne Pathogens
Human Immunodeficiency Virus (HIV)	Mycobacterium tuberculosis (TB)
Hepatitis B	
Diphtheria	
Meningococcal meningitis	
Plague	
Hemorrhagic Fever	
Rabies	

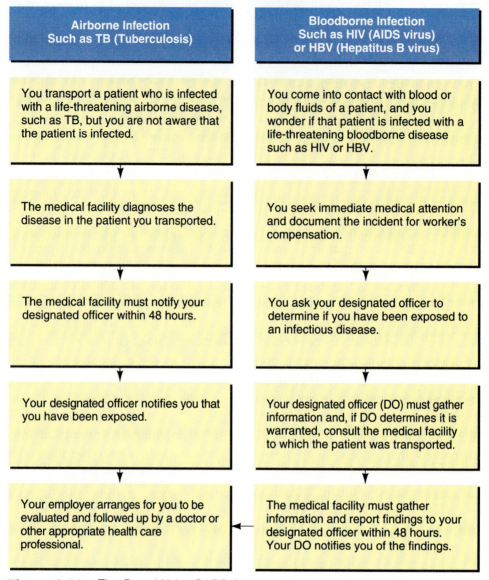

Figure 3-10 The Ryan White CARE Act provides procedures to follow if you suspect that you have been exposed to a life-threatening infectious disease.

tious disease, it still has a responsibility until the patient is discharged or for up to 60 days to inform the DO of the patient's infectious disease status if additional information becomes available. This procedure is followed when an ERE believes that a bloodborne exposure has occurred.

The procedure is different if an EMT has been in contact with a patient with an airborne disease, especially infectious pulmonary TB. The EMT may

have no reason to suspect that the patient has an infectious disease. In such a case, the diagnosis of the patient would be made at the hospital after the EMT has transferred care of the patient. Once diagnosis of an airborne infectious disease is made, the hospital has the obligation of notifying the DO of the department where the EMT works about the possible exposure.

Chapter Review

SUMMARY

Ensuring body substance isolation is a vital part of providing emergency medical care. Always be alert to the possibility of risk from infectious diseases. The use of personal protective devices is essential and must become part of your routine. Your department or agency should provide periodic training in infection control and—whenever possible—use of engineering devices and controls that can lower the risk of exposure. Additionally, knowledge of your health status is important to your well being. You should have a physical exam on a regular basis that includes evaluation for TB and review of immunizations for hepatitis B, influenza, and tetanus. In the event of an occupational exposure, your agency is required to have an exposure control plan that will rapidly provide you with counseling, evaluation, and needed treatment.

REVIEWING KEY CONCEPTS

1. Explain the importance of body substance isolation.
2. List the types of personal protective equipment that should be used for body substance isolation. Describe situations in which each type of equipment should be used.
3. List diseases for which EMTs should receive immunizations or regular screenings.
4. Explain the differences among cleaning, disinfection, and sterilization. Describe when each would be appropriate.
5. Outline the basic elements of an emergency response agency's exposure control plan.

RESOURCES TO LEARN MORE

West, Katherine H. *Infectious Disease Handbook for Emergency Care Personnel*. Philadelphia: J.B. Lippincott, 1987.

Zimmerman, Lynn, Neuman, Mary, and Jurewicz, Deb. *Infection Control for Prehospital Providers, 2nd Edition*. Grand Rapids, MI: Mercy Ambulance, 1993.

INFECTION CONTROL AND PERSONAL PROTECTIVE EQUIPMENT

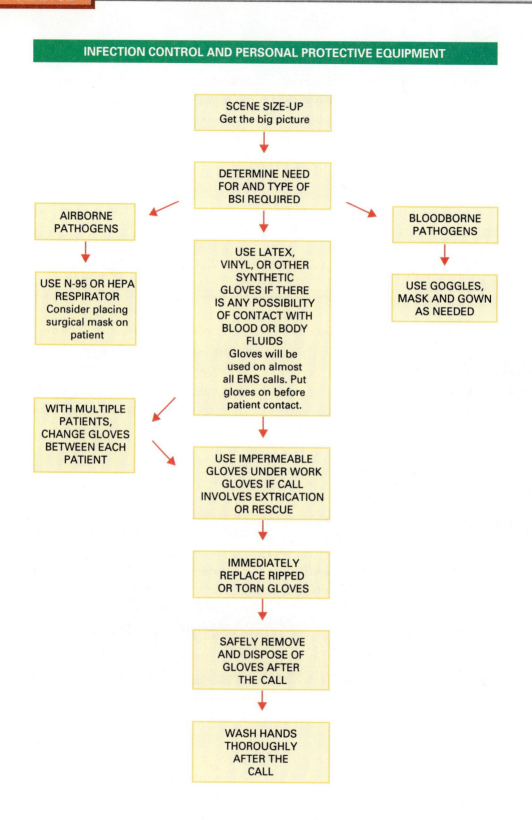

SCENE SIZE-UP
Get the big picture

DETERMINE NEED FOR AND TYPE OF BSI REQUIRED

AIRBORNE PATHOGENS

USE N-95 OR HEPA RESPIRATOR
Consider placing surgical mask on patient

USE LATEX, VINYL, OR OTHER SYNTHETIC GLOVES IF THERE IS ANY POSSIBILITY OF CONTACT WITH BLOOD OR BODY FLUIDS
Gloves will be used on almost all EMS calls. Put gloves on before patient contact.

BLOODBORNE PATHOGENS

USE GOGGLES, MASK AND GOWN AS NEEDED

WITH MULTIPLE PATIENTS, CHANGE GLOVES BETWEEN EACH PATIENT

USE IMPERMEABLE GLOVES UNDER WORK GLOVES IF CALL INVOLVES EXTRICATION OR RESCUE

IMMEDIATELY REPLACE RIPPED OR TORN GLOVES

SAFELY REMOVE AND DISPOSE OF GLOVES AFTER THE CALL

WASH HANDS THOROUGHLY AFTER THE CALL

Medical/Legal Issues

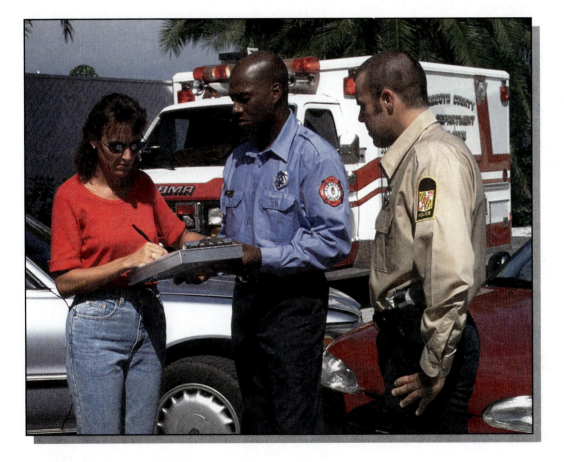

*T*he EMT-Basic must provide appropriate care to patients while respecting their legal rights. The EMT must at the same time also follow a professional code of ethics. Every state has passed laws or regulations that govern, to a greater or lesser extent, the activities of EMTs. Failure to abide by these laws exposes the EMT to criminal or civil penalties, or both. In addition, our system of civil law places special burdens on health care professionals such as EMTs. As you will discover, it is not always easy to balance a patient's legal rights with his or her medical needs!

▶

In this chapter, you'll learn about many important legal concepts that will affect your practice as an EMT every day. Included among these are the EMT's scope of practice, the difference between legal and ethical requirements, advanced directives, refusals of care, and a host of other important issues.

OBJECTIVES

At the completion of this chapter, the EMT student should be able to meet the following objectives:

Knowledge and Understanding

1. Define the EMT-Basic scope of practice. (p. 54)
2. Discuss the importance of Do Not Resuscitate (DNR) orders (advanced directives) and local or state provisions regarding EMS application. (p. 55)
3. Define consent and discuss the methods of obtaining consent. (pp. 54–55)
4. Explain the role of consent of minors in providing care. (p. 60)
5. Discuss the implications for the EMT-Basic in patient refusal of transport. (pp. 55–58)
6. Discuss the issues of abandonment, negligence, and battery and their implcations to the EMT-Basic. (pp. 55–56, 58–60)
7. State the conditions necessary for the EMT-Basic to have a duty to act. (p. 59)

8. Explain the importance, necessity, and legality of patient confidentiality. (pp. 60–61)
9. Discuss the considerations of the EMT-Basic in issues of organ retrieval. (p. 61)
10. Differentiate the actions that an EMT-Basic should take to assist in the preservation of a crime scene. (p. 63)
11. State the conditions that require an EMT-Basic to notify local law enforcement officials. (pp. 61–63)
12. Explain the role of EMS and the EMT-Basic regarding patients with DNR orders. (p. 55)
13. Explain the rationale for the needs, benefits, and usage of advance directives. (p. 55)
14. Explain the rationale for the concept of varying degrees of DNR. (p. 55)

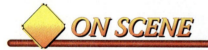 ON SCENE

DISPATCH: *ENGINE 5 AND AMBULANCE 3. RESPOND PRIORITY 1 TO A MALE SUBJECT, 435 HARRIS ROAD. POSSIBLE BEHAVIORAL EMERGENCY. TIME OUT IS 0755.*

You're responding without either of your city's paramedic units, which are busy with other patients. In five minutes, you arrive at a neatly kept blue colonial-style home in a residential neighborhood. After you knock several times, a crying child about 8 years old lets you in. She says, "Daddy is having spells again." As you enter the home, you ask if there is another adult

at home. The child shakes her head and replies, "Mommy's at work."

You enter the living room to find a man in his late 40s lying on a couch, mumbling incoherently. As you survey the room to ensure your safety, you begin your initial assessment. The patient does not answer your questions appropriately and exhibits strange arm movements. Suddenly, he shouts that he wants you to "get out of my house and leave me alone." He tries to stand, but falls back onto the couch mumbling.

You identify yourselves as fire department EMTs and explain that you've come to help him.

The patient waves his arms, shouting for you to leave. He demands, "Where's Colleen?" You back away slowly, explaining again that you're here to help him and that he may be having a medical problem.

His daughter, who is standing in the hallway, says, "He gets like this when his sugar acts up." The patient attempts to stand, but falls back onto the couch and seems to become less responsive.

Your lieutenant, who is also an EMT, has done a quick survey of the home. He states that he has found two used syringes and a vial of "NPH insulin" in the bathroom. The patient meanwhile has begun to snore deeply and responds only to painful stimuli. You now notice a "Medic Alert" bracelet on the patient's arm that reads "Insulin Dependent Diabetic."

Based upon the patient's presentation and the small amount of information you have been able to gather, you decide to proceed with treatment based on the concept of implied consent. While protecting the patient's airway, you complete the initial survey and then restrain the patient prior to packaging him for transport. As you load the patient into your ambulance, a paramedic unit arrives. You brief the paramedics on your findings and treatment and transfer to them responsibility for the patient's care.

LAWS AND ETHICS

Laws are the rules or regulations of a society enacted by government—or in the case of the United States, federal, state, and local governments—that are binding its members. Laws adopted by a society make up its *civil* and *criminal codes*. Generally, such laws either compel or prohibit certain behavior. Violation of a *civil law* (often referred to as a *tort* or *civil wrong*) exposes an individual to civil damages. In our society, civil damages usually translate to a monetary award against the EMT and his agency. Violation of the *criminal laws* (often referred to as the *penal code*) exposes the individual to criminal penalties, which may include fines and/or imprisonment. In most states, violation of the civil or criminal codes may also result in the suspension or revocation of an EMT's license or certification to practice.

Ethics are rules of conduct and behavior recognized by a particular group, for example, the medical profession. Though we live in a society of laws, it is impossible either to write or to enforce laws governing every human interaction. A profession's *code of ethics* supplies a model of behavior to follow in many situations not directly addressed by laws. As an EMT, having a strong set of personal and professional ethics is essential to meeting the expectations of your patients and their families.

For example, not all states have passed laws protecting the confidentiality of medical information about patients, even though confidentiality is one of the cornerstones of medical ethics. In your practice, you will often be entrusted with confidential and sensitive information about your patients, your co-workers, and other heath care professionals. You will sometimes be expected to disclose confidential information to your medical director or to outside agencies—for example, in a quality improvement (QI) review or in the investigation of a suspected child abuse case.

In your professional interactions as an EMT, it is also essential to always tell the "unembellished truth." No amount of technical knowledge or expertise will substitute for a lack of integrity!

At times, government laws and professional ethics can be or seem to be in conflict. Such conflicts are heightened as governments and professional groups struggle to address changes caused by new technologies and social issues. To help sort your way through such conflicts, you must become thoroughly familiar with the laws, regulations, and protocols governing emergency medical services in the jurisdiction where you will practice as an EMT. As part of your training program, you should receive copies of those statutes affecting your practice.

Finally, some basic guidelines may help you in decision making if you face a conflict between the requirements of the law and medical ethics.

1. First, *do no harm* to the patient!

2. When in doubt, always do what is in the *patient's* best interest.

3. Always *document your care,* and the reasons for it, in writing on a detailed patient care report.

4. If available, *consult with medical control on the appropriate care for a particular patient.*

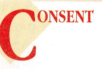

SCOPE OF PRACTICE

The whole body of authorized skills and procedures that an EMT may perform on a patient is referred to as the **scope of practice.** Many states have defined at least portions of the EMT's scope of practice in laws or regulations. Other states permit local or regional protocols to further define it. As an EMT, you work as a designated agent of your system's medical director. The medical director may place additional restrictions on your practice as an EMT, or may be permitted to expand it to include additional responsibilities.

You must become intimately familiar with the laws, regulations, and protocols that define the scope of practice for EMTs in your community. Failure to abide by the requirements of the scope of practice could endanger your patients. It could also expose you to civil damages resulting from a lawsuit.

CONSENT

In a famous legal case known as *Schloendorf* v. *Society of the NY Hospital* (1914), Judge Benjamin

Cardozo declared, "Every human being of adult years and sound mind has a right to determine what shall be done with his own body." In the field of medicine, this means that a competent adult has an absolute right to make informed decisions about his or her medical care. A competent patient can agree, or **consent,** to suggested treatment or refuse to accept that treatment.

For consent to treat (or refusal of treatment) to be legally valid, however, it must be based on the patient's full understanding of the risks, consequences, and available alternatives, if any, to treatment. In the vast majority of prehospital cases, the patient or the patient's family will have requested your response and will clearly accept your care. Nevertheless, in order to prevent misunderstandings and potential problems, you should use the guidelines below when you arrive on scene to provide treatment. If you do, you will have obtained **expressed consent** from the patient.

1. Introduce yourself to the patient and, if present, to the patient's family.

2. Explain that you are there to help the patient.

3. Ask the patient, and the family, to describe the reason(s) they requested EMS assistance.

4. Whenever possible, explain in plain language what you propose to do to the patient *before* beginning treatment.

5. Whenever possible, obtain the patient's verbal consent.

The courts have long recognized that in public safety services, such as EMS, fire, and police agencies, decisions must sometimes be made quickly and without much time to consider all the options. In such circumstances, courts have held that life-sustaining treatment can begin before the patient's formal consent is obtained, if the treatment is not specifically refused by the patient. The courts assume that, given the choice, a competent adult would accept necessary medical care in order to save his life. Thus, **implied consent** can be assumed whenever a patient needs immediate medical care and is incapable of giving either informed consent or informed refusal. For example, patients who are unresponsive, or whose reasoning is impaired by drugs, may be assumed to give consent for necessary medical care and transportation to the hospital.

At times, an EMT may encounter a patient who clearly needs medical care, who may be incapable of making an informed refusal as a result of impairment by head injury, drugs, alcohol, or a pre-existing medical condition, yet who firmly refuses to permit that care. This is one of the most difficult situations an EMT can face. This was the scenario the EMTs had to deal with in On Scene at the beginning of this chapter. There, a patient who was incoherent as a result of his diabetes may have needed immediate medical care and yet was incapable of understanding the need for such care. The EMTs correctly decided to treat and transport this patient based on the concept of implied consent.

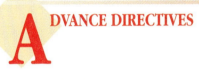

ADVANCE DIRECTIVES

As noted above, a competent adult has an absolute right to make informed decisions about his or her medical care. Such decisions include the right to refuse specific procedures, to refuse transportation, to refuse medical care entirely, or to stop it once it has begun.

An **advance directive** is a written document, executed by a competent adult that specifies what medical care should be provided to him if he is unable to make decisions at some future date. Most states have now adopted some type of legislation defining advance directives and specifying the conditions under which they are valid.

A **Do Not Resuscitate Order (DNR)** is a common type of advance directive (Figure 4-1). DNR orders generally direct EMS personnel to withhold resuscitation in the event of a cardiac arrest. It is very important to note that DNR orders do *not* mean "Do not treat!" It is unethical, and may be illegal, to withhold treatments such as oxygen from a patient simply because that patient has executed a DNR. Never withhold supportive and comforting care (often referred to as *palliative care*) simply because the patient has executed a DNR.

However, most DNR orders prevent an EMT from initiating CPR in the setting of a cardiac arrest.

In some states, **living wills** and **health care proxies** may also be legal forms of advance directives. Such documents may not only specify the extent of care to be provided to the patient but also name a person authorized to make medical decisions on behalf of the patient if he is unable to make them.

You must become familiar with any legislation enabling advance directives in the community where you will practice.

REFUSAL OF CARE/ABANDONMENT

In many EMS systems, 20 percent or more of the responses to calls end with a refusal of medical care or transportation. **Patient-initiated refusals (PIRs)** occur when the patient declines medical care or transportation. **EMS-initiated refusals (EMSIRs)** occur when EMS calls are either screened out of the system or when EMS personnel respond to a call but do not transport the patient. As explained below, these situations are legally very risky for the EMT and his department.

Abandonment is the sudden termination of care by the EMT without the patient's informed consent and without affording the patient an opportunity to secure medical care at a similar or higher level from another source. PIRs and EMSIRs, if not properly obtained, could be seen as abandonment of the patient.

Consider, for example, the following scenario. EMTs respond to a call for medical assistance. When they reach the scene, they find a patient who is in need of, but refuses medical care. However, the patient is unable to give an informed refusal because of apparent drug and/or alcohol use. Nevertheless, the EMTs permit the patient to "sign off," and they then leave the scene. After their departure, the patient's condition worsens. This deterioration is a direct result of the same medical problem for which the EMTs were originally called. The EMTs in this case have exposed themselves to legal liability for abandonment of the patient.

PREHOSPITAL DO NOT RESUSCITATE ORDERS

ATTENDING PHYSICIAN

In completing this prehospital DNR form, please check part A if no intervention by prehospital personnel is indicated. Please check Part A and options from Part B if specific interventions by prehospital personnel are indicated. To give a valid prehospital DNR order, this form must be completed by the patient's attending physician and must be provided to prehospital personnel.

A) _____ **Do Not Resuscitate (DNR):**
No Cardiopulmonary Resuscitation or Advanced Cardiac Life Support be performed by prehospital personnel

B) _____ **Modified Support:**
Prehospital personnel administer the following checked options:
_____Oxygen administration
_____Full airway support: intubation, airways, bag/valve/mask
_____Venipuncture: IV crystalloids and/or blood draw
_____External cardiac pacing
_____Cardiopulmonary resuscitation
_____Cardiac defibrillator
_____Pneumatic anti-shock garment
_____Ventilator
_____ACLS meds
_____Other interventions/medications (physician specify)
_____

Prehospital personnel are informed that (print patient name)_____
should receive no resuscitation (DNR) or should receive Modified Support as indicated. This directive is medically appropriate and is further documented by a physician's order and a progress note on the patient's permanent medical record. Informed consent from the capacitated patient or the incapacitated patient's legitimate surrogate is documented on the patient's permanent medical record. The DNR order is in full force and effect as of the date indicated below.

_____   _____

Attending Physician's Signature   _____

_____   _____

Print Attending Physician's Name   Print Patient's Name and Location
                                          (Home Address or Health Care Facility)

_____

Attending Physician's Telephone

_____   _____

Date   Expiration Date (6 Mos from Signature)

Figure 4-1   An EMS Do Not Resuscitate order.

At one time, filing a lawsuit against EMTs in such a case would have been almost unthinkable. Today, care provided by EMTs is subject to the same scrutiny as that provided by other medical professionals. There are, however, steps you can follow to protect yourself from liability if a patient refuses care (Figure 4-2):

◆ **Be sure the patient is mentally competent and oriented.** Spend time speaking with him

and attempting to reason with him. Remember that informed refusal *cannot* be provided by the following types of patients:

—Those intoxicated by drugs and/or alcohol

—Those suffering from mental disease or defect

—Those suffering from head injury

—Those suffering from severe hypoxia

EMS PATIENT REFUSAL CHECKLIST

PATIENT's NAME: _____ AGE: _____

LOCATION OF CALL: _____ DATE: _____

AGENCY INCIDENT #: _____ AGENCY CODE: _____

NAME OF PERSON FILLING OUT FORM: _____

I. **ASSESSMENT OF PATIENT** (Check appropriate response for each item)

    1.   Oriented to: Person? ☐ Yes ☐ No
    Place? ☐ Yes ☐ No
    Time? ☐ Yes ☐ No
    Situation? ☐ Yes ☐ No

    2.   Altered level of consciousness? ☐ Yes ☐ No

    3.   Head injury? ☐ Yes ☐ No

    4.   Alcohol or drug ingestion by exam or history? ☐ Yes ☐ No

II. **PATIENT INFORMED** (Check appropriate response for each item)

☐ Yes ☐ No   Medical treatment/evaluation needed

☐ Yes ☐ No   Ambulance transport needed

☐ Yes ☐ No   Further harm could result without medical treatment/evaluation

☐ Yes ☐ No   Transport by means other than ambulance could be hazardous in light of patient's illness/injury

☐ Yes ☐ No   Patient provided with Refusal Information Sheet

☐ Yes ☐ No   Patient accepted Refusal Information Sheet

III. **DISPOSITION**

☐ Refused all EMS assistance

☐ Refused field treatment, but accepted transport

☐ Refused transport, but accepted field treatment

☐ Refused transport to recommended facility

☐ Patient transported by private vehicle to_____

☐ Released in care or custody of self

☐ Released in care or custody of relative or friend

    Name:_____ Relationship:_____

☐ Released in custody of law enforcement agency

    Agency: _____ Officer: _____

☐ Released in custody of other agency

    Agency: _____ Officer: _____

IV. **COMMENTS:** _____

_____

_____

_____

_____

Figure 4-2 Some EMS systems have checklists for procedures to follow when a patient refuses care.

—Those who are suicidal or homicidal

—Those who are less than 18 years old

◆ **Be sure the patient is fully informed about the treatment and understands the risks and consequences of refusing it.**

◆ **Be sure the patient signs a "release from liability" form upon refusal of treatment.** Be sure the signing is witnessed by a third party. If the patient refuses to sign the form, document the refusal and have it witnessed by the third party (Figure 4-3).

Even if you've followed all of the steps above, you should not give up on efforts to persuade the patient if you believe he needs treatment. Consider doing the following:

◆ **Try again to persuade him, being absolutely sure he understands the consequences of his decision.**

◆ **Try to determine why the patient is refusing care.** If you know this, you may be able to come up with an argument to overcome his objections to medical care.

◆ **Consult with medical direction.** If the on-line physician is willing, have him speak to the patient.

◆ **Consider contacting family members.** Sometimes their arguments can convince a patient to accept care.

◆ **Consider calling law enforcement personnel.** They can assist with involuntary transport if the patient's condition appears life threatening. In some localities, police may arrest such a patient—on charges of public intoxication, for example. The police might then direct EMTs to treat and transport the patient.

◆ **If everything fails, indicate your willingness to return if the patient changes his mind.**

NEGLIGENCE

Negligence with respect to care provided by an EMT can be defined in several ways. It exists when an EMT performs either of the following types of actions:

◆ Conduct that fails to meet a standard established by statute, regulation, or protocol

◆ Actions that deviate from accepted standards and that other EMTs, acting in similar circumstances, would not have performed

With respect to medical care, negligence must be proven in a court of law. *Simple negligence* has four components that must be proven at trial:

Figure 4-3 Have both the patient and a witness sign a form indicating that the patient has refused treatment or transport.

REFUSAL OF TREATMENT AND TRANSPORTATION

I, THE UNDERSIGNED HAVE BEEN ADVISED THAT MEDICAL ASSISTANCE ON MY BEHALF IS NECESSARY AND THAT REFUSAL OF SAID ASSISTANCE AND TRANSPORTATION MAY RESULT IN DEATH, OR IMPERIL MY HEALTH. NEVERTHELESS, I REFUSE TO ACCEPT TREATMENT OR TRANSPORT AND ASSUME ALL RISKS AND CONSEQUENCES OF MY DECISION AND RELEASE GOLD CROSS AMBULANCE COMPANY AND ITS EMPLOYEES FROM ANY LIABILITY ARISING FROM MY REFUSAL.

_____
SIGNATURE OF PATIENT

_____
WITNESSED BY

_____
DATE SIGNED

◆ ***Duty to act.*** An EMT incurs a **duty to act** when he accepts a call for help and responds to a patient. At least one state court has ruled that *accepting* a call for assistance then obligates the EMS service to respond in a timely manner.

Whether an EMT who renders assistance while off-duty or outside his agency's service area incurs a duty to act varies from state to state. In such situations, the EMT usually acts out of moral or ethical considerations in providing emergency care.

In some states, an off-duty EMT may create a legal duty to act when he stops to offer assistance. The EMT, however, may be protected from liability for negligence in such circumstances by **Good Samaritan laws.** Good Samaritan laws are designed to encourage medical personnel like physicians, nurses, and EMTs to render assistance off-duty by limiting liability that results from providing care. Note, however, that Good Samaritan laws do not provide an absolute shield against lawsuits. In general, to be protected by these laws, the EMT must:

—Render the assistance while off duty

—Not charge the patient for services rendered

—Not commit gross negligence

◆ ***Breach of duty.*** This occurs when the EMT performs an action that is medically inappropriate or performs an appropriate procedure improperly. Such actions involve a **commission.** When an EMT *fails* to take an appropriate action that would normally be performed, an **omission** occurs. An EMT may breach his duty to the patient by either commission or omission.

◆ ***Damages.*** For negligence to be proven, the EMT's commission or omission must result in harm, or **damages,** to the patient. In most states, damages could include both physical and psychological harm to the patient.

◆ ***Proximate cause.*** This means that the EMT's breach of duty had a direct relationship to the damages suffered by the patient.

Here's a simple example of negligence. EMTs respond to a call to assist a child who has fallen off a bicycle. They clearly have a *duty to act* here. The child is complaining of severe pain in his lower leg and the leg is obviously deformed. Nevertheless, the EMTs moves the child onto the ambulance stretcher without first splinting the leg. While the EMTs are moving the child, bone ends come through the skin of the lower leg, creating an open fracture.

The child's parents later sue the EMTs and the EMS system, charging that the EMTs were negligent in moving the child without first splinting the leg. In court, the attorney for the parents introduces expert witnesses who testify that splinting a leg in such a situation is standard procedure. This demonstrates the EMTs *breach of duty*. The witnesses also testify that it is extremely likely that the EMTs' decision to move the child without splinting directly caused the open fracture. This testimony indicates that the EMTs' actions were the *proximate cause* of injury to the child. The child, his parents, and other witnesses also testify to the pain and difficulties the child has faced as a result of the open fracture. This testimony shows the *damages* that resulted for the patient. The jury finds for the parents and awards monetary damages.

Many states have enacted additional legal protections for certain EMS personnel. In New York State, for example, EMTs who voluntarily provide their services in an emergency are given legal exemption from damages alleged to have occurred to a patient, unless **gross negligence** is proven. Though the definition of gross negligence varies from state to state, it is generally held to be conduct that deviates so greatly from acceptable standards that a reasonable EMT would find it offensive.

You should note that, even in states that have granted limited immunity to EMTs who volunteer their services, damages that result from the operation of a motor vehicle are never included.

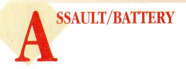

ASSAULT/BATTERY

Legal problems can arise when an EMT attempts to treat a patient who has given an informed refusal of care. In such a case, the EMT may risk criminal charges of assault and battery. **Assault,** in general terms, is unlawfully placing a patient in imminent fear of bodily harm. **Battery** would occur when an EMT touches a patient, without malicious intent, after that patient has given an informed refusal of care. All states have laws that provide their own, more precise definitions of assault and battery. If an EMT were to unlawfully restrain a patient against his will or to illegally transport a patient, other laws such as those regarding kidnaping, could apply.

While it is possible that such serious charges could be filed against EMTs, it is unlikely. In fact, court literature shows not a single legal case in an American court where an EMS provider was convicted of assault, battery, or kidnaping when providing appropriate medical care and transportation. An EMT is far more likely to face a civil lawsuit on the grounds of abandonment or negligence than a criminal trial for assault or battery. Even though as an EMT you are unlikely to face criminal charges, remember that civil penalties can be severe. You have a legal and ethical responsibility to provide appropriate care. Again, refer to the four general rules outlined earlier.

MINORS AND SPECIAL RISK PATIENTS

With some exceptions, the law views children under the age of 18 as minors. A minor can neither legally consent to medical treatment nor make an informed refusal of care. A minor's parents or legal guardians must make decisions regarding the child's medical treatment. In the absence of a parent or legal guardian, the EMTs may and should provide all appropriate treatment and transportation to the hospital. A minor should never be permitted to sign a refusal of treatment form. In some states, however, laws allow *emancipated minors*— those who are married, or of a certain age, or who are pregnant—to provide consent; know the laws in your jurisdiction.

The vast majority of parents will cooperate fully with EMS and will agree to whatever treatment is necessary for their child. However, in rare situa-tions, the EMT may be faced with a parent who refuses to allow an injured or acutely ill child to be treated or transported. This sometimes occurs because the parent is frightened, or worried about the cost. Also, the religious beliefs of some parents may lead them to refuse medical care for a child.

In such cases, the EMT should patiently but firmly explain to the parent why immediate medical care and transportation is necessary. If this fails to win permission to treat the child, the EMT should immediately request the assistance of a law enforcement agency. The EMT should explain to the responding officer that the child needs immediate medical attention and that the parent is refusing such care. No court in the United States has ever upheld the right of a parent to refuse emergency medical care for a child.

There are other *special risk patients* who, for one reason or another, may not be capable of giving either informed consent or informed refusal. The following is a partial list of such patients:

- Certain developmentally disabled patients
- Acute head injury patients, particularly if they suffer a loss of consciousness
- Diabetic patients experiencing very low or very high blood sugar
- Dementia patients, including those with advanced Alzheimer's disease and similar conditions
- Certain psychiatric patients, including those deemed suicidal or homicidal
- Acutely intoxicated patients, whether from drugs or alcohol

Remember that, unless a legal guardian directs otherwise, implied consent to treat and transport can be assumed in all such cases. Remember also that the EMT should always strive to do what is in the *patient's* best interest, though admittedly this is sometimes easier said than done.

CONFIDENTIALITY

One of the cornerstones of medicine is that information shared by the patient with his or her medical care provider is confidential. Such information is said to be **privileged.** Examples of such information include, but are *not* limited to, your documentation of the patient's medical history, your assessment of the patient's illness or injury, and details of the care that you provide. In many states, the prehospital care report or run report cannot be disclosed to anyone other than the patient without the patient's written permission.

Exceptions to confidentiality usually involve legal issues. For example, you may receive a court order (a subpoena) requiring you to provide information at a trial or hearing. Also, confidential information essential to the investigation of a crime or potential crime can generally be disclosed to appropriate legal authorities without the need for written permission from the patient.

Many EMS agencies obtain the patient's written permission to release certain information to third-party insurers. This is often done through use of an information release form signed by the patient or the patient's representative.

You should become familiar with any laws or regulations that affect patient confidentiality in the area where you will practice as an EMT. Each EMS agency should have a written policy detailing how, and under what conditions, confidential patient information can be disclosed.

POTENTIAL ORGAN DONORS

An individual who has willed that his organs be made available for transplant in the event of his death is referred to as a **potential organ donor.** People who wish to become organ donors may carry a card indicating this in a wallet or purse. In many states, the driver's license provides a place where a person's willingness to donate his organs can be recorded (Figure 4-4).

There are a few general rules to keep in mind if you encounter a patient who is a potential organ donor. First, all appropriate medical care must be provided to the patient. *The signing of an organ donor card is not a Do Not Resuscitate (DNR) order!* In the event that efforts to resuscitate the patient fail, *organ supportive care,* includ-

ing oxygen, ventilation, and CPR, should be provided, if appropriate. The patient should be rapidly transported to a hospital for evaluation and potential harvesting of the organs.

Become familiar with any regulations or protocols that address the care of potential organ donors in the jurisdiction in which you will practice.

SPECIAL REPORTING SITUATIONS

Each state has laws requiring EMTs to report to the appropriate authorities when they see or suspect that certain types of crimes have been committed. Situations usually covered by such laws include the following:

◆ Physical or psychological abuse of a child, a spouse, or an elderly person

◆ An injury resulting from a violent crime such as a shooting or stabbing

◆ Sexual assault

◆ An injury that results from a suicide attempt or gesture

◆ Burns

◆ Suspected exposure to an infectious disease

◆ Cases where restraint of a patient was necessary

Figure 4-4 An indication that a person is willing to be an organ donor may appear on the driver's license.

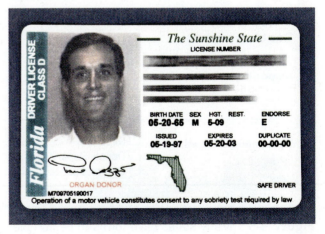

Special Incident Report

Town of Colonie
Department of Emergency Medical Services ————

EMERGENCY MEDICAL SERVICES
TOWN OF COLONIE

Date of Incident: _____ **Time:** _____ **REMO #:** _____

Town Run #: _____ **Reported by:** _____ **Zone:** _____

Type of Incident: ☐ MCI ☐ Rescue ☐ Personnel Matter ☐ Injury ☐ Accident with an EMS vehicle
☐ Infectious Disease Exposure ☐ Scene Conflict ☐ Other _____

Total # of Patients: ☐ #P-1: _____ ☐ #P-2: _____ ☐ #P-3: _____ ☐ #P-0: _____
Elapsed Scene Time: *(First unit arrival to last unit to hospital)* _____
Total Time of Incident: _____

Describe the Incident Below:
Attach any additional documentation such as news clipppings and the pre-hospital care report.
Attach additional sheets if necessary.

_____
_____
_____
_____
_____
_____
_____
_____
_____
_____
_____
_____
_____
_____
_____
_____
_____
_____
_____
_____
_____

Signature: _____ **Date:** _____

- -

Office Use Only
This incident relates to: ☐ Day Operation: TOT ☐ Night Operations: TOT: ☐ Administration: TOT:
_____ _____ _____

Disposition: _____
_____
_____ Date:

Notifications/Copies: ☐ Director ☐ Deputy Director ☐ Supervisors
☐ Deputy Supervisors ☐ Senior Medics ☐ Zone Coordinator(s)
☐ Other _____ Zone: ☐ 2 ☐ 3 ☐ 4

Figure 4-5 Many states have forms to be completed in special reporting situations.

◆ Patients who may be intoxicated or mentally incompetent and are found with injuries

In many of these situations, the EMT is empowered by the law to breach normal patient confidentiality when making a report. Your instructor and your agency should outline the laws about special reporting situations in your jurisdiction (Figure 4-5).

SUSPECTED CRIME SCENES

As an EMT, you may at some point treat patients involved in an apparent or suspected crime. *Your first duty is to provide all appropriate medical care to the patient, including transport to a hospital if appropriate.* If you suspect that a crime has been committed, request that law-enforcement personnel respond to the scene. Potential crimes may include apparent assaults, rapes, alcohol- or drug-related motor vehicle accidents, suspected child or elder abuse, suicides, and homicides. You must become familiar with the laws or regulations in your area that detail what suspected crimes must be reported and to which agencies.

EMTs are often dispatched simultaneously with the police to suspected crime scenes. If you arrive before the police, first determine if the scene is safe to enter as part of your scene size-up. If it is not or if you have any doubts about safety, establish a safe perimeter away from the scene and await the arrival of police. This practice is often referred to as staging. Each EMS agency should have a written policy describing the procedure for the staging of personnel and vehicles at potentially dangerous situations, such as a crime in progress.

If a scene is deemed safe to enter before the police arrive, be sensitive to the need to preserve evidence. While all appropriate medical care should always be provided, the EMT should observe the following general rules at the scene of a potential crime:

◆ **Only essential personnel should enter a potential crime scene.** As the number of rescuers increases, so does the potential for disturbing evidence.

◆ **Disturb as little as possible at the scene.** Do not move furniture, turn lights off or on, or touch anything that is not essential to providing direct patient care. At the scene of an automobile accident, do not move pieces of a vehicle or clothing unless doing so is essential to providing patient care.

◆ **Do not remove or cut through the clothing of a patient at a potential crime scene, unless it is essential to providing appropriate patient care.** You should especially avoid cutting through bullet or knife holes in clothing. Any clothing that is removed should be placed in a plastic bag and given to law enforcement officers. Never leave potential evidence unattended at the scene.

◆ **If possible, make a drawing of the scene or take a photograph of the scene prior to moving the patient and prior to altering the scene.** Such documentation should be given to the responding law enforcement officers.

In many states, patient information that would normally be confidential can be legally disclosed to a law enforcement agency in the event of a crime investigation. You should become familiar with laws that apply where you will practice.

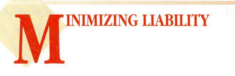

MINIMIZING LIABILITY

No one likes to be sued. Being named in a lawsuit alleging that you harmed a patient by your actions can be psychologically devastating because of the pride you take as an EMT in providing quality care. While you cannot eliminate the possibility of a lawsuit, you can minimize liability by following the basic guidelines cited at the beginning of the chapter. To repeat:

1. First, *do no harm* to the patient!

2. When in doubt, always do what is in the *patient's* best interest.

3. Always *document your care,* and the reasons for it, in writing on a detailed patient care report.

4. If available, *consult with medical control on the appropriate care for a particular patient.*

Finally, studies have shown that by acting in a professional manner, taking the time to speak and listen to the patient, and simply demonstrating kindness and compassion toward the patient you can greatly reduce potential liability.

Chapter Review

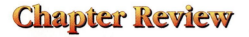

SUMMARY

As an EMT, you will provide prehospital emergency medical care under a wide variety of conditions, some very difficult or even hostile. A strong set of personal and professional ethics will guide you in always doing what is in the *patient's* best interest. However, legal considerations also affect your actions in the field.

You must recognize that competent adults have the legal right to determine what medical care—if any—will be provided to them. For this reason, you must be familiar with the concepts of expressed and implied consent. You must also know how to ensure, when treatment is refused, that the refusal is informed and therefore valid.

You must be familiar with advance directives as forms of expressing either consent or refusal of treatment. You must also understand the concept of duty to act—as well as implications of breaching it. Know the importance of patient confidentiality, as well as the measures you should follow at the scene of a crime.

Remember above all that, from an ethical and legal point of view, it is always better to err on the side of treating and transporting a patient rather than abandoning the patient. Never let undue concern about lawsuits prevent you from providing necessary and appropriate medical care to your patient.

REVIEWING KEY CONCEPTS

1. Define *scope of practice*.
2. Explain what kind of consent must be obtained before you can provide treatment to a patient.
3. Explain how discovering that a patient has a Do Not Resuscitate order might affect your care of the patient.
4. Describe the steps you should follow when a patient refuses treatment or transport.
5. Define *negligence* and list the four elements that must be met for an EMT to be found guilty of simple negligence.
6. List some of the conditions under which an EMT can release confidential information about a patient.
7. Describe how discovering that a patient has an organ donor card would affect your care of the patient.
8. List actions you can take to help preserve evidence at a crime scene.

RESOURCES TO LEARN MORE

George, James E. *Law and Emergency Care.* St. Louis: C.V. Mosby, 1980.

Anatomy and Physiology

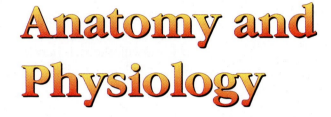

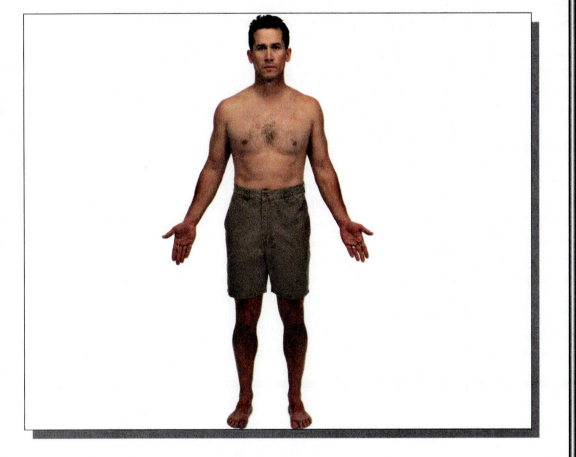

*A*s an EMT, you must understand basic human anatomy and physiology. **Anatomy** is the study of the structure of the human body. If you know normal anatomy, you can more easily recognize injuries in the patients you treat. A knowledge of anatomy will also allow you to describe and document more accurately the findings you make during a physical exam. **Physiology** is the study of the body's functions. If you know how the body normally functions, you can more easily recognize when disease or injury alters those functions.

At the completion of this chapter, the EMT-Basic student should be able to meet the following objectives:

Knowledge and Understanding

1. Identify the following topographic terms: medial, lateral, proximal, distal, superior, inferior, anterior, posterior, midline, bilateral, right, left, bilateral, mid-clavicular, and mid-axillary. (pp. 69–73)

2. Describe the anatomy and function of the following major body systems: respiratory, circulatory, musculoskeletal, nervous, and endocrine. (pp. 73–92)

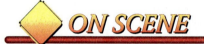

ON SCENE

DISPATCH: *MEDIC AMBULANCE 3, ENGINE 12, RESPOND TO THE CORNER OF LANCASTER STREET AND FOURTH AVENUE FOR A MOTOR VEHICLE CRASH WITH INJURIES.*

You are one of three EMTs assigned to Engine 12. Your unit is first on the scene. On arrival, you find a single patient who has been ejected from a car. He is lying face down on the sidewalk. The patient is alert and speaking, but he has multiple obvious injuries. The other crew members provide manual in-line stabilization , log-roll the patient, and apply a cervical collar. They provide high flow oxygen and position him on a long spine board. Meanwhile, you do a rapid trauma assessment, noting the injuries that the patient has sustained. Your department's

paramedic ambulance is responding from across town, so you radio them with a scene assessment and patient update:

"Engine 12 to Medic 3."

"Medic 3."

"We have an approximately 25-year-old male ejected from a motor vehicle. Upon arrival, we found him lying prone. He is awake and alert with an open airway and adequate breathing. He has sustained the following injuries: a deep laceration of the left parietal scalp; multiple abrasions and lacerations of the anterior and left lateral chest. He also has left upper quadrant abdominal tenderness. He is on a backboard, high flow oxygen is applied, and all bleeding is controlled."

"Copy that, Engine 12. Our ETA is 2 minutes."

HUMAN ANATOMY BASICS

The parts of the human anatomy that you must be most familiar with and able to describe are the parts that you can readily see. The description of this external anatomy of the human body is referred to as **surface** or **topographic anatomy.** Many of the features of topographic anatomy can

be appreciated by touching, or **palpating,** them. The specialized terms of topographic anatomy describe both specific areas of the body and the relationship of one body area to another. People in the medical field use these terms to convey information about patients accurately and concisely, as in the On Scene incident above. By knowing these terms, you will be better able to communicate both orally and in writing with other members of the health care team in your emergency medical system.

Anatomical Terms

EMTs are called to care for patients who have injuries or pains in all parts of their bodies. They discover these patients in a variety of positions. Some are found lying face down, others on their backs or sides. Some are sitting in chairs or hunched over steering wheels. The specialized language of medicine enables EMTs to describe a patient so that other medical personnel can see clearly the conditions in which the patient was found and focus rapidly on the patient's problem.

One of the key terms that will allow you to pass on information about a patient properly is **normal anatomic position.** This is defined as a person standing, facing forward, with the arms at the sides and the palms facing forward (Figure 5-1). Virtually all descriptions of the body are based upon this normal anatomic position.

Now visualize a person standing in the normal anatomical position. Imagine a line drawn vertically through that person's body from the nose through the umbilicus (belly button). That line is called the **midline.** It divides the body into right and left sides. Such a straight-line division is also called an **anatomical plane.**

There are two other anatomical lines or planes commonly used to describe location on the body. On a patient standing in profile, the **mid-axillary line** is an imaginary line drawn from the center of the armpit (the axilla) through the ankle (Figure 5-2). The **mid-clavicular lines** are vertical lines drawn through the centers of each clavicle (collar bone) (Figure 5-2).

The midline and the mid-axillary lines help to define several anatomical terms indicating how parts of the body relate to each other. The normal terms describing such relationships—terms like "above," "next to," and "in front of"—are not precise enough for medical use.

Anterior and **posterior** refer to front and back. The mid-axillary line divides the body into front and back halves. A position in front of this line is called *anterior* and a position in back of the line is considered *posterior.* Thus, you would say that "the tip of the nose is anterior to the eye." This same relationship could also be stated correctly as "the eye is posterior to the tip of the nose." Sometimes the terms **ventral** and **dorsal**

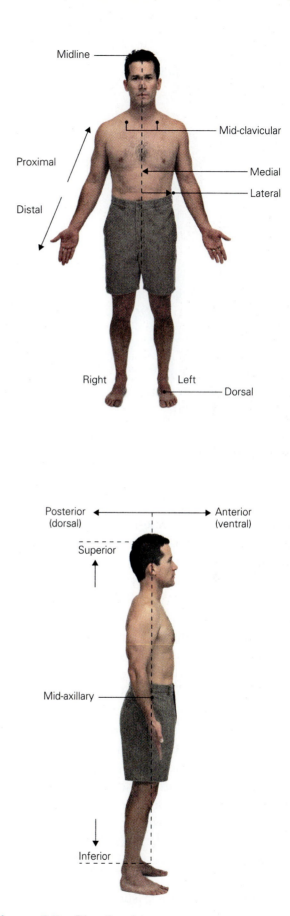

Figure 5-1   Directional terms.

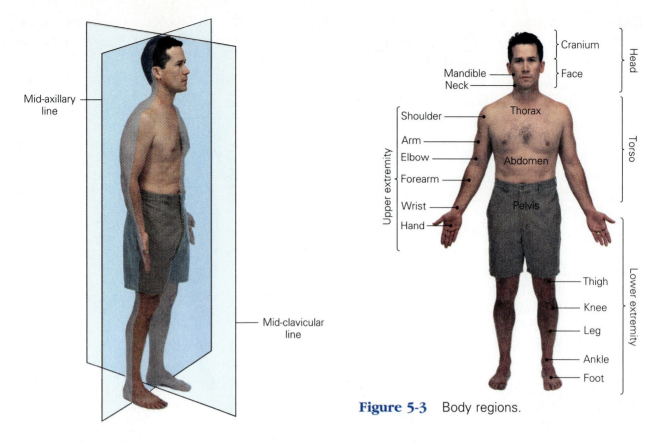

Figure 5-2 Mid-axillary and mid-clavicular planes.

Figure 5-3 Body regions.

are also used to describe the anterior and posterior surfaces of the body (Figure 5-1).

Superior and **inferior** refer to above and below. You would thus say "the head is superior to the chest" or "the chest is inferior to the head" (Figure 5-1).

Medial and **lateral** refer to positions toward the midline and away from the midline. For example, "the eye is medial to the ear" and "the ear is lateral to the eye" (Figure 5-1). **Bilateral** refers to structures or features that occur on both sides of the midline—the eyes, the ears, the arms, etc.

Proximal and **distal** refer to positions toward the trunk of the body and away from it. These terms are generally used to describe positions on the arms and legs. For example, you could say that "the elbow is proximal to the wrist" or that "the wrist is distal to the elbow" (Figure 5-1).

Plantar refers to the surface of the sole of the foot.

Palmar refers to the surface of the palm of the hand.

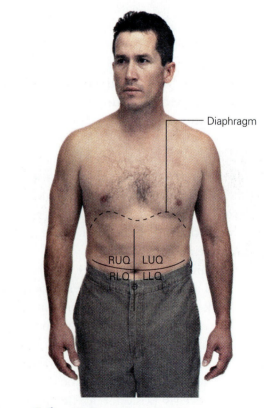

Figure 5-4 Abdominal quadrants.

Right and left are common terms, but their use is standardized in medical practice. When you use the terms to describe some part of a patient's anatomy, it is the *patient's* right and the *patient's* left to which you are referring.

Body Regions

The human body is divided into various general anatomic regions (Figure 5-3).

The **head** includes the face and the cranium, which encloses the brain.

The **neck** connects the superior chest to the head.

The **torso** includes the chest (thorax), the abdomen, and the pelvis. Other terms make referring to positions on or in the abdomen easier. Imagine that straight vertical and horizontal lines are drawn through the umbilicus. These lines divide the abdomen into four parts or **quadrants** (Figure 5-4). These parts are the right upper quadrant (RUQ), the right lower quadrant (RLQ), the left upper quadrant (LUQ), and the left lower quadrant (LLQ). It is usually helpful to describe the location of pain, tenderness to touch, or site of injury in the abdomen by the specific quadrant involved.

The **upper extremities** include the shoulders, arms, elbows, forearms, wrists, and hands.

The **lower extremities** include the thighs, knees, legs, and feet.

Anatomic terms are most often used by the EMT to describe the exact location on the body of injuries or other physical findings. Figure 5-5

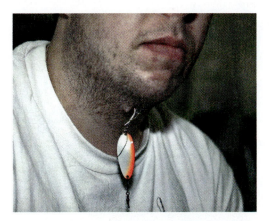

Figure 5-5A A fish hook impaled in the mid-line of the anterior neck just inferior to the chin.

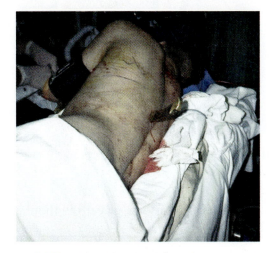

Figure 5-5B A knife impaled in the center of the back just to the left/lateral of the midline.

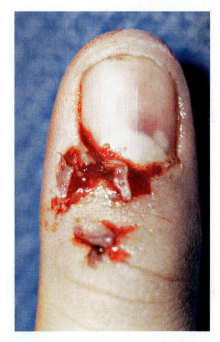

Figure 5-5C A crush injury to the distal finger just proximal to the nail.

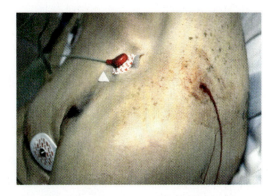

Figure 5-5D A gunshot wound, with an entry wound in the left lateral superior chest and an exit wound in the posterior shoulder.

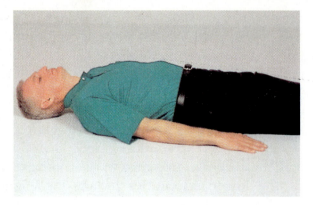

Figure 5-6A   Supine position.

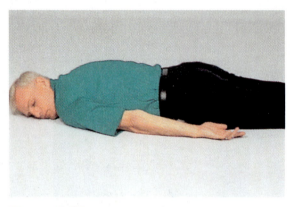

Figure 5-6B   Prone position.

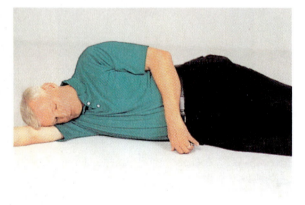

Figure 5-6C   Right lateral recumbent position.

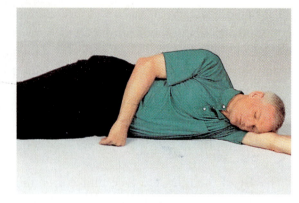

Figure 5-6D   Left lateral recumbent position.

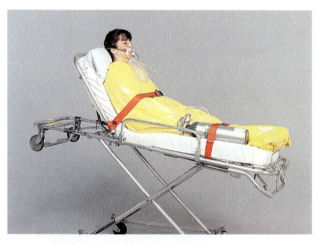

Figure 5-6E   Fowler's position.

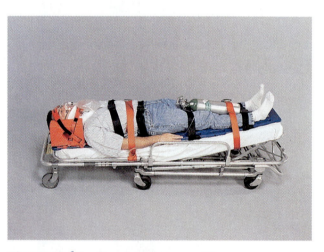

Figure 5-6F   Trendelenburg position.

shows a set of injuries and their locations stated in anatomic terms.

Body Positioning

It is rare for EMTs to find patients standing in the normal anatomical position. Therefore, the EMT must be familiar with the terms used to describe the positions in which patients are found. In addition, there are specific names given to the posi-

tions in which patients are placed by the EMT for transport and treatment.

◆ A patient lying on his back facing upward is in the **supine** position (Figure 5-6A).

- A patient lying face down is in the **prone** position (Figure 5-6B).
- A patient lying on his right side is in the **right lateral recumbent** position (Figure 5-6C), while a patient lying on his left side is in the **left lateral recumbent** position (Figure 5-6D). Another term for the lateral recumbent position is the **recovery position.**

Patients may also be placed in any of the positions above by medical personnel as part of treatment. For instance, many trauma patients are placed supine on a backboard to prevent spinal injury. Women in the advanced stages of pregnancy are often placed in the left lateral recumbent position to allow improved blood flow to the mother and baby. Other common positions in which patients are placed include the following:

- A patient lying on his back with the upper body elevated at an angle of 45° to 60° is in **Fowler's position** (Figure 5-6E).
- A patient lying on his back with the lower part of his body elevated about 12 inches (300 mm) is in the **Trendelenburg position** (Figure 5-6F). This is also sometimes known as the **shock position,** because it is used to treat patients in shock with no suspected head or spine injury.

ANATOMY AND PHYSIOLOGY OF BODY SYSTEMS

The body contains many specialized structures called **organs.** Examples of body organs include the heart, liver, lungs, brain, and kidneys. Organs are in turn made up of millions of smaller living structures called **cells.** Each organ contains many different types of cells with various functions within the organ. For example, the lungs contain some cells that allow the exchange of oxygen and carbon dioxide to take place, other cells that line the air passages, and still other cells that help produce mucus to clear the airways of inhaled debris. It is at the cell level that the body uses oxygen and produces waste products, especially carbon dioxide. Organs or groups of organs and body tissues that have a common function are classified as **body systems.**

The human body's normal functions result from the complex interactions of several body systems. The major body systems include the musculoskeletal, respiratory, cardiovascular, nervous, digestive, and endocrine systems. The various parts of these systems work together to achieve certain body functions. For example, the musculosketetal system includes all of the body's bones, the muscles under voluntary control, the tendons, and the ligaments. These parts of the musculoskeletal system work together to allow the body to move.

As an EMT you should be familiar with the structure (anatomy) and functions (physiology) of the body's major systems.

Musculoskeletal System

The musculoskeletal system comprises the parts described above. It has three major functions:

- It gives the body shape.
- It protects vital internal organs.
- It provides for body movement.

Bones of the Musculoskeletal System

The bones of the musculoskeletal system provide the body's physical structure and serve to protect the internal organs. The bones of the body make up the human skeleton and are sometimes called the skeletal system. The human body contains 206 separate bones. It is not necessary as an EMT to know the names and locations of all these bones. However, since injuries to the musculoskeletal system are common, knowing the names and locations of the major and commonly injured bones is important (Figure 5-7).

The bones of the skull protect the brain. The skull is made up of several bones joined together at seam-like sutures. In infancy and childhood, these sutures are expandable and allow the brain and skull to grow. By adulthood, the sutures become fused, making the skull a rigid capsule enclosing the brain. More important than naming the specific bones of the skull, the EMT should be able to identify the regions of the scalp. The names of the regions of the scalp are named based on the underlying bones of the skull. They

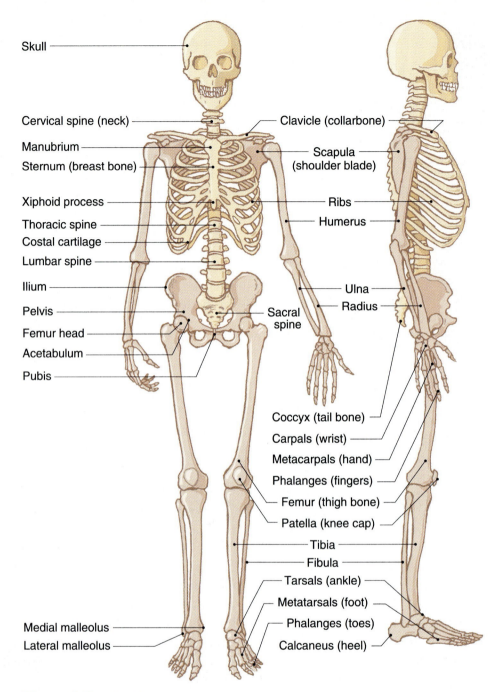

Figure 5-7   The skeleton.

include the **frontal, occipital, parietal,** and **temporal** regions (Figure 5-8).

The bones of the face have several functions. All the facial bones help to protect the brain from frontal impacts. The **orbits** (eye sockets) are made up of several bones that surround and protect the eye. The **mandible** (lower jaw) and the **maxillae** (upper jaw) provide support for the teeth. The **nasal bones** support the nose, which allows for the sense of smell. The **zygomatic bones** (cheek bones) contribute to facial structure by forming the cheeks (Figure 5-9).

The head is supported by the bony **spinal column.** The spinal column extends from the base of the skull into the pelvis and contains and protects the spinal cord. The spinal column or "spine" is the most crucial support structure of the body. The spine is made up of 33 stacked bones

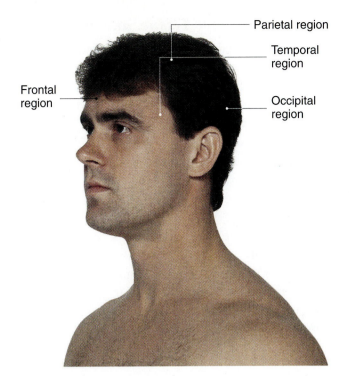

Parietal region

Temporal region

Occipital region

Frontal region

Figure 5-8   Regions of the scalp.

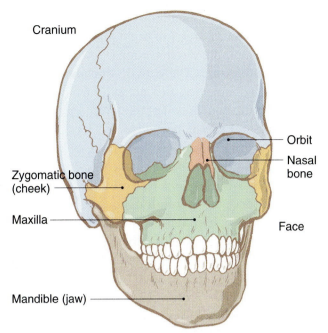

Cranium

Orbit

Nasal bone

Zygomatic bone (cheek)

Maxilla

Face

Mandible (jaw)

Figure 5-9   The skull: cranium and face.

called **vertebrae.** The spinal column is separated into five sections: the seven neck or **cervical** vertebrae, the twelve chest or **thoracic** vertebrae, the five lower back or **lumbar** vertebrae, the five fused **sacral** vertebrae that make up the posterior wall of the pelvis, and the four fused tailbone or **coccyx** vertebrae (Figure 5-10). Because the thoracic spine is supported by the ribs and the sacral and coccyx vertebrae are supported by the pelvis, they are less prone to injury than the unsupported cervical and lumbar vertebrae.

The bones of the **thorax** (chest) include the thoracic spinal column. Twelve pairs of ribs attach posteriorly to the thoracic spine. The ribs are numbered superiorly to inferiorly, with rib 1 the most superior and rib 12 the most inferior. Rib pairs 1 through 10 attach anteriorly to the **sternum** (breastbone). The ribs 11 and 12 are called "floating" because they do not attach anteriorly to the sternum. The sternum itself is divided into three sections. The superior portion is the **manubrium,** the middle portion is the **body,** and the inferior portion is the **xiphoid process.**

The pelvis is made up of two sets of paired bones, the **ilium** and the **ischium.** The pelvis is joined anteriorly at the **pubis** and posteriorly at

the sacral spine. The **iliac crest** of the pelvis can be palpated laterally and the ischium can be palpated inferiorly.

The lower extremities extend from the pelvis, where the head of the femur forms a ball that sits in the indentation or socket of the pelvis called the **acetabulum** to form the hip joint. The femur then angles downward at the **greater trochanter** to form the thigh bone. The knee joint is formed by three bones, the distal femur, the **patella** (knee cap), and the proximal **tibia.** The lower leg is

Figure 5-10   The divisions of the spine.

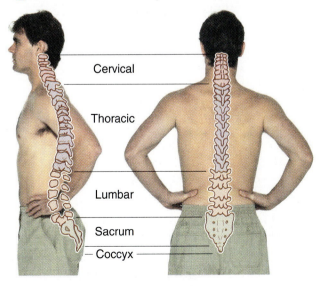

Cervical

Thoracic

Lumbar

Sacrum

Coccyx

formed by the tibia (shin bone) and the **fibula** laterally. The distal portion of the fibula is the **lateral malleolus** and the distal portion of the tibia is the **medial malleolus.** These two structures are the surface landmarks of the ankle joint, which is formed by the connection of the lower leg bones to the **proximal tarsal bones** of the foot. A tarsal bone called the **calcaneus** (heel bone) is the most posterior portion of the foot. In the mid-foot are the **distal tarsal bones** and the **metatarsal bones,** which connect to the **phalanges** (toes). The toes are identified by number, with the great toe being the first toe and the small toe being the fifth.

The upper extremities extend from the shoulders. Each shoulder is made up of a **scapula** (shoulder blade), **clavicle** (collarbone), and **acromion** (which forms the lateral tip of the shoulder). The head of the **humerus** rests in the shoulder joint. The humerus forms the proximal part of the upper extremity (commonly called the "arm"). The elbow joint is the connection between the distal humerus and the two bones of the forearm—the **radius** (lateral and aligning with the thumb) and the **ulna** (medial and aligning with the fifth finger. The bony prominence that you can feel on the posterior side of the elbow is the **olecranon** process of the ulna.

The wrist is made up of the distal radius and ulna and the proximal bones of the hand called the **carpals.** The carpals connect to the **metacarpals,** which form the bones of the palm of the hand. The **phalanges** (fingers) are also identified by numbers, with the thumb being the first finger and the little finger being the fifth.

Figure 5-11 **A.** Ball-and-socket joint. **B.** Hinge joint.

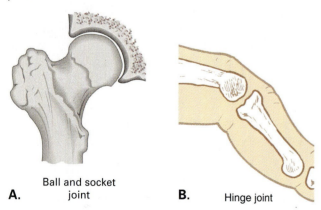

A. Ball and socket joint   **B.** Hinge joint

Joints, Connective Tissue, and Muscles

The human skeleton can move because it has many joints. **Joints** are the places where bones connect to other bones. Joints are held together by strong, band-like connective tissue called **ligaments.** The two most common types of joints are **ball-and-socket joints,** like the hip, and **hinge joints,** like the finger joints (Figure 5-11).

Muscles are attached to bones by **tendons** and cause movement across joints. The muscles that move the body are called **skeletal** or **voluntary muscles** because they can be purposefully, or voluntarily, controlled by the brain to move many of the body's bones (Figure 5-12). These muscles make up the muscular mass of the human body. They include the muscles of the extremities, chest, and abdominal wall.

Figure 5-12 The three types of muscles.

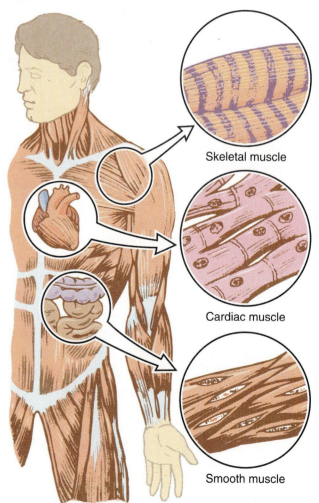

Skeletal muscle

Cardiac muscle

Smooth muscle

There are two other types of muscles in the body (Figure 5-12). **Involuntary (smooth) muscles** line the tubular structures of the body such as the arteries and the walls of the intestines. Smooth muscles are not under the voluntary control of the brain. Smooth muscles respond to stimuli such as stretching, heat, and cold. These muscles work to control flow through the structures in which they are found. For example, involuntary muscles propel food through the digestive tract.

The other type of muscle is **cardiac muscle,** which is found only in the heart. Cardiac muscle is a specialized type of involuntary muscle that cannot be controlled by conscious thought. It is a unique muscle because it has the ability to contract on its own without nerve input. It is cardiac muscle that is damaged in a heart attack or myocardial infarction. (*Myocardial* means "muscle of the heart"; *infarction* means "tissue death from lack of blood flow.") Cardiac muscle can only tolerate brief interruptions of blood flow before permanent damage occurs and the ability of the muscle to contract and pump blood through the heart is impaired.

Respiratory System

Although the musculoskeletal system forms the scaffolding in and upon which the human body is built, it is the respiratory system that supplies the crucial element every cell in the body needs for survival—oxygen (Figure 5-13).

Respiratory Anatomy

The respiratory system allows oxygen-containing air to pass from the environment to the structures of the lungs called **alveoli,** where gases are passed to and from the blood. The passageway through which the air flows is commonly referred to as the **airway.** Maintaining an open airway is essential to life and is the highest priority in patient care.

Air enters the body through the mouth and nose (Figure 5-13). Here the air is warmed and large particles such as soot are filtered out. Air then passes to the back of the nasal and oral cavities called the **pharynx.** Air that enters via the nose passes through the **nasopharynx,** and air

that enters through the mouth passes through the **oropharynx.** The air then passes into the **hypopharynx,** the area directly above the openings of the trachea and the esophagus, or the tube to the stomach.

In the inferior portion of the pharynx is a leaf-like structure called the **epiglottis.** The epiglottis sits atop the entrance to the **larynx** (voice box) and **trachea** (windpipe). The epiglottis covers this entrance during swallowing to prevent food and liquids from passing into the larynx and lower airway. The larynx contains several structures including the vocal cords, the shield-like thyroid cartilage, and the firm **cricoid cartilage,** which encircles the trachea and forms the lowest portion of the larynx.

Air travels from the larynx through the trachea into the chest, where the trachea splits (bifurcates) into the two mainstem **bronchi.** The two mainstem bronchi then carry the air into the **lungs.** The bronchi then subdivide into smaller and smaller air passages until they end in the tiny grape-like clusters of alveoli. It is in the alveoli where gas exchange takes place.

Respiratory Physiology

Breathing, or **respiration,** is not a simple process. Oxygen must be delivered to the alveoli where it can enter the bloodstream and be exchanged for carbon dioxide. Respiration requires not only an open airway but also the interaction of several muscle groups. The major muscle of respiration is the **diaphragm.** The diaphragm is relatively thin, but powerful. It stretches across the body and separates the chest cavity from the organs of the abdominal cavity. Along the ribs is another group of muscles used in breathing called the intercostal muscles.

The process of breathing in is called **inhalation.** Inhalation is an active process. It results from contraction of the diaphragm and the intercostal muscles. As these muscles contract, the diaphragm moves inferiorly and the ribs move upward and outward. These movements increase the size of the thoracic cavity, which causes air to enter the lungs (Figure 5-15A).

The process of breathing out is called **exhalation.** Exhalation is a passive process. It occurs as

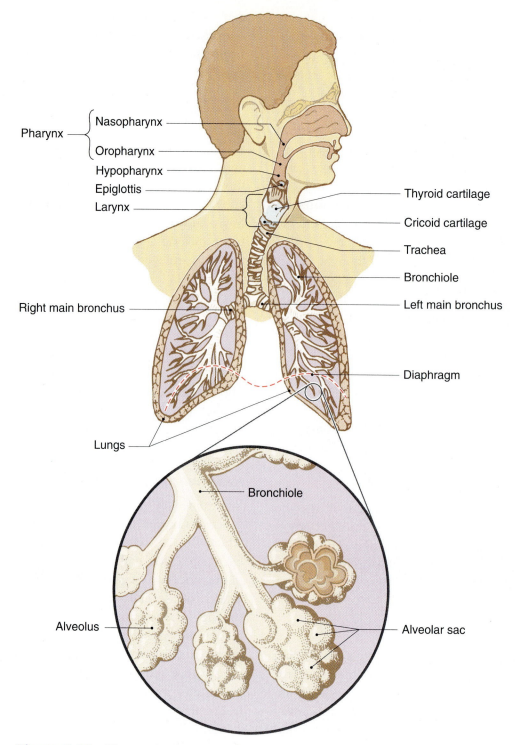

Figure 5-13 The respiratory system.

the diaphragm and intercostal muscles relax. When they do, the diaphragm moves superiorly and the ribs move downward and inward. These movements decrease the size of the thoracic cavity, which causes air to exit the lungs (Figure 5-15B).

After air enters the lungs it travels to the alveoli. Thin-walled capillaries surround the alveolar sacs. It is at this alveolar/capillary level that gas exchange occurs. Air that has just been inhaled is rich in oxygen. Meanwhile, the venous blood

PEDIATRIC NOTE

The anatomy of the respiratory system of infants and children differs in several ways from that of the adult (Figure 5-14).

◆ The mouths and noses of infants and children are smaller and more easily obstructed than those of adults. In infants and children, the tongue takes up more space in the mouth proportionately than it does in adults.

◆ Newborns and infants are *obligate nose breathers.* This means they will not know to open their mouths to breathe when the nose becomes obstructed.

◆ The trachea (windpipe) and the cricoid cartilage are softer and more flexible in infants and children. (This is why you must open their airways gently. Infants can be placed in a neutral neck position and children only require slight extension of the neck. Do not overextend the neck; doing so may collapse the trachea.)

◆ Because children's heads are larger proportionally than those of adults, they tend to shift position easily. When you have properly positioned an infant's or child's head, be sure to recheck the positioning frequently.

◆ The trachea is more narrow in infants and children and is thus more easily obstructed by swelling.

◆ The chest wall is softer in infants and children who therefore tend to depend more on the diaphragm for breathing.

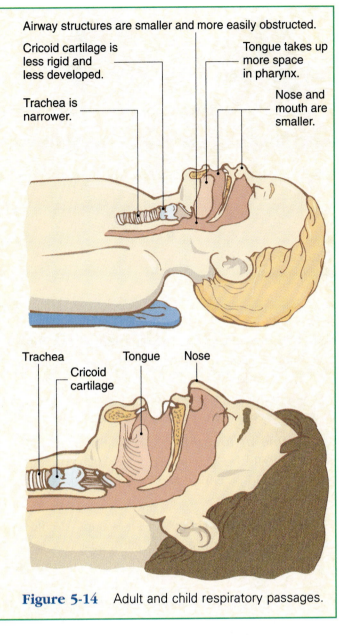

Figure 5-14 Adult and child respiratory passages.

returning to the capillaries is oxygen depleted and high in carbon dioxide, which has been given off as a waste product by the body's cells. At the alveolar/capillary level, the oxygen from the newly inhaled air is exchanged for carbon dioxide from the circulatory system (Figure 5-16).

Normal respiratory system anatomy and physiology provide adequate breathing. This means that a sufficient amount of oxygen is being delivered to the alveoli and that carbon dioxide is being removed from the body. Inadequate breathing occurs when, because of disease or injury, the respiratory system can no longer provide enough oxygen and/or cannot remove carbon dioxide

effectively. During the assessment of a patient's breathing, the EMT should look for the following to determine if breathing is adequate:

◆ **Rate** of breathing

◆ **Rhythm** of breathing

◆ **Quality** of breathing as determined by
  —Breath sounds
  —Chest expansion
  —Effort of breathing

◆ **Depth** of breathing

Rate of breathing Adequate breathing rates vary with age. For a normal adult, the rate is

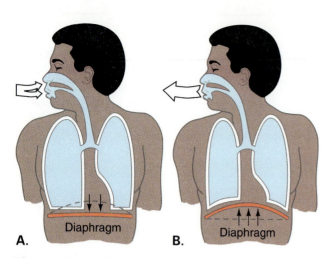

A. **B.**

Figure 5-15 The breathing process. **A.** Inhalation. **B.** Exhalation.

between 12 and 20 breaths per minute. For a normal child, the rate is between 15 and 30 breaths per minute. For a normal infant, the rate is between 25 and 50 breaths per minute. A respiratory rate faster or slower than these norms should be considered a sign of inadequate breathing.

Rhythm of breathing A patient's breathing pattern should be regular. An irregular breathing pattern should be considered a sign of inadequate breathing.

Quality of breathing Breath sounds should be heard equally on both the right and left sides of the chest. Diminished or unequal breath sounds are a sign of inadequate breathing. The chest wall should expand equally and fully with each breath. Diminished or unequal chest rise with inhalation should be considered a sign of inadequate breathing. Breathing should occur with little or no effort. If the patient is struggling to breathe and is using the accessory muscles of the chest, neck, or shoulders not usually used in breathing, the patient should be considered to be exhibiting signs of inadequate breathing.

Depth of breathing The depth of breathing refers to the volume of air entering and exiting the lungs (tidal volume). The volume of air must be large enough to deliver oxygen to the level of the alveoli and to carry carbon dioxide out of the patient's mouth and nose. The patient should breathe in full, deep breaths. Shallow breathing should be considered a sign of inadequate breathing.

The ability to recognize the signs and symptoms of inadequate breathing is one of the most important assessment skills that you can learn. It is a life-saving skill. The sooner you recognize inadequate breathing, the sooner you can begin treatment, which might include administering high flow oxygen to a patient (Chapter 6, "Airway Management") or assisting the patient in taking prescribed breathing medication (Chapter 12, "Res-

Figure 5-16 Alveolar/capillary gas exchange.

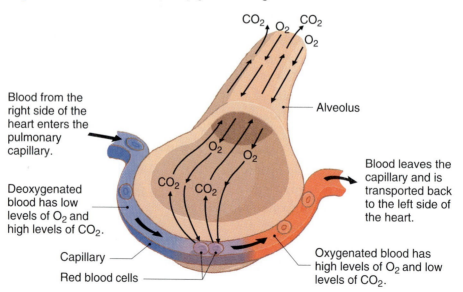

piratory Emergencies"). The signs and symptoms of inadequate breathing include the following:

- Rate of breathing faster or slower than normal range

- Irregular rhythm of breathing

- Poor quality of breathing

  —Breath sounds that are unequal, absent, or diminished

  —Chest expansion with inhalation that is unequal or inadequate

  —Increased effort of breathing with use of accessory muscles, especially in infants and children

- Shallow breathing resulting in an inadequate tidal volume

- Skin changes including:

  —Bluish discoloration (cyanosis)

  —Pale color

  —Cool and moist skin (sometimes called "clammy" skin)

- Agonal respirations, the gasping, irregular breaths often seen just before cardiac arrest.

- Retractions of the skin above the clavicles, between the ribs, and below the rib cage.

Circulatory System

Simply stated, the **circulatory** or **cardiovascular, system** has three major components—the pump (the heart), the pipes (the blood vessels), and the fluid in the system (blood). The system functions to deliver blood to all parts of the body (Figure 5-17). The blood carries oxygen from the lungs and other nutrients from the digestive system to the cells of the body's organs and carries away waste products from the cells.

The Heart

The heart is the center of the circulatory system (Figure 5-18). The heart is a muscular organ about the size of a fist. It sits just to the left of the sternum in the lower chest. The heart has four chambers, the two upper **atria** (which receive blood) and the two lower **ventricles** (which pump blood out of the heart).

PEDIATRIC NOTE

Infants and children share many of the same signs and symptoms of inadequate breathing found in adults, such as retractions. However, there are several special features of inadequate breathing in children:

- **Slow pulse** An abnormally slow pulse in a child should always be considered a sign of inadequate oxygen delivery to the alveoli (hypoxia).

- **Nasal flaring** The pattern of the nostrils collapsing followed by the nostrils flaring open during respirations is an important sign of inadequate breathing in infants and children.

- **"Seesaw" breathing** Normally, the abdomen and the chest expand outward together during inhalation and move inward together during exhalation. In "seesaw" breathing, the abdomen and chest move in opposite directions during breathing. This breathing pattern is very inefficient and rapidly exhausts the infant or child.

- **Retractions** These can be observed in the skin and tissues between and below the ribs and above the clavicles and sternal notch. They are more common in children than in adults.

- **Loud or noisy breathing** This can include high-pitched sounds or grunting.

Functionally, the heart is divided into a right-side pump and a left-side pump. The right atrium and ventricle form a low-pressure pump. This pump takes oxygen-depleted blood in from the major veins and pumps it to the lungs to be reoxygenated. The left atrium receives the blood back from the lungs, and the left ventricle pumps it out of the heart under high pressure into the body's arteries.

The chambers of the heart are separated by valves. These valves allow the forward flow of blood through the heart and prevent backflow.

The pumping action of the heart's muscle is controlled by a specialized **cardiac conduction system** (Figure 5-19). This conduction system generates and carries the electrical impulses that coordinate the rhythmic pumping of the atria and

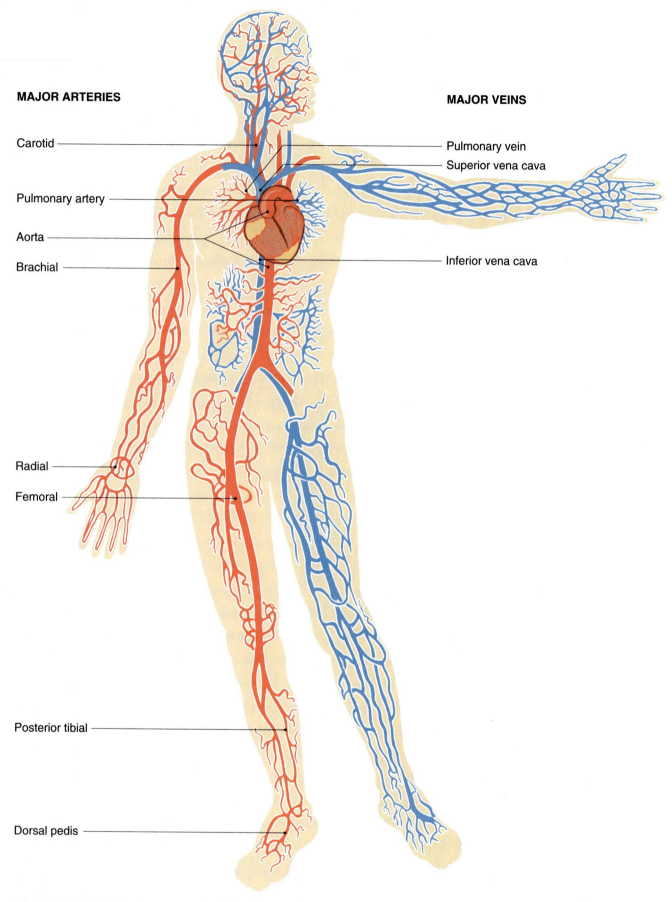

MAJOR ARTERIES

Carotid

Pulmonary artery

Aorta

Brachial

Radial

Femoral

Posterior tibial

Dorsal pedis

MAJOR VEINS

Pulmonary vein

Superior vena cava

Inferior vena cava

Figure 5-17   The circulatory system.

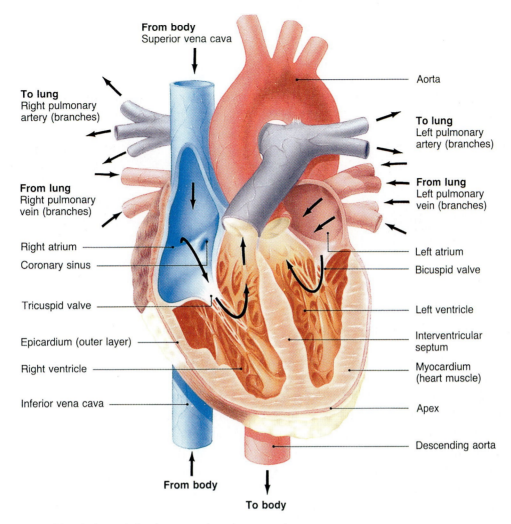

Figure 5-18 Circulation of the heart and major vessels.

ventricles. Specialized groups of cells within the heart act as "pacemakers," setting the rate at which the heart beats. In a normal heart, the sinoatrial (SA) node located in the right atrium sets the normal adult heart rate of 60 to 100 beats per minute. The electrical impulses generated by the SA node are carried down the heart, causing the muscles of the atria and then the ventricles to contract. The heart is made up of specialized cardiac muscle, which contracts when stimulated by the electrical impulses of the cardiac conduction system. In addition, cardiac muscle can by itself generate and carry electrical impulses that cause other surrounding cardiac muscle cells to contract.

The cardiac conduction system and the pumping function of the heart are closely related. If the cardiac conduction system does not function properly, the heart's pumping action may be greatly reduced. It may even stop entirely, resulting in **cardiac arrest.** Many of the cardiac emergencies EMTs encounter are related to diseases that cause abnormal functioning of the cardiac conduction system. When the normal electrical rhythm of the heart is disrupted, the patient is said to have a **dysrythmia** (*dys* meaning "abnormal"). The diagnosis of dysrythmias is usually made in the field by advanced EMTs. They use a cardiac monitor, which shows the patient's heart electrical impulses as an **electrocardiogram (EKG).**

As an EMT, however, you will be expected to treat the most common lethal cardiac dysrythmia, which is called **ventricular fibrillation.** In ventricular fibrillation, the heart loses all normal patterns of cardiac conduction. Uncontrolled elec-

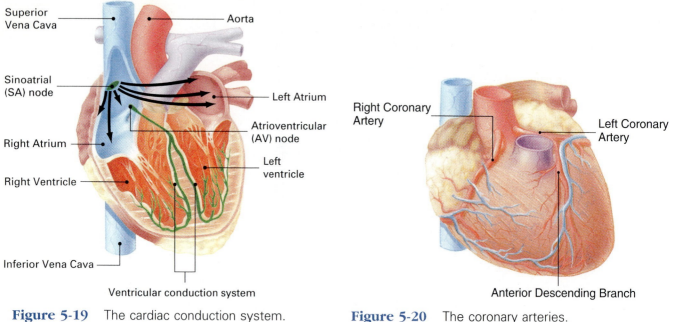

Figure 5-19 The cardiac conduction system.

Figure 5-20 The coronary arteries.

trical impulses then cause the cardiac muscles to quiver or fibrillate. As a result, the heart looses all ability to pump blood to the body. The most effective treatment for ventricular fibrillation is to deliver a sudden, massive electrical shock to the heart in the form of **defibrillation.** In Chapter 13, "Cardiac Emergencies," you will learn how to use an automated external defibrillator to treat ventricular fibrillation.

The Vascular System

Although the heart is truly the center of the circulatory system, it is the body's network of blood vessels that carries blood throughout the body, delivering oxygen and other nutrients and removing the cell's waste products.

Arteries carry blood away from the heart to the organs of the body. With the exception of the **pulmonary artery,** which carries oxygen-depleted blood away from the right ventricle to the lungs, arteries carry oxygen-rich blood. Arteries have thick walls lined with smooth involuntary muscle. Arteries contain blood under pressure from the strong pumping action of the left ventricle. The major arteries of the body include the **aorta,** which is the largest artery in the body and begins at the left ventricle of the heart. All arteries in the body receive their blood from the aorta. The first arterial branches off the aorta are the

coronary arteries, which supply the heart with blood (Figure 5-20). It is the narrowing or blockage of these vessels that cause many cardiac emergencies including heart attack or myocardial infarction. The aorta descends through the chest anterior to the thoracic spine into the abdomen. There, it divides at the level of the navel into the iliac arteries.

There are other major arteries that are important to the EMT because they run close to the body's surface and are used in patient assessment and/or treatment. All these arteries are found bilaterally (on each side of the patient).

The two **carotid arteries** are the major arteries of the neck. They supply blood from the aorta to the head and brain. The pulsation of the carotid artery can be felt on either side of the neck as it travels superiorly into the head.

The **brachial artery** is a major artery of the upper arm. Pulsations of this artery can be felt on the anterior, medial surface of the arm between the elbow and the shoulder. The brachial artery is used when performing a pulse check during infant CPR. It is also the artery used when obtaining a patient's blood pressure with a blood pressure cuff (sphygmomanometer) and stethoscope.

The **radial artery** is the largest artery in the forearm. Pulsations from the radial artery can be felt at the thumb side of the wrist over the distal radius.

Major arteries of the lower extremities include the **femoral artery,** which branches off the iliac artery and supplies blood to the entire lower extremity. The femoral artery is the major artery of the thigh and its pulsations can be felt in the groin in the crease between the lower abdomen and the thigh.

The two major arteries of the foot are the **posterior tibial artery** and the **dorsalis pedis artery.** The pulsations of these arteries are used to assess blood flow to the foot. That blood flow could be compromised by a more proximal lower extremity injury such as a femur fracture that also injured the femoral artery. The pulse of the posterior tibial artery can be felt over the posterior surface of the medial malleolus of the ankle. The pulse of the dorsalis pedis artery can be felt on the dorsal surface of the foot.

As arteries branch out they become progressively smaller. The smallest arteries are called **arterioles.** Arterioles branch down to the smallest blood vessels, which are called **capillaries.**

Capillaries are very thin-walled vessels found throughout the body. It is at the capillary level in the body's organs that the exchange of oxygen and other nutrients for the cells' waste products such as carbon dioxide takes place (Figure 5-21). Capillaries form the connection between the arterial side of the circulatory system and the venous side of the system. Capillaries connect to tiny blood vessels called **venules.** Through venules, oxygen-depleted blood begins the journey back to the heart.

Venules are tiny **veins.** The function of veins is to carry blood back toward the heart. With the exception of the **pulmonary vein,** which returns oxygenated blood back to the left atrium of the heart from the lungs, all veins carry oxygen-depleted blood. Veins carry blood under low pressure and their walls are thin as compared to arteries. Because of the low pressure, veins contain tiny valves, which prevent the backflow of blood. Venules empty into larger veins as blood returns to the heart. Blood eventually flows back

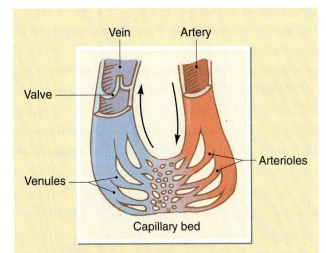

From the heart, oxygen-rich blood is carried out into the body by arteries. The arteries gradually branch into smaller arteries called arterioles. The arterioles gradually branch into tiny vessels called capillaries.

In the capillaries, the blood gives up oxygen and nutrients, which move through the thin walls of the capillaries into the body's cells. At the same time, carbon dioxide and other wastes move in the opposite direction, from the cells and through the capillary walls, to be picked up by the blood.

On its return journey to the heart, the oxygen-poor blood, now carrying carbon dioxide and other wastes, flows from the capillaries into small veins called venules which gradually merge into larger veins.

Figure 5-21   How the arteries, veins, and capillaries work.

to the largest veins of the body, the **inferior** and **superior vena cavae,** which return blood to the right atrium.

Blood

Blood is composed of both solid and liquid material. The major solid component of blood is **red blood cells.** In addition to giving blood its distinctive color, the red blood cells carry oxygen to and carbon dioxide away from the body's organs. Blood also contains white blood cells. **White blood cells** are an important part of the body's immune system, which helps fight off infections. The other solid component of blood is **platelets.** Platelets are essential for the formation of blood clots, which help control both internal and external bleeding. The fluid component of blood is plasma. **Plasma** is the fluid in which blood cells and platelets are suspended. Plasma also contains nutrients, such as sugars, that are essential to cells and organ function.

Circulatory Physiology—Pulse and Blood Pressure

The cardiovascular system is directly responsible for the generation of two important vital signs that are obtained by the EMT during initial patient assessment and ongoing assessment. These vital signs are pulse and blood pressure. The pulse is generated by the strong pumping action of the left ventricle of the heart. When the left ventricle contracts, it sends a wave of blood out through the arteries. It is this wave that can be palpated in a patient's artery as it passes near the skin surface and over a bone (Figure 5-22).

Pulses can be palpated on the extremities (peripherally) at the radial artery on the wrist, the brachial artery at the elbow, at the posterior tibial artery on the medial ankle, and at the dorsalis pedis artery on the dorsal foot. Pulses can also be palpated on the neck and torso (centrally) at the

carotid artery in the neck and the femoral artery in the groin. When you take a patient's pulse, you should record the location of the pulse and its quality and rate. For example, you might report, "The patient has a strong carotid pulse at a rate of 70 per minute."

The **blood pressure** is a measurement of the pressure exerted on the walls of the artery. Blood pressure is usually obtained at the brachial artery at the elbow with a blood pressure cuff (sphygmomanometer) and a stethoscope. The **systolic blood pressure** is the pressure exerted on the artery wall when the left ventricle contracts and sends a pressure wave down the artery. The **diastolic blood pressure** is the pressure the blood exerts against the artery wall when the left ventricle is at rest. In Chapter 7, you will learn how to determine both systolic and diastolic blood pressures during patient assessment.

Circulatory Physiology—Perfusion and Hypoperfusion

The circulatory system delivers oxygen and other nutrients to all the cells of the body's organs and removes waste products from the cells of those same organs. The normal circulation of blood to the body's organs is called **perfusion.** In order for the circulatory system to work properly, all three of its components (the heart, the blood vessels, and the blood) must function properly.

If any part of the system fails—for example, because of severe bleeding from a damaged blood vessel—then the organs will become inadequately perfused. Inadequate perfusion of the body's organs is called **hypoperfusion** (*hypo* meaning "under"). When the body's organs are hypoperfused, they do not receive adequate oxygen and their waste products are not efficiently removed. Lack of perfusion will result in the body's organs ceasing to work properly. Hypoperfusion of the body's organs will cause the patient to show the signs and symptoms of what is commonly known as **shock.** These signs and symptoms usually reflect the problems specific organs have as a result of hypoperfusion (Table 5-1). (Hypoperfusion and shock are discussed in more detail in Chapter 19, "Bleeding and Shock.")

Figure 5-22   Locations of pulses.

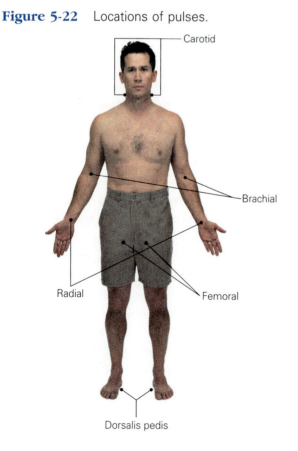

Table 5-1

The Body's Responses to Significant Blood Loss

Organ	Response to Blood Loss	Resulting Signs and Symptoms
Brain	Decrease of perfusion in higher centers of thinking in order to maintain cardiac and respiratory control centers	Altered mental status —Confusion —Restlessness —Anxiety
Cardiovascular system	Heart pumps faster; blood vessels constrict	Increased pulse rate Rapid, weak pulse Low or falling blood pressure Lowered capillary refill time
Gastrointestinal organs	Decrease of perfusion in the digestive tract	Nausea and vomiting
Kidneys	Reduction in function to conserve the body's salt and water	Decreased urine production Increased thirst
Skin	Marked loss of perfusion	Cool, clammy, pale skin Cyanosis
Extremities	Marked loss of perfusion	Weak or absent peripheral pulses Decreased blood pressure

The basic signs and symptoms of shock (hypoperfusion) include the following:

◆ Altered mental status including restlessness or anxiety

◆ Evidence of decreased peripheral perfusion

—Weak, thready, or absent pulse

—Pale, cool, clammy skin

—Delayed capillary refill time in infants and children

◆ Alteration of normal vital signs

—Increased pulse rate (an early sign)

—Increased breathing rate

—Shallow, labored, or irregular breathing

—Decreased blood pressure (a late sign)

◆ Other signs and symptoms

—Dilated pupils

—Marked thirst

—Nausea and vomiting

—Low body temperature

—Pallor (pale or gray skin)

—Cyanosis (bluish discoloration) of lips or conjunctiva of eyes

Nervous System

The function of the nervous system is to control all voluntary and involuntary activity of the body. The nervous system is also responsible for our ability to sense and react to our environment. The nervous system is structurally divided into the central nervous system and the peripheral nervous system (Figure 5-23).

The **central nervous system** is made up of the brain and the spinal cord. The brain is located within the cranium. The brain is responsible for both higher functions, such as thought and memory, as well as the more basic functions, such as breathing. The spinal cord extends from the base of the brain and descends down the back, protected by the vertebrae of the spinal column. The spinal cord carries messages from the brain to the body. Such messages might include directions for the peripheral nervous system to cause movement of voluntary muscles. The spinal cord also carries messages back to the brain from the body. Such messages include information gathered by the peripheral nervous system about the body's environment.

The **peripheral nervous system** includes all the nerve fibers outside of the brain and spinal cord. There are two basic types of peripheral nerves, motor nerves and sensory nerves. Motor nerves carry information *from* the brain and the spinal cord to the body to direct its activity. Sensory nerves carry information from the body *back* to the spinal cord and brain.

The **autonomic nervous system** is a third division of the nervous system that includes certain parts of both the central and peripheral nervous systems. The autonomic nervous system is responsible for specialized body responses such as increasing the heart rate when the body's normal physiology is stressed, as in shock (hypoperfusion). The autonomic nervous system causes changes in the body both directly and by acting upon the endocrine system.

Endocrine System

The **endocrine system** causes changes within the body by producing chemicals called **hormones.** The organs of the endocrine system include the hypothalamus in the brain, the pituitary gland, the thyroid and parathyroid glands, the adrenal glands, and the parts of the pancreas that produce insulin (Figure 5-24). Certain cells within the female ovaries and the male testes are also part of this system. The effects that hormones have on the body are widespread and varied. They include body growth, reproductive changes, and the regulation of sugar (glucose) by insulin.

Gastrointestinal System

The **gastrointestinal (GI) system** is responsible for the digestion of food (Figure 5-25). Food enters the mouth where the first step in digestion is chewing by the teeth. Food travels down the esophagus, into the stomach, and through the small and large intestines. As food is digested, nutrients are taken up into the extensive blood vessels surrounding the GI system. Food left undigested is eventually passed out the rectum as feces. The liver, gallbladder, and parts of the pan-

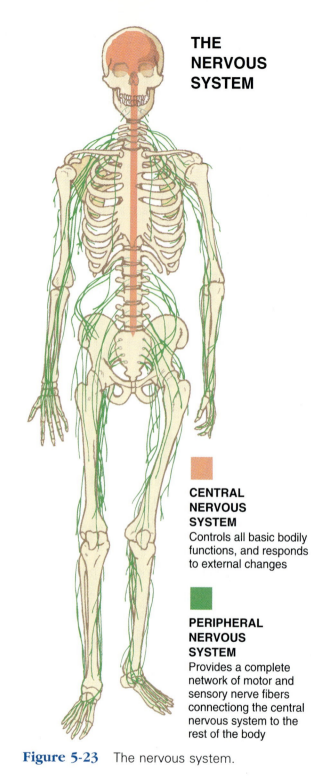

THE NERVOUS SYSTEM

CENTRAL NERVOUS SYSTEM
Controls all basic bodily functions, and responds to external changes

PERIPHERAL NERVOUS SYSTEM
Provides a complete network of motor and sensory nerve fibers connectiong the central nervous system to the rest of the body

Figure 5-23   The nervous system.

creas all contribute chemicals that assist in the digestion of food.

Genitourinary System

The **genitourinary system** includes the reproductive organs and those organs responsible for

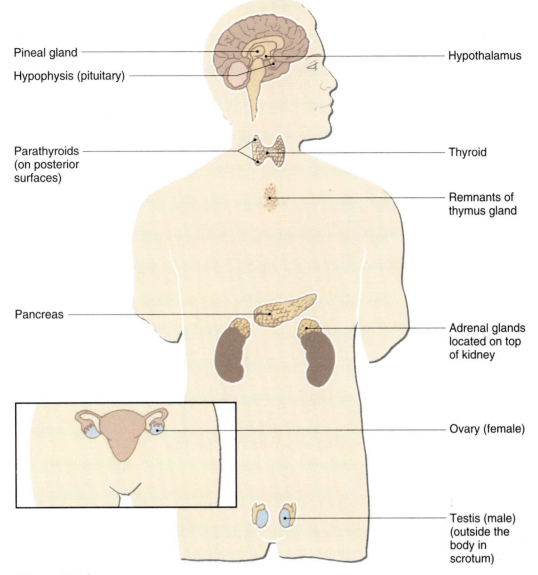

Pineal gland

Hypophysis (pituitary)

Parathyroids (on posterior surfaces)

Pancreas

Hypothalamus

Thyroid

Remnants of thymus gland

Adrenal glands located on top of kidney

Ovary (female)

Testis (male) (outside the body in scrotum)

Figure 5-24 The endocrine system.

the production and excretion of urine. These organs are grouped together because they are in close proximity in the abdomen and pelvis and share common functions. The kidneys filter the blood and produce urine. Urine then travels down the ureters, is stored in the bladder, and is finally passed out of the body through the urethra. The female reproductive organs are located internally, whereas the male reproductive organs are external.

The Skin

The skin is also considered an organ system of the body (Figure 5-26). The skin is the interface between the body and the environment and performs several vital functions. It protects the body from the environment and from bacteria and other organisms. The skin also contains specialized sensory organs that detect heat, cold, pressure, and pain and transmit this information back to the spinal cord and brain. In addition to sensing and relaying information about environmental temperature, the skin is responsible for much of the body's temperature regulation. For example, sweat produced by the sweat glands in the skin helps to cool the body in warm conditions. (See Chapter 16, "Environmental Emergencies," for a more in-depth discussion.) All these varied func-

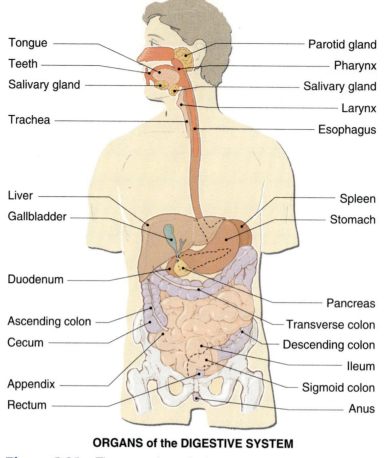

Tongue — Parotid gland
Teeth — Pharynx
Salivary gland — Salivary gland
— Larynx
Trachea — Esophagus

Liver — Spleen
Gallbladder — Stomach

Duodenum

Pancreas
Ascending colon — Transverse colon
Cecum — Descending colon
— Ileum
Appendix — Sigmoid colon
Rectum — Anus

ORGANS of the DIGESTIVE SYSTEM

Figure 5-25   The gastrointestinal system.

tions are so essential, that if too great an area of skin is destroyed, as with major burn injuries, the patient may die.

The skin is made up of three basic layers. The **epidermis** is the outer layer. It contains the pigments that give the skin its color. Beneath the epidermis is the **dermis.** It contains blood vessels, nerves, sweat glands, hair follicles, and oil glands that enable the skin to carry out many of its functions. Beneath the dermis is the **subcutaneous layer.** This is largely made up of fatty tissue that provides insulation and shock absorption.

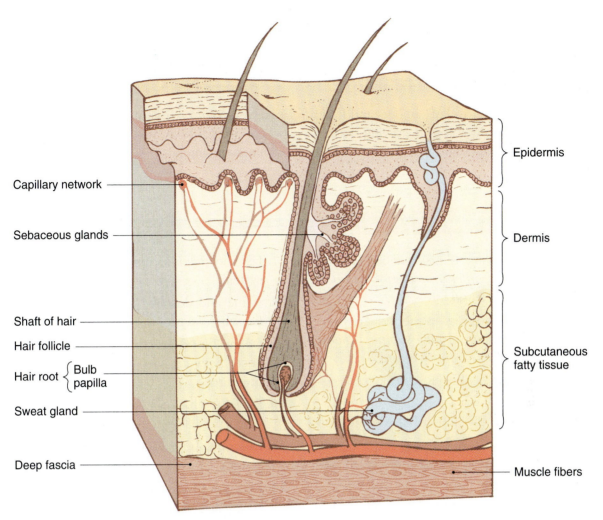

Capillary network

Sebaceous glands

Shaft of hair

Hair follicle

Hair root { Bulb
              papilla

Sweat gland

Deep fascia

Epidermis

Dermis

Subcutaneous
fatty tissue

Muscle fibers

Figure 5-26 The layers of the skin.

Chapter Review

SUMMARY

It is essential that you as an EMT understand basic human anatomy and physiology. Knowing normal anatomy and physiology will allow you to more easily recognize injuries and detect situations where normal body function is disrupted because of illness or injury.

REVIEWING KEY CONCEPTS

1. Define the following terms: *medial, lateral, anterior, posterior, inferior, superior, plantar, palmar, proximal, distal.*

2. Describe the following positions: *normal anatomical position, prone, supine, lateral recumbent, Fowler's, Trendelenburg.*

3. List the functions of the musculoskeletal system.

4. Describe the five divisions of the spine and their locations.

5. Describe the three types of muscle in the human body.

6. Describe the body structures through which air passes as it is inhaled.

7. List the major components of the circulatory system.

8. Name and describe the locations of the arteries where a patient's pulse can be palpated.

9. Define blood pressure and explain the difference between systolic and diastolic blood pressure.

10. Explain what perfusion is and what occurs when perfusion is not adequate.

11. Describe the divisions of the body's nervous system.

12. Describe the functions of the skin and list the layers that make it up.

RESOURCES TO LEARN MORE

Agur, A.M. *Grant's Atlas of Anatomy, 9th Edition*. Baltimore: Williams & Wilkins, 1991.

Fremgen, Bonnie F. *Medical Terminology: An Anatomy and Physiology Systems Approach*. Upper Saddle River, NJ: Brady/Prentice Hall, 1997.

MAJOR BODY SYSTEMS

Musculoskeletal
- Bones
- Ligaments
- Muscles
- Tendons

Respiratory
- Nose and mouth
- Epiglottis
- Bronchi
- Pharynx
- Larynx and trachea
- Lungs

Circulatory
- Heart
- Blood vessels
- Blood

Nervous
- Brain
- Spinal cord
- Nerves

Endocrine
- Glands
- Horomones

Gastrointestinal
- Mouth
- Stomach
- Liver
- Intestines
- Esophagus
- Pancreas
- Gallbladder

Genitourinary
- Kidneys
- Ureters
- Bladder
- Urethra
- Male and female reproductive organs

Skin
- Epidermis
- Dermis
- Subcutaneous layer

Airway Management

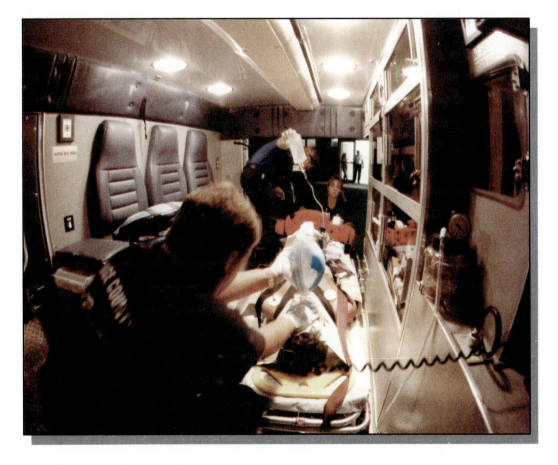

*T*he most important life-saving skills you will learn as an EMT are how to open and maintain a patient's airway, ensure effective ventilation, and provide oxygen to the patient.

The airway is the passageway that allows air to move freely in and out of the lungs. When the airway is blocked, essential oxygen cannot enter the lungs and carbon dioxide, the major waste product of respiration, cannot be exhaled. The resulting lack of oxygen and build-up of carbon dioxide will both pose immediate threats to the patient's life. Similarly, if a patient is not breathing adequately for a

▶

variety of reasons, a lack of oxygen and a build-up of carbon dioxide will also result.

For these reasons, airway management—opening and maintaining the airway and ensuring that the patient receives adequate oxygen—is vital for the EMT to master. Airway skills are taught early in the course because they are skills that EMTs may need during the assessment and emergency medical care of every patient.

OBJECTIVES

At the completion of this chapter, the EMT-Basic student should be able to meet the following objectives:

Knowledge and Understanding

1. Name and label the major structures of the respiratory system on a diagram. (pp. 99–100)
2. List the signs of adequate breathing. (p. 99)
3. List the signs of inadequate breathing. (pp. 99, 101)
4. Describe the steps in performing the head-tilt, chin-lift. (pp. 102–103)
5. Relate mechanism of injury to opening the airway. (pp. 104–105)
6. Describe the steps in performing the jaw thrust. (p. 104)
7. State the importance of having a suction unit ready for immediate use when providing emergency care. (pp. 105, 108)
8. Describe the techniques of suctioning. (pp. 120–123)
9. Describe how to artificially ventilate a patient with a pocket mask. (pp. 106–107)
10. Describe the steps in performing the skill of artificially ventilating a patient with a bag-valve mask while using the jaw thrust. (p. 109)
11. List the parts of a bag-valve-mask system. (pp. 107–108)
12. Describe the steps in performing the skill of artificial ventilation to a patient with a bag-valve mask with one and two rescuers. (pp. 108–110)
13. Describe the signs of adequate artificial ventilation using the bag-valve mask. (pp. 109–110)
14. Describe the signs of inadequate artificial ventilation using the bag-valve mask. (pp. 109–110)
15. Describe the steps in artificially ventilating a patient with a flow-restricted, oxygen-powered ventilation device. (p. 112)
16. List the steps in performing mouth-to-mouth and mouth-to-stoma artificial ventilation. (pp. 110–111)

17. Describe how to measure and insert an oropharyngeal (oral) airway. (pp. 114–116)
18. Describe how to measure and insert a nasopharyngeal (nasal) airway. (pp. 117–118)
19. Define the components of an oxygen delivery system. (pp. 127–131, 134–135)
20. Identify a nonrebreather face mask and state the oxygen flow requirements needed for its use. (pp. 131, 134)
21. Describe the indications for using a nasal cannula versus a nonrebreather face mask. (pp. 134, 135)
22. Identify a nasal cannula and state the flow requirements needed for its use. (pp. 134, 135)
23. Explain the rationale for basic life support artificial ventilation and airway protective skills taking priority over most other basic life support skills. (pp. 95, 98)
24. Explain the rationale for providing adequate oxygenation through high inspired oxygen concentrations to patients who, in the past, may have received low concentrations. (p. 126)

Skills

1. Demonstrate the steps in performing the head-tilt, chin-lift.
2. Demonstrate the steps in performing the jaw thrust.
3. Demonstrate the techniques of suctioning.
4. Demonstrate the steps in providing mouth-to-mouth artificial ventilation with body substance isolation (barrier shields).
5. Demonstrate how to use a pocket mask to artificially ventilate a patient.
6. Demonstrate the assembly of a bag-valve-mask unit.

7. Demonstrate the steps in performing the artificial ventilation of a patient with a bag-valve mask for one and two rescuers.

8. Demonstrate the steps of artificially ventilating a patient with a bag-valve mask while using the jaw thrust.

9. Demonstrate artificial ventilation of a patient with a flow-restricted, oxygen-powered ventilation device.

10. Demonstrate how to artificially ventilate a patient with a stoma.

11. Demonstrate how to insert an oropharyngeal (oral) airway.

12. Demonstrate how to insert a nasopharyngeal (nasal) airway.

13. Demonstrate the correct operation of oxygen tanks and regulators.

14. Demonstrate the use of a nonrebreather face mask and state the oxygen flow requirements needed for its use.

15. Demonstrate the use of a nasal cannula and state the flow requirements for its use.

16. Demonstrate how to artificially ventilate infants and children.

17. Demonstrate oxygen administration for infants and children.

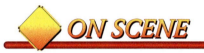

ON SCENE

DISPATCH: *AMBULANCE 1 AND ENGINE 6, RESPOND FOR A PRIORITY 1 CALL. PATIENT IS A 64-YEAR-OLD FEMALE IN RESPIRATORY DISTRESS. THE ADDRESS IS 405 CRANBERRY LANE. TIME OUT IS 1334.*

You are assigned as an EMT to Ambulance 1. As you arrive on the scene, you discover that the address is in a row of townhouses with direct access onto a busy highway. In your scene size-up, you determine that your ambulance and Engine 6 may be creating a hazard by partially blocking one lane of traffic. Before you get out of the ambulance, you leave all your warning beacons on and radio the dispatcher to request police for traffic control.

A man who gives his name as Ralph Hayes meets you at the townhouse door. He states that his wife is in the kitchen and that she is very short of breath. As Mr. Hayes leads you to the kitchen, you note an oxygen cylinder on the living room floor. Tubing from the cylinder leads to the kitchen. In the kitchen, you find a middle-aged woman who appears to be in severe distress. She is sitting in a chair at the kitchen table, leaning forward with her hands on her knees. Her face has a grayish-blue color. You note that the woman has an oxygen cannula in her nose.

You approach the woman and introduce yourself, explaining that you're an emergency medical technician with the fire department and are there to help her. She replies, "I'm . . . Anna . . . Hayes. Please . . . help . . . me."

You note that Mrs. Hayes is so short of breath she can only speak a single word at a time before having to catch her breath. Your partner removes the patient's nasal cannula and provides her with high concentration oxygen by a nonrebreather mask. Meanwhile, you begin your initial assessment of Mrs. Hayes. Your general impression, based on the patient's color and her obvious respiratory distress, is that of a critically ill patient with a high priority for transport. You immediately radio your dispatcher to request that a paramedic unit either respond to the scene or meet you en route to the hospital.

As you continue to assess Mrs. Hayes, she vomits and becomes unresponsive. You and the Engine 6 crew carefully move her to the floor. You then begin to suction her airway with a large-bore, rigid-tip suction device. When Mrs. Hayes' airway has been cleared, you return to your assessment. The patient's mental status is unresponsive, her airway is now clear and being kept open by your partner with a head-tilt, chin-lift maneuver. The patient's breathing is slow and very irregular, and you assess it to be inadequate.

You immediately set up a bag-valve-mask device attached to high concentration oxygen in order to ventilate the patient. You insert a naso-pharyngeal airway and, with your partner holding a two-handed mask seal, you begin to ventilate the patient using the bag-valve-mask device. As you deliver the ventilations, you note that the color of Mrs. Hayes' face changes from grayish-blue to pink. You note that her pulse is rapid and strong. With the aid of the Engine 6 crew, you place Mrs. Hayes on a Reeves stretcher and move her to the ambulance while you continue to pro-

vide ventilations You note that her chest is expanding equally and fully with each ventilation.

As you are loading Mrs. Hayes into your rig, the mutual-aid paramedic unit arrives on scene. Two paramedics from it hop into the back of your ambulance. They begin advanced life support care while you continue to maintain the air-way and ventilate the patient. En route to the hospital, the paramedics perform an endotracheal intubation and establish an IV line. You now ventilate Mrs. Hayes through the endotracheal tube that the paramedics have placed in her air-way. By the time the ambulance arrives at the emergency department, Mrs. Hayes is more alert, opening her eyes when you ask her to do so.

During your EMT-Basic course, you will learn the importance of the ABCs—airway, breathing, and circulation. It is no coincidence that the *A* for Airway in the ABCs is the first priority in treating every patient you will ever take care of as an EMT.

THE IMPORTANCE OF AIRWAY MANAGEMENT

Of all the skills you will learn in your EMT-Basic course and subsequently use on patients in the field, airway management is the most important. Simply stated, *patients without an adequate airway die.* No matter how good the care you may render to a critically ill or injured patient, if you cannot adequately clear and maintain the patient's airway, everything else you've done will be wasted because the patient will not be able to survive.

The cells of the human body must have oxygen to function properly and to survive. The reason the ABCs are so important is that they are the means by which oxygen is brought into the body and carried to the cells. If the **airway**—the passageways that lead from the mouth and nose to the lungs—is not open, air cannot get into the body. If the patient is unable to breathe, air does

not get into the body even if the airway is open. If the heart is not pumping blood through the lungs to pick up oxygen and circulate it around the body, an open airway and the ability to breathe are of no use. (In fact, breathing and the heartbeat are so dependent on each other that if breathing stops first, the heart will stop very soon, or if the heart stops pumping first, breathing will stop almost at once.)

EMT training puts a great deal of emphasis on the airway because it is so easy and so common for a patient's airway to become blocked. It's also very easy for an EMT to forget to monitor the patient's airway in the midst of an emergency when so many other details demand attention.

The EMT's primary responsibilities (although not the only ones) are finding and correcting immediately life-threatening problems—airway, breathing, and circulation problems—and getting the patient to the hospital. As a prerequisite to your EMT-Basic course, you studied basic life support. At that time, you should have learned how to treat airway obstructions, perform rescue breathing, and perform cardiopulmonary resuscitation (CPR). In this chapter, you will learn additional EMT-level skills that relate to the airway, artificial ventilation, and oxygen therapy. (A review of BLS skills will be found in Appendix B.)

RESPIRATION

Another word for breathing is **respiration.** You learned about the respiratory system in Chapter 5. In preparation for this chapter, you should review the following structures of the respiratory system and be able to label them on a blank diagram of the respiratory system (Figure 6-1).

◆ Nose

◆ Mouth

◆ Oropharynx

◆ Nasopharynx

◆ Epiglottis

◆ Trachea

◆ Cricoid cartilage

◆ Larynx (voice box)

◆ Bronchi (right and left mainstem)

◆ Lungs

◆ Alveoli

◆ Diaphragm

Also review in Chapter 5 how oxygen and carbon dioxide are exchanged through the alveoli and the capillaries in the lungs and at the level of the body's cells.

Adequate and Inadequate Breathing

The function of the respiratory system is to enable the body to obtain (through inhalation) oxygen, which is then used by all the cells and organs in the body, and to dispose of (exhale) carbon dioxide, the major waste product of respiration. If either of these vital functions is disrupted, then the patient is likely to develop the sensation of shortness of breath and be at risk of respiratory failure.

Respiratory failure is the reduction of breathing to the point where oxygen intake is not sufficient to support life. When breathing stops completely, the patient is in **respiratory arrest.** Both respiratory failure and respiratory arrest can develop for many reasons including heart attack,

stroke, airway obstruction, drowning, electrocution, drug overdose, poisoning, head injury, severe chest injury, and suffocation.

Assessment of Respiratory Failure or Respiratory Arrest

As an EMT, you must be able to determine whether or not a patient is breathing adequately so that you can provide appropriate airway management. To determine the signs of *adequate breathing*, you should:

◆ **Look** for full and equal expansion of both sides of the chest with inhalation. In addition, observe the skin color: it should have a pink hue. There should be no blue or gray coloration. Note that the rate of breathing is normal, the rhythm is regular, and the depth of breathing is normal for a patient at rest (Table 6-1).

◆ **Listen** for air entering and leaving the nose, mouth, and chest. The breath sounds should be present and equal on both sides of the chest. The sounds from the mouth and nose should be typically free of gurgling, gasping, crowing, and wheezing.

◆ **Feel** for air moving out of the nose or mouth.

The following are signs of *inadequate breathing* (Figure 6-2).

◆ Chest movements are absent, minimal, or uneven.

◆ Movements associated with breathing are limited to the abdomen (abdominal breathing).

◆ No air can be felt or heard at the nose or mouth, or the amount of air exchanged is evaluated to be below normal.

◆ Breath sounds are diminished or absent.

◆ Noises such as high-pitched wheezing, snoring, gurgling, or gasping are heard during breathing.

◆ The rate of breathing is too rapid or slow—above or below normal rates.

◆ Breathing is very shallow, very deep, or appears labored.

◆ The patient's skin, lips, tongue, ear lobes, or nail beds are blue or gray. This is called **cyanosis.** The patient is said to be cyanotic.

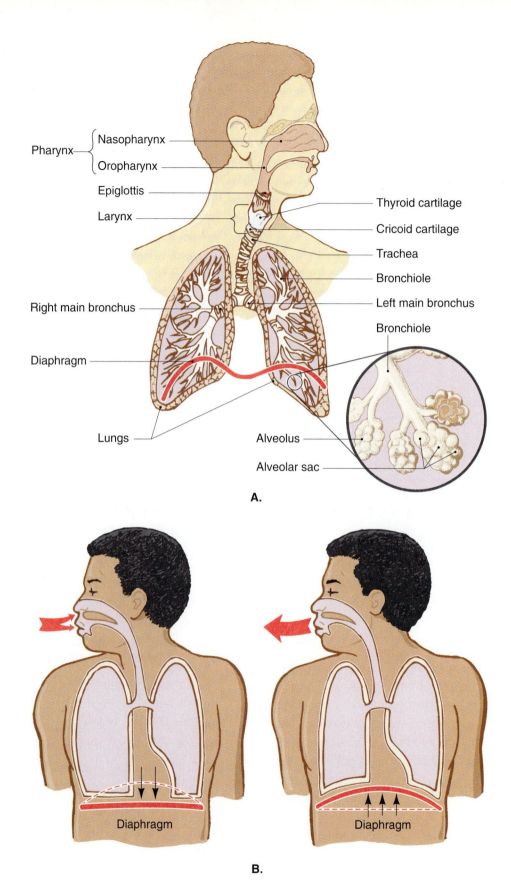

Figure 6-1 **A.** The respiratory system. **B.** The action of the lungs and the diaphragm during inhalation (left) and exhalation (right).

Table 6-1

Adequate Breathing

Normal Rates

Adult—12 to 20 per minute

Child—15 to 30 per minute

Infant—25 to 50 per minute

Rhythm

Regular

Quality

Breath sounds—present and equal

Chest expansions—adequate and equal

Minimum effort

Depth

Adequate

◆ Inspirations are prolonged (indicating a possible upper airway obstruction) or expirations are prolonged (indicating a possible lower airway obstruction).

◆ The patient is unable to speak, or the patient cannot speak full sentences because of shortness of breath.

◆ In children, there may be retractions (a pulling in of the muscles) above the clavicles and sternum and between and below the ribs.

◆ Nasal flaring (widening of the nostrils) may be present, especially in infants and children.

◆ A patient is found in the tripod position (sitting and leaning forward, with hands on knees).

◆ Emergency Care—Respiratory Failure or Respiratory Arrest

When the patient exhibits signs or symptoms that indicate inadequate or no breathing (respiratory failure or respiratory arrest), this is a life-threatening situation. You must promptly take action. The principal procedures with which you will treat life-threatening respiratory problems are as follows:

Figure 6-2 Signs of inadequate breathing and severe respiratory distress.

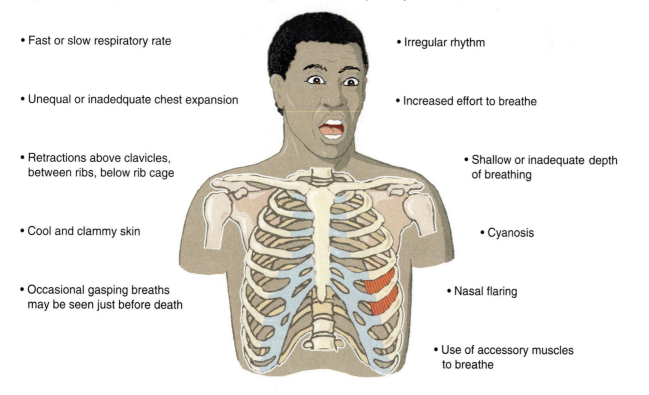

• Fast or slow respiratory rate

• Unequal or inadedquate chest expansion

• Retractions above clavicles, between ribs, below rib cage

• Cool and clammy skin

• Occasional gasping breaths may be seen just before death

• Irregular rhythm

• Increased effort to breathe

• Shallow or inadequate depth of breathing

• Cyanosis

• Nasal flaring

• Use of accessory muscles to breathe

- Opening and maintaining the airway
- Providing supplemental oxygen to the breathing patient
- Providing artificial ventilations to the non-breathing patient and assisting the ventilations of the inadequately breathing patient with a positive pressure device
- Suctioning as needed

OPENING THE AIRWAY

The airway is the passageway by which air enters or leaves the body. The structures of the airway are the nose, mouth, pharynx, larynx, trachea, bronchi, and lungs.

The procedures for airway evaluation, opening the airway, and artificial ventilation are best carried out with the patient lying supine, or flat on his back. Often you will find a patient already supine and you can proceed to perform airway procedures. Patients who are found in positions other than supine or on the ground should be moved to a supine position on the floor or stretcher for evaluation and treatment (Figure 6-3).

Any movement of a suspected trauma (injured) patient before immobilization of the head and spine can produce serious injury to the spinal cord. If injury is suspected, protect the head and neck as you position the patient. Airway and breathing, however, have priority over immobilization of the spine and must be assured as quickly as possible. If the trauma patient must be moved in order to open the airway or to provide ventilations, you will probably not have time to provide immobilization with a cervical collar or head immobilization device on a stretcher. Instead, you should provide as much manual stabilization as possible.

Use the following as indications that head, neck, or spinal injury may have occurred—especially when the patient is unconscious and cannot tell you what happened.

- The mechanism of injury is one that can cause head, neck, or spinal injury. A patient who is found on the ground near a ladder or stairs, for example, may have such injuries. Motor vehicle collisions are common causes of head, neck, and spinal injuries. These injuries are also common in diving incidents and sports activities.

- Any injury at or above the level of the shoulders indicates that head, neck, or spinal injuries may also be present.

- Family or bystanders may tell you that an injury to the head, neck, or spine has occurred or may give you information that leads you to suspect that it did.

As an EMT, you must open and maintain the airway in any patient who cannot do so for himself. This includes patients who have altered mental status, are unconscious, or are in respiratory or cardiac arrest.

Many airway problems are caused by the tongue. As the head flexes forward, the tongue may slide into the airway, causing an obstruction. If the patient is unconscious, the tongue loses muscle tone and muscles of the lower jaw relax. Since the tongue is attached to the lower jaw, the risk of airway obstruction by the tongue is even greater when a patient is unconscious. The basic procedures for opening the airway help to correct the position of the tongue (Figure 6-4).

There are two procedures commonly recommended for opening the airway: the head-tilt, chin-lift maneuver and the jaw-thrust maneuver— the latter being recommended when a head, neck, or spinal injury is suspected.

Head-Tilt, Chin-Lift Maneuver

The **head-tilt, chin-lift maneuver** provides for the maximum opening of the patient's airway (Figure 6-5). It is useful on all patients who need assistance in maintaining an airway or breathing. It is one of the best methods for correcting obstructions caused by the tongue. Follow the steps listed below to perform the head-tilt, chin-lift maneuver.

Warning: *If there are any indications of head, neck, or spine injury, do NOT use the head-tilt, chin-lift maneuver. (Use the jaw-thrust maneuver instead.) Remember that any unconscious and many conscious trauma patients may have an injury to the head, neck, or spine.*

Positioning the Patient for Basic Life Support

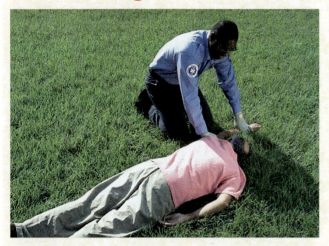

Figure 6-3A Straighten the patient's legs and position the arm closest to you above the head.

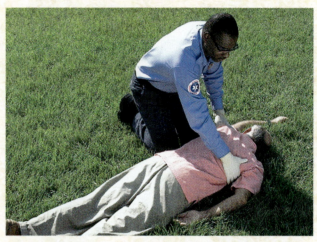

Figure 6-3B Grasp under the armpit that is farther away.

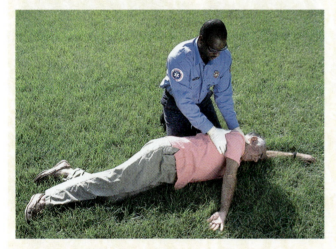

Figure 6-3C Cradling the head and neck, move the patient as a unit onto his side.

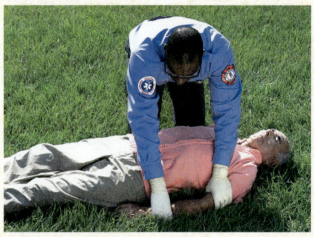

Figure 6-3D Move the patient onto his back and reposition the extended arm.

1. **Once the patient is supine, place one hand on the forehead and place the fingertips of the other hand under the bony area at the center of the patient's lower jaw.**

2. **Tilt the head by applying gentle pressure to the patient's forehead.**

3. **Use your fingertips to lift the chin and to support the lower jaw. Move the jaw forward to a point where the lower teeth are** **almost touching the upper teeth.** *Do not* compress the soft tissues under the lower jaw, which can obstruct the airway.

4. ***Do not* allow the patient's mouth to be closed.** To provide an adequate opening at the mouth, you may need to use the thumb of the hand supporting the chin to pull back the patient's lower lip. *Do not* insert your thumb into the patient's mouth.

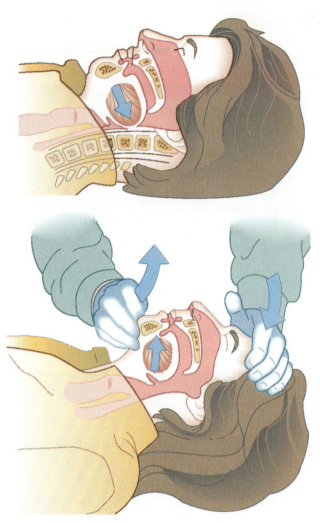

Figure 6-4   The head-tilt, chin-lift maneuver will help to reposition the patient's tongue.

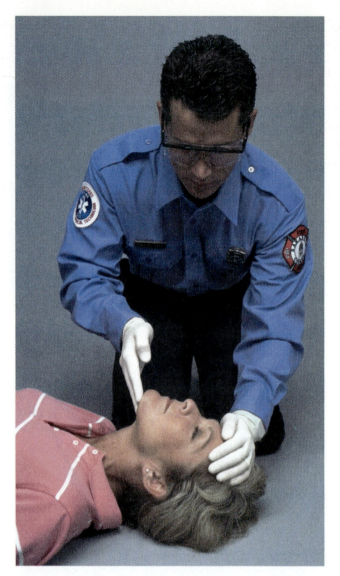

Figure 6-5   The head-tilt, chin-lift maneuver.

Jaw-Thrust Maneuver

The **jaw-thrust maneuver** is most commonly used to open the airway of an unconscious patient or one with suspected head, neck, or spinal injuries (Figure 6-6). All unconscious patients or patients with possible head, neck, or spinal injuries must have their airways opened with the jaw-thrust maneuver rather than the head-tilt, chin-lift maneuver in order to avoid worsening a potential spinal injury. Follow the steps listed below to perform the jaw-thrust maneuver.

1. **Carefully keep the patient's head, neck, and spine aligned, moving him as a unit as you place him in the supine position.**

2. **Kneel at the top of the patient's head, resting your elbows on the same surface on which the patient is lying.**

3. **Carefully reach forward and gently place one hand on each side of the patient's lower jaw, at the angles of the jaw below the ears.**

4. **Stabilize the patient's head with your forearms.**

5. **Using your index fingers, push the angles of the patient's lower jaw forward.**

6. ***Do not*** **tilt or rotate the patient's head.**

Remember, the purpose of the jaw-thrust maneuver is to open a patient's airway *without* moving the head or neck.

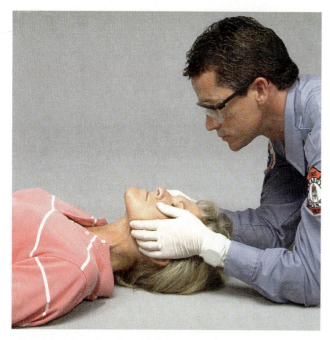

Figure 6-6　The jaw-thrust maneuver.

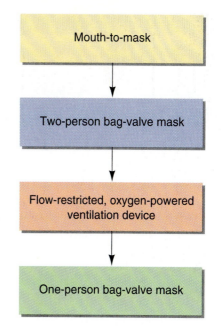

Figure 6-7　The order of preference for techniques to be used in ventilating a patient.

In addition to physically opening the airway with the head-tilt, chin-lift or the jaw-thrust maneuver, you must also be sure to clear the airway of any secretions, blood, or vomitus. The most effective way to clear the patient's airway is with a wide-bore, rigid-tipped (Yankauer) suction device. For this reason, it is crucial that a suction unit be ready for immediate use when you are opening and maintaining the airway. The specific equipment and techniques used for suctioning will be discussed later in this chapter.

TECHNIQUES OF ARTIFICIAL VENTILATION

If you determine that the patient is not breathing or that his breathing efforts are inadequate, you will have to provide artificial ventilation. **Ventilation** is the breathing in of air or oxygen. **Artificial ventilation** (also called **positive pressure ventilation**) is forcing air or oxygen into the lungs when a patient has stopped breathing or has inadequate breathing. There are various techniques for providing artificial ventilations. The 1994 U.S. DOT curriculum lists them as the following order of preference (Figure 6-7):

1. Mouth-to-mask (preferably with high flow supplemental oxygen at 15 liters per minute)

2. Two-person bag-valve mask (preferably with high flow supplemental oxygen at 15 liters per minute)

3. Flow restricted, oxygen-powered ventilation device

4. One-person bag-valve mask

No matter what method is used to ventilate the patient, you should assure that the patient is being adequately ventilated. To determine the signs of *adequate* artificial ventilation, you should:

◆ Watch the chest rise and fall with each ventilation.

◆ See the patient's heart rate return to normal with artificial ventilation.

◆ Assure that the rate of ventilation is sufficient—approximately 12 per minute in adults, 20 per minute in children, a minimum of 20 per minute in infants, and 40 per minute in neonates.

Inadequate artificial ventilation is being provided when

◆ The chest does not rise and fall with ventilations.

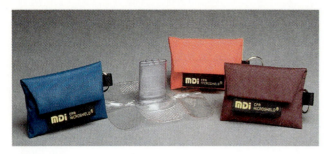

Figure 6-8 Barrier devices for mouth-to-mouth ventilations.

◆ The patient's heart rate does not return to normal with artificial ventilations.

◆ The rate of ventilation is too fast or too slow.

Techniques used for artificial ventilation should also assure adequate isolation of the rescuer from the patient's body fluids, including saliva, blood, and vomit. For this reason, mouth-to-mouth ventilation is not recommended unless there is no alternative method of artificial ventilation available. There are a number of compact barrier devices available for personal use (Figure 6-8).

Mouth-to-Mask Ventilation

Mouth-to-mask ventilation is performed using a **pocket face mask.** When properly used, the pocket face mask will deliver higher volumes of air to the patient than the bag-valve-mask device.

The pocket face mask is made of soft, collapsible material and can be carried in your pocket, jacket, or purse (Figure 6-9). Many EMTs purchase their own pocket face masks for their workplace or automobile first-aid kits.

Face masks have important infection control features. Your ventilations (breaths) are delivered

Figure 6-9 This pocket mask has a one-way valve as an infection control feature and an oxygen inlet for supplemental oxygen.

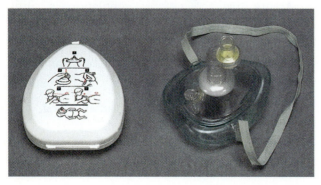

through a port in the mask so that you do not have direct contact with the patient's mouth. Most pocket masks have one-way valves that allow your ventilations to enter but prevent the patient's exhaled air from coming back through the valve and into contact with you.

Some pocket masks have oxygen inlets. When high concentration oxygen is attached to the inlet, an oxygen concentration of approximately 50 percent is delivered. This is significantly better than the 16 percent delivered by mouth-to-mask ventilations without oxygen.

Most pocket face masks are made of a clear plastic. This is important because you must be able to observe the patient's mouth and nose for vomiting or secretions that need to be suctioned. You also need to observe the color of the lips, an indicator of the respiratory status of the patient. Some pocket face masks may have a strap that goes around the patient's head. This strap is helpful during one-rescuer CPR, because it will hold the mask on the patient's face while you are performing chest compressions. However, it does not replace the need for proper hand placement during ventilations as described below.

To provide mouth-to-mask ventilation, you should follow the steps listed below (Figure 6-10):

1. **Position yourself at the patient's head and open the airway.** It may be necessary to clear the airway of obstructions. If necessary, insert an oropharyngeal airway (described later in this chapter) to help keep the patient's airway open.

2. **Connect oxygen to the inlet on the face mask.** Oxygen should be run at 12 to 15 liters per minute. *If oxygen is not immediately available, do not delay in starting mouth-to-mask ventilations.*

3. **Center the ventilation port over the patient's mouth.** This is done by positioning the mask on the patient's face so that the apex (top of the triangle) is over the bridge of the nose and the base is between the lower lip and prominence of the chin.

4. **Hold the mask firmly in place while maintaining the proper head tilt** by:

   ◆ Placing both thumbs on the sides of the mask

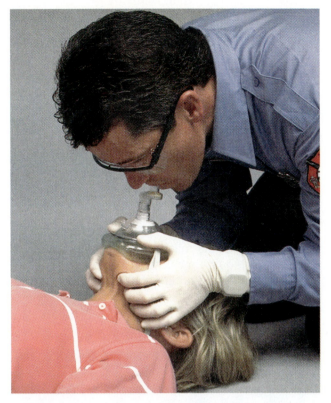

Figure 6-10 Delivering mouth-to-mask ventilations.

◆ Placing the index, third, and fourth fingers of each hand to grasp each side of the lower jaw between the angle of the jaw and the ear lobe and lifting the jaw forward

5. **Take a deep breath and exhale into the mask port or one-way valve at the top of the mask port.** Each ventilation should be delivered over 1½ to 2 seconds in adults and 1 to 1½ seconds in infants and children. Watch for the patient's chest to rise.

6. **Remove your mouth from the port and allow for passive exhalation.** Continue as you would for mouth-to-mouth ventilations or CPR.

The Bag-Valve Mask

The **bag-valve mask** is a hand-held ventilation device. It may also be referred to as a bag-valve-mask unit, system, device, resuscitator, or simply BVM. The bag-valve-mask unit can be used to ventilate a nonbreathing patient. It is also helpful to assist ventilations in the patient whose own respiratory attempts are not enough to support life, such as a patient in respiratory failure or drug overdose. The BVM also provides an infection-control barrier between you and your patient. The use of the bag-valve mask in the field is often referred to as "bagging" the patient.

Bag-valve-mask units come in sizes for infants, children, and adults. Many different types of bag-valve-mask systems are available; however, all have the same basic parts as shown in Figure 6-11. The bag must be a self-refilling shell that is easily cleaned and sterilized. (Some BVMs are designed to be used with a single patient and then disposed of.) The system must have a non-jam valve that allows an oxygen inlet flow of 15 liters per minute. The valve should be nonrebreathing (preventing the patient from rebreathing his own exhalations) and not subject to freezing in cold temperatures. Most systems have a standard 15/22

Figure 6-11 A bag-valve-mask unit.

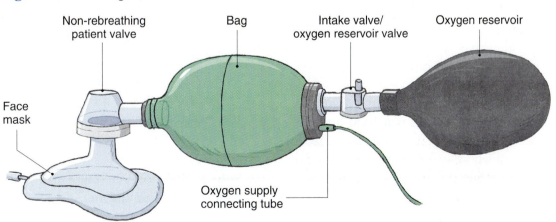

Non-rebreathing patient valve
Bag
Intake valve/oxygen reservoir valve
Oxygen reservoir
Face mask
Oxygen supply connecting tube

mm respiratory fitting to ensure a proper fit with other respiratory equipment, face masks, and endotracheal tubes. A BVM system should also have a clear face mask so that you can observe the lips for cyanosis and monitor the airway in case suctioning is needed.

Warning: *Many older bag-valve masks have "pop-off" valves. These valves were designed to open after certain pressures were obtained. Studies have shown that pop-off valves may prevent adequate ventilations. BVM systems with pop-off valves should be replaced.*

The mechanical workings of a bag-valve-mask device are simple. Oxygen, flowing at 15 liters per minute, is attached to the BVM and enters the reservoir. When the bag is squeezed, the air inlet to the bag is closed, and the oxygen is delivered to the patient. Systems with an oxygen reservoir provide nearly 100 percent oxygen. BVM systems without a reservoir supply approximately 50 percent oxygen. BVM systems used by EMS units should always have an oxygen reservoir.

When the squeeze of the bag is released, a passive expiration by the patient will occur. While the patient exhales, oxygen enters the reservoir to be delivered to the patient the next time the bag is squeezed. The bag itself will hold from 1,000 to 1,600 milliliters of air, depending on the age of the system. Newer models are designed to hold more air. According to American Heart Association guidelines, at least 800 milliliters of air must be delivered. This means that the system must be used properly and efficiently.

The most difficult part of delivering BVM artificial ventilations is obtaining an adequate mask seal so that air does not leak in or out around the edges of the mask (Figure 6-12). It is difficult to maintain a seal with one hand while squeezing the bag with the other, and one-person bag-valve-mask operation is often unsuccessful or inadequate for this reason. Therefore, the American Heart Association recommends that BVM artificial ventilation be performed by two rescuers. In two-person BVM ventilation, one person is assigned to squeeze the bag while the other person uses two hands to maintain a mask seal (Figure 6-13).

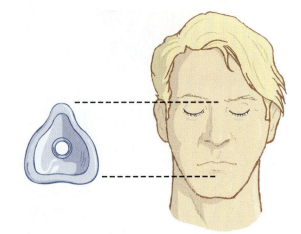

Figure 6-12 Use a mask of the proper size to ensure an adequate mask seal. The mask should fit securely over the bridge of the nose and in the cleft of the chin.

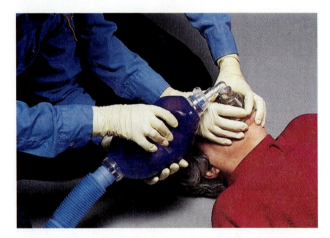

Figure 6-13 Delivering two-person bag-valve-mask ventilations.

The two-person technique can also be modified so that the jaw-thrust can be used during BVM ventilations. This technique is to be used when performing BVM ventilation on a patient with a suspected head, neck, or spinal injury.

Perform two-rescuer BVM ventilation when no trauma (injury) is suspected, as follows:

1. **Open the patient's airway using the head-tilt, chin-lift technique.** Suction and insert an airway adjunct (described later in this chapter) as necessary.

2. **Select the correct bag-valve mask size (adult, child, or infant).**

In-Line Stabilization During BVM Ventilations

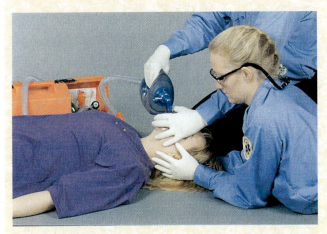

Figure 6-14A Stabilization technique during two-person BVM ventilations.

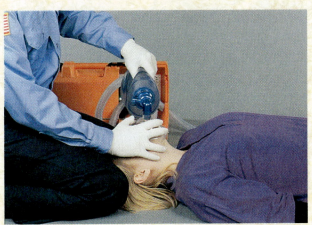

Figure 6-14B If only one rescuer is available, he can provide stabilization by positioning the patient's head between his knees.

3. **Kneel at the patient's head. Position thumbs over the top half of the mask, index and middle fingers over the bottom half.**

4. **Place the apex, or top, of the triangular mask over the bridge of the patient's nose, then lower the mask over the mouth and upper chin.** If the mask has a large, round cuff surrounding a ventilation port, center the port over the patient's mouth.

5. **Use ring and little fingers to bring the patient's jaw up to the mask and maintain the head-tilt, chin-lift.**

6. **The second rescuer should connect bag to mask, if this has not already been done. While you maintain the mask seal, second rescuer should squeeze the bag with two hands until the patient's chest rises.** The second rescuer should squeeze the bag once every 5 seconds for an adult, and once every 3 seconds for a child or infant. If CPR is in progress, the ventilations should be delivered at the end of a cycle of chest compressions.

7. **The second rescuer should release pressure on the bag and let the patient exhale passively.** While this occurs the bag is refilling from the oxygen source.

To perform BVM ventilation on a patient when trauma is suspected, follow the same steps but have one of the rescuers use the jaw-thrust maneuver while stabilizing the head and neck. The second EMT then provides ventilations with a one-hand mask seal (Figure 6-14).

As noted above, use of a bag-valve mask by a single rescuer is the last choice of artificial ventilation procedures behind use of a pocket mask with supplemental oxygen, a two-person bag-valve mask procedure, and use of a flow-restricted, oxygen-powered ventilation device (described below). Its effectiveness is limited because of the difficulties a single rescuer faces in opening the airway, maintaining an adequate mask seal, and simultaneously squeezing the bag enough to deliver adequate ventilations. You should provide ventilations with a one-person bag-valve-mask procedure only when no other options are available (Figure 6-15). When using

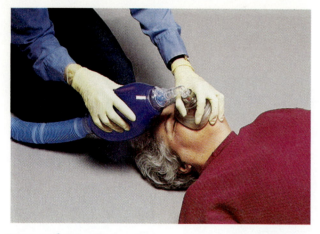

Figure 6-15 Delivering one-person bag-valve-mask ventilations.

the bag-valve mask device alone you should follow these steps:

1. **Position yourself at the patient's head and establish an open airway.** Suction and insert an airway adjunct as necessary.

2. **Select the correct size mask for the patient. Position the mask on the patient's face as described above for the two-person BVM technique.**

3. **Form a "C" around the ventilation port with thumb and index finger. Use middle, ring, and little fingers under the patient's jaw to hold the jaw to the mask.**

4. **With your other hand, squeeze the bag *once every 5 seconds* for adults.** The squeeze should be a full one, causing the patient's chest to rise. For infants and children, squeeze the bag *once every 3 seconds*.

5. **Release pressure on the bag and let the patient exhale passively.** While this occurs, the bag is refilling from the oxygen source.

If the patient's chest does not rise and fall during BVM ventilation, you should follow these steps:

1. Reposition the head.
2. Check for escape of air around the mask and reposition fingers and mask.
3. Check for airway obstruction or obstruction in the BVM system. Suction the patient again if necessary. Consider insertion of an airway adjunct if not already done.

4. If none of the above methods work, use an alternative method of artificial ventilation, such as a pocket mask or a flow-restricted, oxygen-powered ventilation device.

Assisting Ventilations with a BVM

Providing only supplemental high flow oxygen to a patient with inadequate breathing may not be enough to sustain that patient's life. You may at times have to "assist" the patient's breathing with a BVM, either increasing the depth of the patient's own inadequate ventilations or giving additional ventilations to supplement the patient's breathing when he is breathing too slowly.

In order to assist a patient's ventilations, carefully watch the movement of the patient's chest wall. When assisting breathing that is too shallow, you must "squeeze in" the BVM ventilation as soon as you see the chest wall rising. When providing additional ventilations to a patient who is breathing too slowly, provide the BVM ventilation immediately after the patient has completed the exhalation of his own breath as the chest wall falls prior to the next spontaneous inhalation. You can deliver assisted ventilations to both sitting and supine patients.

BVM Use During CPR

The BVM may also be used during CPR. The bag is squeezed once each time a ventilation is to be delivered. In one-rescuer CPR, it is preferable to use a pocket mask with supplemental oxygen rather than a BVM system. A single rescuer would take too much time picking up the BVM and obtaining a face seal each time a ventilation is to be delivered, in addition to the normal difficulty in maintaining a seal with the one-person BVM technique.

BVM-to-Stoma Ventilations

Finally, the BVM can be used to artificially ventilate patients with a **stoma** or **tracheostomy tube** (Figure 6-16). A stoma is a surgical opening in the neck through which a patient breathes. A tracheostomy tube is a short curved tube of rubber, plastic, or metal that is inserted into a stoma to keep it open (Figure 6-17). Patients with stomas who are found to be in severe respiratory distress

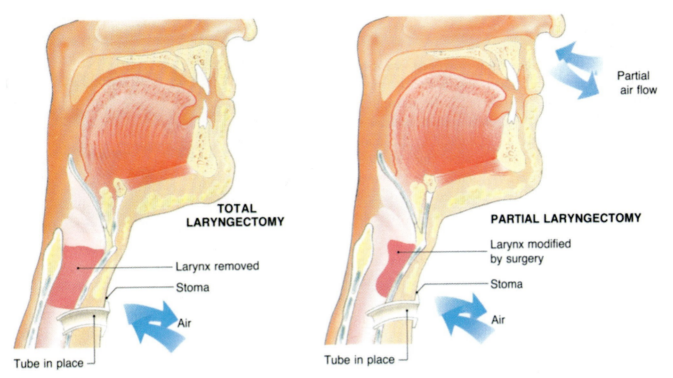

TOTAL LARYNGECTOMY

Larynx removed

Stoma

Air

Tube in place

PARTIAL LARYNGECTOMY

Partial air flow

Larynx modified by surgery

Stoma

Air

Tube in place

Figure 6-16   A neck breather's airway has been changed by surgery.

or respiratory arrest frequently have thick secretions blocking the stoma. It is recommended that you suction the stoma frequently in conjunction with BVM-to-stoma ventilations. As with other BVM uses, a two-person technique is preferred over a one-person technique. To provide artificial ventilation to a stoma breather with a BVM you should follow these steps:

Figure 6-17   The BVM has been designed so that it can connect directly to a tracheostomy tube.

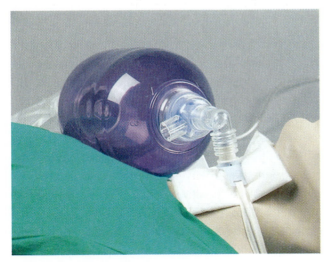

1. **Clear any mucus plugs or secretions from the stoma.**

2. **Leave the patient's head and neck in a neutral position** as it is unnecessary to position the airway prior to ventilations in a stoma breather.

3. **Use a pediatric-sized mask to establish a seal around the stoma.**

4. **Ventilate at the appropriate rate for the patient's age.**

5. **If you are unable to artificially ventilate through the stoma, consider sealing the stoma and attempting artificial ventilation through the mouth and nose.** (This may work if the trachea is still connected to the passageways of mouth, nose, and pharynx—partial laryngectomy. In some cases, the trachea has been permanently connected to the neck opening with no connection to mouth, nose, or pharynx—total laryngectomy.)

Bag-valve-mask devices should be completely disassembled and disinfected after each use. Because proper decontamination is often costly and time consuming, many hospitals and EMS agencies use single-use disposable BVMs.

The Flow Restricted, Oxygen-Powered Ventilation Device

A **flow-restricted, oxygen-powered ventilation device** (FROPVD) uses oxygen under pressure to deliver artificial ventilations through a mask placed on the patient's mouth and nose (Figure 6-18). This device is similar to the traditional demand-valve resuscitator but includes newer features designed to optimize the effectiveness of ventilations and safeguard the patient. Recommended features for the device include the following:

◆ A peak flow rate of 100 percent oxygen at up to 40 liters per minute

◆ An inspiratory pressure relief valve that opens at the pressure of approximately 60 cm of water

◆ An audible alarm when the relief valve is activated

◆ A rugged design and construction

◆ A trigger that enables the rescuer to use both hands to maintain a mask seal while triggering the device

◆ Satisfactory operation in both ordinary and extreme environmental conditions

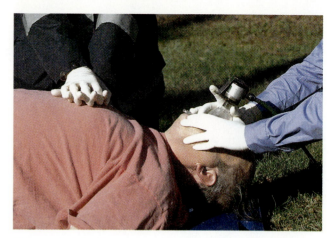

Figure 6-19   Delivering ventilations with a flow-restricted, oxygen-powered ventilation device.

Follow the same procedures for achieving a mask seal as recommended for the BVM. Trigger the device until the patient's chest rises and *repeat every 5 seconds* (Figure 6-19). If the chest does not rise, reposition the patient's head, check the mask seal, check for obstructions, and consider the use of an alternative artificial ventilation procedure.

If you suspect a neck or spine injury, have an assistant hold the patient's head manually or use your knees to prevent movement. Bring the jaw up to the mask without tilting the head or neck using the jaw-thrust maneuver.

The flow-restricted, oxygen-powered ventilation device should be used only on adults.

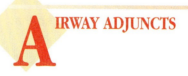

AIRWAY ADJUNCTS

Once you gain access to a patient and begin your initial assessment, your first course of action is to establish an open airway. This airway must be maintained throughout all care procedures.

As noted above, the patient's tongue is a common cause of an obstructed airway. Even though a head-tilt, chin-lift or jaw-thrust maneuver will help open the airway, the tongue may return to its obstructive position once the maneuver is released. Sometimes even when the head-tilt, chin-lift or jaw-thrust is maintained, the tongue will "fall back" into the pharynx.

Figure 6-18   A flow-restricted, oxygen-powered ventilation device.

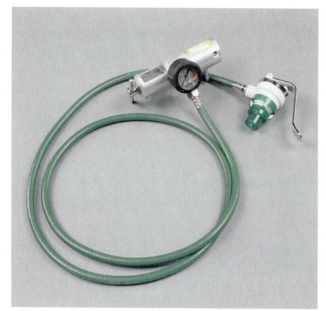

Airway adjuncts, devices that aid in maintaining an open airway, may be used early in the treatment of the unresponsive patient and their use may continue throughout your care. There are several types of airway adjuncts. In this chapter, only the devices that are a part of the standard EMT-Basic course—those whose main function is to keep the tongue from blocking the airway—will be discussed.

The two most common airway adjuncts that EMTs use are the **oropharyngeal airway** and the **nasopharyngeal airway.** The structure and use of these airways can be understood by analyzing their names. *Oro* refers to the mouth, *naso* to the nose, and *pharyngeal* to the pharynx or throat. Oropharyngeal airways are inserted into the mouth and help keep the tongue from falling back into the pharynx. Nasopharyngeal airways are inserted through the nose and rest in the pharynx, also helping keep the tongue from becoming an airway obstruction.

Rules for Using Airway Adjuncts

Some general rules that apply to the use of oropharyngeal and nasopharyngeal airways include the following:

◆ Use an oropharyngeal airway on all unconscious patients who do not exhibit a **gag reflex.** The gag reflex causes vomiting or retching when something is placed in the pharynx. When a patient is deeply unconscious, the gag reflex usually disappears, but it may reappear as a patient begins to regain consciousness. A patient with a gag reflex who cannot tolerate an oropharyngeal airway may be able to tolerate a nasopharyngeal airway.

◆ Open the patient's airway manually before using an airway adjunct.

◆ When inserting the airway, take care not to push the patient's tongue into the pharynx.

◆ Do not continue inserting the airway if the patient begins to gag. Continue to maintain the airway manually and *do not* use an adjunct device. If the patient remains unconscious for a prolonged time, you may later attempt to insert an airway to determine if the gag reflex is still present.

◆ When an airway adjunct is in place, *you must maintain a head-tilt, chin-lift or a jaw thrust and monitor the airway.*

◆ When an airway adjunct is in place, *you must remain ready to suction the patient's airway* to clear vomitus or secretions as necessary.

◆ If the patient regains consciousness or develops a gag reflex, remove the airway immediately. Be prepared to suction the patient again.

◆ Use infection control practices while maintaining the airway. Wear disposable gloves. In airway maintenance, there is a chance of a patient's body fluids coming in contact with your face and eyes. Wear mask and goggles or other protective eyewear to prevent this contact.

Oropharyngeal Airways

Once a patient's airway is opened, an oropharyngeal airway can be inserted to help keep it open. An oropharyngeal airway is a curved device, usually made of plastic, that can be inserted through the patient's mouth. The oropharyngeal airway has a flange that will rest against the patient's lips. The rest of the device holds the tongue as it curves back to the throat. The proper use of an oropharyngeal airway greatly reduces the chances of the patient's airway becoming obstructed.

There are standard sizes of oropharyngeal airways (Figure 6-20). Many manufacturers make a complete line, ranging from airways for infants to large adult sizes. An entire set should be carried to allow for quick, proper selection.

Figure 6-20 A variety of sizes of oropharyngeal airways should be carried on the emergency vehicle.

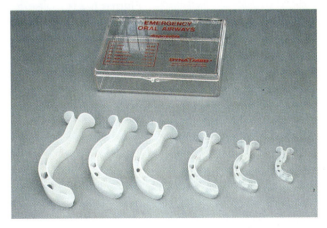

Inserting an Oropharyngeal Airway

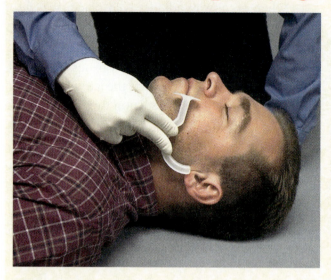

Figure 6-21A Select an airway, measuring from the corner of the patient's mouth to the tip of the earlobe.

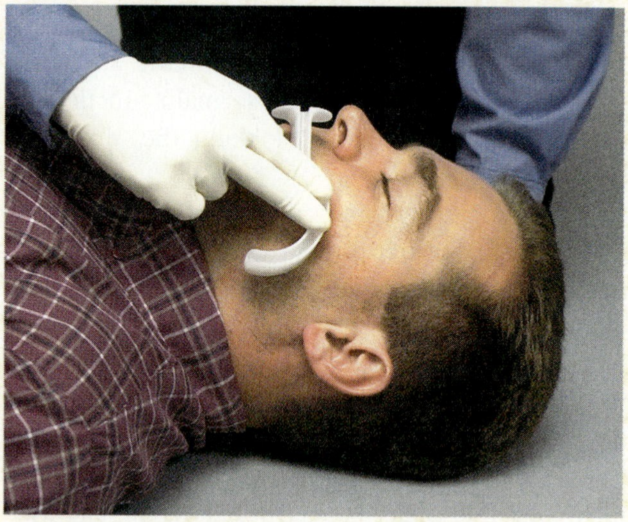

Figure 6-21B An alternative way of ensuring correct size is to measure from the center of the mouth to the angle of the lower jaw bone.

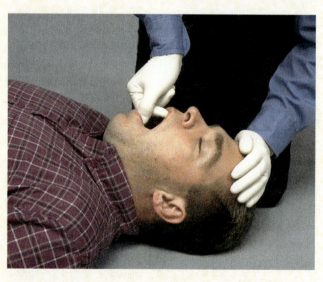

Figure 6-21C Use a crossed-fingers technique to open the mouth.

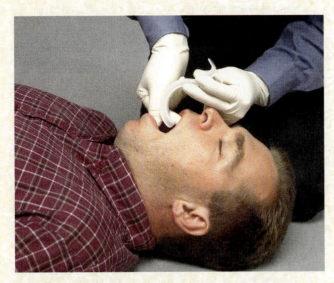

Figure 6-21D Insert the airway with the tip pointing up and rotate into correct position.

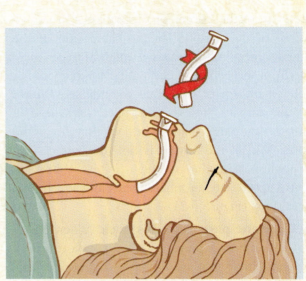

Figure 6-21E Diagram showing the oropharyngeal airway properly positioned.

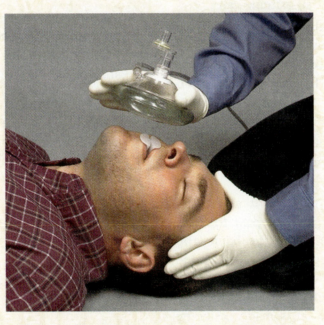

Figure 6-21F When the airway is in place, the patient is ready for ventilations.

The airway adjunct *cannot* be used effectively unless you select the correct airway size for the patient. An airway of proper size will extend from the corner of the patient's mouth to the tip of the earlobe on the same side of the patient's face. An alternative method is to measure from the center of the patient's mouth to the angle of the lower jaw bone (mandible). *Do not* use an airway unless you have measured it against the patient and verified that it is the proper size. If the airway is not the correct size, do not use it on the patient.

To insert an oropharyngeal airway, follow these steps (Figure 6-21):

1. **Place the patient on his back.** When caring for a medical patient with no indications of spinal injury, the neck may be hyperextended. If there are possible spinal injuries, use the jaw-thrust maneuver, moving the patient no more than necessary to ensure an open airway (the airway takes priority over immobilization of the spine). Use extreme care.

2. **Cross the thumb and index finger of one hand and place them on the upper and lower teeth at the corner of the patient's mouth. Spread your fingers apart to open the patient's jaws (the crossed-fingers technique).**

3. **Position the correct size airway so that its tip is pointing toward the roof of the patient's mouth.**

4. **Insert the airway and slide it along the roof of the patient's mouth, past the soft tissue hanging down from the back (the uvula), or until you meet resistance against the soft palate.** Be certain not to push the patient's tongue back into the pharynx. Any airway insertion is made easier by using a tongue blade (tongue depressor). In a few cases, you may have to use a tongue blade to hold the tongue in place. *Watch* what you are doing when inserting the airway. This procedure should not be performed by "feel" only.

5. ***Gently* rotate the airway 180 degrees so that the tip is pointing down into the patient's pharynx.** This method prevents pushing the tongue back. Alternatively, insert the airway with tip already pointing "down" towards the patient's pharynx, using a tongue depressor to press the tongue down and forward to avoid obstructing the airway. *This is the preferred method for airway insertion in an infant or child to prevent damage to the tissues of their oral cavities.*

6. **Place the non-trauma patient in a maximum head-tilt position.** Minimize head movements if there are possible spinal injuries.

7. **Check to see that the flange of the airway is against the patient's lips.** If the airway is too long or too short, remove the airway and replace it with the correct size.

8. **Place the mask you will use for ventilation over the in-place airway adjunct.** If no barrier device is available, provide direct mouth-to-adjunct ventilation as you would provide mouth-to-mouth ventilation.

9. **Monitor the patient closely. If there is a gag reflex, remove the oropharyngeal airway at once.** Remove it by following the anatomical curvature. You do not need to rotate the device when removing it.

Note: Some EMS systems allow an oropharyngeal airway to be inserted with the tip pointing to the side of the patient's mouth. The device is then rotated 90° so that its tip is pointing down the patient's pharynx. Use this approach only if it is part of the protocol of your EMS system.

Any patient who tolerates an oropharyngeal airway in place cannot adequately protect his own airway because the gag reflex is no longer present. Any patient who tolerates an oropharyngeal airway will need ongoing suctioning and protection of the airway by an endotracheal (through-the-trachea) tube. Endotracheal intubation is an advanced life support procedure that can be performed by paramedics, in the emergency department, and, in some jurisdictions, by EMTs. Techniques for endotracheal intubation are discussed in Chapter 29, "Advanced Airway Management," an elective your course may offer.

Inserting a Nasopharyngeal Airway

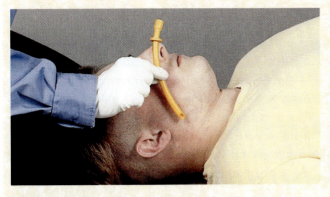

Figure 6-22A Chose a properly sized airway, measuring from the patient's nostril to the earlobe or the angle of the jaw.

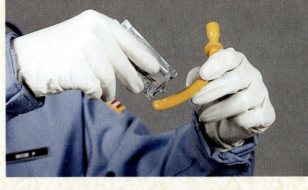

Figure 6-22B Lubricate the airway with a water-based lubricant.

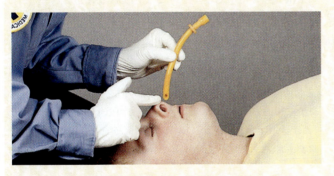

Figure 6-22C Gently push the tip of the patient's nose up, insert the airway (usually into the right nostril), and advance it until the flange rests against the patient's nostril.

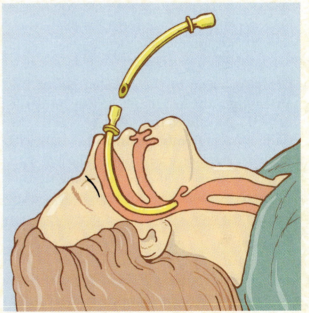

Figure 6-22D Diagram showing the nasopharyngeal airway properly inserted.

Nasopharyngeal Airways

The nasopharyngeal airway has gained popularity because it often does not stimulate the gag reflex. This allows the nasopharyngeal airway to be used in patients who have a reduced level of consciousness but still have an intact gag reflex. Other benefits include the fact that it can be used when the teeth are clenched and when there are oral injuries.

Use the soft flexible latex nasal airway and not the rigid clear plastic airway in the field. The soft ones are less likely to cause soft-tissue damage or bleeding. The typical sizes for adults are 34, 32, 30, and 28 French.

To insert a nasopharyngeal airway, follow the steps listed below (Figure 6-22). Using proper techniques for sizing and inserting the airway will reduce the risk of excessive bleeding from the nose that will further obstruct the airway.

1. **Select the largest nasopharyngeal airway that will fit into the patient's nostril without using any force.** This is approximately the diameter of the patient's little finger.

2. **Lubricate the outside of the tube with a water-based lubricant before insertion.** *Do not* use a petroleum jelly or any other type of non-water-based lubricant. Such substances can damage the tissue lining the nasal cavity and the pharynx and increase the risk of infection.

3. **Gently push the tip of the nose upward. Keep the patient's head in a neutral position.** Most nasopharyngeal airways are designed to be placed in the right nostril. The bevel (angled portion at the tip of the airway) should face toward the septum (wall that divides the two nostrils).

4. **Grasping close to the beveled tip of the airway, gently insert the airway into the nostril. Advance the airway until the flange rests firmly against the patient's nostril.** Never force a nasopharyngeal airway. If you experience difficulty advancing the airway, pull the tube out, rotate it 180°, and try the other nostril.

    Caution: Do not attempt the use of a nasopharyngeal airway if there is evidence of clear (cerebrospinal) fluid coming from the nose or ears. This may indicate a skull fracture in the nasal area through which the airway could pass into the brain.

Oropharyngeal and nasopharyngeal airways can be tremendous assets when used properly. However, no device can replace the well-trained EMT. The proper use of these airways or any other device depends on appropriate use, good judgment, and adequate monitoring of the patient by the EMT.

Oropharyngeal and nasopharyngeal airways prevent blockage of the upper airway by the tongue. To completely ensure an open airway to the level of the lungs, it is sometimes necessary to insert an endotracheal tube.

SUCTION AND SUCTION DEVICES

The patient's airway must be kept clear of foreign materials, blood, vomitus, and other secretions. Materials that are allowed to remain in the airway may be forced into the trachea and eventually into the lungs. This will cause complications ranging from severe pneumonia to complete airway obstruction and death. **Suctioning** is the method of using a vacuum device to remove such materials. A patient who cannot breathe, who is breathing inadequately, or has an altered mental status cannot remove these materials on his own. These types of patients will require at least intermittent suctioning. Suction a patient immediately whenever you hear a gurgling sound in the upper airway.

There are various types of suction equipment. Each suction unit consists of a suction source, a collection container for materials you suction, tubing, and suction tips or catheters. Systems are either mounted in the ambulance or are portable and may be brought to the scene.

Mounted Suction Systems

Suction units are mounted in patient compartments of most ambulances (Figure 6-23). These units are usually installed near the head of the stretcher so they can be used easily. Mounted systems, often called "on-board" units, create a suctioning vacuum using the engine's manifold or an electrical power source. To be effective, suction devices must furnish an air intake of at least 30 liters per minute at the open end of a collection tube. This will occur if the system can generate a vacuum of no less than 300 mmHg (millimeters of mercury) when the collecting tube is clamped.

Portable Suction Units

There are many types of portable suction units. They may be electrically powered (by batteries or household current), oxygen- or air-powered, or manually operated (Figure 6-24). Portable units must provide an amount of suction identical to that of mounted suction unit (30 liters per minute,

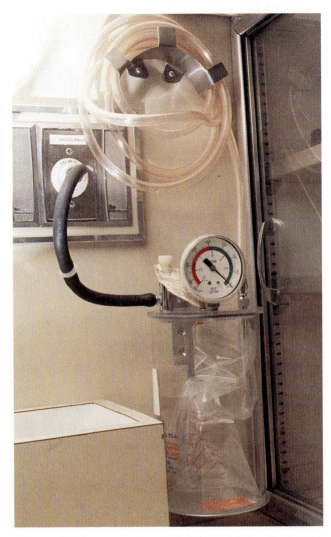

Figure 6-23 A mounted suction unit in the passenger compartment of an ambulance.

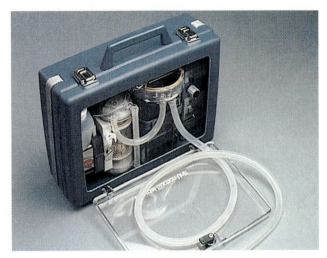

A.

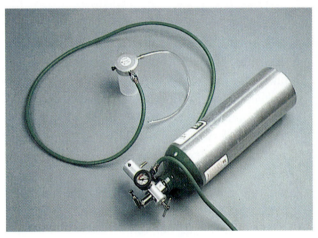

B.

Figure 6-24 **A.** Electric-powered portable suction unit. **B.** Oxygen-powered portable suction unit.

300 mmHg). Portable suction devices give EMTs the ability to suction patients anywhere.

Tubing, Tips, and Catheters

For suctioning to be effective, you must use the proper equipment. While a suction unit might be the most powerful available, it will do no good unless used with the proper attachments.

 Tubing—The tubing attached to a suction unit must be thick-walled, non-kinking, wide-bore tubing. The tubing must not collapse due to the suction, must allow "chunks" of suctioned material to pass, and must not kink, which would reduce the suction. The tubing must be long enough to reach comfortably from the suction unit to the patient.

♦ *Suction Tips*—Currently the most popular type of suction tip is the rigid pharyngeal tip, also called "Yankauer," "tonsil sucker," or "tonsil-tip." This rigid device allows you to suction the mouth and throat with excellent control over the distal end of the device. It also has a larger bore than flexible catheters.

The rigid tip is most successfully used with unresponsive patients. Use it with caution, however, especially with a patient who is not completely unresponsive or may be regaining consciousness. Placing the tip into the pharynx may activate the gag reflex, producing additional vomiting. The tip may also stimulate the vagus nerve in the back of the throat, which can slow the heart rate. Never lose sight of the tip.

- *Suction Catheters*—Suction catheters are flexible plastic tubes. They come in various sizes identified by a number "French." The larger the number, the larger the catheter. For example, a 14 French catheter is larger than an 8 French catheter. These catheters are usually not large enough to suction vomitus or thick secretions and may kink. Flexible catheters are designed for situations in which a rigid tip cannot be used. For example, a soft catheter can be passed through a tube such as a nasopharyngeal or endotracheal tube or used for suctioning the nasopharynx. (A bulb suction device may also be used to suction nasal passages.)

- *Collection containers*—Another important part of a suction device is the collection container. All units should have a non-breakable container for collecting suctioned materials. These containers must be easy to remove and decontaminate. Remember to wear gloves, protective eyewear, and mask not only while suctioning, but also while cleaning the equipment. Most newer suction devices have disposable containers that eliminate the time and risks involved in decontamination.

- *Water containers*—Suction units must also have a container of clean (preferably sterile) water nearby. This water is used to clear matter that is partially blocking the tubing. When a partial blockage of the tube occurs, place the suction tip or catheter in the container of water. This will cause a stream of water to flow through the tip and tubing, usually forcing the clog to dislodge. When the tip or tubing becomes clogged with an item that will not dislodge, replace it with a new tip or catheter.

With copious, thick secretions or vomiting, consider removing the rigid tip or catheter and using the large bore, rigid suction tubing. After you are finished, place the standard tip back on for further suctioning.

Techniques of Suctioning

Although there may be some variations in suction technique (one technique is shown in Figure 6-25 on pages 122–123), a few rules always apply. These include the following:

- *Always use appropriate infection control practices while suctioning.* These practices include the use of protective eyewear, a mask, and disposable gloves. An impervious gown may sometimes be necessary. Proper suctioning requires you to have your fingers around and, in the case of an unresponsive patient, inside the patient's mouth. Disposable gloves prevent contact with the patient's body fluids. Protective eyewear and a mask are also recommended because fluids may splatter, or the patient may gag or cough, sending droplets into your face, eyes, and mouth.

- *Suction for no longer than 15 seconds at a time in an adult; suction for even shorter times in infants and children.* Remember that patients who need airway control and suctioning are often unconscious and may be in cardiac or respiratory arrest. Oxygen delivery to such patients is very important. During suctioning, the ventilations or other method of oxygen delivery are discontinued to allow for the passage of the suction catheter. To prevent prolonged delays in oxygen delivery, limit suctioning to a maximum of 15 seconds in adults and shorter periods in infants and children. Then resume ventilations or oxygen delivery.

  If the patient produces secretions as rapidly as suctioning can remove them, suction for 15 seconds, artificially ventilate for 2 minutes, then suction for 15 seconds, and continue the sequence. Consult medical direction in this situation.

  You may **hyperventilate** a patient before and after suctioning. That is, you may ventilate a patient who is receiving artificial ventilations at a faster rate before and after suctioning to help compensate for the oxygen not delivered during suctioning.

- *Place the tip or catheter where you want to begin the suctioning and suction on the way out.* Most suction tips and catheters do not produce suction at all times; you have to start the suctioning. The tip or catheter will have an open distal end where the suction is delivered. It will also have an opening, or port, in the proximal portion. When you put your finger over the proximal port, suctioning begins from the distal end.

It is not necessary to measure when using a rigid tip. Rather, you should be sure not to lose sight of the tip when inserting it. When using a flexible catheter, however, measure it in a manner similar to measuring for an oropharyngeal airway. The length of catheter that should be inserted into the patient's mouth is equal to the distance between the corner of the patient's mouth and his earlobe.

Carefully bring the tip of the catheter to the area where suctioning is needed. Never "jab" or force the suction tip into the mouth or throat. Then place your finger over the proximal opening to begin the suctioning, and suction as you slowly withdraw the tip from the patient's mouth, moving the tip from side to side.

Suctioning is usually delivered with the patient turned on his side. This allows free secretions to flow from the mouth during suctioning. Use caution when suctioning patients with suspected neck or spinal injuries. If the patient is fully and securely immobilized, the entire backboard may be tilted. With a patient for whom such injuries are suspected but who is not immobilized, suction the best you can without turning the patient. If all other methods have failed, as a last resort you may turn the patient's body as a unit, attempting to keep the neck and spine in line. Suctioning should not be delayed to immobilize a patient.

The rigid suction tip or flexible catheter should be moved into place carefully and not forced. Rigid suction devices may cause tissue damage and bleeding. Never probe into wounds or attempt to suction away attached tissue with a suction device. Certain skull fractures may actually cause brain tissue to be visible in the throat. If this occurs, do not suction near this tissue; limit suctioning to the mouth.

Suction devices may also activate the gag reflex and stimulate vomiting when placed in the posterior mouth or pharynx. In a patient who already has secretions that must be suctioned, vomiting only makes things worse. If you advance a suction catheter or rigid suction tip and the patient begins to gag, withdraw the tip to a position that does not cause gagging and begin suctioning.

The techniques described above apply to suctioning of the upper airway. Techniques for orotracheal deep suctioning to the level of the lungs—an advanced life support procedure that may be performed by EMTs in some jurisdictions—are discussed in Chapter 29.

OXYGEN THERAPY

The Importance of Supplemental Oxygen

Administration of oxygen is often one of the most important and beneficial treatments an EMT can provide. The earth's atmosphere provides approximately 21 percent oxygen. If a person is without illness or injury, that 21 percent is enough to support normal functioning. EMTs, however, usually come in contact with sick or injured people who often require supplemental oxygen. Conditions that may require oxygen include the following:

◆ *Respiratory or cardiac arrest*—CPR is only 25 to 33 percent as effective as normal circulation. High concentration oxygen administration provides a better chance of survival for the patient in respiratory or cardiac arrest.

◆ *Heart attacks and strokes*—These emergencies result from an interruption of blood to the heart or brain. When such an interruption occurs, tissues are deprived of oxygen. Providing extra oxygen is extremely important.

◆ *Chest pain*—All patients with chest pain are presumed to be having a cardiac emergency and should be placed on oxygen.

◆ *Shortness of breath*—All patients who complain of shortness of breath should be placed on oxygen.

◆ *Shock (Hypoperfusion)*—Since shock is the failure of the cardiovascular system to provide sufficient blood to all the vital tissues, all cases of shock reduce the amount of oxygenated

Techniques of Suctioning

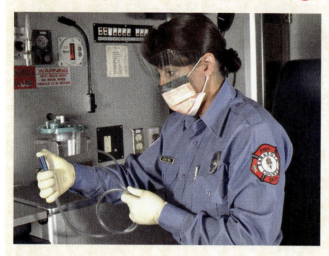

Figure 6-25A Turn the unit on, attach a catheter, and test for suction.

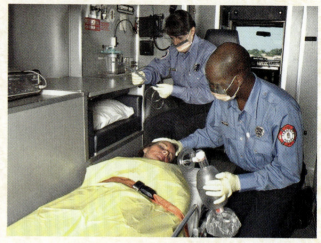

Figure 6-25B The EMT should be positioned at the patient's head for suctioning and the patient's head turned to the side. For trauma patients, turn the entire patient to the side as a unit.

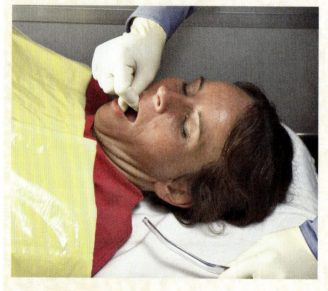

Figure 6-25C Open the patient's mouth with the crossed-fingers technique.

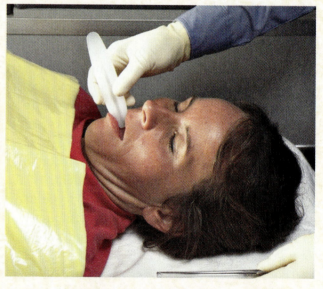

Figure 6-25D Alternatively, a commercially manufactured device can be used to open the mouth.

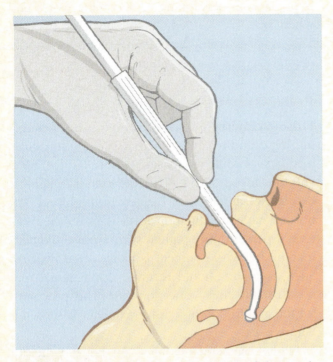

Figure 6-25E Place the convex side of the rigid tip against the roof of the mouth. Insert just to the base of the tongue.

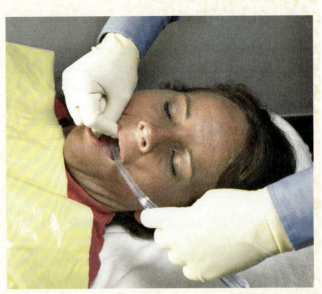

Figure 6-25F It is not necessary to measure the rigid-tip catheter, simply do not lose sight of the tip as you suction. Apply suction only after the rigid tip is properly positioned.

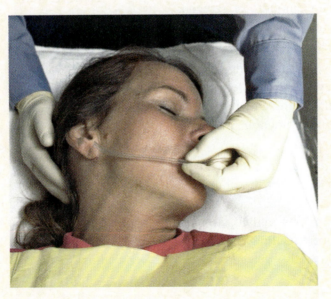

Figure 6-25G When using a flexible catheter, size it by measuring from the patient's earlobe to the corner of the mouth, or from the center of the mouth to the angle of the jaw.

blood reaching the tissues. Administration of oxygen helps the blood that does reach the tissues deliver the maximum amount of oxygen possible.

◆ *Significant blood loss*—Whether the bleeding is internal or external, there is a reduced amount of circulating blood and red blood cells, so the blood that is circulating needs to be saturated with oxygen.

◆ *Lung diseases*—The lungs are responsible for turning oxygen over to the blood cells to be delivered to the tissues. When the lungs are not functioning properly, supplemental oxygen helps assure that the body's tissues receive adequate oxygen.

Hypoxia

Hypoxia is an insufficiency in the supply of oxygen that reaches the body's tissues. There are several major causes of hypoxia. Consider, for example, the following scenarios in which patients develop hypoxia.

◆ A victim is trapped in a fire. The air that the victim breathes contains smoke, carbon monoxide, and reduced amounts of oxygen. Since the victim cannot breathe in enough oxygen, hypoxia develops.

◆ A patient has emphysema. This lung disease decreases the efficiency of the transfer of oxygen between the atmosphere and the body. Since the lungs cannot function properly, hypoxia develops.

◆ A patient overdoses on a drug that has a depressing effect on the part of the brain that controls the respiratory system. The patient's respirations are only 5 per minute. In this case, the victim is not breathing frequently enough to support the body's oxygen needs. Hypoxia develops.

There are many causes of hypoxia in addition to the ones above. They include stroke, shock, and others. The most important thing to know is how to recognize signs of hypoxia so that it may be treated. Hypoxia may be indicated by cyanosis (blue or gray color to the skin). Additionally, when the brain suffers hypoxia, the patient's men-

tal status may deteriorate. Restlessness or confusion may result.

As an EMT, your concern will be to prevent hypoxia from developing or becoming worse and, when possible, to reduce the level of hypoxia. This is done with the administration of supplemental oxygen to the patient.

Pulse Oximetry

Pulse oximetry is a non-invasive way of detecting hypoxia in patients. The use of pulse oximeters has become increasingly popular for EMTs and advanced EMTs. The devices use light to detect the saturation of oxygen in the blood. The normal oxygen saturation level is in the high 90s to 100 percent. Any patient with a pulse oximetry reading below 96 percent is likely to be hypoxic. Such a patient should receive supplemental oxygen (usually high concentration). The procedure for the application of a pulse oximeter is shown in Figure 6-26.

Pulse oximeter readings can be very helpful for more than simply detecting patients with hypoxia. These readings can also help you assess the effectiveness of airway management techniques you are using on a patient. For example, your initial pulse oximeter reading on a patient with shortness of breath revealed an oxygen saturation of 88 percent. A pulse oximeter reading taken after you provide the patient with supplemental high concentration oxygen shows a level of 98 percent. These readings indicate that the patient is becoming less hypoxic and his condition is probably improving. On the other hand, a similar patient whose pulse oximeter reading drops from 93 percent to 84 percent while on supplemental oxygen is deteriorating. You will probably have to provide this patient with assisted ventilations using a BVM because the increasing hypoxia indicates that he is progressing into respiratory failure.

Follow the general guidelines listed below whenever you use a pulse oximeter:

◆ *Always treat the patient, not the pulse oximeter reading.* Just because a person has a good pulse oximetry reading does not mean that the patient does not need oxygen. As you will

Using a Pulse Oximeter

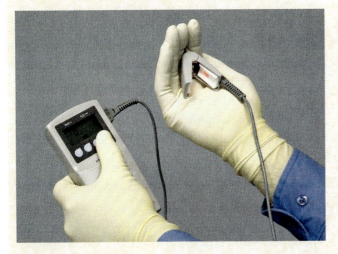

Figure 6-26A Check the pulse oximeter to ensure that it is working.

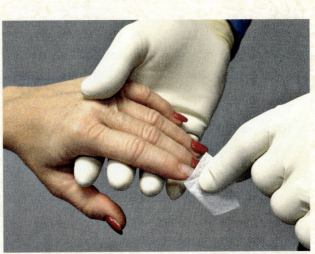

Figure 6-26B If the patient is wearing nail polish, remove the polish using an acetone dampened

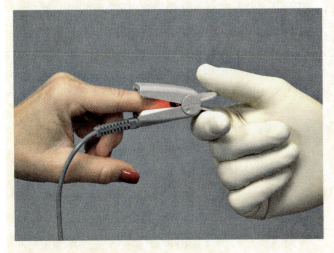

Figure 6-26C Apply the oximeter to the patient's fingertip.

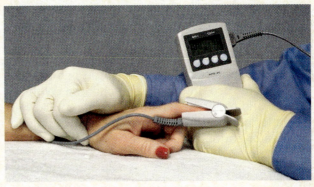

Figure 6-26D Obtain the reading. In this case, the oximeter shows a pulse reading of 100 beats per minute and a blood oxygen level of 76 percent.

learn, all patients with chest pain or shortness of breath or those who have signs of shock must be placed on high concentration oxygen regardless of what the pulse oximeter reading shows.

◆ *Make sure that the pulse oximeter is getting a true reading.* The pulse oximeter can give an accurate reading of oxygen saturation only if it can detect good blood flow. Most pulse oximeters display a pulse rate reading next to the oxygen saturation reading. Make sure the pulse rate indicated by the meter matches the pulse you feel on the patient. If the pulse oximeter's reading does not match the patient's actual pulse rate, the oxygen saturation reading will not be accurate. It is often difficult to get accurate pulse oximeter readings on patients in shock (hypoperfusion) or on those with cold extremities. In addition, nail polish can affect the accuracy of the pulse oximeter's readings. Always carry acetone pads with the pulse oximeter so that you can remove nail polish from a patient's finger when you have to use a pulse oximeter.

- *Certain medical conditions will give a falsely high pulse oximeter reading.* The most common of these conditions you are likely to encounter is carbon monoxide poisoning. Patients with carbon monoxide poisoning will display high oxygen saturation readings. Those patients may, in fact, be very hypoxic. To respond properly in a situation like this, always remember the initial guideline for pulse oximeter use: *treat the patient, not the pulse oximeter reading*.

PEDIATRIC NOTE

Pulse oximetry may also be used with infants and children if authorized by local protocols. Before you try to place the pulse oximeter probe, explain to the patient and parents that the procedure does not hurt. In fact, you can reassure children by making a game of placing the probe with its bright red light. Most manufacturers have specialized pediatric adapters for use on infants and children. With infants and children, you can place the pulse oximeter probe not only on the fingers but also on toes or earlobes.

Hazards of Oxygen Therapy

Although the benefits of oxygen are great, oxygen must be used carefully. The hazards of oxygen therapy may be grouped into two categories, non-medical and medical.

The nonmedical hazards of oxygen include the following:

- The oxygen used in emergency care is stored under pressure, usually 2,000 to 2,200 pounds per square inch (psi) (13,800 to 15,180 kPa) or greater in a full cylinder. If the tank is punctured, or a valve breaks off, the supply tank can become a missile. Damaged tanks have penetrated concrete walls. Imagine what would happen in the passenger compartment of an ambulance if such an accident occurred.

- Oxygen supports combustion, causing fire to burn more rapidly. It can saturate towels, sheets, and clothing, greatly increasing the risk of fire.

- Under pressure, oxygen and oil do not mix. When they come into contact, a severe reaction occurs which, for our purposes, can be termed an explosion. For this reason you should *never* lubricate an oxygen-delivery system or gauge with petroleum products. Also, you should *never* allow contact between oxygen and a petroleum-based adhesive (e.g., adhesive tape).

These nonmedical hazards are extremely rare and can be avoided if oxygen and oxygen equipment are treated properly.

The medical hazards of oxygen involve certain patients who, when exposed to high concentrations of oxygen for prolonged periods, may develop negative side effects. These situations are rare in the field. Some examples include the following:

- *Infant eye damage*—This condition may occur when premature infants are given too much oxygen over a period of days or weeks. These infants may develop scar tissue on the retina of the eye. Oxygen by itself does not cause this condition, which is the result of a combination of factors. Never withhold oxygen from any infant with signs of inadequate breathing.

- *Respiratory depression or respiratory arrest*—Patients with chronic obstructive pulmonary disease (COPD) may, over time, lose the normal ability to use the body's increased blood carbon dioxide levels as a stimulus to breathe. When this occurs, the COPD patient's body may use low blood oxygen as the factor that stimulates breathing. Because of this so-called *hypoxic drive,* EMTs have for years been trained to administer only low concentrations of oxygen to these patients for fear of increasing the patient's blood oxygen levels and "wiping out the drive to breathe." It is now widely accepted that more harm is done by withholding high concentration oxygen from these patients than could be done by administering it.

As an EMT you will probably never see adverse conditions such as those above that can result from oxygen administration. The time required for such conditions to develop is likely too long to cause any problems during emergency care in the field. The bottom line is this: *Never withhold high concentration oxygen from a patient who needs it!*

Oxygen Therapy Equipment

In the hospital setting, oxygen is delivered to the patient from conveniently located oxygen tanks or regulators. In the field, oxygen equipment must be safe, lightweight, portable, and dependable. Some field oxygen systems are very portable so they may be brought almost anywhere (Figure 6-27). Other systems are installed inside the ambulance so that oxygen can be delivered during transportation to the hospital.

Most oxygen delivery systems contain several items: oxygen cylinders, pressure regulators, and a delivery device (face mask or cannula). When the patient is not breathing or is breathing inadequately, additional devices (such as a bag-valve mask) can be used to force oxygen into the patient's lungs.

Oxygen Cylinders

Outside a medical facility, the standard source of oxygen is the oxygen cylinder. This is a seamless steel or lightweight alloy cylinder filled with oxygen under pressure, equal to 2,000 to 2,200 psi (13,800 to 15,180 kPa) when the cylinders are full. Cylinders come in various sizes, identified by letters (Figure 6-28). Those in common use in emergency care include the following:

◆ D cylinder—contains about 350 liters of oxygen

◆ E cylinder—contains about 625 liters of oxygen

◆ M cylinder—contains about 3,000 liters of oxygen

Fixed systems on ambulances, commonly called "onboard oxygen," include the M cylinder and larger cylinders (Figure 6-29):

◆ G cylinder—contains about 5,300 liters of oxygen

◆ H cylinder—contains about 6,900 liters of oxygen.

The United States Pharmacopoeia has assigned a color code to distinguish compressed gases. Green and white cylinders have been assigned to

Figure 6-28 From left to right, jumbo D, D, and E oxygen cylinders.

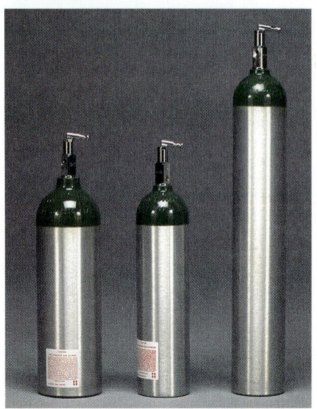

Figure 6-27 An oxygen-delivery system for use in the field.

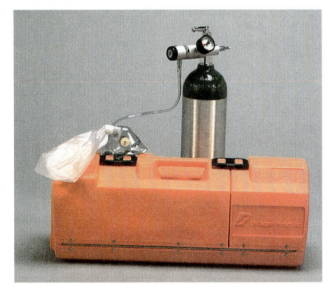

the pressure gauge reads 200 psi (1,400 kPa) or above. Below this point there is not enough oxygen in the cylinder to allow for proper delivery to the patient. Before the cylinder reaches the 200 psi reading, you must switch to a fresh cylinder.

COMPANY OFFICER'S NOTES

Administration of high flow oxygen is an essential part of emergency medical care for critically injured or ill patients. Delivering oxygen at rates of 15 liters per minute using a nonrebreather mask or BVM or even higher using a flow-restricted, oxygen-powered ventilation device can quickly deplete the supply contained in a portable cylinder. Since you will rarely know in advance whether or not a call will require large amounts of oxygen, always presume that large amounts of oxygen will be required. Most departments recommend that the primary portable oxygen cylinder have at least 500 psi (1,400 kPa) at the start of every call. Spare oxygen cylinders should always be readily available on the emergency apparatus or ambulance in case the primary cylinder becomes depleted. Remember, allowing an apparatus that is responsible for EMS calls to be placed in service with its primary oxygen cylinder only one quarter full can be as catastrophic as allowing an engine whose booster tank is only one quarter full to respond on a fire call.

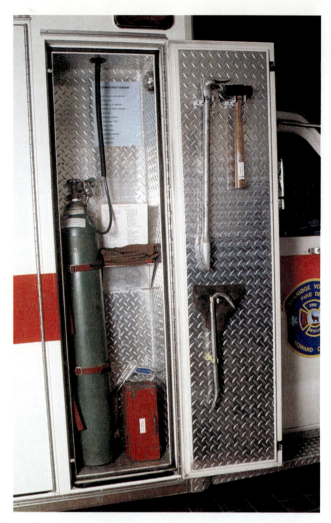

Figure 6-29 A large oxygen cylinder for a fixed system onboard an ambulance.

all grades of oxygen. Unpainted stainless steel and aluminum cylinders are also used for oxygen. Regardless of the color, always check the label to be certain you are using medical grade oxygen.

Part of your duty as an EMT is to make certain that the oxygen cylinders you will use are full and ready before they are needed to provide care. The length of time you can use an oxygen cylinder depends on the pressure in the cylinder and the flow rate of oxygen delivery. You cannot tell if an oxygen cylinder is full, partially full, or empty by lifting or moving the cylinder. Most portable oxygen cylinders containing less than 500 psi (3,500 kPa) after a call should be refilled or replaced.

Never allow oxygen cylinders to empty below the safe residual: doing so may damage the tank. The safe residual for an oxygen cylinder is when

Safety is of prime importance when working with oxygen cylinders. Always keep the following guidelines in mind:

◆ *Never* drop a cylinder or let it fall against any object. When transporting a patient with an oxygen cylinder, make sure the oxygen cylinder is strapped to the stretcher or otherwise secured.

◆ *Never* leave an oxygen cylinder standing in an upright position without being secured.

◆ *Never* allow smoking around oxygen equipment in use. Clearly mark the area of use with signs that read "OXYGEN—NO SMOKING."

◆ *Never* use oxygen equipment around an open flame.

- *Never* use grease, oil, or fat-based soaps on devices that will be attached to an oxygen supply cylinder. Take care not to handle these devices when your hands are greasy. Use greaseless tools when making connections.

- *Never* use adhesive tape to protect an oxygen tank outlet or to mark or label any oxygen cylinders or oxygen delivery apparatus. The oxygen can react with the adhesive and debris and cause a fire.

- *Never* try to move an oxygen cylinder by dragging it or rolling it on its side or bottom.

- *Always* use pressure gauges, regulators, and tubing that are intended for use with oxygen.

- *Always* use nonferrous metal oxygen wrenches for changing gauges and regulators or for adjusting flow rates. Other types of metal tools may produce a spark should they strike against metal objects.

- *Always* ensure that valve seat inserts and gaskets are in good condition. This prevents dangerous leaks. D and E cylinders have disposable gaskets that should be replaced each time a cylinder change is made.

- *Always* use medical grade oxygen. Industrial oxygen contains impurities. The cylinder should be green in color and labeled "OXYGEN U.S.P."

- *Always* open the valve of an oxygen cylinder fully, then close it half a turn to prevent someone else from thinking the valve is closed and trying to force it open. The valve does not have to be turned fully to be open for delivery.

- *Always* store reserve oxygen cylinders in a cool, ventilated room, properly secured in place.

- *Always* have oxygen cylinders hydrostatically tested *every 5 years.* The date a cylinder was last tested is stamped on the cylinder. Some cylinders can be tested every 10 years. These will have a star after the date (e.g., 4M86M☆).

Pressure Regulators

Oxygen is stored in a cylinder at too high a pressure (approximately 2000 psi in a full tank and varying with surrounding temperature) to be delivered directly to a patient. A pressure regulator must be connected to the cylinder to provide a safe working pressure of 30 to 70 psi (210 to 490 kPa).

On cylinders of the E size or smaller, the pressure regulator is secured to the cylinder valve assembly by a yoke assembly. The yoke is provided with pins that must mate with corresponding holes in the valve assembly. This is called a *pin-index safety system.* Since the pin position varies for different gases, this system prevents an oxygen delivery system from being connected to a cylinder designed to contain another gas.

Cylinders larger than the E size have a valve assembly with a threaded outlet. The inside and outside diameters of the threaded outlets vary according to the gas in the cylinder. This prevents an oxygen regulator from being connected to a cylinder containing another gas. In other words, a nitrogen regulator cannot be connected to an oxygen cylinder, and vice versa.

Before connecting the pressure regulator to an oxygen supply cylinder, stand to the side of the main valve opening and open (crack) the cylinder valve slightly for just a second to clear dirt and dust out of the delivery port or threaded outlet.

> ***Note:*** *You must maintain the regulator inlet filter. It has to be free of damage and clean to prevent contamination of and damage to the regulator.*

Flowmeters

A **flowmeter** allows control of the flow of oxygen in liters per minute. It is connected to the pressure regulator. Most jurisdictions keep the flowmeter permanently attached to the pressure regulator. Although several types of flowmeters are available, the one using a constant flow selector valve is the best suited for prehospital care.

A flowmeter with a constant flow selector valve has no gauge. It allows for the adjustment of flow in liters per minute in stepped increments (2, 4, 6, 8, . . . up to 15 liters or more per minute). When using this type of flowmeter, make certain that it is properly adjusted for the desired flow and monitor the meter to make certain that it stays properly adjusted. This type of meter should be tested for accuracy as recommended by the manufacturer.

Humidifiers

A **humidifier** can be connected to the flowmeter to provide moisture to the dry oxygen coming from the supply cylinder. Dry oxygen can dehydrate the mucous membranes of the patient's airway and lungs. In most short-term use, the dryness of the oxygen is not a problem; during long transports, however, the patient is usually more comfortable when given humidified oxygen. This is particularly true if the patient has COPD. Humidified oxygen can also be beneficial with some pediatric patients.

A humidifier is usually no more than a nonbreakable jar of water attached to the flowmeter. Oxygen passes (bubbles) through the water to become humidified. As with all oxygen delivery equipment, the humidifier must be kept clean. The water reservoir can become a breeding ground for algae, harmful bacteria, and dangerous fungal organisms. To avoid this risk, a sterile single-patient-use humidifier should be employed whenever humidified oxygen is given. In many EMS systems humidifiers are no longer used because they are not indicated for short transports and because of the infection risk.

Administering Oxygen

The process of administering oxygen and discontinuing its administration is shown in Figures 6-32, 6-33, and 6-34. Do not attempt to learn on your own how to use an oxygen delivery system. You should work with your instructor and follow your instructor's directions for the specific equipment you will be using.

As you have already learned, high concentration oxygen is used to adequately ventilate nonbreathing patients. Oxygen is also administered to *breathing patients* for a variety of conditions. A number of oxygen-delivery devices and systems are used. Each has benefits and drawbacks. A device that is good for one patient may not be ideal for another. The goal is to use the oxygen delivery device that is best suited for each patient.

Delivering Oxygen to the Breathing Patient

For the patient who is breathing and requires supplemental oxygen due to potential hypoxia, there are various oxygen delivery devices available. In general, however, the nonrebreather mask and the nasal cannula are the two devices most commonly used by the EMT to provide supplemental oxygen (see Table 6-3).

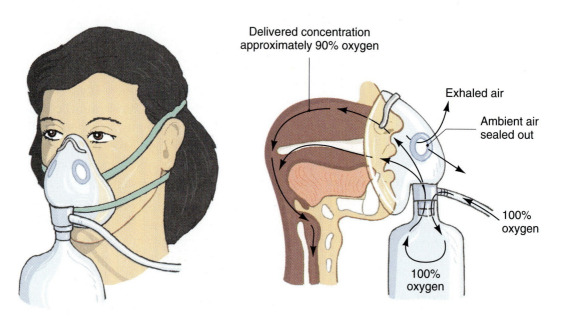

Delivered concentration approximately 90% oxygen

Exhaled air

Ambient air sealed out

100% oxygen

100% oxygen

Figure 6-30 The nonrebreather mask.

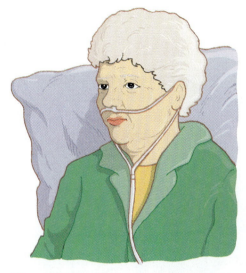
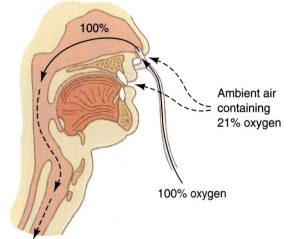

100%

Ambient air containing 21% oxygen

100% oxygen

22% to 44% oxygen concentration delivered

Figure 6-31 The nasal cannula.

Nonrebreather Mask

Excluding the bag-valve mask used with oxygen and flow-restricted, oxygen-powered ventilation devices, the **nonrebreather mask** is the EMT's best way to deliver high concentrations of oxygen (Figure 6-30). This device must be placed properly on the patient's face to provide the necessary seal to ensure high concentration delivery. Nonrebreather masks come in different sizes for adults, children, and infants.

The reservoir bag must be inflated before the mask is placed on the patient's face. To inflate the reservoir bag, use your finger to cover the connection between the mask and the reservoir and allow the bag to inflate. The reservoir must always contain enough oxygen so that it does not deflate by more than one third when the patient takes his deepest inspiration. This can be maintained by the proper flow of oxygen (usually 10 to 15 liters per minute). Air exhaled by the patient

Table 6-3

Oxygen Delivery Devices

Device	Flow Rate	% O$_2$ Delivered	Special Use
Nonrebreather mask	10–15 liters per minute	80–90%	Delivery system of choice for patients with signs of inadequate breathing and patients who are cyanotic, cool, clammy, short of breath or suffering chest pain, suffering severe injuries or displaying altered mental status.
Nasal cannula	1–6 liters per minute	24–44%	Appropriate for patients who cannot tolerate a mask or COPD patients with minimal respiratory distress

Preparing the Oxygen Delivery System

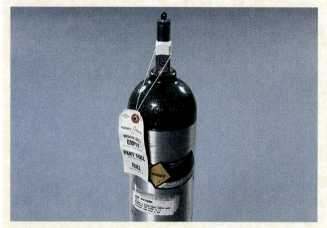

Figure 6-32A Select the desired cylinder and be sure its label reads "Oxygen U.S.P."

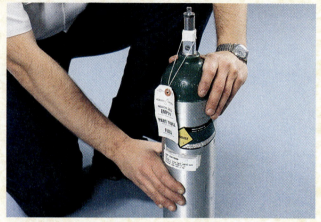

Figure 6-32B Place the cylinder upright and position yourself to one side.

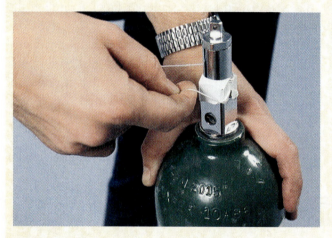

Figure 6-32C Remove the plastic wrapper or cap protecting the cylinder outlet.

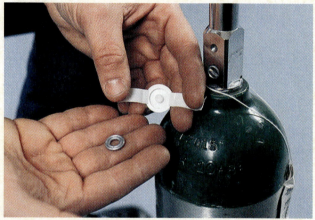

Figure 6-32D With some set-ups, be sure to keep the plastic washer.

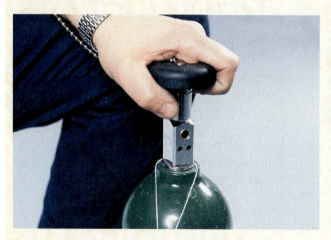

Figure 6-32E "Crack" the main valve for one second.

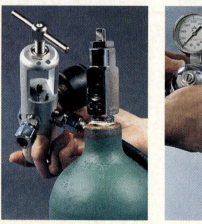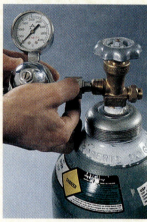

Figure 6-32F Select the correct pressure regulator and flowmeter. Pin yoke is shown on the left, threaded outlet on the right.

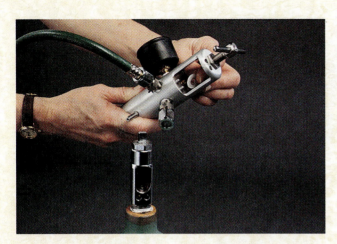

Figure 6-32G Place the cylinder valve gasket on the regulator oxygen port.

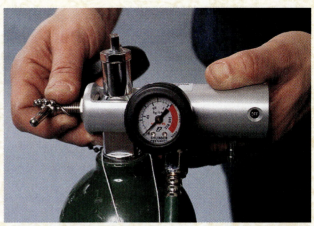

Figure 6-32H Make certain that the pressure regulator is closed.

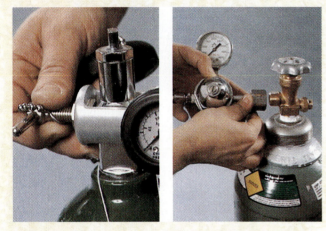

Figure 6-32I Align pins (left) or thread by hand (right).

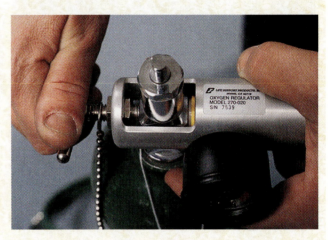

Figure 6-32J Tighten T-screw for a pin yoke.

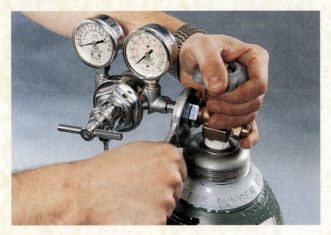

Figure 6-32K Tighten a threaded outlet with a nonferrous wrench.

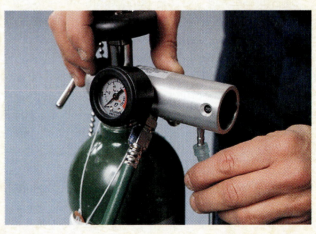

Figure 6-32L Attach tubing and delivery device.

Administering Oxygen

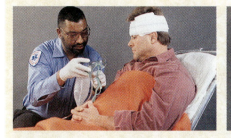

Figure 6-33A Explain the need for administering oxygen to the patient.

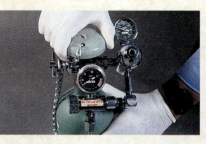

Figure 6-33B Open the main valve and adjust the flowmeter.

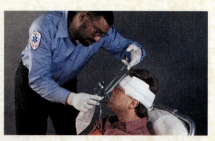

Figure 6-33C Place the oxygen delivery device on the patient.

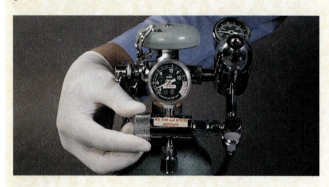

Figure 6-33D Adjust the flowmeter.

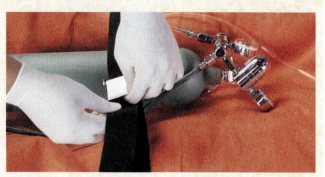

Figure 6-33E Secure the oxygen-delivery system during patient moves and transport.

does not return to the reservoir (is not rebreathed). Instead, it escapes through a flutter valve in the face piece.

This mask will provide concentrations of oxygen ranging from 80 to 90 percent. (Oxygen delivery provided at these levels and up to 100 percent is often referred to as **high concentration oxygen**.) The minimum regulator flow rate for a nonrebreather mask is 8 liters per minute. Depending on the manufacturer and the fit of the mask, the maximum flow can range from 10 to 15 liters per minute. (This is often referred to as **high flow oxygen**.) New design features allow for one emergency port in the mask so that the patient can still receive atmospheric air should the oxygen supply fail. This feature keeps the mask from being able to deliver 100 percent oxygen but is a necessary safety feature. The mask is excellent for use in patients with inadequate breathing or who are cyanotic (blue or gray), cool, clammy, short of breath, or suffering chest pain, shock, or displaying an altered mental status.

Nasal Cannula

A **nasal cannula** provides low concentrations of oxygen (between 24 and 44 percent). Oxygen is delivered to the patient by two prongs that rest in the patient's nostrils (Figure 6-31). The device is usually held to the patient's face by placing the tubing over the patient's ears and securing the slip-loop under the patient's chin.

Patients who have chest pain, signs of shock, hypoxia, or other more serious problems need a higher concentration than can be provided by a cannula. However, some patients will not tolerate a mask-type delivery device because they feel

Discontinuing Oxygen

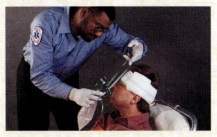

Figure 6-34A Remove the delivery device from the patient.

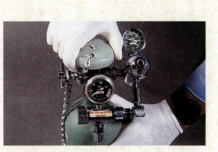

Figure 6-34B Close the main valve.

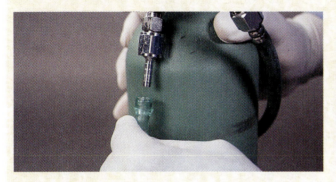

Figure 6-34C Remove the delivery tubing.

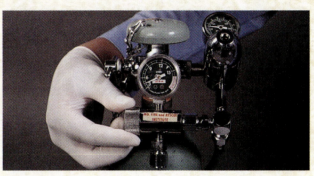

Figure 6-34D Bleed the flowmeter.

"suffocated" by the mask. For the patient who refuses to wear an oxygen face mask, the cannula is better than no oxygen at all. The cannula should generally be used *only* when a patient will not tolerate a nonrebreather mask or in cases of COPD patients within minimal respiratory distress and adequate ventilation.

When a cannula is used, the flow rate should be no more than 4 to 6 liters per minute. (This is often referred to as **low flow oxygen**.) At higher flow rates, the cannula begins to feel more uncomfortable and dries out the nasal mucous membranes.

It is not necessary for a patient to breathe only through his nose when on a nasal cannula. Mouth breathing with a cannula in place will provide adequate oxygen delivery, assuming the nasal passages are clear of obstructions.

SPECIAL CONSIDERATIONS

There are several special considerations in airway management. These include the following:

◆ *Facial injuries and burns*—Take extra care with the airway when there have been facial injuries. Because the blood supply to the face is so rich, blunt injuries to the face frequently result in severe swelling or bleeding that may block or partially block the airway. The airways of patients with facial burns are also apt to swell and close and become partially or completely obstructed (Figure 6-35). Frequent suctioning may be required. Insertion of an

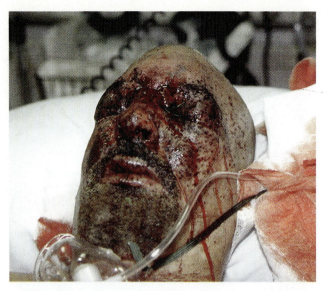

Figure 6-35 Facial injuries can pose a significant risk of airway compromise.

TRANSITION OF CARE

Personnel aboard a non-transporting apparatus who are assigned to EMS first response and who initiate oxygen therapy should act to assure a smooth transition of that therapy to the crew of the transporting ambulance. The oxygen mask or nasal cannula that the first responding crew placed on the patient should remain on the patient. In most jurisdictions, the transporting unit will exchange the first responding unit's mask or cannula for a new one from the ambulance's onboard stock.

The first responding EMT should determine from the transporting crew the oxygen source—onboard ambulance or another portable cylinder—to which they would like the patient's oxygen tubing transferred. Both first responding and transporting EMTs share the responsibility of assuring that the new oxygen source is turned on and is working properly before transfer of the oxygen tubing. If the patient is on a nonrebreather mask, many experienced EMTs will briefly slip it off the patient's face during the oxygen transfer and quickly replace it after the transfer is complete. They do this because, if the transfer is prolonged for any reason, the reservoir bag on the mask will quickly be depleted, making it very difficult for the patient to breathe with the mask snugly attached to his face.

airway adjunct or endotracheal tube may be necessary.

◆ *Obstructions*—Many suction units are not adequate for removing solid objects like teeth and large particles of food or other foreign objects. These must be removed using manual techniques for clearing airway obstructions, such as abdominal thrusts, chest thrusts, or finger sweeps that you learned in your basic life support course. You may need to log roll the patient into a supine position to clear the oropharynx manually.

There are certain medical emergencies such as severe allergic reactions to bee stings or medications that may cause the tongue or lips to swell to the point of obstructing the airway. These patients should be placed in a position of comfort and transported rapidly to the emergency department.

◆ *Dental appliances*—Dentures should ordinarily be left in place during airway procedures. Partial dentures may become dislodged during an emergency. Leave a partial denture in place if possible, but be prepared to remove it if it endangers the airway.

◆ *Pediatric considerations*—These are described in the Pediatric Note on the next page.

PEDIATRIC NOTE

There are several special considerations that you must take into account when managing the airway of an infant or child.

Anatomic Considerations

- The mouth and nose are smaller and more easily obstructed than in adults.

- In infants and children the tongue takes up more space proportionately in the mouth than in adults.

- The trachea (windpipe) is softer and more flexible in infants and children.

- The trachea is narrower and is easily obstructed by swelling.

- The chest wall is softer, and infants and children tend to rely more on the diaphragm for breathing.

- The head is larger and should be monitored and maintained in a "sniffing" position.

Management Considerations

- Open the airway gently. Infants should be placed in a neutral neck position and children only require slight extension of the neck. Do not overextend the neck, because doing so may collapse the trachea.

- When ventilating with a BVM, avoid excessive bag pressure and volume. Use only enough to make the chest rise.

- Use a properly sized face mask when providing BVM ventilations to assure a good mask seal.

- Flow-restricted, oxygen-powered ventilation devices are contraindicated (should not be used) in infants and children.

- Use pediatric-sized nonrebreather masks and nasal cannulas when administering supplemental oxygen.

- Infants and children are prone to gastric distention during ventilations or respiratory distress, which may impair adequate ventilations. (See nasogastric tube insertion in Chapter 29, "Advanced Airway Management.")

- An oral or nasal airway may be considered when other measures fail to keep the airway open.

- In suctioning infants and children, use a rigid tip but be careful not to touch the back of the airway.

- Limit suctioning to less than 15 seconds at a time.

Chapter Review

SUMMARY

The airway is the passageway by which air enters the body during respiration, or breathing. A patient cannot survive without an open airway. Maintaining an open airway is the first priority of emergency care.

Respiratory failure is inadequate breathing that is insufficient to support life. A patient in respiratory failure or respiratory arrest (complete stoppage of breathing) must receive artificial ventilations.

Airway adjuncts—the oropharyngeal and nasopharyngeal airway—can help keep the airway open during artificial ventilation. It may also be necessary to suction the airway or to use manual techniques to remove fluids and solids from the airway before, during, or after artificial ventilation.

Oxygen can be delivered to the nonbreathing patient as a supplement to artificial ventilation. Oxygen can also be administered as therapy to the breathing patient whose breathing is inadequate, who is cyanotic (blue), cool and clammy, short of breath, suffering chest pain, suffering severe injuries, or displaying an altered mental status.

REVIEWING KEY CONCEPTS

1. Name the major structures of the airway.
2. List the signs of adequate breathing.
3. List the signs of inadequate breathing.
4. Describe the two chief manual methods of opening the airway. Explain the circumstances in which each should be used.
5. Name, in order of preference, the methods the EMT can use to artificially ventilate a patient.
6. Explain how to determine if the artificial ventilations being provided to a patient are adequate or inadequate.
7. Name two airway adjuncts, explain their purpose, and describe when it is appropriate to use each type.
8. Explain how to size the two basic types of airway adjuncts.
9. Describe the purpose of suctioning of the upper airway and explain what equipment is needed for successful suctioning.
10. List the time limits for suctioning attempts and explain why they must be observed.
11. List common conditions for which oxygen is administered to patients.
12. Explain the purpose of the pulse oximeter and list general guidelines for its use.
13. List possible medical and nonmedical hazards associated with oxygen therapy.
14. Describe the characteristics of two common oxygen delivery devices and explain when the use of each is appropriate.
15. Describe differences between the airways of adults and those of infants and children. Explain the implications of these differences on opening and securing the airways of pediatric patients.

RESOURCES TO LEARN MORE

Roberts, J. R. and Hedges, J. R. *Clinical Practices in Emergency Medicine, 3rd Edition.* Philadelphia: W. B. Saunders, 1997.

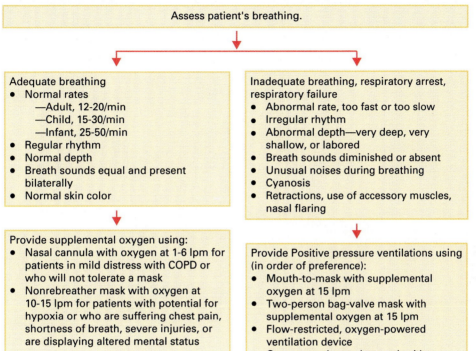

OXYGEN THERAPY GUIDELINES

Assess patient's breathing.

Adequate breathing
- Normal rates
    —Adult, 12-20/min
    —Child, 15-30/min
    —Infant, 25-50/min
- Regular rhythm
- Normal depth
- Breath sounds equal and present bilaterally
- Normal skin color

Inadequate breathing, respiratory arrest, respiratory failure
- Abnormal rate, too fast or too slow
- Irregular rhythm
- Abnormal depth—very deep, very shallow, or labored
- Breath sounds diminished or absent
- Unusual noises during breathing
- Cyanosis
- Retractions, use of accessory muscles, nasal flaring

Provide supplemental oxygen using:
- Nasal cannula with oxygen at 1-6 lpm for patients in mild distress with COPD or who will not tolerate a mask
- Nonrebreather mask with oxygen at 10-15 lpm for patients with potential for hypoxia or who are suffering chest pain, shortness of breath, severe injuries, or are displaying altered mental status

Provide Positive pressure ventilations using (in order of preference):
- Mouth-to-mask with supplemental oxygen at 15 lpm
- Two-person bag-valve mask with supplemental oxygen at 15 lpm
- Flow-restricted, oxygen-powered ventilation device
- One-person bag-valve mask with supplemental oxygen at 15 lpm

Patient Assessment

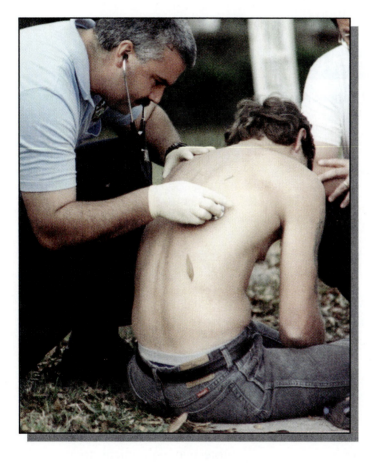

*A*s an EMT, you will provide emergency medical care for sick and injured patients. However, you cannot provide proper care for a patient until you have performed a patient assessment and determined what care he needs. To do this, you must examine and interview the patient. You must also carefully consider the environment in which the patient is found.

SECTION I: An Overview

Patient assessment is a systematic, step-by-step process. In fire suppression, there is a similar, step-by-step assessment of the fire scene called scene size-up. In that assessment, the company officer's priorities are *rescue* followed by *protection of exposures* followed by *fire suppression* and, ultimately, by *overhaul*.

In patient assessment, the EMT performs the steps of *scene size-up* followed by *initial assessment* followed by a *focused history and physical exam* followed by a *detailed physical exam* and continuing with an *ongoing assessment*. This system of patient assessment assures the safety of the EMT first so that he can continue the process. It also assures that the EMT will identify and treat life-threatening conditions immediately as well as identify and evaluate lesser injuries and medical conditions as appropriate.

Table 7-1

Components of Patient Assessment

Scene Size-up
Initial Assessment
Focused History and Physical Examination
Detailed Physical Exam
Ongoing Assessment

Later sections of this chapter will discuss each component of the patient assessment process in depth. First, though, a brief overview will orient you to the steps in the process.

SCENE SIZE-UP

Patient assessment and treatment cannot begin until the EMT's own safety is assured. Thus, **scene size-up** is the first step of the assessment process (Figure 7-1). During the scene size-up, the EMT determines if there are any hazards or potential hazards that could affect his safety or the safety of other crew members and the patient. He then takes steps to eliminate or control those hazards.

It is during scene size-up, for example, that the EMT puts on the appropriate level of personal protective equipment to assure body substance isolation (BSI). The EMT is especially alert at this stage to conditions such as crowd violence, downed power lines, and leaking hazardous materials. Before continuing on with the assessment, the EMT will take steps to assure that such hazards are controlled. For example, he might call for police back-up, assistance from the utility company, or dispatch of the department's or area's hazardous materials team.

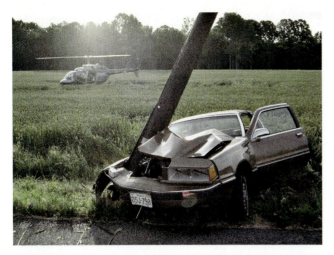

Figure 7-1 During the scene size-up at a motor vehicle crash, you will identify possible hazards and consider the mechanism of injury to the patient.

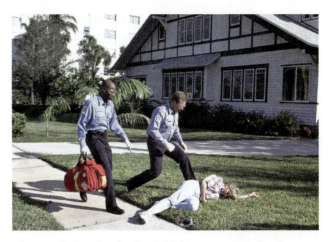

Figure 7-2 Begin the initial assessment by forming a general impression while you approach the patient.

During scene size-up, the EMT will try to determine what caused a trauma patient's injury from physical evidence and the statements of the patient or witnesses. The factors that contribute to an injury are known as the **mechanism of injury (MOI)**. The MOI is an important factor in determining which patients will require stabilization of the spine during initial assessment. With a medical patient, the EMT will attempt to determine the **nature of the illness (NOI)**. In determining this, the EMT will again use statements of the patient, family, or bystanders as well as physical evidence at the scene.

The final stage of the scene size-up requires the EMT to determine if there are adequate resources —ambulances, personnel, specialized equipment —on or en route to the scene to handle the situation. If resources are inadequate, the EMT must request that additional resources be dispatched before moving on to the initial assessment, the next step in the patient assessment process.

INITIAL ASSESSMENT

The chief purpose of the **initial assessment** is for the EMT to discover and immediately treat any life-threatening conditions affecting the patient (Figure 7-2). To achieve this, the EMT should:

◆ Form an overall impression of the patient's condition

◆ Assess the patient's—
　　—Mental status
　　—Airway status
　　—Adequacy of breathing
　　—Circulation status

◆ Treat immediately any life-threatening conditions as soon as they are detected. This may include opening the airway, administering oxygen, providing artificial ventilations, and controlling life-threatening bleeding as appropriate.

◆ Determine the need for expedited versus routine transport of the patient. A patient requiring expedited transport is termed a **priority patient.** Consider requesting advanced life support (ALS) assistance (if it has not been dispatched already) for any priority patient before proceeding to the next assessment step, the focused history and physical exam.

FOCUSED HISTORY AND PHYSICAL EXAMINATION

The purpose of the **focused history and physical examination** is to uncover additional injuries or medical conditions that may also be life threatening. How this step of the patient assessment is carried out will vary depending on whether the patient is a medical or trauma patient. Baseline vital signs and a SAMPLE history are, however, obtained on all patients during this step. Baseline vital signs include the patient's pulse, blood pressure, and respiratory rates, as well as his skin condition. The purpose of the SAMPLE history is to gather data that may reveal the nature of the patient's complaint. Elements of the SAMPLE history include the following:

◆ *S*igns/*S*ymptoms of the present illness

◆ *A*llergies to medications, foods, or environmental factors

◆ *M*edications currently being taken

◆ *P*ertinent past medical history

◆ *L*ast oral intake

◆ *E*vents leading up to the current illness or injury

With the medical patient, the EMT will use the SAMPLE history to determine the signs and symptoms of the present illness as well as the patient's relevant past medical history. The extent of the physical examination performed on the medical patient is largely determined by the patient's signs and symptoms.

With the trauma patient, a careful reconsideration of the mechanism of injury is a key part of this step. A rapid, head-to-toe examination of the patient is also performed to identify and assess injuries. This rapid trauma assessment can be carried out at the scene where the patient is found, unless the scene is hazardous or the patient has been identified as a priority patient during the initial assessment. For the trauma patient, the baseline history and vital signs are obtained after the rapid assessment.

Whenever a patient, either medical or trauma, is identified as a priority patient, then the focused history and physical exam should occur en route to the hospital after essential treatments have been provided.

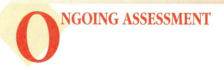

DETAILED PHYSICAL EXAMINATION

The **detailed physical examination** is carried out after life-threatening conditions have been identified and addressed. This detailed, systematic exam usually begins at the patient's head and concludes at his extremities.

The EMT-Basic National Standard Curriculum calls this examination "patient and injury specific." This means that the extent of the detailed physical examination will vary based on the injuries and illnesses of the patients. Indeed, you may never perform a detailed physical examination on some patients. For example, with a patient who has cut the tip of his finger opening a soda can, you would focus your attention on his finger and hand during the focused history and physical exam. Thus, a detailed physical examination would not be necessary. Conversely, with a motorcyclist who has been thrown from his bike at high speed, you would attend to any life-threatening conditions at the scene and then perform a detailed physical exam en route to the hospital. With such a patient, injuries are likely to be extensive, and your examination could reveal important information about them.

In general, the detailed physical examination is more relevant to the assessment of the trauma patient than the medical patient. With a trauma patient, a careful detailed physical examination can provide much more information about injuries than the initial assessment and the rapid trauma assessment reveal. With a medical patient, most relevant physical findings will be identified during the initial assessment, the SAMPLE history, and the rapid, focused medical examination; a detailed physical exam is unlikely to provide more pertinent data.

ONGOING ASSESSMENT

A patient's condition often changes during the time he is in the EMT's care. It may improve or it may deteriorate. For this reason, the **ongoing assessment** (sometimes called *reassessment*) is a crucial part of the patient assessment process. The groundwork for the ongoing assessment is laid during the initial assessment and the focused history and physical exam where the patient's initial, or *baseline,* condition (including vital signs) is established. It is this baseline condition that provides the point of comparison for the EMT during the ongoing assessment.

During the ongoing assessment, the EMT repeats the initial assessment, the taking of vital signs, and relevant portions of the focused examination and compares the results to the patient's baseline condition and vital signs. The EMT also evaluates the patient's response to any care that has been provided. He might, for example, check the effectiveness of bleeding control measures or the adequacy of assisted ventilations.

Stable patients require an ongoing assessment every 15 minutes. Priority patients require re-evaluation at least every 5 minutes because their conditions and their responses to emergency interventions are likely to change rapidly and must be carefully monitored.

SECTION II: Scene Size-up

A proper scene size-up is a crucial first step in providing safe and efficient patient care. Without proper size-up, both the EMT and the patient may be placed at increased risk for serious injury or even death because of failure to recognize scene hazards.

OBJECTIVES

At the completion of this section of the chapter, the EMT-Basic student should be able to meet the following objectives:

Knowledge and Understanding

1. Recognize hazards/potential hazards. (pp. 146–147, 149–152)
2. Describe common hazards found at the scenes of a trauma and a medical patient. (pp. 146–147, 149–152)
3. Determine if a scene is safe to enter. (pp. 146–147, 149–152)
4. Discuss common mechanisms of injury and nature of illnesses. (pp. 152–161)
5. Discuss the reason for identifying the total number of patients at the scene. (pp. 162–163)
6. Explain the reason for identifying the need for additional help or assistance. (pp. 162–163)
7. Explain the rationale for crew members to evaluate scene safety prior to entering. (pp. 146–147, 149–152)
8. Serve as a model for others in explaining how patient situations affect your evaluation of mechanism of injury or illness. (pp. 152–161)

Skills

1. Observe various scenarios and identify potential hazards.

Although the concept of scene size-up is well established in the fire service, it has only recently become a mandatory component of the EMT-B curriculum. As an EMT, your scene size-up will include many of the same components that you are familiar with from the fire scene size-up. As at a fire scene, you will identify special hazards and assure scene safety (Figure 7-3). You will also try at this time to determine the nature of the patient's illness or the mechanism of injury that prompted the initial call for emergency medical assistance. Finally, you will determine the total number of patients and whether adequate resources have been committed to the scene.

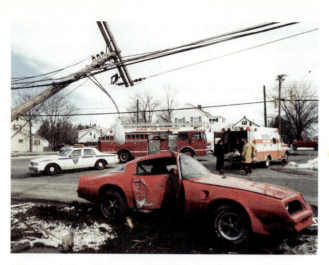

Figure 7-3 The emergency scene can present hazards for rescuers as well as patients.

DISPATCH INFORMATION

Scene size-up can often begin even before you arrive on the scene. Properly trained emergency dispatchers can assist in the process by gathering valuable information from the initial caller, the first-arriving law enforcement personnel, and other sources. The dispatcher should routinely tell responding EMS units the number of patients involved in an incident, any obvious scene hazards, and whether extrication is required. Many dispatchers are trained to evaluate this information and direct appropriate additional units to the scene.

The dispatcher should be particularly careful to determine whether crime scenes or scenes involving behavioral emergencies have been made safe by law enforcement agencies, thus allowing the EMT to proceed into the scene. If for any reason the dispatcher determines the scene is unsafe for EMS, then the responding EMS units should be **staged,** or held, outside the scene until the scene is made safe. In some situations such as fires or hazardous materials incidents, it may be your unit's responsibility both to make the scene safe and to provide patient care.

Remember, however, that the dispatcher is not at the scene himself. He is passing on information that was given to him. That information may be incorrect or incomplete. Also, conditions at the scene may have changed since the dispatcher received the call. Use the dispatch information to prepare for the initial call, but be ready to evaluate the scene yourself.

SCENE SAFETY

Any time you are called to assist a patient, the scene may be hazardous. Sometimes the hazards will be obvious—a building collapse or fighting between rival gangs. At other times, the hazards may be harder to detect—a downed power line at a motor vehicle crash or the contagious disease with which a patient is infected.

As an EMT, you must think seriously about potential hazards during any response and at every scene. Consider not just your own safety but the safety of your patient(s) and bystanders as well. A traditional fire service teaching is to think of the safety of yourself first, your partner second, and then of everybody else. Although the fire service has always rewarded heroism, at no time should you carelessly risk your own personal safety to care for a patient. *You do your patient no good if you too become a victim.*

With these points in mind, you can help assure scene safety in many ways:

◆ *Use the information provided by your dispatcher.* If you are instructed to stage, follow the dispatcher's directions. If it is obvious from the dispatch information or your first view of the scene that additional units will be needed, request dispatch of those units.

◆ *Observe! Keep your eyes open at all times.* Be careful approaching every scene. Scan for hazards such as downed power lines, fuel spills, armed or violent people, or unleashed dogs.

Once on scene, be alert to your environment. Note unstable surfaces such as slopes, ice, and mud. Observe the people around you, being alert for signs of family or crowd hostility.

◆ *Listen! Keep your ears open at all times.* Listen for the sirens of other approaching emergency units as you near the scene.

Once on the scene, listen carefully for sounds of potential violence such as shouting, gun shots, or breaking glass. Be alert to the "hiss" of escaping gases or the "hum" of high-voltage electricity.

◆ *Always assume the worst.* If you identify a hazard or suspect that one may exist, assume the worst danger that the hazard could present is real and act accordingly. For example, assume that all downed power lines are still energized and keep a safe distance from them. Assume that all spilled fuel has the potential to ignite and assure that a charged hose line is ready.

◆ *If you determine a scene is unsafe, make it safe.* If you have been trained in control of a hazard—fire, hazardous materials, fuel spill, etc.—then act to make the scene safe. If you haven't been trained in control of a hazard—a hostage situation, a violent psychiatric patient, etc.—do not enter the scene but instead stage outside it. Then immediately request the dispatch of appropriately trained personnel who can make the scene safe to enter (Figure 7-4).

Body Substance Isolation (BSI)

The proper use of personal protective equipment (PPE) should be part of scene safety on every call. Proper use of this gear will assure body substance isolation to prevent the spread of infectious diseases. The level of BSI required—gloves, eye protection, mask, gown—will be based on the patient's injuries or condition. (BSI precautions and use of PPE are discussed in detail in Chapter 3, "Infection Control and Body Substance Isolation"; you may wish to review that material at this time.)

Dispatch information can give you some idea of the level of BSI that will be needed before you arrive on the scene. In EMS systems that use an emergency priority dispatching system, the dispatcher will always determine whether the bleeding is currently controlled or not. The dispatcher may also be able to learn if a patient has an infectious disease. If the dispatcher can tell you that a patient may have tuberculosis, you can get your N-95 or HEPA respirator ready for use. Whenever dispatch information indicates that specific BSI precautions are required, prepare that equipment while en route to the scene if possible.

Once on the scene, you should always "dress for the occasion" when it comes to BSI. If you discover a patient with spurting, uncontrolled bleeding during the scene size-up, you should be aware that the possibility of coming into contact with his blood is high. That means you should dress for maximum protection with gloves, a mask, eye protection, and a gown or garment impervious to blood. If, on the other hand, the scene size-up reveals a patient with minor bleeding from an elbow abrasion, then gloves may be the only PPE necessary

Personal Safety of the EMT

In addition to blood and body fluids, you may face many other potential on-scene hazards. Some hazardous scenes that EMTs often encounter are discussed below. Remember that on these scenes—and on any others you are called to—you should be prepared to identify the hazards that are present. Identify a danger zone at the scene (Figure 7-5). Then you should take steps to make the scene safe in spite of the hazards. If you are not properly trained to do this, you must request that appropriate resources be dispatched to make the scene safe.

Finally, keep in mind that conditions at a "safe" scene can suddenly change, making the scene hazardous. When on a call then, you must always be alert not only to determine if it is safe

Figure 7-4 Don't hesitate to request additional resources if they are needed to make a scene safe. For example, law enforcement personnel should control traffic at emergency scenes.

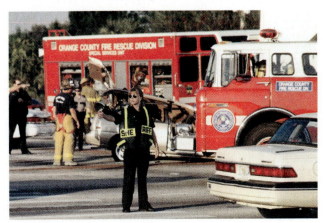

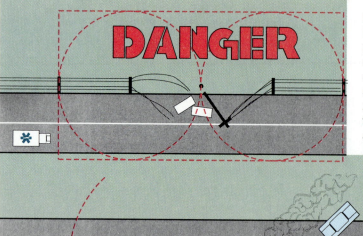

Downed Lines

In accidents involving downed electrical wires and damaged utility poles, the danger zone should extend beyond each intact pole for a full span and to the sides for the distance that the severed wires can reach. Stay out of the danger zone until the utility company has deactivated the wires, or until trained rescuers have moved and anchored them.

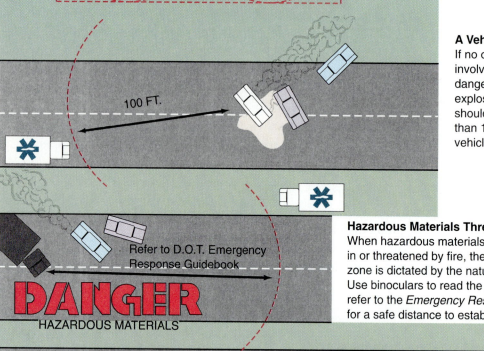

A Vehicle on Fire

If no other hazards are involved–hazards such as dangerous chemicals or explosives–the ambulance should be parked no closer than 100 feet from a burning vehicle.

Hazardous Materials Threatened by Fire

When hazardous materials are either involved in or threatened by fire, the size of the danger zone is dictated by the nature of the materials. Use binoculars to read the placard on the truck and refer to the *Emergency Response Guidebook* for a safe distance to establish your command post.

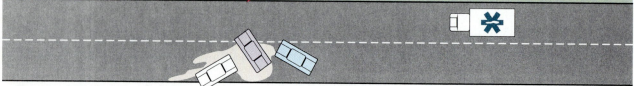

Spilled Fuel The ambulance should be parked uphill from flowing fuel. If this is not possible, the vehicle should be parked as far from the fuel flow as possible, avoiding gutters, ditches, and gullies that may carry the spill to the parking site. Remember, your ambulance's catalytic converter is an ignition source with a temperature over 1000 degrees F.

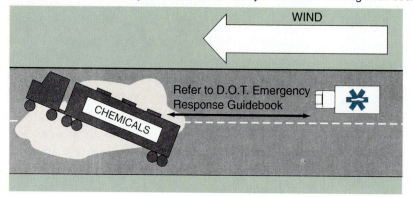

Hazardous Materials

Leaking containers of dangerous chemicals may produce a health as well as a fire hazard. When chemicals have been spilled, whether fumes are evident or not, the ambulance should be parked upwind. If the hazardous material is known, seek advice from experts through the dispatcher or CHEMTREC.

Figure 7-5 At hazardous scenes, establish a danger zone and stay out of it until the scene is secure.

to approach the patient but also to see that the scene remains safe.

Crime Scenes

Almost all crime scenes to which EMTs are called have the potential for violence. Included are scenes of shooting, stabbings, or domestic disputes. An EMT should never enter a crime scene until it has been secured by a law enforcement agency (Figure 7-6). Responding EMS units should be staged a safe distance from the scene until they are advised that the scene is safe to enter.

Motor Vehicle Crash Scenes

Crash scenes are filled with potential hazards such as broken glass, sharp metal, fuel spills, fire, and downed power lines. Many of these hazards may be present at the same scene. Often the assistance of several agencies and multiple units is required to make a scene safe.

Approach all motor vehicle crashes carefully. The risk that an ambulance or other piece of responding apparatus might accidentally run over a crash victim—or another rescuer—as it enters the scene is quite real.

Always observe some basic rules before attempting to aid a patient still trapped in the wreckage of a vehicle. One of the most important is assuring that the vehicles involved in the crash are properly stabilized before patient care begins.

You will learn more about reaching and assisting patients involved in crashes in Chapter 26.

Another way of avoiding injuries at a crash scene is through use of proper personal protective equipment. This includes turnout gear, heavy leather gloves, protective eyewear, and a helmet. In addition, the use of bright reflective trim or gear at night (Figure 7-7A) or colorful bibs during the day (Figure 7-7B) can be a life-saver for the rescuer at the crash scene, greatly reducing the risk of being struck by a passing vehicle. If the hazards of passing traffic pose too great a threat to rescuers, then Command should assure that the road is shut down to civilian traffic to make the scene safe.

Figure 7-7 **A.** Gear should have reflective trim for nighttime operations. **B.** Colorful bibs make rescue personnel more visible during daytime operations.

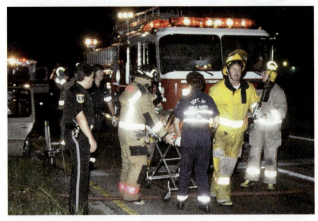

A.
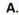

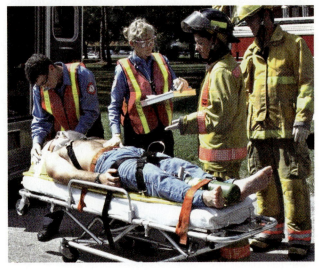

B.

Figure 7-6 Enter a crime scene or a potential crime scene only after it has been secured by law enforcement personnel.

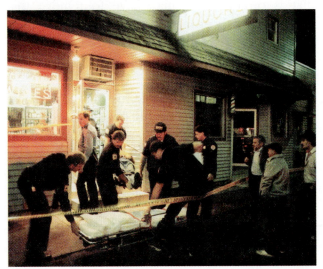

Hazardous and Toxic Materials

Hazardous and toxic materials may be present at any emergency scene. Sometimes their presence may have caused the emergency. At other times, they represent a potential threat that may become real if caution is not used. Sometimes their presence is obvious—a leaking tanker truck that has placards warning "CORROSIVE." At other times, the threat is more subtle—in a home kitchen where a helpful teenager's attempt to make a "super" cleaning solution by mixing ammonia and bleach has instead created a poisonous gas.

If it is known at the time of dispatch that the call involves a hazardous or toxic substance, a hazardous materials, or "hazmat," team should also be dispatched. Arriving EMS units should stage until they are cleared to enter the scene.

In some situations, the first-arriving EMTs may discover the presence of hazardous materials during the scene size-up. In calls involving trucks, vans, or railroad cars, always check the vehicles for placards indicating that hazardous materials are on board. The U.S. Department of Transportation requires such placards (Figure 7-8). In crashes involving tractor trailers without placards, always try to determine what the cargo is. You may be able to do this either by asking the driver or by checking the shipping manifest.

Keep in mind that toxic materials can cause multiple casualties in unexpected settings such as office buildings or factories. Whenever you are called to the scene of a medical emergency where multiple patients share the same complaints, assume that hazardous materials may be involved. For example, you are dispatched to an office building for a single patient who is complaining of headache, nausea, and weakness. Upon arrival, you size up the scene and discover that a dozen of his co-workers share the same complaints. This is a common scenario for carbon monoxide poisoning caused by a heating system malfunction. This scene is obviously unsafe and you, too, are at risk for becoming ill from the gas. Rapidly evacuate the patients—it may be necessary to don self-contained breathing apparatus (SCBA)—and call for additional units to help care for the multiple patients and to make the scene safe.

(Responses to calls involving hazardous materials will be discussed at greater length in Chapter 28, "EMS Special Operations.")

Natural Hazards

Natural hazards such as unstable surfaces (ice, mud, slopes, running water, etc.), extremes of weather (heat, cold, wind, snow), and dangerous animals (dogs, snakes, scorpions, spiders) are common causes of injury and illness. When performing a scene size-up, always keep in mind that the environmental conditions that disabled the patient can also threaten your well being (Figure 7-9). Although there is little you can do to alter the environment, there are steps you can take to make a scene involving natural hazards as safe as possible.

If necessary, request that specialized teams—water rescue, confined space, and high-angle rescue, for example—be dispatched to the scene. In cases of severe weather, remove yourself and the patient from exposure to the elements as quickly as possible. Do this even if it means making transport of the patient from the scene a higher priority than it would be under better weather conditions.

Patient Safety

Taking steps to assure the safety of the patient is also part of the scene size-up. Be on the alert for conditions that pose an immediate threat to a patient's life. As you will learn in later chapters, it may be necessary to rapidly remove patients from the dangers of such scenes. At one scene you may find a badly injured patient unconscious in a car that is on fire. You may have to remove that patient from the car without taking all the precautions you normally would to avoid aggravating a potential spinal injury (see Chapter 22, "Head and Spine Injuries").

As you size-up the scene, try also to think of what may have happened before you arrived. If you are called to treat a patient found outdoors in extreme weather (heat, cold, rain, etc.), consider how long the patient may have been exposed to those conditions before your arrival. Take, for example, a call to help a patient with a broken leg who fell while taking out the garbage. If the temperature was in the teens and the patient was

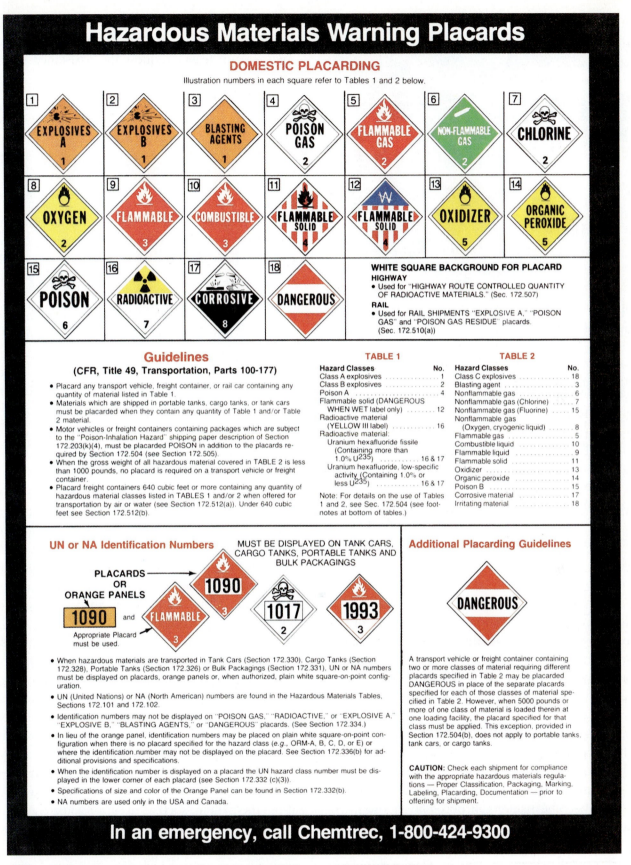

Hazardous Materials Warning Placards

DOMESTIC PLACARDING

Illustration numbers in each square refer to Tables 1 and 2 below.

1 EXPLOSIVES A — 1	2 EXPLOSIVES B — 1	3 BLASTING AGENTS — 1	4 POISON GAS — 2	5 FLAMMABLE GAS — 2	6 NON-FLAMMABLE GAS — 2	7 CHLORINE — 2
8 OXYGEN — 2	9 FLAMMABLE — 3	10 COMBUSTIBLE — 3	11 FLAMMABLE SOLID — 4	12 FLAMMABLE SOLID W — 4	13 OXIDIZER — 5	14 ORGANIC PEROXIDE — 5
15 POISON — 6	16 RADIOACTIVE — 7	17 CORROSIVE — 8	18 DANGEROUS			

WHITE SQUARE BACKGROUND FOR PLACARD

HIGHWAY
- Used for "HIGHWAY ROUTE CONTROLLED QUANTITY OF RADIOACTIVE MATERIALS." (Sec. 172.507)

RAIL
- Used for RAIL SHIPMENTS "EXPLOSIVE A," "POISON GAS" and "POISON GAS RESIDUE" placards. (Sec. 172.510(a))

Guidelines
(CFR, Title 49, Transportation, Parts 100-177)

- Placard any transport vehicle, freight container, or rail car containing any quantity of material listed in Table 1.
- Materials which are shipped in portable tanks, cargo tanks, or tank cars must be placarded when they contain any quantity of Table 1 and/or Table 2 material.
- Motor vehicles or freight containers containing packages which are subject to the "Poison-Inhalation Hazard" shipping paper description of Section 172.203(k)(4), must be placarded POISON in addition to the placards required by Section 172.504 (see Section 172.505).
- When the gross weight of all hazardous material covered in TABLE 2 is less than 1000 pounds, no placard is required on a transport vehicle or freight container.
- Placard freight containers 640 cubic feet or more containing any quantity of hazardous material classes listed in TABLES 1 and/or 2 when offered for transportation by air or water (see Section 172.512(a)). Under 640 cubic feet see Section 172.512(b).

TABLE 1

Hazard Classes	No.
Class A explosives	1
Class B explosives	2
Poison A	4
Flammable solid (DANGEROUS WHEN WET label only)	12
Radioactive material (YELLOW III label)	16
Radioactive material: Uranium hexafluoride fissile (Containing more than 1.0% U235)	16 & 17
Uranium hexafluoride, low-specific activity (Containing 1.0% or less U235)	16 & 17

Note: For details on the use of Tables 1 and 2, see Sec. 172.504 (see footnotes at bottom of tables.)

TABLE 2

Hazard Classes	No.
Class C explosives	18
Blasting agent	3
Nonflammable gas	6
Nonflammable gas (Chlorine)	7
Nonflammable gas (Fluorine)	15
Nonflammable gas (Oxygen, cryogenic liquid)	8
Flammable gas	5
Combustible liquid	10
Flammable liquid	9
Flammable solid	11
Oxidizer	13
Organic peroxide	14
Poison B	15
Corrosive material	17
Irritating material	18

UN or NA Identification Numbers

MUST BE DISPLAYED ON TANK CARS, CARGO TANKS, PORTABLE TANKS AND BULK PACKAGINGS

PLACARDS OR ORANGE PANELS

1090 and FLAMMABLE 3 — 1090 3 — 1017 2 — 1993 3

Appropriate Placard must be used.

- When hazardous materials are transported in Tank Cars (Section 172.330), Cargo Tanks (Section 172.328), Portable Tanks (Section 172.326) or Bulk Packagings (Section 172.331), UN or NA numbers must be displayed on placards, orange panels or, when authorized, plain white square-on-point configuration.
- UN (United Nations) or NA (North American) numbers are found in the Hazardous Materials Tables, Sections 172.101 and 172.102.
- Identification numbers may not be displayed on "POISON GAS," "RADIOACTIVE," or "EXPLOSIVE A," "EXPLOSIVE B," "BLASTING AGENTS," or "DANGEROUS" placards. (See Section 172.334.)
- In lieu of the orange panel, identification numbers may be placed on plain white square-on-point configuration when there is no placard specified for the hazard class (e.g., ORM-A, B, C, D, or E) or where the identification number may not be displayed on the placard. See Section 172.336(b) for additional provisions and specifications.
- When the identification number is displayed on a placard the UN hazard class number must be displayed in the lower corner of each placard (see Section 172.332 (c)(3)).
- Specifications of size and color of the Orange Panel can be found in Section 172.332(b).
- NA numbers are used only in the USA and Canada.

Additional Placarding Guidelines

DANGEROUS

A transport vehicle or freight container containing two or more classes of material requiring different placards specified in Table 2 may be placarded DANGEROUS in place of the separate placards specified for each of those classes of material specified in Table 2. However, when 5000 pounds or more of one class of material is loaded therein at one loading facility, the placard specified for that class must be applied. This exception, provided in Section 172.504(b), does not apply to portable tanks, tank cars, or cargo tanks.

CAUTION: Check each shipment for compliance with the appropriate hazardous materials regulations — Proper Classification, Packaging, Marking, Labeling, Placarding, Documentation — prior to offering for shipment.

In an emergency, call Chemtrec, 1-800-424-9300

Figure 7-8 The U.S. Department of Transportation requires warning placards on vehicles carrying hazardous materials.

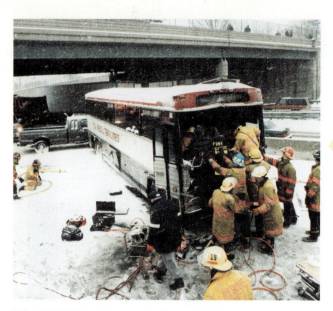

Figure 7-9 Environmental conditions can cause and then complicate rescue operations.

lightly dressed and had gone unnoticed for a long time, exposure to the cold may present a greater threat to his life than the broken leg. You must think about how such conditions can affect the patient during your scene size-up.

In balancing the need to make the scene safe for both yourself and the patient, remember that your personal safety comes first. When your safety is assured, you can then provide better patient care.

Bystander Safety

You may at times have to assure the safety of on-lookers at emergency scenes. Crowds often gather to watch the "action" at fire scenes, exposing themselves to the dangers of drifting smoke and falling debris. Bystanders will cluster at motor vehicle crashes, blocking the access of emergency vehicles while putting themselves at risk of being hit by passing traffic.

Whenever possible, you should take steps during the scene size-up to assure that bystanders do not become patients. If necessary, request the dispatch of law enforcement personnel to the scene to provide crowd control. You and your crew can also keep bystanders from getting too close to the scene by using barrier tape, road-blocks, or public address systems. If bystanders are interfering with your work, they should be asked, politely but firmly, to leave the scene. If they do not leave, request the assistance of law enforcement personnel.

SCENE ASSESSMENT

Once you have assured safety at the scene, the next step is to assess the scene and its surroundings. Doing this will provide information relevant to the patient care you provide. For a call involving a medical emergency, you will quickly determine the nature of the illness that prompted the call for EMS assistance. When the call involves trauma, you will quickly assess the mechanism of injury to determine how the patient was hurt. During scene assessment, you must also determine the total number of patients involved and whether resources adequate to handle them have been dispatched to the scene.

Nature of Illness

Simply stated, the nature of the illness is what condition(s) a medical patient is suffering from. Often the emergency medical dispatcher can tell you the nature of a patient's illness when you are sent out on a call. In such cases, you should confirm from the patient, family members or bystanders that the dispatch information which you received was correct.

Usually, most of the information about the nature of the illness will be gathered directly from the patient. In doing this, you will rely heavily on the patient's **chief complaint.** This is a statement, in the patient's own words, of the reason that EMS was called to the scene. For example, a patient's chief complaint might be "I can't breathe" or "My chest hurts" or "I'm vomiting blood." During scene assessment, you should also note obvious facts about the patient, such as his approximate age and the level of his distress. You will continuously gather information throughout the phases of the assessment process, including the initial patient assessment and the focused history and physical exam.

At times, you will encounter patients who are unresponsive or unable to answer questions. In such cases, you may have to question family members or bystanders to discover the nature of illness.

Mechanism of Injury

Whenever you are called to assist a trauma patient, you must attempt to determine the mechanism of injury (MOI) as part of the scene size-up. The mechanism of injury is what physically caused the patient to become injured. Examples of mechanisms of injury include motor vehicle crashes, falls, and shootings.

Determining the mechanism of injury is important for two reasons. The first reason involves scene safety. The mechanism of injury that caused trauma to the patient may still pose a threat to you on the scene. Determining the mechanism of injury will help you assure that the scene is truly safe.

The second reason for determining MOI involves patient care. Many mechanisms of injury produce predictable patterns of injury. Knowing the mechanisms and the injuries they produce can help you provide proper prehospital care. Information about the MOI passed along to the emergency department physician will also help assure the highest level of hospital care.

Often, the mechanism of injury may be obvious, as when you are called to a scene where a car has gone through a guardrail and down an embankment or where a patient has fallen from a ladder while painting a house. At other times, the mechanism of injury is not immediately apparent. In such case, you must question the patient, family members, or bystanders and study the physical evidence to determine what happened.

Trauma is frequently separated into two general categories—blunt and penetrating. Examples of blunt trauma include falls and motor vehicle crashes. Shootings, impalements, and stabbings are considered penetrating trauma.

Blunt Trauma

Certain principles of physics govern the mechanisms of injury that produce blunt trauma. When you think about your own experiences with injuries, the following should seem logical.

◆ *Force is a function of mass (size) and velocity (speed).* The bigger something is and the faster it is moving, the greater the force that is created.

◆ *The greater the force acting on a person the greater the potential for injury.* Consider some real-life examples. The injuries to a pedestrian who is struck by a bicycle traveling at 15 miles (24 km) per hour with a 140-pound (64-kg) teenager aboard would tend to be less severe than those that would result if the pedestrian were struck by a 3,000 lb. (1,360 kg) car traveling at 40 miles (64 km) per hour. Similarly, a person who falls 30 feet (10 m) from a roof builds up more speed and is likely to be more severely injured than a person who falls 4 feet (1.4 m) from a step ladder.

◆ *Anything that is moving contains a certain amount of energy.* When the moving object collides with something, that energy of motion is either absorbed by the object or passed along to what the object strikes. For example, when a person falls off a ladder and suddenly stops by hitting the ground, the energy generated in the fall travels back through the person causing injuries. When a moving car strikes a pedestrian, however, the car absorbs a relatively small amount of energy (as in a dented hood). Far more of the energy is passed along to and acts on the pedestrian, resulting in multiple injuries (Figure 7-10).

Certain mechanisms of injury tend to produce predictable patterns of injury. You should be on the lookout for these mechanisms and their related injury patterns as you conduct your scene size-up.

Motor Vehicle Crashes EMS providers have traditionally referred to motor vehicle crashes as "motor vehicle accidents" or "MVAs." Medical research and police investigations have demonstrated, however, that MVAs are very rarely "accidents." Instead, most crashes result from preventable, non-accidental factors such as driving while intoxicated, driving at an unsafe speed, and

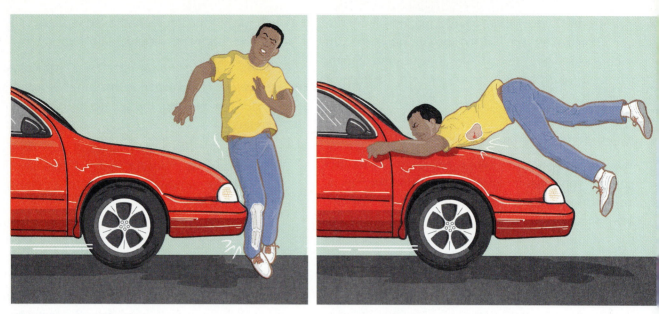

Figure 7-10 The forces that may act on pedestrians in pedestrian vs. vehicle collisions.

following too closely. For this reason, experts in injury prevention now recommend that the term "motor vehicle accident" or MVA no longer be used and that it be replaced with the term "motor vehicle crash" or MVC.

A key to understanding the mechanisms of injury involved in MVCs is to realize that every crash actually results in *three* distinct collisions (Figure 7-11). In the first collision, the car strikes an object such as a tree. In the second collision, the patient's body strikes the vehicle's interior. In the third and final collision, the patient's internal organs strike surfaces within the body. Although this triple-impact pattern is common in MVCs, there are several types of crashes that result in even more specific patterns of patient injury.

◆ **Head-on crashes.** These crashes are the most likely to result in patient death. Upon impact, the occupant is thrown forward as the vehicle suddenly decelerates below him. Two injury patterns are especially common in head-on crashes (Figure 7-12). In the *up-and-over pattern,* the unrestrained occupant is projected forward, over the steering wheel and into the windshield. Injuries to the head, neck, chest, and abdomen are likely to result. In the *down-and-under pattern,* the unrestrained occupant is projected forward, but under the

steering wheel. Injuries to the hips, knees, and legs are common with this pattern. In both patterns, injuries result from impact with structures in front of the occupant such as the dashboard, steering wheel, and windshield (Figure 7-13). Seat belts (when worn) and airbags are especially helpful in reducing injuries during head on collisions.

◆ **Rear-end collisions.** A patient in a vehicle that is rear-ended is subjected to a sudden backward force as the vehicle accelerates beneath him. These crashes often result in neck, head, and chest injuries (Figures 7-14 and 7-15).

The integrity of the vehicle's seat and headrest play an important role in reducing rear-end mechanism injuries. In the photo shown in Figure 7-16, the front seats of the mini-van failed, collapsing backwards. The two occupants were thrown through the interior of the vehicle striking their heads on the tailgate (note blood on cargo deck).

The occupant of the rear-ended vehicle may receive additional, "head-on" type injuries if his car is pushed into additional vehicles or objects. This "battering ram" effect is evident in the fatal crash shown in Figure 7-17.

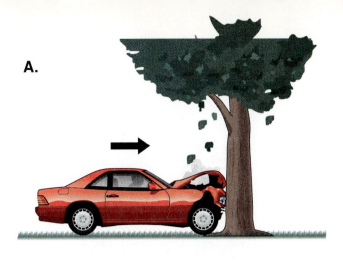

A.

B.

C.

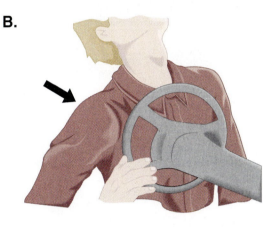

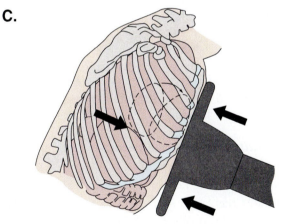

Figure 7-11 There are three collisions in a motor vehicle crash. **A.** The vehicle strikes an object. **B.** The person's body strikes the vehicle's interior. **C.** The person's organs strike the interior surfaces of the body.

A.

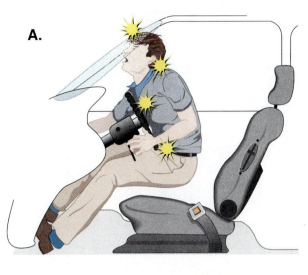

B.

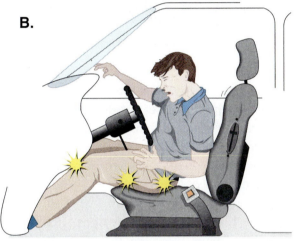

Figure 7-12 Injury patterns in head-on collisions. **A.** The up-and-over pathway is likely to cause head, neck, chest, and abdominal injuries. **B.** The down-and-under pathway is likely to cause hip, knee, and leg injuries.

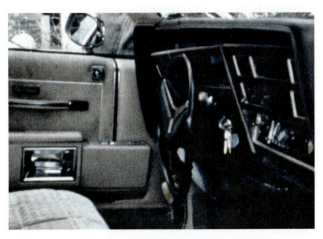

Figure 7-13 Suspect serious injury when you observe a steering wheel that has been deformed, a common occurrence in head-on crashes.

◆ ***Side-impact collisions.*** Most automobiles offer little protection against side-impact collisions (Figure 7-18). During size-up, it is important to determine whether the patient was seated on the same side as the impact or on

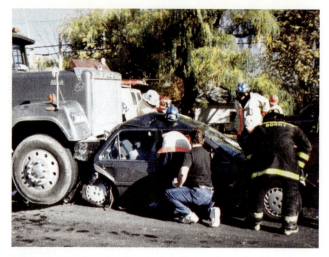

Figure 7-14 A rear-end collision between a truck and a small car.

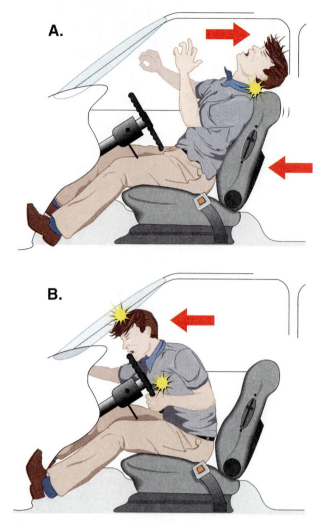

Figure 7-15 Injury patterns in rear-end collisions. The unrestrained passenger's head is **(A)** jerked violently backward and then **(B)** forward causing neck, head, and chest injuries.

the opposite side. Patients seated on the same side as the impact can suffer significant head, neck, chest, abdominal, and pelvic trauma, more so than patients seated on the opposite side (Figure 7-19). Another factor in such collisions is that the occupant's head tends to remain stiff while the body is pushed laterally. This results in neck injuries. Side-impact airbags have recently been introduced by some auto makers to provide additional protection in these crashes.

◆ *Rollover collisions.* Rollover collisions can cause multiple injuries (Figure 7-20). This is especially true if the patient is not using a seat belt because he will sustain multiple impacts as the vehicle rolls. Even patients wearing seatbelts can receive serious injuries if the vehicle's roof collapses while the car is inverted (Figure 7-21).

◆ *Ejections from vehicles.* Patients thrown from a vehicle during a crash can sustain injuries at any or all of three different times: when inside the vehicle before being ejected; upon impact after ejection; and upon being struck by the same or another vehicle after impact. Because of this complex mechanism of injury, patients ejected from vehicles are always considered high-priority trauma patients.

◆ *Fatality in the same vehicle.* Evaluate carefully any patient found in the same vehicle in which another person has been killed. Such a patient has been subjected to the same forces that killed the other occupant. This means that the chances the patient has received life-threatening injuries are increased.

◆ *Seatbelts and airbags.* Efforts to make automobiles safer have led to many design innovations over the years. Seat belts and airbags are two of the best-known. These devices have greatly reduced the incidence of death and serious injury in MVCs. Yet in certain cases, both seat belts and airbags can themselves produce injuries. Always consider these

(text continues, page 159)

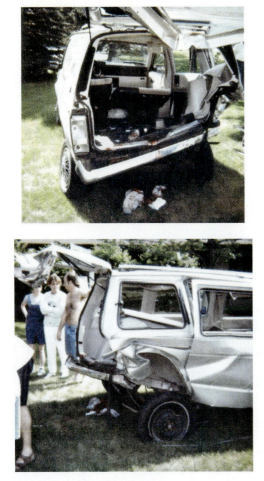

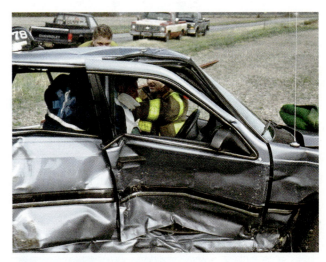

Figure 7-18 A side-impact collision.

Figure 7-16 The seats failed when this mini-van was rear-ended, and its occupants were propelled backward through the vehicle. Note the blood on the cargo deck in the top photo.

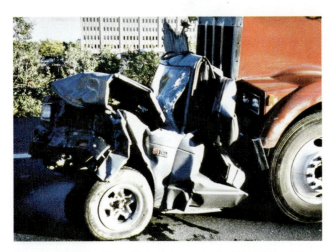

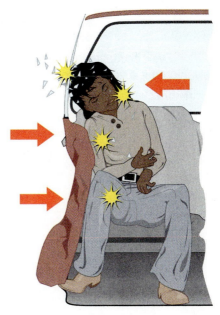

Figure 7-19 Side-impact collisions may cause head and neck injuries, as well as injuries to the chest, abdomen, pelvis, and thighs.

Figure 7-17 The "battering-ram" effect in a fatal rear-end collision.

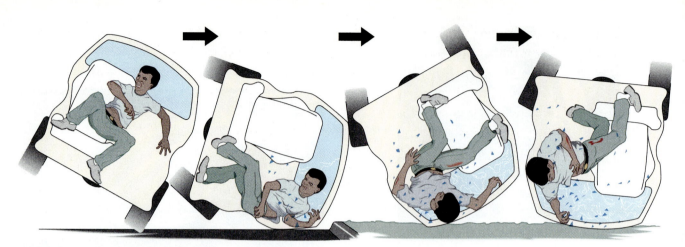

Figure 7-20 In a rollover collision, the unrestrained passenger will suffer multiple impacts and injuries.

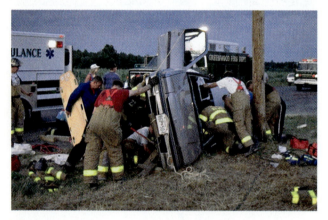

Figure 7-21 Even occupants using restraints may be seriously injured if a vehicle's roof is collapsed during a rollover.

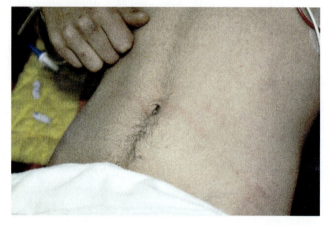

Figure 7-22 Suspect the possibility of serious injuries if you observe lap-belt bruises like these during your assessment of a patient.

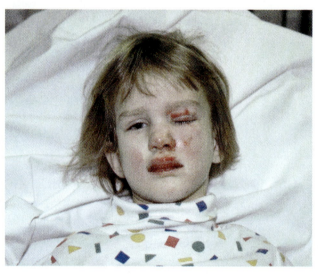

Figure 7-23 This child suffered facial injuries when a passenger-side airbag deployed.

devices when evaluating the mechanism of injury for a patient injured in an MVC.

Although shoulder and lap belts are now standard in cars, older models may have only lap belts, especially in the rear seats. When used alone, lap belts may cause both internal and spinal injuries, especially during head-on collisions. If you observe lap-belt bruising across a patient's abdomen, be alert to the possibility of serious injuries (Figure 7-22).

Steering column and dashboard airbags deploy when a car's front bumper impacts an object. These devices have been very effective in reducing injuries during collisions. However, airbags can cause serious injury—even death—to children in the front seat (Figure 7-23). Especially at risk are infants in rear-facing car seats. In these cases, the force of the airbag deployment propels the car seat and the infant backward into the vehicle's seat (Figure 7-24). Children and small adults riding in the front seat can also suffer severe facial and head injuries when air bags deploy. These injuries occur because air bags are designed to cushion the chests of larger adults. With children and shorter adults, airbags tend to deploy directly in their faces. It is currently recommended that no child under 12 years old ride in the front seat of a vehicle with a passenger-side airbag.

Penetrating Trauma Penetrating trauma results when an object passes through body tissue. Penetrating trauma is often categorized by the speed, or velocity, of the object that passed through the skin (Table 7-2).

Table 7-2	
Classification of Penetrating Trauma by Velocity	
Velocity Category	**Examples of Trauma**
Low	Stabbed by knife Struck by arrow Impaled by fence post
Medium	Shot with handgun or shotgun
High	Shot with assault rifle or high-powered rifle

Figure 7-24 A deploying airbag can propel a child safety seat back into the vehicle's seat, seriously injuring the child secured in it.

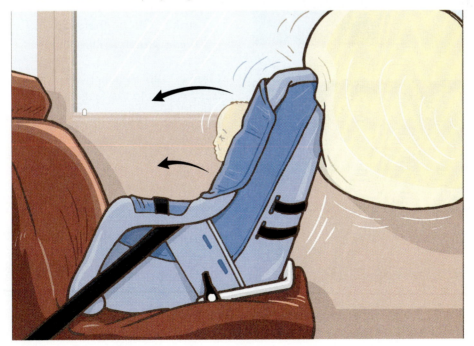

When determining the mechanism of injury in cases of penetrating trauma, remember that the first priority in scene size-up is your personal safety. Most penetrating traumas are the result of violence. Do not enter the scene until it has been made safe by the police.

A bullet can produce especially damaging penetrating injuries. In fact, it can cause damage in two ways:

◆ *The bullet itself damages anything it contacts as it passes through the body.* This type of damage varies depending upon the size of the bullet, whether or not the bullet breaks into fragments, and the course the bullet follows through the body. A bullet can easily be deflected once it enters the body and may damage tissue in unexpected areas.

◆ *The bullet produces a pressure wave as it passes through body tissue.* This pressure wave can damage tissues and organs not physically struck by the bullet itself.

Never underestimate the seriousness of penetrating trauma to the head, neck, torso, or proximal extremities. The entry wound you detect may be small, but the internal damage may rapidly lead to the patient's death (Figure 7-25).

Blast Injuries

Blast injuries occur when a patient is subjected to an explosion and the debris it generates (Figure 7-26). Blast injuries are common in combat situations. They can also occur in civilian settings as a result of explosions of fireworks, grain elevators, industrial plants, or terrorist bombs. Several different mechanisms of injury are at work in the primary, secondary, and tertiary types of blast injuries (Figure 7-27).

◆ *Primary blast injuries* result when the patient is subjected to the sudden change in environmental pressure created by the blast wave. Hollow organs, like the lungs and bowels, and fluid-filled organs, like the eyes and bladder, can rupture as a result of the blast wave strike. Often, there are no external signs of these primary phase injuries.

Figure 7-25 Damage caused by a bullet wound. **A.** Entry wound in the upper arm. **B.** The bullet exited the upper arm and entered the chest.

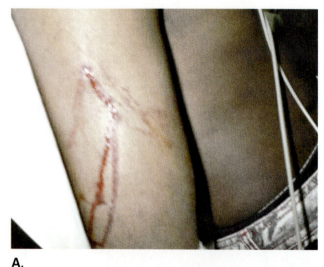

A.

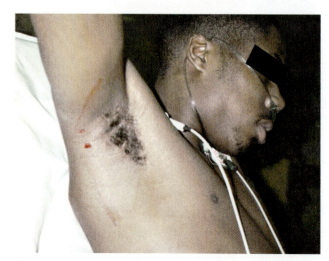

B.

Figure 7-26 Patient with primary and secondary blast injuries to the face as well as facial burns.

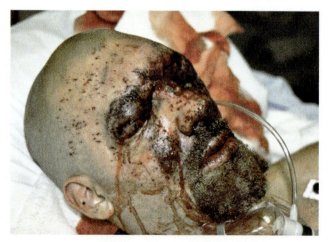

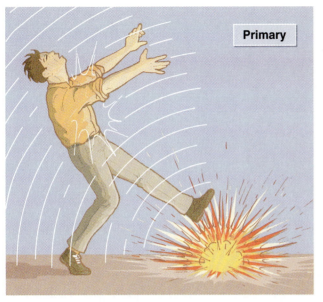

Primary

A.

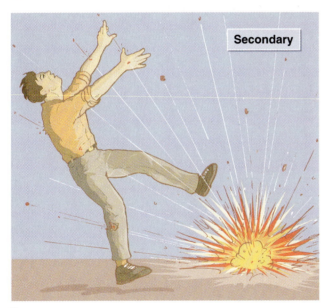

Secondary

B.

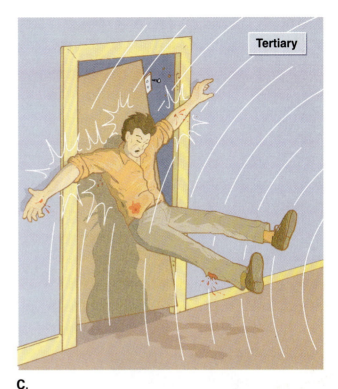

Tertiary

C.

Figure 7-27 Mechanisms of blast injury. **A.** Primary blast injuries are caused by the blast wave. **B.** Secondary blast injuries are caused by flying debris. **C.** Tertiary blast injuries are caused when the patient, who has been propelled by the blast, comes into contact with the ground or some object.

◆ *Secondary blast injuries* result when the patient is struck by flying debris propelled by the explosion. The wounds produced can include medium-velocity penetrating trauma, lacerations, fractures, and burns. These injuries are usually more obvious than those produced by the primary type.

◆ *Tertiary blast injuries* result when a patient is picked up and thrown by the blast wave. The injuries occur when the patient impacts a stationary object like a door frame or the ground. The injuries produced are similar to those seen in a patient ejected from a vehicle in a crash.

Some authorities consider the burns or the effects of heated gases that result from blasts to be *quarternary* or *miscellaneous blast injuries.*

Falls

Falls are one of the most common mechanisms of injury (Figure 7-28). The trauma that results from them will vary depending on the height a person fell from, the surface on which he landed, and the part of the body that first came in contact with the surface. Falls from greater than 20 feet (6 m) should be considered severe with adults. Falls from 10 feet (3 m) or more should be considered severe in children. Internal organ damage and spinal injuries are commonly associated with falls from height.

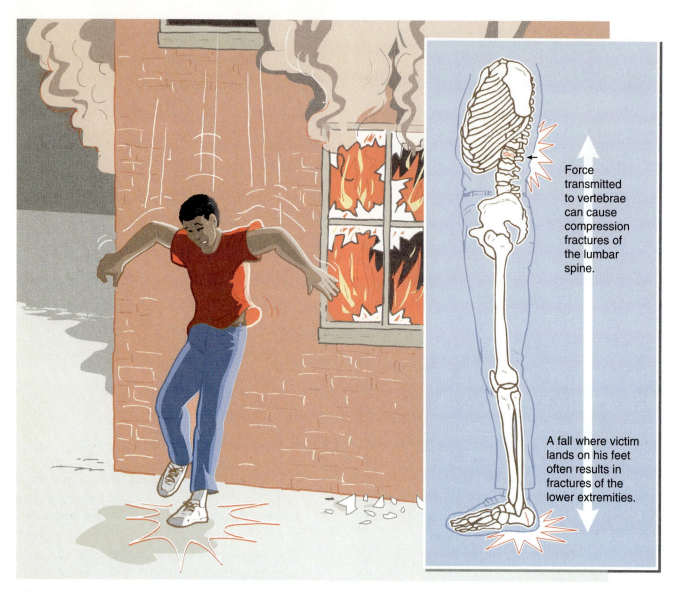

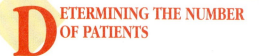

Force transmitted to vertebrae can cause compression fractures of the lumbar spine.

A fall where victim lands on his feet often results in fractures of the lower extremities.

Figure 7-28 In a fall, the energy of impact is transmitted through the skeletal system. This can cause injuries in parts of the body that did not initially contact the surface on which the person landed.

DETERMINING THE NUMBER OF PATIENTS

During the scene size-up, you must determine the number of patients involved in the incident. You must then judge whether the resources currently assigned to the scene are adequate to care for those patients. If you determine that there are too many patients for the on-scene resources to care for, then you must request that additional resources be dispatched to the scene. It is important to make this determination during the scene size-up. Once you begin assessing and treating patients, it will be harder to take time to call for additional resources. Also, the longer you delay the request for resources, the longer the patients on the scene will be without adequate care.

Most often, the number of patients involved in an incident will be obvious as you perform the size-up. On occasion, however, the exact number of patients can not be easily determined, as might be the case in a large incident such as a train or airliner crash (Figure 7-29). At other times, the number of patients may increase after you perform the

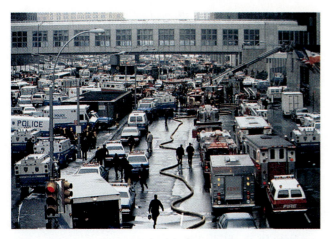

Figure 7-29 In large incidents, such as the World Trade Center bombing, it may be difficult to rapidly determine the number of patients.

initial size-up, as might be the case with a hazardous materials spill or a carbon monoxide poisoning in a large office building. With all cases, you must continuously reassess the scene and the available resources. Request or release additional resources to the scene as the situation evolves.

SECTION III: Initial Assessment

The initial assessment is a rapid way of evaluating the patient's condition, while identifying and treating any immediately life-threatening conditions.

OBJECTIVES

At the completion of this section of the chapter, the EMT-Basic student should be able to meet the following objectives:

Knowledge and Understanding

1. Summarize the reasons for forming a general impression of the patient. (pp. 165–167)
2. Discuss methods of assessing altered mental status. (pp. 168–170)
3. Differentiate between assessing the altered mental status in the adult, child, and infant patient. (pp. 173, 175)
4. Discuss methods of assessing the airway in the adult, child, and infant patient. (pp. 170–171, 173–175)
5. State reasons for management of the cervical spine once the patient has been determined to be a trauma patient. (p. 165)
6. Describe methods used for assessing if a patient is breathing. (pp. 171–172)
7. State what care should be provided to the adult, child, and infant with adequate breathing. (p. 171)
8. State what care should be provided to the adult, child, and infant without adequate breathing. (pp. 171–172)
9. Differentiate between a patient with adequate and inadequate breathing. (pp. 171–172)
10. Distinguish between the methods of assessing breathing in the adult, child, and infant patient. (pp. 173–175)

11. Compare the methods of providing airway care to the adult, child, and infant patient. (pp. 173–175)

12. Describe the methods used to obtain a pulse. (pp. 172, 180)

13. Differentiate between obtaining a pulse in an adult, child, and infant patient. (pp. 172, 180–182)

14. Discuss the need for assessing the patient for external bleeding. (p. 172)

15. Describe normal and abnormal findings when assessing skin color. (p. 172)

16. Describe normal and abnormal findings when assessing skin temperature. (pp. 172–173)

17. Describe normal and abnormal findings when assessing skin condition. (pp. 172–173)

18. Describe normal and abnormal findings when assessing skin capillary refill in the infant and child patient. (pp. 173, 174)

19. Explain the reason for prioritizing a patient for care and transport. (pp. 175–176)

20. Explain the importance of forming a general impression of the patient. (pp. 165–167)

21. Explain the value of performing an initial assessment. (pp. 165–167)

Skills

1. Demonstrate the techniques for assessing mental status.

2. Demonstrate the techniques for assessing the airway.

3. Demonstrate the techniques for assessing if the patient is breathing.

4. Demonstrate the techniques for assessing if the patient has a pulse.

5. Demonstrate the techniques for assessing the patient for external bleeding.

6. Demonstrate the techniques for assessing the patient's skin color, temperature, and condition and for assessing capillary refill in infants and children.

7. Demonstrate the ability to prioritize patients.

The initial assessment is based upon an essential concept in emergency medical care—the priorities in patient assessment and care are the "ABCs"—airway, breathing, and circulation. Because an open airway, adequate breathing, and sufficient circulation of blood are essential to life, any inadequacies in these areas that are identified during the initial assessment must be immediately treated and corrected. Once the status of the patient's ABCs have been assessed, the EMT can then determine the patient's priority for treatment and transport.

STEPS OF INITIAL ASSESSMENT

The initial assessment is carried out in a logical series of steps. Following these steps will assure that patients receive proper assessment, immediate care of life threatening conditions, and appropriate prioritization. The steps of the initial assessment are summarized in Table 7-3 and illustrated in Figure 7-30, page 166.

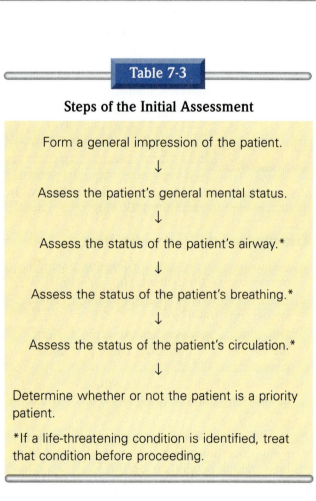

Table 7-3

Steps of the Initial Assessment

Form a general impression of the patient.

↓

Assess the patient's general mental status.

↓

Assess the status of the patient's airway.*

↓

Assess the status of the patient's breathing.*

↓

Assess the status of the patient's circulation.*

↓

Determine whether or not the patient is a priority patient.

*If a life-threatening condition is identified, treat that condition before proceeding.

During the initial assessment, you will identify immediately life-threatening conditions and immediately treat those conditions. *Immediately treat* means that the problem must be corrected before continuing any further with the initial assessment. Managing the "A""B""C"s *in that order* is essential to the survival of seriously ill or injured patients. It makes no sense, for example, for you to proceed with assessing a patient's breathing or circulation if his airway is obstructed because without an adequate airway there can be no effective breathing or circulation.

FORMING A GENERAL IMPRESSION

The first step in the initial assessment is to form a general impression of the patient. This general impression will help you determine how seriously ill or injured the patient is and what immediate care he will require. The general impression will also help you gauge the patient's priority for transport to the hospital.

The general impression is based upon the patient's chief complaint and the environment in which the patient is found, including the mechanism of injury. The patient's age and gender will also play parts in forming the general impression.

The chief complaint is what prompted the patient or others to call EMS for assistance. For patients who are able to speak to you, the chief complaint is what the patient tells you his problem is. Examples might include "chest pain," "shortness of breath," and "high fever." Later during your patient assessment, you may detect other conditions that are more serious than the one the patient gave as his chief complaint. However, the chief complaint remains whatever the patient first told you the problem was. When a patient is unresponsive, you may need to document the chief complaint as "unresponsive" or "cardiac arrest." When the patient is an infant or young child, the parent or caretaker will frequently provide the chief complaint.

Note the patient's age and gender as you form your impression. Both can impact on determining priority for transport and the care of the patient. For example, infants and the elderly are often more prone to severe complications of illness and injury (see Chapter 23, "Infants and Children," and Chapter 24, "Geriatric Patients"). Another example might be a female patient whose chief complaint of abdominal pain might indicate a gynecological emergency (see Chapter 17, "Obstetrics and Gynecology").

Part of your general impression will be based on whether a patient appears ill (a medical patient) or seriously injured (a trauma patient). With a medical patient, you will begin to assess the nature of the illness that prompted the call for assistance. When the initial assessment reveals a trauma patient, then the mechanism of injury must be determined. *If you suspect that the mechanism of injury may have caused a neck or spine injury, manually stabilize the patient's cervical spine immediately (Figure 7-31, page 168). Prompt manual spinal stabilization will help assure that spinal injuries are not worsened during further assessment and treatment. Remember that even a simple nodding of the patient's head in response to a question can cause serious spinal cord injury in certain circumstances.*

Experienced EMS providers often refer to the general impression as the "look test." Simply put, with experience and proper training, emergency care providers develop a sense of which patients "look OK" (pass the look test) and which "don't look OK" (fail the look test). Patients who fail the look test are those who require immediate interventions for life-threatening problems and will be candidates for immediate transport and possible ALS assistance.

You can develop such a sense. To do so, you must make the forming of a general impression an active process, using your senses—looking, listening, touching, smelling—to take in clues about a patient's condition. You must learn to recognize patterns in patient responses. For example, you will note that patients with certain illnesses position themselves in certain ways.

Developing this sense takes time. While you are developing it—and once you have developed it—always follow the specific steps of the initial assessment. Doing so will assure that the patient

The Initial Assessment

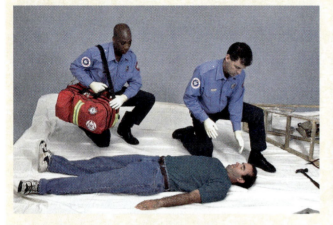

Figure 7-30A Form a general impression of the patient and the circumstances that led to the call to EMS.

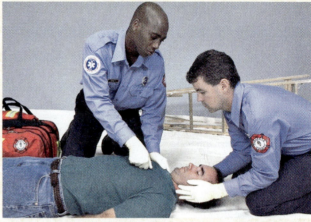

Figure 7-30B Assess the patient's mental status. Provide manual stabilization of the cervical spine throughout the initial assessment if the mechanism of injury suggests the possibility of trauma to the head, neck, or spine.

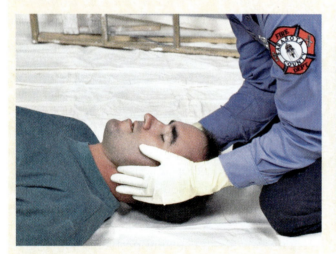

Figure 7-30C Assess the patient's airway. If necessary, open or clear the airway using manual maneuvers, suctioning, or insertion of an oro- or nasopharyngeal airway.

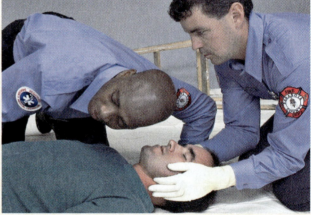

Figure 7-30D Assess the patient's breathing. If breathing is inadequate, provide high concentration oxygen via nonrebreather mask or positive pressure ventilations as necessary.

is properly assessed and that life-threatening conditions are identified and treated.

As you form your general impression, you may discover obviously life-threatening conditions. For example, you may observe that the patient's blood-filled mouth has obstructed his airway or you may detect that a patient is in respiratory or cardiac arrest. Whenever you discover

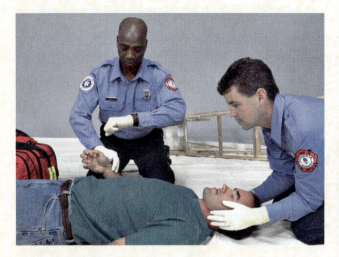

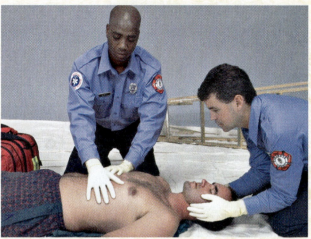

Figure 7-30E Assess the patient's circulation. Take the patient's pulse and assess skin color, temperature, and condition. In infants and children, check capillary refill (See Figure 7-37, page 174.)

Figure 7-30F As part of the assessment of circulation, check for and control any serious bleeding. Cut away clothing from areas of bleeding to better assess wounds.

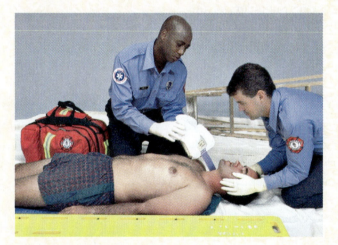

Figure 7-30G Make a decision about the patient's priority for further assessment, treatment, or immediate transportation.

such a life-threatening condition, immediately treat and correct the problem before proceeding with the assessment.

Once you have formed a general impression of the patient, you will then move on to more carefully assess the patient's mental status and ABCs (the adequacy of the airway, breathing, and circulation).

Manual Stabilization of the Head and Spine

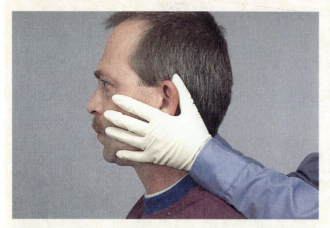

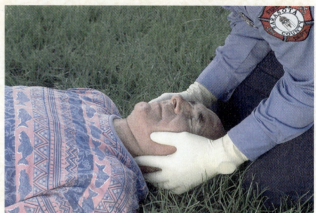

Figure 7-31A When the patient is sitting up, position yourself behind him and hold his head by spreading your fingers over the sides of the head and placing your thumbs on the back of the head. Hold the head in a neutral, in-line position without any twisting or turning. You can rest your arms by supporting them on the patient's shoulders or the back of the seat he is sitting in.

Figure 7-31B When the patient is supine, kneel behind him and spread your fingers and thumbs around the sides of his head to hold it steady. Rest your elbows on the ground for support. Manual stabilization must be maintained until the patient is fully immobilized to a long spine board.

ASSESSMENT OF MENTAL STATUS

The term **mental status** refers to a patient's level of responsiveness. Under normal circumstances, a person's brain receives messages, or stimuli, both from other parts of the body and from the surrounding environment. When a person is alert and has a normal mental status, he will respond to all types of stimuli. He will respond to visual stimuli (seeing and reacting to what is going on around him), verbal stimuli (hearing and reacting to what is going on around him), and tactile stimuli (feeling and reacting to pain when it is inflicted). When a person is not responding normally to such stimuli, he is said to have an **altered mental status.**

If during your initial assessment you note that the patient is less than fully alert, you must presume that the patient's brain is not functioning properly. It may be helpful to ask anyone present if he knows what the patient's normal mental status is. Common causes of an altered mental status include the following:

◆ Inadequate blood flow to the brain because of compromised circulation

◆ Inadequate oxygen delivered to the brain because of compromised airway or breathing

◆ Excessive carbon dioxide delivered to the brain because of inadequate breathing

◆ Inadequate sugar delivered to the brain, usually because of diabetes-related problems

If a patient has an altered mental status, you don't have to determine the cause—your task at this time is simply to record that the mental status is altered and to what degree it is altered. If the cause of the altered mental status is an inadequate airway, breathing, or circulation, you will identify the problem immediately and correct it before proceeding further with the initial assessment.

Assessment of mental status begins when you introduce yourself to the patient. Always introduce yourself to a patient, giving your name and identifying yourself as an Emergency Medical Technician. You should reassure the patient by telling him that you are there to help.

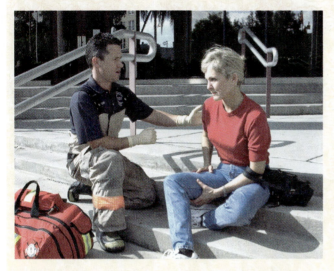

Figure 7-32A When the patient is *A*lert, she can talk or otherwise respond appropriately to your questions.

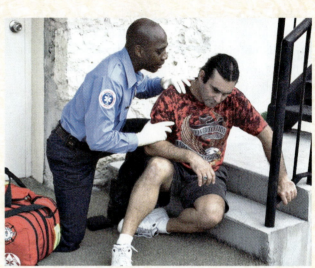

Figure 7-32B The next lowest level on the AVPU scale is responsive to *V*erbal stimulus. The patient does not respond appropriately to your questions, but he still reacts to spoken or shouted statements.

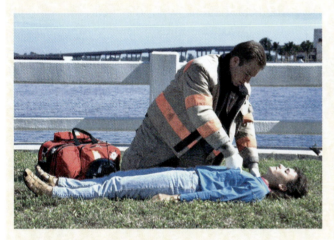

Figure 7-32C At the next lowest level, the patient does not react at all to spoken statements, but will respond to a *P*ainful stimulus such as a pinch or a brisk rubbing of the sternum (breastbone) by pulling away, flinching, or groaning.

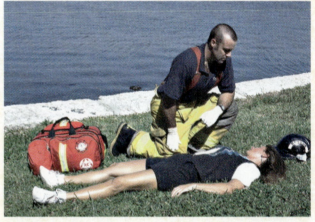

Figure 7-32D At the lowest level, the patient is *U*nresponsive to spoken or painful stimuli.

If you earlier formed a general impression that the patient may have a neck or spine injury, be sure that the cervical spine is manually stabilized now if that has not already been done. If the patient is conscious, explain what is happening. Ideally, a second EMT should provide the manual cervical stabilization while you conduct the assessment.

There is a standard, four-category scale that is used to describe a patient's mental status (Figure 7-32). It is based on the stimuli to which the patient can respond. Its categories can be remembered by using the letters "AVPU" as a memory aid. Each succeeding letter on this AVPU scale represents a lower level of responsiveness.

- *Alert*. Most patients you treat will be able to speak to you when you speak with them. Their eyes are open and they appear awake and aware of their surroundings. However, a patient can be awake and alert but confused or disoriented. You can check the mental status of an alert, speaking patient by asking him to tell you his name (orientation to person), where he is (orientation to place), and the day, date, or time (orientation to time).

- *Verbal*. These patients may not appear awake but do respond to verbal stimuli such as talking or shouting. If a patient cannot speak, ask him to respond to a command such as "blink your eyes" or "squeeze my hand."

- *Pain*. These patients appear unconscious and only respond to noxious, painful stimuli such as pressure on the nail beds or a brisk rubbing of the sternum (breastbone). Look for a response such as a facial grimace or a movement of some part of the body.

- *Unresponsive*. These patients are truly unconscious and do not respond to any stimuli. They lack a gag reflex and are very likely to suffer airway compromise. An unresponsive patient should be considered a priority patient.

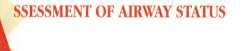

ASSESSMENT OF AIRWAY STATUS

Simply put, without an open airway a patient will die. During the initial assessment, you must determine whether the patient's airway is open and clear. In the responsive patient, evaluation of the airway may be relatively simple. If the patient is speaking, screaming, or crying (in the case of infants), then the patient has an open airway.

If a responsive patient cannot speak or cry, assume that his airway is not open. You must then immediately open or clear the airway. To do this, you may have to use a head-tilt, chin-lift maneuver or, in a patient with a suspected neck or spine injury, a jaw-thrust maneuver. In some cases, you may have to provide aggressive suctioning of the upper airway. If the airway is completely obstructed, then follow BLS procedures for clearing a foreign body airway obstruction.

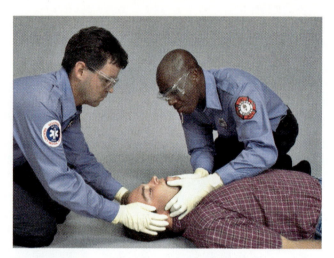

Figure 7-33 When opening the airway of a trauma patient, maintain manual stabilization and use a jaw-thrust maneuver. If no trauma is suspected, use the head-tilt, chin-lift maneuver.

With an unresponsive patient, you will always have to open the airway manually. (You may wish to review those techniques in Chapter 6, "Airway Management.") Open the airway of an unresponsive medical patient with the head-tilt, chin-lift maneuver. With an unresponsive trauma patient, assume that a spinal injury is present. Provide manual stabilization of the cervical spine, and open the airway using the jaw-thrust maneuver (Figure 7-33).

When caring for unresponsive patients, you will likely have to clear the airway once it is open. Loose teeth, blood, and vomitus can all compromise the airway. To remove such obstructions, provide aggressive suctioning while continuing to use manual maneuvers to open the airway (Figure 7-34).

Figure 7-34 During the initial assessment, clear the airway by suctioning if necessary.

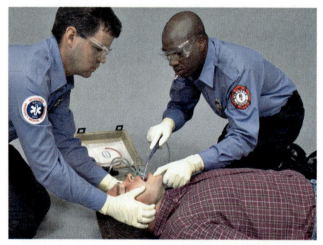

Once the airway is open and clear, you may insert an oro- or nasopharyngeal airway to maintain it.

Remember: it makes no sense to continue on in your assessment until the airway is clear and secure. Without an open airway, all other efforts will be futile since the patient will die.

ASSESSMENT OF BREATHING STATUS

Once the airway is clear, you must determine if the patient's breathing is adequate. If you discover that it is inadequate, you will have to provide treatment such as administering supplemental oxygen or providing assisted ventilations with a pocket mask or bag-valve-mask device (BVM). In cases where breathing has stopped altogether (respiratory arrest), you will have to provide positive pressure ventilations.

Assessment of Breathing—Responsive Patient

With a responsive patient, immediately determine if his respirations are adequate or inadequate. With some patients—for example, a patient with an isolated ankle injury who is speaking to you calmly and distinctly—it will be immediately clear that breathing is adequate and that no treatment is required. Other responsive patients may display signs of inadequate breathing. These signs include:

◆ Rate of breathing faster (more than 24 per minute) or slower (less than 8 per minute) than normal

◆ Irregular rhythm of breathing

◆ Poor quality of breathing

　　—Breath sounds that are unequal, absent or diminished

　　—Unequal or inadequate chest expansion upon inhalation

　　—Increased effort of breathing with use of accessory muscles in the neck, shoulders, chest, and abdomen, especially in infants and children

◆ Shallow breathing resulting in an inadequate tidal volume

◆ Altered mental status

◆ Bluish or grayish skin (cyanosis)

◆ Retractions of the skin above the clavicles, between the ribs, and below the rib cage

◆ "Agonal respirations," gasping irregular breaths often seen just before cardiac arrest.

All responsive patients who display *any* signs of inadequate breathing should be given high concentration oxygen via a nonrebreather mask. If respirations are absent, agonal, or do not improve with the supplemental oxygen, then provide positive pressure ventilations using an adjunct such as a pocket mask or BVM.

You should provide high concentration oxygen to certain responsive patients whether their breathing is adequate or not. In general, give supplemental high concentration oxygen during the breathing assessment to any patient with one of these chief complaints or presenting problems:

◆ Chest pain

◆ Shortness of breath

◆ Possible carbon monoxide poisoning

◆ Alteration in normal mental status

Assessment of Breathing—Unresponsive Patient

All unresponsive patients must have their airways opened and maintained using airway adjuncts and suctioning as needed. All should receive high concentration supplemental oxygen. Continuously assess the adequacy of the breathing in these patients:

◆ If breathing is adequate:

　　—Maintain the airway and administer high concentration oxygen via nonrebreather mask at 15 liters per minute.

◆ If breathing is inadequate:

　　—Maintain the airway and administer high concentration oxygen via nonrebreather mask at 15 liters per minute. If breathing efforts are minimal, agonal, or do not immediately improve on high concentration oxygen, provide positive pressure ventilations using a pocket mask or BVM attached to high concentration oxygen.

♦ If the patient is not breathing:

—Maintain the airway and provide positive pressure ventilations using an adjunct such as a pocket mask or BVM attached to high flow oxygen.

ASSESSMENT OF CIRCULATION STATUS

Circulation, or perfusion, is the process through which the body's organs receive adequate blood flow to function properly. During the initial assessment, you must assess three aspects of a patient's circulation:

♦ Assess for the presence of a pulse.

♦ Determine if the patient has any major external bleeding.

♦ Assess the general adequacy of perfusion by evaluating the patient's skin.

Assessment of the Pulse

When assessing the pulse in an adult or child check first for the presence of a radial pulse. If the radial pulse is absent, then check for a carotid pulse. In infants less than 1 year of age palpate for a brachial pulse (see page 181).

If you determine that a patient has no pulse, then begin CPR. If the patient is a medical patient older than 12 years of age, apply and use an automated external defibrillator (AED).

Assessment for External Bleeding

Because blood loss will reduce the body's ability to maintain adequate circulation, any major external bleeding must be identified and controlled during the initial assessment. This does not mean you must dress every wound found during the initial assessment. You should, instead, control sites of active bleeding where blood loss is significant and ongoing.

To assess for external bleeding, perform a rapid head-to-toe exam using appropriate BSI precautions. Cut away any blood-soaked clothing and check for an underlying wound. Carefully reach behind the patient's back to feel for the wetness of blood. If necessary, log roll the patient (see Chapter 22) to better assess his back. When feeling for the presence of blood, be careful of broken glass and other debris that could puncture your gloves and cause injury.

If you discover major bleeding, control it through use of direct pressure and other methods described in Chapter 19, "Bleeding and Shock."

Assessment of the Skin

The skin is one of the first of the body's organ systems to show signs of inadequate circulation (perfusion). The condition of the skin can also give indications of other problems that may be affecting the patient. The skin is readily accessible and should be checked for color, temperature, and condition as the final step in assessment of the patient's circulation status. Skin condition refers to the amount of moisture on the skin's surface. In infants and children, the skin will also be assessed for capillary refill as a measure of the adequacy of perfusion.

Skin Color

Normal skin should have a pink hue. In all patients, including dark-skinned individuals, the best places to assess skin color are the nail beds, the lips, and the mucous membranes that line the eyelids. Abnormal skin colors include:

♦ *Pale*—often associated with poor perfusion, especially from blood loss

♦ *Blue-gray* (cyanotic)—indicates lack of adequate oxygen

♦ *Red or flushed*—can be associated with heat-related emergencies and severe carbon monoxide poisoning

♦ *Yellow or jaundiced*—associated with liver diseases (Figure 7-35)

Skin Temperature and Condition

In order to properly assess skin temperature and condition, use the back of your hand. If conditions found during scene size-up or department policy require that gloves be worn, partially remove a glove during this portion of the assessment (Figure 7-36). Avoid assessing skin tempera-

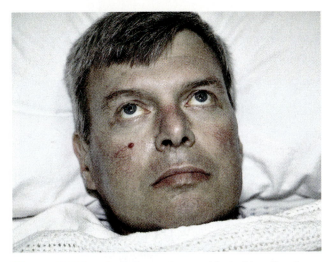

Figure 7-35   A patient whose skin is jaundiced.

ture and condition on parts of the patient's skin wet with blood or other body fluids.

Normal skin should be warm and dry to the touch. Abnormal skin temperature and conditions include the following:

◆ *Cool and moist ("clammy") skin*—occurs when perfusion is inadequate and blood flow to the skin is reduced. May also occur in some heat-related emergencies and shock (hypoperfusion).

◆ *Cold skin*—may occur in situations of exposure to low environmental temperatures.

Figure 7-36   Use the back of your hand to assess skin color and temperature. When doing this, roll down your glove without removing it completely.

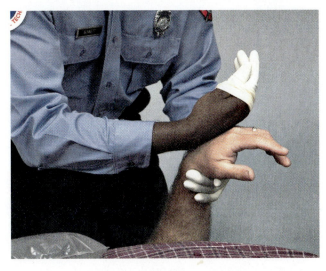

◆ *Hot and dry skin*—may occur with fevers and certain life-threatening heat-related emergencies.

Assessment of Capillary Refill

In infants and children, another way to check for adequate circulation is by testing capillary refill time. This test is not reliable in adult patients and should not be used in their assessment.

To test capillary refill, press either the top of the patient's foot or the back of his hand with your thumb for several seconds (Figure 7-37). When you remove your thumb, normal skin will briefly show a blanched (white) appearance where your thumb had been before returning to its normal color within 2 seconds. If the return of normal color takes longer than 2 seconds, then capillary refill is said to be "prolonged" or "delayed." This may indicate inadequate perfusion.

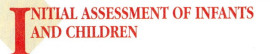

INITIAL ASSESSMENT OF INFANTS AND CHILDREN

Assessment and treatment priorities for the initial assessment are the same with all patients regardless of age. Yet because infants and children differ from adults in anatomy, physiology, and stages of development, these differences mean that there are special considerations to take into account when performing an initial assessment on them (Table 7-3, page 175). Some of the most important of these considerations include:

◆ When assessing the mental status of an infant or child, flick the soles of his feet with your finger to provide a painful stimulus. Crying is considered an appropriate response; quiet whimpering is not.

◆ Open the airway more carefully in infants and children to avoid hyperextending the neck, which can itself obstruct the airway.

◆ A child should have normal muscle tone; a flaccid, "floppy" child should be considered abnormal.

◆ Be aware that normal respiratory rates are faster in infants and children.

Assessing Capillary Refill

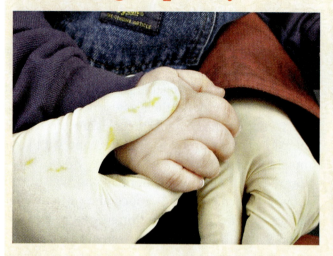

Figure 7-37A When assessing capillary refill, press your thumb down on the back of the child's hand (or the top of his foot) for several seconds.

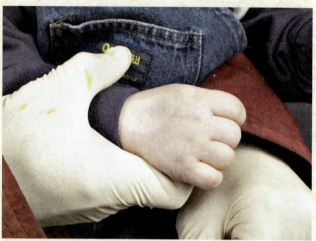

Figure 7-37B Release your thumb and observe the whitened (blanched) area where you had been pressing.

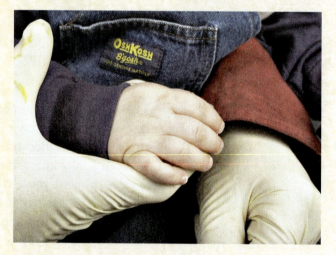

Figure 7-37C Normal color should return to the area in 2 seconds or less. If it takes longer, capillary refill is said to be delayed, a sign of inadequate circulation.

◆ Be aware that normal pulse rates are faster in infants and children.

◆ When assessing the pulse in infants, assess at the brachial pulse.

◆ Be aware that a slower-than-expected pulse rate in an infant or child is likely to be the result of an inadequate airway or inadequate breathing.

◆ Assess capillary refill only in infants and children, not in adults.

◆ Note respiratory patterns/quality of breathing (crowing, stridor, etc.).

◆ Note unusual patient positioning. For example, the "tripod" position, in which a sitting patient leans forward with hands on knees, may be a sign of respiratory distress.

Table 7-3

Initial Assessment of Adults, Infants, and Children

	Adults	Children, 1–5 Yrs.	Infants to 1 Yr.
Mental Status	AVPU: Is patient alert? Responsive to verbal stimulus? Painful stimulus? Unresponsive?	As for adults	If not alert, is infant responsive to shouting as stimulus? to flicking of the soles of its feet as painful stimulus? (Response would be crying.)
Airway	Opening the airway: trauma, use jaw thrust; medical, use head-tilt, chin-lift. Both: Suction an oro- or nasopharyngeal airway.	As for adults, but avoid hyperextending the neck when opening the airway. (See Chapter 6, "Airway Management," for other concerns with infants and children.)	As for children. (See Chapter 6 for special concerns with infants.)
Breathing	With patient in respiratory distress, provide positive pressure ventilations. If patient is unresponsive and breathing adequately, provide high concentration oxygen. If breathing inadequately—responsive or unresponsive—provide high concentration oxygen via nonrebreather mask; provide positive pressure ventilations if necessary.	As for adults, but normal rates are faster for children than for adults. (See Section IV of this chapter.) Consider letting parent hold mask if oxygen is needed.	As for children, but normal rates are faster for infants than for children. (See Section IV of this chapter.)
Circulation	Assess pulses and skin condition. Immediately control external bleeding. If patient in cardiac arrest, perform CPR. Apply AED as soon as possible. Treat for bleeding and shock if necessary (see Chapter 19).	Assess skin, radial pulse, bleeding, capillary refill. (See Section IV of this chapter for child pulse rates.) If cardiac arrest, provide CPR. Treat for bleeding and shock if necessary (see Chapter 19).	Assess skin, brachial pulse, bleeding, capillary refill. (See Section IV of this chapter for infant pulse rates.) If cardiac arrest, provide CPR. Treat for bleeding and shock if necessary (see Chapter 19).

IDENTIFICATION OF PRIORITY PATIENTS

The final component of the initial assessment is determining which patients are to be identified as priority patients. Priority patients should receive immediate transport to a hospital, with further assessment and emergency care being provided in the ambulance en route. With priority patients, you should also request advanced life support (ALS) assistance if available. With non-priority patients, you will usually continue the assessment and provide care on the scene before transporting the patient, if he requires transport at all.

There are no firm rules requiring that a patient be labeled "priority." Generally, however, if a patient shows signs of a potentially life-threatening condition for which little or nothing can be done in the field, he should be considered a priority patient. In general, if your initial assessment of a patient reveals any of the following, you should identify him as a priority patient:

◆ Poor general impression (i.e. fails the "look test")

◆ Unresponsive patient

- Patient with altered mental status
  - —Status less than alert
  - —Responsive, but not following commands
- Difficulty in breathing
- Inability to establish or maintain an open airway
- Signs of inadequate circulation (perfusion)
- Uncontrolled bleeding

- Complicated childbirth
- Respiratory and/or cardiac arrest
- Chest pain with systolic blood pressure less than 100
- Severe pain anywhere
- Extremely high body temperature
- Poisoning or overdose with unknown substance

SECTION IV: SAMPLE History and Vital Signs

After the initial assessment, you begin a more detailed assessment of the patient. Two important parts of this assessment are obtaining a medical history of the patient and taking his vital signs. These skills are used extensively in the focused history and physical exam. In addition, taking of vital signs is a key part of the ongoing assessment. This section of Chapter 7 explains how to do both.

OBJECTIVES

At the completion of this section of the chapter, the EMT-Basic student should be able to meet the following objectives:

Knowledge and Understanding

1. Identify the components of vital signs. (p. 180)
2. Describe the methods used to obtain a breathing rate. (pp. 182–183)
3. Identify the attributes that should be obtained when assessing breathing. (pp. 182–183)
4. Differentiate between shallow, labored, and noisy breathing. (pp. 182–183)
5. Describe the methods to obtain a pulse rate. (pp. 180–182)
6. Identify the information obtained when assessing a patient's pulse. (pp. 180–182)
7. Differentiate between a strong, weak, regular, and irregular pulse. (pp. 180–182)
8. Describe the methods to assess the skin color, temperature, condition (capillary refill in infants and children). (pp. 185–186)
9. Identify the normal and abnormal skin colors. (pp. 172, 185–186)
10. Differentiate between pale, blue, red, and yellow skin color. (pp. 172, 185–186)
11. Identify the normal and abnormal skin temperatures. (pp. 172–173, 185–186)
12. Differentiate between hot, cool, and cold skin temperature. (pp. 172–173, 185–186)
13. Identify normal and abnormal skin conditions. (pp. 172–173, 185–186)
14. Identify normal and abnormal capillary refill in infants and children. (pp. 173–174)
15. Describe the methods to assess the pupils. (pp. 186–187)
16. Identify normal and abnormal pupil size. (p. 186)
17. Differentiate between dilated (big) and constricted (small) pupil size. (p. 186)
18. Differentiate between reactive and nonreactive pupils and equal and unequal pupils. (p. 186)
19. Describe the methods to assess blood pressure. (pp. 184–185)
20. Define systolic pressure. (p. 183)
21. Define diastolic pressure. (p. 183)
22. Explain the difference between auscultation

and palpation for obtaining a blood pressure. (p. 184)

23. Identify the components of the SAMPLE history. (pp. 177–178)

24. Differentiate between a sign and a symptom. (p. 178)

25. State the importance of accurately reporting and recording the baseline vital signs. (p. 180)

26. Discuss the need to search for additional medical information. (pp. 177–180)

27. Explain the value of performing the baseline vital signs. (p. 180)

28. Recognize and respond to the feelings patients experience during assessment. (p. 177)

29. Defend the need for obtaining and recording an accurate set of vital signs. (p. 180)

30. Explain the rationale of recording additional sets of vital signs. (p. 180)

31. Explain the importance of obtaining a SAMPLE history. (pp. 177–180)

Skills

1. Demonstrate the skills involved in assessment of breathing.

2. Demonstrate the skills associated with obtaining a pulse.

3. Demonstrate the skills associated with assessing the skin color, temperature, condition, and capillary refill in infants and children.

4. Demonstrate the skills associated with assessing the pupils.

5. Demonstrate the skills associated with obtaining blood pressure.

6. Demonstrate the skills that should be used to obtain information from the patient, family, or bystanders at the scene.

The medical history that you will gather at this time is called the SAMPLE history. Its purpose is to pull together information about the patient's present problem and any pre-existing conditions that may possibly have a bearing on it.

The vital signs include the patient's pulse, blood pressure, respirations, and skin condition. The first set of these readings is called the **baseline vital signs.** You will obtain baseline vital signs on all patients. Measuring these signs early in the assessment process provides a set of readings that indicate the patient's current condition. By comparing these baseline readings against sets of vital signs gathered later in the process, you can detect trends that may indicate if the patient's condition is improving or deteriorating.

Exactly when you will gather the SAMPLE history and the baseline vital signs in the next assessment stage will be based on the patient's condition. For example, with responsive medical patients, the SAMPLE history is obtained before the baseline vital signs. With unresponsive medical patients, the opposite order is followed. In reality, however, vital signs and a SAMPLE history are frequently obtained simultaneously. You will learn more about *when* to gather this information in Sections V and VI of this chapter. This section will focus on *how* to gather the information.

THE SAMPLE HISTORY

When you obtain a patient's medical history, you are gathering information that will help shape your subsequent assessment and treatment. That information will also be valuable to the caregivers to whom you transfer the patient's care. In fact, if the patient becomes unresponsive, the history that you gather may be the only source of much vital information. Try to gather as much pertinent information as you can when obtaining a patient's history. Be sure to write down your findings.

With responsive adult patients, you can usually obtain the history from the patient himself. With unresponsive patients and patients with altered mental status, you must try to determine the history from family, friends, or bystanders; also be sure to see if the patient is wearing a medical identification device (Figure 7-38). With infants and younger children, you can usually turn to a parent or caregiver for the patient's history.

The most effective way of taking a patient's history is to use the SAMPLE format. The letters of word SAMPLE will help you to remember the information you must gather in a patient history. The elements of the SAMPLE history are as follows:

- ◆ *S*igns/*S*ymptoms
- ◆ *A*llergies
- ◆ *M*edications being taken
- ◆ *P*ertinent past history
- ◆ *L*ast oral intake
- ◆ *E*vents leading up to the illness or injury

Whenever you take a SAMPLE history, speak clearly in a normal tone of voice. Make eye contact with the patient when talking to him. If the patient is seated or if you are assessing a child, get down to his eye level. If you haven't done so earlier, introduce yourself and explain why you are there and why you will be asking questions. Learn the patient's name and how he would like to be addressed. You can also ask the patient's specific age at this time. (You should have obtained an approximate idea of the age when you formed your general impression of the patient.)

If there is difficulty in communicating or the patient misunderstands a question, repeat the question or rephrase it. Avoid the use of slang terms or medical jargon when speaking to a patient. Most importantly, *listen* to the patient's response and *record* your findings.

Signs and Symptoms

In medical terms, **signs** are "objective" findings that you can see, hear, feel, or smell without having to question the patient. For example, you might see that a patient is using accessory muscles as he breathes, hear wheezing as he exhales, feel that his skin is cool and clammy, and smell an acetone-like odor on his breath.

Symptoms are "subjective." You can't observe them; you only know about them because the patient tells you. Examples of symptoms include a patient's report of chest pain, shortness of breath, or nausea. To determine what symptoms the patient is having, ask questions like "What's wrong?" or "What problems are you having that you needed to call us today?" Try to avoid questions that can be answered "yes" or "no."

Allergies

Determine if the patient is allergic to any medications, foods, or environmental agents, such as bee

venom or molds. Ask, "Do you have any allergies? Are you allergic to any medications?" It is important to ask the patient a specific question about allergies to medications because many patients assume that "Do you have any allergies?" refers only to environmental allergies. Also check to see if the patient is wearing a medical identification device that might list an allergy (Figure 7–38).

Medications

Determine what, if any, medications a patient is currently taking. This information can give important clues about the patient's past history and the reasons for his present illness. As you gain more experience as an EMT, you will begin to recognize the names of some prescription drugs and the conditions for which they are taken (see Chapter 11, "General Pharmacology"). You will also learn that certain medications can cause side effects that can trigger medical emergencies or change the way the patient's body responds to medical conditions.

Figure 7-38 **A.** A medical identification device. **B.** The back of the device can give important information about the patient's condition including allergies and past medical history.

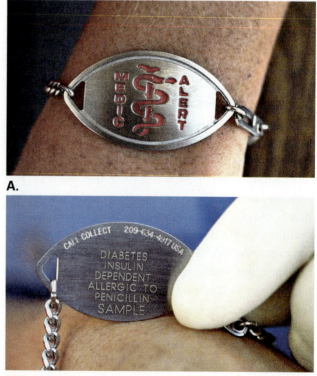

A.

B.

To determine what medications the patient has taken or normally takes, ask: "Do you take any medications on a regular basis?" and "Have you taken any medications today." Ask specifically about prescription medications. Also ask about over-the-counter medications and "holistic" (herbal) preparations because some patients may not consider these to be "real" medications. If the patient is a woman, ask if she uses birth-control pills.

As a rule, avoid using the word "drugs" when questioning the patient about medications. A question like "Are you taking any drugs?" can be easily misinterpreted as an accusation about the use of illegal street drugs. If, however, you strongly suspect that a patient may have taken illicit drugs, ask specifically about their use, reminding the patient that you are an EMT, not a police officer, and are there to help with his medical problem.

In some cases, as with an unresponsive medical patient, the medications the patient is taking may not be readily found. Look for medical identification devices on the patient. Also, assign one crew member to search the home quickly for pill bottles (Figure 7-39). Common places where patients store their medications are in the kitchen, on the nightstand, and in the bathroom. Always check the refrigerator for medications. Patients may also keep lists of their medications and schedules of when to take them. Document any medications that are found.

Patients with several medical conditions often have entire drawers filled with boxes and bottles

Figure 7-39 When checking a patient's medications, look for both prescription and over-the-counter medications.

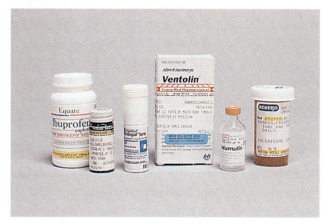

of prescription medications. Rather than sort through these large collections, gather them in a bag and bring them to the emergency department with the patient. Make sure they are given to the nurse who will be caring for the patient.

Pertinent Past Medical History

To obtain the patient's past medical history, ask questions such as these:

◆ "Have you had any medical problems in the past?"

◆ "Have you had any recent injuries?"

◆ "Have you ever been hospitalized?"

◆ "Are you currently under the care of a doctor for any problems? Have you recently seen a doctor? What is your doctor's name?"

◆ "Have you ever had _____ (chest pain, shortness of breath, etc.) like this in the past?"

The patient with a known past medical history is assessed somewhat differently than a patient without a significant past history. As a general rule, past history tends to repeat itself. That is, patients who have had shortness of breath from asthma in the past, tend to call EMS again for assistance with the same problem. Patients with an established past medical history may also have with them certain medications, such as nitroglycerin for chest pain, inhalers for shortness of breath, and epinephrine auto-injectors for allergic reactions. You may be able to assist the patient in taking such medications if authorized to do so by medical direction. Patients without a past medical history who call for assistance with new signs and symptoms are sometimes more difficult to assess because of their lack of past history.

Last Oral Intake

To determine the patient's last oral intake, ask: "When was the last time you had anything to eat or drink today? What did you eat or drink then?"

Of all the SAMPLE history you will gather, this information is probably the least crucial to out-of-hospital care. However it can be helpful, even vital, to the hospital personnel to whose care the patient is transferred. Knowing this information can help a physician make a preliminary diagnosis in some patients who present with abdominal and chest pain. The information may also help surgeons and anesthesiologists determine how soon they can take a patient to the operating room. In general, it is preferable to wait at least 6 hours after the last oral intake prior to surgery to reduce the risk of complications such as aspiration of stomach contents.

Events Leading Up to the Illness or Injury

Determining the events that led up to the onset of a medical emergency or injury is a crucial part of the patient history. Knowing what a medical patient was doing when his symptoms began can be very helpful in a patient assessment. For example, all patients with chest pain will receive the same emergency treatment of high flow oxygen and consideration of ALS intervention. However, a patient who was wakened from his sleep with chest pain at 3 A.M. is more likely to be having a myocardial infarction than the patient who just bench pressed 230 pounds (104 kg) in the gym.

To determine from the patient the events that led up to the present illness, ask questions like, "What were you doing just before the _____ (chest pain, abdominal pain, shortness of breath, etc.) started?"

VITAL SIGNS

Vital signs include the patient's respiratory rate, pulse rate, and blood pressure. Whenever you obtain vital signs, you should also reassess the patient's mental status using the AVPU scale. Closely monitoring for changes in mental status is especially important with patients who are unresponsive or have severely altered mental status. It is also routine to assess condition of the skin and pupils as part of a "full set of vital signs."

This first set of vital signs you obtain is called the "baseline." It is this set to which you will compare measurements of vital signs gathered later during the ongoing assessment. By noting the findings of sequential sets of vital signs, you can

detect changes, or trends, in the vital signs. These trends may indicate important changes in the patient's condition.

To understand the importance of recording trends in vital signs, consider the following examples. As you are transporting a patient, you take his vital signs and discover that, compared to the baseline readings, the patient's pulse rate is rising and his blood pressure is falling. This indicates that the patient's condition is deteriorating, since this trend in vital signs is often associated with worsening shock or hypoperfusion. On the other hand, consider a patient who complained of difficulty breathing and whose baseline vital signs revealed elevated pulse and respiratory rates. You placed the patient on oxygen; later measurement of vital signs shows that pulse and respiratory rates have returned to normal. This trend in vital signs indicates that your treatment has been effective and the patient's condition is improving.

Remember, however, that you can't detect trends if you don't take baseline readings. Also remember that, whenever you take vital signs, you must record your findings.

Pulse

A pulse is the pulsation felt where an artery passes over a bone near the surface of the skin. The pulsation that is felt is the pressure wave of blood created by the pumping of blood out of the left ventricle.

First try to assess the radial pulse (Figure 7-40). Palpate for this over the patient's anterior wrist on the thumb side where the radial artery is located. If no pulse is felt at the wrist, then try to find the carotid pulse (Figure 7-41). Palpate on either side of the neck over the carotid artery. In infants and young children, assess the brachial pulse at the brachial artery in the upper arm (Figure 7-42).

Although you determined the presence of a pulse in the initial assessment, when you obtain baseline vital signs as part of the focused history and physical exam, you will determine the *rate* and the *quality* of the pulse.

The pulse rate is recorded as the number of beats felt per minute. To determine the rate, count pulsations for 30 seconds and multiply by 2. Many factors can affect a pulse rate. These may include

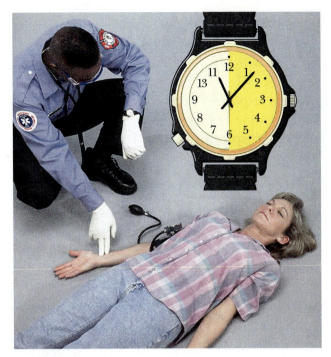

Figure 7-40 Assess the rate and quality of the patient's pulse. Try the radial pulse first. Count the pulsations for 30 seconds, then multiply by 2.

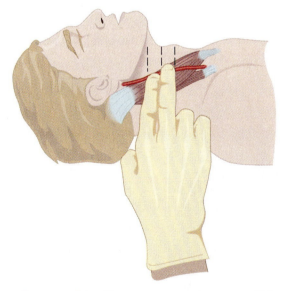

Figure 7-41 If you cannot palpate a radial pulse, detect and assess the carotid pulse.

patient age, level of anxiety, underlying heart disease, and the use of medications. Normal pulse rates are listed in Table 7-4.

Rates above or below the ranges given in Table 7-4 are considered rapid or slow. A pulse rate more rapid than normal is called a **tachycardia.** In adults, any heart rate greater than 100 beats per

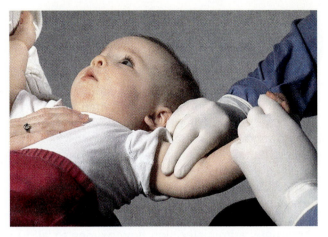

Figure 7-42 Assess the brachial pulse in infants and young children.

minute is called a tachycardia. Tachycardias can be caused by a variety of conditions ranging from emotional upset to a life-threatening problem with the heart's electrical conduction system. A pulse rate that is slower than normal is called a **bradycardia.** The causes of bradycardia include use of medications prescribed for heart disease or high blood pressure as well as heart disease itself.

The quality of the pulse is described in terms of strength and regularity (Table 7–5). The strength of the pulse is usually described as either normal or weak (sometimes called "thready"). Since the pulse is created by the pumping action of the heart, a weak pulse may indicate a problem with the heart and the circulatory system, as is the case in shock (hypoperfusion).

The regularity of the pulse is important because it may indicate underlying problems with

| Table 7-4 |

Normal Pulse Rates

Patient	Pulse rate (beats per minute, at rest)
Adult (older than 10 years)	60 to 100
2 years to 10 years	60 to 140
3 months to 2 years	100 to 190
Newborn to 3 months	85 to 205

the heart's electrical conduction system. Those problems can produce abnormal heart rhythms known as **dysrhythmias.** Under normal conditions, you should note a regular pattern as you palpate a patient's pulse. If you detect an irregular pulse pattern, especially in a patient who is unresponsive or has an altered mental status, assume that the patient is experiencing a life-threatening dysrhythmia. Immediately request ALS assistance if not already dispatched.

Respirations

Assessing the patient's respirations is important because doing so can help you determine the adequacy of his breathing. You will determine the patient's respiratory rate as well as the quality and rhythm of the respirations.

The **respiratory rate** is the number of breaths the patient takes per minute. Determine the respiratory rate either by observing the rise and fall of the patient's chest or by gently placing a hand on it for 30 seconds (Figure 7-43). Count the number of breaths (one rise and one fall of the chest is a complete breath) and double that number to find the respiratory rate. Normal respiratory rates are shown in Table 7-6.

You may have noticed earlier in the assessment that the patient seemed to be breathing faster or slower than normal. If you are determining the respiratory rate of an unresponsive patient and note no breathing in the first 15 seconds, assume that the patient has inadequate or absent

Figure 7-43 Assess the rate and quality of the patient's respirations. You can gently place a hand on the patient's chest, count each rise-and-fall for 30 seconds, then multiply by 2.

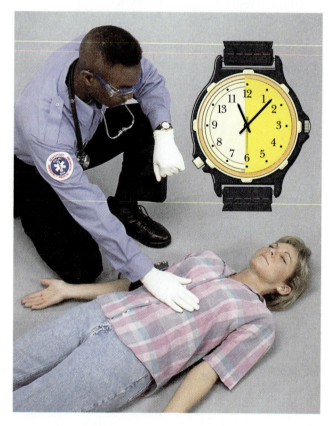

Table 7-5

Pulse Quality and Possible Problems

Pulse	Possible Problem
Rapid, regular, strong (full or bounding)	Exertion, fright, fever, high blood pressure, first stages of blood loss (increased pulse rate may be normal in pregnancy)
Rapid, regular, weak (thready)	Shock (hypoperfusion), later stages of blood loss
Slow	Head injury, medications, some poisons, some cardiac problems, lack of oxygen in children
Irregular	Problems with the heart's electrical conduction system
No pulse	Cardiac arrest, severe hypoperfusion, severe hypothermia

Table 7-6

Normal Respiratory Rates

Patient	Normal Respiratory Rate
Adult	12 to 20 breaths per minute
Child	15 to 30 breaths per minute
Infant	25 to 50 breaths per minute

breathing. Immediately begin ventilations with a device such as a pocket mask or BVM and consider insertion of an oro- or nasopharyngeal airway. Patients with respiratory emergencies usually breathe at rates higher than normal. Patients with slower than normal respiratory rates generally need aggressive management including high flow oxygen and assisted ventilations with a ventilatory adjunct.

In addition to rate, you must note the quality of the patient's respirations. There are four basic categories for the quality of respirations.

◆ *Normal breathing* The patient breathes easily, with no use of accessory muscles or any signs of inadequate breathing.

◆ *Labored breathing* The patient shows signs of increased effort to breathe. Such signs include grunting, stridor (a harsh, high-pitched sound on inhaling), nasal flaring (widening of the nostrils during exhalation), the use of accessory muscles, and retractions (pulling in of skin around the collarbone and between the ribs, especially in children).

◆ *Shallow breathing* The patient's chest and abdomen rise and fall only slightly during breathing.

◆ *Noisy breathing* There is increased sound when the patient inhales or exhales. Types of noisy breathing include snoring, wheezing, gurgling, crowing. Noisy breathing indicates some type of airway obstruction. You may have to open or reopen the airway or provide suctioning.

Finally, you should observe the rhythm of the patient's respirations. Patients normally breathe in a regular rhythm. Patients with an irregular breathing pattern may have lost the ability to control their respirations as can happen with strokes and certain diabetic emergencies. Such patients may have inadequate breathing; observe them carefully and be prepared to supply supplemental oxygen or positive pressure ventilations.

Blood Pressure

The human circulatory system delivers blood to all parts of the body. The heart is the pump that drives the blood through the system. The force of the blood against the walls of the blood vessels is called **blood pressure.** If the blood pressure is too low—for example, from blood loss or a heart attack—the body's organs will not get enough blood. This can lead to severe organ damage and death. If the blood pressure is too high, arteries in the brain may rupture causing a stroke and the heart, kidneys, and other organs may be damaged.

Normally there is always pressure in the body's blood vessels, much like a charged hoseline. The blood pressure rises whenever the left ventricle of the heart pumps blood out of the heart. The pressure exerted on the walls of the arteries when the left ventricle pumps is called the **systolic pressure.** The pressure in the arteries when the left ventricle is at rest is called the **diastolic pressure.** Blood pressure is measured in units of millimeters of mercury or "mmHg." (Hg is the chemical symbol for mercury.)

Blood pressure (often abbreviated BP) is normally written and stated as the systolic pressure "over" the diastolic pressure. For example, you determine that a patient has a systolic blood pressure of 138 mmHg and a diastolic pressure of 82 mmHg. On a report form, you could write this as "BP is 138/82." If you were passing the information on orally, you would say "BP is 138 over 82". It is not usually necessary for the EMT to write or state the units of measure when reporting blood pressure.

The normal ranges of blood pressure by age are listed in Table 7-7. Many people normally run blood pressure above and below the normal ranges. In adults, a systolic blood pressure of less than 90 mmHg is generally considered low. The

Table 7-7

Normal Blood Pressure Ranges

Patient	Systolic	Diastolic
Adult male	Patient's age + 100 (up to 150 mmHg)	60 to 90 mmHg
Adult female	Patient's age + 90 (up to 140 mmHg)	50 to 80 mmHg
Infants and children Adolescent (11-14 yrs) Child (6-10 yrs) Child (3-5 years)	Approx. 80 × 2 age (yrs) average 114 average 105 average 99	Approx. 2/3 systolic average 59 average 57 average 55

definition of "high" blood pressure is a systolic blood pressure greater than 140 mmHg and/or a diastolic blood pressure greater than 90 mmHg.

High blood pressure is rarely immediately life threatening in the prehospital setting until the systolic blood pressure exceeds 200 mmHg or the diastolic pressure exceeds 120 mmHg. Whenever you obtain an abnormally high or low blood pressure, be sure to *look carefully at the patient.* Try to determine if the abnormal blood pressure is having any effect on the patient. An athletic young woman with no medical complaints who walks up to a blood pressure screening in the mall and has a blood pressure of 86/60 is a very different case than the unresponsive geriatric patient with the same low blood pressure.

To measure blood pressure, you will use of an instrument called a **sphygmomanometer,** commonly called a "blood pressure cuff." The device has three basic parts—the cuff that wraps around the upper arm; the hand bulb with thumb valve that inflates and deflates the cuff, and the gauge that allows for measurement. When measuring blood pressure, you inflate the cuff on the patient's upper arm to a pressure that is greater than the pressure in the brachial artery. When the cuff is properly inflated, normal pulses and arterial blood flow distal to the cuff in the anterior elbow and wrist are temporarily lost. As the cuff is deflated, blood flow will return. You should record the pressure showing on the gauge at the point at which the blood flow returns. This is equal to the systolic pressure Detecting the point at which blood flow returns can be done in two ways: by listening with a stethoscope over the brachial artery (called *auscultation*) or by feeling the brachial pulse (called *palpation*).

Determining Blood Pressure

The procedure for determining a patient's blood pressure is as follows (Figure 7-44):

1. Have the patient sit or lie down, depending on his condition. For the sitting patient, have the patient's arm slightly flexed at the elbow and supported at the level of his heart. (Note that obtaining a blood pressure from a standing patient is very awkward for both the patient and the EMT.)

2. Place the cuff snugly around the upper arm just above the elbow. The lower edge of the cuff should be about 1 inch (25 mm) above the crease of the elbow. For most patients, a standard adult-size cuff may be used. With pediatric or particularly large patients, select a cuff width that will cover about two-thirds of the upper arm above the elbow. Cuffs that are too small will give falsely high readings.

3. Palpate for the brachial pulse, which is located medially on the surface of the anterior

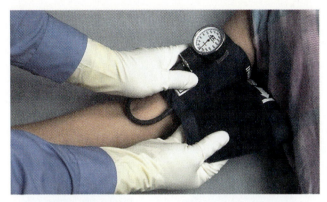

A.

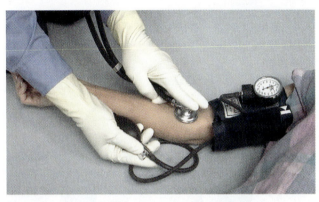

B.

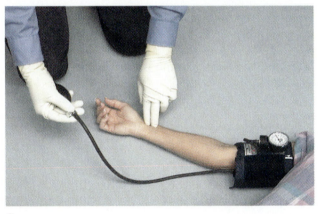

C.

Figure 7-44 When taking the patient's blood pressure, **(A)** position the cuff properly and inflate. You can then determine the blood pressure either by **(B)** auscultation or by **(C)** palpation of the brachial or radial pulse.

elbow at the crease (antecubital fossa). With the thumb or two fingers of one hand on the brachial pulse, inflate the cuff to about 30 mmHg above the pressure at which the pulse disappears. (You can also perform this procedure by palpating the radial pulse.)

4. Without moving your fingers from the area where the brachial pulse was felt, slowly deflate the cuff. Keeping an eye on the sphygmomanometer's gauge, note the pressure at which the pulse in the brachial artery returns. This is the systolic blood pressure as determined by palpation. Deflate the cuff completely.

5. Place the bell of the stethoscope over the brachial artery at the same place you felt the pulse. Make sure the ear pieces of the stethoscope are pointed forward into your ear canals. Reinflate the cuff to about 30 mmHg above the palpated systolic pressure.

6. Slowly deflate the cuff at a rate of no more than 3 to 5 mmHg per second. As the cuff deflates, watch the gauge and listen to the stethoscope for the sound of pulse beats in the stethoscope. The pressure at which the first two consecutive beats (or clicks or taps) are heard is the systolic pressure by auscultation.

7. Continue to allow the cuff to deflate and note the pressure at which the pulse sounds disappear (or the sounds change from clicks or taps to dull thuds). The pressure on the gauge when the pulse sounds disappear is the diastolic blood pressure.

8. Record your findings. It is generally not necessary to report or document the systolic pressure both by palpation and by auscultation unless there is a difference of greater than 10 to 20 mmHg between the two.

Often at a noisy scene or in a moving ambulance, it is only possible to determine the systolic blood pressure by palpation. If you can only obtain the palpated systolic pressure, report your finding as "by palpation." If, for example, you obtain a systolic pressure of 140 mmHg by palpation, write this as "BP is 140/palp" or "BP is 140/P."

Skin

The skin should be assessed again as it was in the initial assessment. Assess for the color, temperature, and condition of the skin. When assessed along with the other vital signs, changes in skin condition often indicate improvement or deterioration in the patient's condition. A patient whose skin was initially pale, cold, and clammy but who now has warm and dry skin is likely improving; the changes in skin condition indicate better circulation (perfusion). Indications of a worsening condition might be seen in a patient whose skin was initially pink, warm, and dry but who later presents with pale, cool, and clammy skin.

Remember that skin color is best assessed around the nail beds, lips, and mucous membranes inside the eyelids. When you assess skin temperature and condition, use the back of an ungloved portion of your hand. Be careful to avoid blood and other body fluids on the patient's skin. You can review the possible meanings of the various skin colors and conditions on page 172.

Pupils

The dark center area of the eye is known as the pupil. In a normal eye, the pupil will become larger (dilate) in low light conditions. It will get smaller (constrict) in bright light conditions. In a normal patient, the pupils of both eyes will constrict and dilate together, maintaining equal size in relation to each other. For example, if the light from a penlight is shined into one eye, both pupils will constrict to the same smaller size. When pupils react properly to light conditions they are said to be "reactive."

During your assessment of the pupils, you will check to see that both pupils are reactive and that both pupils are of equal size and shape (Figure 7-45). (Many systems use the memory aid PERRL when assessing the pupils. It stands for *P*upils *E*qual, *R*ound, and *R*eactive to *L*ight.) Pupils should be tested as follows:

1. Note the size of both pupils before you shine any light in them. The pupils should be of equal size. A small number of people normally have unequal pupils; if you observe this, ask the patient whether this condition is normal for him. Otherwise, you should assume a finding of unequal pupils in a patient to be new and important. The pupils should be an appropriate size for the light conditions. If the

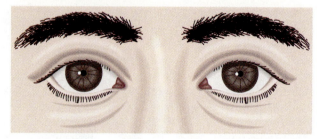

Constricted pupils

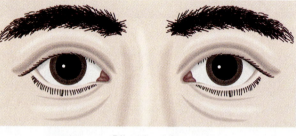

Dilated pupils

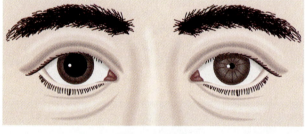

Unequal pupils

Figure 7-45 Assess the pupils for size and equality.

pupils are abnormally small ("pinpoint") or abnormally dilated, this should also be considered an important physical finding. Such findings may be related to a patient's unresponsiveness or altered mental status.

2. Shine a penlight in one eye while observing that same eye. The pupil should constrict when the light is shining into it and dilate when the light is removed. Wait 1 to 2 seconds. Then shine the light in the same eye again and remove it, but this time check the reaction in the other eye. The pupil should constrict when the light is shining in the other eye and dilate when it is removed.

3. Repeat the procedure above, this time shining the light in the other eye. Check first for its direct reactivity and then for the reactivity of the other eye.

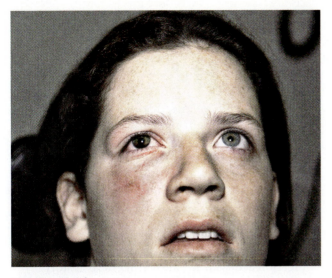

Figure 7-46 When assessing the eyes, note the presence of any abnormal collection of blood.

Table 7-8

Abnormal Findings in the Pupils

Pupil Appearance	Possible Cause
Constricted	Toxic exposure to pesticides; narcotic overdose; glaucoma medication; treatment with eye drops
Dilated	Fright; treatment with eye medication
Unequal	Stroke; head injury; eye injury; artificial eye (rare); normal condition (rare)
Lack of reactivity	Severe lack of oxygen to brain; local eye injury; drug use
Irregularly shaped	Acute injury, chronic disease, postoperative condition

When you are checking for pupil response and equality, you will sometimes note an abnormal collection of blood in the eye (Figure 7-46). If you detect an abnormal collection of blood, protect the eye from further injury (see Chapter 20).

SECTION V: Focused History and Physical Exam/Detailed Physical Exam—Medical Patients

After the initial assessment, the next step in patient assessment is the focused history and physical examination. During this assessment phase, you will use the skills of obtaining a SAMPLE history and taking vital signs that you learned in Section IV. In the scene size-up, you assured your safety as well as the patient's and began to put together information about his problem. In the initial assessment, you identified and managed immediately life-threatening problems.

In the focused history and physical exam, you will look more closely at the patient's problem and other information relevant to it. You'll identify any other life-threatening injuries or illnesses. Based on what you learn, you will provide appropriate prehospital medical care. The focused history and physical exam for the medical patient will differ from that for the trauma patient. Similarly, whether the patient is responsive or unresponsive will affect the specific steps to follow during assessment.

After completing the focused history and physical exam, you may perform a detailed physical exam to identify and treat other injuries and conditions. When and how to perform a detailed physical exam will be based on the type of patient you are caring for.

At the completion of this section of the chapter, the EMT-Basic student should be able to meet the following objectives:

Knowledge and Understanding

1. Describe the unique needs for assessing an individual with a specific chief complaint with no known prior medical history. (pp. 194–197)
2. Differentiate between the history and physical exam that are performed for responsive patients with no known prior history and responsive patients with a known prior history. (pp. 194–197)
3. Describe the needs for assessing an individual who is unresponsive. (pp. 189–194)
4. Differentiate between the assessment that is performed for a patient who is unresponsive or has an altered mental status and other medical patients requiring assessment. (pp. 188–197)

5. Attend to the feelings that medical patients might be experiencing. (pp. 194–195)
6. Distinguish between the detailed physical exam that is performed on a trauma patient and that of the medical patient. (pp. 194, 196–197)

Skills

1. Demonstrate the patient assessment skills that should be used to assist a patient who is responsive with no known medical history.
2. Demonstrate the patient assessment skills that should be used to assist a patient who is unresponsive or has an altered mental status.

Most of your calls as an EMT will be for medical patients. You will perform a focused history and physical examination on all of them as part of the patient assessment process. With these patients, it has been said that 85 percent of the assessment is based on the patient's *history* (both of past and present illnesses). That is, most of the vital information you will gather about a medical patient will come from the questions you ask and what you observe about the patient's chief complaint and past history. This differs from the trauma patient, where most vital information after you determine the mechanism of injury will come from the *physical examination*. Any physical findings that are made during the focused examination of the medical patient can be further investigated during the detailed physical examination if the situation permits.

APPROACHES TO THE FOCUSED HISTORY AND PHYSICAL EXAM

The "focus" of the focused history and physical exam for medical patients will be the chief complaint and the present illness—in other words, the reason the patient or someone else called EMS.

During this phase of the medical patient's assessment, you will gather information about the present illness, obtain a SAMPLE history, and determine baseline vital signs. The rapid physical assessment performed on the medical patient is

Table 7-9

Steps in the Focused History and Physical Exam—Medical Patients

Unresponsive Medical Patient	Responsive Medical Patient
Perform rapid physical assessment (head to toe.)	Obtain a history of the present illness and SAMPLE history (from patient).
↓	↓
Assess baseline vital signs.	Perform focused physical exam (based on the present illness).
↓	↓
Obtain SAMPLE history (from family or bystanders).	Assess baseline vital signs.

designed to detect physical findings related to the chief complaint and present illness.

The order in which you perform the steps of the focused history and physical exam with medical patients varies depending on whether the patient is unresponsive or responsive (see Table 7-9). Whether the patient has a past medical history related to the chief complaint will also influence the approach you take.

(see Table 7-9)

THE UNRESPONSIVE MEDICAL PATIENT

Before reading about the actual steps of the focused history and physical exam, consider the following case study that describes a call for an unresponsive medical patient.

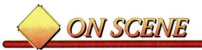

ON SCENE

DISPATCH: *PRIORITY 1—DELTA RESPONSE FOR AN UNCONSCIOUS FEMALE. ADDRESS IS 75 VAL VERDE DRIVE. TIME OUT IS 1534.*

You and two other EMTs are on duty for your fire department's rapid response BLS team. As your light rescue unit is en route, the emergency medical dispatcher updates you that the patient is unresponsive but breathing. You arrive at the scene 2 minutes later.

The house is located on a quiet residential street. There appear to be no hazards as you and your crew approach the front door. A teenaged girl meets you there. She gives her name as Jamie Taylor and tells you, "My sister Becky and I got home from school a few minutes ago. Mom was lying on the living room floor when we came in the door. We tried to wake her up, but she didn't say anything or move or open her eyes. Becky stayed with Mom then, and I called 9-1-1."

Jamie leads you into the house to a neatly kept living room. Another teenaged girl is kneeling beside a woman lying supine on a rug in the center of the room. Your general impression of the patient is that of an unresponsive female in her early 40s found in an environment that does not immediately explain why she is unconscious. You quickly determine Mrs. Taylor's mental status as unresponsive (U on the AVPU scale) because she does not respond when you say her name loudly or when you pinch her earlobe. You open her airway with a jaw-thrust maneuver and note that the airway is clear. You observe the patient's equal and full chest rise and a respiratory rate of about 15 breaths per minute and determine that her breathing is adequate.

As your partners apply high flow oxygen with a nonrebreather mask, you quickly assess Mrs. Taylor's circulation. You note that she has a weak and rapid radial pulse and that her skin is cool and clammy to the touch. You determine that Mrs. Taylor is a high priority for transport. You radio the in-coming ambulance and advise its crew of the patient's condition. You also request that the dispatcher arrange an ALS intercept while the patient is en route to the hospital. While one of your partners monitors the airway, you begin the focused history and physical exam of this unresponsive patient.

The Rapid Physical Examination— Unresponsive Patient

During the initial assessment, you determine a patient's mental status. This status helps decide the order in which you perform the focused history and physical exam for the medical patient. Whenever you determine that a patient either is unresponsive or has an altered mental status, you should perform an immediate rapid physical examination. The purpose of this exam is to identify any possible physical causes for the patient's mental status. Perform this examination in a systematic, head-to-toe order (Figure 7-47).

Rapid Physical Exam—Unresponsive Medical Patient

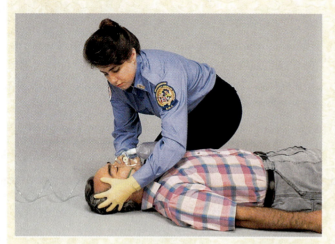

Figure 7-47A Assess and palpate the head.

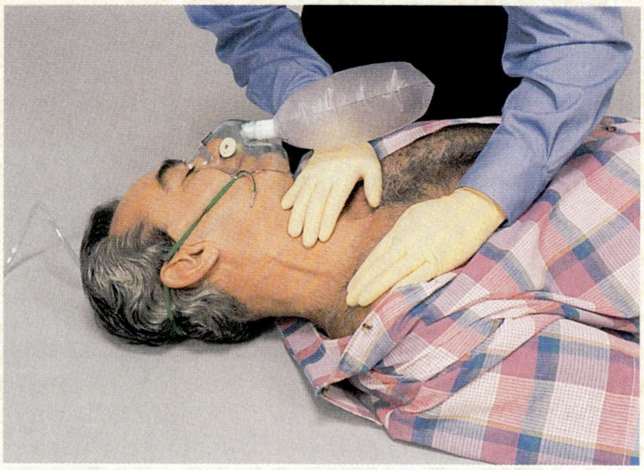

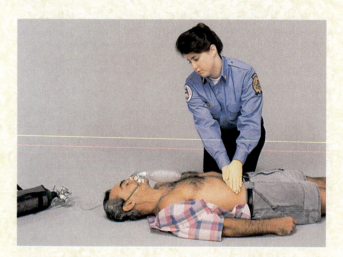

Figure 7-47B Assess the neck. Look for jugular vein distention, excessive use of neck muscles in breathing, a tracheostomy tube, or a medical identification device.

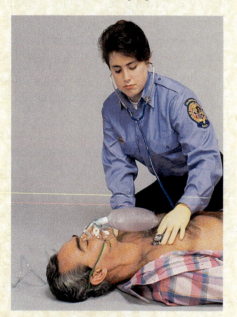

Figure 7-47C Assess the chest. Look for adequate rise and fall during respirations. Look for accessory muscle use during respirations. Auscultate breath sounds.

Figure 7-47D Assess the abdomen. Look for scars, discoloration, or distention. Palpate for tenderness, rigidity, distention, and pulsating masses.

1. Assess the head.

Look (inspect) and feel (palpate) for any signs of trauma. These signs might include bruising, lacerations, swellings, depressions, or blood in the ears. Trauma to the head is a common cause of patient unresponsiveness. If you find signs of trauma, assume that a neck injury also occurred and immediately provide manual stabilization for the cervical spine.

Open the mouth to assess for any new airway problems including obstruction by vomitus, loose teeth, or bleeding. If the airway is not open, discontinue the rapid examination. Instead, clear the airway through positioning—

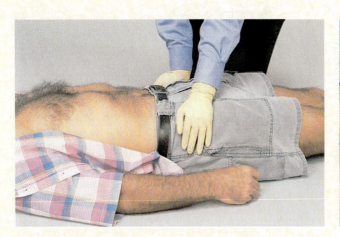

Figure 7-47E Assess the lower abdomen and pelvic region. palpate for distention and tenderness.

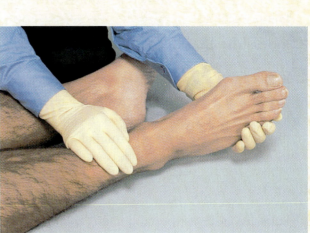

Figure 7-47F Assess all extremities. Inspect for swelling and discoloration.

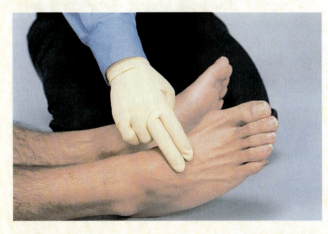

Figure 7-47G Assess pulses in all extremities.

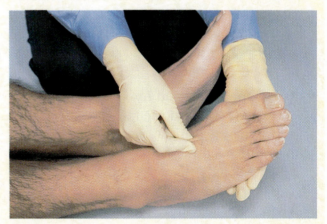

Figure 7-47H Assess motor function and sensation in all extremities. Conclude the rapid physical exam by inspecting and palpating the patient's posterior body.

with the head-tilt, chin-lift maneuver or the jaw-thrust maneuver in patients with suspected neck or spine injury—or through use of suction, before proceeding with the examination.

2. Assess the neck.

Inspect for the presence of a medical identification device such as a necklace. It may

indicate that the patient has diabetes, a seizure disorder, or some other medical condition that may account for the change in mental status.

Look also for the presence of **jugular vein distention** (JVD). You can best assess this bulging of the veins when the patient is found in a sitting position. JVD may indicate that the patient's heart cannot pump effectively, a condition known as congestive heart failure (CHF).

3. Assess the chest.

Look for adequate and equal rise of both sides of the chest as the patient breathes. Watch for any use of accessory muscles in the chest and lower neck during breathing. Quickly listen to the chest anteriorly at the mid-clavicular line to determine if breath sounds are present and equal.

4. Assess the abdomen.

Look to see if the abdomen is distended (swollen) or discolored. Palpate the abdomen to determine if it is tender. Feel for any masses. An **aneurysm** (weakening and bulging of the wall) of the abdominal aorta may be felt as a pulsating mass in the center of the abdomen. Blood loss from an aortic aneurysm may account for altered mental status or unconsciousness.

5. Assess the pelvis and lower abdomen.

Check the lower abdomen for distention. Also palpate that region and the pelvic bones and hips for tenderness. Lower abdominal tenderness in young women may indicate a gynecological emergency. Hip fractures are common in elderly patients who pass out and fall.

6. Assess the extremities.

Assess the upper extremities first, and then the lower extremities. Look again for medical identification bracelets. (Teenagers often wear them around the ankle.) Look for swelling, deformity, or discoloration. Observe for needle marks over the anterior upper extremities (usually from injection of street drugs) and over the thighs (a site often used by diabetics for insulin injections). Check that pulses are present and equal in all extremities.

Check also for motor function and sensation in each of the patient's extremities. A deeply unconscious patient may have no response at all, whereas a patient with altered mental status may move the extremities when stimulated by touch. Pinch the hands and feet to see if the patient reacts.

7. Assess the posterior body.

Carefully roll the patient onto his side. Use spinal precautions if head or neck trauma has been detected earlier in the examination. Observe any wounds, deformities, or contusions.

In the On Scene case described above, the only significant physical finding during the focused history and physical exam was a medical identification bracelet Mrs. Taylor was wearing. It identified her as a diabetic.

Determining Baseline Vital Signs

Obtain a set of baseline vital signs on the unresponsive medical patient as soon as you complete the rapid physical exam. Follow the procedures described above in Section IV of this chapter. Remember that vital signs include the patient's respiratory rate, skin condition, pulse rate, condition of the pupils, and blood pressure. Whenever you take vital signs, you should also reassess the patient's mental status using the AVPU classifications described in the initial assessment. It is especially important to monitor closely for changes in mental status with patients who are unresponsive or who have severely altered mental status.

In Mrs. Taylor's case, the findings were as follows: respiratory rate—30; skin—cool and clammy; pulse rate—100; pupils—equal and reactive; blood pressure—120/70. The patient's mental status remained unresponsive.

Positioning the Patient

An unresponsive patient cannot protect his own airway. You must do it for him. Monitor the airway of any unresponsive patient continuously. Clear the airway as necessary.

If you have not already done so, place the patient on the stretcher and ready him for transport in a position that helps assure that the airway remains open. The left lateral recumbent, or recovery, position is usually ideal for this purpose (Figure 7-48). In it, the patient is placed on stretcher lying on his the left side. You can then more easily monitor and suction his airway during transport because the patient will be facing the bench where you will be sitting in the ambulance.

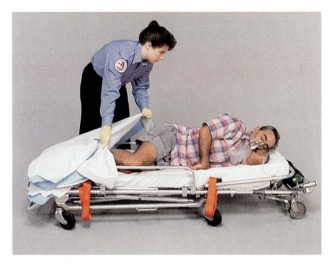

Figure 7-48 Place an unresponsive medical patient in the recovery position. This will help protect the airway and prevent aspiration of secretions, blood, or vomitus.

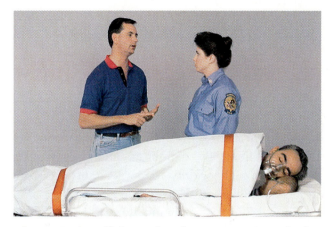

Figure 7-49 If the patient is unresponsive, obtain as much of the SAMPLE history as possible from family members or bystanders.

In some cases, use of the recovery position will not maintain an open airway. When it does not, move the patient into a supine position and open the airway with a head-tilt, chin-lift or a jaw-thrust maneuver. Continue to suction the patient's mouth and pharynx as needed. Insertion of an oro- or nasopharyngeal airway may be necessary to secure the airway.

Mrs. Taylor is placed on the stretcher in the recovery position.

Obtain a SAMPLE History

With an unresponsive medical patient, you will obtain the SAMPLE history after the rapid physical exam because that examination is of higher priority. When a patient is unresponsive, try to obtain the history by asking family members, friends, or bystanders about the patient and the events that led up to the current problem. Be aware, however, that there are times when you will be unable to get a complete SAMPLE history on an unresponsive patient. Perhaps no one was around when the emergency began. Or the people who are on hand simply don't know much about the patient or the events leading up to the emergency. When a patient is initially found unresponsive, ask anyone present when was the last time the patient was seen and if there appeared to be any problems at that time (Figure 7-49).

In the case of Mrs. Taylor, for example, you would try to find out about the patient's current problem and her past medical history from her daughters. The girls might be able to provide some information about their mother's past medical problems. In fact, after you mentioned the finding of the medical identification bracelet, the girls did confirm Mrs. Taylor's diabetes. However, it's unlikely that they could tell you much about the events leading up to the emergency since it occurred while they were in school or traveling to or from school. Under these circumstances, you should ask the daughters if their mother appeared ill or complained of any symptoms in the morning when they left for school.

In cases like these, EMS personnel should conduct a quick search of the premises for anything that might shed light on the patient's condition. In the On Scene case, an EMT searching the house for medications Mrs. Taylor might be taking found a supply of insulin in the refrigerator.

When adequate EMS personnel are available, the rapid physical examination and the taking of a SAMPLE history from family, friends, or bystanders can usually be done at the same time. When you don't have enough personnel to permit this, remember that the rapid physical examination takes priority over the SAMPLE history with the unresponsive medical patient.

Always assign an unresponsive medical patient a high priority for transport from the scene. Such patients warrant ALS evaluation and intervention. However, ALS assistance should be obtained only when it would not delay the patient's arrival at the emergency department.

The Detailed Physical Examination—Unresponsive Medical Patient

Do not waste time on the scene conducting a detailed physical examination on an unresponsive medical patient. By definition, an unresponsive patient is a high priority for rapid transport. You are far more likely to help such a patient by maintaining his airway, initiating transport, and performing an ongoing assessment than by performing a detailed physical exam on the scene.

There are, however, times when you may perform a detailed physical exam on an unresponsive medical patient en route to the hospital. Do so when the patient's condition is relatively stable and adequate personnel are present. The exam is especially appropriate if the cause of the patient's unresponsiveness remains unknown. When you perform the detailed exam, you will seek any additional information that may help emergency department staff determine the cause of the unresponsiveness. (See page 210 for how to perform this exam.)

THE RESPONSIVE MEDICAL PATIENT

With responsive medical patients, the order of the steps in the focused history and physical exam is different than with unresponsive patients. Before studying those steps, consider this case study.

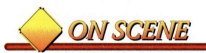
ON SCENE

DISPATCH: *AMBULANCE 621, PRIORITY 1. ELDERLY WOMAN WITH CHEST PAIN. ADDRESS IS BARDWELL TOWERS, 232 PALMER AVENUE. TIME OUT, 0412.*

You are one of two EMTs on your department's ambulance. You recognize the address as an apartment building that is home to many senior citizens. The building's night manager meets you at the front door when you pull up. The street outside and the halls of the building are as quiet as you'd expect this early in the morning, and you detect no obvious scene hazards.

The manager takes you up to the patient's apartment and lets you in. You proceed to the bedroom, where you begin your initial assessment.

Your general impression is that the patient is an elderly female who appears uncomfortable. She is sitting on the edge of the bed, dangling her feet over its side and holding her chest. You introduce yourself, and she responds weakly but appropriately, giving her name and thanking you for coming. You assess her mental status as normal and alert. Because she is speaking, her airway is open. However, you do notice that her breathing appears slightly labored, with a respiratory rate of about 30 breaths per minute. Your partner immediately provides Mrs. Cannon with high flow oxygen via nonrebreather mask.

You, meanwhile, begin to assess Mrs. Cannon's circulation by palpating her radial pulse. Although her skin appears normal, warm, and dry, you note that her pulse is very irregular, with many skipped beats. The patient's complaint of chest pain, her shortness of breath, and the irregular pulse that may indicate a cardiac arrhythmia lead you to assign Mrs. Cannon a high priority for rapid transport. You know that the ALS paramedic ambulance will be on the scene momentarily, so you begin to conduct your focused history and physical exam of this responsive medical patient.

History of the Present Illness—OPQRST

The conscious medical patient can provide you with a great deal of information. Obtaining a SAMPLE history with careful attention to the signs and symptoms of the present illness is the first step in the focused history and physical examination with a responsive medical patient.

Recall that the S in SAMPLE stands for Signs and Symptoms. Try to determine as much as possible about the patient's current signs and symptoms as you begin to take the SAMPLE history. The letters OPQRST can serve as memory aids for the questions to ask a patient about his signs and symptoms. These aids are particularly useful when the patient's symptoms are related to pain or shortness of breath. What the letters stand for and some questions you might use with patients follow:

◆ *Onset*—"What were you doing when the symptoms started?

◆ *Provocation*—"Is there anything that makes the symptoms worse

◆ *Quality*—"What does the pain feel like?"

◆ *Relief*—"Is there anything that makes the problem better?" "Have you moved to any position or taken medications that have made the problem better?"

◆ *Radiation (of pain)*—"Where do you feel the pain?" "Has the pain spread from where it started?" If the patient has chest pain, ask: "Does the pain go from your chest into your neck, jaw, shoulder, or arm?

◆ *Severity*—"How bad is the pain? How would you rate the pain on a scale of 1 to 10, with 10 being the worst pain you've felt in your life?"

◆ *Time*—"For how long has the problem been going on?"

You can see how the format is used by looking back at Mrs. Cannon, the patient in On Scene. When she was asked the questions above, she responded as follows:

Onset—"The chest pain woke me out of a sound sleep."

Provocation—"No, nothing makes the pain worse. But I just can't get comfortable."

Quality—"It feels dull, like a big dog is sitting on my chest."

Radiation (of pain)—"The pain started in my chest. It's spread. It goes up into my left arm like a terrible ache."

Severity—"The pain is bad. From 1 to 10, it's about 7."

Time—"The problem's been going on since I woke up, about 40 minutes ago."

A good general rule to follow when asking OPQRST questions is to make the questions as open ended as possible. Try not to ask questions that the patient can answer with a single word or a simple "Yes" or "No." For example, the question to Mrs. Cannon about the quality of the pain was "What does the pain feel like?" rather than "Is the pain sharp or dull?" You want to find out as much as possible about the problem, and open-ended questions encourage the patient to talk.

Completing the SAMPLE History

Having learned a great deal about the patient's symptoms with the OPQRST questions, you must go on to complete the SAMPLE history. Remember that, in addition to the *S* of *Signs/Symptoms* you must determine the following:

◆ *Allergies*—Does the patient have any allergies? Any allergies to medications?

◆ *Medications*—Is the patient taking any medications?

◆ *Pertinent past history*—Does the patient have any past medical history that relates to the current problem?

◆ *Last oral intake*—When was the last time the patient ate or drank anything?

◆ *Events leading up to the illness*—What events led up to today's emergency?

Determining a responsive medical patient's past medical history and whether he takes any medications can be extremely important. A patient with a past medical history may be taking a medication like nitroglycerin for chest pain or an albuterol inhaler for breathing difficulty. You may be able to assist a patient with taking certain prescribed medications.

Always remember to record the patient's answers to OPQRST and SAMPLE questions.

With Mrs. Cannon, the remaining SAMPLE responses give you this additional information. She denies any allergies. She has a prescribed pain reliever for arthritis and prescribed nitroglycerin for chest pain. She acknowledges previous episodes of chest pain "every few months." She had chicken breast with rice and broccoli and a cup of herbal tea for dinner at about 7 P.M. and a glass of water with her pain reliever about 11 P.M. She had done nothing special the previous day and was asleep when the pain woke her.

The Focused Physical Examination—Responsive Medical Patient

With an unresponsive medical patient, you performed a rapid, head-to-toe physical assessment, looking for possible causes of his altered mental status. With a responsive medical patient, the physical exam is usually much more limited. This exam is *focused*. You should direct it to the part(s) of the body that relate to the patient's current complaint.

For example, in On Scene, Mrs. Cannon's chief complaint was chest pain. Therefore, her physical exam should focus on things related to chest pain—checking the neck for JVD, palpating the center of the chest to check for tenderness, observing her chest wall movement and auscultating her lungs (because of her increased respiratory rate noted on the initial assessment). The exam might also include a rapid palpation of her left arm for signs of injury because she complained of the pain radiating to that arm.

Sometimes, a responsive patient's complaints will be too vague or general to help you focus on a certain area or areas of the body. A patient might, for example, complain of "aching all over." In such cases, you should perform a rapid physical assessment like the one you would perform on an unresponsive medical patient.

Assessing Baseline Vital Signs

Once the focused physical exam of the patient has been completed, you should obtain a full set of baseline vital signs. Follow the same procedures that were described in Section IV of this chapter.

In the case of Mrs. Cannon, the findings were as follows: respiratory rate—30; skin—warm and dry; pulse—100, irregular and thready; pupils—equal and reactive; blood pressure—180/90. The patient remained alert and oriented.

Providing Emergency Care

What you learn in the initial assessment and the focused history and physical examination, should give you enough information to provide appropriate emergency medical care for the patient. That care might be simply providing supplemental oxygen and transporting a patient. Or it might involve rewarming a patient suffering from exposure to the cold or cooling a patient with a heat-related emergency. In some EMS systems, you might assist certain patients with administration of their prescribed medications, such as nitroglycerin for chest pain, prescribed inhalers or nebulizers for shortness of breath, and the epinephrine auto-injector for allergic reaction. You will learn the specifics of the care you can provide in later chapters.

Keep in mind, however, that some responsive medical patients are high priority for immediate transport and possible ALS intervention. Among them are patients with symptoms of chest pain, altered mental status, severe pain, and shortness of breath. In addition, patients who present a poor general impression or who are breathing inadequately should also be considered high priority.

If you have any questions about transport priority or treatment of a patient, contact medical direction.

In Mrs. Cannon's case, you determine that she has nitroglycerin spray that is prescribed for her. You contact medical direction, which authorizes you to assist the patient with administration of the nitroglycerin. You help Mrs. Cannon, following procedures that will be described in Chapter 13, "Cardiac Emergencies."

The Detailed Physical Examination—Responsive Medical Patient

The focused physical examination of the responsive medical patient is somewhat limited in scope.

The same is true of the detailed physical examination. In these physical exams, the chief complaint and signs and symptoms of the present illness determine what parts of the body you examine. If time allows, you may examine areas related to the chief complaint, signs, and symptoms. On the other hand, it is equally acceptable not to perform a detailed examination at all on many medical patients, but instead to initiate transport and begin the ongoing assessment.

SECTION VI: Focused History and Physical Examination/Detailed Physical Examination—Trauma Patients

The assessment of the trauma patient differs somewhat from that of the medical patient. Although the scene size-up and initial assessment are largely the same for both types of patients, after those steps the assessment of the trauma patient is largely based on the findings from the physical examination. This is unlike the assessment of the medical patient, where the greater emphasis is usually placed on the patient history.

As was the case with medical patients, you will sometimes also perform a detailed physical examination on trauma patients. When and how to perform that exam are described below.

OBJECTIVES

At the completion of this section of the chapter, the EMT-Basic student should be able to meet the following objectives:

Knowledge and Understanding

1. Discuss the reasons for reconsideration concerning the mechanism of injury during the focused history and physical examination. (pp. 198–199)
2. State the reasons for performing a rapid trauma assessment. (p. 201)
3. Recite examples and explain why patients should receive a rapid trauma assessment. (pp. 200–201)
4. Describe the areas of the body included in the rapid trauma assessment and discuss what should be evaluated in each area. (pp. 205, 206–209)
5. Differentiate when the rapid trauma assessment may be altered in order to provide patient care. (pp. 200–201)
6. Discuss the reasons for performing a focused history and physical exam. (pp. 216–217)
7. Discuss the components of the detailed physical exam. (pp. 210, 211–215, 217)
8. State the areas of the body that are evaluated during the detailed physical exam. (pp. 211–215)
9. Explain what additional care should be provided while performing the detailed physical exam. (p. 210)
10. Distinguish between the detailed physical exam that is performed on a trauma patient and that of the medical patient. (pp. 194, 196–197, 210)
11. Recognize and respect the feelings that patients might experience during assessment. (p. 201)
12. Explain the rationale for the feelings that these patients might be experiencing. (p. 201)

Skills

1. Demonstrate the rapid trauma assessment that should be used to assess a patient based on the mechanism of injury.
2. Demonstrate the skills involved in performing the detailed physical exam.

In the last section, you learned that how you perform the focused history and physical exam with medical patients depends on whether the patients are responsive or unresponsive. There are also different ways of performing the focused history and physical exam with trauma patients. With these patients, the differences depend on the severity of the patients' mechanisms of injury.

RECONSIDERING THE MECHANISM OF INJURY

You initially determined the mechanism of injury during the scene size-up. Reevaluating that mechanism is the first step in the focused history and physical exam of the trauma patient. By determining how serious the mechanism of injury is, you will know how to proceed with the focused history and physical examination. With a patient who has a significant mechanism of injury—one that has the potential to result in serious injuries—you will carry out a rapid trauma assessment. This is an aggressive head-to-toe search for serious or potentially life threatening injuries. With a trauma patient who does not have a significant mechanism of injury, you will instead perform a focused physical exam and gather a history related to the specific injury.

The experiences of EMS personnel and medical research have demonstrated that certain mechanisms of injury are more likely to result in serious patient injuries. These mechanisms include the following:

◆ Motor vehicle crashes where the patient was:

—ejected from the vehicle

—in the same passenger compartment where a death of another occupant occurred

—involved in a rollover

—involved in a high speed crash

—unrestrained

—propelled with enough force to deform the steering wheel (remember to lift and look at the steering wheel under a deployed airbag to check for deformity)

◆ Pedestrians struck by vehicles

◆ Motorcycle crashes

◆ Falls of greater than 20 feet (6 m)

◆ Blast injuries from explosions

◆ Penetrating injuries (gunshot wounds or stabbings) to the head, chest, abdomen, or proximal extremities.

With pediatric patients, significant mechanisms would include the following:

◆ Falls greater than 10 feet (3 m)

◆ Motor vehicle crash in which the child was wearing only a lap belt—especially if seat belt marks are seen across the abdomen

◆ Medium speed collisions

◆ Bicycle collisions—especially those in which the child was struck in the abdomen by the handle bar

Not all the patients that you encounter with these mechanisms of injury will have serious injuries. However, these patients are at such an increased risk that a rapid trauma assessment aimed at uncovering signs and symptoms of serious injury is warranted.

You should also presume that serious injury exists in any trauma patient found during the initial assessment to be unresponsive or to have an altered mental status, inadequate breathing, or inadequate circulation. You should perform a rapid trauma assessment on these patients as well.

Fortunately, many of the injuries trauma patients receive result from minor mechanisms of injury. Examples of such mechanisms would include the following:

◆ A cut to the finger received when picking up a broken drinking glass

◆ An ankle injury received when stepping in a hole

◆ A cut on a toddler's face received when he ran into a coffee table

Patients with mechanisms of injury like these do not need the extensive evaluation and rapid trauma assessment required by patients with significant mechanisms of injury. When a trauma patient has no significant mechanism of injury, you will need to perform a trauma assessment that is focused on the site of the injury and gather history related to that injury.

The differences in how to carry out the focused history and physical exam for trauma patients based on mechanisms of injury are summarized in Table 7-10.

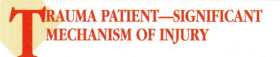

TRAUMA PATIENT—SIGNIFICANT MECHANISM OF INJURY

Begin study of the focused history and physical exam in a trauma patient with a significant mechanism of injury, by reading the case study below.

Table 7-10

Focused History and Physical Examination—Trauma Patients

Significant Mechanism of Injury	No Significant Mechanism of Injury
After scene size-up and initial assessment:	After scene size-up and initial assessment:
Reconsider the mechanism of injury.	Reconsider the mechanism of injury.
↓	
Continue spinal stabilization.	↓
↓	
Consider a request for ALS assistance.	↓
↓	
Reconsider the transport decision.	↓
↓	
Reassess mental status.	↓
↓	
Perform rapid trauma assessment.	Perform focused physical exam based on chief complaint and mechanism of injury.
↓	↓
Assess baseline vital signs.	Assess baseline vital signs.
↓	↓
Obtain a SAMPLE history.	Obtain a SAMPLE history.

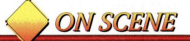

DISPATCH: *COUNTY DISPATCH TO STATION 4. RESPOND TO REPORTED ROLLOVER ON SHORE ROAD JUST EAST OF STONE MILL. STATE POLICE ARE ON SCENE. TIME OUT IS 0235.*

Jack Ball, who is the district chief and also an EMT, responds to the call. He arrives and sizes up the scene. As he examines the vehicle, which is resting at the bottom of an embankment, he speaks to the state police officer, who saw the accident. The trooper says the car drifted across the center line, went off the road, and rolled over several times before coming to rest on its wheels. As Chief Ball makes his way down the embankment, he observes an unconscious person who has been partially ejected from the passenger-side door. Chief Ball radios Fire Control his general impression that the incident involves a serious trauma. He requests that a LifeGuard helicopter respond directly to the scene.

The patient is showing signs of responsiveness as Chief Ball and the trooper reach his side. The chief asks the trooper to manually stabilize the patient's neck while the chief continues with the initial assessment. The patient's airway is open, but he seems to be having some difficulty breathing, and there is unequal expansion of his chest during inspiration. Chief Ball immediately places the patient on high concentration oxygen via nonrebreather mask.

Rescue 4 arrives on scene, and the chief instructs its crew to bring down a basket stretcher, a cervical collar, head blocks, and a long spine board. One EMT takes over manual cervical stabilization from the trooper as another firefighter-EMT places a cervical collar on the patient. As the patient is immobilized on the spine board, the chief completes the initial assessment, noting that the patient's pulse is present but rapid and that his skin is cool and clammy.

Using a low-angle rescue technique, the Rescue 4 crew moves the patient to the roadside to await the arrival of the helicopter. As they wait, Chief Ball conducts a rapid trauma assessment. It reveals severe deformity of the right chest wall, a very tender abdomen, and a deformity of the patient's right forearm. It is also apparent that the patient is now fully awake. He gives his name as Aaron Bartfield and complains of trouble in breathing and abdominal pain. Just as the chief finishes taking baseline vital signs, the Life-Guard crew arrives on the scene.

Chief Ball gives an oral report and a copy of the just-obtained vital signs to the flight crew. The patient is then loaded onto the helicopter. Four minutes later, LifeGuard is in-bound to the trauma center. Chief Ball radios Fire Control and places all fire-rescue units back in service.

PRIORITIES WITH THE TRAUMA PATIENT WITH SIGNIFICANT MECHANISM OF INJURY

A seriously injured trauma patient requires care at the hospital—preferably a trauma center. Your role as an EMT is to rapidly identify this patient, detect and correct life-threatening conditions during the initial assessment, and identify specific signs, symptoms, and injuries during the focused history and physical exam. The steps of the focused history and examination of trauma patients with significant mechanisms of injury are designed to allow you to provide the best possible care on the scene while minimizing the time you spend there. Review the steps listed in Table 7-10. Each of those steps is described below.

Continuing Spinal Stabilization

You initially identified the mechanism of injury during the scene size-up. You should also reevaluate the mechanism as you begin the focused history and physical exam. You should have provided the patient with manual spinal stabilization as soon as you identified a significant mechanism of injury in the scene size-up. Manual stabilization should have continued throughout the initial assessment. You will continue to provide manual stabilization throughout the focused history and physical exam until the patient is fully immobilized for transport.

Requesting ALS Support

With seriously injured trauma patients, always consider a request for ALS support, if available. ALS personnel can provide advanced airway management and other life-saving interventions that you as an EMT are not trained or authorized to carry out. Often, ALS personnel can reach a seriously injured patient in less time than it would take to get the patient to a hospital. In such cases, an ALS intercept would be appropriate. Do not, however, allow waiting for an ALS intercept to delay transport of a patient to a receiving facility.

Reconsidering the Transport Decision

Never forget that the priority with the severely injured patient is to get him off the scene and to the hospital as quickly as possible. The patient's survival depends on rapidly reaching definitive care. Be prepared to transport the patient at any time during the rapid trauma assessment if you discover critical injuries or note that the patient's condition is deteriorating.

Remember, you may carry out the rapid trauma assessment and the history taking either on the scene or en route to the hospital. Your decision about where to perform these steps will depend on the hazards at the scene, the availability of a transport unit, and the patient's condition.

Reassessing Mental Status

Repeat the mental assessment of the patient using the AVPU scale as you did in the initial assessment. Be particularly alert to deterioration in mental status—for example, a patient who had responded to a verbal stimulus but now only responds to a painful one. This is a sign that the patient's condition is worsening. In such cases of altered mental status or unresponsiveness, consider transport a high priority.

Performing the Rapid Trauma Assessment

The physical exam portion of focused history and physical exam for the trauma patient with a significant mechanism of injury is also called the "rapid trauma assessment." During the rapid trauma assessment, you will gain more specific information about the patient's injuries while continuing to manage any life-threatening conditions.

The rapid trauma assessment is done in a head-to-toe fashion. It begins with assessment of the head and ends with an examination of the extremities. Remember that significant mechanisms of injury can often cause damage to more than one part of the body. The rapid trauma assessment is designed to ensure that you check all parts of a patient's body for significant injuries.

During the rapid trauma assessment, you will search for signs or symptoms of injuries in the following ways:

◆ By inspecting (looking)

◆ By palpating (feeling)

◆ By auscultating (listening with a stethoscope)

You will be searching for the many different types of injuries trauma produces. They include *d*eformities, *c*ontusions, *a*brasions, *p*unctures and *p*enetrations, *b*urns, *t*enderness, *l*acerations, and *s*welling (Figure 7-50). The first letters of these injuries make up the memory aid DCAP-BTLS, pronounced "dee-cap, b-t-l-s." During the rapid trauma assessment, you will inspect each part of the body for DCAP-BTLS injuries. Most of these injuries can be identified by inspection or palpation; one, tenderness, can only be discovered by palpation. Characteristics of the DCAP-BTLS injuries are given in Table 7-11.

When you perform a rapid trauma assessment, you will rapidly and systematically inspect and palpate all regions of a patient's body (Figure 7-51, page 206). In addition to DCAP-BTLS injuries, you will also check for other signs of injury that are specific to different regions. The body regions and what you should be examining for in each of those areas are shown in Table 7-12. Once you have examined the anterior surface of the body, you should log-roll the patient onto his side, observing spinal precautions, so you can examine the back for injuries. You can examine injuries found during the rapid trauma assessment more carefully during the detailed physical examination if time and the patient's condition permit.

As you identify injuries during the rapid trauma assessment, begin to form a plan for treatment for those injuries. Think of how you will dress lacerations or punctures and how you might immobilize tender, swollen, or deformed extremities. You can begin to treat these non-life-threatening injuries after completing the focused history and physical examination if all life-threatening injuries are controlled.

Assessing Baseline Vital Signs

As you complete the rapid trauma assessment, obtain a full set of baseline vital signs following the procedures in Section IV of this chapter. As with medical patients, you will determine respiratory rate, skin condition, pulse rate, condition of the pupils, and blood pressure.

In assessment of a trauma patient with a significant mechanism of injury, the vital signs are a
(text continues, page 204)

Identifying DCAP-BTLS Injuries

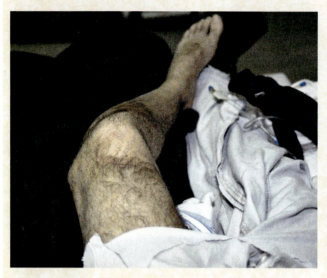

Figure 7-50A Deformity

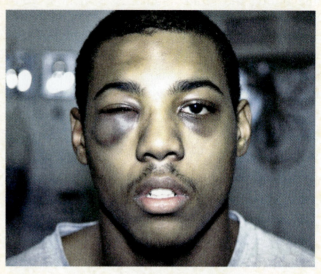

Figure 7-50B Contusion.

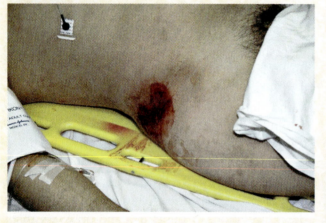

Figure 7-50C Abrasion.

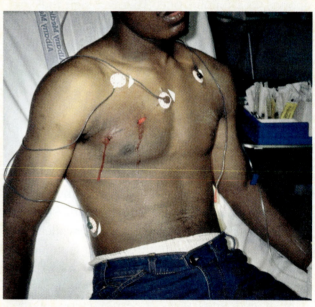

Figure 7-50D Puncture/penetration.

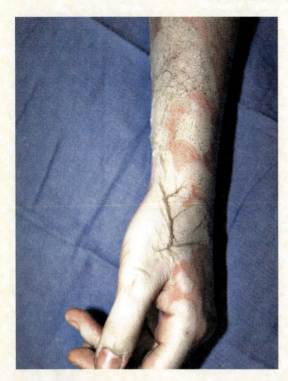

Figure 7-50E Burn.

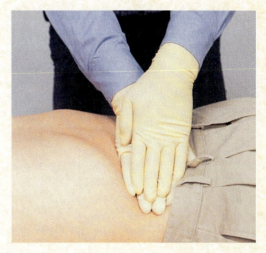

Figure 7-50F Palpate for tenderness.

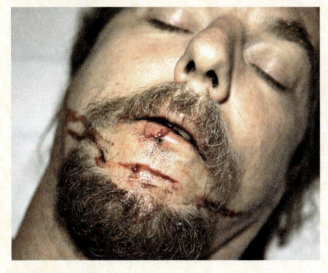

Figure 7-50G Laceration.

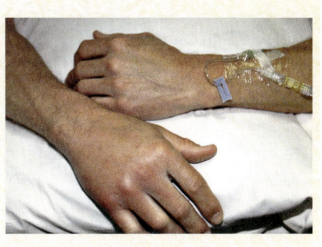

Figure 7-50H Swelling.

Table 7-11

Characteristics of DCAP-BTLS Injuries

Injury	Description	How Discovered
Deformity	Any appearance of a body part where the normal contours of the anatomy are distorted	Inspection, palpation
Contusion	Body area with bruising, characterized by bluish-red discoloration	Inspection
Abrasion	Body area where skin has been scraped off	Inspection
Puncture/penetration	Wound where a sharp object has stabbed into the skin and possibly into deeper structures; the object may or may not still be present in the wound	Inspection
Burn	Area where the skin has been injured by contact with chemicals, heat, or radiation. .	Inspection
Tenderness*	Areas that when touched produces complaints of pain, moaning, or a pulling away by the patient	Palpation
Laceration	Wounds or cuts to the skin	Inspection
Swelling	Area where skin and tissue bulge out due to injury	Inspection, palpation

*Tenderness is an objective *sign* that you can observe. Pain is a subjective *symptom* that the patient must tell you about (complain of). In cases of trauma, areas that the patient complains of as being painful are usually found to be tender on palpation, but this is not always the case.

particularly important indicator of the patient's condition. Abnormal findings in the baseline vital signs or a deteriorating trend discovered when later sets of vital signs are taken may help detect signs of shock (hypoperfusion). You should be very concerned when you discover persistent or increasing tachycardia (a pulse rate greater than 100 beats per minute in an adult) in a trauma patient. As you will learn in Chapter 19, "Bleeding and Shock," this early and important sign of shock appears long before the patient's blood pressure begins to fall. Pale, cool, and clammy skin may be another indication of shock.

Obtaining the SAMPLE History

Because the primary focus in trauma assessment is determining the nature and extent of injuries, obtaining the SAMPLE history is the last step in the focused history and physical examination. As you remember, this is in contrast to the focused history and physical exam of the medical patient, where the history is often the primary focus.

As with a medical patient, if the trauma patient is responsive, ask him the SAMPLE questions. If he is unresponsive, ask family, friends, or bystanders.

(*text continues, page 208*)

Table 7-12

Rapid Trauma Assessment by Body Region

Body Region	DCAP-BTLS	Also Assess For
Head	DCAP-BTLS	*Crepitation*—palpable or audible crunching or grating on palpation of the scalp and/or face
Neck*	DCAP-BTLS	*Crepitation* *Jugular vein distention*—may indicate heart failure or life-threatening chest injury
Chest	DCAP-BTLS	*Crepitation* *Paradoxical motion*—movement of a section of the chest wall inward when the patient inhales and outward when he exhales (opposite, or paradoxical, to normal motion); indicates multiple rib fractures *Breath sounds*—auscultate on the mid-clavicular line on both sides at the tops and bases of the lungs to determine if breath sounds are absent, present, and equal on both sides (Figure 7-54)
Abdomen	DCAP-BTLS	*Distention*—bloating *Rigidity*—the abdomen is firm to the touch upon palpation *Seatbelt marks*—can be a sign of serious injury, especially in children
Pelvis	DCAP-BTLS	*Stability*—if motion is felt or the patient reports pain when the pelvis is gently compressed, it is an indicator of a likely pelvic fracture *Signs of bowel or bladder incontinence*
Extremities	DCAP-BTLS	*Distal pulses*—check dorsalis pedis pulses on both feet, radial pulses on both wrists; determine equality of pulses on each side of body *Sensation*—with responsive patient, ask if he can feel your touch on each extremity; with unresponsive patient, compress nail beds or pinch web between fingers and toes to see if patient reacts *Motor function*—with responsive patient, ask him to wiggle fingers and toes; with unresponsive patient, observe for any spontaneous movement
Posterior (back)	DCAP-BTLS	

*Apply a cervical collar once the neck has been assessed during the rapid trauma assessment.

The Rapid Trauma Assessment

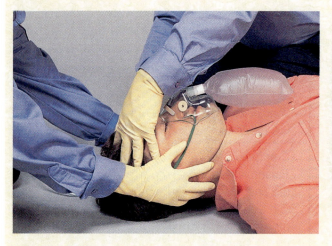

Figure 7-51A Inspect and palpate the scalp and skull.

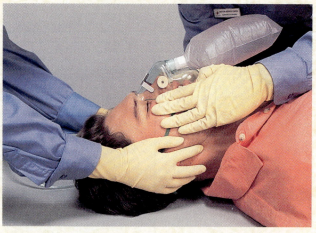

Figure 7-51B Inspect and/or palpate the face, including the ears, pupils, nose, and mouth. Watch for injuries that could block the airway with blood, bone, teeth, or tissue.

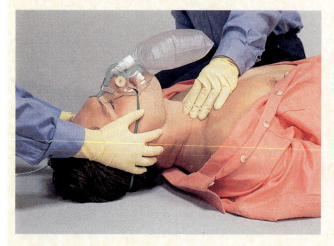

Figure 7-51C Inspect the neck. Look for jugular vein distention, excessive use of neck muscles in breathing, deformities, lacerations, and punctures.

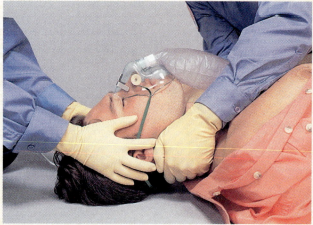

Figure 7-51D Palpate both anterior and posterior aspects of the neck. Note any posterior bony tenderness that may indicate injury to the cervical spine.

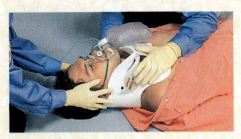

Figure 7-51E Apply a cervical collar.

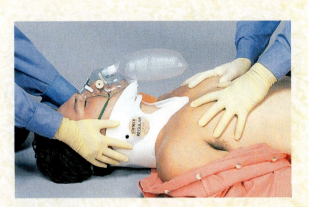

Figure 7-51F Expose the chest. Inspect and palpate for open wounds, flail segments, muscle retractions, and asymmetrical chest movement.

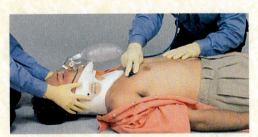

Figure 7-51G Perform a quick four-point auscultation of the chest, listening for the presence and equality of breath sounds.

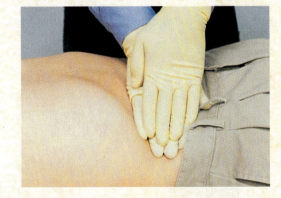

Figure 7-51H Inspect the abdomen for any evidence of trauma or distention. Palpate for tenderness and rigidity.

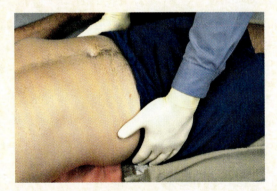

Figure 7-51I Inspect the pelvic area for evidence of instability. Palpate by gently pushing in on the wings of the pelvis.

(continued)

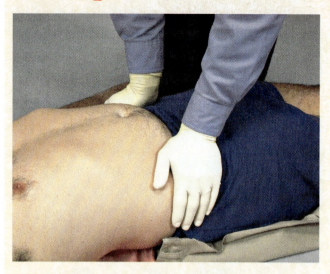

Figure 7-51J   Then gently push out on the wings.

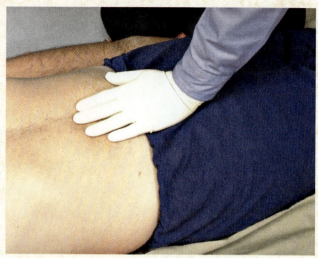

Figure 7-51K   Complete the pelvic assessment by pushing down with a flat hand just above the pubis.

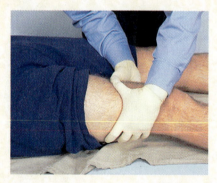

Figure 7-51L   Inspect and palpate each lower extremity.

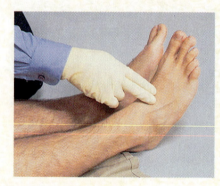

Figure 7-51M   Assess pedal pulses in both lower extremities.

With a conscious trauma patient, the *S*igns/*S*ymptoms portion of the SAMPLE history can be obtained while the rapid trauma assessment is going on. With these patients, ask questions that relate to the ongoing part of the assessment. For example, as you examine the chest, ask the patient if he has any chest pain or shortness of breath.

Although you usually will have determined the mechanism of injury by this stage, it is very important to find out as much as you can about the *E*vents that led up to the injury. For example, in the case of a motor vehicle crash, try to find out how fast the car was going and whether the patient was wearing a seat belt. In the case of a shooting, try to determine what kind of gun and caliber of ammu-

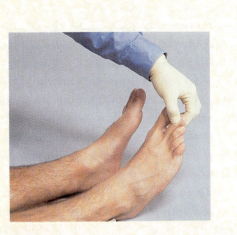

Figure 7-51N Assess motor and sensory function in each foot.

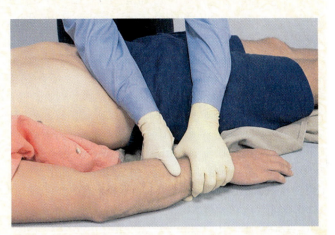

Figure 7-51O Inspect and palpate each upper extremity.

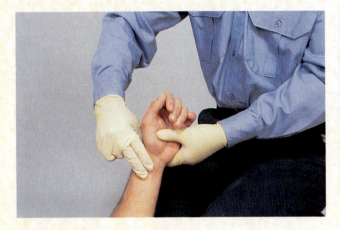

Figure 7-51P Assess pulses and motor and sensory function in each upper extremity.

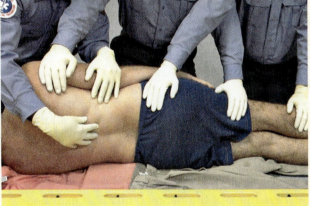

Figure 7-51Q Log-roll the patient and inspect and palpate the posterior body. Carefully palpate the spine for tenderness. Be sure to maintain in-line manual stabilization as you do this.

nition was used, the number of shots fired, and how far the patient was from the gun.

Trying to determine events leading up to a trauma can be especially crucial with older patients. Such patients often experience medical events that can cause the trauma-producing event. For example, you may be called to treat a patient injured in a motor vehicle crash. But the patient may have had a seizure, passed out (syncope), or suffered a cardiac arrest while driving. Your careful scene size-up should have provided you with clues to such situations. Crashes involving a single vehicle and the absence of skid marks at a crash site may point to a medical event before the crash. You should consider rapid transport and a request for ALS assistance whenever you encounter such patients. Remember that they may have potentially life-threatening medical conditions in addition to the injuries sustained in the crash.

Detailed Physical Examination— Trauma Patient with a Significant Mechanism of Injury

When you've completed the focused history and physical exam portion of the assessment, you may be able to perform a detailed physical exam. The purpose of this exam for the trauma patient with a serious mechanism of injury is to gain information about his non-life-threatening injuries and conditions and to provide care for them.

Undertake this exam only *after* you have managed *all* life-threatening injuries and conditions. Indeed, there will be many times when you never perform a detailed physical examination on a seri-

COMPANY OFFICER'S NOTES

The detailed physical exam of the seriously injured trauma patient is a luxury, to be conducted only if time permits. It should only be done while the patient is en route to the hospital. Its performance should never delay transport of the patient to the hospital. Always think of the detailed physical examination as something to be done "on-the-fly." (An exception to this rule would be a situation where the apparatus that is to transport the patient has not yet arrived on scene. At such times, the detailed physical exam can be performed as long as life-threatening conditions have been controlled.)

ously injured trauma patient. In some cases, the run time to the hospital may be too short for an exam, or the patient's condition may be so serious that all efforts in the back of the rig will be directed toward immediate patient care rather than additional examination.

The detailed physical exam is, like the rapid trauma assessment, performed in a systematic, head-to-toe order (Figure 7-52, page 212). If you have not already exposed the patient, do so now. You will examine the same body regions that you did in the earlier rapid assessment; in addition, you will more carefully assess the ears, eyes, nose, and mouth. During the exam you will be looking for DCAPS-BTLS injuries. Other things to assess for during the detailed physical exam are indicated in Table 7-13.

Remember, the search for any of these findings is of lesser priority than assuring that a patient's life-threatening conditions are treated and monitored. When time is short and the patient's condition is serious, it is likely that the detailed physical examination will not be completed.

TRAUMA PATIENT—NO SIGNIFICANT MECHANISM OF INJURY

When a trauma patient has no significant mechanism of injury, you will perform the focused history and physical exam differently than you would on a patient with a significant mechanism. Before exploring how the assessments differ, consider the case study on page 216.

Table 7-13

Detailed Physical Exam by Body Region

Body Region	Assess For
Head	DCAP-BTLS and *Crepitation*
Face	DCAP-BTLS
Ears	DCAP-BTLS and *Drainage*—drainage of blood may indicate local injury; drainage of clear fluid (cerebrospinal fluid) or clear fluid streaked with blood may indicate basilar skull fracture
Eyes	DCAP-BTLS and *Discoloration* *Unequal pupils* *Foreign bodies* *Blood in the anterior chamber (hyphema)*—sign that eye experienced considerable force (Figure 7-46, page 187)
Nose	DCAP-BTLS and *Drainage*—see Ears above
Mouth	DCAP-BTLS and *Teeth*—whether any are loose, whether they permit the mouth to close properly *Obstructions or potential obstructions in oral cavity* *Unusual breath odors*—alcohol, fruity breath odor (may indicate diabetes), accidentally or purposely ingested poisons (cleaners, solvents, cologne, etc.) *Discoloration of the oral cavity*—may include bluish color (cyanosis), pale discoloration (severe blood loss), and yellow discoloration (liver diseases and alcohol abuse)
Neck	DCAP-BTLS and *Jugular vein distention* *Crepitation* *Medical identification device*
Chest (anterior/posterior)	DCAP-BTLS and *Crepitation* *Paradoxical motion* *Breath sounds*—present, absent, equal on both sides *Medical identification device*
Abdomen	DCAP-BTLS and *Distention* *Rigidity (firmness)*
Pelvis	DCAP-BTLS and *Stability* *Incontinence*
Extremities	DCAP-BTLS and *Distal pulses* *Sensation* *Motor function* *Medical identification device*
Posterior (back)	DCAP-BTLS

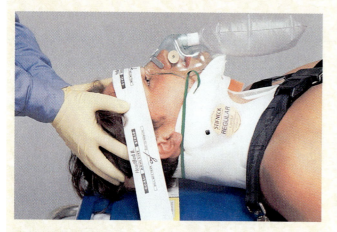

Figure 7-52A Inspect the head for signs of trauma. Carefully palpate the skull for abnormalities.

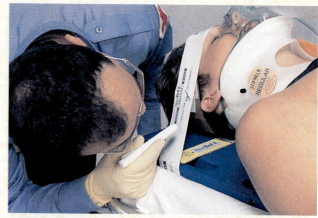

Figure 7-52B Inspect and palpate the ears. Note any leakage of blood or fluids.

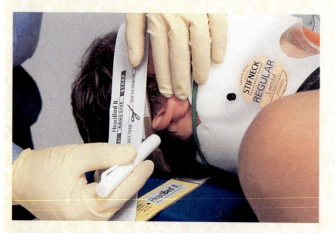

Figure 7-52C Inspect behind the ears for discoloration.

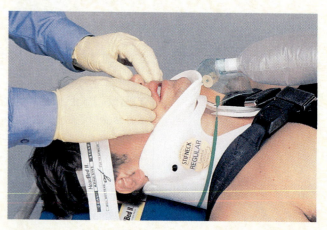

Figure 7-52D Inspect and palpate the face. Note any deformity, instability, burns, or swelling.

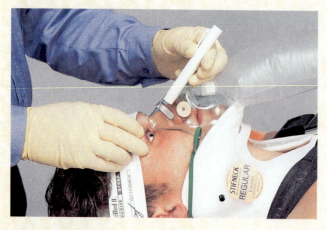

Figure 7-52E Assess pupils for equality of size and reactivity to light.

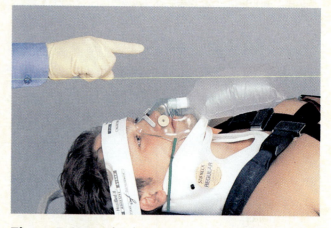

Figure 7-52F Check eye movement by having the patient follow your finger. Note gazes in one direction or jerky eye movements.

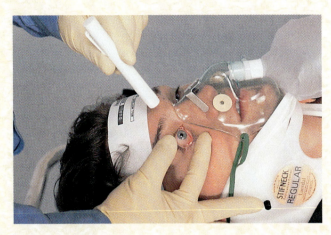

Figure 7-52G Inspect the conjunctiva by pulling the lower eyelid down.

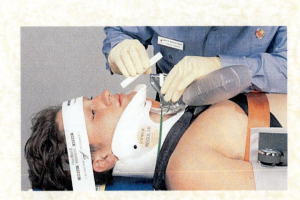

Figure 7-52H Inspect and palpate the nose for signs of trauma, burns, bleeding, or fluid leakage.

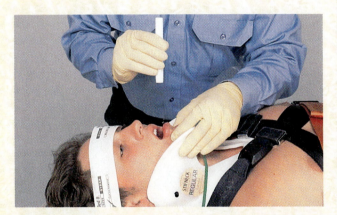

Figure 7-52I Inspect the inside of the mouth for signs of trauma, burns, and discoloration. Note the color of the mucous membranes. Smell the breath for unusual odors.

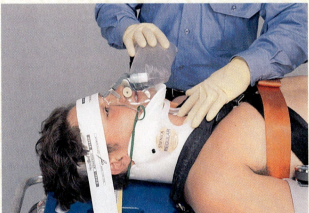

Figure 7-52J Assess the neck for jugular vein distention and use of accessory muscles in breathing. Note any lacerations or punctures.

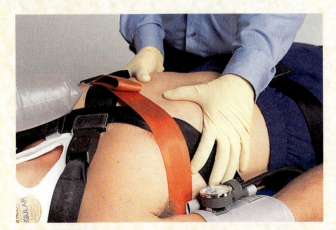

Figure 7-52K Inspect and palpate the entire chest. Check for paradoxical chest wall movement. Palpate the sternum, clavicles, and shoulders.

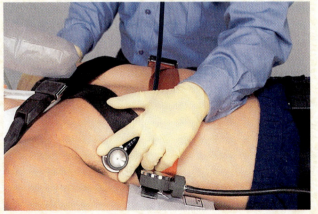

Figure 7-52L Auscultate breath sounds, comparing one side to the other.

(continued)

The Detailed Physical Exam (continued)

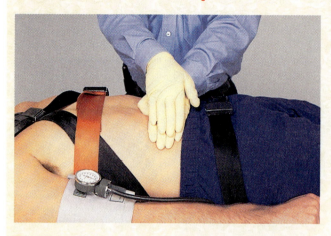

Figure 7-52M Inspect and palpate each quadrant of the abdomen. Note any guarding, tenderness, or rigidity.

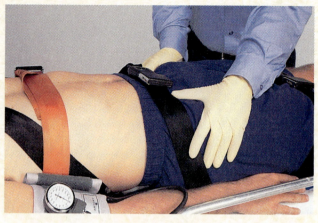

Figure 7-52N Assess the stability of the pelvis in a patient who is unresponsive or who has no noted pain in that area.

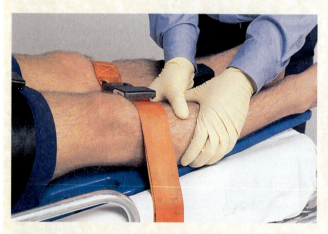

Figure 7-52O Inspect and palpate each lower extremity. Look for signs of wounds, bleeding, deformity, swelling, and discoloration.

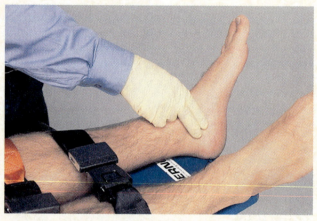

Figure 7-52P Assess distal pulses in each lower extremity. Also note skin color, temperature, and condition.

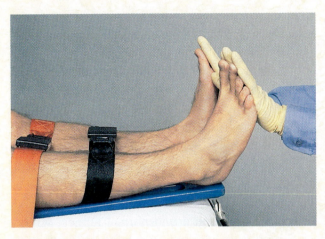

Figure 7-52Q Check motor response of both extremities by having the patient push both feet against your hands. Compare and note the equality of strength.

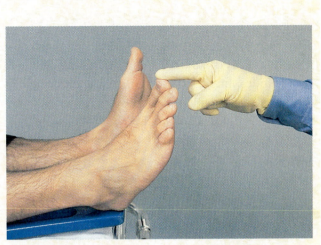

Figure 7-52R Assess sensation by lightly touching a toe and asking the patient to identify which toe you are touching. If the patient is unresponsive, pinch the foot and note the patient's response.

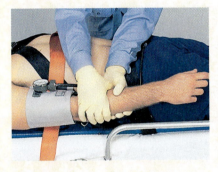

Figure 7-52S Inspect and palpate each upper extremity.

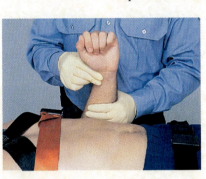

Figure 7-52T Assess the radial pulse on each upper extremity. Note skin color, temperature, and condition.

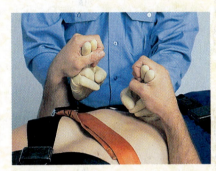

Figure 7-52U Assess motor function by having the patient grip the fingers of both of your hands simultaneously. Note equality of strength. Assess sensory function by asking the patient to identify which finger you are touching. If the patient is unresponsive, pinch the hand and note the patient's response. Conclude the exam by inspecting and palpating the posterior body to the extent that immobilization of the patient allows.

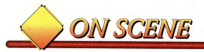
Paul Fink is helping to prepare dinner at Station 1. He is peeling potatoes with a knife when the blade suddenly slips and he cuts a chunk out of his left index finger. The wound is bleeding heavily, so Paul wraps a kitchen towel around his hand. Walking into the TV room, he finds Wendy Williams, one of two EMTs assigned to Station 1 for the shift.

Wendy asks her partner to grab a jump kit out of the ambulance while she begins the assessment of her fellow firefighter. The only hazard that Wendy can identify is the risk of contamination from the patient's blood, so she puts on a pair of latex exam gloves.

She notes that Paul has a normal mental status and is speaking easily, thus confirming both an adequate airway and adequate breathing. She then carefully peels back the towel and notes a 2-centimeter avulsion laceration of the tip of Paul's left index finger. The bleeding has slowed considerably and is not life threatening. While checking the bleeding, she notes that Paul has a

strong radial pulse and warm, dry skin. Paul denies any other injuries and has no complaints other than feeling very embarrassed.

The focused history and physical exam that Wendy performs centers around the injured hand. She notes that the remainder of Paul's fingertip is pink in color. There is normal capillary refill in the nail bed of the finger, and both the motor function and the sensation on the intact skin are normal.

Wendy's partner takes a set of baseline vital signs, all of which are in normal ranges. While her partner is taking the vital signs, Wendy obtains a SAMPLE history, which reveals no allergies or other problems. Wendy records the vital signs and SAMPLE history results on the patient care report she has begun. She then dresses the wound and applies a bandage.

The battalion chief then drives Paul to the Memorial Hospital emergency department. There the wound is sutured by the on-duty physician assistant.

Not all trauma involves a significant mechanism of injury. Patients injured by a "minor" mechanism do not require an assessment with the same aggressive, head-to-toe search for injuries as do patients with potentially life-threatening injuries.

PRIORITIES WITH THE TRAUMA PATIENT—NO SIGNIFICANT MECHANISM OF INJURY

You evaluated the patient's mechanism of injury in both the scene size-up and the initial assessment. With any trauma patient, you begin the focused history and physical exam by reconsidering whether the mechanism of injury is significant or not significant. If you ever have any doubts about whether a mechanism is significant or not, err on the side of caution and consider the mechanism to be significant. You are less likely to overlook significant

injuries when you perform the rapid trauma assessment as needed with a significant mechanism of injury.

Once you determine that the mechanism of injury is not significant, you will then perform a modified physical examination, take the baseline vital signs, and obtain a sample history.

The Focused Physical Examination

The major difference in this process for the patient with no significant mechanism of injury is that the focused physical exam truly is "focused." It is modified to concentrate on the region of the body where the injury occurred or where the patient is complaining of pain.

Once you complete the initial assessment and assure that there are no immediately life-threatening conditions present, you will direct your full attention to examining the site of the injury. Inspect and palpate the body region of the injury. You will look for the same types of DCAP-BTLS injuries that you looked for in the rapid trauma assessment. Check also for any signs of trauma specific to the region of injury (see Table 7-12, page 205). Remember, you perform the focused physical exam in the same way that you perform a rapid trauma assessment; the difference is that the focused physical exam is not head-to-toe, but aimed at a specific body region (or regions).

Vital Signs and SAMPLE History

Once you have completed the focused physical exam, obtain a set of baseline vital signs. Then take a SAMPLE history. Remember to document all this data in addition to the findings of the focused physical examination.

Detailed Physical Examination— Trauma Patient with No Significant Mechanism of Injury

Normally, you do not have to perform a detailed physical examination on a patient with a minor mechanism and injury. You should have examined the area of the injury thoroughly during your focused physical exam. You will also reexamine the area of the injury during the ongoing assessment. Remain alert, however, for any changes at the site of the injury—increased bleeding, the patient's complaint of pain or numbness, etc.

SECTION VII: The Ongoing Assessment

The patient assessment does not end when the patient is loaded into the ambulance for transport to the emergency department. It continues in the form of an ongoing assessment that is conducted intermittently during transport. This ongoing assessment allows you to detect any changes in a patient's condition as well as to monitor the effectiveness of treatments you may have provided. With critically ill or injured patients, performing the ongoing assessment is usually a higher priority in patient care than performing the detailed physical examination.

OBJECTIVES

At the completion of this part of the chapter, the EMT-Basic student should be able to meet the following objectives:

Knowledge and Understanding

1. Discuss the reasons for repeating the initial assessment as part of the ongoing assessment. (p. 218)
2. Describe the components of the ongoing assessment. (p. 218)
3. Describe trending of assessment components. (pp. 218–219)
4. Explain the value of performing an ongoing assessment. (pp. 218–219)

5. Recognize and respect the feelings that patients might experience during assessment. (p. 218)
6. Explain the value of trending assessment components to other health professionals who assume care of the patient. (pp. 218–219)

Skills

1. Demonstrate the skills involved in performing the ongoing assessment.

A patient's condition can change while he is in your care. Often it will improve, but it can also deteriorate. You must observe your patient carefully in order to detect these changes. The phase of the patient assessment process in which you watch for changes in the patient's condition after your initial evaluation and treatment is the ongoing assessment. By following the steps of the ongoing assessment, you can discover both obvious and subtle signs indicating how the patient is doing. What you observe can also lead you to adjust interventions you have provided or to provide additional care.

The ongoing assessment is usually performed in the ambulance en route to the hospital. However, if transport is delayed for any reason, begin the ongoing assessment on the scene and continue it once transport begins.

STEPS OF THE ONGOING ASSESSMENT

During the ongoing assessment, you will repeat components of the initial assessment and of the focused history and physical examination. To these, you will add an assessment of the effectiveness of any emergency medical interventions that you provided. The steps of the ongoing assessment are as follows (Figure 7-53, page 220):

1. **Reassess mental status.** If the patient is talking, check for changes in his speech patterns or the appropriateness of the content. Use the AVPU scale.

2. **Maintain and monitor the open airway.** Open the mouth of an unresponsive patient and check for obstructions. Provide suctioning if necessary.

3. **Monitor breathing for rate and quality.** Look, listen, and feel for adequate breathing. If breathing is inadequate, provide positive pressure ventilations.

4. **Reassess pulse for rate and quality.**

5. **Monitor skin color and condition.** Look and feel for changes in skin condition. Check capillary refill in infants and children.

6. **Confirm and, if necessary, reestablish patient priorities.** If you begin the ongoing assessment of a non-priority patient on the scene and its results indicate that the patient's condition is deteriorating, reconsider your emergency care and transport decisions. Make the patient a high priority and transport immediately.

7. **Reassess and record vital signs.** Take a complete set of vital signs following the procedures that are described in Section IV of this chapter.

8. **Repeat a focused assessment regarding patient complaint or injuries.** Reassess the original body regions where the patient was injured or complained of pain. If the patient has new complaints of pain or discomfort, assess those regions.

9. **Check the effectiveness of interventions.**

   ◆ Assure adequacy of supplemental oxygen delivery or artificial ventilations.

   ◆ Assure that the management of bleeding is effective.

   ◆ Assess the patient's response to any interventions such as your assistance with a prescribed inhaler, nitroglycerin, or an epinephrine auto-injector.

10. **Record your findings as you carry out the steps of the ongoing assessment.**

Trending of Assessment Components

The first set of vital signs you obtain during the focused history and physical exam are called "baseline vital signs." They have this name because they are the baseline, or reference point, to which you will compare later sets of vital signs. Following and documenting changes from set to set of vital signs is called **trending.** In addition to vital signs, trending is also done for other objective signs and subjective symptoms that are initially identified during the initial assessment and focused history and physical examination (see Table 7-14).

Using a 1-to-10 scale can be particularly helpful when you are trending symptoms. For example, when first asking the OPQRST questions

Table 7-14

Signs and Symptoms to Record During Ongoing Assessment

Signs	Symptoms
Vital signs	Shortness of breath
Mental status	Chest pain
Adequacy of breathing	Other pain

during the focused history and physical exam, ask the patient to describe how severe his pain is. Tell him to do this by using a 1-to-10 scale, with 1 being the mildest and 10 the most severe pain. During the ongoing assessment, ask the same question. A chest pain patient who answered "9" the first time and who answers "4" on reassessment after you provide oxygen is likely improving. As you can see, trending is a very important tool for measuring both the patient's condition and the effectiveness of your treatment.

WHEN TO PERFORM THE ONGOING ASSESSMENT

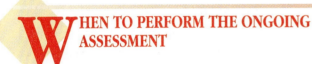

You should perform an ongoing assessment on all patients, both medical and trauma. The ongoing assessment is performed after completion of critical interventions to assure an open airway, adequate breathing, and control of any life-threatening bleeding. It is usually performed after the detailed physical, if one is performed. If a detailed physical exam is not done, the ongoing assessment usually comes after the focused history and physical exam.

How often you repeat the ongoing assessment is based on the condition of your patient. The recommended intervals for performing it are as follows:

◆ **At least every 5 minutes with unstable patients.** Unstable patients include patients who are unresponsive, who have an altered mental status, who have a significant mechanism of injury, or who required life-saving interventions during the assessment process.

◆ **Every 15 minutes with stable patients.** Stable patients include those who are alert, who have vital signs in the normal ranges, and have no serious injury.

When performing ongoing assessments, however, be guided by the patient's condition, not your wristwatch. Whenever a patient's condition suddenly changes (for example, a loss of consciousness), perform a reassessment immediately. If you ever have any doubts about a patient's condition, perform a reassessment. Whenever you perform a reassessment, be sure to document your findings.

THE ONGOING ASSESSMENT IN PRACTICE

To better understand how the ongoing assessment is carried out in the field, consider the cases of the four patients presented earlier in this chapter.

Unresponsive Medical Patient— Mrs. Taylor (Diabetic)

Because the patient remains unresponsive, she is a high priority for transport. An intercept with a paramedic unit has already been requested. Because of her serious condition and the need to maintain an open airway, no detailed physical examination can be conducted. Mrs. Taylor requires nearly constant reassessment of her ABCs and vital signs as part of the ongoing assessment. Airway and breathing are of particular concern. She remains in the recovery position on the stretcher. You open her mouth from time to time to check for obstruction and have a rigid-tip suction device ready to suction if necessary. You pay particular attention to the rise and fall of her chest and the trending of her respiratory rate. If they reveal that her spontaneous breathing on the non-rebreather mask is not adequate, you will have to begin positive pressure ventilations with a pocket mask or bag-valve-mask device.

The Ongoing Assessment

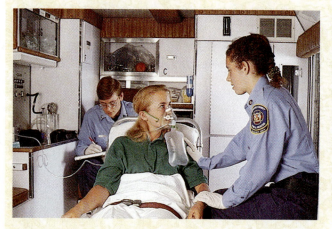

Figure 7-53A Repeat the steps of the initial assessment, reevaluating mental status, airway, breathing, and circulation. Confirm or if necessary reestablish patient priorities.

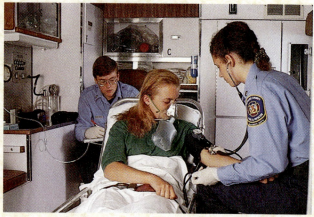

Figure 7-53B Reassess and record vital signs.

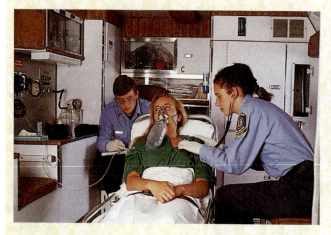

Figure 7-53C Repeat the focused assessment.

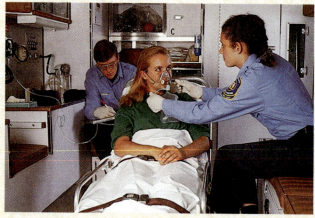

Figure 7-53D Check the effectiveness of all interventions. Remember to record all your findings during the ongoing assessment.

Responsive Medical Patient—Mrs. Cannon (Chest Pains)

After completing your focused history and physical exam, you contact medical direction, which authorizes you to assist Mrs. Cannon in taking one dose of her prescribed nitroglycerin spray. Because of her potentially life-threatening complaint of chest pain, you will provide an ongoing assessment at least every 5 minutes until you transfer her care to the in-coming paramedic unit. On the first reassessment, you note that her men-

tal status, airway, and breathing remain the same as during the initial assessment. Her pulse, which you had initially determined to be irregular and thready, now seems strong and regular. When you ask how severe her chest pain is now, after the oxygen and nitroglycerin have been administered, she states it is now a "1 or 2," down from the "7" she had first described. You document these trends in the patient's condition and will report them to the paramedics upon their arrival.

Trauma Patient with Significant Mechanism of Injury—Aaron Bartfield (Rollover)

Because of his serious multiple injuries, Aaron does not receive a detailed physical examination in the field. Also, because the flight crew assumes his care immediately after the rapid trauma assessment is completed, the EMTs who initially cared for him cannot perform the ongoing assessment. However, the two paramedics on board the helicopter constantly monitor the patient while en route to the trauma center. Using Chief Ball's assessment as a baseline, the flight crew follows the trends in Aaron's ABCs and vital signs. By comparing their findings against Chief Ball's initial set, they determine that Aaron's breathing is becoming inadequate and that his condition is rapidly worsening. Because they detect this downward trend, they perform an endotracheal intubation and provide assisted ventilations until they reach the trauma center.

Trauma Patient with No Significant Mechanism of Injury—Paul Fink (Cut Finger)

Because Paul's injury was minor and the injured finger was carefully examined during the focused physical exam, an extensive ongoing assessment is not necessary. Because the trip to the hospital takes less than 15 minutes, a second set of vital signs is not obtained. Monitoring of the dressing on Paul's finger to assure that bleeding remains controlled is an appropriate part of the ongoing assessment in this case.

Chapter Review

SUMMARY

Patient assessment is a skill that you will use on every call in your career as an EMT. No effective treatment can be provided and no appropriate priority of care and transport decisions made without a proper assessment. The scene size-up and initial assessment phases are carried out in similar fashion with all patients. The way you conduct the focused history and physical examination, the detailed physical examination, and the ongoing assessment will vary based on the patient's condition and, in the case of trauma, the mechanism of injury.

REVIEWING KEY CONCEPTS

1. Explain the chief purposes of the patient assessment.

2. List the basic components of the patient assessment.

3. List the goals you should attempt to accomplish during the scene size-up.

4. Define mechanism of injury and nature of illness.

5. List the six steps of the initial assessment.

6. Explain the purpose of the AVPU scale and how it is used.

7. Explain how to assess the ABCs during the initial assessment. Explain what steps to take to correct problems with airway, breathing, or circulation at this time.

8. Define the term *priority patient*. List some categories of patients who might automatically be considered priority patients.

9. Identify the components of a SAMPLE history.

10. List the elements that make up the vital signs.

11. Explain how and why the focused history and physical exam stage of the patient

assessment is different for medical and trauma patients.

12. Explain how and why the focused history and physical exam for the responsive medical patient differs from that for the unresponsive medical patient.

13. Explain what the OPQRST memory aid means and describe the phase of the patient assessment process in which it is most useful.

14. Explain when and how to perform a rapid physical examination with an unresponsive medical patient.

15. List some common significant mechanisms of injury for adult and pediatric patients.

16. Explain how the focused history and physical exam for a trauma patient with a significant mechanism of injury will differ from that for the trauma patient with no significant mechanism. Give reasons for this difference.

17. Name the signs and symptoms for which the letters DCAP-BTLS stand.

18. List the steps of the rapid trauma assessment.

19. Describe additional areas assessed in the detailed physical exam that are not evaluated in the rapid trauma assessment.

20. Explain when it is and when it is not appropriate to perform a detailed physical exam.

21. Describe the steps for carrying out an ongoing assessment.

22. Explain how often an ongoing assessment should be performed (a) on a stable patient and (b) on an unstable patient.

RESOURCES TO LEARN MORE

Book

Bates, Barbara et al. *A Guide to Physical Examination and History Taking/A Guide to Clinical Thinking, 6th Edition*. Philadelphia: Lippincott-Raven, 1995.

Video

Patient Assessment. Upper Saddle River, NJ: Brady/Prentice Hall.

PATIENT ASSESSMENT

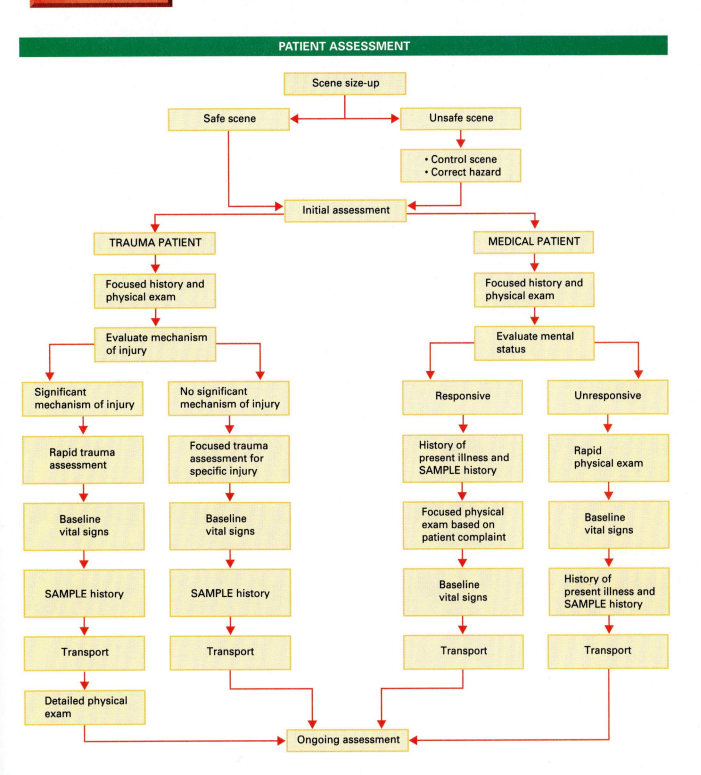

Communication and Documentation

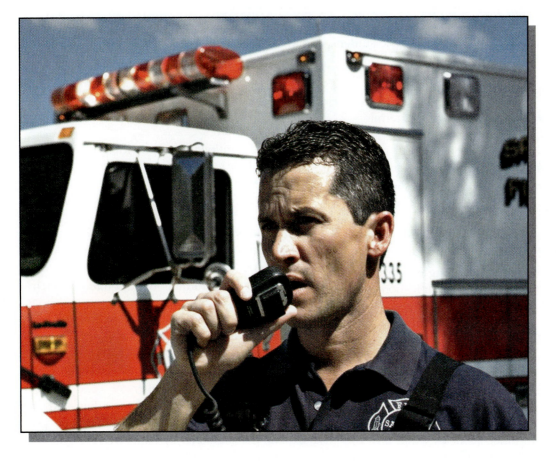

*I*n many ways, communication is the key to providing good
emergency medical services. That communication starts with the
call for EMS assistance. The EMS dispatcher must communicate
with the caller to find out, at a minimum, where the patient is and what
is wrong with him. That first contact starts a chain of communications—

◆ Between the dispatcher and the responding EMS unit

◆ Between the members of the responding unit and the patient, family
members, and bystanders

- *Between the EMS unit and medical direction*
- *Between the unit and the receiving facilities.*

Good communication at all these stages can assure that a patient receives appropriate treatment and transport as rapidly as possible. Poor communication, on the other hand, can delay that treatment and transport and ultimately affect overall patient care.

Documentation of a call continues the process of communication. Written patient reports contain information that can be used not only by medical personnel treating the patient both during the emergency and after but also by your EMS system to improve the quality of its care. In this chapter, you will learn the basics of both good communications and proper documentation.

OBJECTIVES

At the completion of this chapter, the EMT-Basic student should be able to meet the following objectives:

Knowledge and Understanding

1. List the proper methods of initiating and terminating radio calls. (pp. 234–235)
2. State the proper sequence for delivery of patient information. (pp. 236–237)
3. Explain the importance of effective communication of patient information in the verbal report. (pp. 234–236)
4. Identify the essential components of the verbal report. (pp. 236–237)
5. Describe the attributes for increasing effectiveness and efficiency of verbal communications. (pp. 229–230, 236–237)
6. State legal aspects to consider in verbal communication. (p. 235)
7. Discuss the communication skills that should be used to interact with the patient. (pp. 229–230)
8. Discuss the communication skills that should be used to interact with the family, bystanders, and individuals from other agencies while providing patient care and the differences between skills used to interact with the patient and those used to interact with others. (pp. 229–230)
9. List the correct radio procedures in the following phases of a typical call: (pp. 235–237)
   —To the scene
   —At the scene
   —To the facility
   —At the facility
   —To the station
   —At the station
10. Explain the rationale for providing efficient and effective radio communications and patient reports. (pp. 235–237)
11. Explain the components of the written report and list the information that should be included in the written report. (pp. 239, 243–245)
12. Identify the various sections of the written report. (pp. 239, 243–245)
13. Describe what information is required in each section of the prehospital care report and how it should be entered. (pp. 239, 243–245)
14. Define the special considerations concerning patient refusal. (pp. 246–248)
15. Describe the legal implications associated with the written report. (pp. 246–250)
16. Discuss all state and/or local recording and reporting requirements. (pp. 249–250)
17. Explain the rationale for patient care documentation. (pp. 237–239)
18. Explain the rationale for the EMS system gathering data. (pp. 238–239)
19. Explain the rationale for using medical terminology correctly. (p. 245)
20. Explain the rationale for using an accurate and synchronous clock so that information can be used in trending. (pp. 243)

Skills

1. Perform a simulated, organized, concise radio transmission.
2. Perform an organized, concise patient report that would be given to the staff at a receiving facility.
3. Perform a brief, organized report that would be given to an ALS provider arriving at an incident scene at which the EMT-Basic was already providing care.
4. Complete a prehospital care report.

◆ ON SCENE

DISPATCH: *SQUAD 3, ENGINE 9, AND BATTALION 2 REPORT OF PEDESTRIAN STRUCK BY A VEHICLE ON WEST AVENUE BETWEEN 3RD AND 4TH STREETS. THIS IS A THIRD PARTY CALL. NO PATIENT INFORMATION AVAILABLE AT THIS TIME. AMBULANCE HAS BEEN DISPATCHED. TIME OUT 1530.*

As the EMT on Squad 3, you'd like more information but understand that the dispatcher probably wasn't able to get much from the caller. The call location is at the end of your district, and you expect a run time of 3 to 4 minutes. Two minutes into your run, you hear, "Dispatch to Squad 3" over the radio.

You respond, "Go ahead, dispatch, this is Squad 3."

"Squad 3, the police are now on the scene and advise that there is one male patient, approximately 8 years old, who was struck by a motor vehicle at low speed. There appears to be a head injury. The patient is breathing on his own."

You acknowledge the transmission and, based on it, plan how you should approach a pediatric head trauma call. You arrive on the scene a minute later and inform dispatch. Dispatch responds, "Squad 3 arriving at 1535."

Because police are on the scene, you know that it is secure. As you get out of your vehicle, a police officer approaches. He tells you that the patient, named Henry, was skateboarding and ran into a parked truck at the end of his driveway. He was not wearing a helmet. Henry was conscious when the police arrived, but now seems less alert.

As you kneel by Henry's side and start your assessment, his mother, who had not been home, pulls up in a car. Seeing Henry lying by the side of the road, she dashes over from the car, obviously very upset. While you focus on Henry's assessment, your partner attempts to calm the mother. Talking slowly in a normal tone of voice, he gives her an overview of what has happened. He tells her firmly that the best way to help Henry right now is to get next to her son, hold his hand, and calmly reassure him that everyone is trying to help him. The mother takes your partner's advice and kneels down across from you as you continue the assessment.

You observe that the patient's breathing is becoming increasingly labored and that he is no longer responding to voice commands. You and your partner begin to ventilate Henry with a bag-valve mask with high concentration oxygen and package him onto a backboard. Henry is ready for transport when the ambulance arrives. You help the ambulance crew load him aboard their vehicle. Because of Henry's condition, you and your partner climb into the patient compartment to ride along and assist on the way to the hospital. Squad 3 will join you at the hospital.

Your partner had earlier contacted dispatch to ask if a paramedic unit would be available to intercept you en route to the hospital. He had been told to stand by as dispatch checked on the status of the nearest unit. As you leave the scene, the ambulance personnel inform the dispatcher that the vehicle is en route to County Receiving Hospital. Dispatch acknowledges the transmission at 1545 hours and adds that the closest available paramedic unit is

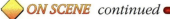

approximately 10 minutes away. You determine that Henry's ventilations are adequate and that the ALS intercept might delay definitive treatment for him. You decide not to intercept and instead to proceed red lights and siren directly to the hospital.

About 5 minutes before estimated arrival, your partner radios a full patient report to the hospital. The report gives Henry's chief complaint, his mechanism of injury, the observed changes in vital signs and level of consciousness, and the treatment being provided. The hospital acknowledges receipt of the patient report and indicates personnel will be awaiting your arrival.

There are no changes in Henry's vital signs and level of consciousness for the rest of the trip. When you arrive at the hospital, Henry is taken directly to the trauma room where, because of the information provided in the radio report, a neurosurgeon is waiting. You give an oral update on Henry's condition to the emergency department staff and answer any questions they have.

You and your partner leave the trauma room. Your partner begins to clean and restock your equipment, while you complete a prehospital care report. You leave a copy of the report with the nurse in charge of the emergency department and rejoin your partner. You radio the dispatcher that Squad 3 is back in service. The dispatcher acknowledges at 1625 hours.

The next week, you and your partner are at the station when the fire department's medical director stops by. He received a call from the neurosurgeon who operated on Henry. The neurosurgeon wanted to let you know that Henry was expected to make a full recovery. The medical director states that he, too, has reviewed the call. He says that the decision about ALS intercept, the way you got off the scene as quickly as possible, and your early radio report to the hospital really helped Henry. He adds that the prehospital care report showed that you had taken frequent vital signs and continually monitored the patient's level of consciousness. As he leaves, he says, "You put it all together, and that is quality EMS."

Too often, people think that communications in an EMS context refers only to equipment like two-way radios, base stations, and repeaters. EMS communications certainly involves those things. But beyond that, communications is about people interacting with other people. How people in an EMS system interact, with patients and with other members of the system, directly affects the quality of the service the system provides.

INTERPERSONAL COMMUNICATION

Interpersonal communication is vital to all aspects of emergency medical care. As an EMT, you must be able to communicate well with a patient. Doing this will allow you to gather vital informa-

tion about his condition. Using good communications skills can also help you calm and reassure patients and their families, making it easier to provide care. You must also be able to communicate well with other EMS personnel. You must be able to explain, clearly and concisely, what you have learned about a patient's condition and what you did to treat it during a call. This is especially crucial when you are assigned to a first-responding unit and will be handing the patient over to other prehospital care providers for transport. You must also be able to listen, understand, and carry out directions that you receive.

Like the skills of lifting and moving patients, effective communication is a vital EMS skill that you can learn. As with other EMS skills, you will need to work on it continually. Remember that good communication can improve every phase of emergency medical care, from outside the hospital through the emergency department and into the care and treatment provided afterwards.

General Guidelines

You will face a variety of stresses and pressures on an emergency call—precautions to take, equipment to prepare, procedures to remember, reports to fill out. With all this, it could be too easy to forget that the *patient* is the reason you're on the scene. Pay attention to him and his needs, both as a patient and as a customer who has summoned you for assistance. Keep in mind that being the focus of an emergency response is a unique situation for most patients. Most never expected to need EMS and may feel very vulnerable, and possibly even embarrassed. For some patients, you will be their first contact with a medical provider. In most cases, patients will place a great deal of trust in you as a provider of emergency medical care. Therefore, it is important to always present yourself in a professional manner.

Interpersonal communications under normal circumstances can be difficult. Communicating with people caught up by the emotions surrounding a disaster, accident, or medical emergency can be even more difficult.

There are some basic guidelines that can aid you in communicating with patients at these times. Be warned, however, that the guidelines below will not work for all situations. It is important to be flexible. Think about what you say and how it might be heard *before* you say it. Remember that good communication is essential to good patient care.

◆ *Introduce yourself to the patient.* When you first make contact with the patient, introduce yourself as an EMT, and state what fire department you are affiliated with. For example, you might say, "Good evening. My name is Mark. I'm an Emergency Medical Technician with the Lyons Fire Department and I'm here to help you." Note that some agencies suggest that personnel not use their surnames (last names); follow your local protocols in this matter. This is a good time to look over the scene as part of the scene size-up.

Then find out the patient's name and how he wishes to be addressed. Do this, whenever possible, by asking the patient directly. Never assume that the patient wants to be called by his first name. In many instances, patients may prefer that their last name be used. Deciding how to address the patient is a judgment call, but keep in mind that your decision can set the tone for a call. Informality when talking with a patient may be mistaken for disrespect, which could lead to mistrust and a lack of communication. Always display courtesy and respect when communicating with patients.

◆ *Use eye contact, position, and body language.* Once you are next to the patient, you should make every effort to establish good eye contact. This shows that you are interested in the patient and his problem. (Note that in some cultures eye contact is considered rude; be alert to this possibility if the patient is avoiding eye contact.)

Getting down to the patient's eye level can help you make good eye contact. You may need to sit or kneel next to the patient in order to accomplish this. Many patients will be uncomfortable if the EMT stands while they are sitting or lying down. In fact it is recommended, when practical, to be at a level lower than the patient. This may help to make conversation with the patient easier. Getting yourself down to or below eye level is especially important when the patient is a child (Figure 8-1).

Touching a patient—holding his hand, patting his back, placing a hand on his forearm—can soothe and reassure patients. However, not all patients will welcome such contact. If a patient draws back or stiffens at your touch, you should not continue physical contact.

◆ *Speak directly to the patient whenever possible.* Try not to talk around the patient. Don't ask a relative or friend to answer for a patient who is capable and willing to respond for himself. At times you will have to turn to others for important information, but make every effort to find out what you can from the patient

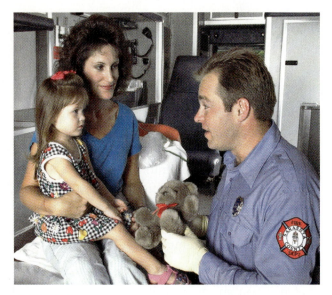

Figure 8-1 Getting down to the child's eye level can help improve communications on a pediatric call.

himself, even if it takes a little more effort on your part.

◆ *Be aware of your language and tone of voice.* Try to keep communication with the patient as clear and simple as possible. Avoid medical terms or EMS jargon as much as possible unless the patient has indicated he wants you to provide information this way. Don't be condescending—the patient expects that you will talk on his level and be respectful at all times.

Don't rush the interview and assessment process, unless doing so is medically indicated. Always speak slowly and clearly. Be sure that the patient is not confused by your questions. Don't be impatient. Give the patient time to answer. At times, you may have to repeat questions or phrase them a different way to help the patient understand.

When asking questions of a patient, try to phrase them in a way that encourages the patient to provide more information. For example, don't just ask if a patient has pain, but ask where the pain is located and how intense it is. One common technique is to ask a patient to identify pain on a scale of 1-to-10, with 10 being the most intense. (This technique also provides a gauge for determining to what degree the patient's pain has lessened, become worse, or stayed the same

when you later question him during the ongoing assessment.)

◆ *Be honest.* Always be honest when talking with a patient. If you don't know the answer to a question, let the patient know. Remember, most patients will trust what you say. If you believe that providing an answer might confuse or incite a patient, try to defer the response by suggesting the patient speak to the doctor at the emergency department or say, "I am not sure."

◆ *Listen to the patient.* Communication is a two-way street. Merely asking questions of a patient and telling him what you are doing or what he should do is not enough. You must *listen* to what the patient is saying. If you don't take enough time to listen to a patient's answers, the patient might think you don't care. Listening is as much a skill as interviewing. If you don't understand what a patient is telling you, repeat back what you think you heard and ask if that is what he meant.

◆ *Be calm and professional.* How you act during a medical emergency can directly affect how the patient, his family members, and your colleagues respond. Excitement is contagious, so stay calm and collected. You have a professional responsibility to act and speak confidently; doing so can help reassure your patients.

Confused or Mentally Disabled Patients

Confused or mentally disabled patients are some of the more difficult to communicate with. Use simple terms and phrases when asking questions. Be especially sure to allow adequate time for the patient to respond. Whenever you must perform a procedure, explain what you are going to do before you do it. If possible, demonstrate the procedure first. For example, if you need to take a blood pressure, apply the cuff to your own arm or your partner's and inflate it. Be alert to the possibility that, even if you show the procedure in advance, actually doing it may confuse or scare the patient.

If a caregiver is present, ask him to assist you. The caregiver probably knows the most effective way to communicate with the patient and already has his trust.

Agitated or Disturbed Patients

Some patients you encounter may be agitated or emotionally disturbed. With some of these patients, communication may be impossible, even using the strategies suggested earlier. Techniques such as touching and making eye contact may anger these patients instead of comforting them.

If you fear that such a patient may become violent, think of your own safety first. Don't get too close to the patient. Position yourself so you can move away from him quickly. Do not allow the patient to position himself between you and your route of escape. Contact a law enforcement agency for help with such a patient if necessary. Be prepared to wait for assistance before trying to care for the patient.

Pediatric Patients

Children involved in accidents and medical emergencies are likely to be scared, confused, and in pain. The arrival of a uniformed stranger carrying unfamiliar equipment may frighten them even more. They may cry, act out, or withdraw when you attempt to talk to them or treat them.

Try to keep the child's parents present during assessment and care. Make sure the parents understand that if they remain calm, their child will be more likely to stay calm as well. If the situation permits, let the parent hold the child or have the child sit on the parent's lap.

Be especially sure to get down to or below the child's level when you speak to him. Make good eye contact, but don't give the child the feeling you are staring at him. Speak to the child in a calm tone, using simple language to explain what you are doing. Show him any instruments you will use and explain what they are for. If you have to talk with the child's parents, try to make the child feel that he is a part of the conversation.

Never lie to a child. If you are going to do a procedure that may hurt, tell him the truth—that he may feel pain. When a child is in pain, acknowledge the pain. Show that you understand that the child may be scared. Emphasize the positive. Praise the child for his cooperation. Try and reassure both the child and the parents as you provide assessment and care.

Geriatric Patients

Be prepared to spend extra time with older patients. Older patients may not respond as quickly to your questions. Ask one question at a time. If you aren't sure you understand a response, repeat it back to the patient. Use soothing tones and remember that touching can be very reassuring. Be respectful and sensitive to the patient's sense of modesty. Always treat the elderly with dignity.

Don't assume that elderly patients have difficulty hearing and seeing because of age. Don't automatically raise your voice. Many elderly people hear perfectly well or have hearing aids that can compensate for hearing loss. Speak slowly and clearly, positioning yourself so that the patient can see your lips. If the patient still has difficulty hearing you, you may try speaking more loudly.

The vision of older patients can likewise vary from excellent to poor. Many older patients, however, do wear glasses. If you encounter an older patient who is not wearing glasses, ask if he normally wears them. If the patient says he does, try to convince him to put them on. Wearing the glasses may make the patient more comfortable and improve communication if the patient can see you and see what is being done.

Patients with Hearing Difficulties

There are a number of ways to improve communication with patients who have difficulty hearing. First, many hearing-impaired patients know how to read lips. Position yourself where the patient can easily see your face and lips. Second, you can exchange information by writing your questions on a note pad and letting the patient use it to write his response. Third, many hearing-impaired patients know American Sign Language (ASL). If the patient indicates that he does, see if family members or bystanders are available to interpret for you.

Patients with Visual Deficits

With a patient who is blind or has a visual deficit, make sure that you explain everything that you are doing during assessment and treatment. Try and stay in direct contact with the patient by keeping a hand on his arm. Remember that a visual deficit is not a hearing deficit; don't raise your voice unnecessarily with these patients. If the patient has a Seeing Eye dog, keep patient and dog together whenever possible. This may mean bringing the animal along in the ambulance. Do not make any sudden movements around a Seeing Eye dog or attempt to pet it. Note that most hospitals allow Seeing Eye dogs on their premises. Finally, remember that the dog's presence will provide a great deal of comfort and security to the patient.

Non-English-Speaking Patients

You may encounter patients who either do not speak English or do not understand it well. In these cases, check to see if there is a relative, friend, or bystander on the scene who can act as interpreter. If someone on the scene does act as interpreter, keep in mind the possibility that his translation may not be accurate. Be cautious in acting on what you are told unless you can somehow verify the information provided.

If no one at the scene can help, check with dispatch or medical direction. They may have someone available who can interpret for you over the radio.

If you work in an area where many residents speak a language other than English, consider learning some basic phrases in that language or carrying a manual or phrase book in that language. Doing so might help you in evaluating a patient and obtaining a history when no translator is available.

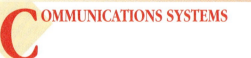

COMMUNICATIONS SYSTEMS

An effective communications system is vital for providing good emergency medical services. That system will link you as an EMT to the dispatcher,

other field personnel, medical control, and the hospital emergency department.

Communications System Components

The communications system is made up of several components, including the following:

◆ *Base station* is a two-way radio located at a fixed site, such as a dispatch center or emergency department. A base station radio usually has a relatively high power output (80 to 150 watts). It is, therefore, able to transmit over a greater distance than a mobile or portable radio.

◆ *Mobile radios* are transmitter/receivers that are mounted in a vehicle (Figure 8-2). They are usually less powerful (20 to 50 watts) than a base station. Their range is typically 10 to 15 miles (16 to 23 kilometers) depending on the surrounding terrain and the frequency being used. These devices are commonly mounted in the patient compartment of an ambulance so that an EMT caring for a patient can transmit a care report to the emergency department or talk to an online medical control physician.

◆ *Portable radios* are usually hand-held transmitter/receivers with about 1 to 5 watts of power. With their lesser power, their range is shorter than a mobile radio's. A portable radio can give an EMT who is away from the ambulance

Figure 8-2 A mobile two-way radio.

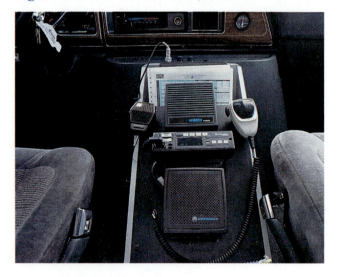

with a patient access to the dispatcher or other EMS personnel to request help.

◆ *Repeaters* are devices that pick up signals from lower-power units, such as portable radios, and retransmit them at a high power (Figure 8-3). They make communications possible in EMS systems that spread over a large territory.

◆ *Digital radio equipment* encodes, or translates, sounds into digital code for broadcast. A decoder, set to recognize that code, receives the broadcast. Because digital messages are transmitted in condensed form, they help ease crowding of radio frequencies. Also, digital transmissions can't be monitored by scanners and are considered secure. Many mobile telephones now use this technology.

◆ *Cellular telephones* are becoming a common and reliable way to transmit patient care information. Most urban and suburban areas have cellular service, and cellular systems are continually expanding. Cellular phones are an efficient way of transmitting information. In systems that use digital technology, conversations are considered protected and confidential. In some systems cellular phones are the standard way of contacting medical control. (Note, however, that analog cellular phone transmissions can be monitored and should not be considered secure.)

◆ *Mobile computer or data terminals* are now used in many EMS systems. A terminal is placed in the ambulance or other emergency response unit. The terminal can receive elec-

Figure 8-3 With a repeater system, signals from relatively low-powered mobile and portable radios are picked up and rebroadcast at higher power, enabling good communications over a wide area.

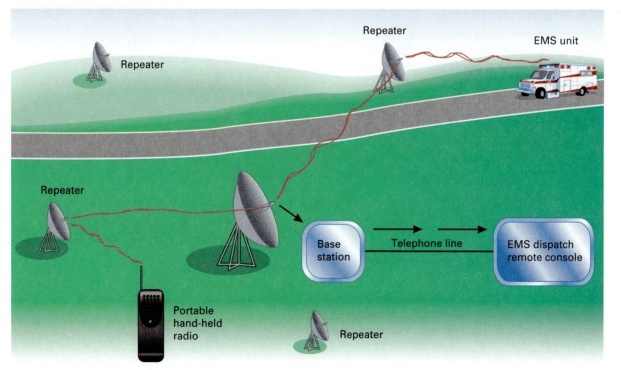

tronic data transmitted to it and display it on a screen. These transmissions are considered secure and confidential. The terminals can reduce air time for transmissions to fractions of a second, allowing busy systems to have more space for voice transmissions available on their frequencies.

System Maintenance

Because so much depends on the proper operations of an EMS communications system, the equipment must be carefully checked and maintained. Crews should check mobile and portable radios at the beginning of each shift. Extra batteries should be available for portable radios. The EMS communications system should also provide some means of back up in case of power or equipment failure. For example, the base station might have a portable generator in case the power goes out, while ambulances and emergency vehicles might carry cellular phones in the event that the radio system goes down.

Communications equipment should be handled with care. It should be cleaned regularly and not exposed unnecessarily to harsh weather con-

ditions. Equipment should receive regular maintenance according to manufacturer's specifications or local requirements.

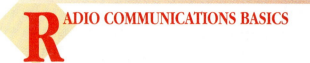

RADIO COMMUNICATIONS BASICS

The Federal Communications Commission (FCC) has jurisdiction over radio operations in the United States. The FCC assigns and licenses radio frequencies. It approves equipment for use and sets limits on transmitter power output. The FCC also establishes regulations aimed at preventing interference with emergency radio broadcasts and prohibiting the use of profanity and offensive language on the air.

General Rules

An EMS communications system must work smoothly and effectively. EMS personnel need access to the system and delays must be avoided. There are some basic guidelines that you should follow when making radio transmissions to assure the efficient working of your system. There may be minor variations to these rules, but the basic principles are the same for any EMS radio system.

◆ Make sure that your radio is on and that the volume is adjusted properly.

◆ Reduce background noise by closing the vehicle window when possible.

◆ Listen to the frequency and ensure that it is clear before beginning a transmission.

◆ Press the "press to talk" (PTT) button on the radio, then wait one second before speaking. This prevents cutting off the first few words of your transmission.

◆ Speak with your lips about 2 to 3 inches (50 to 75 mm) from the microphone.

◆ Hold the microphone at a 45°-angle to your mouth (Figure 8-4).

◆ When calling another unit or base station, use their unit number or name, followed by yours. "Dispatch, this is Engine 3."

◆ The unit being called will signal that the transmission should start by saying "go ahead" or

COMPANY OFFICER'S NOTES

Properly working radios are vital to providing good emergency medical care. To ensure that they will work when needed, do the following:

◆ Be sure that there is a program for checking and maintaining your agency's radio equipment on a regular basis.

◆ Check on all radios—base station, mobile, and portable—by performing test transmissions.

◆ Recharge and exchange batteries regularly. Replace them according to manufacturer's recommendations.

◆ Always be sure spare batteries are available for any radio.

◆ Ensure that a qualified technician performs maintenance on radios following a regular schedule and records that maintenance in a logbook.

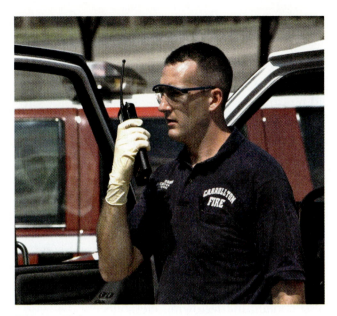

Figure 8-4 When using a mobile or portable radio, hold the microphone about 2 or 3 inches away from and at a 45°-angle to your lips.

another regionally accepted term: "Engine 3, this is Dispatch. Go ahead." If the unit you are calling tells you to "stand by," wait until they tell you they are ready to take your transmission.

◆ Speak slowly, clearly, and distinctly.

◆ Keep transmissions brief. If a transmission takes longer than 30 seconds, stop at that point and pause for a few seconds so that emergency traffic can use the frequency if necessary.

◆ Use plain English. Avoid codes, other than standard ones approved in department protocols.

◆ Do not use phrases like "be advised." These are implied and serve no purpose.

◆ Courtesy is assumed, so there is no need to say "please," "thank you," and "you're welcome."

◆ When transmitting a number that might be unclear (15 may sound like 16 or 50), give the number, then repeat the individual digits. Say "15, one-five."

◆ Anything said over the radio can be heard by the public on a scanner. Avoid using the patient's name over the radio. For the same reason, do not use profanities or statements that tend to slander any person. Use objective, impartial statements.

◆ Use "we" instead of "I." As an EMT, you will rarely be acting alone.

◆ "Affirmative" and "negative" are preferred over "yes" and "no" because the latter are difficult to hear.

◆ Give assessment information about your patient, but avoid offering a diagnosis of the patient's problem. For example, say "Patient complains of chest pain," but not "Patient probably having a heart attack."

◆ After transmitting, wait for acknowledgment that the person to whom you were speaking heard your message.

◆ Avoid slang or abbreviations that are not authorized.

◆ Use EMS frequencies only for authorized EMS communication.

Communication and Dispatch

EMS dispatch is often the public's first contact with the EMS system. Dispatch usually answers calls to 9-1-1 or some other emergency access phone number (Figure 8-5). Dispatch questions the caller to find out as much as possible about the nature of the emergency. More systems are

Figure 8-5 Dispatchers at an EMS communications center receive emergency calls from the public and direct appropriate resources to the scene.

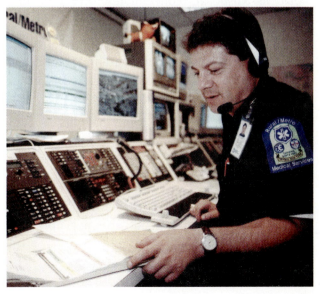

using certified Emergency Medical Dispatchers (EMDs). EMDs are specially trained in obtaining information and in providing instructions to the caller on how to care for the patient before the arrival of EMS.

With the information obtained, dispatch directs appropriate EMS units to the scene. Dispatch may also provide responding units with updated information about the call or response to it. Dispatch gives the time after most communications with responding EMS units. This helps the unit crews by providing times for their written care reports.

As an EMT on a responding EMS unit, you will have the responsibility of providing dispatch with some information. This information will enable dispatch to keep track of the whereabouts of emergency units and will help the system work more efficiently. You should usually communicate with dispatch in order to do the following:

◆ To acknowledge dispatch information.

◆ To estimate arrival time on scene and to note any special road conditions encountered.

◆ To announce arrival on the scene and to request additional resources if needed. For example, if your BLS unit finds a patient in cardiac arrest, you should notify dispatch so other units, particularly ALS units, can be directed to the scene. With the notification, you are free to concentrate on patient care while dispatch, which has more information at its disposal, concentrates on contacting and directing appropriate resources to the scene.

◆ To advise dispatch that your first-responding unit is back in service after transition of patient care to a transporting ambulance.

◆ If your unit is transporting patients, to announce your departure from the scene, your destination hospital, the number of patients, and estimated time of arrival.

◆ To announce your unit's arrival at the hospital.

◆ To announce that you are available for another assignment.

◆ To announce your return to quarters.

Communication with Medical Direction

In many systems, EMTs must contact medical direction to receive approval for assisting with the administration of certain medications or for providing specific types of treatment to a patient. The physician who provides medical direction may be located at the base station radio at a hospital emergency department or at a separate site.

Whenever you contact medical direction, be concise, organized, and accurate in the information you provide. Be sure that the information you provide is pertinent to the patient's condition. Specifically state the reason for contacting medical direction. Your report to medical direction should also contain the following elements:

◆ Your unit's identification and level of service: BLS (Basic Life Support) or ALS (Advanced Life Support)

◆ The patient's age and sex

◆ The patient's chief complaint

◆ A brief history of the present illness

◆ Pertinent past major illnesses

◆ Current medications the patient is using

◆ Allergies the patient may have

◆ The patient's mental status

◆ The patient's baseline vital signs

◆ Pertinent findings from your physical examination of the patient

◆ Any emergency care you (or first responders) have provided

◆ The patient's response to that emergency care

◆ Your unit's estimated time of arrival (ETA) at the receiving facility

Once you receive an order from medical direction, repeat the order back word for word to ensure that you understood it correctly. If you do not understand an order, ask medical direction to repeat it and then repeat it back yourself, word for word.

If an order from medical direction seems inappropriate, question medical direction before carrying it out. Medical direction may have misunderstood information you provided or may have misspoken. By questioning the order, you may prevent administration of a harmful medication or application of a procedure that is inappropriate for the patient.

Communications En Route to the Hospital/Receiving Facility

An important part of your patient care is providing information by radio about the patient's condition to the staff at the receiving facility before your arrival there. This information helps the emergency department get ready for the patient and, when necessary, to assemble or prepare any additional personnel or special equipment that may be needed. Your radio report to the receiving facility includes much of the same information you would provide to medical direction:

◆ Your unit's identification
◆ The patient's age and sex
◆ The patient's chief complaint
◆ A brief, pertinent history of the present illness
◆ Major past illnesses
◆ The patient's mental status
◆ The patient's baseline vital signs and any later readings you obtained
◆ Pertinent findings from your physical examination of the patient
◆ Any emergency care you (or first responders) have provided
◆ The patient's response to that emergency care
◆ Your ETA at the facility

Your transmissions to the receiving facility should be relatively short. Those transmissions should not take priority over patient care. If you have a patient who needs constant attention, ask the driver to have dispatch alert the hospital and provide it with as much information as possible.

During transport, you will reassess the patient and record your findings. If you note any change in the patient's condition—for better or worse—contact the receiving facility and provide an update.

Communications After Arrival at the Hospital/Receiving Facility

When you arrive at the receiving facility, you should provide the staff there with an oral report on the patient's condition. This report is basically a summary of the information you provided in your radio report. It is necessary to provide this information in an oral report because emergency department physicians and nurses may not have heard your radio report directly. Be sure to include in the oral report any reassessment findings made after your last radio transmission. Begin the report, whenever possible, with an introduction of the patient, by name, to the receiving facility's medical staff. Your report should include at least the following information:

◆ The patient's chief complaint
◆ Pertinent history and information that was not given in your earlier radio report
◆ Additional treatment given to the patient while en route and his response to it
◆ Additional vital signs taken en route

Your oral report is a way of ensuring that staff members at the receiving facility receive all the patient data they require. Delivery of the oral report allows for interaction among EMS crew members, receiving facility personnel, and—when possible—the patient. You should be prepared to answer the staff's questions about the call to supplement the information already provided.

Transferring patient care responsibility to the receiving facility's staff does not complete your part in the call. You must fill out a written prehospital care report and leave a copy of it at the facility.

DOCUMENTATION

Written documentation is another of your professional obligations and responsibilities in providing patient care. The documentation that you must complete is known by a number of names—prehospital care report, ambulance run report, ambulance call report, EMS encounter form, and run sheet to name a few. (This book will use "prehospital care report" or PCR.) Whatever name your jurisdiction uses for the report of a call, you will be expected to complete the report thoroughly and accurately. You will also be expected to keep the information contained in the report confidential.

For many EMTs, documentation is the least-liked part of the job. Keep in mind, though, that good documentation of patient care is vital for the patient, for you as an EMT, and for your EMS system as a whole.

Reasons for Documentation

There are a number of reasons for documenting a call. First and most important, documentation helps the patient and the medical personnel who are caring for him by providing a permanent record of patient information. Documentation can do more than this, however:

◆ It can serve as a legal document if any proceedings arise as a result of the call.

◆ It can help the organizations that cared for the patient carry out administrative functions.

◆ It can help your EMS system improve the quality of care it provides.

◆ It can provide data that may be used by scientists in research projects.

Medical Functions

The chief reason for documentation is that it helps provide high-quality patient care. During your contact with a patient, you gather valuable information about his condition. You must record what you discover during that contact—the patient's presenting problems, his vital signs and pertinent history, other physical findings, and the care that has been provided.

Your documentation will remain with the patient after you complete a transfer of his care. The hospital staff can see, through your report, what the patient's condition was before he entered the hospital. Your documentation serves as a baseline against which the staff can measure his improvement or deterioration. Referring to your documentation, they will know what med-

ications and treatments have been provided. This will help them decide what additional medications and treatment to give the patient.

Even after the patient leaves the emergency department, your documentation, as a part of the patient's permanent medical record, remains available to other medical personnel who may treat him. The documentation thus helps assure continuity of care for the patient.

In order for your documentation to become a part of the patient's medical record, you must give a copy to the hospital before you return to service. Your original report should be kept on file, in a secure area, with your agency.

Legal Functions

Your documentation may become a legal document. This can happen in several ways:

◆ A patient you cared for might have been injured while committing a crime.

◆ A patient might have been injured by someone else who was committing a crime.

◆ A patient may have been injured and claim that someone else's negligence caused his injury.

In any of these situations, you might be called as a witness in a legal proceeding, even for an event that took place months or years earlier. As a witness, you will refer to the documentation you prepared at the time of the event. That documentation can help refresh your memory of the event. Also, if your documentation is entered as evidence in the case, it may help the judge or jury decide what really happened during the event. For these reasons, you should be accurate, thorough, and neat when documenting a call.

There is another thing to keep in mind whenever you prepare documentation. EMTs can also be sued. If you are ever sued, good documentation can be a vital part of your defense. Sloppy, incomplete, or inaccurate documentation can only hurt your case.

Administrative Functions

Your documentation may be used to determine costs and prepare bills. Insurance companies may refer to it in determining payments. Depending on your jurisdiction, you may have to gather insurance and billing information as part of your documentation.

In addition, most EMS agencies employ some type of Quality Improvement or Quality Assurance program. Review and evaluation of patient care documentation is a routine part of such a program. The review reveals how well agency personnel are meeting the agency's performance goals. The review may suggest areas in which the agency should provide additional training for its personnel.

The agency's medical director should periodically review patient care documentation for assurance of the quality of care being given by agency personnel. Senior EMS personnel should also routinely check the documentation to see that it is being filled out properly.

Educational and Research Functions

Scientists and researchers may use your documentation long after the call. For example, researchers might study your report along with thousands of others while looking for ways to shorten response times or cut costs of providing services. Other scientists might analyze documentation to determine how effective certain treatments or medications are at different stages of the patient care process.

Documentation can be used to create a "picture" of EMS service on a statewide or regional basis. In fact, some states require that data from prehospital documentation forms be submitted to designated organizations or agencies for review and analysis. The data is studied in hopes of finding ways to improve the quality of service while holding down costs. Be sure to follow any state or regional distribution or reporting requirements regarding documentation.

The Prehospital Care Report

As you can see, documentation is important. The major piece of documentation you complete will be the prehospital care report. Always be sure to fill out this vital report as completely and carefully as you can.

Prehospital Care Report Formats

Prehospital care reports can vary from one jurisdiction to another. The greatest variation comes in the formats in which the data is recorded.

The *written report* usually combines several different elements (Figures 8-6 and 8-7). There are check boxes and write-on lines for information that can be entered briefly, like the patient's name, age, sex, and vital signs. Larger areas are also provided in which the EMT can write out the more detailed information called the patient narrative.

In the *computerized report,* most vital information about a patient is recorded by filling in boxes. The completed form is then scanned by a computer and the data stored for easy access (Figure 8-8). This format is easy to use. However, the space available for writing a narrative is often very limited. If you use a computerized format, be sure to fill in the appropriate boxes completely and avoid stray marks. Be sure to use only the specific type of pen or pencil recommended.

The *electronic clipboard* is a different type of computerized report. It is a computer in the form of a clipboard (Figure 8-9). The computer recognizes handwriting done on its screen with a special pen. It converts the writing into electronic data and stores it. The data can later be printed out or downloaded to a larger computer.

In some systems, EMTs enter data directly into computer terminals to generate and store patient records.

Prehospital Care Report Data

The same basic types of information are generally required on prehospital care reports. However, there are different requirements from state to state and jurisdiction to jurisdiction.

The Minimum Data Set In an attempt to standardize the types of data collected, the National Highway Traffic Safety Administration of the U.S. Department of Transportation issued a report in 1994. That report recommended a *minimum data set* of elements that should be documented on prehospital care reports. The belief was that a standard set of elements would make analysis of large numbers of reports easier and

(text continues, page 243)

MAINE EMS

PRESS DOWN, YOU ARE MAKING THREE COPIES.

RUN REPORT #	Mo.	Day	Year	M T W Th	F S Sun	SERVICE NAME		SERVICE NO.	VEHICLE NO.	ALS ☐ Performed ☐ Back-up called	SERVICE RUN NO.
746118											

NAME | BILLING INFORMATION

STREET OR R.F.D.

CITY/TOWN | STATE | ZIP

AGE/DATE OF BIRTH | ☐ Male ☐ Female | PHONE

INCIDENT LOCATION: | ADDRESS | CITY/TOWN

TRANSPORTED TO: | TREATING/FAMILY PHYSICIAN | CREW LICENSE NUMBERS

TRANSPORTATION/COMMUNICATIONS PROBLEMS

☐ Medical
  ☐ Cardiac
  ☐ Poisoning/OD
    ☐ Respiratory
  ☐ Behavioral
    ☐ Diabetic
  ☐ Seizure
    ☐ CVA
  ☐ OB/Gyn
    ☐ Other _____

☐ Trauma
  ☐ Multi-Systems Trauma
  ☐ Head
    ☐ Spinal
  ☐ Burn
    ☐ Soft Tissue Injury
  ☐ Fractures
    ☐ Other _____

☐ Code 99

☐ MEDICATIONS   ☐ ALLERGIES

CHIEF COMPLAINT:

R L LUNG SOUNDS
☐ ☐ CLEAR
☐ ☐ ABSENT
☐ ☐ DECREASED
☐ ☐ RALES
☐ ☐ WHEEZE
☐ ☐ STRIDOR

TYPE OF RUN
☐ Emergency Transport
☐ Routine Transfer
☐ Emergency Transfer
☐ No Transport
☐ Refused Transport

	TIME	CODE		ODOMETER
Call Received				
Enroute				
At Scene				
From Scene				
At Destination				
In Service				

TIME	PULSE	RESP	BP	PUPILLARY RESPONSE	SKIN	VERBAL RESPONSE	MOTOR RESPONSE	EYE-OPENING RESPONSE	CAPILLARY REFILL
						5 4 3 2 1	6 5 4 3 2 1	4 3 2 1	☐ Normal ☐ None ☐ Delayed
						5 4 3 2 1	6 5 4 3 2 1	4 3 2 1	☐ Normal ☐ None ☐ Delayed
						5 4 3 2 1	6 5 4 3 2 1	4 3 2 1	☐ Normal ☐ None ☐ Delayed

☐ MVA   ☐ Concern AOB/ETOH   SEAT BELTS: ☐ Used ☐ Not Used ☐ N/A ☐ Helmet Used

MUTUAL AID: Assisted/Assisted by Service # _____ Time Called: _____

PATIENT'S SUSPECTED PROBLEM:		746118

☐ Medication Administered   ☐ Defib Lic.# _____

☐ Monitor   ☐ Chest Decomp

☐ Pacing   ☐ Caricothyrotomy

MEDICAL CONTROL ☐ Written Order/Protocol ☐ Verbal Order/Protocol

IV   ☐ SUC LIC.# _____   Total Attempts _____
   ☐ UNSUC LIC.# _____

		EOA		ET		Total Attempts

Cleared Airway	Extrication
Artificial Respiration/BVM	Cervical Immobilization
Oropharyngeal Airway	KED/Short Board
Nasopharyngeal Airway	Long Board
CPR–Time:	Restraints
Bystander CPR	Traction Splinting
AED	General Splinting
Suction	Cold Application
Oxygen–LPMin ___ ☐ Nasal ☐ Mask	MAST Inflated
Pulse Oximetry	
Autovent	

EOA ☐ SUC LIC.# _____ Total Attempts ___
   ☐ UNSUC LIC.# _____

ET ☐ SUC LIC.# _____ Total Attempts ___
   ☐ UNSUC LIC.# _____

LIC #	EKG RHYTHM	TIME	MEDS/DEFIB/C-VERT	DOSE W/S	ROUTE

NAME OF E.D. TREATING PHYSICIAN | SIGNATURE OF CREW MEMBER IN CHARGE | COPY 1 HOSPITAL

Figure 8-6 One version of a prehospital care report with fill-in boxes and spaces for a narrative.

Prehospital Care Report
FOR BLS FR USE ONLY

M D Y DATE OF CALL RUN NO. AGENCY CODE VEH. ID.

Name
Address
Ph #
AGE DOB M D Y SEX M F
Physician

CARE IN PROGRESS ON ARRIVAL:
☐ None ☐ Citizen ☐ PD/FD/Other First Responder ☐ Other EMS

MECHANISM OF INJURY
☐ MVA (✓ seat belt used →) ☐ Fall of ___ feet ☐ GSW ☐ Machinery
☐ Struck by vehicle ☐ Unarmed assault ☐ Knife ☐ _____

Agency Name
Dispatch Information
Call Location
CHECK ONE ☐ Residence ☐ Health Facility ☐ Farm ☐ Indus. Facility ☐ Other Work Loc. ☐ Roadway ☐ Recreational ☐ Other
LOCATION CODE

CALL TYPE AS REC'D.
☐ Emergency
☐ Non-Emergency
☐ Stand-by

COMPLETE FOR TRANSFERS ONLY
Transferred from ___
☐ No Previous PCR
☐ Unknown if Previous PCR
Previous PCR Number ___ – ___

☐ Extrication required ___ minutes
Seat belt used? ☐ Yes ☐ No ☐ Unknown
Seat Belt Use Reported By ☐ Crew ☐ Patient ☐ Police ☐ Other

MILEAGE END BEGIN TOTAL

USE MILITARY TIMES
CALL REC'D
ENROUTE
ARRIVED AT SCENE
FROM SCENE
AT DESTIN
IN SERVICE
IN QUARTERS

CHIEF COMPLAINT
SUBJECTIVE ASSESSMENT

PRESENTING PROBLEM
If more than one checked, circle primary
☐ Airway Obstruction
☐ Respiratory Arrest
☐ Respiratory Distress
☐ Cardiac Related (Potential)
☐ Cardiac Arrest

☐ Allergic Reaction
☐ Syncope
☐ Stroke/CVA
☐ General Illness/Malaise
☐ Gastro-Intestinal Distress
☐ Diabetic Related (Potential)
☐ Pain _____

☐ Unconscious/Unresp.
☐ Seizure
☐ Behavioral Disorder
☐ Substance Abuse (Potential)
☐ Poisoning (Accidental)

☐ Shock
☐ Head Injury
☐ Spinal Injury
☐ Fracture/Dislocation
☐ Amputation

☐ Major Trauma
☐ Trauma-Blunt
☐ Trauma-Penetrating
☐ Soft Tissue Injury
☐ Bleeding/Hemorrhage

☐ OB/GYN
☐ Burns
Environmental
☐ Heat
☐ Cold
☐ Hazardous Materials
☐ Obvious Death

☐ Other _____

PAST MEDICAL HISTORY		TIME	RESP	PULSE	B.P.	LEVEL OF CONSCIOUSNESS	GCS	R PUPILS L	SKIN	STATUS
☐ None ☐ Allergy to___ ☐ Hypertension ☐ Stroke ☐ Seizures ☐ Diabetes ☐ COPD ☐ Cardiac ☐ Other (List) ☐ Asthma Current Medications (List)	V I T A L S I G N S		Rate: ☐ Regular ☐ Shallow ☐ Labored	Rate: ☐ Regular ☐ Irregular		☐ Alert ☐ Voice ☐ Pain ☐ Unresp.		☐ Normal ☐ Dilated ☐ Constricted ☐ Sluggish ☐ No-Reaction	☐ Unremarkable ☐ Cool ☐ Pale ☐ Warm ☐ Cyanotic ☐ Moist ☐ Flushed ☐ Dry ☐ Jaundiced	☐ C ☐ U ☐ P ☐ S
			Rate: ☐ Regular ☐ Shallow ☐ Labored	Rate: ☐ Regular ☐ Irregular		☐ Alert ☐ Voice ☐ Pain ☐ Unresp.		☐ Normal ☐ Dilated ☐ Constricted ☐ Sluggish ☐ No-Reaction	☐ Unremarkable ☐ Cool ☐ Pale ☐ Warm ☐ Cyanotic ☐ Moist ☐ Flushed ☐ Dry ☐ Jaundiced	☐ C ☐ U ☐ P ☐ S
			Rate: ☐ Regular ☐ Shallow ☐ Labored	Rate: ☐ Regular ☐ Irregular		☐ Alert ☐ Voice ☐ Pain ☐ Unresp.		☐ Normal ☐ Dilated ☐ Constricted ☐ Sluggish ☐ No-Reaction	☐ Unremarkable ☐ Cool ☐ Pale ☐ Warm ☐ Cyanotic ☐ Moist ☐ Flushed ☐ Dry ☐ Jaundiced	☐ C ☐ U ☐ P ☐ S

OBJECTIVE PHYSICAL ASSESSMENT

COMMENTS

TREATMENT GIVEN
☐ Moved to ambulance on stretcher/backboard
☐ Moved to ambulance on stair chair
☐ Walked to ambulance
☐ Airway Cleared
☐ Oral/Nasal Airway
☐ Esophageal Obturator Airway/Esophageal Gastric Tube Airway (EOA/EGTA)
☐ EndoTracheal Tube (E/T)
☐ Oxygen Administered @ ___ L.P.M., Method _____
☐ Suction Used
☐ Artificial Ventilation Method _____
☐ C.P.R. in progress on arrival by: ☐ Citizen ☐ PD/FD/Other First Responder ☐ Other
☐ C.P.R. Started @ Time ▶ Time from Arrest Until C.P.R. ▶ ___ Minutes
☐ EKG Monitored (Attach Tracing) [Rhythm(s) _____]
☐ Defibrillation/Cardioversion No. Times ___ ☐ Manual ☐ Semi-automatic

☐ Medication Administered (Use Continuation Form)
☐ IV Established Fluid _____ Cath. Gauge ___
☐ Mast Inflated @ Time _____
☐ Bleeding/Hemorrhage Controlled (Method Used: _____)
☐ Spinal Immobilization Neck and Back
☐ Limb Immobilized by ☐ Fixation ☐ Traction
☐ (Heat) or (Cold) Applied
☐ Vomiting Induced @ Time ___ Method _____
☐ Restraints Applied, Type _____
☐ Baby Delivered @ Time ___ In County _____
☐ Alive ☐ Stillborn ☐ Male ☐ Female
☐ Transported in Trendelenburg position
☐ Transported in left lateral recumbent position
☐ Transported with head elevated
☐ Other _____

DISPOSITION (See list) DISP. CODE CONTINUATION FORM USED YES ←

CREW	IN CHARGE	DRIVER'S NAME	NAME	NAME
	☐ EMT ☐ AEMT #	☐ CFR ☐ EMT ☐ AEMT #	☐ CFR ☐ EMT ☐ AEMT #	☐ CFR ☐ EMT ☐ AEMT #

AGENCY COPY/WHITE
EMS 100 (11/86) provided by NYS-EMS PROGRAM
DOH 3822 (6/94)

Figure 8-7 One system's prehospital care report for first-responding EMTs.

Do Not Staple or Fold

| AGENCY CODE | UNIT # | UNIT TYPE | DATE | PERSONNEL INFORMATION | RESPONSE/ TRANSPORT MODE | RESPONSE OUTCOME |

UNIT TYPE: AMBULANCE, RESCUE, OTHER

DATE: Jan, Feb, Mar, Apr, May, Jun, Jul, Aug, Sep, Oct, Nov, Dec — DAY — YR (91, 92, 93, 94, 95)

PERSONNEL INFORMATION: ATTENDANT #1, ATTENDANT #2, ATTENDANT #3

RESPONSE/TRANSPORT MODE:
To Scene: (2) Non-Emerg (3) Emergency
From Scene: (2) Non-Emerg (3) Emergency

RESPONSE OUTCOME:
- Transported By This Unit
- Care Transfer/Another Unit
- Cancelled Enroute
- Cancelled On Scene
- False Call/No Patient Found
- Dead on Scene
- Refused Treatment
- Treated, Refused Transport
- P.O.V.
- Standby
- Unknown
- Other

| CALL RECEIVED | ENROUTE | ARRIVE SCENE | DEPART SCENE | ARRIVE HOSPITAL | RETURN TO SERVICE | INCIDENT LOCATION | DISPATCH/INCIDENT TYPE |

(Each time field labeled MILITARY TIME)

INCIDENT LOCATION:
- Residence
- Interstate
- Highway
- Street/Road.
- Public Access
- Industrial/Off.
- HMO/Clinic/Doctors Office
- Hospital
- Other

DISPATCH/INCIDENT TYPE:
- Abdominal Pain
- Asphyxiation/Choke
- Chest Pain
- Diff. Breathing
- Drowning
- Heat/Cold Problems
- Ill Person
- OB/GYN
- OD/Poison
- Person Down/Unconsc.
- Psych/Behavioral
- Seizures
- Other Medical
- MVA
- MVA - Motorcycle
- MVA - Ped/Bike
- Assault
- Assault - Sexual
- Bite/Sting
- Burn/Elect.
- Fall
- Person Trapped
- Stab/Gunshot
- Other Trauma
- Standby
- InterFacility Transfer

SUSPECTED MEDICAL ILLNESS (None)
(P=Primary, S=Secondary)
- Abdom. Pain
- Airway Obstr
- Allergic React
- Cancer Compli
- Cardiac Arrest
- Cardiac Sympt.
- Chest Pain
- Childbirth
- COPD
- Diabetes Comp.
- Drug Reaction
- Heat/Cold Problems
- Inhalation
- OB/GYN
- OD/Poison
- Psych/Behv
- Resp. Arrest
- Resp. Dist
- Seizures
- Stroke
- Syncope
- Unconscious
- Other

INJURY SITE/TYPE (Amputate, Bite/Sting, Blunt-Major, Burn/Elec, Frac/Disloc., Penetrate, Soft-Closed, Soft-Open) — None
- Head
- Face
- Eye
- Neck
- Chest
- Back
- Upper Ext
- Abdomen
- Pelvis
- Lower Ext

MECHANISM OF INJURY:
- Flail Chest
- Burns 10+%/face/arwy
- Fall 20+ feet
- Speed 40+ mph
- 20+ speed change
- Deformity 20+"
- Intrusion 12+"
- Rollover
- Ejection
- Death same MV
- Pedest.vs. MV 5+mph
- Pedst. thrown/run over
- Mtcycle 20+mph/sep.
- Extrication >15 min.

GLASGOW COMA SCALE

EYES	VERBAL	MOTOR
(4) Spontaneous	(5) Oriented	(6) Obeys Comm.
(3) To Voice	(4) Confused	(5) Pain-Local.
(2) To Pain	(3) Inappropriate	(4) Pain-Withdraws
(1) Unresponsive	(2) Garbled	(3) Pain-Flexion
	(1) None	(2) Pain-Extends
		(1) None

PRIOR AID (None) — CPR, Extricate, Wound Mgt
- Fire
- Police
- 1st Resp.
- Rescue
- Bystander

THIS PATIENT LOCATION/PROTECTION:
- Driver
- Front Pass
- Rear Pass
- Other
- Unknown
- Shldr/Lap Belt
- Shoulder Belt
- Lap Belt
- Safety Seat
- Helmet
- Not Used
- Not Available
- Unknown
- Airbag (Deployed) Yes

SEX: (F) (M)

AGE — Months, Apprx.

INITIAL VITAL SIGNS: Unable to Take, Not Taken, Pt. Refused
SYSTOLIC, DIASTOLIC, PULSE, RESP, PUPILS (L, R: N, D, C, NR)

This Patient Resident of: City, County, Arizona, Out of State, Unknown

BLS TREATMENT (A1 A2 A3 O)
- Assessment
- C-Spine Precautions
- Oxygen
- CPR
- Crisis Intervention
- Defibrillation (AUTO)
- Extrication
- Fracture Stabilize
- Hemorrhage Control
- Ipecac/Charcoal Admin.
- MAST Application
- MAST Inflation
- Monitor IV
- Oral Care/Airway
- Oral Glucose
- Restraints Applied
- Suction
- Traction Splint
- Wound Management
- Other

CPR INFORMATION:
Time: Minutes (<4, 4-10, >10, Unk)
- Arrest to CPR
- Arrest to Defib
- Arrest to ALS
- Witnessed Arrest? (Y) (N) Unk
- Pulse/Rhythm Restored? (Y) (N)
- Traumatic Cardiac Arrest? (Y) (N)

ALS TREATMENT (A1 A2 A3 O)
- Cardiac Monitoring
- Cardioversion
- Cricothyroidotomy
- Defibrillation
- EOA
- Intubation - Nasal
- Intubation - Oral
- IV-Central
- IV-Peripheral
- Medication Admin
- NG Tube
- Needle Thoracostomy
- Phlebotomy
- SVN
- Other

ATTEMPTS: IV, ET, OTH (1) (2) (3) (U)

MEDICATIONS:
- Albuterol
- Aminoph.
- Atropine 1/10
- Atropine 8/20
- Bretylium
- Calcium Chl.
- D50
- Diazepam
- Diphenhydram.
- Dopamine
- Epi 1:1000
- Epi 1:10,000
- Furosemide
- Isoetharine
- Isoproterenol
- Lidocaine-Bolus
- Lidocaine Drip
- Methylprednisone
- Morphine
- Naloxone
- Nifedipine
- Nitrostat. Tab.
- Nitrous Oxide
- Oxytocin
- Phenobarbital
- Sodium Bicarbonate
- Thiamine
- Verapamil
- Other
- HAZMAT

EKG INITIAL/LAST (I, L):
- Nrml Sinus
- Sinus Tach
- Sinus Brady
- Asystole
- AV Block
- Atrial Fib
- Atrial Flut
- EMD
- Junctional
- Paced
- SV Tach
- Vent Tach
- Vent Fib
- Other
- PVC's

IV TYPE/RATE (TKO, Bolus, Wide, Other):
- D5W
- Normal Saline
- Ringers Lact.
- Other

 # LINES: # Peripheral (1 2 3 4), # Central (1 2 3 4)

MEDICAL CONTROL: First, Hospital
- Radio/Good
- Radio/Poor
- Protocol
- Telephone
- Radio/Phone Patch
- Cellular
- Phys On-Scene
- None Required
- Unable

ORDERS BY:
- Protocol
- Standing
- Verbal

PT. RECEIVED BY / **RESEARCH CODE**

PATIENT DISPOSITION:
- Improved
- Worsened
- Unchanged
- Died in ER

MISCELLANEOUS:
If Multiple Pts On Scene, How Many?
If Transport to Level 1 Receiving Facility, Due to:
- Pt. Condition
- Mechanism

2002094

PLEASE DO NOT MARK IN THIS AREA

EMS FIRST CARE FORM - ARIZONA DEPARTMENT OF HEALTH SERVICES
Return to State EMS Office

SCANTRON® FORM NO. F-3087-EMS   0792-C 671-5 4 3 2 1
© 1992 EMS DATA SYSTEMS

Figure 8-8 The format of an Arizona prehospital care report allows its information to be scanned into a computer.

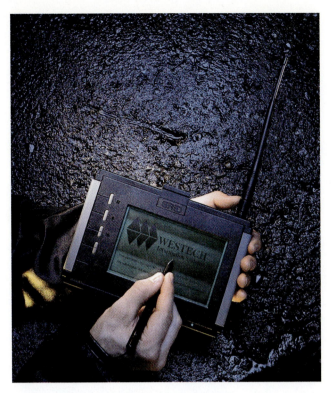

Figure 8-9 The electronic clipboard is a handheld computer into which patient information can be entered with a special pen.

more meaningful. This could make it easier to find out what is being done right in emergency medical care and where there is need for improvement. The elements of the minimum data set are as follows:

Patient Information Gathered by the EMT

◆ Chief complaint

◆ Level of consciousness (AVPU)—mental status

◆ Systolic blood pressure for patients greater than 3 years old

◆ Skin perfusion (capillary refill) for patients less than 6 years old

◆ Skin color and temperature

◆ Pulse rate

◆ Respiratory rate and effort

Administrative Information

◆ Time the incident was reported

◆ Time the EMS unit was notified

◆ Time of the unit's arrival at patient

◆ Time the unit left the scene

◆ Time the unit arrived at its destination (emergency department, etc.)

◆ Time of transfer of patient care

Note that the administrative information calls for the times at which different things happen during a call. This points out the need for an EMS system to use *accurate and synchronous clocks.* This term means that all watches and time-keeping devices in the system must be set to the same, correct time. Generally speaking, use the times given by the dispatcher as much as possible when you are filling out a prehospital care report.

An accurate time-keeping system will help provide accurate data about the patient. When you are dealing with human life, minutes can make a difference. For example, medical personnel at the receiving facility will need to know how long a patient has been in cardiac arrest. An accurate time-keeping system also makes it easier to determine how efficiently EMS units are responding to calls.

Many EMS systems already collect information required in the minimum data set. Often that information is found in several different sections of the prehospital care report.

Administrative Information This section is also referred to as *run data.* It usually consists of the administrative information listed above in the minimum data set. It also might include the following:

◆ The name of the EMS agency

◆ The EMS unit number

◆ The run or call number

◆ The names of unit crew members and their levels of certification

◆ The address to which the unit is dispatched

Patient Data This section is the heart of the prehospital care report. It usually includes information required in the minimum data set plus additional facts and observations. A typical prehospital care report might expect you to provide the following:

◆ The patient's name, address, age, date of birth, sex

◆ Billing and insurance information

- The location of the call
- The patient's chief complaint and presenting problem(s)
- The mechanism of injury (if applicable)
- Treatment provided to the patient before the arrival of the EMTs (by first responders or bystanders)
- The patient's signs and symptoms
- The patient's level of consciousness (AVPU)
- The patient's vital signs (baseline and later readings)
    —Pulse
    —Respiratory rate and effort
    —Blood pressure (for patients greater than 3 years of age)
    —Skin temperature and condition
    —Pupil response
- The patient's SAMPLE history
- Treatment provided to the patient by the EMT and the patient's response to that treatment
- Changes in the patient's condition throughout the call
- The patient's regular/family physician

Many prehospital care report forms are designed so that you use check boxes or a combination of check boxes and short write-on lines to record this information in a brief, easy-to-read format.

Patient Narrative Some patient data is too complex to be summed up in check boxes or a few blank lines. This material goes in the section of the prehospital care report called the *patient narrative*. There you have the space to write out more detailed descriptions of the patient and his condition. The patient narrative section usually contains the patient's chief complaint and his SAMPLE history.

In the patient narrative, you are trying to "paint a picture" of the patient for other medical personnel who become involved in his care. You want them to be able to know what you observed about the patient during your time with him. Do not use the narrative section to present your conclusions about the patient and his condition. Instead, use it to record accurate and pertinent information about

the patient that others can use as evidence in making diagnoses and providing treatment.

Below are some guidelines to follow when writing the patient narrative:

- *Include both objective and pertinent subjective information. Objective* information can be measured and verified in some way. For example, if you observe that a patient is bleeding from the ears and has a blood pressure of 135/80, another EMT could examine the patient and confirm your observations.

    Remember that observations about the scene are objective information that should be included in the narrative. For example, you should note the presence of an open and empty pill bottle by the bedside of an unresponsive patient. (In that case, you would also bring the pill bottle to the hospital when you transport the patient.)

    Subjective information is information based on an individual's perceptions or interpretations. In the narrative, you might include information based on the patient's perceptions: for example, "I feel dizzy." You might also include information based on your perceptions: for example, "Patient appears to be in pain."

    Try to use objective statements as much as possible. If you do include subjective statements, be sure they are pertinent, or relevant to the patient's medical condition. The patient's statement "I feel dizzy" is pertinent because dizziness can be a symptom of a medical condition. On the other hand, your statement "Patient is probably having a heart attack" is not pertinent; it is a conclusion that you are not qualified to make. Likewise, your statement "Patient's wife was rude" is not pertinent because it isn't directly relevant to the patient's medical condition.

    When you do include subjective statements from the patient, family members, or bystanders, put them in quotation marks. Do this with any information you did not directly observe yourself. Note that the patient's chief complaint is a type of subjective information that is usually placed in quotation marks. Be sure to include the source of that information in the narrative—for example, "Patient states, 'My right arm aches.'" or "Patient's wife states, 'Harry said he had a bad headache.'"

◆ *Include pertinent negatives in your report.* **Pertinent negatives** are things you might expect to find based on the patient's chief complaint or the mechanism of injury but that are not present. For example, in patients with chest pain, difficulty in breathing is common. If a patient with chest pain denies having difficulty in breathing, that is a pertinent negative and should be included in your report. Or if a patient has fallen in such a way that injury to his left leg or hip would be expected but the patient denies having any pain there, you should include the denial in your report. Including pertinent negatives assures medical direction and staff at the receiving facility that you performed a thorough assessment. Don't *assume,* but document what you want the reader to know.

◆ *Avoid using radio codes and non-standard abbreviations in your report.* Hospital personnel may not know radio codes and may be confused by them. Using abbreviations in your report can save time and space, but they must be standard abbreviations. Use of non-standard abbreviations can lead to confusion and errors on the part of the reader of the report. Many EMS systems issue lists of standard abbreviations approved for use on their prehospital care reports. Table 8-1 lists some standard abbreviations.

◆ *Use medical terminology correctly.* Improper use of medical terms can cause confusion and possible errors by people who must use the report. Check spellings and definitions of terms in a medical dictionary. If you are unsure about a specific term and its application, use everyday language instead.

◆ *Be neat.* Neatness does count. Write legibly. Remember that other people will be relying on the information in the report and they must be able to read it.

◆ *Be thorough.* Always keep in mind that in the report you are trying to present as complete and accurate a picture of the patient and his

Table 8-1

Standard Abbreviations

$\bar{a}$	before
$\bar{c}$	with
NTG	nitroglycerin
O_2	oxygen
OB	obstetrics
$\bar{p}$	after
PE	physical exam, pulmonary edema
po	orally, by mouth
Pt	patient
q	every
QID	four times a day
R/O	rule out
Rx	prescription
$\bar{s}$	without
s/s	signs/symptoms
SL	sublingual (under the tongue)
SOB	shortness of breath
STAT	immediately
Sx	symptoms
TIA	transient ischemic attack
TID	three times a day
Tx	treatment
×	times
y/o	years old
↑	increased
↓	decreased

condition as you can. There are two things you should always remember when filling out a prehospital care report:

"If it's not written down, you didn't do it." This means that you should record everything pertinent that you observe about a patient and everything that you do for him. Without the written documentation, hospital personnel may not know important facts about a patient. Also, unless you record what you saw or did in the report, you may not be able to prove it in court.

"If it wasn't done, don't write it down." In your report, only include what you actually observed, did, or learned from someone else. Including anything else is falsification, which can lead to errors in treatment and harm to the patient. (You will read more about falsification below.)

Legal Issues

Prehospital care reports are legal documents. Working with them involves a number of legal issues that you should be aware of.

Confidentiality

Confidentiality is a cornerstone of medicine. The patient has a legal right to confidentiality. This means that you should not distribute the prehospital care report or discuss information on it with unauthorized individuals. Nor should you discuss treatment of the patient or statements made by the patient during treatment with anyone other than health care professionals who need the information to provide proper care.

Naturally, you will have to discuss the patient and share the report with some people to ensure proper care. You may have to give information to the ambulance crew that is transporting the patient or to doctors or nurses at the emergency department that is receiving the patient.

Information about the patient may also be distributed to other organizations for reasons other than direct patient care. For example, the patient's insurance company may need information so that it can reimburse the patient's expenses. The police may request information about a call if they are investigating a crime. Your agency's Quality Improvement committee may also study your report as it looks for ways to improve service.

State and local regulations describe who may have access to a prehospital care report and information about a patient. Some areas even set regulations on what patient information can be transmitted over the radio. Learn the regulations that apply to your agency and follow them.

When you document information of a sensitive nature, be sure to note the source. If you discover that a patient has attempted suicide or has a communicable disease, record who provided that information—the patient, a spouse, a relative, or someone else. Write the information and its source in the appropriate section of the prehospital care report. Do not highlight it or otherwise identify it as unique or special. Of course, you must treat this information as confidential.

Patient Refusal of Treatment

In Chapter 4, "Medical/Legal Issues," you learned about what to do if a patient refuses to accept the treatment or transport you believe is necessary. That chapter also gave suggestions for ways to convince patients to accept treatment. You may wish to review that material now.

In the end, competent adults do have the right to refuse care and treatment. However, legal questions may arise after the fact about whether or not the adult was really competent to refuse care.

Make extra efforts to be sure that the patient is competent to refuse care. Is he under age? Is he under the influence of alcohol or drugs? Is his medical condition interfering with his ability to make a competent decision? If the answer to any of these questions is "yes," the patient is not competent to refuse care. He can be treated and transported. However, you must document all the evidence that led you to decide he was not competent. If you decide he is competent to refuse care, document your reasons for that decision as well.

If the patient is competent to refuse care, still try to persuade him to accept it. Explain what may happen to him if he refuses treatment. Document your attempts to convince him.

Perform as much of an assessment as you can on the patient. Try to learn at least something about his chief complaint, presenting problems, and medical history. You may also be able to persuade the patient to let you take his vital signs. What you discover during the assessment may give you addi-tional information that you can use to change the patient's mind about refusing care. Don't forget to gather additional information from family, friends, or bystanders if they are present. Document every-thing you learn during the assessment.

Contact medical direction or your supervisor, if required by local protocols. Explain what you have observed about the patient's competency, what actions you have taken to convince him to accept care, and what you found during your assessment. Medical direction or the supervisor may be able to provide additional reasons why the patient should change his mind. If the patient still refuses, med-ical direction may have suggestions for additional care that you can give on the scene.

If the patient rejects all of your efforts to change his mind, you must document that by having him sign a form. There are many names for the form: "release from liability," "refusal of treatment/trans-port," "release from responsibility," and "refusal of medical assistance" are just a few (Figure 8-10). By

Figure 8-10 One example of a refusal of care form.

RELEASE FROM RESPONSIBILITY

DATE _____ 19 _____ TIME _____ a.m. / p.m.

This is to certify that _____

is refusing ☐ TREATMENT ☐ TRANSPORTATION

against the advice of the attending Emergency Medical Technician and of the Phoenix Fire Department, and when applicable, the base hospital and the base hospital physician.

I acknowledge that I have been informed of the following:

1. The nature and potential of the illness or injuries.
2. The potential risks of delaying treatment and transportation, up to and including death.
3. The availability of ambulance transportation to a hospital for treatment.

Nevertheless, I assume all risks and consequences of my decision, including further physical deterioration, loss of limb, paralysis, and even death, and hereby release the attending Emergency Medical Technician and the Phoenix Fire Department, and when applicable, the base hospital and the base hospital physician from any ill effects which may result from my refusal.

Witness _____ Signed: **X** _____

Witness _____ Relationship to Patient _____

Refusal must be signed by the patient; or by the nearest relative or legal guardian in the case of a minor, or when patient is physically or mentally incompetent.

☐ Patient refuses to sign release despite efforts of attending Emergency Medical Technician to obtain such signature after informing patient of concerns listed in numbers 1, 2, and 3 above.

GUIDELINES — Patient Refusal Documentation

In addition to those items normally documented (chief complaint, history of present illness, mechanism of injury, physical assessment, etc.) the following items should be recorded, regardless of patient's cooperation:

- Mental Status (orientation, speech, etc.)
- Suspected presence of alcohol or drugs
- Patient's exact words (as much as possible) in the refusal of care OR the signing of the release form
- Circumstances or reasons (including exact words of patient, if possible) for INCOMPLETE ADVISEMENT (risk of injury, abusiveness, unruliness, risk of injury other than from patient, etc.)
- Advice given to patients' guardian(s)

Table 8-2

Refusal of Care Information

Include as much of the following information as possible in the prehospital care report when a patient refuses treatment and/or transport.

- ◆ Patient assessment, including indications that the patient was competent to refuse care

- ◆ Treatment/transport you thought was necessary and that the patient refused

- ◆ Your statement explaining to the patient the possible consequences of refusing treatment/transport, including the possibility of death

- ◆ Your suggestions for alternative methods of accessing care

- ◆ Your statement of willingness to return to treat/transport the patient

- ◆ Your formal statement that the patient appears to have understood the statements and suggestions described above and appears competent to refuse care based on that understanding

signing the form, the patient indicates that you have told him he should get medical care, that you have explained the dangers of refusing care, and that he is refusing care anyway.

Make sure the patient reads the form before signing it. If you have any doubts about his ability to read, read it to him. Have a family member, police officer, or other bystander sign the form as a witness. Obtain the addresses of any witnesses in case they must be contacted.

Sometimes a patient may refuse to sign the form. In that case, have a family member, police officer, or bystander sign a statement saying the patient refused treatment and would not sign the refusal form.

Before you leave the scene, suggest other places the patient can go for medical help—a clinic, an emergency department, a private physician. Make it clear to the patient that he can call EMS back if he changes his mind about accepting treatment. Document your actions and the state-ments you made to the patient on the prehospital care report.

Falsification

The prehospital care report is supposed to record what was actually observed or done on a call. At times, however, EMTs make mistakes during their assessment or care of a patient. They make errors of *omission,* not doing something they should have. Or they make errors of *commission,* doing something inappropriate or wrong. Some EMTs try to hide errors, either by leaving information about what they did out of the prehospital care report or by putting incorrect information into the report.

Falsifying a prehospital care report is a serious act that can have grave consequences. The false information in the report may result in the patient receiving unnecessary, inappropriate, or harmful treatment. If the falsification is discovered, the EMT may have his license or certification suspended or revoked. The EMT may also face civil or criminal charges in court.

Never falsify the prehospital care report or any document you may have to complete on the job. If you become aware that you made an error during a call, notify a physician at the receiving facility or talk with the your agency's medical director. No matter what your error was, never claim to have observed or done something that you didn't. For example, if you had time to take only one set of vital signs, don't make up additional readings because you know you should have taken another set. Likewise, if you provided the patient with incorrect medication or inappropriate treatment, record that fact so that other medical personnel will be alert to possible problems. For example, if you meant to assist the patient with taking his nitroglycerin, but accidentally gave him a different pill, write down what you did.

Correcting Errors

Even if you are very careful in filling out the pre-hospital care report, you may still make mistakes from time to time. You may check the wrong check box or you may write "left" when you meant "right" or you may transpose numbers, writing "37" when you meant to write "73."

PATIENT COMPLAINS OF PAIN IN HIS ~~RIGHT~~ ^{DL} LEFT SHOULDER THAT RADIATES TO THE LEFT ARM.

Figure 8-11   To correct an error on a prehospital care report, draw a single line through the error and write in the correct information. Initial the correction.

Whenever you discover an error on a prehospital report you must correct it. If you find the error while you are still writing the report, draw a single horizontal line through the error, initial it, and write in the correct information (Figure 8-11). (Some systems require EMTs to write the word "error" near the line drawn through the error.) Do not try to erase or write over the incorrect information; it may look like you are trying to falsify the report.

If you discover the error after you have submitted the form, draw a single line through the error and initial and date that line. Then add the correct information to the end of the report or supply it on a separate sheet of paper, signing and dating the addition. Use a different color ink for these changes. If copies of the report have already been sent to other agencies, be sure that each of them receives a corrected copy of the report.

If you have omitted information that you wish to add after the report has been submitted, write the information on a different form or sheet of paper. Provide identifying information, such as date of the call, the run number, and the patient's date of birth on the supplement. Then give the information you wish to add. When you are done, sign and date the supplement. Submit the document to the person responsible for maintaining the department's PCRs.

Special Situations

At times, you may be involved in situations where the prehospital report is not the appropriate documentation or you are required to use other forms in addition to it. Such situations might include the following:

◆ Possible occupational exposure to an infectious disease

◆ Injury in the line of duty

◆ Suspected child or elder abuse

Figure 8-12   Triage tags are commonly used to document patient information at multiple-casualty incidents.

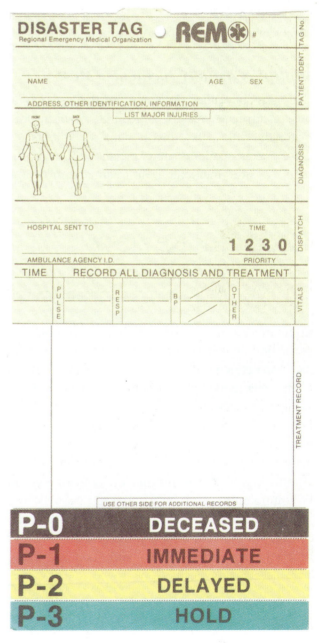

◆ A patient who must be referred to a social service agency

State laws and local protocols will set the requirements for filling out this documentation. Whenever you must provide additional documentation, however, keep in mind the basic principles for completing a prehospital care report. Be thorough and accurate in describing what happened. Be objective in your descriptions. Be neat. Cross reference the document to your prehospital care report for the call if you completed one by including information such as the run number and date of call. Attach a copy of the document to the prehospital care report and/or keep a copy for your agency's records. Submit an incident report in a timely manner. Never falsify a report.

Multiple Casualty Incidents (MCIs)

You may be called to some incidents, such as bus or airplane crashes, large fires, or hazardous materials leaks, that involve many patients. In these cases, patients may be moved from the scene of the incident to a treatment area and then to a hospital. Their care may be transferred to different EMS providers several times. During these multiple-casualty incidents, it may be difficult to provide thorough documentation for every patient, but it is important that medical information stay with the patient as he moves through the system.

Every EMS system should have a plan for handling MCIs. That plan should describe procedures for patient documentation. Most systems use some form of triage tag (Figure 8-12). Basic medical information—for example, the chief complaint and injuries, patient priority, vital signs, and treatment provided—is written on the tag. The tag is then attached to the patient and stays with him during his EMS care. A prehospital care report will still be required, but it may be less detailed than a normal report. Information from the triage tag can be used to complete the report.

You will find out more about procedures to follow during MCIs in Chapter 28, "EMS Special Operations." You must become familiar with your EMS system's plans for MCIs and documentation of them.

Chapter Review

SUMMARY

Communication and documentation are vital to good prehospital patient care. From the moment the dispatcher is notified until the patient arrives at the emergency department, you will need to communicate well with patients and with other EMS personnel. Being able to communicate well means using interpersonal skills to gather information from other people. It also means being able to organize that information both orally and in writing and pass it on to others.

Communication on a call may involve radio contact with system dispatch, medical control, and hospital personnel. Clear and concise radio reports are essential to ensuring a smooth continuity of care for the patient from the field to the hospital.

Communication continues even after care of the patient is transferred to the receiving facility. Then, communication takes the form of documentation. You must prepare a complete, well-written prehospital care report on the patient. That report will become part of the patient's permanent medical records. The report serves administrative, research, and quality improvement functions, but its main purpose is to assure the best possible patient care.

1. List five of the basic guidelines that EMTs should follow to assure good interpersonal communications with patients.

2. List some special considerations to keep in mind to assure better communications with pediatric patients.

3. List some special considerations to keep in mind to assure better communications with geriatric patients.

4. Describe standard components of an EMS communications system.

5. List ten of the basic guidelines to follow whenever you make radio transmissions.

6. List the information an EMT is expected to supply when communicating with EMS dispatch.

7. List the information an EMT is expected to supply when communicating with the receiving facility while en route with a patient.

8. Describe the information that an EMT should provide in an oral report when transferring care of a patient to the staff at the receiving facility.

9. Explain the various ways in which the information in a prehospital care report may be used.

10. Explain what the minimum data set is and why it is important.

11. Describe basic formats for prehospital care reports.

12. Describe the types of objective and subjective information that might be included in the patient narrative section of a prehospital care report.

13. Explain what pertinent negatives are and why they are important.

14. Describe the steps that an EMT should follow if a patient refuses treatment or transport.

15. Describe how to correct an error in a prehospital care report.

16. List some of the situations in which an EMT might be expected to file special reports in addition to or instead of the prehospital care report.

RESOURCES TO LEARN MORE

Bevelacqua, A.S. *Prehospital Documentation: A Systematic Approach*. Upper Saddle River, NJ: Brady/Prentice Hall, 1992.

Perez-Sabido, Jesus. *Spanish English Handbook for Medical Professionals, 4th Edition*. Los Angeles: Practice Management Information Corp., 1994.

Stanford, Todd. *EMS Report Writing: A Pocket Reference*. Upper Saddle River, NJ: Brady/Prentice Hall, 1992.

Steele, Susi B. *Emergency Dispatching: A Medical Communicator's Guide*. Upper Saddle River, NJ: Brady/Prentice Hall, 1992.

KEY INFORMATION IN COMMUNICATION AND DOCUMENTATION

RADIO REPORTS

Standard basic information in radio reports to medical direction or a receiving facility includes the following

- The unit's identification and level of service: BLS (Basic Life Support) or ALS (Advanced Life Support)
- The patient's age and sex
- The patient's chief complaint
- A brief history of the present illness
- Pertinent past major illnesses
- Current medications the patient is using
- Allergies the patient may have
- The patient's mental status
- The patient's baseline vital signs
- Pertinent findings from the physical examination of the patient
- Any emergency care EMTs (or first responders) have provided
- The patient's response to that emergency care
- The unit's estimated time of arrival (ETA) at the receiving facility

PREHOSPITAL CARE REPORTS

Standard basic information expected in prehospital care reports includes the following:

- The name of the EMS agency
- The EMS unit number
- The run or call number
- The names of unit crew members and their levels of certification
- Time the incident was reported*
- The address to which the unit is dispatched
- Time of dispatch*
- The location of the call
- Time of arrival at the scene*
- The patient's name, address, age, date of birth, sex
- Billing and insurance information
- The patient's chief complaint and presenting problem(s)*
- The mechanism of injury (if applicable)
- Treatment provided to the patient before the arrival of the EMTs (by first responders or bystanders)
- The patient's signs and symptoms
- The patient's level of consciousness (AVPU)*
- The patient's vital signs (baseline and later readings)
  - —Pulse*
  - —Respiratory rate and effort*
  - —Blood pressure for patients greater than 3 years of age; capillary refill time for those younger*
  - —Skin temperature and condition*
  - —Pupil response
- The patient's SAMPLE history
- Treatment provided to the patient by the EMT and the patient's response to that treatment
- Changes in the patient's condition throughout the call
- The patient's regular/family physician
- Time the unit left the scene*
- Time of arrival at the receiving facility*
- Time of transfer of patient care*

*Elements of the minimum data set

Transition of Prehospital Care

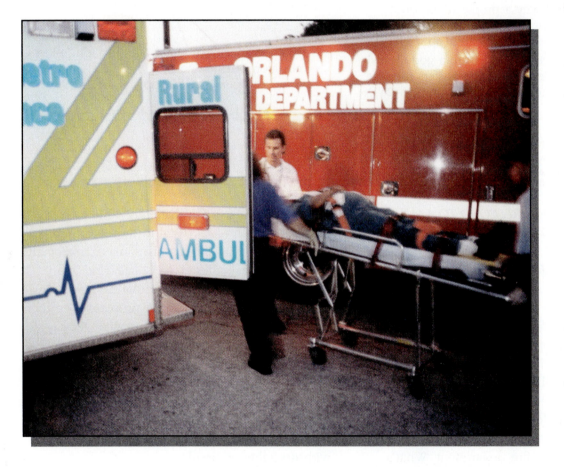

*A*s an EMT, you are a key part of the Emergency Medical Services system. It is important to keep in mind that this system works only through the efforts of many people at different levels of training. Your EMS system may include Emergency Medical Dispatchers, Certified First Responders, EMT-Basics, EMT-Paramedics, physicians, nurses, and physician assistants. In many areas, prehospital care of patients may be provided by many EMS system members working not only for the fire department but also for other municipal or private agencies. The goal of all members of the EMS system is to provide the best possible care for the ▶

patient from the moment the emergency call is received through the patient's arrival in the emergency department and beyond. Because a single patient can be cared for by so many care providers, it is essential that the hand-off, or transition of care, from one EMS provider to another be accomplished in a way that assures the best possible treatment of the patient.

OBJECTIVES

At the completion of this chapter, the EMT-Basic student should be able to meet the following objectives. These objectives are supplemental to the U.S. DOT 1994 EMT-Basic Curriculum.

Knowledge and Understanding

1. State the reasons why a proper transition of prehospital care from one provider to the next is essential to good patient care. (pp. 255–256)

2. List the steps necessary to assure a good transition of care as the EMT-Basic transfers the care of a patient to another provider. (pp. 256–257)

3. List the steps necessary to assure a good transition of care as the EMT-Basic assumes the care of a patient from another provider. (pp. 257–258)

4. Describe special circumstances that can affect transition of care and how to adjust procedures in those circumstances. (pp. 258–259)

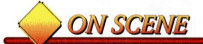

ON SCENE

DISPATCH: *ENGINE 5, RESPOND TO A REPORTED MAN DOWN ON THE CORNER OF ADDISON AND 4TH STREETS. COUNTY AMBULANCE HAS ALSO BEEN DISPATCHED. TIME OUT IS 0847.*

Your engine company is quartered only 3 blocks away and you are on the scene 2 minutes after the dispatch. On arrival, you detect no unusual scene hazards on what you know to be a usually quiet street. You see a middle-aged man sitting on the curb holding his right ankle and approach him, introducing yourself and saying, "I'm an EMT with the fire department. What's your name and what happened?"

"My name is Jack and—stupid me—I missed the step off the curb. I think I broke my ankle."

"Did you hurt yourself anywhere else?"

"No."

You quickly palpate Jack's neck, back, and hips and find them to be without any tenderness. Meanwhile, another EMT on the crew stabilizes Jack's lower leg, which shows an area of

obvious deformity. The patient is able to move his toes, and the foot distal to the deformity is pink in color with intact pulses. Your assessment is that Jack has suffered an isolated leg injury. You confirm with the patient that he agrees to be transported for care of the problem. You then radio the inbound county ambulance: "Engine 5 to county ambulance inbound to Addison and 4th streets."

"Go ahead, Engine 5."

"To advise you, patient is a 34-year-old male, stable with an isolated lower leg injury. You can downgrade to a cold response [non-emergency, with no lights or siren]."

"County copied."

After speaking with the ambulance, you tell the patient, "Jack, the ambulance that will be taking you to the hospital will be here in a couple of minutes. We're going to put your leg into a splint to immobilize it. I'm also going to ask you some medical questions".

By the time the ambulance arrives 4 minutes later, your crew has splinted the injured leg and obtained a complete set of vital signs. The two EMTs from the county ambulance crew approach you with their stretcher and you greet them by saying, "Guys, this is Jack. Jack is 34 years old. He missed his step off the curb here and injured his left ankle. He denies other injuries and denies loss of consciousness. His neck and back are non-tender. He is a previously healthy person with no medications and no allergies. His vital signs are stable, and we've splinted the leg with intact motor function and pulses both before and after applying the splint. He seems more comfortable now that the splint has been applied."

One of your partners hands the county EMT a copy of your first-response form, which includes the patient's vital signs, medical history, and documentation of his injuries and of the treatment provided by your crew. After quickly looking over your paperwork and checking out the splinted leg, the county EMT nods to you that he's all set. Your crew assists the county crew in placing the patient onto the ambulance stretcher.

When you are finished at the scene, you contact the dispatcher: "Dispatcher, Engine 5 clearing the scene and back in service."

"Copied Engine 5. Back in service 0902."

As noted above, the goal of all emergency medical care is to provide the best possible care, optimizing the patient's chances of survival and complete recovery. This goal holds true for all medical and trauma-related emergencies. One of the greatest challenges in EMS is to assure excellent patient care in spite of the fact that there are often several hand-offs of a patient from one set of care providers to another as he passes through the system.

TRANSITION OF CARE

Whenever care of a patient passes from one provider to another, a **transition of care** takes place. In such a transition, both the provider handing over care of the patient and the provider assuming that care share the responsibility of assuring that the patient's care is not compromised because of the transition. To assure a proper transition, all relevant aspects of patient history, assessment, reassessment, treatment, and response to treatment must be conveyed from one provider to the next through oral communication and written documentation.

TIERED EMS SYSTEMS

Transition of care is a common occurrence in the fire service because many fire departments provide EMS as part of a **tiered response system.** A tiered EMS system means that multiple units and, possibly, multiple agencies respond to emergency calls. Most tiered systems also include care providers with various levels of training. This assures that the appropriate resources can be directed to patients depending on their conditions. Examples of responses in tiered systems would include the following:

◆ An engine company staffed by EMTs arrives first on scene. The engine company EMTs initiate care until the fire department paramedic unit reaches the scene. When a non-fire department ambulance service arrives, the patient is then transported by the ambulance service either with the fire department paramedics on board or—if the patient is stable—with care having been turned over to the ambulance's EMT crew.

- A local fire department engine company staffed by EMTs responds to an emergency scene. They provide care until a mutual-aid fire department paramedic ambulance arrives to assume patient care during transportation.

- The rescue unit of a rural volunteer fire department responds to an accident scene. That unit, staffed by Certified First Responders, begins patient care until the neighboring village's ambulance corps, staffed by EMTs, arrives on the scene. The EMTs assume care and initiate transport. En route to the hospital, the ambulance meets with the county sheriff's paramedic unit. A paramedic from the unit gets on board the ambulance and takes over patient care during transport to the hospital.

- A fire department dispatches its nearest unit (truck or engine company), staffed by EMTs, and the fire department ambulance, staffed by paramedics, to all calls. If the EMTs arrive first, they assess the patient and begin care. When the firefighter paramedics arrive, care of the patient is turned over to them.

Transitions such as these are daily occurrences in EMS systems. In these systems, specific policies should be in place to assure smooth patient hand-offs. If you are an EMT in such a system, it is your professional responsibility to know these policies and to carry them out in order to provide a proper transition of care.

TRANSITION OF CARE PROCEDURES

Exactly what occurs during a transition of care will depend on both the type of EMS system in which you work and the type of illness or injury you encounter. Some hand-offs will be very simple—for example, a child who cuts his lower leg sliding into second base but sustains no other injuries. Other hand-offs will be more complicated—for example, the patient stung by a bee who has a life-threatening allergic reaction that requires the first responding EMT to assist in administering the patient's Epi-Pen®.

As a rule, the more seriously ill or injured the patient is, the more difficult the assessment, the more extensive the treatment interventions, and the more complicated the transition of care. In addition, the sicker the patient is, the more important it is that the transition of care takes place smoothly. In cases of seriously ill or injured patients, conveying an accurate history, assessment, and description of the patient's response to treatment to the EMS personnel assuming care takes on added importance. This is true because those personnel need the information not only for their care of the patient but also because they will eventually pass that information along to emergency department personnel. The steps described below can help you to assure a good transition of care.

When you are the initial EMT on the scene, you should prepare to turn care over to another unit by doing the following:

- *Conduct a careful scene size-up.* You should advise in-coming units by radio of any unique circumstances or hazards. Request additional resources if they are required.

- *Conduct an initial assessment of the patient.* A key part of this assessment will be a determination of patient priority.

- *Initiate appropriate treatment.*

- *Provide any in-coming units with a brief radio report about the patient.* A concise radio report can assist in-coming units in preparing needed equipment. It is also the first step in passing along patient information during a transition of care. In some EMS systems, the first unit on the scene may also have the authority to upgrade or downgrade the response of in-coming units based on its initial patient assessment as was the case in the On Scene above.

Another sample report might be transmitted as follows: "Engine 6 to Medic Ambulance 2. We have a 31-year-old male with a laceration to his anterior leg. The bleeding is minor and is controlled with a bandage. No other visible injuries. You may downgrade your response to non-emergency priority."

- *Gather pertinent information from the patient, family members, or bystanders.* Such information might include prescription medications the patient is taking, any drug allergies, and any relevant past medical history.

- *Briefly document the information you gather.* Include as much of the following data as possible:

  —Patient's name

  —Patient's age

  —Chief complaint

  —Initial vital signs

  —Patient medications and allergies to drugs or other substances

  —Patient's pertinent past medical history

  —Treatment rendered

  If time allows:

  —Subsequent vital signs

  —Patient's response to treatment

Written documentation will save time for the crew members to whom you transfer care. It will also reduce the risk of oral miscommunication during the patient hand-off. Ideally, a standardized form that generates multiple copies will be used for this documentation (Figure 9-1). To reduce the risk of miscommunication, use common terminology and accepted abbreviations when preparing patient reports.

- *Explain to the patient that other EMS personnel will be arriving on the scene and that a transition of care will be taking place.*

- *Deliver an oral report and written documentation to the EMS personnel assuming care.*

As an EMT who is assuming patient care from another EMS provider you should do the following:

- *Allow the initial provider to complete any procedure in progress such as application of splints, etc.*

- *Introduce yourself to the patient.*

- *Listen carefully to the oral report given by the EMS personnel who arrived on the scene first.*

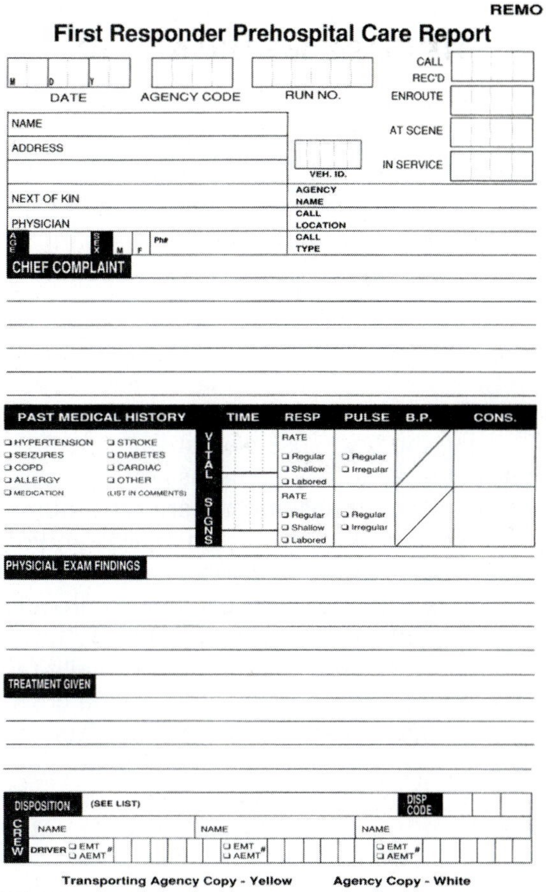

Figure 9-1 A standardized form for documenting patient information that is used during transition of care in one regional EMS organization.

Ask for clarification of any unclear statements.

- *Obtain a copy of the initial unit's documentation and quickly review it.*

- *Briefly assess the patient to make sure the oral report and written documentation you receive appear consistent with your observations.* Discuss with the other provider any of your observations that differ from what was reported to you.

As the EMT who assumes responsibility for a patient's care, you must be "comfortable" with accepting the transition of care from another provider. If you feel that you and your unit will need additional assistance with patient care, say so. For example, with a high priority, unstable patient, it may be necessary to request that the first-arriving EMS crew accompany you and the patient to the hospital.

A similar case might occur in a tiered EMS system where an ALS paramedic unit performs an assessment and determines that the patient does not require ALS care. The paramedics then transfer the patient's care to an EMT crew. If the EMTs

nevertheless feel that the patient's condition warrants continued ALS monitoring or care or if they feel uncomfortable caring for the patient, they should request that a paramedic ride in with the patient and the EMT crew.

COMPANY OFFICER'S NOTES

The goal of any EMS system is to provide the best possible patient care. To meet that goal, it may be necessary at times to vary the normal transition of care procedures in your system. Tactical circumstances and/or considerations of the patient's condition are common reasons for such changes in procedure. Most often, these changes involve having personnel from units that do not normally take part in patient transport accompany the crew transporting a patient to the hospital. For example, if a patient is potentially or clearly unstable, additional personnel might ride with the transporting crew to facilitate better patient care. Other cases in which additional personnel might be required are those of multiple-trauma patients whose airways need constant suctioning or those in which CPR is in progress.

When making decisions about whether to assign additional personnel to assist a patient, remember that it is better to place a first-responding unit temporarily out of service because its personnel are needed than it is to allow a patient's care to be compromised.

PEDIATRIC NOTE

It is not unusual for injured and ill children to rapidly form strong emotional bonds with an EMS provider whom they feel they can trust during an emergency situation. In such a circumstance, it may be necessary to have that "special" provider accompany the patient to the hospital, even if the provider belongs to a unit that would normally transfer care to a transporting unit. Providing this continuity of psychological support may prevent the child from becoming severely upset at an already highly stressful time.

SPECIAL CIRCUMSTANCES IN TRANSITION OF CARE

There are certain circumstances in which transition of care procedures will not proceed in the ways discussed above. Two of these special circumstances are described below.

Bystander Care

It is not unusual for EMTs to arrive at a scene to find that some level of care is being provided by a citizen. In EMS systems with Emergency Medical Dispatchers (EMDs), the care being provided by family members or bystanders may be based on *pre-arrival instructions*. Pre-arrival instructions are specific, step-by-step directions given to a caller by an EMD for providing first aid prior to an EMS unit's arrival on scene. These instructions may include steps to control bleeding, to assure an open airway, or to assist in childbirth.

In general, bystanders carrying out EMD-directed care will readily allow you to assume patient care upon your arrival. It is appropriate, however, to ask the family member or bystander what response the patient has had to the treatment advised by the EMD over the phone.

At other times, the treatment of a patient by family members or bystanders that is in progress upon your arrival on scene may not be medically appropriate or may even be harmful. In such situations, take immediate control of the situation as part of the scene size-up. You must halt the improper treatment and begin appropriate care. A common situation of this type occurs when bystanders try to remove a patient from the wreckage of a motor vehicle crash without concern for stabilizing the patient's cervical spine.

On occasion, EMTs arrive at a scene to find a medically trained bystander providing patient care. Physicians, nurses, off-duty EMTs, and other health care professionals often render assistance out of a sense of ethical and professional duty. Sometimes interactions between the EMT and the bystander health care professional can be awkward. There are specific steps that the EMT can take to help assure a smooth transition of care in these situations:

◆ Introduce yourself and give your affiliation and your level of training—"Hello, I'm Stan. I'm an EMT with the fire department."

◆ If the bystander provider does not identify himself, ask his name and determine his level of training. Ask to see some identification if it seems appropriate.

◆ Obtain information about the bystander's findings upon his arrival, the treatment he has given, and the patient's response to treatment.

In some situations, the medically trained bystander care provider may be reluctant to completely transfer the patient's care to you. This tends to be more common when the bystander is a physician, nurse practitioner, physician's assistant, or other more highly trained provider. In some circumstances, as with unstable patients, it may be appropriate for the bystander to continue to assist in patient care and even to accompany the patient to the hospital with the transporting unit.

In fact, the health care professional may be obligated to continue to provide care. By law, such professionals cannot hand over care to EMS personnel with a lower level of training. This could be considered abandonment of the patient (see Chapter 4, "Medical/Legal Issues"). Remember, however, that at no time should you allow a bystander health care professional, regardless of level of training, to provide care that is harmful or inappropriate.

Most EMS systems have specific policies and protocols in place that govern on-scene interactions with bystander health care professionals. As long as both the EMT and the bystander professional keep the patient's well-being as their primary goal, these on-scene interactions should proceed without difficulty.

Aviation Crews

Another special transition of patient care occurs when a helicopter is dispatched to a scene to transport a patient. In this setting, which usually involves a seriously injured trauma patient, conditions at the scene may hamper the oral communication that is so important to a good transition of care. Noise from hydraulic rescue tools and helicopter rotors can easily drown out the EMT's attempt to give an oral report to the helicopter crew (Figure 9-2).

In these conditions, pass on to the flight crew, if at all possible, a brief written report of your patient assessment, the patient's vital signs, your treatment, and the patient's response to the treatment. The oral report to the flight crew should be brief and extremely focused, reinforcing the points covered in the brief written report. (You will learn more about operations involving helicopters in Chapter 25, "Emergency Vehicle Operations," and Chapter 28, "EMS Special Operations.")

Figure 9-2 When transition of patient care is to a helicopter crew, be aware that aircraft noise can interfere with communication of patient information.

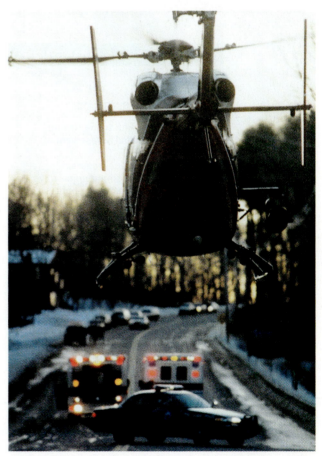

Chapter Review

Because many firefighter EMTs operate as part of a tiered EMS system, transitions of patient care from one EMS provider to another are common prehospital occurrences. When such hand-offs do take place, it is essential that accurate and relevant information about the patient and his condition be passed from one provider to the next to assure the best possible care.

REVIEWING KEY CONCEPTS

1. Define *transition of care.*

2. Describe how a tiered response system works in EMS.

3. List the steps that an EMT who is turning care of a patient over to another unit should perform.

4. List the steps that an EMT who is assuming care of a patient from another unit should perform.

5. Describe some of the special considerations in the transition of care when a helicopter is the transporting vehicle.

AT A GLANCE

TRANSITION OF CARE PROCEDURES

EMT TRANSFERRING CARE	EMT ASSUMING CARE
• Conduct a careful scene size-up. • Conduct an initial assessment of the patient. • Initiate appropriate treatment. • Provide any in-coming units with a brief radio report about the patient. • Gather pertinent information from the patient, family members, or bystanders. • Briefly document the information you gather. • Explain to the patient that other EMS personnel will be arriving on the scene and that a transition of care will be taking place. • Deliver an oral report and written documentation to the EMS personnel assuming care.	• Allow the initial provider to complete any procedure in progress such as application of splints, etc. • Introduce yourself to the patient. • Listen carefully to the oral report given by the EMS personnel who arrived on the scene first. • Obtain a copy of the initial unit's documentation and quickly review it. • Briefly assess the patient to make sure the oral report and written documentation you receive appear consistent with your observations.

Lifting and Moving Patients

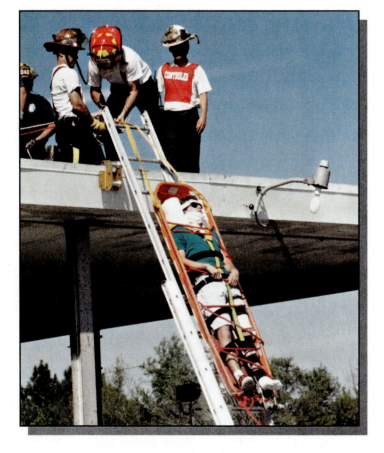

*A*s an EMT, you are responsible for assessing a patient and seeing that he receives appropriate care. If the scene in which you find the patient is unsafe, you may, however, have to move him before providing a complete assessment. Also, the definitive care that the patient needs will only be available at a hospital, which means he must be moved to an ambulance and transported. You must therefore be prepared to lift and move patients as part of your job. You must also be prepared so that you can carry out these tasks safely, without injuring yourself or doing further harm to the patient.

At the completion of this chapter, the EMT-Basic student should be able to meet the following objectives:

Knowledge and Understanding

1. Define body mechanics. (p. 264)
2. Discuss the guidelines and safety precautions that need to be followed when lifting a patient. (pp. 264–265)
3. Describe the safe lifting of cots and stretchers. (pp. 264–265)
4. Describe the guidelines and safety precautions for carrying patients and/or equipment. (p. 266)
5. Discuss one-handed carrying techniques. (p. 266)
6. Describe correct and safe carrying procedures on stairs. (p. 266)
7. State the guidelines for safe reaching and their application. (pp. 266–267)
8. Describe correct techniques for log rolls. (pp. 267–268)
9. State the guidelines for pushing and pulling. (pp. 266–267)
10. Discuss the general considerations of moving patients. (pp. 268–276)
11. State three situations that may require the use of an emergency move. (p. 268)
12. Identify the following patient carrying devices:
    —wheeled ambulance stretcher (pp. 276–277)
    —portable ambulance stretcher (pp. 277, 279)
    —stair chair (pp. 279–280)
    —scoop stretcher (p. 280)
    —long spine board (p. 280)
    —basket stretcher (p. 281)
    —flexible stretcher (pp. 281–282)
13. Explain the rationale for properly lifting and moving patients. (pp. 263–264)

Skills

1. Working with a partner, prepare each of the following devices for use, transfer a patient to the device, properly position the patient on the device, move the device to the ambulance, and load the patient into the ambulance:
    —wheeled ambulance stretcher
    —portable ambulance stretcher
    —stair chair
    —scoop stretcher
    —long spine board
    —basket stretcher
    —flexible stretcher
2. Working with a partner, the EMT-Basic will demonstrate techniques for the transfer of a patient from an ambulance stretcher to a hospital stretcher.

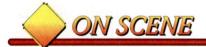

ON SCENE

DISPATCH: *AMBULANCE 10 AND ENGINE 10. PROCEED TO 73 PALMER ROAD, PRIORITY 1, SUBJECT FALLEN. TIME OUT IS 2330.*

As you are en route to the scene on this late summer night, dispatch contacts you with more details about the call. The subject is an elderly male who has fallen in the bathroom and cannot stand. He is conscious and alert.

You arrive at the Palmer Road address, a single-family house, about 5 minutes after receiving the call. The scene appears secure, so you and your partner approach the house. At the front door, an elderly woman greets you and gives her name as Mrs. Casivant. She says that her husband started shouting for help a few minutes after he went to the toilet.

You proceed through the house to a small bathroom at its rear. In the bathroom, you find an elderly male patient lying on his left side, next to the toilet. Mr. Casivant is conscious and alert. He complains of severe pain in his lower back and left hip. Assessment of his vital signs indicates the following: pulse—130, strong and regular; respirations—28; blood pressure—168/98; skin—warm and dry. Your physical exam reveals

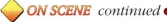

an 82-year-old male with deformity of the left hip and tenderness of the lower back. The patient's left hip is flexed and his knee bent. The findings of the physical exam are otherwise unremarkable.

The bathroom is located at the end of a long, narrow hallway. Two 90-degree turns must be negotiated to get to the only door leading out of the home. You complete your assessment of Mr. Casivant and decide to use a long spine board to move him safely. Since the patient's leg is flexed and cannot be straightened without causing additional pain, you decide that a pillow is needed to stabilize the leg. You send a firefighter to the ambulance to get the appropriate equipment.

After properly immobilizing Mr. Casivant to a long spine board and stabilizing the injured leg with a pillow splint, you request the help of two additional firefighters from the engine company. Under your direction, Mr. Casivant is moved safely down the narrow hallway, around the two sharp turns and down the front steps of the home. The ambulance stretcher has been set up outside the front door and the patient is transferred to it. After loading the stretcher into the ambulance and securing it properly, you transport Mr. Casivant to the hospital while performing an ongoing assessment.

Lifting and moving of patients are parts of almost every call you will answer as an EMT. You will also have to **"package"** patients, or prepare them so they can be transported safely. You must learn how to carry out these tasks efficiently and *safely*. Poorly planned or poorly executed lifting, moving, and packaging can lead to unwanted results. These include injuries to the patient or to fire and EMS personnel and lawsuits on behalf of the injured parties against the fire or EMS agency and its personnel. This chapter will outline basic information you need to know to lift, move, and package patients properly.

PLANNING FOR LIFTING AND MOVING

Lifting and moving a patient is serious business. When you are performing these tasks, the patient is particularly vulnerable. A patient restrained in a carrying device will probably be unable to protect himself if the device is dropped or banged against a wall. Nationally, lawsuits against emergency care providers alleging injuries from improper patient packaging and transport are second in number only to those arising from motor vehicle crashes. In addition, far too many EMS personnel

suffer career-ending injuries while attempting to move patients. The total costs to the EMS community of workman's compensation, disability payments, and litigation associated with such injuries are staggering.

There are specific techniques to follow when lifting patients in different situations or using different types of patient-carrying equipment. These will be discussed later in the chapter. However, there are guidelines you should keep in mind for any situation that involves the lifting and moving of patients.

1. **Devise the plan before packaging the patient.** Nothing is more frustrating than packaging a patient with a specific device and beginning the move, only to discover that you cannot negotiate a narrow turn in a hallway with that device. Make your decisions based on the patient's medical needs and the logistics of removing him to the ambulance. Take a moment to devise a logical plan for extracting the patient, packaging him, and then moving him safely to the ambulance.

2. **Summon adequate help before moving the patient.** If the patient is large or if extricating him will be difficult or complicated, make sure that you have enough help before attempting to move him. Two EMTs who

attempt to package and move a 400-hundred-pound (181 kg) patient out of a small bathroom and down a set of narrow stairs are asking for trouble. If the patient were to be dropped and injured, the EMTs' behavior would likely be viewed as grossly negligent. If you need more manpower or equipment, summon additional fire companies immediately after your initial scene size-up.

3. **Perform your initial assessment and begin appropriate medical care before packaging the patient.** Patients should receive appropriate medical care *before* being packaged for transport. Whether the patient should receive *immediate life support* only, or *all appropriate care* before packaging, is a medical decision that must be based on the patient's condition. The exception to this rule about assessing and treating the patient before packaging him is when the patient is found in a situation hazardous either to himself or to his rescuers—when there is the threat of toxic gases or a possible explosion, for example. These situations will be discussed in detail later in this chapter.

BODY MECHANICS AND LIFTING AND MOVING

The science of physics deals with properties of physical bodies in motion. The principles of physics govern what happens to your body as you lift and move patients. **Body mechanics** refers to the application of these principles to ensure safe and efficient lifting and moving. Whenever you must lift or move a patient or a piece of equipment, have the following basics of body mechanics in mind:

◆ *Keep the weight of the object to be lifted as close to your body as possible.* The farther the weight is away from your body, the greater the strain that will be placed on your lower back.

◆ *Keep your back straight, using the muscles of your legs, hips, and buttocks to do the lifting.* The muscles of the lower back are almost always weaker than those of the thigh and lower legs.

◆ *Make sure your feet are properly positioned, firmly planted, and secure before lifting or moving the patient.* While on duty, use appropriate safety footwear with non-slip soles.

◆ *Never twist or attempt to make other moves while lifting.* Twisting and turning while lifting are major causes of injury.

◆ *Be realistic in how much weight you can safely lift.* Summon more help, if needed, to lift the patient safely. If the patient is very heavy, consider whether he can be placed safely on a rolling stretcher instead of being carried.

◆ *Communicate well and often with your partners.* Do this both before and during the move. This practice will help assure that all members of the crew are working together. If you become tired during a move, tell your partners and stop to rest. The patient can usually be lowered to the ground, if necessary, to give carriers a momentary rest.

◆ *Avoid sudden moves, particularly those that twist your back or limbs.* Jerking and twisting movements are more likely to cause injuries to EMTs than smooth movements are.

◆ *Never hyperextend the back.* This typically occurs when the EMT leans backward from the waist while lifting or lowering the weight. Because the muscles of the lower back tend to be weak, such poor technique is the source of many occupational injuries.

The Power Lift and Power Grip

Two useful techniques have been developed to help the rescuer move a patient while observing the principles described above.

The **power lift** was first developed by weight lifters and is known to them as the dead lift (Figure 10-1A to C). When lifting, get as close to the object to be lifted as possible. Straddle it and squat, with your feet planted firmly and comfortably apart. This will permit maximum distribution of the weight, which should be shifted to the heels and arches of the feet. Keep your back locked-in. Place your hands a comfortable dis-

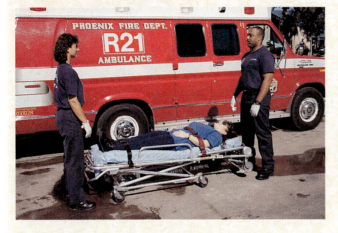

Figure 10-1A Get in position as close to the object as possible. Plant your feet firmly, about shoulder width apart, turned slightly outward.

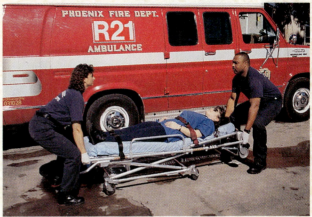

Figure 10-1B Squat, keeping the back locked-in and the feet flat. Hands should be a comfortable distance apart on the object to be lifted.

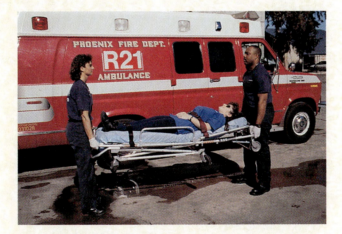

Figure 10-1C Lift with the arms locked, raising the upper body by extending the back. The back should remained locked in. Never bend from the waist when lifting.

tance apart on the object to be lifted. Lift with your arms locked, raising your upper body by extending your back. Never bend from the waist when lifting.

The **power grip** helps to ensure that your hands work efficiently and that an object does not slip as you lift it (Figure 10-2). Curve your fingers *under* the device being lifted. Grip the object with your hands about 10 to 12 inches (200-300 mm) apart. Use as much of the surface area of your fingers and palms as possible. All of your fingers should be bent at the same angle. Neither the device nor your hands should be slippery or wet. Lift with both arms in unison.

Special Lifting and Carrying Considerations

There are special techniques that you should apply when lifting or moving patients or equipment in certain circumstances.

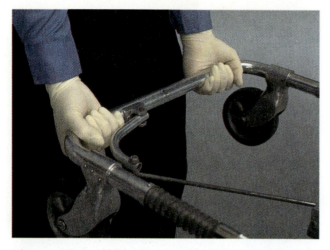

Figure 10-2 With the power grip, curl the fingers *under* the device being lifted. Grip the object a comfortable distance apart, using as much of the surface area of the fingers and palms as possible. Bend the fingers at the same angle.

One-Handed Carrying Techniques

When four or more rescuers are used to carry a backboard or a stretcher, they may chose to walk facing the same direction, each using *one hand* to carry the device (Figure 10-3). Also, you may at times have to carry equipment with one hand (Figure 10-4). When carrying with one hand, remember to do the following:

◆ *Initially lift and then lower the device with both hands,* using proper lifting and lowering technique.

Figure 10-3 When using one hand technique in carrying an object, maintain an erect posture and avoid leaning to one side.

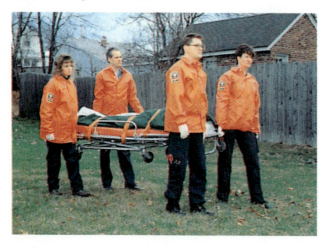

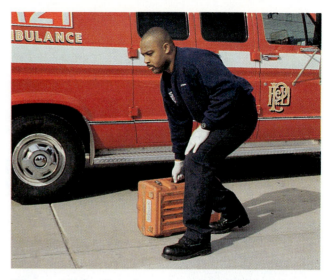

Figure 10-4 Get close to an object that is to be lifted to reduce the distance through which it must be moved. Reposition yourself if necessary before lifting.

◆ *Have someone take the lead during the lift,* coordinating it by saying, "One, two, three, lift!"

◆ *Avoid leaning to either side,* in an attempt to compensate for the use of only one extremity.

Carrying Techniques on Stairs

Firefighter-EMTs frequently need to move patients up or down flights of stairs. In such cases, whenever it is possible and medically appropriate, you should use the special carrying device called a **stair chair** instead of a stretcher or backboard for such moves. As in all lifting situations, keep your back *straight* and bend with your knees, *not* your lower back. Remember to keep your arms (and thus the weight of the load) as close to the vertical axis of your body as possible. Whenever possible, use a spotter positioned behind the firefighter who is walking backwards up or down the stairs (Figure 10-5). The spotter can help guide the move and count out the number of steps to be negotiated. Potential obstacles or hazards, such as loose throw rugs, should be moved from the path before beginning the move.

Reaching and Pulling Techniques

Although carrying of heavy loads accounts for many line-of-duty injuries, improper *reaching* or

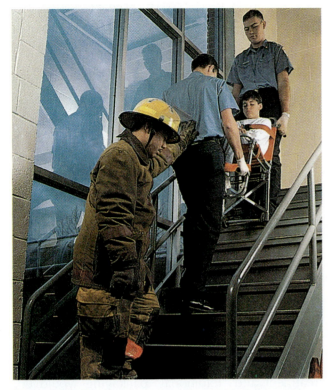

Figure 10-5 Position a spotter behind the rescuer walking backwards up or down stairs with a patient-carrying device to help to guide the move.

pulling can also cause serious damage to joints and muscles.

Follow these guidelines when reaching for an object:

- *Keep your back locked-in.*
- *Avoid twisting from side to side while reaching.*
- *When reaching above the level of your shoulders, never hyperextend your back.*
- *Avoid reaching for an object more than 15–20 inches (380–500 mm) away from you.* Keep the weight as close to the vertical axis of your body as possible. If necessary, move closer to the object before reaching.
- *Avoid prolonged reaching under strenuous conditions.*

Follow these guidelines for pushing/pulling an object:

- *Push rather than pull an object whenever possible.*
- *Use the weight of your whole upper body, not just your arms, when pushing.* Push using the

area between the waist and the shoulders, so as to minimize stress to the lower back.

- *Keep your back locked-in.*
- *Keep your elbows bent and your arms close to your sides as you push.*
- *Keep the weight close to your body as you push.* Push and then, if necessary, move closer to the object before pushing again.
- *Never bend over from a standing position to push or pull an object on the ground.* Instead, kneel in front of it and then push or pull.
- *Avoid pushing or pulling on objects that are overhead.*

Log-Rolling Techniques

A special technique that involves both reaching and pulling is the log roll. It is a maneuver commonly used to move a patient onto or off a sheet or backboard (Figure 10-6). With it, three or four rescuers usually work as a team to minimize movement of the patient's spine. When log rolling a patient, a rescuer should do the following:

- Keep the back as straight as possible.
- Lean over the patient from the hips, not from the waist.
- Use the arms and shoulders to roll the patient.
- Avoid using the lower back as a fulcrum.

Figure 10-6 When log-rolling a patient, keep the back as straight as possible and lean over the patient from the hips, using the arms and shoulders to roll the patient.

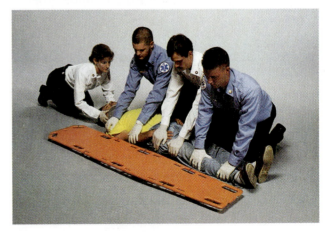

The log roll is one of several techniques for safely moving a patient with a suspected spinal injury. Important general considerations of such moves are discussed below.

PATIENT SAFETY CONSIDERATIONS

As noted above, when EMTs lift and move patients they should avoid injuring themselves. However, they must also avoid injuring the patient or making existing injuries worse. Perhaps the most difficult situations involving patient moves you will face are cases in which the patient has an actual or suspected neck or spine injury. Moving the patient improperly in such a case can lead to permanent injury or even death.

Normally, such patients should be fully immobilized and completely packaged before they are moved. (The techniques for immobilizing and packaging such patients are discussed in Chapter 22, "Head and Spine Injuries.") However, there are times when safety considerations require that you move a patient before he is completely immobilized. The circumstances of such moves are discussed below. Whenever circumstances call for a patient to be moved before he is completely immobilized, you should ensure that the following three sections of the patient's body move as a unit: the *head,* the *shoulder girdle,* and the *pelvic girdle.* If an EMT is assigned to each of these three locations, the patient with a suspected neck or spine injury can be safely evacuated from a wide variety of locations, including vehicles (such as in rapid extrication, discussed below), out of stair wells, or off the ground.

Types of Patient Moves

As a general rule, patients should be immobilized (when appropriate) and packaged before they are moved. Patients should be moved before they are fully immobilized and packaged only under the following conditions:

◆ There is an immediate hazard to the patient or the rescuers

◆ The patient has a medical condition requiring emergency care and immediate transportation.

The types of patient moves fall into three categories.

An **emergency move** is called for when there is an immediate danger to the patient—or rescuers—if he is not moved. Circumstances that would call for an emergency move include the following:

◆ Fire or the imminent danger of fire

◆ Explosives or other hazardous materials at the scene

◆ Other immediate environmental hazards (such as high speed traffic that cannot be diverted)

◆ The patient's position or location restricts access to other more seriously injured patients

◆ The patient's position or location prevents you from providing life-saving emergency care

An **urgent move** is indicated when the patient's condition is so unstable that continued treatment and "traditional" packaging would endanger the patient's chances of survival. Such patients might include unstable trauma patients in shock or those with inadequate breathing due to chest injuries. Such cases require a rapid *risk–benefit analysis.* If the potential *benefits* of moving the patient prior to complete immobilization and packaging *outweigh* the potential *risks* of immediate transportation, then an urgent move is medically justified.

A **non-urgent move** is indicated for the vast majority of patients treated by EMTs. In such patients, no immediate life-threat is present. All appropriate medical care can be provided and the patient properly secured to a stretcher, stair chair, or similar device before being moved.

Emergency Moves

When you use an emergency move, you do not have time to employ an interim immobilization device like a spine board. Thus, it is almost impossible to carry out an emergency move without aggravating an existing spinal injury. For this reason, the patient—or rescuer—*must* be in immediate danger before an emergency move is used. Remember, the convenience of the EMT or others is *never* a justification for using an emergency move.

You can take steps to give the patient's spine as much protection as possible when carrying out an emergency move. For example, make every effort to move the patient in the direction of the *long axis* of his body (the line running down the center of the body from the top of the head and along the spine). Always try to move the patient's head, shoulder girdle, and pelvic girdle as a unit.

Examples of emergency moves include various drags, carries, and assists (Figures 10-7 and 10-8). Among these are the blanket drag, the clothes drag, the foot drag, the incline drag, the firefighter's carry, and variations on these moves. Practice these techniques with other members of your crew *before* they are needed.

Urgent Moves

If the patient's condition is so unstable that taking time for full immobilization and packaging would endanger the patient's survival, an urgent move is appropriate. Unlike the emergency move, an urgent move permits some precautions to prevent spinal injury.

Rapid Extrication
One of the most common urgent moves is called **rapid extrication.** It is used to remove sitting patients from vehicles when there is not enough time to immobilize the patient to a short spine board or a vest-type extrication device. Using those devices, it often can take 10 minutes or more to remove a patient with a suspected spinal injury from a vehicle, which is acceptable if the patient's injuries are not life-threatening. Using rapid extrication techniques, removal of the patient can be done in 1 to 2 minutes. However, use of this technique poses a greater risk of damage to the spine. Perform a quick risk–benefit analysis to determine if the threat to the patient is great enough to outweigh the possible damage that rapid extrication may cause.

There are, of course, many variations of this technique, but the basic principles are always the same. At least three EMTs are required for this move. A general description of the process follows. Remember that it must be modified depending upon the type of vehicle, extent of crash damage, location of the patient, etc.

1. EMT #1 gains access to the patient and applies manual stabilization (*not* traction) of the patient's head, either from behind or from the side of the patient, placing the head in a neutral, in-line position. This ensures an open airway and permits the application of a rigid cervical collar. Since EMT #1 is responsible for protecting the patient's cervical spine, he usually functions as the team leader.

2. EMT #2 sizes and applies a rigid extrication collar. EMT #2 is then responsible for stabilizing the patient's shoulder girdle and chest during the move.

3. EMT #3 places a long backboard near the vehicle's door. He then frees the patient's lower extremities (if necessary) and then grasps the pelvic girdle. EMT #3 is responsible for ensuring that the pelvis moves in alignment with the shoulders and the head and for keeping the long axis of the patient's body as straight as possible.

4. Working together, the three EMTs slowly rotate the patient on the seat and lower him to the seat. Depending upon the vehicle and the amount of access available to the EMTs, this may require several "mini-rotations" of the patient. The EMTs may also have to switch positions in order to keep the patient's spine in alignment. The patient may be rotated so that either his feet or his back are at the vehicle's open doorway; the position will depend upon the size of the patient compartment and the amount of damage it received in the crash.

5. The end of the backboard is placed on the seat next to the patient and he is maneuvered onto it in short, coordinated moves.

6. The board is removed from the vehicle and the patient is properly immobilized to it.

The importance of excellent communication among the three EMTs to assure that the patient's head, chest, and pelvis move as a unit cannot be overemphasized. (The rapid extrication procedure is illustrated in Chapter 22, "Head and Spine Injuries.")

Emergency Moves—One-Rescuer Drags

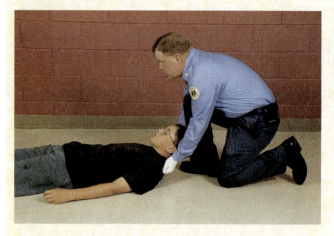

Figure 10-7A. With the **clothes drag,** as with all emergency moves, pull in the direction of the long axis of the patient's body. Do not pull sideways or twist the patient's trunk.

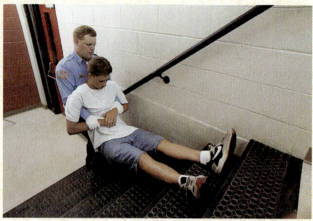

Figure 10-7B With the **incline drag,** always move the patient head first on the incline.

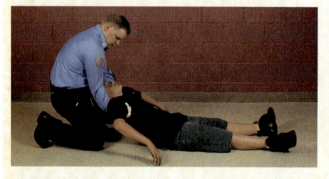

Figure 10-7C Grip under the patient's armpits with the **shoulder drag** and be careful not to bump his head.

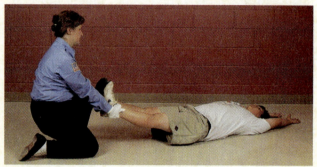

Figure 10-7D With the **foot drag,** grip the patient's ankles and be very careful not to bump his head.

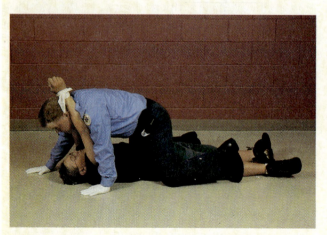

Figure 10-7E With the **fireman's drag,** tie the patient's wrists together. Straddle the patient and pass your head through his bound wrists, then raise your body and crawl on your hands and knees.

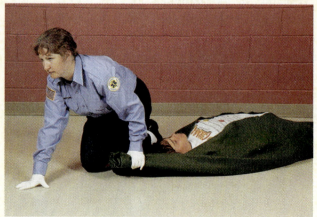

Figure 10-7F With the **blanket drag,** arrange a blanket along the side of the patient and bunch the blanket up against the patient. Roll the patient toward your knees and move the blanket material under him. Gently roll the patient back down onto the blanket and drag him by grasping the blanket.

Emergency Moves—One Rescuer Assists and Carries

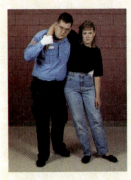

Figure 10-8A For the **one-rescuer assist,** place the patient's arm around your neck, grasping that hand in yours. Place your other hand around the patient's waist. Help the patient walk to safety.

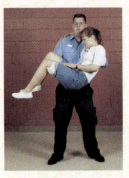

Figure 10-8B For the **cradle carry,** place one of your arms across the patient's back with your hand under the patient's arm. Place the other hand behind the patient's knees and lift, remembering principles of body mechanics as you lift. If conscious, the patient should place her near arm around your neck.

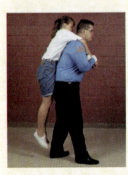

Figure 10-8C For the **pack strap carry,** turn your back to a standing patient and bring the patient's arms over your shoulders, crossing them over your chest. Keep the patient's arms as straight as possible so that her armpits are over your shoulders. Grasp the patient's wrists, bend, and pull the patient onto your back.

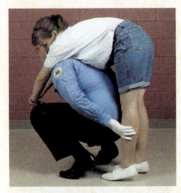

Figure 10-8D For the **piggy back carry,** turn your back to a standing patient and bring the patient's arms over your shoulders, crossing them over your chest. Bend and lift the patient. While the patient holds on with her arms, crouch and grasp each thigh. Then lift her onto your back and pass your forearms under her thighs and grasp her wrists.

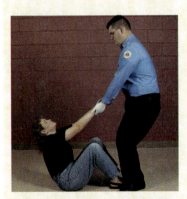

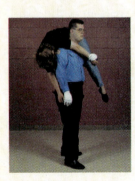

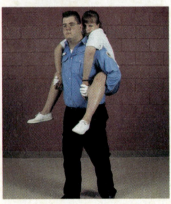

Figure 10-8E For the **fireman's carry,** place the patient's feet against yours, grasp her wrists, and pull her towards you. Bend at the waist and flex your knees. Duck and pull her across your shoulders, keeping hold of one wrist. Use your free arm to reach between her legs and grasp her thigh, transferring the patient's weight onto your shoulders. Stand up, shifting your grip from the patient's thigh to her wrist.

Non-Urgent Moves

The vast majority of patients treated by the EMT will qualify for a non-urgent move. When there is no immediate threat to life, complete the assessment and any needed on-scene treatment. Only then should you move the patient from the location in which he was found by using an appropriate patient-carrying device. In non-urgent moves, the priorities are as follows:

◆ To permit continued medical treatment, as appropriate

◆ To protect the patient from aggravation of his injuries or from any additional injury

◆ To minimize the possibility of injury to a rescuer while moving the patient

Take time to plan the move correctly. Select an appropriate patient-carrying device (see below). Choose an appropriate non-urgent move and coordinate it properly. Position the patient properly on the device. Perform a quick assessment of the route you will follow with the device. Remove any obstacles (such as throw rugs and toys) from your path. Assure adequate lighting for areas through which you will move, if possible.

While there are many non-urgent move techniques, the direct ground lift, the extremity lift, and the supine patient transfer are among the most commonly used.

The **direct ground lift** is useful for supine patients in whom no spinal injury is suspected and when two (or three) EMTs are available (Figure 10-9). The patient is essentially scooped up into the EMTs' arms. The EMTs kneel on one side of the patient. One EMT is responsible for the patient's head and back. The second EMT is responsible for the patient's buttocks and thighs (see the annotated illustration). On signal, the EMTs lift the patient to their knees, roll him to their chests, and then stand. (If a third rescuer is available, he should slide both arms under the patient's waist while the other EMTs move their arms up and down appropriately.)

The **extremity lift** is used when no spinal injury is suspected and two EMTs are available (Figure 10-10). With this technique, one EMT kneels behind the patient and reaches across the patient's chest to grasp his wrists. The second EMT, kneeling at the patient's feet, slips his hand under the patient's knees. On signal, the EMTs move to a crouching position, then stand.

When using either the direct ground lift or the extremity lift, be very careful to lift with your legs. Keep your lower back locked-in. Avoid using either of these techniques to carry an extremely heavy patient if more manpower and equipment are available for use of a different method.

To move a patient from a bed to the stretcher or from your stretcher to the hospital gurney, a **supine patient transfer** is necessary. This can be accomplished either with the draw sheet method or with a direct carry.

Using the **draw sheet method** the stretcher is positioned next to the patient's bed and adjusted to the bed's height. The stretcher's rails should be down and its straps unfastened. The bed sheet underneath the patient is loosened and gathered up at each side. Two EMTs position themselves on one side of the stretcher and two additional personnel position themselves on the side of the patient's bed. The four rescuers grasp the sheet on each side of the patient in a way that provides support to his head, chest, hips, and legs. The patient is then slid either onto the bed or onto the stretcher. When using this method, be sure not to "over reach" and strain your lower back, particularly if the patient is heavy. Both bed and stretcher should be locked into position before moving the patient.

Alternatively, two EMTs can place the stretcher between themselves and the bed, reach across the stretcher to grasp the loosened sheet, then pull the sheet and patient onto the stretcher (Figure 10-11).

When using the **direct carry method** (Figure 10-12), the ambulance stretcher is placed at a 90° angle to the patient's bed at either its head or its foot and adjusted to the height of the bed. Two or three EMTs then slide their arms under the patient's head, neck, chest, hips, and legs. On command, the patient is then "rolled" upward and curled against the EMTs' chests. The EMTs then pivot and carry the patient to the hospital stretcher. The procedure is then reversed to gently place the patient on the hospital bed. When

(text continues, page 276)

Direct Ground Lift

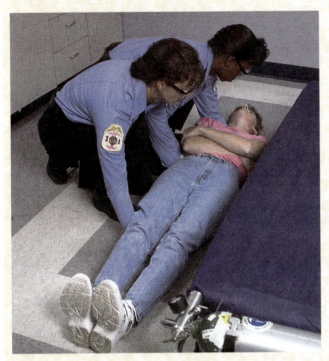

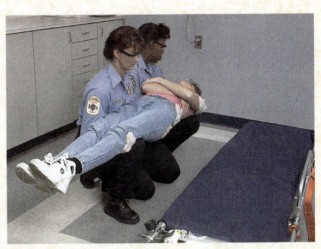

Figure 10-9B On a signal, the EMTs lift the patient to their knees.

Figure 10-9A Set stretcher at its lowest position on the side opposite the patient. EMTs drop to one knee facing patient, whose arms are crossed on chest if possible. The EMT at patient's head cradles the head and neck by sliding one arm under the patient's neck to grasp the shoulder and slides the other arm under the patient's lower back. The other EMT slides one arm under the patient just above the buttocks and slides the other arm under the patient's knees. If a third rescuer is available, he places both arms under the patient's waist while the other two EMTs slide their arms up to the mid back or down below the buttocks accordingly.

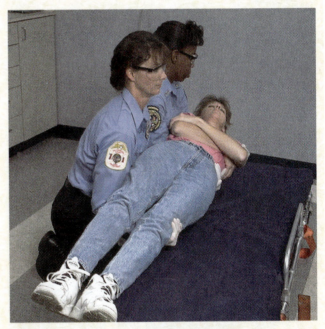

Figure 10-9C On a signal, they stand and carry the patient to the stretcher, drop to one knee, and roll forward to place the patient on the stretcher.

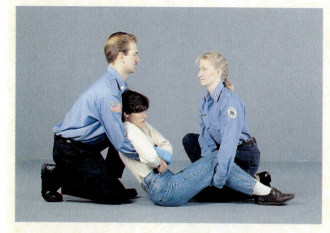

Figure 10-10A One EMT places a hand under each of the patient's arms and grasps her wrists. The other EMT slips hands under the patient's knees.

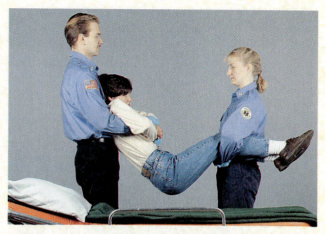

Figure 10-10B On signal, both EMTs move to a crouching and then a standing position.

SKILL SUMMARY
Draw Sheet Method

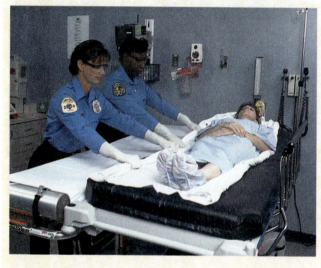

Figure 10-11A Loosen bottom sheet of bed and roll it toward patient on both sides. Place the stretcher with its rails lowered parallel to the bed and touching it. EMTs place themselves on one side of the stretcher, anchoring against the bed with their bodies.

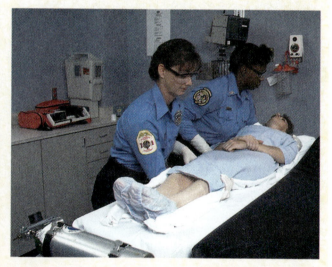

Figure 10-11B EMTs pull on sheet to move the patient to the side of the bed. They then reach under patient and sheet to provide support while drawing the patient onto the stretcher.

Note: This maneuver can also be performed with two EMTs on each side of the patient, cradling the patient in the sheet during transfer.

Direct Carry

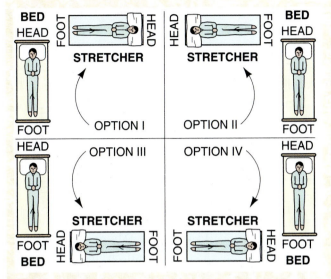

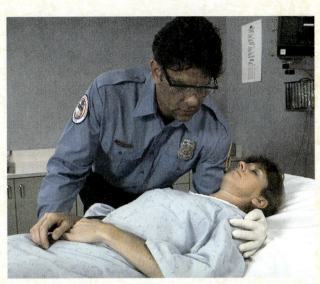

Figure 10-12A Lower rails on stretcher and unloosen straps. Place stretcher at foot of the bed at 90° angle to the bed. EMTs position themselves in the angle between the stretcher and the bed.

Figure 10-12B The EMT at the patient's head cradles the patient's head and neck by sliding an arm under the patient's neck to grasp a shoulder.

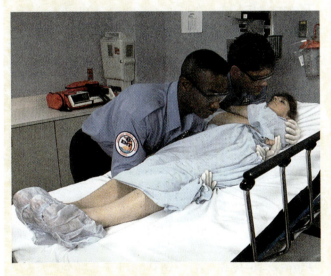

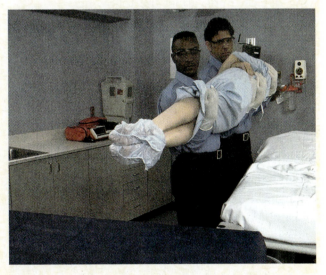

Figure 10-12C The EMT at the patient's feet slides a hand under the patient's hips and lifts slightly to allow the head-end EMT to slide his other arm under the patient's back. The foot-end EMT then slides his arms under the patient's hips and legs.

Figure 10-12D EMTs slide patient to the edge of the bed and bend toward the patient with their knees slightly bent. On signal, they lift and curl the patient to their chests and return to standing position. They rotate as a unit and place the patient gently onto the stretcher.

performing this maneuver, be careful to lock your lower back to prevent muscle strain.

Remember that using improper technique during any type of lift or move can cause a career-ending, life-long injury.

PATIENT-CARRYING EQUIPMENT

There are a number of devices that can be used to move a patient from the scene where he is found to the ambulance and from the ambulance to the hospital. The device you use will vary with the circumstances of the call. Among the factors that can affect your choice are the following: the condition of the patient, the working space available around the patient, the physical features of the building in which the patient is found, and the terrain over which the patient must be carried.

Whenever you are going to use a patient-carrying device, think about the following:

◆ *When carrying a patient, use the lightest device that will do the job safely.* A typical ambulance stretcher, loaded with a patient, oxygen cylinder, and cardiac monitor or automated external defibrillator can easily weigh in excess of 250 pounds (112 kg); a portable folding stretcher will usually do the job with much less weight. Remember that a typical firefighter-EMT will see thousands of patients in his career and that the movement of each one is a potential source of injury.

◆ *When it's feasible and medically appropriate to roll the patient instead of carrying him, don't hesitate to do so!*

◆ *When lifting cots or stretchers, a minimum of two people is required.* If more are available, use an even number of people so that weight is evenly distributed.

◆ *When possible, partners on opposite sides of the load should have similar heights and strengths.* This permits a more even distribution of weight.

◆ *Move the patient feet first whenever feasible.* Few things are more frightening to a patient than being immobilized to a board and then carried, head first, down a set of stairs.

Most patient-carrying devices are mechanical equipment. You must be familiar with how they are assembled and used before you attempt to carry patients with them. The devices must also be properly maintained if they are to be used safely. Follow the manufacturers' guidelines for maintenance as well as for the weight each device can safely carry. Practice using each type of carrying device frequently.

Wheeled Ambulance Stretcher

The wheeled stretcher, also called "the cot" or "the gurney," is found in the back of every ambulance (Figure 10-13A and B). There are a number of different models in common use, and each works a little differently from the others. Most, however, do have some features in common. For example, the head of the stretcher can be ele-

Figure 10-13A A lift-in wheeled stretcher.

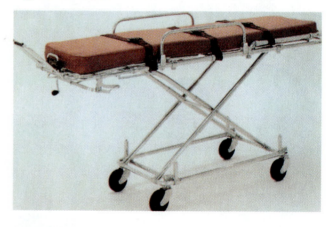

Figure 10-13B A roll-in wheeled stretcher.

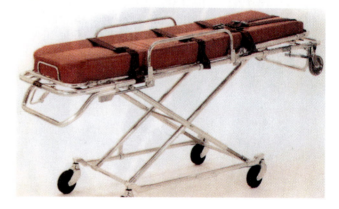

vated. The height of the stretcher can usually be adjusted to different levels. You should become thoroughly familiar with the operation and safe handling of the types of wheeled ambulance stretchers you will be using.

There are some general recommendations for use that apply to all types of wheeled stretchers. These include the following:

◆ *Patients should always be strapped safely into the stretcher.* If the patient's arms are not strapped in, carefully instruct the patient not to reach out and grab anything while the stretcher is being moved.

◆ *Whenever the stretcher is being moved with a patient on it, the stretcher should be adjusted to the lowest practical position.* With the weight of a patient and associated medical equipment on them, stretchers can quickly become top heavy and prone to tipping over. Lowering the stretcher lowers the device's center of gravity, increasing its safety and decreasing the chances of a tip-over.

◆ *Roll the stretcher whenever possible,* pulling from the foot end with the person at the head end guiding (Figure 10-14). Be aware that rough terrain can easily cause the stretcher to tip.

◆ *If the stretcher must be moved over rough terrain, use four EMTs whenever possible.* Position one rescuer at each corner of the stretcher. This produces greater stability,

Figure 10-14   Whenever possible, roll the wheeled stretcher.

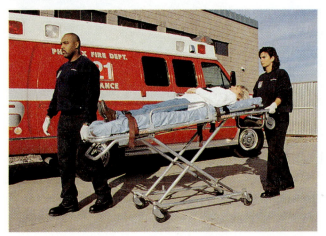

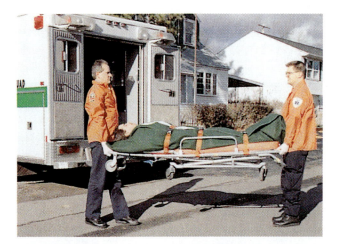

Figure 10-15   When two rescuers carry a stretcher, they should face each other.

requires less strength from each of the EMTs, and is ultimately safer for the patient.

◆ *When two EMTs move a stretcher, one should be at its foot and the other at its head.* The EMTs should face each other (Figure 10-15). This arrangement is somewhat awkward for the EMT who must walk backwards. However, it ensures good communication between the two EMTs, which is essential for the safe moving of patients. Remember that stretchers moved with only two rescuers can easily become unbalanced. Use extreme caution when moving a patient in this manner. This technique is recommended only to negotiate tight spaces.

◆ *Once in the ambulance, secure the stretcher to the wall or floor of the patient compartment using a stretcher mount* (Figure 10-16). Before beginning to transport the patient, recheck to ensure that the stretcher is properly secured in the mount.

Portable Ambulance Stretcher

Portable stretchers of aluminum, canvas, heavy plastic, or coated fabric are also standard equipment on ambulances (Figure 10-17A and B). Most models fold or collapse, and they are easily stored and cleaned.

Portable stretchers can be used to evacuate supine patients from locations where the wheeled ambulance stretcher is impractical or impossible to use. They are particularly helpful in mass casu-

Loading the Wheeled Stretcher

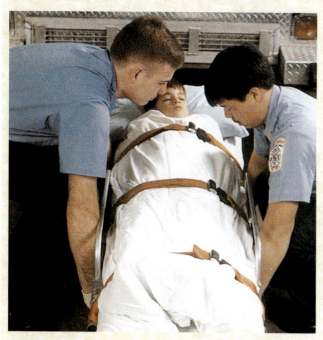

Figure 10-16A Clear the ambulance interior and lift rear step if necessary. Lower stretcher to its lowest level and lock it in that position. EMTs, who are positioned on both sides of the stretcher, bend at the knees and grasp the lower bar of the stretcher frame using the power grip.

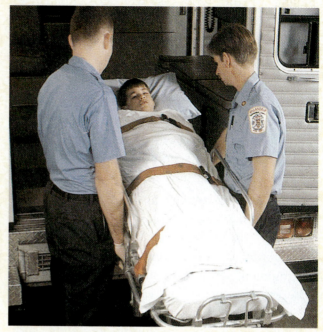

Figure 10-16B The EMTs rise to a full standing position and move the stretcher onto the ambulance using small sideways steps.

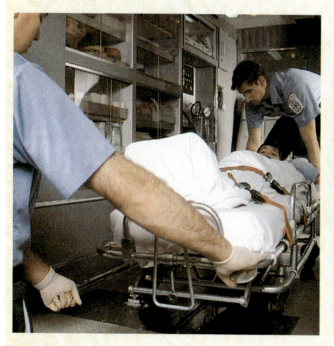

Figure 10-16C The EMTs move the stretcher into the securing device.

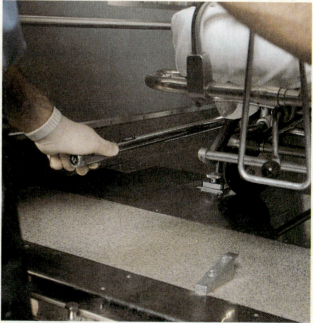

Figure 10-16D EMTs should be sure that both forward and rear catches are engaged.

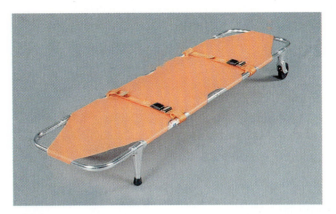

Figure 10-17A Portable stretcher with a continuous tubular metal frame.

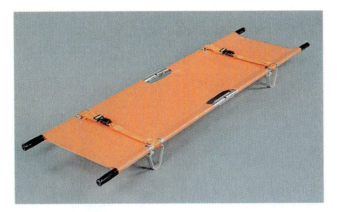

Figure 10-17B Portable pole stretcher, also known as a canvas litter.

alty incidents where there are more patients than wheeled ambulance stretchers.

Properly secured to the crew bench or hanging hardware, portable stretchers can be used to transport additional patients in the back of an ambulance. Perhaps the only disadvantage of portable stretchers is that most models lack wheels and thus require that an adequate number of EMTs be available if the patient is to be carried for any distance.

Stair Chair

The stair chair is, as its name implies, an extremely useful device for moving seated patients up and down stairs (Figure 10-18). It is also helpful in narrow hallways, small elevators, and other tight, confined spaces. Since the device has wheels, it can be rolled, making it less tiring for EMTs to use. Because patients with breathing difficulty often breathe more easily when sitting

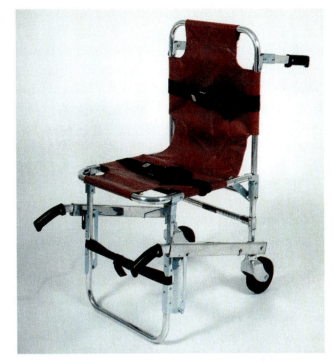

Figure 10-18 A stair chair.

up, the stair chair can be particularly effective when carrying them.

There are circumstances in which the stair chair should *not* be used. As noted, patients on it are placed in a sitting position. Thus, the device is contraindicated for patients with suspected spinal injuries or injuries to the lower extremities. Also avoid the device for patients with an altered level of consciousness who may not be capable of maintaining an open airway.

When going down a set of stairs, carry the patient feet first down the stairs. It is *extremely* important that the EMT at the foot of the stair chair (that is, lower on the stairs) lift the device upwards so that the patient's knees are approximately at the level of that EMT's chest. Doing this will lessen the strain on the lower back of the EMT at the head of the device. It will also help prevent that EMT from losing his or her balance.

A third rescuer, if available, should act as a spotter when the stair chair is used. He should stand behind the EMT who is moving backward and help guide that EMT. All belts on the stair chair should be securely fastened. In addition, the patient's arms should be gently restrained while he is in the stair chair. He should be cautioned not to reach out and grab anything while being carried.

It may be good idea to *temporarily* disconnect some medical monitoring equipment from the patient while moving him up or down stairs. Exceptions should be made for portable oxygen equipment (which should be administered continuously if its use is indicated) and lightweight devices such as pulse oximeters. These should be carried by another rescuer during the move. Any equipment that is disconnected should immediately be reconnected once the patient is off the stairs.

Scoop Stretcher

The scoop stretcher is sometimes called an orthopedic stretcher (Figure 10-19). The device is most commonly used at sporting events and for patients with hip injuries. The device can sometimes be used in places where other stretchers will not fit. Constructed of aluminum or lightweight steel, this stretcher splits apart into two or four pieces along its long axis. Its pieces are laid out on both sides of a supine patient. They are then pushed together and secured under the patient (Figure 10-20A and B). The patient is then "scooped up" for transfer to the wheeled ambulance stretcher or other device.

The scoop stretcher alone offers no support under the patient's spine. It is not recommended for a patient with suspected spinal injury.

Spine Boards

Spine boards or backboards are standard equipment on emergency vehicles. They are used to

Figure 10-19 A scoop (orthopedic) stretcher.

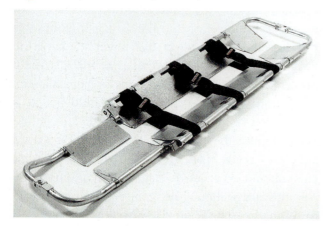

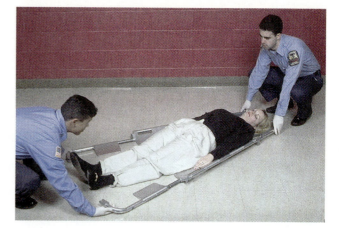

Figure 10-20A When using the scoop stretcher, one EMT assures that the patient's head is supported while the lower part of the stretcher is positioned.

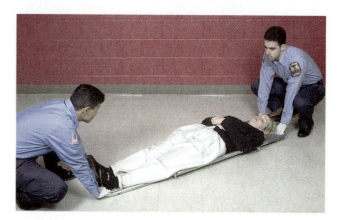

Figure 10-20B The EMTs lock the two halves of the stretcher together, continuing to assure proper support for the head.

immobilize patients with suspected neck or spine injuries.

Long spine boards can be made of wood, aluminum, or plastic polymer (Figure 10-21). They are used to package patients who are found lying down or standing. They also help protect patients from rocky or uneven ground. Many of the more popular models have molded handholds. Straps and head-immobilizing devices can be secured easily to the boards.

Short spine boards (Figure 10-22) and vest-type extrication devices (Figure 10-23) are used to immobilize patients with suspected neck or spine injuries who are found in a sitting position, as in a vehicle. The devices are most often applied so

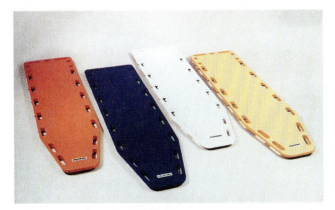

Figure 10-21 Long spine boards.

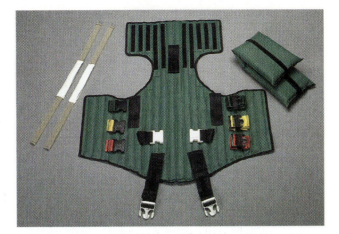

Figure 10-23 A vest-type extrication device.

that the patient can be moved from a sitting to a supine position on a long spine board.

It is essential that you practice frequently with the specific devices that your EMS agency uses for spinal immobilization. A crushed automobile containing a critically injured patient on a sub-zero winter's night is *not* the time or place to learn how to use a vest-type extrication device! (You will learn more about backboards in Chapter 22, "Head and Spine Injuries.")

Basket Stretcher

A basket stretcher, often called a Stokes litter or basket, can be made of wire mesh with a metal frame or of plastic polymer (Figure 10-24A). The basket stretcher is most commonly used in high-angle and low-angle rescues and to carry patients over rough terrain (Figure 10-24B). Specialized training beyond the EMT curriculum is required to use this piece of equipment safely. The patient is

usually immobilized on a long spine board, which is then secured in the basket. Because plastic stretchers will eventually deteriorate if exposed to ultraviolet radiation, basket stretchers should be stored away from direct sunlight.

Flexible Stretcher

The flexible stretcher is particularly useful when evacuating patients through narrow hallways or other tight passageways. Examples of these

Figure 10-24A A basket stretcher.

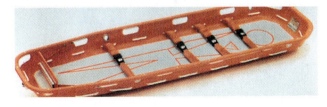

Figure 10-24B The basket stretcher is often used to carry patients over rough terrain.

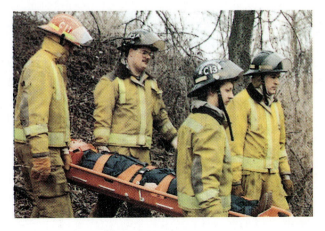

Figure 10-22 Short spine boards.

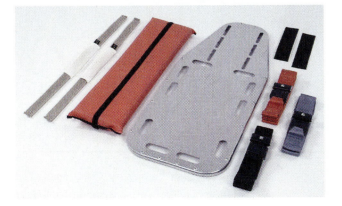

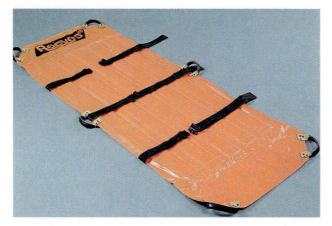

Figure 10-25 A flexible stretcher.

devices include the Reeves and SKED stretchers. They are made of canvas or some other heavy-duty flexible material and have three carrying handles attached to each side (Figure 10-25). The devices are easily rolled up or folded for storage when not in use. Flexible stretchers, when used alone, do *not* provide adequate immobilization for a patient with suspected neck or spine injury.

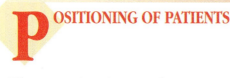

POSITIONING OF PATIENTS

When a patient is moved to a carrying device, he must be properly positioned on it for transport. The position in which he is placed will depend upon his condition and the equipment you are using. There are some basic rules to follow when positioning patients:

◆ An unresponsive patient with no suspected head, neck, or spine injury should be placed on his side in the left lateral recumbent, or recovery, position (Figure 10-26). This positioning should be done without twisting the patient's body. When the patient is in this position, fluids or vomitus can drain from the mouth more easily. Having the patient face left will also make it easier for the EMT seated on the ambulance bench to monitor the airway during transport.

◆ A patient with chest pain or discomfort or with difficulty breathing should be placed in a position of comfort. Most often this will mean

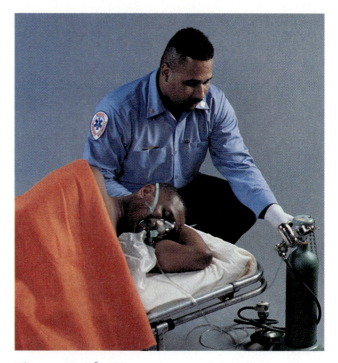

Figure 10-26 Place unresponsive patients with no suspected head, neck, or spine injury on the carrying device in the left lateral recumbent, or recovery, position.

a sitting or semi-sitting position (Figure 10-27). Do not, however, transport a patient with hypoperfusion in a sitting position.

◆ A patient with suspected head, neck, or spine injury should be fully immobilized to a long backboard for transport. Tilt the board as a unit onto its left side if necessary for drainage of fluids or vomitus from the patient's mouth.

Figure 10-27 For patients with breathing difficulty or chest pain, a semi-sitting position is often the position of comfort.

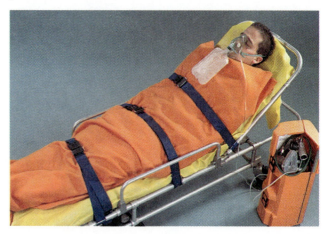

- A patient suffering from shock should be transported in a supine position with his feet or the foot of the backboard elevated 8 to 12 inches (200 to 300 mm) (Figure 10-28). Do *not* elevate the legs of a patient with suspected head, neck, or spine injury.

- Transport a woman more than 6 months pregnant on her left side. If she is immobilized on a spine board, you can place a pillow or rolled towel under the right side of the board to tip her to the left.

- An alert patient who is nauseated or vomiting should be transported in a position of comfort. This will often be the recovery position. If a sitting or semi-sitting position is used, monitor the airway carefully and be prepared to transfer the patient to the recovery position if his level of consciousness decreases.

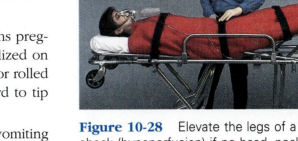

Figure 10-28 Elevate the legs of a patient in shock (hypoperfusion) if no head, neck, or spine injuries are suspected.

Chapter Review

SUMMARY

You must be able to lift and move patients safely to assure that they receive appropriate care. The word *safely* in the previous sentence refers to the patient's safety—improperly executed lifts or moves can easily harm the patient. The word refers to the EMT's safety as well—improperly executed moves can mean needless pain and career-ending injury for the EMT. To lift and move safely, you must understand body mechanics, so that you can use your body's strength efficiently. You must know different types of moves and when each is appropriate. You must be familiar with the types and characteristics of different patient-carrying devices. Finally, you must understand how to position patients properly on those devices.

REVIEWING KEY CONCEPTS

1. Describe basic guidelines you should follow whenever you must lift or move a patient.

2. Define "body mechanics." Explain some basics of body mechanics that you should follow when lifting or moving patients or objects.

3. Describe the circumstances in which an emergency move should be used. Give some examples of emergency moves.

4. Describe the circumstances in which an urgent move should be used.

5. Describe the circumstances in which a non-urgent emergency move can be used. Give some examples of non-urgent moves.

6. List the steps of a rapid extrication.

7. List basic points to keep in mind whenever a patient-carrying device is used.

8. List basic rules to follow when positioning a patient on a carrying device.

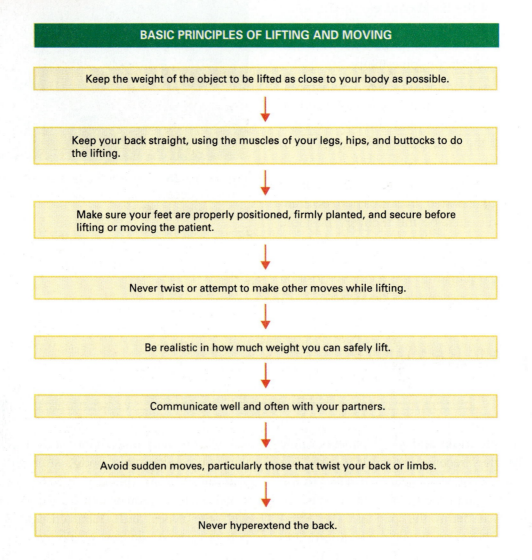

BASIC PRINCIPLES OF LIFTING AND MOVING

Keep the weight of the object to be lifted as close to your body as possible.

Keep your back straight, using the muscles of your legs, hips, and buttocks to do the lifting.

Make sure your feet are properly positioned, firmly planted, and secure before lifting or moving the patient.

Never twist or attempt to make other moves while lifting.

Be realistic in how much weight you can safely lift.

Communicate well and often with your partners.

Avoid sudden moves, particularly those that twist your back or limbs.

Never hyperextend the back.

PART
2

MEDICAL AND TRAUMA EMERGENCIES

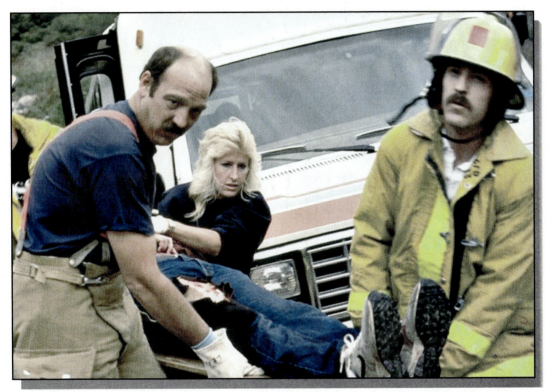

I n Part 1, you learned about the essential components of patient
assessment and care. This knowledge will empower you to
approach systematically the types of emergencies you will
encounter on the job. These emergencies fall into two broad categories,
those involving patient illness—medical emergencies—and those
involving patient injury—trauma emergencies.

The chapters of Part 2 describe the assessment and care of specific
types of medical and trauma emergencies. You will learn about a wide
range of illnesses and injuries—from the care of infants to the care of ▶

geriatric patients, from the treatment of minor cuts to that of life-threatening head injuries, and from behavioral emergencies to childbirth. This variety reflects the reality of prehospital care itself—you never know what the next call will involve.

As you read this part of the textbook, always keep in mind the fundamentals of patient assessment and care that you have already studied. Combining those basics with a knowledge of the specific conditions you are about to study will assure that you provide the best possible patient care no matter what illness or injury you are faced with. How you can accomplish this is discussed in the chapters of Part 2.

Chapter 11   *General Pharmacology*
Chapter 12   *Respiratory Emergencies*
Chapter 13   *Cardiac Emergencies*
Chapter 14   *Altered Mental Status Emergencies—Diabetes and Other Causes*
Chapter 15   *Poisoning and Allergic Reactions*
Chapter 16   *Environmental Emergencies*
Chapter 17   *Obstetrics and Gynecology*
Chapter 18   *Behavioral Emergencies*
Chapter 19   *Bleeding and Shock*
Chapter 20   *Soft Tissue Injuries*
Chapter 21   *Musculoskeletal Injuries*
Chapter 22   *Injuries to the Head and Spine*
Chapter 23   *Infants and Children*
Chapter 24   *Geriatrics*

General Pharmacology

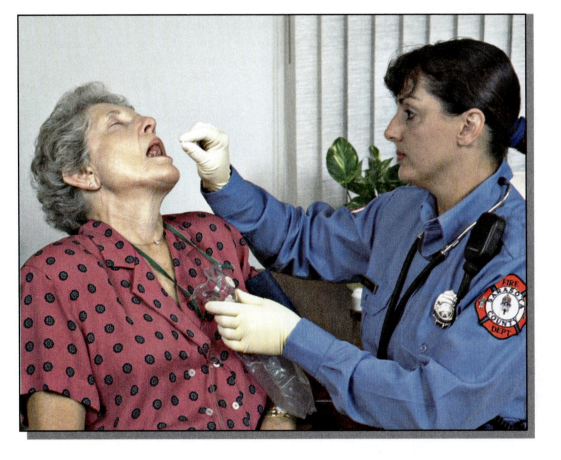

*I*n the past, administering medications in the out-of-hospital setting
was a role reserved for advanced EMTs. In 1994, however, the U.S.
Department of Transportation adopted its new curriculum for EMT-
Basics. Under it, local EMS systems may permit EMT-Basics to administer
or assist in administering certain medications or drugs.

    This new role brings with it new responsibilities for the EMT-Basic.
Medications may have negative as well as positive effects on patients.
Anyone who is authorized to administer medications to patients must be
aware of the effects of those medications. In addition, having a general ▶

knowledge of the names and types of common medications as well as their effects may enhance the ability to assess certain patients.

*This chapter deals with basic **pharmacology**—the study of drugs and their effects. In it, you will study common forms of medications, their names, and the ways in which they are administered. You will pay particular attention to medications that EMTs are authorized to administer or assist in administering.*

OBJECTIVES

At the completion of this chapter, the EMT-Basic student should be able to meet the following objectives:

Knowledge and Understanding

1. Identify which medications will be carried on the unit. (pp. 295–297)
2. State the medications carried on the unit by the generic name. (pp. 295–297
3. Identify the medications with which the EMT-Basic may assist the patient with administering. (pp. 293–295)
4. State the medications the EMT-Basic can assist the patient with by generic name. (pp.293–295)

5. Discuss the forms in which the medications may be found. (p. 290)
6. Explain the rationale for the administration of medications. (pp. 291–293)

Skills

1. Demonstrate the general steps for assisting patients with self-administration of medications.
2. Read the labels and inspect each type of medication.

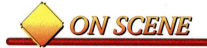

ON SCENE

DISPATCH: *HAMILTON FIRE RESCUE. HAMILTON, RESPOND TO THE NAUTILUS SANDWICH SHOP ON BROAD STREET FOR AN 18-YEAR-OLD FEMALE WITH POSSIBLE ALLERGIC REACTION. PATIENT IS CONSCIOUS, BUT BREATHING WITH SEVERE DIFFICULTY. VILLAGE AMBULANCE IS ON ANOTHER CALL. MUTUAL AID AMBULANCE HAS BEEN DISPATCHED. 1301.*

You are the Rescue Company Lieutenant on Rescue 195. As you turn into Broad Street, your scene size-up reveals a quiet street with the owner of the sandwich shop standing on the curb to flag you down. The owner escorts you and your crew into the shop, saying as he does, "She ate some of her friend's shrimp salad by

mistake. Two minutes later, she was gasping and saying she couldn't catch her breath."

As you enter the shop, you note a young woman lying on the floor. Two women about her age are beside her, trying to assist her. The young woman's face is very red and swollen. Your initial assessment reveals that she is poorly responsive, with a weak and thready radial pulse and with severe respiratory distress. While your crew places her on high flow oxygen, you introduce yourself and say, "My crew and I are here to help you. What is your name?"

With great difficulty the young woman responds, "Jo . . . dy . . . I can't . . . breathe . . . allergic . . . shrimp . . . need Epi-Pen® . . .

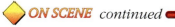
my purse." One of the women with Jody reaches to the counter for a purse and hands it to you.

In it, you find the Epi-Pen® auto-injector. You look at the label and confirm that the auto-injector has, in fact, been prescribed to Jody. You also note that the auto-injector contains epinephrine and that the medication has not expired.

Your assessment is that Jody is having a life-threatening allergic reaction and needs to have her Epi-Pen® administered immediately. You use the shop's phone and call the emergency department physician at Community Hospital. As you do, one of the other firefighter EMTs obtains vital signs that include a pulse of 130 and a blood pressure of 80/40. You report those findings as part of your brief patient assessment to the emergency room physician. She gives you permission to administer the patient's epinephrine auto-injector.

You prepare the Epi-Pen® for use and inject the medication by pressing the pen against Jody's thigh. By the time the mutual aid ambulance arrives 5 minutes later, Jody is already breathing more comfortably and her facial swelling has decreased. The paramedics initiate an IV line and administer an additional medication prior to transport. As Jody is wheeled out on the stretcher, she thanks you and the crew for saving her life.

ESSENTIALS OF PHARMACOLOGY

Medications

As an EMT, you will be administering, assisting in the administration of, and coming into contact with people who are using various medications. A **medication** is defined as a drug or other substance that is used as a remedy for illness. EMTs and other medical personnel often use the terms "medications" and "drugs" interchangeably. When you are dealing with the public as an EMT, it is better to use the terms "medication" or "medicine" because there can be negative associations with the word "drug."

Medication Names

There are thousands of different medications available in the United States, with and without a prescription. Each of these drugs has at least three names, which can make the subject of pharmacology seem hopelessly overwhelming.

No one, however, will expect you as an EMT to know all the names and types of medications. It is important, though, that you understand the basic naming systems used to identify medications.

First, each drug has a **chemical name.** This indicates the drug's chemical make-up.

Next, the drug has a **generic name.** This is usually a shortened form of the chemical name. The generic names are used in the U.S. Pharmacopoeia, a government publication listing all drugs officially approved by the U.S. Food and Drug Administration.

Pharmaceutical companies manufacture and market the drugs listed in the U.S. Pharmacopoeia. When they do, the companies give each drug they produce a **trade name** or **brand name.** Sometimes different companies produce the same generic drug, but each sells it under a different trade or brand name.

As an EMT, you might be authorized to assist a patient in taking a nitroglycerin tablet for chronic chest pain. The chemical name for this medication is 1,2,3-propanetriol trinitrate. Its generic name is nitroglycerin tablet. One trade name for this medication is Nitrostat®. Examples of the generic and trade names of other common medications are given in Table 11-1.

Table 11-1

Medication Names

Generic Name	Trade Name
acetaminophen	Tylenol®
ibuprofen	Motrin®, Advil®
albuterol	Ventolin®
diazepam	Valium®

Routes of Administration

Medications can enter the body through several **routes of administration.** The route affects the rate at which the medication enters the bloodstream and the speed with which it reaches the target organ to produce the desired effect.

Most medications are taken orally in pill or capsule form and absorbed into the bloodstream from the intestinal tract. Medications can also be administered by injection either into the subcutaneous tissues of the skin or the muscles or injected directly into a vein.

Still other medications in the form of either fine powders or sprays are inhaled by the patient directly into the respiratory tract. In cases of breathing difficulty, this route permits administration of the medications as close as possible to the area in which they are to act.

The various routes of administration are summarized in Table 11-2.

Forms of Medication

Medications come in various forms. These forms ensure proper administration of the medications as well as their correct controlled release. Among the different forms of medications you are likely to encounter as an EMT are the following:

◆ Gases, such as oxygen
◆ Compressed powders or tablets, such as nitroglycerin pills
◆ Liquids for injection, such as the epinephrine in an auto-injector
◆ Gels, such as an oral glucose paste
◆ Suspensions, such as activated charcoal in water
◆ Fine powders for inhalation, such as those in metered dose inhalers
◆ Sublingual sprays, such as nitroglycerin sprays
◆ Liquids for vaporization, such as those in nebulizers

Prescription Labeling

It is very important that you be able to read the labels of a patient's prescription medications. This is especially true when you are assisting a patient in taking a medication at the direction of medical

---

Table 11-2

Routes of Drug Administration

Route	Example
Oral—taken by mouth	Pills and syrups
Parenteral—injected	Epinephrine auto-injector
Rectal—inserted in rectum	Medications for vomiting
Transdermal—through skin	Nitroglycerin patch
Inhalation—through lungs	Oxygen
Sublingual—under the tongue	Nitroglycerin tablets or spray

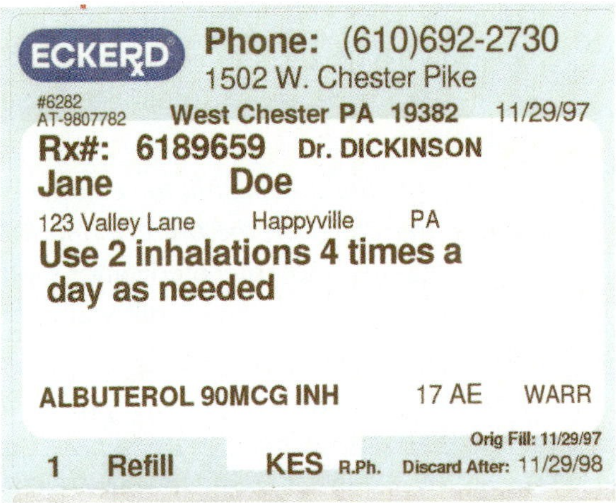

Figure 11-1 The prescription label gives important information about a medication. Read it carefully.

control. Figure 11-1 shows a typical prescription label as prepared by a pharmacist. From a prescription label, you should be able to identify the following:

◆ The patient's name

◆ The medication name (either the generic or the trade name)

◆ The strength of the medication (usually in milligrams)

◆ The date the prescription was filled

◆ The expiration date of the medication

◆ The prescribing health professional's name

◆ How often the medication should be taken

Sometimes prepackaged medications will have a pharmacist's label applied over the manufacturer's or will have only the manufacturer's label (Figure 11-2). Such labeling is especially common in the three types of prescription medications EMTs are allowed to assist patients in taking— inhaled bronchodilators, nitroglycerin, and epinephrine auto-injectors.

Understanding Medications

Administering medications and assisting patients with the administration of their own prescription medications is a great responsibility. As an EMT, you must have a thorough practical knowledge of the medications with which you are working. Because the administration of any medication always carries with it certain risks, you must know

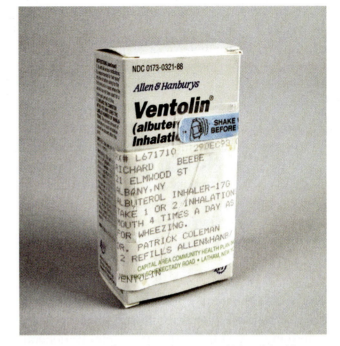

Figure 11-2 Sometimes a prescription label is pasted over the manufacturer's label on the package containing the medication.

the following facts about drugs you administer or assist in administering.

◆ **Indications** These are the circumstances in which it is appropriate to administer a medication to a patient. For example, life-threatening allergic reaction or anaphylactic shock is an indication for use of a patient's epinephrine auto-injector.

◆ **Contraindications** These are the circumstances in which or reasons why a medication should not be administered because doing so may harm the patient. For example, low blood pressure is a contraindication for administration of a patient's nitroglycerin tablets. Nitroglycerin lowers blood pressure and could, in this case, result in stroke or other serious complications.

◆ **Dose** This is the amount of a medication that should be administered to a patient. For example, with oral glucose a typical dose is one tube.

◆ **Route of Administration** This refers to the route and form of administration (discussed above).

◆ **Actions** These are the desirable effects a medication produces in a patient. For example, the action of albuterol (a common medication in metered dose inhalers) is to relax the smooth muscle in the bronchioles to open the airways of a wheezing asthma patient.

◆ **Side effects** These are the undesirable responses that a medication may cause in a given patient. For example, administration of albuterol can produce side effects of shakiness or tremors in some patients. Side effects are not the same thing as an allergic reaction to a medication.

Administration of Medications

The exact procedures for administering medications or assisting patients in taking medication are determined by your local EMS system. In general, however, the procedures below should be followed when assisting a patient with the administration of medication:

1. **Initiate assessment and treatment of the patient as indicated by signs and symptoms.** (Usually a patient who requires assistance with administration of nitroglycerin, metered dose inhalers, or epinephrine should be on high flow oxygen.) Obtain baseline vital signs.

2. **Verify that the patient has medication with him and has the signs and symptoms for which the medication is prescribed:**

Signs and Symptoms	Medication
Chest pain	Nitroglycerin
Shortness of breath Wheezing	Metered dose inhaler
Severe allergic reaction	Epinephrine

3. **Verify the following:**

◆ *That the medication has been prescribed by a physician for the patient.* Frequently patients borrow prescribed medications from family or friends who have had sim-

ilar signs and symptoms. In such cases, medical direction will most likely refuse to allow you to assist in administering the medication.

◆ *That the medication inside the container is the one indicated on the prescription label.* Patients taking multiple medications often combine them into a single pill vial to simplify carrying the medicines.

◆ *That the medication has not passed the expiration date on the prescription label.* Drugs like nitroglycerin frequently lose potency over time.

4. **Determine the last time that the patient self-administered the medication and the number of doses taken.**

5. **Contact medical direction.** Present a brief history and assessment, including baseline vital signs. Inform the physician exactly which medication in what strength the patient has with him and when the last self-administered dose of the medication was taken.

6. **If the physician orders you to assist the patient in taking the medication, verify the order** by repeating it back to the physician word-for-word.

7. **Administer the medication as directed.**

8. **Document the administration** of the medication by recording the drug, dose, route of administration, and time of administration.

COMPANY OFFICER'S NOTES

If your local EMS system permits EMTs to assist patients in the administration of their medications, a communications link with the ability to rapidly access the local emergency department for physician consultation is vital. Such communication systems using radios or cellular technology are well established for advanced life support EMT units. However, you may need to develop such a system to ensure scene-to-hospital communications for the engine or ladder companies who are often first responders and who may need to assist in administration of a medication prior to the arrival of ALS providers.

TRANSITION OF CARE

If you assist a patient in taking medications, it is mandatory that you document the following information and pass it along to the arriving advanced EMTs or to the transporting unit:

◆ The physician or authority ordering the medication
◆ The medication administered
◆ The dosage of that medication
◆ The exact time of administration
◆ Vital signs before and after administration
◆ Response of the patient to the medication

9. **Five minutes after administration of the medication, reassess** the patient's vital signs and any changes in his condition. Document your reassessment findings.

10. **Advise medical direction of your post-medication reassessment.**

MEDICATIONS ADMINISTERED BY EMTs

There are six medications that EMTs may be trained to administer (Figure 11-3). Three of these are medications prescribed by physicians for spe-

Figure 11-3 The medications that an EMT may be able to administer or assist in administering to a patient include oral glucose, inhaled bronchodilators, epinephrine, nitroglycerin, activated charcoal, and oxygen.

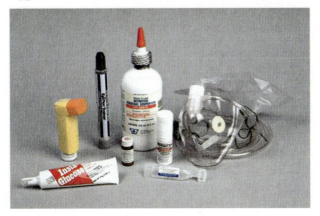

cific patients and with whose administration the EMT may assist. Three others are carried on the EMS unit for administration by the EMT under specific circumstances.

Medications that you may administer are discussed in greater depth in these chapters: inhaled bronchodilators in Chapter 12, "Respiratory Emergencies"; nitroglycerin in Chapter 13, "Cardiac Emergencies"; oral glucose in Chapter 14, "Altered Mental Status Emergencies—Diabetes and Other Causes"; epinephrine in Chapter 15, "Poisonings and Allergic Reactions": oxygen in Chapter 6, "Airway Management"; and activated charcoal in Chapter 15, "Poisonings and Allergic Reactions."

Medications the EMT May Assist in Administering

Depending on local protocols, EMTs may be authorized to assist patients in the administration of the following prescription medications under the direction of medical control: inhaled bronchodilators, nitroglycerin, epinephrine.

Inhaled Bronchodilators

This group of medications is prescribed to patients with asthma or chronic obstructive pulmonary diseases (COPD) such as chronic bronchitis and emphysema. The medications are inhaled from a metered dose inhaler (MDI) or via a nebulizer directly into the respiratory tract. The medications are designed to relax the smooth muscles in the bronchioles that have caused the airways to narrow, resulting in shortness of breath. When a patient is having difficulty breathing, you may be authorized by medical control to assist in administering his prescribed MDI (Table 11-3).

Nitroglycerin

Nitroglycerin is a drug commonly prescribed to patients with angina pectoris, or chest pain resulting from inadequate blood flow to the heart (Table 11-4). Nitroglycerin dilates the coronary blood vessels, allowing more oxygenated blood to reach the heart. The medication is generally prescribed with instructions to take one tablet or spray under the tongue when experiencing chest

Table 11-3

Inhaled Bronchodilators

Indications	Shortness of breath or respiratory distress as a result of asthma or chronic obstructive pulmonary disease
Contraindications	Known allergy to the medication (unlikely if the medication is prescribed by a physician to a particular patient)
Actions	Relaxes smooth muscles in the bronchioles causing the airway passages to widen or dilate
Side effects	Increased heart rate, shakiness
Names: Generic (brand)	Albuterol (Ventolin®, Proventil®), ipratropium bromide (Atrovent®), metaproterenol (Alupent®)
Dosage	Albuterol: 90 micrograms per spray, usual dose 2 sprays; ipratropium bromide: 18 micrograms per spray, usual dose 2 sprays

pain. (Some patients are prescribed nitroglycerin patches to wear at all times.) Usually the patient is told to use the medication every 3 to 5 minutes until the pain ends, up to a maximum of three doses. If the third dose fails to relieve the pain, the patient is usually told to contact EMS. As an EMT, you may be authorized to assist patients in taking their tablets or using their spray.

Epinephrine

Epinephrine is prescribed to patients who are at risk for severe allergic reaction or anaphylactic shock from exposure to certain allergens such as bee venom. Epinephrine is usually prescribed in a self-contained auto-injector system (Table 11-5). The patient is instructed to give himself an injection of epinephrine if signs of a severe allergic

Table 11-4

Nitroglycerin

Indications	Chest pains from angina pectoris
Contraindications	Low blood pressure
Actions	Dilates blood vessels
Side effects*	Headache, lowered blood pressure
Names: Generic (brand)	Nitroglycerin (Nitrostat®, Nitrobid®, Nitrolingual® Spray)
Dosage	0.4 mg per tablet or spray

*The side effects of nitroglycerin may also affect an EMT who absorbs nitroglycerin through his skin. Always wear gloves when assisting with nitroglycerin administration.

Table 11-5

Epinephrine

Indications	Severe allergic reactions
Contraindications	No contraindications when used in a life-threatening situation
Actions	Dilates bronchioles to improve breathing; constricts blood vessels to improve blood pressure
Side effects	Anxiety, palpitations, chest pain (rare), irregular heart beats (dysrhythmias)
Names: Generic (brand)	Epinephrine (Adrenalin®; names of auto-injectors—EpiPen®, EpiPen Jr.®)
Dosage	Adult: 0.3 mg injected subcutaneously; Child: 0.15 mg injected subcutaneously

reaction, such as facial swelling, throat tightening, or shortness of breath develop after an exposure such as a bee sting.

Medications Carried on the EMS Unit

There are several medications that may be carried on board EMS units. All units should carry oxygen, which is considered an inhaled medication and which EMTs may administer. In addition, local EMS protocols may permit EMS units to carry and EMTs to administer activated charcoal and oral glucose.

Oxygen

Oxygen is essential to life. The air we breathe contains about 21 percent oxygen. This percentage is sufficient for healthy, uninjured people. However, people who are ill or injured may not have adequate respirations or circulation and may need oxygen at higher concentrations. The administration of oxygen at higher concentrations is a routine part of emergency medical care for many traumatic injuries and many medical emergencies (Table 11-6). Often, the EMT will administer high

Table 11-6

Oxygen

Indications	Any patient with shortness of breath, chest pain, signs of hypoperfusion or serious injury
Contraindications	No contraindications to the short-term use of oxygen
Actions	Essential for proper organ metabolism and function
Side effects	Dry mouth and nose
Name	Oxygen (no brand name)
Dosage	High flow: 90–100% concentration via nonrebreather mask at 15 liters per minute; low flow: 25–40% concentration via nasal cannula at 1 to 6 liters per minute

flow oxygen (15 liters per minute). For other patients like those with COPD and mild respiratory distress, local protocols may require that low flow oxygen (1 to 6 liters per minute) be administered through a nasal cannula.

Oral Glucose

Diabetic patients can develop low blood sugar (hypoglycemia) when they take too much of the medication designed to lower their blood sugar in relation to the amount of food they eat. Hypoglycemia can be life threatening, with symptoms ranging from mild confusion and sweats to complete unresponsiveness. Administration of supplemental glucose is essential for treatment of hypoglycemia (Table 11-7).

Activated Charcoal

Local protocols may allow the EMT to administer activated charcoal in certain cases of poisoning or drug overdose (Table 11-8). Activated charcoal is administered orally to patients with the aim of absorbing poisons from the gastrointestinal tract. As the charcoal travels through the intestines, it binds to the toxin, and both the charcoal and the toxin are passed out of the body with the stool rather than being absorbed by the body. Activated charcoal is usually combined with a drug called sorbitol, which speeds passage of the charcoal and toxin out of the intestines, further reducing the body's absorption of the toxin.

Medical studies have shown that the administration of activated charcoal is more effective in reducing absorption of toxins than the inducing of vomiting in patients. For this reason, activated charcoal has replaced ipecac, a drug that induces vomiting, as the preferred medication for EMTs in treatment of poisonings.

Although activated charcoal is effective in the gastrointestinal tract, introduction of the substance into the lungs and respiratory system can prove fatal. For that reason, activated charcoal should only be administered to cooperative patients who are awake and alert and have a normal gag reflex.

Commonly Encountered Medications

Many of the patients you will contact as an EMT take prescription medications under the direction of their doctors. Remembering the generic and brand names and uses of all the medications you will encounter is a monumental task. Having a basic knowledge of why patients take the most common prescription drugs may be more helpful to you when performing your patient assess-

Table 11-7

Oral Glucose

Indications	Diabetic patients with altered mental status and suspected hypoglycemia
Contraindications	Patient lacks gag reflex (which could lead to aspiration of glucose into the lungs)
Actions	Restores lack of blood sugar necessary for normal functioning of organs (especially the brain)
Side effects	None
Names: Generic (brand)	Oral glucose (Insta-Glucose®, Glutose®)
Dosage	One tube administered gradually into the mouth (tongue blade may be used to apply gel to inside of mouth and cheeks)

Table 11-8

Activated Charcoal

Indications	Oral ingestion of poisons or drugs (especially if prolonged transport is expected)
Contraindications	Lack of gag reflex or rapidly decreasing mental status
Actions	Binds to drugs or toxins which are then passed with the stool
Side effects	Dark stools, constipation
Names: Generic (brand)	Activated charcoal (Liqui-Char, InstaChar)
Dosage	Adult: one 50-gram container. Child: 1 gram per kilogram of body weight

ments. For example, a patient with altered mental status who is taking Humulin® insulin may benefit from the administration of oral glucose. On the other hand, the altered mental status of a patient taking Dilantin® is more likely to result from a seizure disorder than from the hypoglycemia that oral glucose can benefit.

Remember, however, that you should not attempt to diagnose patients based on their medications. Instead, be alert to the implications of those medications and be sure to record and pass on any medications that a patient is taking as part of the SAMPLE history. Be sure that this information is passed on to any other care providers as part of a transition of care. Table 11-9 on the next page lists medical conditions you will frequently encounter and some of the medications commonly prescribed for those conditions. At the scene of a call, you should try to gather any medications that a patient may be taking and bring them to the hospital.

Table 11-9

Medications Prescribed for Common Medical Conditions

Purpose of Medication	Generic Name	Trade Name®
To control diabetes	insulin glyburide metformin	Humulin Micronase/Diabeta Glucophage
To control high blood pressure	nifedipine captopril diltiazem atenolol hydrochlorothiazide	Procardia Capoten Cardizem Tenormin Hydrodiuril/Esidrix
To control congestive heart failure	furosemide bumetanide hydrochlorothiazide	Lasix Bumex Hydrodiuril/Esidrix
To control rapid heart rate	digoxin verapamil diltiazem	Lanoxin Calan Cardiazem
For angina	nitroglycerin isosorbide	Nitro-stat Isordil
To control seizures	phenytoin carbamazepine valproic acid phenobarbital	Dilantin Tegretol Depakote —
For asthma and COPD	albuterol ipratropium theophylline terbutaline	Ventolin Atrovent Theo-dur Brethine
To control pain	ibuprofen oxycodone hydrocodone	Motrin/Advil Percocet Lortab
For digestive problems	ranitidine cimetidine cisapride	Zantac Tagamet Propulsid

Chapter Review

SUMMARY

Assisting a patient in the administration of certain prescribed medications is one of the most serious responsibilities you will have as an EMT. You must be aware of the indications, contraindications, actions, side effects, dosages, and routes of administration of those medications prior to their use. In addition, your ability to assess certain patients will be enhanced by a knowledge of the names and types of medications they take and by a knowledge of basic facts of pharmacology.

REVIEWING KEY CONCEPTS

1. Describe the different kinds of names a medication can have.
2. Describe the various routes by which medications can enter the body.
3. Describe the steps to be followed when administering or assisting with administration of a medication to a patient.
4. Name three medications an EMT may administer or assist in administering with if they have been prescribed for a patient.
5. Name three medications that are carried on the emergency vehicle and that the EMT may administer to patients under certain circumstances.

RESOURCES TO LEARN MORE

Physicians' Desk Reference. Montvale, NJ: Medical Economics Data Production Company, published yearly.

Brian Bledsoe et al. *Prehospital Emergency Pharmacology,* 4th Edition. Upper Saddle River, NJ: Brady/Prentice Hall, 1996.

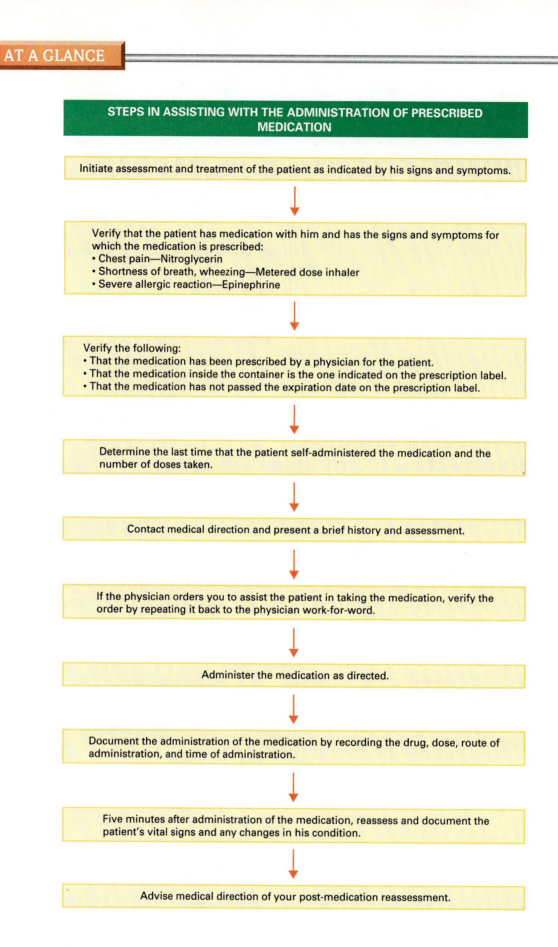

STEPS IN ASSISTING WITH THE ADMINISTRATION OF PRESCRIBED MEDICATION

Initiate assessment and treatment of the patient as indicated by his signs and symptoms.

Verify that the patient has medication with him and has the signs and symptoms for which the medication is prescribed:
• Chest pain—Nitroglycerin
• Shortness of breath, wheezing—Metered dose inhaler
• Severe allergic reaction—Epinephrine

Verify the following:
• That the medication has been prescribed by a physician for the patient.
• That the medication inside the container is the one indicated on the prescription label.
• That the medication has not passed the expiration date on the prescription label.

Determine the last time that the patient self-administered the medication and the number of doses taken.

Contact medical direction and present a brief history and assessment.

If the physician orders you to assist the patient in taking the medication, verify the order by repeating it back to the physician work-for-word.

Administer the medication as directed.

Document the administration of the medication by recording the drug, dose, route of administration, and time of administration.

Five minutes after administration of the medication, reassess and document the patient's vital signs and any changes in his condition.

Advise medical direction of your post-medication reassessment.

Respiratory Emergencies

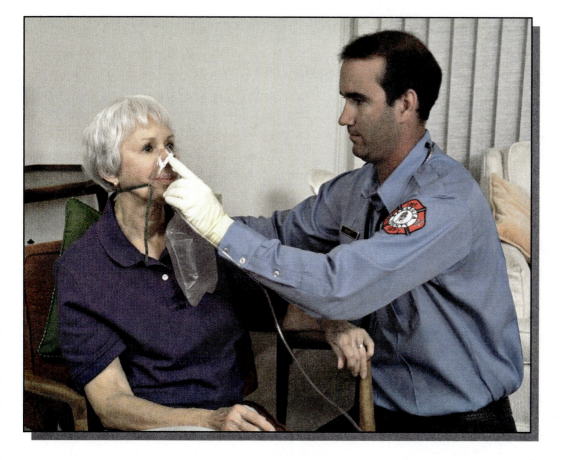

*C*alls to assist patients with difficulty breathing are among the most common for EMTs. The sensation of not being able to breathe adequately can be terrifying for patients. Their fears are often justified. Difficulty in breathing can often be life threatening. As an EMT, you must learn to assess adequate and inadequate breathing in patients. You must also be ready to take appropriate action when you meet a patient with signs and symptoms of inadequate breathing.

At the completion of this chapter, the EMT-Basic student should be able to meet the following objectives:

Knowledge and Understanding

1. List the structure and function of the respiratory system. (pp. 303–304)
2. State the signs and symptoms of a patient with breathing difficulty. (pp. 306–308)
3. Describe the emergency medical care of the patient with breathing difficulty. (pp. 309–310, 312)
4. Recognize the need for medical direction to assist in the emergency medical care of the patient with breathing difficulty. (pp. 311, 312)
5. Describe the emergency medical care of the patient with breathing distress. (pp. 309–310, 312)
6. Establish the relationship between airway management and the patient with breathing difficulty. (pp. 305–306)
7. List signs of adequate air exchange. (pp. 305–306)
8. State the generic name, medication forms, dose, administration, action, indications, and con-traindications for the prescribed inhaler. (pp. 311, 312–314)
9. Distinguish between the emergency medical care of the infant, child, and adult patient with breathing difficulty. (pp. 311, 314–315)
10. Differentiate between upper airway obstruction and lower airway disease in the infant and child patient. (pp. 314–315)
11. Defend EMT-Basic treatment regimens for various respiratory emergencies. (pp. 306–307, 310, 311, 315)
12. Explain the rationale for administering an inhaler. (pp. 311, 312)

Skills

1. Demonstrate the emergency medical care for breathing difficulty.
2. Perform the steps in facilitating the use of an inhaler.

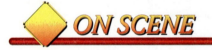

ON SCENE

DISPATCH: *ENGINE 405, RESPOND TO THE CITY SENIOR CITIZEN CENTER FOR A PATIENT WITH DIFFICULTY BREATHING. TIME OUT, 1344.*

The company officer acknowledges the call as the engine responds to the scene. The engine company crew is familiar with the center. There are several calls a week to the location for everything from falls to cases of cardiac arrest.

All crew members survey the scene as the engine pulls up. Everything appears calm. A resident caseworker meets your crew at the door and directs you to the first-floor apartment of Mrs. Phyllis Thompson, the patient. As you enter, you see the patient sitting on the couch, propped almost fully upright by several pillows. Your general impression is that the woman is in her 70s and is having considerable difficulty breathing. Recognizing this, your company officer directs you to begin the patient assessment while another EMT provides the patient with oxygen via a nonrebreather mask.

You introduce yourself and the crew and explain that you have come to help her. Your initial assessment reveals that the patient is alert. She has considerable respiratory distress, but her respirations are adequate. She has a rapid radial pulse. There is no external bleeding or any signs of trauma. You assign the patient a high priority for transport and provide her with oxygen via nonrebreather mask at 15 liters per minute. By radio, the company officer updates the ambulance crew on the situation. They advise that their ETA is 5 minutes.

You reassure the patient as you ask questions about her complaint and medical history using the SAMPLE and OPQRST mnemonics. She tells you that she didn't sleep at all last night and can't breathe if she lies flat. Her difficulty breathing has been getting worse since about two days ago. She has a history of heart problems and takes a "water pill." She has no allergies and hasn't eaten since last night. Your physical examination reveals noisy but equal lung sounds and adequate breathing. She has obvious swelling in her ankles.

You notice that the patient is less anxious and breathing a little more easily as the ambulance crew arrives. You suspect that the patient's improvement is from oxygen and from the reassurance you have been giving in large quantities. You have not had time to perform an ongoing assessment. Since you had the most communication with the patient, you provide the report to the ambulance crew during the transition of care.

With Mrs. Thompson packaged and transported, you return to the station. After cleaning and restocking the engine, you are again ready for service. Later that day you work with the same ambulance crew. They advise you that Mrs. Thompson suffers from congestive heart failure. Her heart had weakened and couldn't pump like it used to. This caused fluid to accumulate in her lungs and body, leading to her breathing problem. The hospital administered medications to Mrs. Thompson to rid her of the excess fluid and admitted her to monitor her condition and readjust her medications.

The crew in On Scene above recognized the signs and symptoms of a patient with breathing difficulty. Because they did, they were able to provide appropriate care promptly. As an EMT, you will meet many such patients. One of the most important skills you will develop is assessing them to determine if their breathing is adequate or inadequate.

To understand what is involved in adequate and inadequate breathing, you should review some basic information about the respiratory system. Look back at material on respiratory anatomy and physiology in Chapter 5, "Anatomy and Physiology," and Chapter 6, "Airway Management." Then read the section below.

 ## ANATOMY AND PHYSIOLOGY OF THE RESPIRATORY SYSTEM

The respiratory system is vital to life. Knowledge of airway structures and the function of the respiratory system will help you identify and treat life-threatening conditions.

Air enters the body through the mouth and nose. Immediately behind these structures is the *pharynx*. The area immediately behind the nose is called the *nasopharynx*. The area behind the mouth is the *oropharynx*. You will recall from Chapter 6 that one adjunct used to help maintain the airway is the oropharyngeal airway. This airway is so named because it is placed in the mouth (oro) and rests in the pharynx, thus oropharyngeal airway. In layperson's terms, the pharynx may be called the throat.

The lowest part of the pharynx is called the *hypopharynx*. Just below the hypopharynx, two passageways begin that air, food, and other materials can follow. The *esophagus* is the path by which food and liquids enter the stomach. The *trachea,* or windpipe, is the pathway to the lungs. Obviously it would be bad if food or liquid were to enter the trachea and the lungs. To prevent this, a leaf-shaped structure called the *epiglottis* covers the trachea during swallowing to prevent food and liquids from entering. Just below the epiglottis and just above the trachea is the *larynx*. Another name for this structure is the voice box. The vocal cords are located here. The *cricoid cartilage* forms the lower portion of the larynx.

The trachea splits into two main tubes called the *bronchi*. One bronchus goes to each of the lungs. The large main bronchi gradually subdivide into increasingly smaller air passages called *bron-*

chioles. The bronchioles eventually end at the thousands of tiny air sacs in the lungs called *alveoli.* The alveoli are where gas exchange takes place with the blood. Oxygen is turned over to the bloodstream, which gives up carbon dioxide to be excreted by the lungs.

There are two lungs. The right lung has three lobes and the left lung has two lobes. Separating the chest cavity from the abdominal cavity is the *diaphragm.* Inhalation occurs when the diaphragm and the *intercostal muscles* (the muscles between the ribs) contract. This causes the ribs to move up and outward and the diaphragm to move downward. This increases the size of the chest cavity and causes air to flow into the lungs. Exhalation occurs when these muscles relax. During relaxation, the size of the chest cavity decreases as the ribs move down and inward and the diaphragm rises. Air is then forced out of the lungs (Figure 12-1).

The airway structures of infants and children differ somewhat from those of adults. Those differences include the following:

◆ The airway structures of infants and children are smaller and more easily obstructed than those of adults.

◆ The tongues of infants and children take up proportionately more space in the mouth than the tongues of adults and can more easily block the airway.

◆ The trachea in infants and children is smaller, softer, and more flexible than in adults. It is more easily obstructed by swelling, trauma, and flexion or extension of the neck.

◆ The cricoid cartilage is less rigid in infants and children than in adults.

◆ Because the chest wall is softer in infants and children, they depend more heavily on the diaphragm for respiration than adults do.

A DEQUATE AND INADEQUATE BREATHING

Simply stated, adequate breathing will support life. Inadequate breathing will not. Perhaps one of the most important functions you will perform as an EMT is to evaluate breathing. Without adequate breathing, your patient will surely die. Whenever you encounter a patient who is breath-

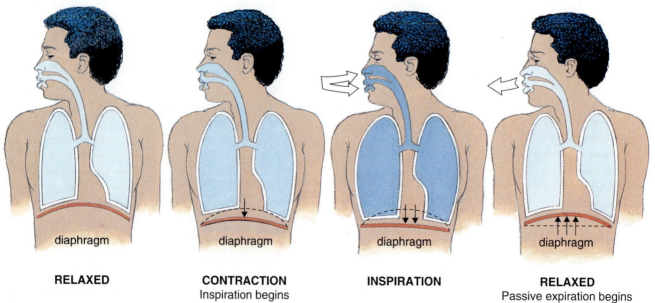

Figure 12-1   The process of respiration. During inhalation, the diaphragm and intercostal (rib) muscles contract, causing air to flow into the lungs. During exhalation, the muscles relax, causing air to flow out of the lungs.

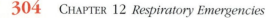

| **RELAXED** | **CONTRACTION**
Inspiration begins | **INSPIRATION** | **RELAXED**
Passive expiration begins |

ing inadequately, you must begin to treat the condition immediately.

Adequate Breathing

Since breathing does not require conscious effort, it is sometimes taken for granted. The brain directs the body to breathe a certain number of times per minute. The normal rate and depth of respiration will vary depending on a person's age and level of activity. Diseases may also change the characteristics of breathing.

Adequate respirations are identified by evaluating rate, rhythm, and quality. *Rate* is the number of respirations in a set period. *Rhythm* refers to the pattern of breathing. *Quality* refers to the effectiveness of the breathing. Table 12-1 lists the characteristics of adequate breathing.

Inadequate Breathing

If you took a CPR class before your EMT training, you learned to check for breathing. This was taught as a "yes-or-no" question. In reality, many patients for whom you might answer "Yes, they

are breathing" are not breathing *adequately* to support life. It is during this period between normal breathing and when breathing stops totally that your care will mean the most for the patient with a respiratory emergency.

To help such a patient, however, you must learn to recognize inadequate breathing. Table 12-2 lists the characteristics of inadequate breathing.

Agonal respirations are occasional gasping respirations that are seen just before respiratory or cardiac arrest. These breaths are shallow and infrequent. Due to the gasping nature of these respirations, they may appear to be adequate. Do not be deceived. Careful examination will reveal the inadequate nature of these breaths.

Adequate and Inadequate Artificial Ventilation

The treatment for absent or inadequate breathing is providing artificial ventilation. As discussed in Chapter 6, "Airway Management," there are many means of providing this ventilation. They include, in order of preference: pocket face mask with supplemental oxygen; two-person bag-valve mask

Table 12-1

Adequate Breathing

Rate	Adult 12–20 breaths per minute Child 15–30 breaths per minute Infant 25–50 breaths per minute
Rhythm	Usually regular (equal time between breaths) but may be irregular when patient talks or is conscious of his breathing efforts
Quality	Breath sounds—present in both lungs; equal when the lungs are compared to each other Chest expansion—adequate expansion; both sides of the chest expand equally Breathing effort—breathing does not appear labored or difficult; accessory muscles not used Depth (volume)—adequate

Table 12-2

Inadequate Breathing

Rate	Outside normal ranges (see Table 12-1), either higher or lower
Rhythm	May be irregular
Quality	Breath sounds—diminished or absent; noisy or high-pitched sounds; may be unequal when the lungs are compared to each other Chest expansion—inadequate expansion; sides of the chest may expand unequally Breathing effort—breathing appears labored or difficult; accessory muscles may be used Depth (volume—inadequate or shallow) Skin—may be pale or cyanotic (blue), cool and clammy

with supplemental oxygen; flow-restricted, oxygen-powered ventilation device; and one-person bag-valve mask with supplemental oxygen. Whatever device is used, you must check to ensure that the ventilations delivered by it are adequate.

The signs of adequate artificial ventilation include the following:

◆ Chest rise and fall with each ventilation

◆ Administration of ventilations at the proper rate (12 per minute for adults, 20 per minute for infants and children)

◆ The patient's heart rate slowing or returning to normal (in pediatric patients, the heart rate increasing to normal)

Signs of inadequate artificial ventilation include the following:

◆ Lack of chest rise or inadequate chest rise with ventilation

◆ Improper rate (either slower or faster than 12 per minute for adults and 20 per minute for infants and children)

◆ Failure of the heart rate to return to normal

If signs indicate that artificial ventilations are inadequate, take corrective action. Check that the patient's airway is open. If it is not, readjust the patient's head position; or insert an oropharyngeal or nasopharyngeal airway; or suction or otherwise clean the airway. Check that the mask seal is adequate and adjust if it is not. Check to assure that the mask is properly hooked up to a source of high flow oxygen and that the oxygen is flowing. Check the force with which ventilations are being delivered; adjust if they are too forceful or—more likely—not forceful enough. Check the rate at which ventilations are being delivered and adjust accordingly if the rate is too fast or too slow.

RESPIRATORY DISTRESS

As noted above, EMTs are called to assist many patients who have some type of breathing difficulty. A general term for this condition is **respiratory distress.** This term covers a wide variety of conditions ranging from shortness of breath to complete respiratory arrest, or stoppage of breathing. There are many conditions that can cause respiratory distress. Illnesses, allergic reactions, cardiac problems, and injuries to the head, face, neck, or chest can lead to respiratory distress. There are also many respiratory diseases that cause respiratory distress (Figure 12-2). For example, you may have heard of or know people with diseases such as asthma and emphysema. Table 12-3 describes several common respiratory conditions and diseases.

Fortunately it is not necessary in most cases to distinguish among diseases or conditions that cause respiratory distress. When you encounter

Figure 12-2 Changes observed at the level of the bronchioles and alveoli as a result of chronic bronchitis and emphysema.

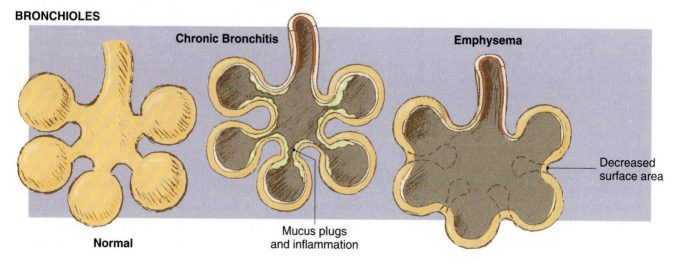

BRONCHIOLES

Chronic Bronchitis

Emphysema

Decreased surface area

Normal

Mucus plugs and inflammation

Table 12-3

Common Respiratory Diseases or Conditions

Disease or Condition	Description
Emphysema	A chronic obstructive pulmonary disease (COPD) that causes the walls of the alveoli to break down and lose elasticity. Excess secretions and damaged alveoli trap stale air in the lungs.
Chronic Bronchitis	A COPD in which the linings of the bronchioles are inflamed. Excessive production of mucus prevents the cilia (small hairs that provide a sweeping motion) from clearing the mucus from the bronchioles.
Asthma	Asthma is *not* a COPD. Triggered by an allergen, exercise, or emotional stress, bronchioles in the lungs constrict and mucus is produced. This causes high-pitched breath sounds (wheezing) and severe difficulty breathing. Asthma effects young and old patients. Asthma is episodic, with attacks occurring at irregular intervals. The patient is free of symptoms between attacks.
Congestive Heart Failure	This is a condition that is caused by the heart but also affects the lungs. The heart fails to pump properly and blood backs up into the pulmonary circulation and into the lungs (pulmonary edema). A patient will have difficulty breathing, noisy breathing, rapid pulse, moist skin that is pale or cyanotic, and swollen ankles. In extreme cases the patient may cough up pink, frothy sputum.

Note: The diseases and conditions presented in this chart are for your information only. Having some knowledge of them may be helpful when you are talking to patients or medical personnel. Patients with respiratory distress all receive similar treatment in the field. It is not necessary to diagnose specific conditions to provide proper treatment.

the signs and symptoms or respiratory distress, your priorities are to ensure an open airway and to facilitate adequate breathing by administering oxygen (Figure 12-3).

Assessment of the Patient in Respiratory Distress

Respiratory distress may range from minor to life threatening. One thing is certain, a patient who is experiencing respiratory distress is often anxious and literally afraid of dying. There are few feelings more frightening than not being able to breathe. A calm demeanor will help during your patient assessment. It will also provide an important part of your treatment—calming the patient.

Look for clues to the nature of the breathing difficulty during the scene size-up. Look for mechanisms of injury that might suggest the problem is trauma related. Also look for inhalers, oxygen tanks, and other medications and devices that might indicate the patient has a respiratory disease.

Proceed with the initial assessment. As you approach the patient to form your general impression, note his position. Many patients with breathing difficulty assume a **tripod position** to ease their breathing efforts (Figure 12-4). They sit upright in a chair leaning slightly forward and supporting themselves with their arms, which rest on the front of the chair between their dangling legs. Note if the patient is restless, agitated, or unresponsive. Such conditions often result from inadequate oxygen reaching the brain. Can the patient talk? Lack of oxygen can cause a patient to mumble or talk incomprehensibly. Or the patient may be able to get only enough air to speak just a word or two at a time.

When assessing the ABCs, pay particular attention to airway and breathing. Are there any sounds—crowing, gurgling, snoring, or stridor—that might indicate airway obstruction? If the airway is obstructed, clear and secure it using suction, repositioning of the patient's head, and airway adjuncts as needed.

Assess the patient's breathing, keeping in mind the signs of adequate and inadequate breathing (Tables 12-1 and 12-2). If the signs indicate the patient is breathing inadequately, stop the assessment and correct this life-threatening condition by

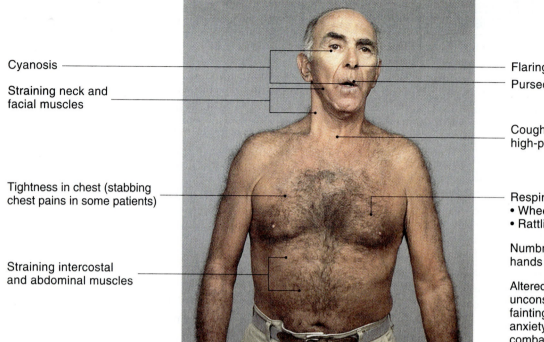

Cyanosis

Straining neck and
facial muscles

Tightness in chest (stabbing
chest pains in some patients)

Straining intercostal
and abdominal muscles

Flaring nostrils
Pursed lips

Coughing, crowing,
high-pitched barking

Respiratory noises
• Wheezing
• Rattling

Numbness or tingling in
hands and feet

Altered levels of awareness,
unconsciousness, dizziness,
fainting, restlessness,
anxiety, confusion,
combativeness

Figure 12-3 Signs and symptoms of respiratory distress.

Figure 12-4 Patients in respiratory distress are
often discovered in a "tripod" position.

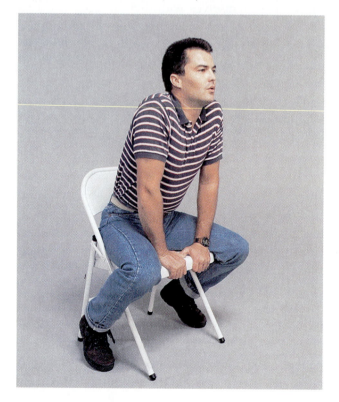

assisting ventilations or by providing artificial ventilations with supplemental oxygen. If the signs indicate the patient is breathing adequately, continue with the assessment.

With responsive patients, conduct a focused history and physical exam. For medical patients, the largest part of this step usually consists of taking the patient's history. Use the OPQRST mnemonic to help you remember the important questions to ask (Table 12-4). Be sure to ask about any treatments or medications that the patient may have taken for the respiratory distress.

Signs and Symptoms of Respiratory Distress

At all the various stages of the assessment process, you should remain alert to the signs and symptoms of respiratory distress. They include the following:

◆ Abnormal rate of breathing (either higher or lower than normal)

◆ Irregular breathing patterns

◆ Shallow breaths

◆ Noisy breathing—wheezing (a musical, high-pitched sound best heard during exhalations),

Table 12-4

OPQRST for Patients with Difficulty Breathing

Use these questions when obtaining information from a breathing difficulty patient.

Onset	When did the difficulty breathing begin? What were you doing?
Provocation	Is there anything that makes your breathing better? Worse?
Quality	Can you describe what the breathing difficulty feels like?
Radiation	Is there pain associated with the difficulty breathing? Has the pain spread to other parts of your body?
Severity	On a scale of 1 to 10, with 10 being the worst, how bad is your breathing difficulty?
Time	How long has this incident of breathing difficulty been going on?

crowing, stridor (a harsh, high-pitched sound usually heard during inhalations), gurgling, snoring

◆ Retractions from use of accessory muscles in the neck, upper chest, and between the ribs

◆ Increased pulse rate in adults

◆ Decreased pulse rate in children

◆ Shortness of breath

◆ Restlessness, anxiety, or other altered mental status

◆ Pale, cyanotic (blue or gray), or flushed skin

◆ Patient positioning

—Tripod position

—Sitting with feet dangling, leaning forward

◆ Barrel chest (common in patients with emphysema)

◆ Inability to speak in full sentences or even to speak a few words without catching a breath

◆ Emergency Care—Respiratory Distress, Breathing Absent or Inadequate

1. **If the scene size-up and initial assessment reveal absent or inadequate breathing,** **establish an open airway.** Use an oropharyngeal or nasopharyngeal airway if necessary to maintain the airway. Consider use of advanced airway techniques, if permitted locally.

2. **Provide artificial ventilations with high concentration oxygen.** If you are uncertain whether the patient's breathing is adequate or inadequate, provide artificial ventilations.

3. **Request an ALS unit meet you en route to the hospital if available.**

4. **Provide rapid transport to the hospital.**

◆ Emergency Care—Respiratory Distress, Breathing Adequate

1. **If the scene size-up and initial assessment reveal the patient is breathing adequately, provide high concentration oxygen via nonrebreather mask.** Use a nasal cannula if the patient will not tolerate a mask.

2. **Complete a focused history and physical examination and obtain baseline vital signs.**

3. **Request that an ALS unit be sent to the scene or to intercept you en route to the**

hospital. Balance your time at the scene with the need for treatment at the hospital. Prompt transportation may be the best care you can provide to the patient.

4. **Provide rapid transport to the hospital.**

5. **If the patient has a prescribed inhaler you may be able to facilitate the use of this medication.** See the section on use of the prescribed inhaler below. Always follow local protocol for medication administration.

6. **Perform the ongoing assessment en route to the hospital.** Monitor the patient closely. Be alert to the possibility that the patient may develop inadequate breathing en route. Begin artificial ventilations with high concentration oxygen if this happens.

Hypoxic Drive

Breathing occurs without conscious control. We do not have to think about breathing 12 times per minute. This is because the brain monitors the level of carbon dioxide in the blood through the use of receptors in the body. If the level of carbon dioxide increases, respirations increase.

In some patients with chronic obstructive pulmonary disease (COPD), the level of carbon dioxide in the blood is at a consistently high level. The receptors in the body can no longer get a proper feel for when the body needs to breathe. When this occurs, the brain looks to the receptors to determine the oxygen content of the blood. The stimulus to breathe then comes from low levels of oxygen in the blood. When oxygen levels decrease, the brain instructs the body to breathe faster and deeper. This condition is known as **hypoxic** (no- or low-oxygen) **drive.**

If a patient has this condition and is given oxygen, the receptors tell the brain that there is plenty of oxygen. The brain directs the body's respiratory efforts to slow or even to stop. Fortunately, hypoxic drive is very rare. Some patients with chronic obstructive pulmonary diseases (emphysema, chronic bronchitis, and black lung) have hypoxic drive, but not all.

In the past, it was recommended that oxygen not be administered to patients with COPD because of the risks associated with the hypoxic

COMPANY OFFICER'S NOTES

It is sometimes difficult to determine the difference between adequate and inadequate breathing. It is even more challenging to assist the ventilations of someone who is breathing inadequately. It is not inconceivable that there will be patients who are still responsive who will require artificial ventilations. Such a situation is rare but intimidating to EMTs.

In these cases, the EMT should explain to the patient what will be done. Then the EMT should attempt to administer the assisted ventilations timed to the patient's natural respiratory efforts. If the patient's respiratory rate is very slow, ventilations should be administered in between the patient's own breaths.

Although assisting the ventilations of a breathing patient may seem awkward, this care can prevent hypoxia, respiratory arrest, and eventual cardiac arrest.

drive. More recently, those who evaluate emergency medical practices have come to believe that withholding oxygen from such patients certainly does more harm than administering it. *Never withhold oxygen from a patient in respiratory distress.*

If a patient with COPD requires oxygen therapy due to severe respiratory distress, chest pain, trauma, or another serious condition, high concentration oxygen should be provided via nonrebreather mask. Monitor the patient's respirations carefully throughout your care. If the patient's respirations slow or cease, be prepared to provide artificial ventilations to the patient immediately.

THE PRESCRIBED INHALER

Many patients with respiratory problems carry inhalers prescribed by their physicians. The prescribed inhaler is one of the medications that you may be allowed to assist the patient in using.

Respiratory diseases such as asthma cause constriction in the bronchioles within the lungs. This causes wheezing and a reduced flow of oxygen to the lungs. Many prescribed inhalers contain medications called **bronchodilators.** Bronchodilators cause the constricted air passages to dilate or widen, thus improving oxygenation and making breathing easier.

Some types of inhalers contain medications other than bronchodilators. In general, EMTs should not assist with the use of these types of inhalers in the prehospital setting.

The prescribed bronchodilator inhaler, or metered dose inhaler (MDI), is constructed to deliver a precisely measured dose of medication to the patient. The generic names of some of the medications that can be found in prescribed inhalers are albuterol, isoetharine, metaproterenol, and ipratropium bromide. Trade names for these medications include Proventil®, Ventolin®, Bronkosol®, Bronkometer®, Metaprel®, Alupent®, and Atrovent®. See the Prescribed Inhaler section on the next page for more information about assisting with MDI.

As noted above, the prescribed inhaler contains a medication that, when used at appropriate doses, opens air passageways and is very beneficial to the patient. That medication, however, may also stimulate the heart, causing an increased pulse rate as well as nervousness and tremors. Because of these potential side effects, it is very important to determine how much, if any, of the medication the patient has taken before your arrival. Medical direction can then determine how many doses, if any, should be administered. Medication administration is a major responsibility that must be taken seriously. Follow local protocols when administering or assisting all medications.

Figure 12-5 A metered dose inhaler with a spacer.

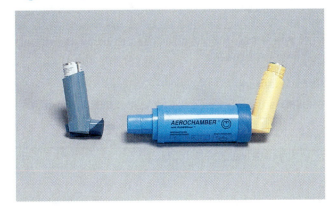

Some inhalers are connected to a device called a **spacer.** The spacer is a chamber into which the medication is delivered before the patient inhales it (Figure 12-5). The spacer prevents any loss of medication to the outside air and permits more effective use of the medication. If the patient has a spacer with his inhaler, be sure to use it.

THE HOME NEBULIZER

With the increase in home care as opposed to hospital-based care, many patients with chronic breathing problems have nebulizer devices in their homes. These devices use either oxygen or air to **nebulize** medications. This means that the devices convert medications like albuterol or ipratropium into a fine vapor mist that the patients then breathe in over several minutes. Nebulizer devices, sometimes called SVNs or small volume nebulizers, are usually more effective in treating acute shortness of breath than standard inhalers. Your medical control physician may authorize you to assist patients in the use of home nebulizers. Follow your local protocols.

INFANTS AND CHILDREN WITH RESPIRATORY COMPLAINTS

Respiratory emergencies are the most common medical cause of death in infants and children in North America. Take all respiratory complaints in this age group seriously.

Children exhibit signs of respiratory distress somewhat differently than adults. For example, children will display retractions (in the neck, upper chest, and between the ribs) more frequently than adults. They may display nasal flaring, in which the nostrils "flare" open with exhalation and clamp down with inhalation. They may also show "seesaw" breathing, in which the abdomen and chest move in opposite directions during breathing.

Children also show signs of severe hypoxia differently than adults. Children with breathing diffi-

(*text continues, page 314*)

PRESCRIBED INHALER

Medication Name

Generic: albuterol, isoetharine, metaproterenol, ipratropium bromide
Trade: Proventil®, Ventolin®, Bronkosol®, Bronkometer®, Metaprel®, Alupent®, Atrovent®

Indications for Administration

All of the following must apply:

1. The patient exhibits signs of respiratory distress.
2. The patient has an inhaler prescribed to him by a physician.
3. Medical direction (either on-line or off-line) has authorized you to assist the patient with use of the medication.

Contraindications

Use of an inhaler is contraindicated if *any* of these conditions exist:

1. The patient is not conscious or otherwise able to use the device.
2. The inhaler is not prescribed for the patient (someone else's inhaler).
3. Medical direction has not authorized use of the inhaler.
4. The patient has already met the maximum prescribed dose before you arrived.

Medication Form

Aerosolized medication in inhaler that delivers pre-measured dose.

Dosage

Number of inhalations based on physician's or medical director's order. Two MDI "puffs" are often prescribed as a normal dose.

Actions

Bronchodilator dilates bronchioles, reducing resistance in the airway.

Side Effects

1. Increased pulse rate
2. Nervousness
3. Tremors

Administration

When you encounter a respiratory distress patient with a prescribed inhaler, follow the steps below to assist him in its use (Figure 12-6 shows steps in administering an inhaler; Figure 12-7 shows the use of an inhaler with a spacer.):

1. **Obtain authorization from medical direction (either on-line or off-line) to assist with administering the medication.**
2. **Determine if the patient has taken any doses of the medication prior to your arrival and, if he has, how many.**
3. **Assure that the medication is the correct one and that it has been prescribed for the patient.**
4. **Assure that the patient is able to use the device.**
5. **Check the expiration date on the inhaler.**
6. **Assure that the inhaler is at room temperature or warmer.**
7. **Shake the inhaler vigorously for at least 30 seconds.**
8. **Remove the oxygen delivery device from the patient.**
9. **Have the patient hold the inhaler upright in his hand, exhale deeply, and put his lips around its opening.** If the patient is unable to hold the inhaler, hold it for him by placing your index finger on the top of the metal canister and your thumb on the bottom of the plastic canister.
10. **Instruct the patient to depress the inhaler as he inhales deeply or to inhale deeply while you depress it.** Usually, two MDI "puffs" are prescribed as a normal dose.
11. **Coach the patient to hold his breath for as long as he comfortably can so that the medication can be absorbed.**
12. **Replace the oxygen delivery device on the patient.**
13. **If medical direction, either on-line or off-line, authorizes a second dose of the medication, repeat steps 7–12 after the patient has taken several breaths.**

Reassessment

Reassess the patient's respiratory distress and vital signs; record your findings. If the patient's breathing becomes inadequate, provide artificial ventilations.

Assisting with a Prescribed Inhaler

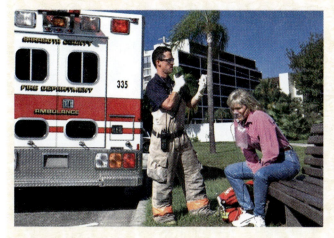

Figure 12-6A Consult with medical direction for authorization to use the inhaler and check the inhaler to make sure it is properly prescribed for the patient and has not reached its expiration date.

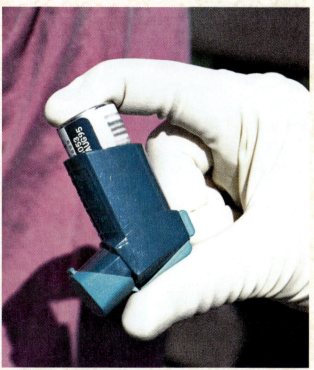

Figure 12-6B Shake the inhaler vigorously for at least 30 seconds.

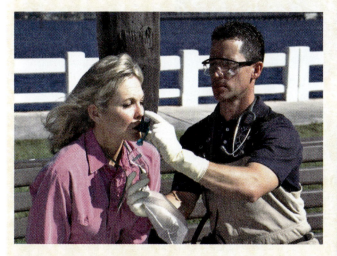

Figure 12-6C Remove the oxygen delivery device. Instruct the patient to inhale deeply and hold her breath while you depress the inhaler to deliver the dose.

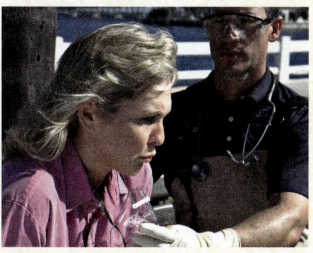

Figure 12-6D Instruct the patient to hold her breath as long as comfortably possible and then to exhale slowly through pursed lips.

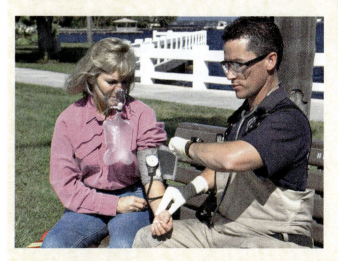

Figure 12-6E Replace the oxygen delivery device. Reassess the patient.

Assisting with a Prescribed Inhaler with a Spacer

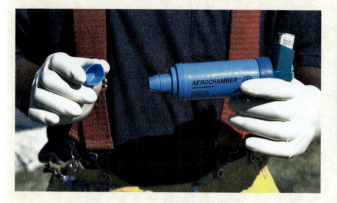

Figure 12-7A Remove the spacer cap and attach the spacer to the inhaler mouthpiece.

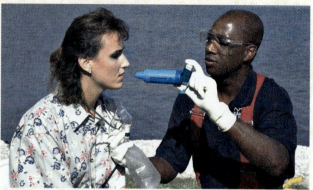

Figure 12-7B Depress the medication canister to fill the spacer with medication.

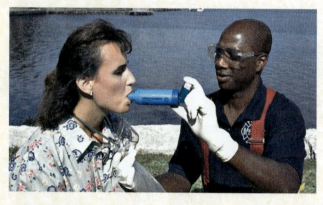

Figure 12-7C Instruct the patient to inhale slowly and deeply. The spacer may whistle if the patient is inhaling too fast.

culty will develop cyanosis much later than adults. A child's pulse will also drop as a result of severe hypoxia. In an adult, a pulse rate that lowers in response to your treatment is a good sign. In a child, it may be a sign that the child is about to suffer cardiac arrest. Any child with signs of inadequate breathing and a decreased heart rate should receive immediate ventilations with high flow oxygen.

If you are delivering artificial ventilations and the infant or child's pulse rate is below expected levels, reevaluate your efforts. Check to be sure the cylinder has not run out of oxygen and that the tubing is not kinked. Check to be sure the airway is open and clear. As necessary, reposition the child's head, suction the airway, or insert an oro- or nasopharyngeal airway.

With infants and children, it is important to distinguish between upper airway obstruction and lower airway disease whenever possible. The *upper airway* is formed by the mouth, nose, pharynx, and epiglottis. Its delicate, narrow structures can easily swell as a result of minor trauma or disease. The *lower airway* is made up of all the structures below the larynx and includes the trachea, the bronchi, the lungs, and all the air passages they contain.

Both upper airway obstruction and lower airway disease can result in pediatric respiratory distress. In both cases, it is important to administer oxygen to the infant or child and place him in a position of comfort. Upper airway obstruction can result from either a foreign object—for example, a piece of a hot dog or a peanut—or from a disease—for example, epiglottitis, which causes a swelling of the epiglottis that can block the airway. In either case, it is crucial that the EMT *not* probe the upper airway unless a foreign object can be clearly seen. Clumsy probing of the mouth and pharynx in children with existing upper airway obstruction can cause complete closure of the airway either from trauma caused by the probing or from reflexive spasming of the larynx.

It may be very difficult to determine whether the cause of a child's breathing problems is upper airway obstruction or lower airway disease. The harsh, high-pitched sound of stridor, usually heard while the patient breathes in, is a clue that the patient may have an upper airway obstruction. In addition, scene size-up evidence, such as a half-eaten hot dog or small pieces of toys lying about, may be clues pointing to upper airway obstruction as the cause of the problem.

As a general emergency care guideline, *never probe the oral cavity or pharynx of an infant or child with breathing difficulty unless a foreign object is visible and reachable in the upper airway*.

Children with respiratory diseases frequently have prescribed inhalers or home nebulizers. Indications for use of a prescribed inhaler or nebulizer for children are the same as for an adult. Remember that child patients have special considerations when it comes to consent. If the child is at school or a camp, health personnel there may have information and consent forms on file. Those personnel may help the child with inhaler use.

Also remember that children become anxious in the presence of strangers, and you and other members of your crew will be seen as strangers. Be prepared to calm the child as you assist him in using the inhaler.

All children in respiratory distress should be placed in a position of comfort. This is usually in the parent's arms with blow-by oxygen provided. (Figure 12-8)

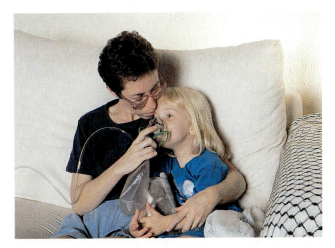

Figure 12-8 A child with respiratory distress may be more likely to tolerate a mask when seated on a parent's lap with the parent holding the mask near the child's face.

SMOKE INHALATION

The use of self-contained breathing apparatus (SCBA) has helped reduce cases of smoke inhalation and lessen the effects of the toxic byproducts of combustion on firefighters. Nevertheless, there may still be situations where firefighters are affected by smoke. In addition, there will always be civilians attempting rescues as well as other victims of fire who may also require care for smoke inhalation.

There are three main components of respiratory injury in fire:

- ◆ *Inhalation of smoke* This causes a reduction of oxygen content in inspired air, respiratory irritation, and—possibly—burns. Depending on the atmosphere and the materials that are burning, carbon monoxide is usually present at high levels.

- ◆ *Inhalation of toxic products of combustion* These products include substances such as hydrogen sulfide or potassium cyanide. They may cause chemical burns of the airway and introduce toxic substances into the bloodstream. The signs and symptoms of toxic inhalation may not show for hours after the inhalation.

Burns These can result as superheated air, steam, and flames enter the airway causing burns to the respiratory tract. The burns can lead to swelling and possible airway obstruction.

Signs and Symptoms of Smoke Inhalation or Heat-Related Airway Injury

In addition to the signs and symptoms of respiratory distress described earlier in the chapter, look for these additional signs and symptoms if smoke inhalation is suspected:

◆ The patient's presence in an area where there was a fire. Enclosed spaces make inhalation of super-heated air more likely.

◆ Soot around the mouth or nose

◆ Singed facial or nasal hair

◆ Stridor or wheezing

◆ Increasing hoarseness

◆ Coughing

COMPANY OFFICER'S NOTES

As a company officer, remember to observe not only patients but also crew members for signs of smoke inhalation.

◆ Emergency Care—Smoke Inhalation or Heat-Related Airway Injury

1. **Perform a thorough scene size-up. Do not attempt a rescue unless properly trained and equipped.**

2. **Remove the patient from the fire or the smoke-filled area.**

3. **Perform an initial assessment and provide artificial ventilations or assisted ventilations as necessary.** Use high concentration oxygen and an appropriate delivery device (pocket face mask, bag-valve mask, flow-restricted, oxygen-powered ventilator, nonrebreather mask).

4. **Perform a focused history and physical exam, remaining alert to the possibility of other injuries.**

5. **Transport the patient promptly to an appropriate facility.**

Chapter Review

SUMMARY

Learning how to evaluate breathing is one of the key skills you must master as an EMT. If you can recognize when a patient is breathing inadequately, you can act quickly to correct this life-threatening situation by providing artificial ventilation with high concentration oxygen.

When you recognize a patient who is experiencing respiratory distress but is breathing adequately, you can reassure him and act to relieve that distress. You can provide high concentration oxygen via nonrebreather mask. If the patient has a prescribed inhaler, you can, with the authorization of medical direction, assist him in using it.

REVIEWING KEY CONCEPTS

1. List the normal breathing rates for adults and for infants and children.
2. List the signs of adequate breathing.
3. List the signs of inadequate breathing.
4. List the signs of inadequate artificial ventilations.
5. Describe corrective actions that might be taken if artificial ventilations are inadequate.
6. List the signs and symptoms of respiratory distress.
7. List the indications and contraindications for assisting in the administration of a prescribed inhaler.
8. Describe the procedure for assisting in the administration of a prescribed inhaler.
9. Describe some of the special considerations in assessing and treating respiratory problems in infants and children.
10. List signs and symptoms of smoke inhalation or heat-related injury.

RESOURCES TO LEARN MORE

"Dyspnea" in Harwood-Nuss, A. L. et al., *The Clinical Practice of Emergency Medicine, 2nd Edition*. Philadelphia: Lippincott-Raven, 1995.

"Dyspnea, Hypoxia, and Hypocapnea" in Tintinalli, J. E. et al., *Emergency Medicine: A Comprehensive Study Guide, 4th Edition*. New York: McGraw-Hill, 1995.

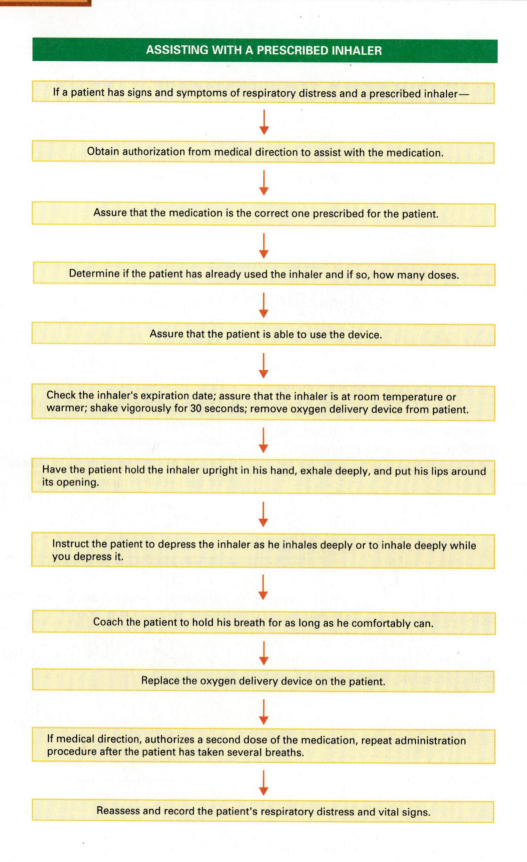

ASSISTING WITH A PRESCRIBED INHALER

If a patient has signs and symptoms of respiratory distress and a prescribed inhaler—

Obtain authorization from medical direction to assist with the medication.

Assure that the medication is the correct one prescribed for the patient.

Determine if the patient has already used the inhaler and if so, how many doses.

Assure that the patient is able to use the device.

Check the inhaler's expiration date; assure that the inhaler is at room temperature or warmer; shake vigorously for 30 seconds; remove oxygen delivery device from patient.

Have the patient hold the inhaler upright in his hand, exhale deeply, and put his lips around its opening.

Instruct the patient to depress the inhaler as he inhales deeply or to inhale deeply while you depress it.

Coach the patient to hold his breath for as long as he comfortably can.

Replace the oxygen delivery device on the patient.

If medical direction, authorizes a second dose of the medication, repeat administration procedure after the patient has taken several breaths.

Reassess and record the patient's respiratory distress and vital signs.

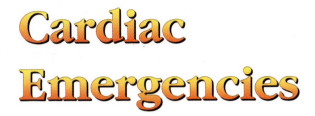

Cardiac
Emergencies

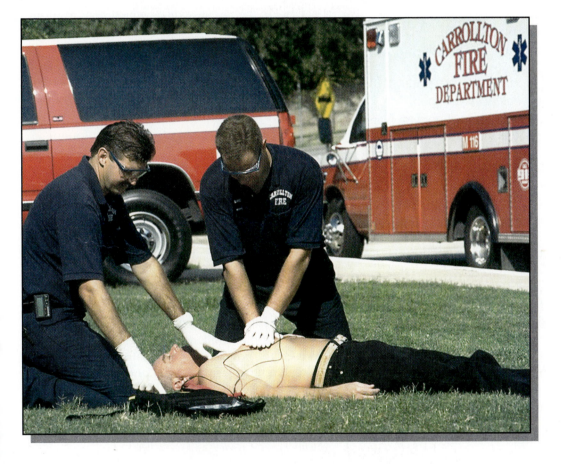

*A*mong the most common calls for EMTs are those from patients with chest pain. Over 600,000 Americans die each year from cardiovascular disease, and half of these deaths occur in the field. You must be able to recognize the warning signs of cardiac emergencies and be prepared to treat patients with them before any significant deterioration can occur. In this chapter, you will learn how and when to provide supplemental oxygen, appropriate medications, and early defibrillation for patients with cardiac emergencies. If properly performed, your interventions in these cases can be truly life saving.

At the completion of this chapter, the EMT-Basic student should be able to meet the following objectives:

Knowledge and Understanding

1. Describe the structure and function of the cardiovascular system. (pp. 322–324)

2. Describe the emergency medical care of the patient experiencing chest pain/discomfort. (pp. 325–342)

3. List the indications for automated external defibrillation. (p. 336)

4. List the contraindications for automated external defibrillation. (p. 336)

5. Define the role of the EMT in the emergency cardiac care system. (pp. 332–335)

6. Explain the impact of age and weight on defibrillation. (p. 336)

7. Discuss the position of comfort for patients with various cardiac emergencies. (p. 327)

8. Establish the relationship between airway management and the patient with cardiovascular compromise. (pp. 323, 327–328)

9. Predict the relationship between the patient experiencing cardiovascular compromise and basic life support. (p. 332)

10. Discuss the fundamentals of early defibrillation. (p. 333)

11. Explain the rationale for early defibrillation. (p. 333)

12. Explain that not all chest pain patients result in cardiac arrest and do not need to be attached to an automated external defibrillator. (pp. 325, 342)

13. Explain the importance of prehospital Advanced Cardiac Life Support intervention if it is available. (pp. 332, 342)

14. Explain the importance of urgent transport to a facility with ACLS if it is not available in the prehospital setting. (pp. 333, 342)

15. Discuss the various types of automated external defibrillators. (pp. 334–336)

16. Differentiate between the fully automated and the semiautomated defibrillators. (p. 334)

17. Discuss the procedures that must be taken into consideration for standard operations of the various types of automated external defibrillators. (pp. 334–336)

18. State the reasons for assuring that the patient is pulseless and apneic when using the automated external defibrillator. (p. 336)

19. Discuss the circumstances which may result in inappropriate shocks. (p. 336)

20. Explain the considerations for interruption of CPR, when using the automated external defibrillator. (p. 337)

21. Discuss the advantages and disadvantages of automated external defibrillators. (pp. 334–336)

22. Summarize the speed of operation of automated external defibrillation. (pp. 334–336)

23. Discuss the use of remote defibrillation through adhesive pads. (p. 335)

24. Discuss the special considerations for rhythm monitoring. (pp. 335–336)

25. List the steps in the operation of the automated external defibrillator. (pp. 338–341)

26. Discuss the standard of care that should be used to provide care to a patient with persistent ventricular fibrillation and no available ACLS. (pp. 342–343)

27. Discuss the standard of care that should be used to provide care to a patient with recurrent ventricular fibrillation and no available ACLS. (pp. 342–343)

28. Differentiate between the single rescuer and multi-rescuer care with an automated external defibrillator. (p. 343)

29. Explain the reason for pulses not being checked between shocks with an automated external defibrillator. (p. 339)

30. Discuss the importance of coordinating ACLS trained providers with personnel using automated external defibrillators. (pp. 332, 342)

31. Discuss the importance of post-resuscitation care. (pp. 342–343)

32. List the components of post-resuscitation care. (pp. 342–343)

33. Explain the importance of frequent practice with the automated external defibrillator. (p. 344)

34. Discuss the need to complete the Automated Defibrillator Operator's Shift Checklist. (p. 344)

35. Discuss the role of the American Heart Association (AHA) in the use of automated external defibrillation. (pp. 332–333)

36. Explain the role medical direction plays in the use of automated external defibrillation. (p. 344)

37. State the reasons why a case review should be completed following the use of the automated external defibrillator. (p. 344)

38. Discuss the components that should be included in a case review. (p. 344)

39. Discuss the goal of quality improvement in automated external defibrillation. (p. 344)

40. Recognize the need for medical direction of protocols to assist in the emergency medical care of the patient with chest pain. (p. 344)

41. List the indications for the use of nitroglycerin. (p. 329)

42. State the contraindications and side effects for the use of nitroglycerin. (p. 329)

43. Define the function of all controls on an automated external defibrillator, and describe event documentation and battery defibrillator maintenance. (pp. 334–335, 344)

44. Defend the reasons for obtaining initial training in automated external defibrillation and the importance of continuing education. (p. 344)

45. Defend the reason for maintenance of automated external defibrillators. (p. 344)

46. Explain the rationale for administering nitroglycerin to a patient with chest pain or discomfort. (pp. 328–329)

Skills

1. Demonstrate the assessment and emergency medical care of a patient experiencing chest pain/discomfort.

2. Demonstrate the application and operation of the automated external defibrillator.

3. Demonstrate the maintenance of an automated external defibrillator.

4. Demonstrate the assessment and documentation of patient response to the automated external defibrillator.

5. Demonstrate the skills necessary to complete the Automated Defibrillator: Operator's Shift Checklist.

6. Perform the steps in facilitating the use of nitroglycerin for chest pain or discomfort.

7. Demonstrate the assessment and documentation of patient response to nitroglycerin.

8. Practice completing a prehospital care report for patients with cardiac emergencies.

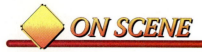

DISPATCH: *ENGINE 15, MEDIC SQUAD 1. RESPOND TO A LIFELINE MEDICAL ALARM. THE ADDRESS IS 442 ELM STREET, APARTMENT 4B. TIME OUT IS 0922.*

You are the EMT assigned to Engine 15. You arrive at 442 Elm and discover that the address is an apartment complex. There are no obvious hazards at the scene, so you and your partner take the medical jump kit and the automated external defibrillator (AED) and proceed to the main door. A man who identifies himself as Mr. Weber, building superintendent, greets you there.

Mr. Weber leads you up to a fourth floor apartment. On the way he says, "It's Mrs. Gordon again. Don't you know her? She's always calling with chest pain. Here's her apartment." He opens the door to let you in and asks, "Can I do anything else?"

You thank him and suggest that he return to the ground floor to guide the paramedic crew to the apartment. Then you and your partner enter the apartment. There you see a woman sitting in a living room armchair. Your first impression is that she is in her 60s and in obvious discomfort. You approach the woman and introduce yourselves, adding, "We're Emergency Medical Technicians with the fire department and we're here to help you. What seems to be the problem?"

Mrs. Gordon replies, "I can't sleep because of this pain in my chest. I put those little white pills that my doctor gave me under my tongue, but the pain just doesn't go away. I keep going to my doctor, but he says nothing is wrong!"

You say, "I'm going to ask you some questions about the pain. Is that okay?"

Before Mrs. Gordon can answer, she suddenly becomes very pale and sweaty and unresponsive. You and your partner help her from the chair to a supine position on the floor to avoid any possibility of injury. You check her ABCs and note that she has no pulse or respiratory effort.

Your partner immediately begins CPR while you prepare the automated external defibrillator (AED). You attach the electrode pads to Mrs. Gordon and direct your partner to stand clear as you push the button to start the AED's analysis of her heart rhythm. The AED indicates that a shock should be delivered and begins to charge. Once the AED is charged, you assure that your partner is still clear of the patient and press the button to deliver the shock.

Immediately after the shock is delivered, Mrs. Gordon wakes up and asks what happened. While explaining to her what happened, you slip a nonrebreather mask on her and supply her with high concentration oxygen. As you do, the paramedics from Squad 1 enter the apartment. You give them a report of your observations of Mrs. Gordon and the care you provided to her. You then assist the paramedics in moving her to the ambulance for transport to the hospital.

Several weeks later, Mrs. Gordon sends a thank-you letter. She explains that her doctors told her that if you hadn't arrived and given the care that you did, she would have died. You saved her life. A homemade chocolate cake accompanies the letter.

ANATOMY AND PHYSIOLOGY OF THE CARDIOVASCULAR SYSTEM

The basic anatomy and physiology of the heart and blood vessels were discussed in Chapter 5. You may wish to review that material at this time.

The discussion below adds to what you have already learned in Chapter 5.

The heart is made up of four chambers, two *atria* and two *ventricles* (Figure 13-1). They work together to pump blood to the entire body. These chambers are connected by valves that prevent

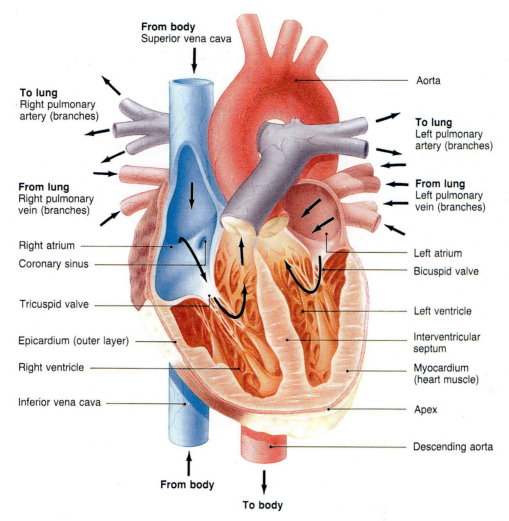

Figure 13-1   The heart.

From body
Superior vena cava

To lung
Right pulmonary
artery (branches)

From lung
Right pulmonary
vein (branches)

Right atrium
Coronary sinus

Tricuspid valve

Epicardium (outer layer)

Right ventricle

Inferior vena cava

From body

To body

Aorta

To lung
Left pulmonary
artery (branches)

From lung
Left pulmonary
vein (branches)

Left atrium
Bicuspid valve

Left ventricle

Interventricular
septum

Myocardium
(heart muscle)

Apex

Descending aorta

blood from flowing backwards. The right side of the heart pumps blood to the lungs and the left side pumps blood to the body.

The major artery coming from the left ventricle is called the *aorta*. Smaller arteries, called the *coronary arteries,* come off the aorta and supply blood to the heart (Figure 13-2). Oxygen for the heart is supplied by these external coronary arteries and not by the blood that flows inside the chambers of the heart. Anything that decreases blood flow to the coronary arteries and heart muscle (for example, a clot or low blood pressure) can cause **ischemia** (lack of oxygen) of the muscle. Remember that all muscles need oxygen to survive and oxygen is carried by the red blood cells. If the heart muscle remains ischemic for too long, the muscle will start to die (**infarction,** or death of tissue). This is why you must give supplemental oxy-

Figure 13-2   The coronary arteries.

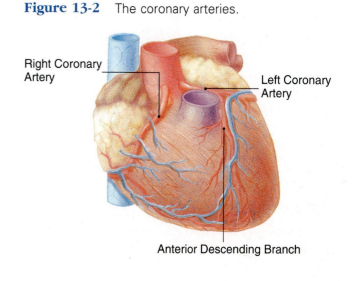

Right Coronary
Artery

Left Coronary
Artery

Anterior Descending Branch

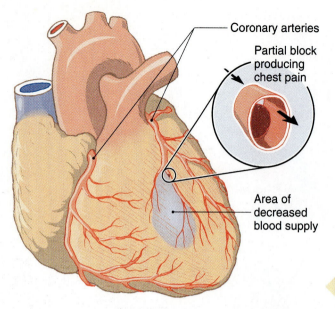

Figure 13-3 Blockage of a coronary artery deprives an area of the heart muscle (myocardium) of oxygen and results in chest pain, or angina pectoris.

gen to patients with suspected heart problems. The pain associated with ischemia is called **angina** (Figure 13-3). If angina progresses due to further narrowing of the coronary arteries it may result in **myocardial** (heart muscle) **infarction** (death), or, as it is commonly called, a heart attack (Figure 13-4). By providing oxygen early on to a patient with a suspected heart problem, you may prevent ischemia from progressing to infarction.

Figure 13-4 Complete blockage of a coronary artery will lead to the death of heart muscle due to lack of oxygen and a resulting heart attack or myocardial infarction.

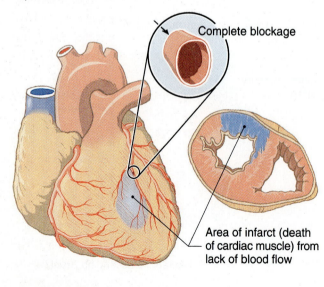

Within the heart muscle is a specialized type of tissue that conducts electrical impulses that enable the heart to contract. Any injury along the paths that carry these impulses can cause a "short circuit," making the heart beat irregularly. These irregular heart rhythms are called **dysrhythmias.** Some heart dysrhythmias may cause the heart to stop pumping, resulting in cardiac arrest. The use of the automated external defibrillator (AED), which will be discussed later in this chapter, may correct these problems and return the heart beat to its normal electrical rhythm.

CARDIAC COMPROMISE

In general, any problem with the heart that causes symptoms such as chest pain or shortness of breath is referred to as **cardiac compromise.** Patients with cardiac compromise may present in many ways. One patient may appear healthy and have normal vital signs; another may be in full cardiac arrest with no vital signs. A patient having a heart attack may complain of chest pain or have no pain at all and just feel "sick." Some signs and symptoms of cardiac compromise may be signs and symptoms of other medical conditions as well. Deciding whether the signs and symptoms result from cardiac compromise or another condition is beyond the scope of your training. Instead, you must treat any patient with signs and symptoms of cardiac compromise as if the problem is the heart.

Assessment of the Cardiac Compromise Patient

When you arrive at the scene, perform a scene size-up to assure that the scene is secure. Be sure to use appropriate body substance isolation equipment and procedures.

Perform an initial assessment. If the patient is unresponsive and pulseless and weighs less than 90 pounds, start CPR. If the patient is unresponsive and pulseless and weighs more than 90 pounds, start CPR and apply an automated external defibrillator (AED) as soon as possible. (Use of the AED is discussed later in this chapter.)

With a responsive patient, take a focused history and perform a physical examination. It is important to ask OPQRST questions like those in Table 13-1. You should also assess and document baseline vital signs.

Signs and Symptoms of Cardiac Compromise

As noted above, cardiac compromise patients can present with a variety of signs and symptoms. These include the following:

◆ Pain, pressure, or discomfort in the chest, upper abdomen, neck, or left shoulder

◆ Difficulty breathing (dyspnea)

◆ Palpitations

◆ Sudden onset of heavy sweating (diaphoresis)

◆ Nausea and/or vomiting

◆ Anxiety or irritability

◆ Feelings of impending doom

◆ Abnormal pulse

◆ Abnormal blood pressure

The most well-known symptom of cardiac compromise listed above is chest pain (Figure 13-5). The pain is often described as "crushing," "aching," or "squeezing." Some patients may deny

pain and instead use some other term such as "discomfort." The pain may radiate (move) to the arm or neck. Encourage the patient to describe the pain in his own words; do not ask leading questions. If a patient has experienced chest pain in the past, ask him to compare the current pain to previous episodes. For instance, if the patient has had a major heart attack and tells you that this pain is very similar, then you should strongly suspect that this pain is associated with a heart problem.

The relationship of pain to the patient's exertion is very important. As you read earlier, heart muscle needs oxygen or it will begin to die. Exertion leads to an increased need for oxygen throughout the body, including the heart muscle. If the additional oxygen is not available, the muscle becomes ischemic and the patient experiences chest pain (angina). The patient may tell you that in recent weeks the pain has come after he has walked short distances; this indicates a reduced blood flow to the heart. The situation may decline to the point where the patient feels pain even when at rest. This progression of angina symptoms is called "unstable" or "pre-infarction" angina. If the patient does not get treatment, infarction may result.

Another common symptom of a heart problem is **dyspnea** (difficulty breathing). Some cardiac compromise patients—especially diabetics—may have dyspnea and no chest pain. Usually, these patients are very anxious and have feelings of impending doom. They may complain of **diaphoresis** (severe sweating), nausea, and vomiting. Again, remember that not all patients have classic symptoms but that all patients with any of the symptoms above must be suspected of having heart problems.

Vital signs, especially pulse and blood pressure, can be important indicators of cardiac compromise. Always check a patient's pulse, particularly its strength and regularity. A normal pulse rate is between 60 and 100. This is only a range, however, and patients may have rates outside of these limits that may still be normal for them. For example, a marathon runner might have a resting pulse of 50, but his health would not be in danger. You must examine these measurements in the context of what is happening

---

Table 13-1

OPQRST for Cardiac Compromise Patients

Use these questions when obtaining information from a cardiac compromise patient.

Onset	When did the pain start and what were you doing when it started?
Provocation	What makes the pain worse?
Quality	What does the pain feel like?
Radiation	Does the pain move anywhere?
Severity	On a scale of 1 to 10, with 10 being the worst, how bad is your pain?
Time	How long have you had this pain?

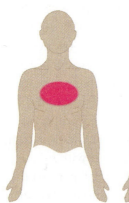
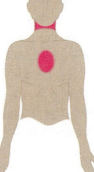
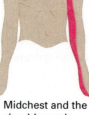
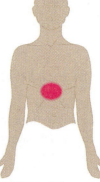
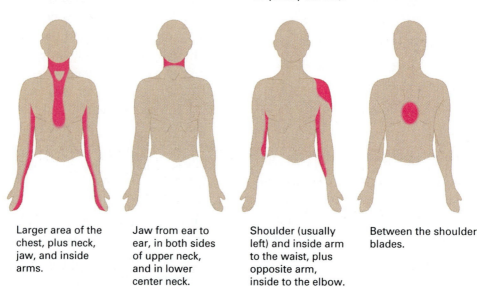

Just under sternum, midchest, or the entire upper chest.

Midchest, neck, and jaw.

Midchest and the shoulder and inside arms (more frequently the left).

Upper abdomen, often mistaken for indigestion.

Larger area of the chest, plus neck, jaw, and inside arms.

Jaw from ear to ear, in both sides of upper neck, and in lower center neck.

Shoulder (usually left) and inside arm to the waist, plus opposite arm, inside to the elbow.

Between the shoulder blades.

Figure 13-5 Typical locations and radiation of chest pain associated with cardiac emergencies.

with the patient. Signs of cardiac compromise include a slow pulse of less than 60 beats per minute, called **bradycardia,** and a fast pulse of more than 100 beats per minute, called **tachycardia.** An irregular pulse, which indicates the presence of a dysrhythmia, may be another sign.

A cardiac compromised patient's blood pressure may be normal. It may also be high, with a systolic pressure greater than 150 mmHg or a diastolic pressure greater than 90 mmHg (a condition called **hypertension**). In another patient, the blood pressure may be low, with a systolic pressure less than 90 mmHg (a condition called **hypotension**). Hypotension is a sign of severe

hypoperfusion, or shock. This is likely due to the loss of the heart's ability to pump effectively. When the body is in shock, there is inadequate blood flow to all tissues of the body including the heart. This condition can cause ischemia and can also lead to infarction. Inadequate blood flow to the brain may cause a patient to pass out and lose consciousness, a condition called **syncope.**

◆ *Emergency Care—Cardiac Compromise*

1. **Place the patient in a comfortable position.** This will usually be sitting up. If the patient is *hypotensive* (has low blood pres-

sure), lay him down and elevate his feet above the level of his heart, if possible. Doing this will cause more blood flow to go to the heart and brain. The patient who is having difficulty breathing or has fluid in the lungs (congestive heart failure) will feel better sitting up. The rule here is to make the patient comfortable—that is, to find a position that causes the patient the least discomfort.

2. **Administer high flow oxygen (15 lpm) via a nonrebreather mask.** You will hear people talk about the need to withhold oxygen to patients with certain lung diseases (for instance, emphysema) and say that if you give it, the patient may stop breathing. You must remember that a cardiac compromise patient desperately needs oxygen; without it, irreversible damage to the heart or even death may occur. Use a nonrebreather mask only if the patient is breathing. If the patient is not breathing, no air exchange will take place. In this case, you must manually ventilate a non-breathing patient using a pocket mask, bag-valve-mask device, or other similar device.

3. **Continually monitor the patient's ABCs.** Be ready for the possibility that your patient's heart may stop beating (cardiac arrest). Be prepared to begin CPR and apply an automated external defibrillator.

4. **If the patient has been prescribed nitroglycerin, if it is available, if your department's protocols permit, and if there are no contraindications to its use, you may assist him in taking this medication.** Nitroglycerin is usually administered only to patients with chest pain. Procedures for assisting with administration of nitroglycerin are described below.

5. **Transport the patient promptly.** Consider calling for Advanced Life Support (ALS) assistance, if it has not already been dispatched.

Nitrogylcerin

Nitroglycerin is a potent medication that is used to treat chest pain in patients with angina (Figure 13-6). It works by relaxing (dilating) blood vessels and decreasing the workload of the heart. Your local protocols may allow you to administer or assist a patient with his prescribed nitroglycerin. Always be sure that the nitroglycerin a patient has in his possession has actually been prescribed for him. Nitroglycerin is a powerful drug. It is never appropriate and is potentially dangerous for a patient to take a family member's or friend's pills. To use the drug properly, you must also become

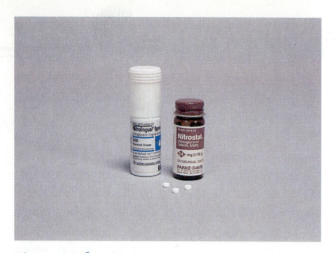

Figure 13-6 Nitroglycerin spray (left) and nitroglycerin tablets (right).

familiar with its indications, contraindications, actions, and method of administration.

Nitroglycerin does not retain its effectiveness for very long in storage. Patients often possess outdated medication. Check the label on the medication to confirm that it was prescribed for your patient and that its expiration date has not passed. If you suspect that the medicine is no longer effective, ask the patient if he got a headache or felt a tingle under his tongue after you gave the medication. The absence of a headache or tingling sensation may indicate that the medicine has lost its potency.

CARDIAC ARREST

The most serious form of cardiac compromise is **cardiac arrest.** When a patient is in cardiac arrest, his normal heart beat stops or is replaced by a different kind of electrical activity. Sometimes the activity may produce an extremely fast rhythm. Sometimes it may result in twitching, or **fibrillation** of the heart muscle. These abnormal heart actions do not support an adequate flow of blood to the body. A patient in cardiac arrest is unresponsive, with no pulse or respirations. When the heart's pumping action stops, the body's cells begin to die. Within 4 to 6 minutes, brain cells begin to die. Without rapid and effective treatment, the patient will die.

The American Heart Association has identified four key factors that affect the chances of successful resuscitation of cardiac arrest patients in an out-of-hospital setting. The association calls them the "chain of survival" (Figure 13-8):

◆ **Early access**—This means that when people see someone having a cardiac problem, a system is in place that allows them to contact EMS rapidly to summon help. Local EMS systems should publicize their 9-1-1 or other access numbers so that people know where to call in cases of cardiac emergency. The EMS system must also be well organized so that appropriate resources reach the scene swiftly.

◆ **Early CPR**—Early CPR can increase a cardiac arrest patient's chances of survival. EMTs are trained in CPR and can begin to provide it as soon as they arrive on the scene. But EMS systems should try to assure that police and other likely first responders also have CPR training. Systems should provide training so that dispatchers can instruct callers over the phone on how to perform CPR prior to EMS arrival. Finally, EMS systems should offer courses so that as much of the general public as possible knows how to perform CPR.

◆ **Early defibrillation**—As noted previously, in cases of cardiac arrest the heart's normal electrical impulses may be replaced by extremely rapid rhythms or by uncoordinated fibrillation. The heart can, in many cases, be restored to its normal rhythms, however, by the application of an external electrical shock. This is known as **defibrillation.** Since sudden cardiac death claims an estimated 350,000 lives each year and many victims experience no prior symptoms, and since the likelihood of successful resuscitation decreases by approximately 10 percent with each minute following the onset of sudden cardiac arrest, early defibrillation is critical. The American Heart Association estimates that as many as 100,000 deaths could be prevented each year through the widespread use of defibrillators.

(text continues, page 334)

NITROGLYCERIN

Medication Name

Generic: nitroglycerin (NTG)
Trade: Nitrostat®, Nitrobid®, Nitrolingual® Spray

Indications for Administration

All of the following conditions must be met:

1. The patient has signs and symptoms of cardiac chest pain.
2. The patient has a history of heart problems.
3. The patient's physician has prescribed the nitroglycerin for him.
4. The patient has a systolic blood pressure greater than 100 mmHg.
5. Medical direction, either on-line or off-line, authorizes administration of the medication.

Contraindications

Do not administer nitroglycerin if any of the following conditions apply:

1. The patient has a systolic blood pressure less than 100 mmHg.
2. The patient is an infant or child.
3. The patient has taken the maximum prescribed dose prior to your arrival.

Medication Form

Sublingual (under-the-tongue) tablets or a sublingual spray

Actions

Relaxes blood vessels
Decreases the workload of the heart

Side Effects

Hypotension (low blood pressure)
Headache
Changes in pulse rate

Dosage

One dose (one tablet or one spray) given under the tongue (sublingually). The dose may be repeated in 5 minutes if the patient's pain is not relieved and his systolic blood pressure remains above 100 mm Hg. Obtain authorization from medical direction for each dose administered. In general, a total of three doses of nitroglycerin may be administered (the total should include any doses that the patient took before arrival of EMS). Follow specific local protocols when assisting with the administration of nitroglycerin.

Administration

Follow the steps below when administering nitroglycerin to a patient (Figure 13-7):

1. **Perform a focused cardiac assessment and determine that the patient has his own nitroglycerin.**
2. **Take the patient's blood pressure to assure that it is greater than 100 mmHg systolic.**
3. **Obtain an order from medical direction either on-line or off-line.**
4. **Check that the nitroglycerin is prescribed for the patient now under your care.**
5. **Check the expiration date of the nitroglycerin.**
6. **Check that the patient is alert and responsive.** Do not administer nitroglycerin to a patient who is not alert.
7. **Ask the patient when he last took the medication and how much he used.**
8. **Ask the patient to lift his tongue and place the tablet or spray a dose under the tongue, or have the patient place the medicine under his tongue.** Do not touch the medicine with your bare skin as it will be absorbed by your body and may adversely affect you. Wear gloves!
9. **Have the patient keep his mouth closed and not swallow until the tablet is dissolved.**
10. **Recheck the patient's blood pressure within 2 minutes after the tablet has dissolved or the spray was administered.** Document the results, including dosage, time of administration, route, and the patient's response.
11. **Reassess the patient.**
    a. Monitor blood pressure.
    b. Monitor pain relief.
    c. Monitor pulse rate.
    d. Record measurements.
    e. Contact medical direction before administering another dose of the drug.

Administration of Nitroglycerin

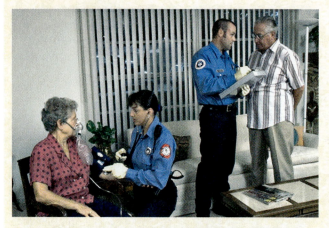

Figure 13-7A   After placing the cardiac compromise patient in a position of comfort and providing high flow oxygen, determine during the focused history and physical exam if the patient has prescribed nitroglycerin.

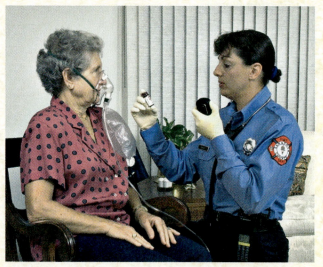

Figure 13-7B   If the patient meets the criteria for nitroglycerin, consult with medical direction or follow standing orders on administering the medication.

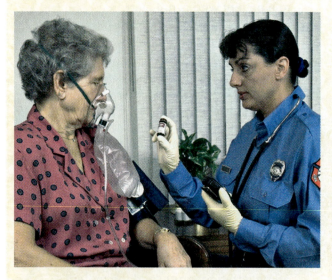

Figure 13-7C   Check the medication to assure right patient, right drug, right dose, right route. Also check the medication's expiration date.

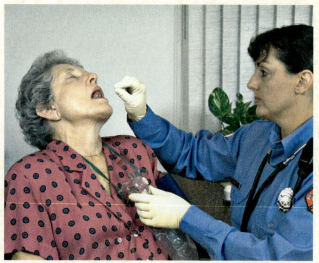

Figure 13-7D   Remove the oxygen mask and ask the patient to open mouth and lift tongue.

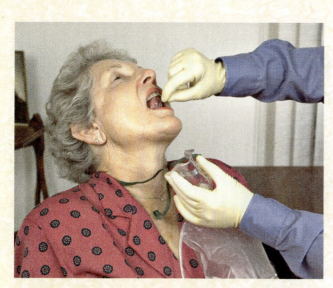

Figure 13-7E Place the nitroglycerin tablet under the patient's tongue. Then direct the patient to close mouth and hold the tablet under it until the tablet dissolves and the medication is absorbed.

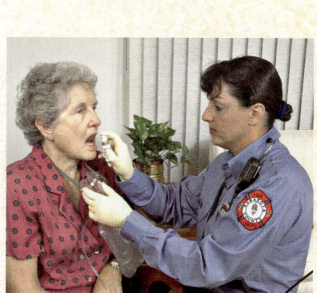

Figure 13-7F If the patient's nitroglycerin is in spray form, spray a dose under the tongue following package instructions. Then direct the patient to close mouth as the medication is absorbed.

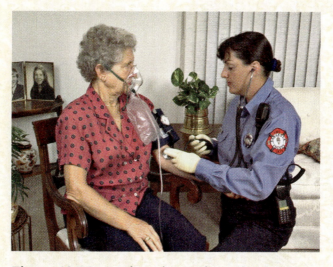

Figure 13-7G Replace the mask on the patient and assess the patient's response to the medication, monitoring blood pressure, pain relief, and pulse rate. If another dose of nitroglycerin is required, check with medical direction or follow standing orders.

Chain of Survival

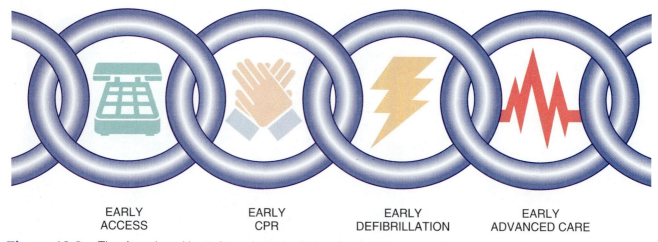

EARLY ACCESS   EARLY CPR   EARLY DEFIBRILLATION   EARLY ADVANCED CARE

Figure 13-8   The American Heart Association's chain of survival.

New, more sophisticated **automated external defibrillators** (AEDs) are in fact becoming increasingly available. For example, some airlines have begun to carry AEDs aboard their planes. In addition, more people are being trained in defibrillation, a skill that once took hundreds of hours to master. Defibrillation became a part of the EMT curriculum in 1994, thus ensuring that thousands more EMS personnel would know how to perform the procedure. To be effective, however, defibrillation must be done early. To ensure this, more AEDs must be on board more emergency vehicles, such as engines or rescue companies, so that first responders can use them in time.

◆ *Early Advanced Cardiac Life Support (ACLS)*—Even though EMT-Bs are now trained to defibrillate patients, they are not authorized to provide additional types of lifesaving care such as starting an intravenous (IV) line and administering medications through it. Complete control of the cardiac patient's airway by endotracheal intubation is also a critical part of ACLS (see Chapter 29). Those advanced skills can be performed by doctors, paramedics, and EMT-Intermediates. As an EMT-B, you have a responsibility to see that your patient gets needed ACLS care as

rapidly as possible. This means you must recognize conditions requiring ACLS care and request that care early, if it is not automatically dispatched in your system. You must also make every effort to transport a cardiac arrest patient rapidly, either to a rendezvous with an ACLS unit or to definitive hospital care. Your EMS system will have protocols about ACLS care; know them and follow them.

DEFIBRILLATION

Defibrillators save lives by converting uncoordinated or abnormal electrical heart rhythms that are deadly into stable ones. As mentioned earlier, the heart contains an electrical conduction system that causes it to beat. A defibrillator uses electrodes placed on a patient's chest to study the heart's electrical activity. Automated defibrillators can analyze that activity and determine if certain abnormal rhythms can be converted to normal ones by delivery of an electric shock.

When working with an AED, there are two heart rhythms considered "shockable"—ventricular fibrillation and ventricular tachycardia.

- **Ventricular fibrillation (VF or V-Fib)** is found in about half of all cardiac arrest victims when EMS personnel arrive in the first 8 minutes after the patient goes into arrest. This rhythm represents very disorganized electrical activity originating from many different sites in the heart. The heart is "shaking" and cannot pump blood adequately. When caught early, defibrillation can be very effective with this rhythm.
- **Ventricular tachycardia (V-Tach)** is an organized heart rhythm, but one that is too fast. The heart pumps so rapidly that it doesn't have time to fill, with the result that not enough blood is pumped to the heart and brain. V-Tach is found in about 10 percent of cardiac arrest patients. Patients with V-Tach who are unresponsive and have no pulse or respirations can receive shocks from the defibrillator. However, some V-Tach patients may be responsive and have both a pulse and respirations. *DO NOT* deliver a shock to these patients. Attach the AED only to unresponsive patients with no pulse and no respirations. Remember: if a patient is talking and awake he *must* have a pulse, and therefore the AED should not be used to shock.

DEFIBRILLATORS

There are several types of defibrillators. They fall into two broad categories, internal and external.

Internal Defibrillators

A cardiac arrest patient who survives a first episode and is at risk for another in the future may have an internal defibrillator implanted at the hospital. Known as an **automatic implantable cardioverter defibrillator** (AICD), the device is placed under the skin and functions like the external types. If you see signs of one of these devices under the skin of the chest wall in a cardiac arrest patient, you may still use an automated defibrillator on the patient. However, you should be sure to place electrode pads at least 5 inches from the site of the AICD. The same spacing considerations apply if you see signs of a pacemaker (a device which controls the rate of a patient's heart beat) on the patient's chest wall.

External Defibrillators

External defibrillators can be manual or automated. The manual type is used by paramedics and in hospitals. With it, the operator studies the patient's heart rhythm on a screen and decides if the rhythm shown can be corrected by a shock. If it can, the operator places two lubricated paddles on the patient's chest and delivers a shock. In newer manual defibrillators, large electrodes (like those used with AEDs) can be applied to the chest wall to deliver shocks without the use of paddles. Use of the manual defibrillator requires extensive training to ensure that the operator knows how to recognize a shockable heart rhythm.

Automated external defibrillators and their use will be the focus of the rest of the chapter.

AUTOMATED EXTERNAL DEFIBRILLATORS (AEDS)

Automated external defibrillators (AEDs) use computer technology to analyze a patient's heart rhythms and determine when administering a shock is appropriate. There are two types of AEDs, fully automated and semi-automated.

Fully Automated AEDs

With the fully automated AED, the EMT need only attach the device to the patient and turn it on. The AED analyzes the patient's heart rhythms and, if it determines a shock is appropriate, charges up and delivers the shock automatically.

Semi-Automated AEDs

Most AEDs that EMTs will use are semi-automated (Figure 13-9). With the semi-automated AED, the EMT attaches the device to the patient, turns it on, and pushes a button to begin rhythm analysis. The AED analzyes the heart rhythms and then advises the EMT, either through a voice synthesizer or a computer display, about whether or not

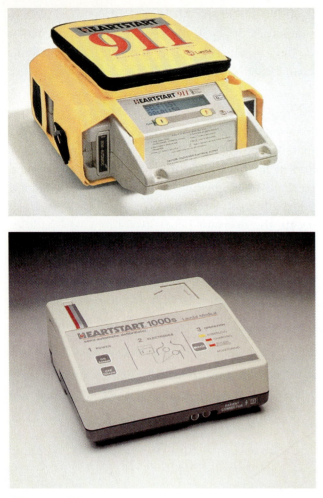

Figure 13-9 Two examples of semi-automated external defibrillators.

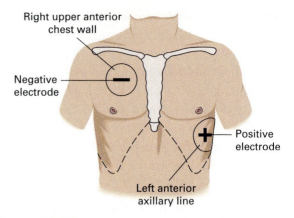

Figure 13-10 Proper placement of electrode pads for automated external defibrillation.

to deliver a shock. The EMT must push another button to deliver the shock. Since minimal operator training is necessary for the fully automated AED, this discussion will focus on use of the semi-automated AED.

Advantages of AEDs

Technological improvements in recent years have added to the benefits of using AEDs in emergency medicine. Because the devices can automatically evaluate a patient's heart rhythms and determine if a shock is needed through the electrodes attached to the patient's chest, the initial training and continuing education are much simpler for operators of those devices than for manual defibrillation. Generally, most EMTs are more comfortable with this procedure because the defibrillation is "hands-off"—pushing a button on a device

away from the patient rather than holding charged paddles against the patient's chest as is necessary with most manual defibrillators.

AEDs offer other advantages over manual defibrillation through their use of electrode pads rather than paddles to read the heart rhythms and deliver the shock. The pads are secured to the patient's chest with adhesive; this assures better placement and provides a greater surface area in contact with the patient's chest than paddles can provide (Figures 13-10 and 13-11). Because the pads are secured to the chest, there is less of a chance of the electrical "arcing" and patient burns that can result from not putting enough pressure against the chest wall with paddles.

Figure 13-11 An alternative placement of electrode pads for defibrillation has the positive (+) pad placed anteriorly over the apex of the heart and the negative (–) pad placed posteriorly, near the center of the back and 1″ to 2″ (25 to 50 mm) above the anterior pad.

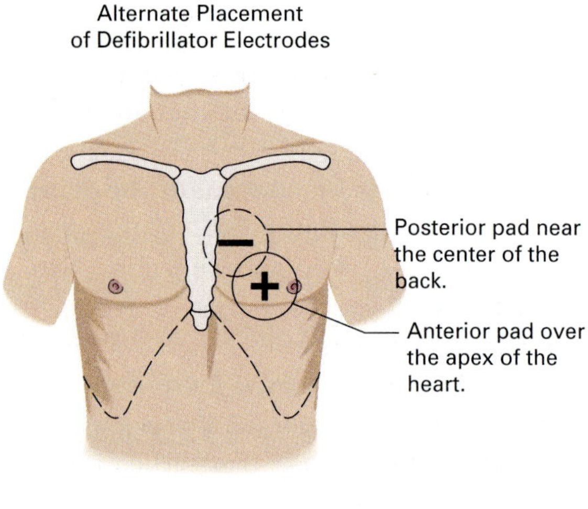

Alternate Placement
of Defibrillator Electrodes

Posterior pad near the center of the back.

Anterior pad over the apex of the heart.

Another advantage of the AED is the speed with which it can be used. The first shock can be delivered within 1 minute of the EMT's arrival at the patient's side with the device! Because time is such a critical factor in cases of cardiac arrest, this is truly a major advantage.

AEDs are extremely reliable devices. Their sophisticated computer microprocessors enable them to analyze cardiac rhythms and deliver shocks while making very few errors. Even some of the mechanical errors that occur with AEDs are at least partly the fault of humans. Those errors result from failure to maintain the AED properly. To decrease the risk of mechanical error, keep the AED in good operating condition, follow the manufacturer's instructions for operation and maintenance, and always be sure the AED is equipped with fresh, fully charged batteries.

Most mistakes in AED operation result from other types of human error. For example, the operator used the device on a patient for whom its use was contraindicated (such as a patient who is awake) or the operator failed to follow instructions while operating the device. To reduce the chance of human error, AED operators should practice with the device frequently, become comfortable with how the AED works, and always follow local protocols for its use.

When and When Not to Use the AED

The AED can save the lives of patients in cardiac arrest. However, it should not be used with *every* cardiac arrest patient. Follow your department's protocols on when and how to use the AED. Generally, however, the AED should be used with a patient only when *ALL* of the conditions listed below are met:

- The patient is an adult (over 12 years of age) in cardiac arrest.
- The patient weighs more than 90 pounds (40 kg).
- The patient is unresponsive, has no pulse, and is not breathing.

Do *NOT* use an AED with a patient if *ANY* of the following conditions apply:

- The patient is responsive, has a pulse, and is breathing. Do not even attach the AED to

such a patient. Shocking such a patient is dangerous and may even cause his death.

- The patient is an infant or child. This is defined as someone under age 12 or who weighs less than 90 pounds (40 kg).

  AED use is not appropriate with infants and children because the device may generate and deliver too much energy. (The electric charge needed to convert a heart rate is based on the patient's weight.) Also, the pads may be too large for a child or infant's chest.

  Note that it is very rare for a child to present with a cardiac rhythm that is susceptible to shock. Cardiac arrest in infants and children usually is the result of respiratory problems. Appropriate care is more likely to be airway management and artificial ventilation rather than defibrillation.

- The patient is a victim of trauma. Trauma patients in cardiac arrest do not usually develop rhythms that may be converted by defibrillation, but when they do, it is usually too late for electrical shock to be helpful. In these cases, the use of an AED may delay transport and should not be used.

Safety Concerns with AEDs

Although the AED is a proven life saver, thoughtless use of the device can be dangerous. Never forget that the AED uses electricity and can deliver a strong shock not only to the patient but also to you if you are careless. Keep the following safety tips in mind whenever you use an AED (Figure 13-12):

- If it is raining, move the patient inside or to a dry area before using the AED. Likewise, if the patient is wet—for example, if he has been pulled from a swimming pool—move him to a dry spot and dry his chest before using the AED.

- If the patient is on a metal stretcher or a metal surface—for example, the bleachers at a football field or a catwalk—make sure that no one is touching the patient or the metal before using the AED. If necessary, move the patient off the metal surface before using the AED.

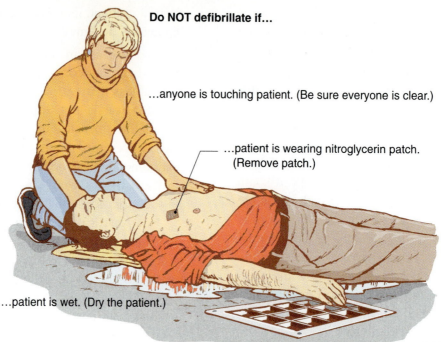

Do NOT defibrillate if...

...anyone is touching patient. (Be sure everyone is clear.)

...patient is wearing nitroglycerin patch. (Remove patch.)

...patient is wet. (Dry the patient.)

...patient is touching metal. (Move away from metal.)

Figure 13-12 Be alert for possible safety hazards when using an AED.

◆ Always remember to say "Clear!" loudly and to look the patient over from head to toe before beginning a rhythm analysis or delivering a shock. This will help assure that no one is in contact with the patient.

◆ If a patient has a nitroglycerin patch on his chest, remove it with a gloved hand before applying the defibrillator electrodes and wipe the area clean with a towel or gauze pad before delivering a shock. The shock could melt the plastic or ignite it. Also, be careful not to touch the medicated surface of the patch with your bare hands; because you are not used to the nitroglycerin, you could pass out or get a severe headache.

◆ If the AED has loose or exposed wires, remove the unit from service immediately and obtain a replacement unit.

CPR and AEDs

Early defibrillation can significantly increase a patient's chance for resuscitation and should be performed as soon as possible. However, basic CPR is still a key part of the defibrillation procedure. Remember that when a patient is in cardiac arrest, the heart cannot deliver blood to the vital organs. Until the patient's heart begins beating on its own, CPR is the only way blood and oxygen will reach the heart and brain.

CPR is important, but use of the AED has been proven more effective in saving the lives of cardiac arrest patients. Therefore, CPR and use of the AED must be carefully coordinated. You will have to stop CPR at certain points to allow the AED to work properly. However, if the AED does not immediately restore the patient's pulse, you

COMPANY OFFICER'S NOTES

Family members or bystanders may have started CPR before your arrival on the scene. Since they are probably not familiar with the protocols and use of the AED, you must make sure that no one is touching the patient when the computer is analyzing the rhythm. It is common for some bystanders or family members to feel frustrated when the AED is working because they feel that "everyone is standing around doing nothing." Someone may begin CPR without authorization. This situation requires firm control and guidance. No one can touch a patient when the AED is analyzing or shocking!

may have to provide an interval of CPR before trying to defibrillate again.

Basically, your partner or another rescuer will provide CPR while the AED is being prepared. Once the device is ready and attached to the patient, CPR must stop and no rescuer should touch the patient. If a CPR provider remained in contact with the patient, the device could give incorrect readings, and the provider would also risk receiving a shock. CPR may be halted for up to 90 seconds while a sequence of analyses and shocks is delivered, but it should be restarted after the sequence is completed. CPR may be interrupted again for further analyses and shocks. Details of when to stop and start CPR during defibrillation are given in "Emergency Care—Cardiac Arrest Patients" below.

Assessment of the Cardiac Arrest Patient

Perform the scene size-up to assure that the scene is secure. Be sure to use body substance isolation equipment and procedures appropriate to the conditions you discover.

Once the scene is secure, begin the initial assessment. If the patient with a suspected cardiac problem is responsive, you would proceed with the assessment and emergency care of the cardiac compromise patient described earlier in this chapter.

When the patient with a suspected cardiac problem is unresponsive and an AED is not available, you will provide CPR and follow the Basic Cardiac Life Support procedures that you learned as a prerequisite to this course. (You may review those procedures in Appendix B, pages 805–832).

When the patient with a suspected cardiac problem is unresponsive and an AED is available, follow this procedure. If a family member or a bystander is performing CPR, direct him to stop. Then, personally verify that the patient is pulseless and not breathing (apneic). If the patient is unresponsive, pulseless, and not breathing, he is in cardiac arrest. In this case, have your partner resume CPR including ventilations with high concentration oxygen.

If the cardiac arrest patient is a child or an adult victim of trauma, do not use the AED unless

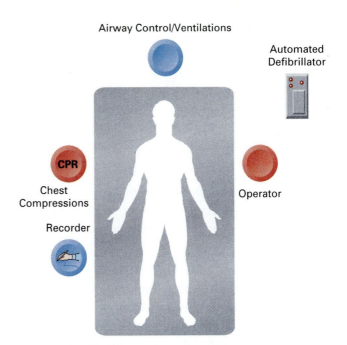

Figure 13-13   A layout of personnel and equipment for automated external defibrillation. Field conditions may not always permit use of this layout, so practice with alternative arrangements as well as this one.

instructed to do so by medical direction or local protocols. Instead, continue CPR and transport the patient rapidly.

If the cardiac arrest patient is an adult, prepare to deliver emergency care using the AED. Have your partner continue CPR while you set up the AED (Figure 13-13).

If another crew member is available, he can try to perform the focused history and physical exam. Since the patient is unresponsive, he will have to question family members or bystanders to learn what he can about the onset of the problems and any signs and symptoms the patient may have displayed before collapsing. Do not, however, let obtaining a focused history and physical exam delay efforts at providing optimal CPR or defibrillation.

◆ *Emergency Care—Cardiac Arrest Patient*

Follow the steps below to use the AED on an unresponsive, pulseless, apneic adult patient (Figure 13-14).

1. **Begin or continue CPR.** Ventilations should deliver high concentration oxygen.

2. Prepare the patient:

   a. Expose the chest. Try to respect the patient's privacy, but do not let this courtesy cause any delay in defibrillation.

   b. Quickly shave the patient's chest if there is too much hair and you think that it will keep the electrode pads from making good contact with the chest.

   c. Use towels or gauze rolls to dry patients who have been sweating heavily, been in the rain, or have otherwise gotten wet so that the electrode pads will adhere better.

   d. Place the pads on the chest so that one cable is situated in the angle between the sternum and right clavicle and the other one is attached over the lower left ribs. Alternatively, the pads may be applied anteriorly and posteriorly. (See Figures 13-10 and 13-11 on page 336.) Since there are several different manufacturers of these machines, each with different instructions, make sure you are familiar with your department's unit.

3. Turn on the AED power.

4. Begin the narrative if the machine has a tape recorder. Give your name and unit, the time, and the situation as you found it. Describe what you have done and continue to describe your actions as you go on with the defibrillation procedure.

5. Stop CPR and make sure that no one is touching the patient. If people are touching the patient, the AED's analysis of heart rhythms may be faulty.

6. Press the "Analyze" button to begin an analysis of the rhythm.

If you get a "Deliver shock" message when you press the "Analyze" button, proceed with steps 7 to 11. If you get a "No shock" message, proceed to step 12:

7. When you get a "Deliver shock" message, loudly say "Clear!" while looking the patient over from head to toe to make sure no one is touching him and do the following:

   a. Press the "Shock" button to deliver a shock.

   b. Press the "Analyze" button to re-analyze the rhythm.

   c. If the machine advises "Deliver shock" again, check to make sure everyone is clear, call "Clear!," and press the button to deliver a second shock.

   d. Re-analyze the rhythm.

   e. If the machine advises "Deliver shock" once again, check to make sure everyone is clear, call "Clear!," and press the button to deliver a third shock.

You have now delivered what is called a "set of three stacked shocks." They are called "stacked" because they are given with no pauses between the shocks to check the patient's pulse or to perform CPR.

8. Check the patient's pulse. If the patient has a pulse, check the breathing and proceed as follows:

   a. If the patient is not breathing adequately, begin artificial ventilations with high concentration oxygen via bag-valve mask and transport.

   b. If the patient is breathing adequately, give high flow oxygen using a nonrebreather mask and transport.

9. If the patient has no pulse, resume CPR for 1 minute.

10. After one minute of CPR, repeat the analysis and shock sequence (steps 7 and 8 above) for up to three more shocks (a second set of three stacked shocks).

11. Assuming that an ACLS unit is not on the scene, you should resume CPR and transport the patient to the hospital if he has not regained a pulse after six shocks.

If you get a "No Shock" message when you press the "Analyze" button, proceed as below:

12. When you get a "No shock" message, check the patient's pulse and proceed as follows:

   a. If the patient has a pulse but is not breathing or not breathing adequately, begin artificial ventilations with high concentration oxygen via BVM and transport.

b. If the patient has a pulse and is breathing adequately, provide high concentration oxygen via nonrebreather mask, and transport.

c. If no the patient has no pulse, resume CPR for 1 minute and repeat an analysis of the rhythm.

    i. If you get a "Deliver shock" message, follow steps 7 to 11 above and deliver up to six shocks (two sets of three stacked shocks).

    ii. If you get a "No shock" message, resume CPR for 1 minute. Re-analyze again. If you receive three "No shock" messages (with 1 minute of CPR between analyses), then resume CPR and transport.

Key Ideas in AED

Always keep the following basic points in mind when using an AED:

◆ Make sure you know how to operate the type of AED used by your department.

◆ Remember that defibrillation comes first. Do it before hooking up oxygen or performing other interventions. If you have a partner, have him initiate CPR while you get the defibrillator ready.

◆ Make sure that one EMT operates the defibrillator while the other performs CPR.

◆ During computer analysis of the rhythm, make sure no one touches the patient. Don't perform CPR while the machine is analyzing.

◆ Say "Clear!" very loudly and look the patient over from head to toe to make sure no one is touching him or any metal in contact with him before administering a shock.

◆ When the heart is not beating by itself, the only way to bring oxygenated blood to it is by performing CPR. Perform 1 minute of CPR between sets of three stacked shocks or after three consecutive "No shock" messages.

◆ Transport a cardiac arrest patient after any of the following conditions is met:

TRANSITION OF CARE

    Always coordinate your defibrillation efforts with your local Advanced Life Support (ALS) units in order to give your patients access to Advanced Cardiac Life Support, the vital fourth link in the American Heart Association's chain of survival. Your local EMS system has established protocols for this coordination of care: follow them.

    Remember, the use of the AED does not require ALS personnel to be on scene, but it does require the participation of medical direction. If possible, notify the responding ALS crew via radio that CPR and/or defibrillation is in progress. When the ALS team arrives, inform the members about all the interventions you have undertaken to that point. If you used the AED, be sure to include the number of shocks delivered as well as any pertinent information obtained from bystanders in your report. The early minutes of the resuscitation are very important and you are a key witness. An accurate relay of the information you have collected and the interventions you have made is essential for a smooth and safe transition of care to the accepting ALS crew.

◆ Six shocks have been administered.

◆ You have received three consecutive "No shock" messages.

◆ The patient regains a pulse.

◆ Do not defibrillate or analyze in a moving vehicle. The movement may cause an incorrect reading by the AED.

◆ Keep batteries well charged. Check the batteries at the beginning of every shift and always carry extras.

Post-Resuscitation Care

After using the AED following the steps outlined above, three basic outcomes are possible. Those outcomes and the actions you should take with each are as follows:

◆ The patient may have pulses. In this case, you will provide high concentration oxygen either via a nonrebreather mask if the patient is breathing adequately or through artificial respiration with a bag-valve-mask device if he is not.

Using A Semi-Automated AED

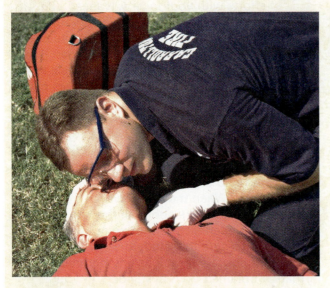

Figure 13-14A Perform the initial assessment, verifying that the patient is pulseless and not breathing.

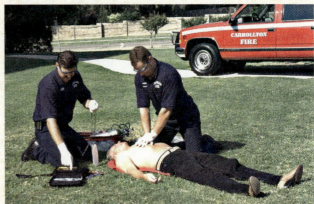

Figure 13-14B One rescuer performs CPR while the other prepares the AED.

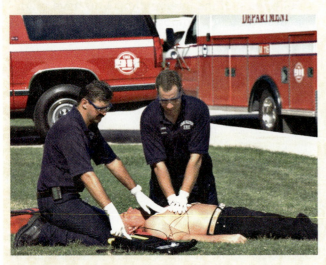

Figure 13-14C The AED operator places the defibrillator pads on the patient's chest.

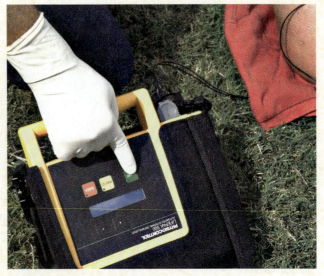

Figure 13-14D The operator turns on the AED and begins the narrative.

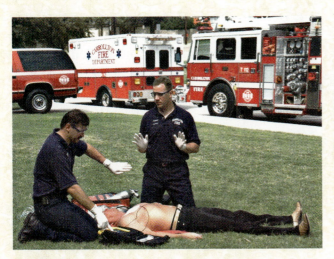

Figure 13-14E CPR is stopped and the operator pushes the button to begin rhythm analysis.

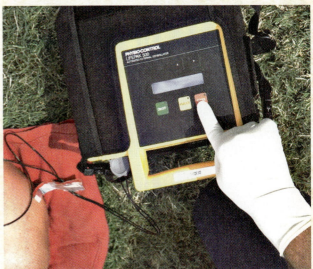

Figure 13-14F If the machine advises "Deliver shock," the operator loudly says "Clear!" and pushes the button to deliver the shock.

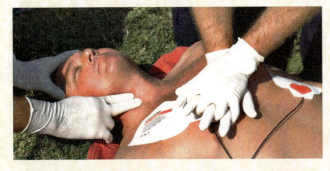

Figure 13-14G If the AED advises "No shock" when you re-analyze the patient's heart rhythm or after you have delivered a set of three stacked shocks, check the patient's pulse.

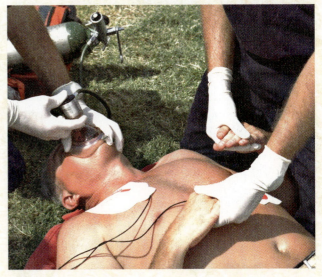

Figure 13-14H If the patient has a pulse, provide high flow oxygen if he is breathing adequately or begin artificial ventilations if he is not. Transport. If the patient has no pulse, resume CPR for 1 minute, then repeat the analysis and shock sequence for up to three more shocks. If the patient still has not regained a pulse, provide CPR and transport.

Many studies have shown that successful AED use must be combined with excellent airway management in order for the patient to survive. Follow procedures described in Chapter 6, "Airway Management." Transport the patient rapidly if ACLS is not immediately available. During transport, watch the patient carefully because there is a good chance that he may go back into cardiac arrest. Do not remove the defibrillator pads from the patient's chest in case you must use the AED again. Check the pulse frequently (every 30 seconds). Have suction ready because cardiac arrest victims are likely to vomit. If possible, perform a focused history and physical exam during transport.

◆ The patient may have no pulse, with the machine giving a "No shock" message. In this case, resume CPR and transport the patient to the hospital or follow your local protocols.

◆ The patient may have no pulse, with the machine giving a "Shock" message (persistent V-Fib). If you have given six shocks, you should not deliver any more shocks unless advised to do so by medical direction. In this case, you should resume CPR and transport the patient to the hospital or follow your local protocols. There is an exception to the rule of not giving more than six shocks. It applies when the patient is resuscitated, regains a pulse, and then loses it again. In that case, follow the procedure described below.

Recurring Cardiac Arrest

It is common for patients who have been resuscitated with an AED to go back into cardiac arrest. Resuscitated patients are often unconscious and being supplied with assisted ventilations. If can be very easy to miss the fact that the patient no longer has a pulse. You should therefore be sure to check a resuscitated patient's pulse every 30 seconds. If you discover that the patient has lost his pulse, follow these procedures:

1. **If you are en route to the hospital, stop the vehicle.** Its motions can interfere with the operation of the AED.

2. **If the defibrillator is not still attached to the patient, have someone perform CPR**

while the device is prepared and re-attached to the patient.

3. **Analyze the rhythm.**

4. **Deliver shock(s) if indicated, up to a maximum of two sets of three shocks separated by 1 minute of CPR or as directed by local protocols.**

Single Rescuer Use of the AED

There may be times when you are alone with a cardiac arrest patient or waiting for help to arrive. If you did not have an AED, you should notify the emergency dispatcher and then begin CPR. If you have an AED available, however, you should use the device on the patient before contacting the dispatcher or beginning CPR. As stressed earlier, defibrillation is the most effective way of saving the lives of patients in cardiac arrest. CPR is only a bridge until the defibrillator is ready for use. Follow these steps when you have an AED and are alone with a cardiac arrest patient:

1. **Perform the initial assessment.**

2. **Make sure the patient is unresponsive and has no pulse or respirations.**

3. **Turn on the AED and begin a narrative if the device has a voice recorder.**

4. **Attach the defibrillator pads.**

5. **Begin the rhythm analysis.**

6. **Deliver shock(s) as indicated by the AED.** Give up to three shocks or whatever local protocols prescribe.

7. **Notify the dispatcher of your situation. If you don't have a radio or help has not yet been summoned, leave the patient to call for EMS help only when one of the following things occurs:**

   ◆ The machine displays a "No shock" message.

   ◆ The patient regains a pulse.

   ◆ You have delivered three shocks.

8. **If the patient is still pulseless, provide 1 minute of CPR and repeat steps 5 and 6 above or follow local protocols.**

Using a Fully Automated AED

The procedures above are for a semi-automated AED. Using a fully automated AED to defibrillate a patient is quite similar. However, once the device is attached to the patient and turned on, it analyzes rhythms and delivers shocks automatically, without the EMT having to push any buttons. The AED will give instructions like "Stop CPR," "Clear the patient," and "Check breathing and pulse" as it goes through the defibrillation process. The machine is programmed to prompt checks of breathing and pulse if shocks are not appropriate or to deliver up to two sets of three stacked shocks with a minute of CPR if necessary. Instructions for operating the devices vary from model to model. If your system has fully automated AEDs, follow manufacturer's instructions and local protocols for their use.

AED Maintenance

To keep AEDs in top working order, service and maintain your unit's devices according to manufacturer's instructions. Generally, defibrillator problems are most often due to battery failure. Therefore, always keep extra batteries available, follow a replacement schedule, and allow adequate charging time before each use.

To help assure the proper working of AEDs, a panel of experts developed an Operator's Shift Checklist (Figure 13-15). The list contains items that AED operators should inspect or try out before going into the field with the AED. The EMTs who may use the unit's AED should complete an Operator's Shift Checklist at the beginning of each shift.

AED Training and Quality Assurance

During an actual resuscitation is no time to learn about the operations of your AED. To avoid problems, schedule regular practice sessions. Most systems set a maximum of 90 days between practice drills to reassess competencies in AED use. Follow your local protocols for practice and retraining. Also remember that the American Heart Association is a good source of information and guidelines that can help keep you up to date on AED use.

Successfully completing an EMT course will teach you how to use the AED. However, you must have the approval of local medical direction under state laws and regulations before you can operate the device on a patient in the field.

Analysis of incidents involving AED use should be a part of your department's quality improvement (QI) or total quality management (TQM) program. The medical director should review all incidents of AED use to assure that operators are using the AEDs properly and to determine what are the outcomes for patients from use of the AEDs. To carry out a thorough review, the medical director should have access to the following:

◆ Written prehospital care reports

◆ Voice ECG tape recorders attached to some models of AEDs

◆ Memory modules and magnetic tape recordings stored in the AED

A careful review can suggest ways of improving AED training for EMTs, ways of cutting down on the time it takes to get AEDs to cardiac arrest patients, and ways of improving coordination between EMT-Bs and ACLS personnel.

AUTOMATED DEFIBRILLATORS: OPERATOR'S SHIFT CHECKLIST

Date: _____ **Shift:** _____ **Location:** _____

Mfr/Model No.: _____ **Serial No. or Facility ID No.:** _____

At the beginning of each shift, inspect the unit. Indicate whether all requirements have been met. Note any corrective actions taken. Sign the form.

	Okay as found	Corrective Action/Remarks
1. Defibrillator Unit		
Clean, no spills, clear of objects on top, casing intact		
2. Cables/Connectors		
a. Inspect for cracks, broken wire, or damage b. Connectors engage securely		
3. Supplies		
a. Two sets of pads in sealed packages, within expiration date * g. Spare charged battery b. Hand towel * h. Adequate ECG paper c. Scissors * i. Manual override module, key, or card d. Razor * j. Cassette tape, memory module, and/or event card plus spares * e. Alcohol wipes * f. Monitoring electrodes		
4. Power Supply		
a. Battery-powered units (1) Verify fully charged battery in place (2) Spare charged battery available (3) Follow appropriate battery rotation schedule per manufacturer's recommendations b. AC/Battery backup units (1) Plugged into live outlet to maintain battery charge (2) Test on battery power and reconnect to line power		
5. Indicators/*ECG Display		
* a. Remove cassette tape, memory module, and/or event card * e. "Service" message display off b. Power-on display * f. Battery charging; low battery light off c. Self-test ok g. Correct time displayed — set with dispatch center * d. Monitor display functional		
6. ECG Recorder		
a. Adequate ECG paper b. Recorder prints		
7. Charge/Display Cycle		
* a. Disconnect AC plug — battery backup units * e. Manual override functional b. Attach to simulator f. Detach from simulator c. Detects, charges, and delivers shock for "VF" * g. Replace cassette tape, module, and/or memory card d. Responds correctly to non-shockable rhythms		
8. *Pacemaker		
a. Pacer output cable intact c. Inspect per manufacturer's operational guidelines b. Pacer pads present (set of two)		
☐ **Major problem(s) identified** (OUT OF SERVICE)		

*** Applicable only if the unit has this supply or capability**

P/N CL6721-00
rev 1.6 auto, 8/8/91

Signature: _____

Figure 13-15   An Operator's Shift Checklist for AEDs.

Chapter Review

SUMMARY

You can make a difference between life and death by early recognition and treatment of patients with cardiac compromise. Patients with cardiac problems may have a wide variety of signs and symptoms: it is your job to recognize what signs and symptoms may indicate a heart problem and initiate treatment and transport.

The most serious cases of cardiac compromise involve cardiac arrest. If a patient experiences cardiac arrest and you are able to apply and use an AED quickly and properly, you may save his life. Time is critical in cases of cardiac arrest. Familiar-

ity with your department's AED and with local protocols and frequent practice will enable you to defibrillate a patient more rapidly and increase his chances of survival. Participation in your department's QI process can also help to provide more rapid care to cardiac patients.

Cardiac compromise is potentially treatable if recognized early. Your commitment to continuing study and to ongoing practice will greatly improve your patient's chances of survival as well as your job satisfaction.

REVIEWING KEY CONCEPTS

1. Describe the basic elements of the cardiovascular system.

2. Explain why providing supplemental oxygen is so important to a patient with suspected heart problems.

3. List common signs and symptoms of cardiac compromise.

4. Describe the general steps in the emergency care of the cardiac compromise patient.

5. Describe the steps that should be followed when administering nitroglycerin.

6. Identify the four links in the American Heart Association's chain of survival.

7. Describe situations in which use of the AED is appropriate and those in which it is not.

8. Explain how the delivery of CPR should be coordinated with use of the AED.

9. Explain why it is important that no one be touching the patient during AED use and describe how to ensure that no one does.

10. Explain when a patient's pulse should be checked during use of the AED.

11. Explain steps to follow if a resuscitated patient rearrests during transport.

12. Identify materials that a medical director needs to assure a proper review of cases involving use of the AED.

RESOURCES TO LEARN MORE

American Heart Association. *Textbook of Advanced Life Support*. Dallas: American Heart Association, 1993.

Graves, J. R. et al. *RapidZap: Automated Defibrillation*. Upper Saddle River, NJ: Brady/Prentice Hall, 1989.

Weigel, Al et al. *Automated Defibrillation*. Upper Saddle River, NJ: Brady/Prentice Hall, 1988.

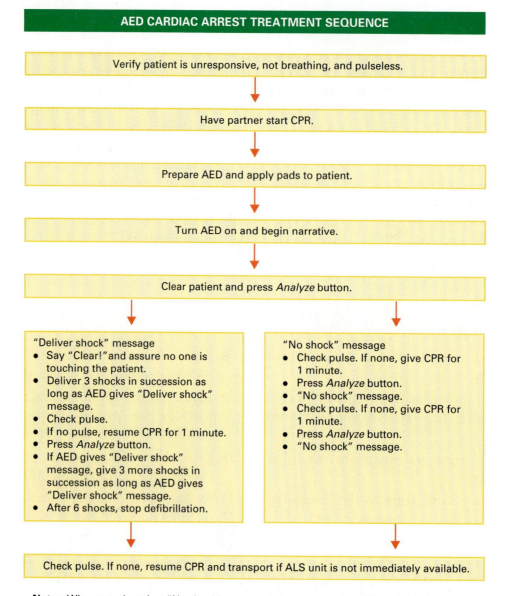

AED CARDIAC ARREST TREATMENT SEQUENCE

Verify patient is unresponsive, not breathing, and pulseless.

↓

Have partner start CPR.

↓

Prepare AED and apply pads to patient.

↓

Turn AED on and begin narrative.

↓

Clear patient and press *Analyze* button.

"Deliver shock" message
- Say "Clear!" and assure no one is touching the patient.
- Deliver 3 shocks in succession as long as AED gives "Deliver shock" message.
- Check pulse.
- If no pulse, resume CPR for 1 minute.
- Press *Analyze* button.
- If AED gives "Deliver shock" message, give 3 more shocks in succession as long as AED gives "Deliver shock" message.
- After 6 shocks, stop defibrillation.

"No shock" message
- Check pulse. If none, give CPR for 1 minute.
- Press *Analyze* button.
- "No shock" message.
- Check pulse. If none, give CPR for 1 minute.
- Press *Analyze* button.
- "No shock" message.

Check pulse. If none, resume CPR and transport if ALS unit is not immediately available.

Notes: Whenever there is a "No shock" message, check for a pulse. If the patient has a pulse, provide oxygen via nonrebreather mask or positive pressure ventilations with high concentration oxygen as needed.

If you initially shock the patient and then receive a "No shock" message before giving 6 shocks, follow the steps in the right-hand column above.

If you initially receive a "No shock" message and then on a subsequent analysis receive a "Deliver shock" message, follow the steps in the left-hand column above.

Occasionally, you many need to shift back and forth between the two columns. If this happens, follow the steps until you receive one of the following indications for transport:

- You have administered 6 shocks.
- You have received 3 consecutive "No shock" messages (separated by 1 minute of CPR).
- The patient regains a pulse.

If the patient is resuscitated and rearrests, start the sequence of shocks from the beginning.

Altered Mental Status Emergencies— Diabetes and Other Causes

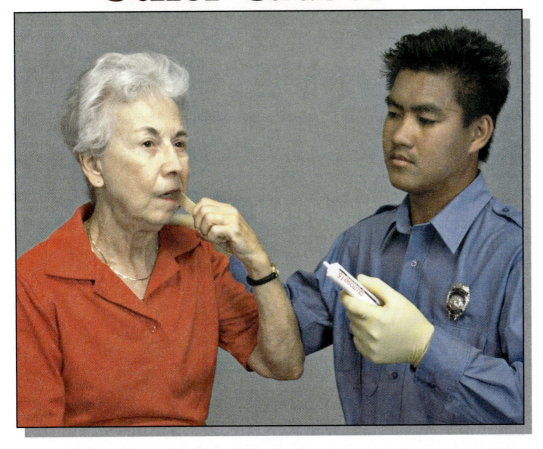

A ltered mental status is a condition in which a patient displays a change in his normal mental state. These changes can range from mild confusion and disorientation to complete unresponsiveness. Many factors may cause these changes, among them a lack of blood flow, sugar, or oxygen to the brain as well as seizures. Because the brain is such a vital organ and because it can be quickly and permanently damaged, any condition that causes an altered mental status should be considered life threatening. All patients with an altered mental status should be made high priority for transport as soon ▶

*as possible. As you will learn in this chapter, you may also be able to
provide treatment in the field that can rapidly improve the condition of a
patient whose altered mental status is a result of diabetes.*

OBJECTIVES

At the completion of this chapter, the EMT-Basic student should be able to
meet the following objectives:

Knowledge and Understanding

1. Identify the patient with altered mental status taking diabetic medications and the implications of a diabetes history. (pp. 351–353)
2. State the steps in the emergency medical care of the patient taking diabetic medications with an altered mental status and a history of diabetes. (pp. 354–355)
3. Establish the relationship between airway management and the patient with an altered mental status. (pp. 349–351, 354, 357)
4. State the generic and trade names, medication forms, dose, administration, actions and contraindications for oral glucose. (pp. 354–355)
5. Evaluate the need for medical direction in the emergency medical care of the diabetic patient. (p. 354)

6. Explain the rationale for administering oral glucose. (pp. 354–355)

Skills

1. Demonstrate the steps in the emergency medical care for the patient taking diabetic medication with an altered mental status and a history of diabetes.
2. Demonstrate the steps in the administration of oral glucose.
3. Demonstrate the assessment and documentation of patient response to oral glucose.
4. Demonstrate how to complete a prehospital care report for patients with diabetic emergencies.

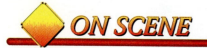

ON SCENE

DISPATCH: *STATION 14, RESPOND WITH THE POLICE TO 34 HAMPTON WAY FOR AN UNKNOWN EMERGENCY. CALL IS SECOND PARTY FROM A NEIGHBOR. TIME OUT 1714.*

You are the captain on Engine 14, which arrives on the scene simultaneously with the police. A woman crosses the lawn from the house next door as you pull up. She says that she called 9-1-1. "I heard breaking glass. Lots of it. It just didn't seem to stop. Finally, I went over to see what was going on. I can see in the kitchen window from the driveway, and there was Mr. Warren, stumbling around, knocking plates off the shelves. That's when I came back and called 9-1-1."

While you wait at the curb, the two police officers approach the house. They find the front door unlocked and enter. After a few moments, one of them reappears at the doorway. He indicates that the scene is secure and that you should enter the house. You pass through a living room, which is in disarray and proceed to the kitchen. There you and the two other firefighter EMTs see a male in his 30s sitting at the table.

You approach the man and introduce yourself, adding, "I'm an EMT with the fire department. What seems to be the problem, sir?"

The patient does not respond to you, but instead stares blankly at the police officer. You determine that the patient has an altered mental status but that his airway and breathing appear adequate. You note that his skin appears pale and his clothes are soaked in sweat. You reach out and feel for a radial pulse, which is rapid.

"Looks like he's a diabetic, Cap," one of your EMTs reports, holding up a bottle of insulin that he found in the refrigerator. "The label says his name is Aaron Warren and his address checks out."

You turn to the patient and ask, "Mr. Warren, are you a diabetic?"

As you say his name, Mr. Warren immediately turns his head toward you but still does not speak.

You try again. "Mr. Warren, are you a diabetic?"

"Since I was six," he responds sluggishly.

As one of the other EMTs obtains a blood pressure, you confirm that Mr. Warren has a gag reflex present by using a tongue depressor. Following your department's protocol, you administer one tube of oral glucose by squeezing the contents onto the tongue depressor. You then place the tongue depressor between the patient's teeth and gums.

Within 10 minutes, Mr. Warren is speaking freely and is fully alert. The ambulance crew arrives on the scene. You give the transporting crew a report that covers your initial assessment of the patient, your use of glucose, and the patient's immediate and excellent response to therapy.

ALTERED MENTAL STATUS

As noted in the introduction, altered mental status may occur as a result of various conditions. Among these conditions are the following:

◆ Head injury

◆ Infection, with or without fever

◆ Seizure

◆ Post-seizure (postictal) state

◆ Hypoperfusion (shock)

◆ Poisoning

◆ Abuse of drugs or alcohol

◆ Hypoxia, or low levels of oxygen in the blood

◆ Build up of excessive carbon dioxide from inadequate ventilation

◆ Stroke

◆ Diabetes

It is not your job as an EMT to diagnose the cause of a patient's altered mental status. Your task is to assure the patient's airway, breathing, and circulation and to transport him to definitive care at the emergency department. However, if you are able to determine during your assessment that the patient has a history of diabetes, you may be able to provide care that can bring a rapid improvement in his condition. For this reason, performing a careful, accurate assessment on the altered mental status patient is vital.

Assessment of the Patient with Altered Mental Status—No History of Diabetes

Perform a scene size-up. Remember that an altered mental status can result from trauma as well as a medical condition. Be alert for any mechanism of injury that may have caused injury to the head. Look also for evidence of a medical condition. This might include medical identification devices or medicine boxes or bottles. Look in the refrigerator of an altered mental status patient because insulin, a medication prescribed for diabetes, may be stored there. If you do discover evidence that the patient is diabetic, proceed as in "Assessment of the Altered Mental Status Patient—History of Diabetes" below.

Perform an initial assessment. Your assessment of the patient's mental status should reveal whether or not it is altered. If your initial assess-

COMPANY OFFICER'S NOTES

If the patient has an altered mental status and neither he nor anyone else can provide a history of diabetes, have crew members search the scene for evidence that might indicate the patient has diabetes. The evidence might include the following:

◆ A medical identification device worn or carried by the patient

◆ Insulin in the refrigerator

◆ Medications prescribed for diabetics (see Table 14-1)

◆ Insulin syringes

◆ A glucometer (a machine used by diabetics to test blood glucose levels)

◆ Chemical reagent strips in the bathroom (used by diabetics to test for sugar and ketones in their urine)

ment indicates an altered mental status and the patient's airway, breathing, and circulation are adequate, proceed to perform the focused history and physical exam. Because of his altered mental status, the patient may not be able to assist you or may even resist you. You may have to gather the history from family members or bystanders. The following are among the important questions to ask as you gather the history:

◆ What events preceded the episode?

◆ Does the patient have a history of diabetes?

◆ Was the onset of the episode rapid or gradual?

◆ How long has the patient had the altered mental status?

◆ Has the patient ever had this happen before?

◆ Is there any evidence or history of trauma?

◆ Did the patient appear to have a seizure?

◆ Has the patient had a fever or other recent or current illness?

◆ Does the patient have any symptoms associated with this episode?

◆ Does the patient take any medications?

◆ When was the patient's last meal?

If you have not already done so, have a crew member search for medications. Medications commonly used by diabetics include insulin (whose trade names include Humulin and Lente) and other oral medications (see Table 14-1). If answers to any of your questions or the presence of medications indicates that the patient has a history of diabetes, proceed as in "Assessment of the Altered Mental Status Patient—History of Diabetes" below. If there is no indication of a history of diabetes, follow the steps in "Emergency Care—Patient with Altered Mental Status and No History of Diabetes" below.

Table 14-1

Brand Names of Oral Medications Prescribed for Diabetics

Diabinese®
Orinase®
Micronase®
Glucotrol®
Glucophage®

◆ Emergency Care—Patient with Altered Mental Status and No History of Diabetes

1. **Assure an open airway.** Consider the possibility that the altered mental status is due to trauma and if that possibility does exist, use the jaw-thrust maneuver. Be prepared to suction.

2. **Administer high concentration oxygen.** An altered mental status may be the result of hypoxia.

3. **Be prepared to artificially ventilate the patient and to suction the airway as needed.**

4. **Transport the patient.** All patients with a persistent alteration in mental status should be transported for further evaluation in the emergency department. Perform an ongoing assessment en route. Continually monitor airway and

breathing and be prepared to suction or provide ventilations if necessary.

DIABETES AND ALTERED MENTAL STATUS

To function normally, the human brain needs a constant supply of both oxygen and **glucose,** a form of sugar. Both oxygen and glucose are delivered to the brain in the blood. The brain's nerve cells use oxygen and glucose to generate the fine electrical impulses that allow all the normal functions of the brain to occur. Any reduction in the flow of blood to the brain or in the amount of oxygen or glucose in the blood can alter a person's mental status.

The condition known as **diabetes mellitus,** commonly referred to as "diabetes," directly affects glucose levels in the blood. Over 15 million people in North America have some form of

diabetes. It is a common cause of altered mental status because patients with diabetes have difficulty maintaining normal levels of blood sugar.

Physiology of Diabetes

Sugars enter the body through the digestion of food and are converted to glucose. Glucose and other nutrients are absorbed from the intestines into the blood. In order for glucose to pass from the bloodstream into the brain and other body tissues, a hormone called **insulin** must be present. The insulin enables glucose to move from the bloodstream into the cells. Once the glucose enters the cells, it helps to power cell function. When people have diabetes, they lose the ability to pass glucose from the blood into the body's cells (Figure 14-1).

In some diabetic patients, this failure occurs because the body stops producing adequate levels of insulin. These patients, or *Type I* diabetics, require insulin injections to provide the missing insulin that enables sugars to pass into the cells.

Figure 14-1   Normal and Type I and Type II diabetic uses of sugar from the digestion of food.

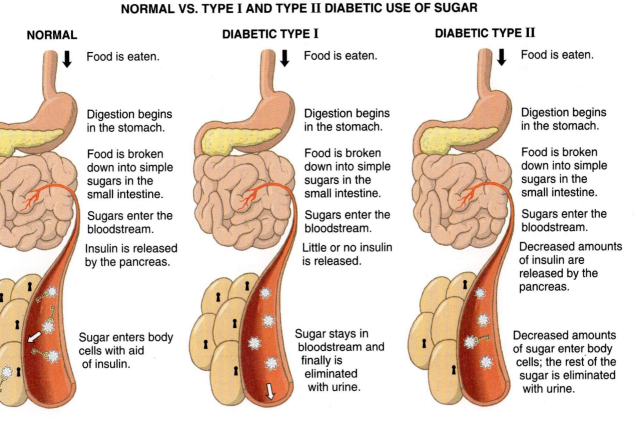

NORMAL VS. TYPE I AND TYPE II DIABETIC USE OF SUGAR

NORMAL

Food is eaten.

Digestion begins in the stomach.

Food is broken down into simple sugars in the small intestine.

Sugars enter the bloodstream.

Insulin is released by the pancreas.

Sugar enters body cells with aid of insulin.

DIABETIC TYPE I

Food is eaten.

Digestion begins in the stomach.

Food is broken down into simple sugars in the small intestine.

Sugars enter the bloodstream.

Little or no insulin is released.

Sugar stays in bloodstream and finally is eliminated with urine.

DIABETIC TYPE II

Food is eaten.

Digestion begins in the stomach.

Food is broken down into simple sugars in the small intestine.

Sugars enter the bloodstream.

Decreased amounts of insulin are released by the pancreas.

Decreased amounts of sugar enter body cells; the rest of the sugar is eliminated with urine.

The majority of diabetic patients, however, do not lack insulin. For them, the problem is that the cells of their bodies do not respond properly to insulin. These patients are termed *Type II* diabetics. To treat their condition, these patients usually take oral medications that help their cells take on insulin from the bloodstream (see Table 14-1).

Both Type I and Type II diabetics usually have an increased blood glucose level, called **hyperglycemia,** because of their diseases. Insulin and oral medications prescribed for diabetic patients act to lower blood glucose levels by helping to move sugar from the bloodstream into the cells. Diabetics can sometimes develop altered mental status from elevated blood sugar levels. These changes in mental status tend to be more gradual in onset than those that occur when blood glucose levels become too low.

When blood sugar levels are abnormally low, the condition is called **hypoglycemia.** Hypoglycemia is the most common cause of altered mental status in diabetic patients. The condition can occur when the insulin and oral medications diabetic patients take are too effective and blood sugar levels drop too rapidly.

Diabetic patients who take insulin injections are far more likely to develop altered mental status than patients who take oral medications. This is because insulin can lower blood sugar levels more rapidly and effectively than oral medica-

tions. Common ways diabetics develop low blood sugar leading to altered mental status include:

- Taking insulin and then missing a meal
- Taking insulin but then vomiting up a meal
- Engaging in far more exercise or physical labor than usual without decreasing the normal insulin dose or increasing the amount of food ingested

Be aware, however, that an altered mental status in a diabetic patient may occur with no readily identifiable explanation.

Assessment of the Altered Mental Status Patient with a History of Diabetes

Determine that the scene is secure during the scene size-up. As you perform the scene size-up, remain alert for clues that might give information about a patient's altered mental status, such as a medical identification device (Figure 14-2). Other evidence that a patient is diabetic might include insulin in the refrigerator, medications such as Orinase® or Micronase® that are prescribed for diabetes, and/or a glucometer (Figure 14-3). Be on the lookout for syringes and other sharp objects that diabetics may use with their medications. These devices represent both clues that the patient is a diabetic and risks of injury to EMTs.

Perform an initial assessment. If your initial assessment indicates an altered mental status, you must rapidly determine if the patient has a history of diabetes. This determination is important because you may be able to treat a diabetic with altered mental status by administering oral glucose.

Diabetics with altered mental status may present with a variety of signs and symptoms. These include the following:

- Intoxicated appearance, slurred speech, and staggering gait
- Complete unresponsiveness
- Combative, violent behavior
- Anxiety
- Uncharacteristic behavior
- Seizures

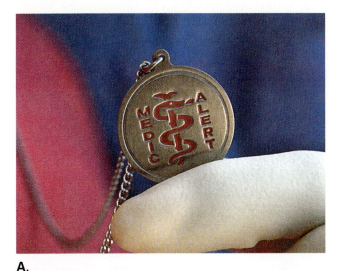

A.

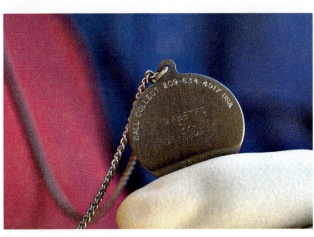

B.

Figure 14-2   The front **(A)** and back **(B)** of a medical identification bracelet.

Figure 14-3   Many diabetics use home glucometers to test their blood glucose levels.

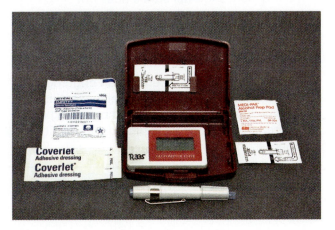

◆ Complaints of hunger

◆ Cold and clammy skin

◆ Elevated heart rate

Perform the focused history and physical exam. Obtain information by questioning the patient, bystanders, or family members. Even if you already know or suspect a history of diabetes, ask the following questions during the focused history and physical exam:

◆ What events preceded the episode?

◆ Does the patient have a history of diabetes?

◆ Was the onset of the episode rapid or gradual?

◆ How long has the patient had the altered mental status?

◆ Has the patient ever had this happen before?

◆ Is there any evidence of trauma?

◆ Did the patient appear to have a seizure?

◆ Has the patient had a fever or other recent or current illness?

◆ Does the patient have any symptoms associated with this episode?

◆ Does the patient take any medications?

If you suspect or if it is reported that the patient has a history of diabetes, be sure to ask:

◆ Did the patient take his medication as usual before the episode?

◆ What time did the patient last have something to eat or drink? Do you know what he ate or drank?

◆ Did the patient vomit after eating a meal?

◆ Did the patient do any unusual exercise or physical activity before the episode?

Obtain baseline vital signs. (Remember that an elevated heart rate and cool clammy skin are common findings in hypoglycemic diabetics with altered mental status.) Complete the SAMPLE history. Also carefully assess whether the patient is able to swallow. Diabetic patients with altered mental status who retain the ability to swallow can be considered for the administration of oral glucose by the EMT.

◆ Emergency Care—Patient with Altered Mental Status and a History of Diabetes

1. **Assure an open airway.** Consider the possibility that the altered mental status is due to trauma and if that possibility does exist, use the jaw-thrust maneuver. Be aware that diabetics with altered mental status often require frequent suctioning of the airway because of secretions and vomiting.

2. **Administer high flow oxygen.**

3. **Determine if the patient is alert enough to swallow. If he is not, maintain his airway, provide high flow oxygen and, if necessary, artificial ventilations, and initiate transport.**

4. **If the patient is alert enough to swallow and local protocols permit, administer oral glucose.** Follow your local protocols or the procedures described in Oral Glucose below.

ORAL GLUCOSE ℞

Medication Name
Generic: Oral glucose
Trade: Glutose®, Insta-glucose®

Indications for Administration
Altered mental status patient with a known history of diabetes controlled by medications who has the ability to swallow.

Contraindications
An unconscious patient or a patient who lacks a gag reflex (is unable to swallow) because aspiration of the glucose into the lungs could occur.

Medication Form
Gel, in toothpaste-like tubes.

Dosage
Typically, one tube administered gradually into the mouth. A tongue blade may be used to apply the glucose paste to the inside of the mouth and cheek.

Actions
Raises the blood glucose level. Restores level of sugar necessary for normal organ function, especially of the brain.

Side Effects
None, if used properly. Could be aspirated into the lungs of a patient without a gag reflex.

Administration

1. Obtain an order from medical direction either on-line or off-line (by standing orders).

2. Assure that the signs and symptoms of altered mental status are present and that the patient has a history of diabetes controlled by medication (either insulin or an oral agent).

3. Assess and assure that the patient is:
   —Conscious
   —Able to swallow
   —Able to protect his own airway (has a gag reflex present)

4. Administer the oral glucose (Figure 14-4). Squeeze oral glucose from a tube onto a tongue depressor. Then place the tongue depressor between the patient's cheek and gum. Alternatively, you can squeeze the glucose directly from the tube into the mouth between the patient's cheek and gum.

5. Reassess the patient. Carefully document vital signs and mental status and the response of the patient to the oral glucose administration. If the patient's mental status does not improve, consult with medical direction about whether to administer more glucose. If the patient loses consciousness, remove the tongue depressor and suction the airway.

6. Transport the patient. Perform an ongoing assessment en route to the receiving facility. Continually monitor airway and breathing and be prepared to suction or provide ventilations if necessary.

Administering Oral Glucose

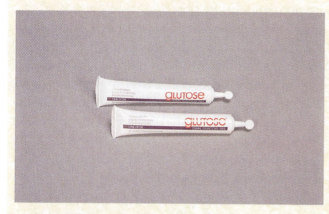

Figure 14-4A Tubes of oral glucose.

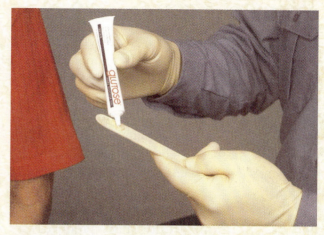

Figure 14-4B One method of administering oral glucose is to first squeeze the glucose onto the end of a tongue depressor.

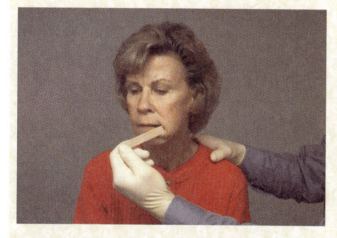

Figure 14-4C Place the tongue depressor with glucose between the patient's cheek and gum.

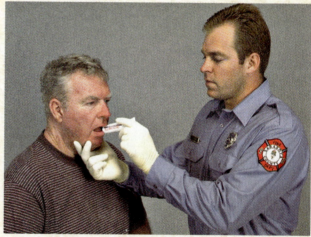

Figure 14-4D An alternative method of administering oral glucose is to squeeze the glucose between the patient's cheek and gum directly from the tube.

GERIATRIC NOTE

Most elderly patients with diabetes developed the disease later in life as what is known as Type II, or "adult onset," diabetes. Most Type II patients take prescribed oral medications for their diabetes. Episodes of hypoglycemia resulting in altered mental status are less common in these Type II patients than in Type I diabetic patients who take insulin.

When caring for older patients with altered mental status, always consider other causes for their condition beside diabetes. Low blood oxygen (hypoxia), stroke, infections, poisonings, and head trauma are all frequent causes of altered mental status in geriatric patients. All geriatric patients with altered mental status should receive supplemental oxygen.

SEIZURES

Seizures are a common cause of altered mental status. A **seizure** is a sudden and temporary alteration in normal neurological function as a result of abnormal electrical activity in the brain. Patients have an altered mental status during most seizures and during the minutes following a seizure (the postictal period). After the seizure, the patient's mental status should gradually return to normal.

A wide variety of conditions can trigger the abnormal electrical activity that produces a seizure. The most common cause of seizures in children is a fever that has risen quickly. The most common cause of seizures in adults is the failure of patients who have a history of seizure disorder to take prescribed medications properly. Other causes of seizures include head injuries, poisonings (including drug and alcohol abuse), epilepsy, heat stroke, hypoglycemia, and hypoxia.

Seizures can cause a wide variety of altered mental status and abnormal body movement. In the seizures that prompt the most calls for emergency assistance (called grand mal or tonic/clonic seizures), patients suddenly lose consciousness and begin to have uncontrolled body movements. Other types of seizures, however, cause more subtle changes. Patients may stare off blankly for brief periods of time, or behave erratically, or experience repeated twitching in one part of the body.

Seizures may be brief, lasting only a few seconds, or prolonged, persisting for more than 15 minutes. Prolonged seizures can be life threatening. Seizures lasting more than 15 minutes or occurring one after another are particularly dangerous. The term for such seizures is *status epilepticus*.

Most seizures only last a few minutes. Although brief seizures, especially those in patients with a known history of seizures, are usually not life threatening, they may have been triggered by potentially life threatening conditions. Therefore, consider any seizure patient to be having a medical emergency.

Assessment of the Seizure Patient

Remember that head injuries can trigger seizures. During scene size-up, be alert for mechanisms of injury that suggest potential head injury.

Form a general impression of the patient as you begin the initial assessment. Usually, patients will no longer be actively seizing by the time you reach them. Your main concern with these patients will be assuring that airway and breathing are adequate.

Assess and record baseline vital signs. Conduct a focused history and physical exam. If the patient is responsive, gather information from him. If he is not, obtain a SAMPLE history and history of the present illness from family or bystanders. A description of the seizure can be very helpful to hospital personnel, so try to find out what the seizure was like by asking:

- What was the patient doing before the seizure?
- What did the person do during the seizure?
- Was there a loss of bowel or bladder control?
- Was the patient responsive during the seizure?
- How long did the seizure last?
- Did the patient bite his tongue?

There are many types of seizures. Signs and symptoms will vary, but may include:

- Tingling, stiffening, or jerking in one part of the body
- An *aura,* a sensory perception—an odor, a visual disturbance, a rising sensation in the stomach—indicating onset of a seizure
- Confusion
- Unresponsiveness
- Muscle rigidity
- Convulsions alternating with relaxation
- Loss of bowel or bladder control
- Biting of the tongue

◆ Emergency Care—Seizure Patient

1. **Do not try to physically restrain the patient or force anything into his mouth while he is seizing.** Avoid further trauma during the seizure if possible. Protect the

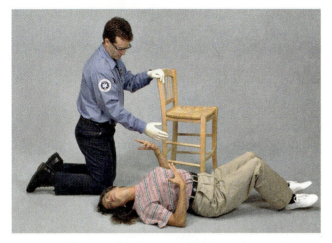

Figure 14-5 Protect an actively seizing patient from further injury by moving furniture and other objects out of the patient's way.

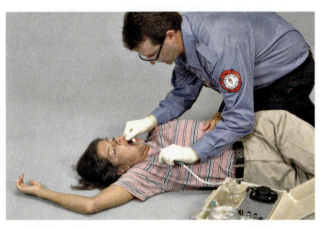

Figure 14-6 Be prepared to suction the airway of the seizure patient.

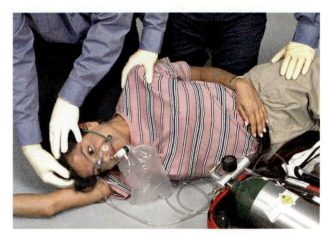

Figure 14-7 Place a seizure patient with no suspected head or spine injury in the recovery position to allow better drainage of fluids from the mouth and supply high concentration oxygen. If a mechanism of injury suggests possible head or spine injury, provide manual spinal stabilization.

actively seizing patient by moving objects like chairs and tables away from him (Figure 14-5).

2. **Assure an open airway.** This may be difficult to do while the patient is actively seizing. Be prepared to suction the airway (Figure 14-6). Administer high concentration oxygen. If trauma is suspected as a cause of the seizure, use the jaw-thrust maneuver to open the airway.

3. **If no neck injury is suspected, place the patient on his side in the recovery position.** (Figure 14-7)

4. **If the patient is cyanotic, assure an open airway and provide artificial ventilations with high concentration oxygen.**

COMPANY OFFICER'S NOTES

Patients with altered mental status who refuse treatment or transport can pose significant legal risks to EMTs (and their departments) who attempt to provide care. Diabetic patients whose mental status returns to normal after the administration of glucose and patients who waken after a seizure are two groups of patients who commonly refuse transport. Review material on refusal of treatment (especially the chapter-closing algorithm) in Chapter 4, "Medical/Legal Issues." Remember that a patient who is not completely alert *cannot* refuse medical care and/or transport because he is unlikely to be able to fully understand the consequences of such a refusal. A patient who is alert and oriented and has a normal mental status after an episode of altered mental status, however, is likely to be within his rights in refusing care. Whenever you have questions about whether a patient's refusal of treatment or transport is appropriate, follow your local protocols or consult medical direction. If it is finally decided that the patient is competent to refuse care, be sure to document the refusal following the guidelines provided in Chapter 4.

5. Transport the patient. Continue to monitor ABCs and vital signs closely. Note, however, that seizure patients who become responsive often refuse further treatment and transport. Follow department protocols with such patients.

CEREBROVASCULAR ACCIDENTS

The 1994 U.S. Department of Transportation EMT-Basic National Standard Curriculum does not specifically include **cerebrovascular accidents** (CVAs), also called strokes, in its discussion of altered mental status. However, the National Institutes of Health (NIH) have developed guidelines for the assessment and care by EMTs of patients with CVAs. To understand the importance of following these guidelines, you should be aware of recent advances in the treatment of acute CVAs.

CVAs most commonly result from the blockage of a cerebral artery in the brain. A small clot or blockage that has traveled through the bloodstream blocks an artery supplying blood to a certain part of the brain, much like what happens during a heart attack. Blood flow to parts of the brain normally supplied by that artery will then be quickly affected, resulting in the loss of the normal brain function controlled by that area. Some CVAs result from the bursting of weakened blood vessels (aneurysms) within the brain. These CVAs also disrupt blood flow to parts of the brain. CVAs of either type can cause permanent disability, even death.

The major advance in CVA therapy has been the use of thrombolytics (like those used in acute heart attacks) to reopen blocked arteries in the brain, resulting in the return of normal brain function. Currently, stroke patients may qualify to receive thrombolytics if they reach the hospital for treatment within 3 hours of the onset of their symptoms. At the hospital, patients undergo a rapid screening process. This includes a CAT (computerized axial tomography) scan of the brain before the final decision as to whether the patient should receive the "clot-busting" drugs.

Remember that these new therapies for CVAs can only be used during a short time window after the onset of symptoms. It is essential, therefore, that you be able to recognize signs of stroke quickly. You must also keep on-scene times short and provide rapid transport to the emergency department, being sure to notify the hospital while you are en route so that the staff can prepare for the patient.

Be alert for the possibility of a CVA whenever you are called to assist a patient with an altered mental status. Look for the signs and symptoms of a CVA as you conduct the initial assessment and the focused history and physical exam (Figure 14-8). The signs and symptoms you encounter in a CVA patent will vary depending on the area of the brain to which blood flow has been interrupted. A common sign is a drooping on one side of the face and a weakness of the arm and or leg on the opposite side of the body. Patients with acute CVAs often have difficulty speaking. Their speech may be slurred, garbled, or incomprehensible, or they may be unable to get the right words out, despite the wish to do so. When assessing a possible CVA patient, remember that, even though he may be unable to communicate, he may still be able to understand what is being said to him and around him.

Other signs and symptoms of CVAs include the following:

◆ Altered mental status ranging from dizziness or confusion to complete unresponsiveness

◆ Paralysis or weakness on *one* side of the body

◆ Paralysis, weakness, or loss of expression on *one* side of the face

◆ Numbness or loss of sensation on *one* side of the body

◆ Loss of motor function without a history of trauma

◆ Unequal pupils

◆ Loss of vision in one eye

◆ Double vision or other visual disturbances

◆ Eyes turned away from the paralyzed side of body

◆ Nausea and vomiting

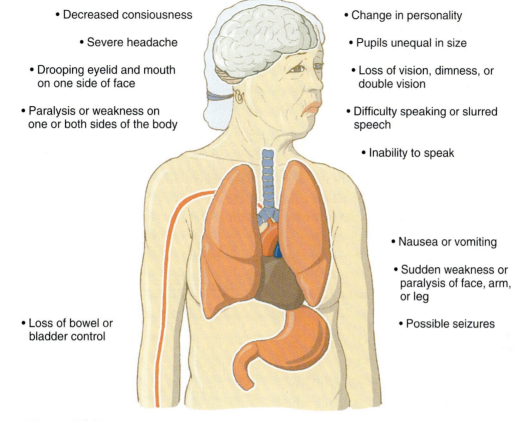

- Decreased consiousness
- Severe headache
- Drooping eyelid and mouth on one side of face
- Paralysis or weakness on one or both sides of the body

- Change in personality
- Pupils unequal in size
- Loss of vision, dimness, or double vision
- Difficulty speaking or slurred speech
- Inability to speak

- Nausea or vomiting
- Sudden weakness or paralysis of face, arm, or leg

- Loss of bowel or bladder control
- Possible seizures

Figure 14-8   Signs and symptoms of cerebrovascular accidents (strokes).

- Severe headache
- Complaints of a severe headache or stiff neck prior to onset of altered mental status
- Patient *may* have a past history of stroke

◆ Emergency Care—Patients With CVAs

1. **Take BSI precautions.**

2. **Maintain the patient's airway and administer oxygen via nasal cannula.** If signs of respiratory distress are present, administer high concentration oxygen via nonrebreather mask. Be prepared to assist ventilations with a bag-valve-mask device. If the patient is breathing inadequately, proceed with intubation if you are permitted to do so by your local protocols.

3. **Place the stroke patient with an altered mental status in the left lateral recumbent position with the head and chest elevated.** If the patient has an affected or paralyzed extremity, place it in a safe and secure position when you move and transport the patient.

4. **Transport the patient to the hospital rapidly.**

5. **Request ALS backup, if available, when the patient is unresponsive or has a compromised airway.**

6. **Notify the receiving hospital of your projected time of arrival and the time of the onset of the patient's symptoms.**

7. **Perform an ongoing assessment en route.**

   Note: In some patients, the signs of CVAs can resolve quickly, in times ranging from several minutes up to 24 hours. These patients must also be transported to the hospital so that they can receive further evaluation.

Chapter Review

SUMMARY

To function normally, the human brain needs a constant supply of oxygen and glucose. Both oxygen and glucose are delivered to the brain in the blood. The brain's nerve cells use oxygen and glucose to generate the fine electrical impulses that allow all the normal functions of the brain to occur. Any reduction in the blood flow to the brain, any reduction in the amount of oxygen or glucose in the blood, or any interruption in the brain's normal electrical activity may result in an altered mental status. Because all episodes of altered mental status involve the functioning of the brain, they should be considered serious. Assure the ABCs of these patients, assess them quickly and thoroughly, and transport them to the hospital. If your assessment reveals a patient with history of diabetes, you may be able to assist him by administering oral glucose, following your local protocols.

REVIEWING KEY CONCEPTS

1. Describe the steps in the emergency care of the patient with an altered mental status and no history of diabetes.

2. List common signs and symptoms displayed by a patient with an altered mental status who has a history of diabetes.

3. Name the indications for use of oral glucose.

4. Name the contraindications for use of oral glucose.

5. Describe the steps in administering oral glucose.

6. List common signs and symptoms of seizures.

7. Describe the steps in the emergency care of the seizure patient.

8. Explain the importance of rapid assessment and transport of patients with cerebrovascular accidents (strokes).

9. List common signs and symptoms of CVAs.

10. Describe the steps in the emergency care of the patient with a CVA.

RESOURCES TO LEARN MORE

Henry, G. L. "Coma and Altered States of Consciousness" in Tintinalli, J. E. et al. *Emergency Medicine: A Comprehensive Study Guide, 4th Edition*. New York: McGraw-Hill, 1995.

Rapid Identification and Treatment of Acute Stroke. NIH Publication No. 97-4239. August 1997.

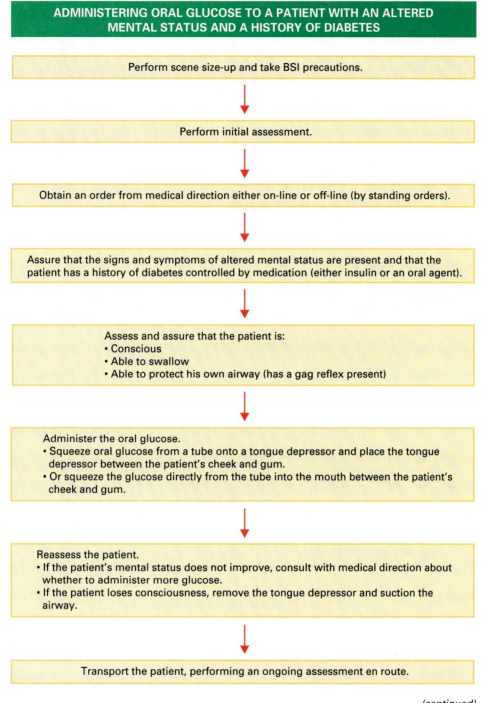

ADMINISTERING ORAL GLUCOSE TO A PATIENT WITH AN ALTERED MENTAL STATUS AND A HISTORY OF DIABETES

Perform scene size-up and take BSI precautions.

Perform initial assessment.

Obtain an order from medical direction either on-line or off-line (by standing orders).

Assure that the signs and symptoms of altered mental status are present and that the patient has a history of diabetes controlled by medication (either insulin or an oral agent).

Assess and assure that the patient is:
• Conscious
• Able to swallow
• Able to protect his own airway (has a gag reflex present)

Administer the oral glucose.
• Squeeze oral glucose from a tube onto a tongue depressor and place the tongue depressor between the patient's cheek and gum.
• Or squeeze the glucose directly from the tube into the mouth between the patient's cheek and gum.

Reassess the patient.
• If the patient's mental status does not improve, consult with medical direction about whether to administer more glucose.
• If the patient loses consciousness, remove the tongue depressor and suction the airway.

Transport the patient, performing an ongoing assessment en route.

(continued)

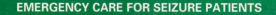

EMERGENCY CARE FOR SEIZURE PATIENTS

Do not physically restrain the patient or force anything into his mouth while he is seizing; protect the actively seizing patient by moving objects like chairs and tables away from him.

Assure an open airway, administer high concentration oxygen, and be prepared to suction the airway.

If no neck injury is suspected, place the patient on his side in the recovery position.

If the patient is cyanotic (bluish-gray), assure an open airway and provide artificial ventilations with high concentration oxygen.

Transport the patient, monitoring ABCs and vital signs closely.

EMERGENCY CARE FOR PATIENTS WITH CVAs

Perform scene size-up and take BSI precautions.

Perform initial assessment.

Maintain the patient's airway and administer oxygen via nasal cannula. If signs of respiratory distress are present, administer high concentration oxygen via nonrebreather mask. If patient is in respiratory arrest, provide ventilations via BVM.

Place the patient with an altered mental status in the left lateral recumbent position with the head and chest elevated.

Transport the patient to the hospital rapidly.

Request ALS backup, if available, when the patient is unresponsive or has a compromised airway.

Notify the receiving hospital of your projected time of arrival and the time of the onset of the patient's symptoms.

Perform an ongoing assessment en route.

Poisonings and Allergic Reactions

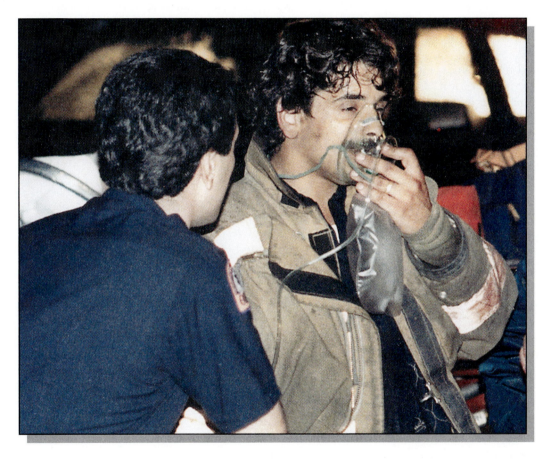

*P*atients can be exposed to many types of substances that will make them ill. The generic term for this type of exposure is **poisoning.** When the poisoning results from a patient's taking an excessive amount of a legal or illegal drug or medication, it is termed an **overdose.** When the body's own immune system reacts to the introduction of a chemical into the body, then this is termed an **allergic reaction.**

As an EMT, you must learn how to recognize poisonings, overdoses, and allergic reactions. If you can promptly recognize these conditions and rapidly begin to provide appropriate emergency medical care, you may save a patient's life.

At the completion of this chapter, the EMT-Basic student should be able to meet the following objectives:

Knowledge and Understanding

1. List various ways that poisons enter the body. (pp. 366–368)
2. List signs and symptoms associated with poisoning. (pp. 369, 371, 372, 374)
3. Discuss the emergency medical care for the patient with possible overdose. (p. 372)
4. Discuss the emergency medical care for the patient with suspected poisoning. (pp. 369, 370, 371–375)
5. Establish the relationship between the patient suffering from poisoning or overdose and airway management. (p. 368)
6. State the generic and trade names, indications, contraindications, medication form, dose, administration, actions, side effects and reassessment strategies for activated charcoal. (pp. 369, 370)
7. Recognize the need for medical direction in caring for the patient with poisoning or overdose. (pp. 369, 370)
8. Explain the rationale for administering activated charcoal. (pp. 369, 370)
9. Explain the rationale for contacting medical direction early in the prehospital management of the poisoning or overdose patient. (p. 369)
10. Recognize the patient experiencing an allergic reaction. (pp. 376–378)
11. Describe the emergency medical care of the patient with an allergic reaction. (pp. 378–381)
12. Establish the relationship between the patient with an allergic reaction and airway management. (pp. 377–381)
13. Describe the mechanisms of allergic response and the implications for airway management. (pp. 376–377)
14. State the generic and trade names, indications, contraindications, medication forms, dose, administration, actions, side effects, and reassessment strategies for the epinephrine auto-injector. (p. 379)
15. Evaluate the need for medical control in the emergency medical care of the patient with an allergic reaction. (pp. 378–381)
16. Differentiate between the general category of those patients having an allergic reaction and those having an allergic reaction and requiring immediate medical care, including immediate use of an epinephrine auto-injector. (pp. 376–378)
17. Explain the rationale for administering epinephrine using an auto-injector. (pp. 378, 379)

Skills

1. Demonstrate the steps in the emergency medical care for the patient with possible overdose.
2. Demonstrate the steps in the emergency medical care for the patient with suspected poisoning.
3. Perform the necessary steps required to provide a patient with activated charcoal.
4. Demonstrate the assessment and documentation of patient response following the administration of activated charcoal.
5. Demonstrate the proper disposal of the equipment used for the administration of activated charcoal.
6. Demonstrate completing a prehospital care report for patients with a poisoning/overdose emergency.
7. Demonstrate the emergency medical care of the patient experiencing an allergic reaction.
8. Demonstrate the use of an epinephrine auto-injector.
9. Demonstrate the assessment and documentation of patient response to an epinephrine injection.
10. Demonstrate the proper disposal of an epinephrine auto-injector.
11. Demonstrate completing a prehospital care report for patients with allergic emergencies.

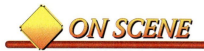
DISPATCH: *AMBULANCE 21, RESPOND WITH THE POLICE TO A REPORTED OVERDOSE AT 1342 EAST SHERMAN STREET. PATIENT IS REPORTED TO HAVE TAKEN AN ENTIRE BOTTLE OF EXTRA-STRENGTH TYLENOL®. TIME OUT IS 1756.*

You and your EMT partner begin preparing for this call while you are en route to the scene. When you are about six blocks from the location, the dispatcher advises you that the police are on the scene and that it is now safe to enter the residence.

You pull up in front of a neatly kept split-level ranch home, grab your jump kit, and proceed to the house. Inside, you find several people, including two county police officers, standing in front of a couch in the living room. Seated on the couch is a teenage woman who appears to be in no acute distress.

You introduce yourself and explain, "I'm an EMT with the Mill Creek Fire Department. What's your name?"

"I'm Amanda," she answers.

"Amanda, what seems to be the matter?"

"Nothing much. I want to kill myself, so I took this whole bottle of Tylenol®." She holds up an empty pill container that, according to the label, had contained fifty 500-milligram tablets.

At this point, your partner Janis explains to Amanda that she is going to take Amanda's vital signs while you continue to gather some necessary information. You then ask Amanda, "How long ago did you take these pills and was the bottle full?"

"I took them an hour ago. I just bought the pills on the way home from school."

"How much do you weigh, Amanda?"

"About 120 pounds, I think."

You contact medical direction by phone. The base station physician orders you to administer 50 grams of activated charcoal to the patient. You shake up the solution and pour it into a Styrofoam cup and cover it with a lid before inserting the straw. You explain to Amanda that you want her to drink the charcoal solution in order to help absorb the medication she has taken. You warn her that it does not taste very good and will feel gritty in her mouth.

You and your partner package Amanda for transportation on the stretcher as she begins to drink the solution. Following your department's policy, one of the police officers accompanies you to the emergency department. You provide an ongoing assessment during transportation. By the time you arrive at the hospital, Amanda has finished her charcoal.

You give a report to the receiving nurse at the bedside and return your unit to service.

A **poison** is any substance that can harm the body. Many of these substances are manufactured—for example, as cosmetics, cleaners, or pesticides—and cause poisoning when they are used improperly or are accidentally consumed. Other poisonous substances occur naturally—for example, some types of mushrooms or plants.

Some substances, known as **allergens,** set off an exaggerated response in the body's immune system. This natural response is intended to defend the body from foreign materials but, when over-exaggerated, can itself harm the body. This exaggerated response is called an **allergic reaction** and can be a life-threatening emergency.

POISONING

Our environment is filled with thousands of substances that are potentially poisonous. As a firefighter, you are exposed to many such poisons in the course of fire suppression duties. Carbon monoxide, hydrogen sulfide, and cyanide are common products of the combustion of modern building materials.

Poisonous materials are also common in the home. They are found as cleaners or bleaches under kitchen sinks or as fuel additives and anti-freeze solutions in the garage. Even substances such as aspirin that are normally thought of as benign or helpful can, when taken in excess, result in a life-threatening poisoning. Children,

with their natural curiosity, account for the largest number of poisoning victims, but anyone at any age can be a victim of poisoning.

You must learn to recognize when a poisoning has occurred and be prepared to provide the appropriate emergency medical care. However, you must always assure your own personal safety when you are called to the scene of a poisoning. The substance that made the patient ill may still be present in a quantity or form that poses a threat to you. In addition, a patient who has attempted to commit

Figure 15-1   Routes by which poisons enter the body.

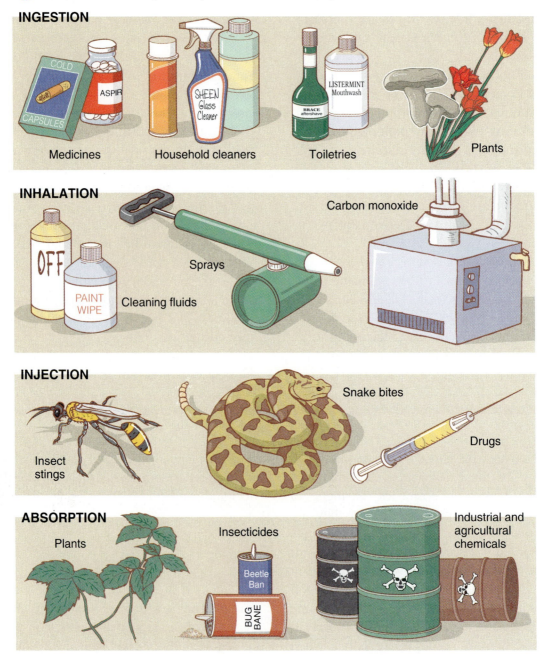

suicide through the use of a poison may be or become violent toward those who may attempt to help him. Always size up the scene of a suspected poisoning carefully, and remain alert at all times.

Routes of Exposure

In order to do harm to a patient, a poison must make contact with and enter the body. There are four general routes through which poisons enter the body (Figure 15-1):

◆ **Ingestion** (swallowing a poison) Ingestion of pills or other medications is a common means of poisoning. Children frequently swallow

medications and other household substances (Figure 15-2). Adults frequently ingest intentional overdoses of pills in suicidal gestures.

◆ **Inhalation** (breathing in a poison) The most common cause of inhalation poisoning is carbon monoxide. Use of self-contained breathing apparatus (SCBA) by firefighters helps to reduce the risk of inhaling toxic substances during structural and vehicle fire suppression activity.

◆ **Injection** (inserting a poison through the skin through use of a sharp object) Intravenous drug abuse and the injection of venom by

Figure 15-2 Poisoning is a common cause of accidental death in children. Always be alert to the possibility of poisoning with these patients.

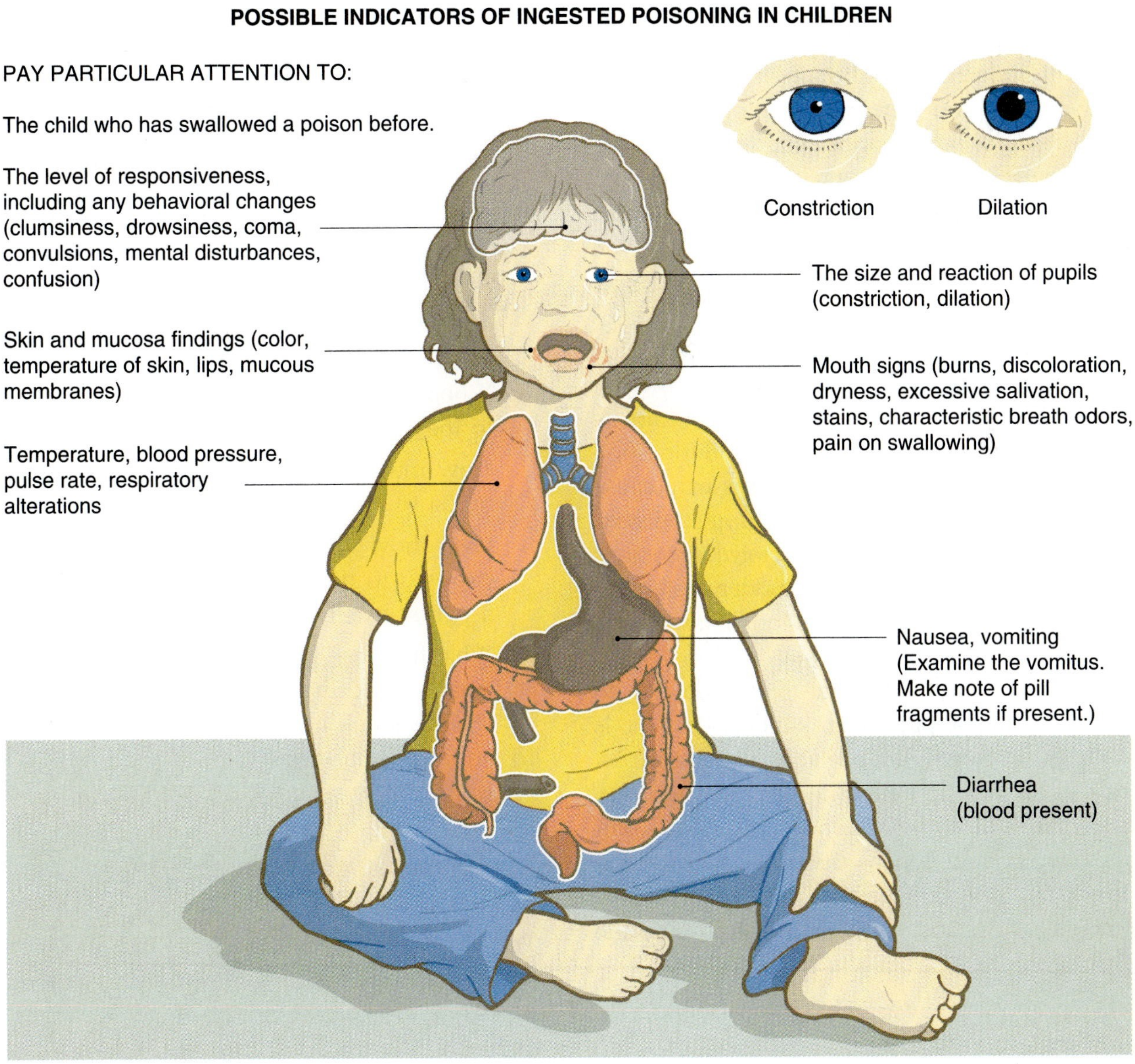

POSSIBLE INDICATORS OF INGESTED POISONING IN CHILDREN

PAY PARTICULAR ATTENTION TO:

The child who has swallowed a poison before.

The level of responsiveness, including any behavioral changes (clumsiness, drowsiness, coma, convulsions, mental disturbances, confusion)

Skin and mucosa findings (color, temperature of skin, lips, mucous membranes)

Temperature, blood pressure, pulse rate, respiratory alterations

Constriction   Dilation

The size and reaction of pupils (constriction, dilation)

Mouth signs (burns, discoloration, dryness, excessive salivation, stains, characteristic breath odors, pain on swallowing)

Nausea, vomiting (Examine the vomitus. Make note of pill fragments if present.)

Diarrhea (blood present)

insects (via stingers) and snakes (via fangs) are common types of injection-related poisonings.

♦ ***Absorption*** (taking a poison in through the unbroken skin or mucous membranes including the nose, eyes, and mouth) Certain chemicals such as organophosphates and solvents can be absorbed directly through intact skin and cause poisoning. Other agents cause direct chemical burns to the body surface.

Some substances such as insecticides can enter the body simultaneously by more than one of the routes described above.

Assessment of the Poisoning Patient

Scene size-up is the first step in the assessment of a potential poisoning patient. It is also an essential step in assuring your personal safety. Remember that inhaled and absorbed poisons that harmed the patient can also pose a risk to your well being. If you determine during the scene size-up that the substance that rendered the patient ill is still present and poses a hazard to rescuers, then request that a hazardous materials unit be dispatched. Do not enter a scene that you think may be unsafe unless you are properly trained and equipped.

As with any patient, control of the poisoned patient's airway is the top priority during the initial assessment and subsequent care. The airway can be particularly difficult to manage during poisonings. For example, chemical burns may cause swelling of the structures of the upper airway. Poisonings can also lead to excessive secretions that may obstruct the airway. Sudden deterioration in the patient's mental status may also cause the tongue to obstruct the airway.

One of the most important things you can do when assessing a poisoning/overdose patient is to obtain a thorough and accurate history. A good history can help medical direction, the poison center, and the emergency department staff make correct and timely decisions about treatment of the patient. Question the patient, family members, or bystanders and try to determine the following:

♦ What substance was the source of the poisoning?

COMPANY OFFICER'S NOTES

Many departments have protocols directing that emergency medical personnel contact the local poison control center for any case of suspected poisoning. In such systems, the poison control center is usually allowed to provide medical direction to the EMT, including approval of the use of activated charcoal. Poison control centers have been established across the United States and Canada. Most are staffed 24 hours a day and can be reached via a toll-free telephone number. The experienced professionals at the centers have access via computers to information on a wide variety of poisons, treatment options, and antidotes. They can answer almost any question about poisonings that you are likely to encounter. Memorize the phone number or be sure it is easily accessible aboard every emergency vehicle.

If you call a poison control center, be prepared to provide as much detail as possible about the patient and the circumstances of the poisoning. This will include the following: the patient's estimated age and weight; the patient's condition, including level of responsiveness, skin color, presence or absence of vomiting, etc.; and as many specifics as you can on the poison itself.

♦ When did the patient ingest/become exposed to the substance?

♦ How much of the substance did the patient ingest (if an ingestion)?

♦ Over how long a period was the patient exposed to the substance? Or over how long a period was he ingesting the substance?

♦ What has been done in an attempt to help the patient since the poisoning? Has he washed? Has he drunk milk or water? Has he received artificial ventilations?

♦ What is the patient's estimated weight?

Assessment and Management Techniques

The specific steps in assessing and managing a poisoning/overdose patient will vary, depending in a large measure, upon the route by which the exposure occurred.

◆ Assessment and Emergency Care—Poisoning by Ingestion

Ingestions are either accidental (a toddler eating an entire bottle of colorful, sweet-tasting children's vitamins) or intentional (a suicidal person taking an overdose of sleeping pills). Specific signs and symptoms associated with poisoning by ingestion include the following:

◆ History of ingesting a poisonous substance (gathered from patient, family members, bystanders, or evidence on the scene)

◆ Nausea

◆ Vomiting

◆ Abdominal pain

◆ Altered mental status

◆ Chemical burns around and inside the mouth

◆ Unusual odors on the breath

The emergency medical care for poisoning by ingestion includes the following steps:

1. **Assure that the patient's airway is open.**

2. **Provide supplemental oxygen if signs of altered mental status or shortness of breath are present.**

3. **Assure adequate breathing.** If breathing is inadequate, ventilate using a BVM. (Use of the pocket mask is not generally recommended for ventilating a poisoning patient.)

4. **Remove any visible pills, tablets, or fragments from the patient's mouth with a gloved hand.** (Do not attempt to remove material from a patient's mouth if there is a risk that you will be bitten.)

5. **Consult medical direction to determine if the administration of activated charcoal is appropriate.** If it is, follow the steps for administration in "Activated Charcoal" on the next page. If administration of activated charcoal is not appropriate, proceed to the next step.

6. **Transport the patient with all containers, bottles, and labels from the substance** (Figure 15-3).

7. **Perform the ongoing assessment en route.** Carefully monitor the patient's airway and

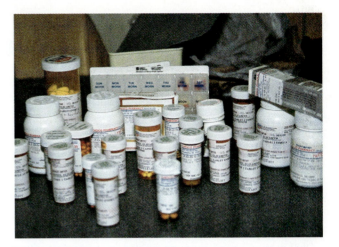

Figure 15-3 If you suspect that a patient has taken an overdose of medications, collect medication containers and transport them with the patient.

breathing and be prepared to suction and provide positive pressure ventilations.

◆ Assessment and Emergency Care—Poisoning by Inhalation

Inhaled toxic agents can harm patients in a variety of ways. Some agents cause direct irritation and injury to the airway. Other inhaled agents displace oxygen and cause severe disruption at the cellular level of the body.

Whenever you are called to the scene of an inhalation poisoning, remember that you, too, are at risk of becoming ill (or worse) from exposure to inhaled toxic agents. NEVER enter a scene without appropriate personal protective equipment including SCBA if there is any chance of coming in contact with the toxic substances that harmed the patient. If necessary, request that a hazardous materials unit be dispatched to the scene to secure it.

Specific signs and symptoms associated with poisoning by inhalation include the following:

◆ History of inhalation of toxic substances (gathered from the patient, family members, bystanders, or evidence at the scene)

◆ Difficulty breathing

◆ Chest pain

◆ Cough

◆ Hoarseness

◆ Dizziness

ACTIVATED CHARCOAL

Medication Name

Generic: Activated Charcoal
Trade*: SuperChar, InstaChar, Actidose, Liquidose

Note: Different types/brands of activated charcoal are more effective in binding ingested poisons than others. Consult with medical direction before purchasing activated charcoal for prehospital use.

Indications for Administration

Oral ingestion of poisons or drugs, especially if a prolonged transport will be required

Contraindications

1. Patient with an altered mental status
2. Patient who has ingested acids or alkalis
3. Patient who is unable to swallow

Medication Form

1. Pre-mixed as a suspension in water—often available in plastic bottles containing 12.5 grams of activated charcoal (Figure 15-4)
2. Dry powder (not for prehospital use)

Dosage

Adults and children: 1 gram of charcoal per kilogram (approximately 2 pounds) of body weight.
Usual adult dose: 25 to 50 grams
Usual infant/child dose: 12.5 to 25 grams

Figure 15-4 Several brands of activated charcoal are available.

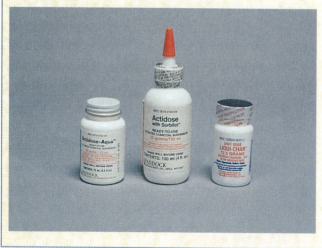

Actions

Binds to certain poisons that are then passed from the body with the stools rather than being absorbed into the body.

Side Effects

1. Dark stools
2. Constipation
3. May cause vomiting
4. Activated charcoal does not bind all poisons. Follow local protocols, which may include consulting with medical direction or the poison control center prior to use.

Administration

1. **Obtain an order from medical direction either on-line or off-line, by standing orders** (Figure 15-5A).
2. **Confirm that the patient is alert, without an altered mental status, and is able to swallow.**
3. **Shake the container thoroughly.**
4. **Because the solution looks like mud, many patients may hesitate to drink it. For best compliance, do the following:**
   a. Place the contents in a covered opaque container with a straw so that the patient cannot see what he is drinking (Figure 15-5B).
   b. Be prepared to spend some time convincing the patient of the need to drink the charcoal.
5. **If the patient takes a long time to drink the solution, the charcoal may settle and you will need to shake or stir it again.**
6. **Record the name, dose, route, and time of administration** (Figure 15-5C).
7. **Transport the patient, monitoring his condition carefully and performing an ongoing assessment en route to the receiving facility.** A poisoning patient may suddenly vomit up the charcoal or his condition may deteriorate rapidly because of the ingested poison. If the patient vomits soon after administration of the initial dose, one additional dose may generally be administered. (Check with medical direction or follow local protocols.)
8. **Bring all pill containers, bottles, and labels of the ingested substance to the receiving facility.**

Administering Activated Charcoal

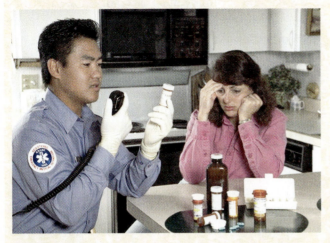

Figure 15-5A Obtain an order from medical direction to administer activated charcoal.

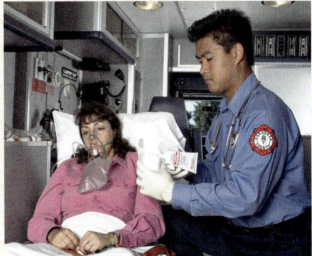

Figure 15-5B Shake the container of activated charcoal thoroughly and pour it into an opaque cup with a lid and a straw. Be prepared to encourage the patient to drink all of the charcoal.

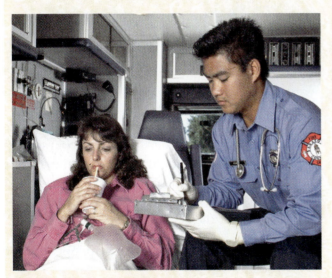

Figure 15-5C Record the dose and the time it was administered. If the patient takes a long time to drink the charcoal, shake or stir the solution again.

◆ Headache

◆ Altered mental status

◆ Seizures

The emergency care for poisoning by inhalation includes the following steps (Figure 15-6, page 373).

1. **Have appropriately trained and equipped rescuers remove the patient from the poisonous environment.**

2. **Provide the patient with high concentration oxygen if you have not already done so during the initial assessment.**

3. **Be prepared to provide positive pressure ventilations with high concentration oxygen via a BVM.** (Do not use a pocket mask when ventilating a patient poisoned by an inhaled agent.)

4. **Transport the patient to the receiving facility.** Bring whatever information—bottles, labels, etc.—is available on the scene about the inhaled substance to the receiving facility.

5. **Perform the ongoing assessment en route.** Carefully monitor the patient's airway and breathing and be prepared to suction and to provide positive pressure ventilations.

COMPANY OFFICER'S NOTES

As a company officer, it will likely be your responsibility to determine when a "poisoning" crosses a line of magnitude to become a "hazardous materials incident" requiring the use of additional resources. Most cases of ingestion and injection can be managed as poisonings. Incidents where illnesses are caused by absorbed or inhaled toxic substances are potentially more likely to require a hazardous materials response. (See Chapter 28, "EMS Special Operations.")

◆ Assessment and Emergency Care—Poisoning by Injection

Among the most common forms of poisoning by injection are intravenous drug overdoses and the stings and bites of animals such as spiders and snakes. (Stings and bites will be discussed in detail in Chapter 16, "Environmental Emergencies," and later in this chapter under Allergic Reactions.) The most commonly injected street drugs are cocaine and narcotic drugs such as heroin. Narcotic overdoses can produce a classic picture of unresponsiveness, inadequate breathing, and pinpoint—or very small—pupils (Figure 15-7, page 374).

Be especially careful of your own safety when called to the scene of a potential drug overdose (Figure 15-8, page 374). Some drug abusers may be calm when you first arrive, but grow more agitated as time passes. If you think there is a potential for violence at a scene, retreat from it and request law enforcement back-up. Do not return until the scene is secure.

Also remember that drug abusers often use hypodermic needles. An accidental puncture with a used needle can transmit infectious diseases. Always take appropriate body substance isolation precautions and watch where you put your hands (Figure 15-9, page 375).

Specific signs and symptoms associated with poisoning by injection include the following:

◆ A history of injection of a harmful substance (gathered from the patient, family members, bystanders, or evidence at the scene)

◆ Weakness

◆ Dizziness

◆ Chills

◆ Fever

◆ Nausea

◆ Vomiting

◆ Tiny, pinpoint pupils

◆ Altered mental status

◆ Chest pain

◆ Inadequate breathing

The emergency medical care for poisoning by injection includes the steps below. Always exercise extreme caution when performing these steps in order to avoid punctures from contaminated needles that the patient may have on him or that are lying about the scene.

1. **Assure scene safety. Take appropriate BSI precautions.**

2. **Maintain an open airway.**

3. **Provide oxygen and assist ventilations as necessary.**

4. **Be alert for vomiting and be prepared to suction the airway.**

5. **Transport the patient to the receiving facility.** Bring whatever information—bottles, vials, etc.—is available on the scene about the injected substance to the receiving facility.

6. **Perform the ongoing assessment en route.** Carefully monitor the patient's airway and breathing and be prepared to suction and to provide positive pressure ventilations.

Inhaled Poisoning

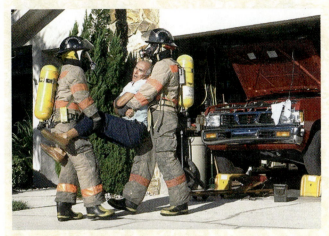

Figure 15-6A Properly equipped rescuers should remove the patient from the scene of the inhalation poisoning.

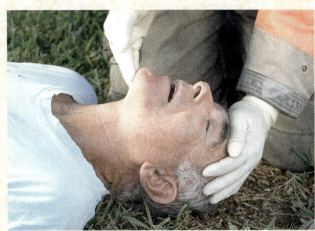

Figure 15-6B Open the patient's airway. Use an oropharyngeal airway if necessary to secure the airway.

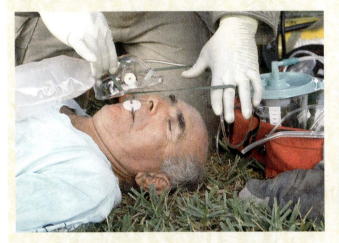

Figure 15-6C Provide high concentration oxygen via nonrebreather mask. If breathing is inadequate, provide positive pressure ventilations via a BVM device.

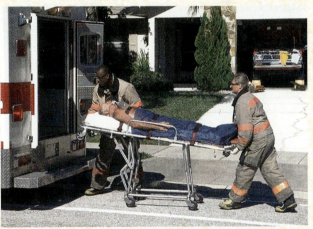

Figure 15-6D Transport the patient, providing an ongoing assessment en route. Be prepared to suction the patient's airway and to provide positive pressure ventilations if his breathing becomes inadequate.

◆ Assessment and Emergency Care—Poisoning by Absorption

Absorbed poisons can pose significant risks to both the patient and the EMT. Many absorbed poisons, such organophosphate insecticides, are highly toxic and can be fatal rapidly. Other absorbed toxic agents can cause severe chemical burns. Take all necessary precautions during scene size-up. Use appropriate personal protective equipment (Figure 15-10, page 375). If the amount of poisonous material released poses a significant threat, request that a hazardous materials unit be dispatched to the scene.

COMPANY OFFICER'S NOTES

Carbon monoxide (CO) is by far the most common cause of death in inhalation poisonings. CO poisoning can result from structural fires, malfunctioning heating systems, and accidental or intentional exposure to automotive exhaust. The use of residential CO detectors has further increased the relevance of assessment and treatment of potential CO poisoning patients for the fire service. Calls prompted by CO detectors account for a growing percentage of fire department responses.

The symptoms of CO poisoning can be subtle and non-specific. They may include headache, nausea, dizziness, and slight alteration in mental status. With such non-specific symptoms, it can be difficult to determine whether a patient has sustained a dangerous exposure to CO. The most reliable indicator of potentially serious CO poisoning is any loss of consciousness. Cases of serious CO poisoning may require specialized care such as treatment in a hyperbaric chamber.

All patients with symptoms that may be related to CO exposure—based on activation of a home CO detector or a history of having been in an atmosphere that contained high levels of CO—should be placed on high concentration oxygen and transported to the hospital for further evaluation. Identify on the scene any patients who are found unconscious or who have a history of loss of consciousness and be sure this information is relayed to the emergency department staff. Identifying these high-risk patients is especially important when caring for multiple patients with potential CO exposure as in a multiple-occupancy dwelling. In these cases, vital information about high-risk patients can too easily get misplaced or overlooked as a dozen or more CO poisoning patients suddenly pour into the emergency department.

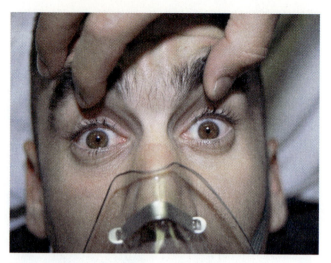

Figure 15-7 A patient with pin-point pupils from a narcotic overdose.

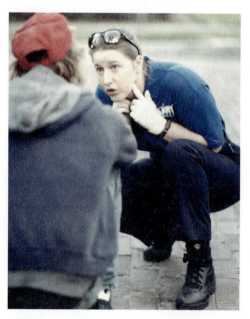

Figure 15-8 A drug overdose patient may appear calm at first but can rapidly turn violent. Position yourself so that you can retreat rapidly if you perceive any possible danger.

Specific signs and symptoms associated with poisoning by absorption include the following:

◆ History of exposure (gathered from the patient, family members, bystanders, or evidence at the scene)

◆ Liquid or powder on the patient's skin

◆ Excessive saliva production

◆ Excessive tear production

◆ Uncontrolled diarrhea

◆ Burns

◆ Itching

◆ Skin irritation

◆ Redness of the skin

The emergency medical care for poisoning by absorption includes the steps described below. Be sure to use appropriate personal protective equipment.

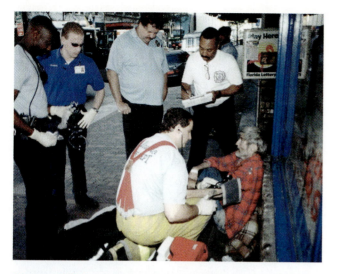

Figure 15-9 Drug overdose patients may carry hypodermic needles with them. If you suspect a drug overdose, exercise caution when performing any procedure to avoid a needle puncture.

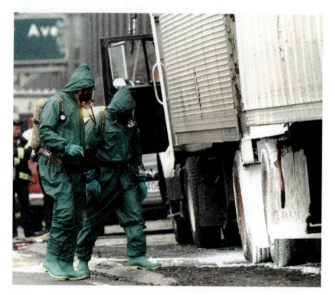

Figure 15-10 Encapsulating suits and SCBA are often required for rescuers at scenes of chemical leaks or spills.

1. **Maintain an open airway.**

2. **Provide oxygen and assist ventilations as necessary**

3. **Remove the substance from the patient in the following ways:**

—*Clothing.* Remove contaminated clothing.

—*Powders.* Carefully brush as much of the powder as possible off the patient. When doing so, be careful not to make the substance airborne and cause wider contamination. Irrigate with clean water for at least 20 minutes at the scene. Continue irrigating en route to the receiving facility if possible.

—*Liquids.* Irrigate with clean water for at least 20 minutes at the scene.

—*Eyes.* Irrigate with clean water for at least 20 minutes (Figure 15-11). Position the patient so that the water drains away from the affected eye and does not wash back into that eye or into the other eye. Continue irrigating en route to the receiving facility if possible.

4. **Transport the patient to the receiving facility.** Bring whatever information—containers, bottles, labels, etc.—is available on the scene about the absorbed substance to the receiving facility. Do not, however, transport potentially hazardous materials.

5. **Perform the ongoing assessment en route.** Carefully monitor the patient's airway and breathing and be prepared to suction and to provide positive pressure ventilations.

Figure 15-11 If a poisonous substance has gotten into a patient's eye, irrigate the eye with clean water for at least 20 minutes. Eyewash stations are ideal for initial irrigation. Position the patient so that the run-off does not drain into the unaffected eye.

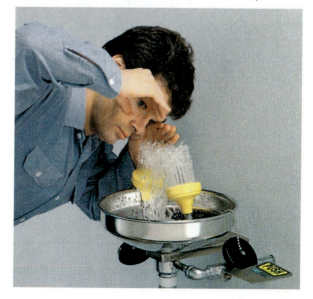

A LLERGIC REACTIONS

The body's immune system is designed to fight off infections and other substances that it identifies as not belonging within the body. When functioning normally, this system controls minor infections, prevents future infections (by developing immunities), and in general, polices the body to assure that it "reacts" to potentially harmful substances that are not naturally occurring. Sometimes, however, the immune system's response to a substance is exaggerated, resulting in a release of chemicals from the cells of the immune system. These chemicals cause the physiologic events that make up an allergic reaction.

A severe allergic reaction can be a life-threatening event. The major physiologic change that makes the event so potentially dangerous is that the body's blood vessels lose their normal tone and ability to contain fluids. "Leaking" from these vessels produces the swelling of the face, neck, and tongue characteristic of severe allergic reaction as fluids seep into the tissues (Figure 12A and B). The leaking can also cause swelling in the linings of the bronchioles of the lungs and upper airway structures, leading to narrowing of the airways as well as fluid loss sufficient to cause hypoperfusion (shock). Hypoperfusion that results from a severe allergic reaction is commonly referred to as **anaphylactic shock.** Shock may be worsened by the dilation of blood vessels.

Allergic reactions can range from the watery eyes and runny nose of hay fever to severe hypoperfusion and respiratory failure that can accompany a bee sting. A wide variety of different substances can cause allergic reactions in people (Figure 15-13). Some of the most common causes include:

♦ Venom from insect bites and stings, especially those of bees, wasps, hornets, and yellow jackets

♦ Foods, including nuts, shellfish/crustaceans, peanuts, milk, eggs, chocolate, etc.

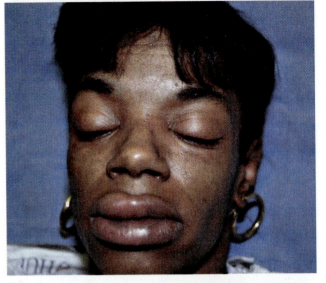

A.

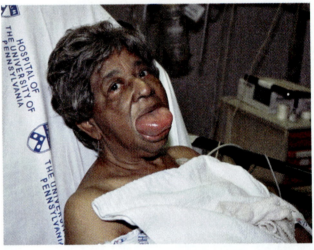

B.

Figure 15-12 **A.** Allergic reaction with swelling of the lips and eyelids. **B.** Swelling of the tongue compromising the airway of a patient with a severe drug reaction.

♦ Plants, including contact with poison ivy, poison oak, and pollen from ragweed and grasses

♦ Medications, including penicillin and other antibiotics, aspirin, seizure medications, muscle relaxants, etc.

♦ Others causes include dust, latex, glue, soaps, make-up, etc.

It is severe allergic reactions that you must be prepared to recognize and treat. One highly effective treatment you may be able to provide in cases of severe allergic reaction is assistance in administering a prescribed epinephrine auto-injector.

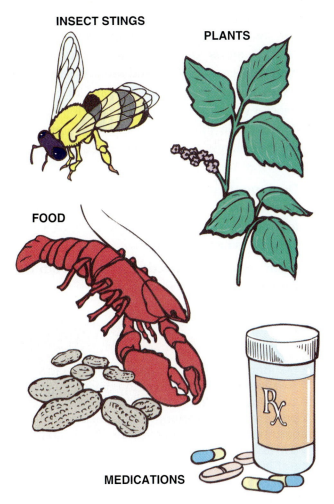

INSECT STINGS

PLANTS

FOOD

MEDICATIONS

Figure 15-13 Some common causes of allergic reactions.

Many patients will know from previous experiences that they have severe allergies to certain substances. Although the patients try to avoid contact with these substances, accidental exposures do sometimes occur. For example, a bee may sting a patient or a patient allergic to peanuts may unknowingly eat a dish prepared with a minute amount of peanuts. A patient with a history of severe allergic reaction may wear a medical identification device with information about his condition. Such a patient may also have an epinephrine auto-injector that has been prescribed by his physician.

Assessment of the Patient with an Allergic Reaction

Control of the allergic reaction patient's airway is the top priority during the initial assessment and subsequent care. The airway can be particularly dif-

ficult to manage during allergic reactions because of swelling of the structures of the upper airway and sudden deterioration in the patient's condition.

Follow all appropriate steps to size up the scene and assure your safety and the patient's. Be sure to scan the scene for signs of an agent that may have produced the allergic reaction. Be aware that the agent that produced the allergic reaction can be dangerous to you as well. For example, a patient may have experienced an allergic reaction after being stung by yellow jackets. Swarms of the insects may still be near the patient and ready to sting anyone who approaches.

During the initial assessment be alert for signs of airway obstruction due to swelling. Administer high flow oxygen during the initial assessment if signs of obstruction or inadequate breathing are present. Assess for signs of hypoperfusion. Also look the patient over for a medical identification device that gives information about his allergies.

During the focused history and physical exam quickly obtain the following information about the allergic reaction along with a SAMPLE history. If the patient is unable to assist you, try to obtain the information from family members or friends.

◆ Does the patient have a previous history of allergies/allergic reactions?

◆ What substance was the patient exposed to?

◆ How long ago did the exposure occur?

◆ What symptoms has the patient experienced (shortness of breath, tightness in the throat/chest, warm, tingling sensations of the skin or face, facial swelling, light-headedness, etc.)?

◆ Have the symptoms progressed? (What happened first? Next? How rapidly?)

◆ Has the patient taken any medications such as Benadryl® (diphenhydramine) or an epinephrine auto-injector? Has any other care been provided to him?

Obtain baseline vital signs and perform a physical examination. Physical exam findings that may indicate an allergic reaction include any of those listed below. Findings that indicate a patient with a severe allergic reaction are marked with an asterisk (*).

- Skin:
  - —Swelling of the face, lips, tongue*, neck, hands
  - —Itching
  - —Hives
  - —Red skin (flushing)
- Respiratory system:
  - —Cough*
  - —Rapid breathing*
  - —Labored/inadequate breathing*
  - —Noisy breathing*
  - —Hoarseness (change or loss of voice)*
  - —Stridor (high pitched noise during inhalation heard at the neck and upper chest)*
  - —Wheezing*
- Cardiovascular system:
  - —Increased heart rate*
  - —Decreased blood pressure*
  - —Signs of hypoperfusion (cool, clammy skin)*
- Decreased mental status *
- Generalized symptoms
  - —Itchy, watery eyes
  - —Headache
  - —Sense of impending doom*
  - —Runny nose

◆ *Emergency Care—Patient with Severe Allergic Reaction, History of Allergic Reaction, and a Prescribed Auto-Injector*

If the patient has come in contact with a substance that has caused allergic reactions in the past and complains of respiratory distress or exhibits signs of hypoperfusion (shock), then proceed as follows:

1. **Administer high flow oxygen if you have not already done so during the initial assessment.** If the patient is not breathing adequately, open his airway and provide positive pressure ventilations.
2. **Determine if the patient has a prescribed epinephrine auto-injector available.**

3. **If the patient has a prescribed auto-injector available, proceed with the administration steps described in "Epinephrine Auto-Injector" below and shown in Figure 15-14.** If he does not have a prescribed auto-injector or it is not available, provide care as described in "Emergency Care—Patient with Severe Allergic Reaction Without a Prescribed Auto-Injector" below.
4. **Document administration of the auto-injector and transport the patient, monitoring closely and reassessing vital signs at least every 5 minutes.**
5. **Remove any constricting jewelry from the fingers, wrists, or neck.**

COMPANY OFFICER'S NOTES

Because an epinephrine auto-injector system uses a needle, the device must be properly handled and disposed of after use to prevent an inadvertent needle stick to a department member. Any vehicle that is staffed by EMTs authorized to assist patients with the use of auto-injectors should carry a biohazard "sharps box" for the safe disposal of the devices.

◆ *Emergency Care—Patient with Severe Allergic Reaction Without a Prescribed Auto-Injector*

If the patient has come in contact with a substance that has caused allergic reactions in the past and complains of respiratory distress or exhibits signs of shock (hypoperfusion), then proceed as follows:

1. **Administer high flow oxygen if you have not already done so during the initial assessment.** If the patient is not breathing adequately, open his airway and provide positive pressure ventilations.
2. **If you determine that the patient does not have a prescribed auto-injector or it is not available, transport him immediately.** Request an ALS intercept if available.

(continued)

EPINEPHRINE AUTO-INJECTOR

Medication Name

Generic: Epinephrine
Trade: Adrenalin®
Delivery system: EpiPen®, EpiPen Jr.®

Indications for Administration

When an EMT assists with/administers an epinephrine auto-injector, a patient must meet *all* of the following three criteria:

1. The patient must exhibit signs of a severe allergic reaction such as respiratory distress or shock (hypoperfusion).
2. The epinephrine auto-injector must be prescribed by a physician for this specific patient.
3. Medical direction must authorize use for this patient.

Contraindications

There are no contraindications when used in a life-threatening situation.

Medication Form

Liquid administered via an automatic needle-and-syringe system designed to administer a predetermined dose (Figure 15-15)

Dosage

Adult: One adult auto-injector dose of 0.3 mg
Child: One pediatric auto-injector dose of 0.15 mg

Actions

Dilates the bronchioles
Constricts blood vessels

Side Effects

Anxiety, palpitations, chest pain (rare), irregular heart beats (dysrhythmias), pale skin, headache, dizziness

Administration

1. **Contact medical direction and obtain an order either on-line or off-line as per local protocol.**
2. **If permission for use of epinephrine is obtained, then ensure the following:**
   a. That the prescription is written for the patient having the allergic reaction
   b. That the medication is clear and not discolored (if you are able to see into the syringe)
3. **Remove the safety cap from the injector.**
4. **Place the tip of the injector against the patient's bare lateral thigh midway between the waist and the knee.**
5. **Push the injector firmly against the thigh until the spring-loaded needle is activated.**
6. **Hold the injector in place until all the medication is injected.**
7. **Record the time of injection on your care report.**
8. **Dispose of the empty auto-injector in an appropriate biohazard sharps container.**
9. **Transport the patient to a receiving facility.**

Reassessment

1. **Reassess the patient 2 minutes after the epinephrine injection.**
2. **If patient's condition worsens (increased breathing difficulty, decreased mental status, worsening signs of hypoperfusion), do the following:**
   - Contact medical control
   - Consider an additional epinephrine dose if approved by medical direction
   - Request an ALS intercept, if available
   - Treat the patient for shock (hypoperfusion).
   - Prepare to initiate life support measures:
     —Ventilation with 100 percent oxygen
     —CPR
     —Application of an AED if the patient suffers a cardiac arrest
   - Document all changes in patient's condition
3. **If patient's condition improves, do the following:**
   - Provide supportive care:
     —High flow oxygen
     —Treatment for shock (hypoperfusion)
4. **Continue to perform the ongoing assessment en route to the receiving facility.** Carefully monitor the patient's airway, breathing, and circulation.

Administering an Epinephrine Auto-Injector

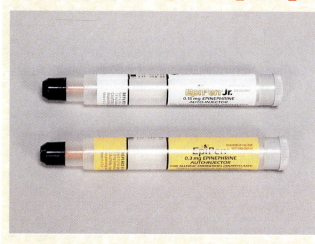

Figure 15-14A Infant/child (white label) and adult (yellow label) epinephrine auto-injectors.

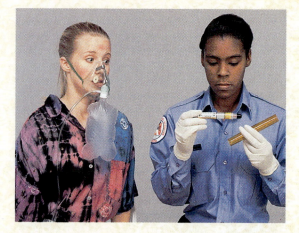

Figure 15-14B If medical direction authorizes use of the auto-injector, check to assure that it is one prescribed for the patient. Also check that the fluid is not discolored (if you can see into the syringe).

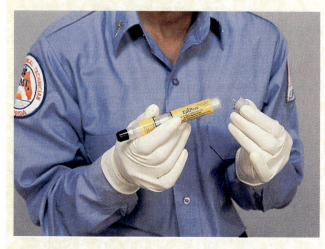

Figure 15-14C Remove the auto-injector's safety cap.

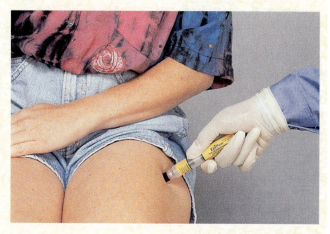

Figure 15-14D Place the tip of the injector on the patient's lateral thigh, midway between waist and knee. Push the auto-injector firmly until it activates. Hold the auto-injector firmly in place until the full dose of medication is delivered.

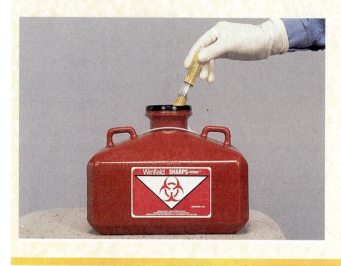

Figure 15-14E Dispose of the used auto-injector in a biohazard sharps container. Record the time you administered the injection on the care report.

3. Remove any constricting jewelry from the fingers, wrists, or neck.

4. **Perform an ongoing assessment en route to the hospital.** Continue to monitor the status of the patient's airway, breathing, and circulation.

5. **If patient's condition worsens (increased breathing difficulty, decreased mental status, worsening signs of hypoperfusion), do the following:**

   ◆ Contact medical control

   ◆ Treat for hypoperfusion (shock)

   ◆ Prepare to initiate life support measures including the following:

   —Ventilation with 100 percent oxygen

   —CPR

   —Application of an AED if patient suffers a cardiac arrest

6. **Document all changes that may occur in the patient's condition.**

◆ *Emergency Care—Patient with an Allergic Reaction but No Signs or Symptoms of Severe Reaction*

If the patient has come in contact with a substance that has caused past allergic reactions but *does not* complain of respiratory distress or exhibit signs of shock (hypoperfusion), then proceed as follows:

1. **Continue the focused assessment.**

2. **Remove any constricting jewelry from the patient's fingers, wrists, or neck.**

3. **Do *NOT* administer an epinephrine auto-injector.**

4. **Initiate transport to a receiving facility.**

5. **Conduct an ongoing assessment. Monitor the patient's airway, breathing, and circulation closely. If signs of a severe allergic reaction develop, then follow the steps outlined above.**

6. **Document any changes in the patient's condition en route to the receiving facility.**

TRANSITION OF CARE

If an epinephrine auto-injector is used by a first-responding EMT who will not be accompanying the patient in the ambulance, then assure that the following information is accurately and concisely conveyed to the transporting crew:

◆ The substance the patient was exposed to

◆ How long ago the exposure occurred

◆ The symptoms the patient reported (shortness of breath, tightness in the throat/chest, facial swelling, light-headedness, etc.) before epinephrine administration

◆ The EMT's assessment findings, including baseline vital signs prior to epinephrine administration

◆ The name of the physician or other authorized health professional who was contacted to authorize epinephrine administration

◆ The time and dosage of epinephrine administered

◆ The patient's response to treatment

Chapter Review

SUMMARY

It is important that you learn how to recognize poisonings, overdoses, and allergic reactions. Prompt recognition and the initiation of appropriate emergency medical care of these medical emergencies including the administration of activated charcoal or epinephrine may be life saving for the patient.

REVIEWING KEY CONCEPTS

1. List four routes by which poisons enter the body.

2. Describe basic elements you should try to establish when gathering a history of a patient who has been poisoned.

3. Describe the steps in the emergency care for poisoning by ingestion.

4. List the indications, contraindications, dosage, and procedures for administration of activated charcoal.

5. Describe the steps in the emergency care for poisoning by inhalation.

6. Describe the steps in the emergency care for poisoning by absorption.

7. Describe common causes of allergic reactions.

8. List common signs and symptoms of allergic reactions. Describe which of those signs and symptoms are associated with acute allergic reaction.

9. Describe the indications and contraindications for use of the epinephrine auto-injector.

10. Describe possible side effects of using an epinephrine auto-injector.

11. Describe steps in administering an epinephrine auto-injector.

RESOURCES TO LEARN MORE

Poisoning

Goldfranks, L. R. et al., eds. *Toxicologic Emergencies, 5th Edition*. Norwalk, CT: Appleton-Lange, 1994.

"Toxicology" in Tintinalli, J. E. et al. *Emergency Medicine: A Comprehensive Study Guide, 4th Edition*. New York: McGraw-Hill, 1995.

Allergic Reactions

Salomone, J. A. "Anaphylaxis and Acute Allergic Reactions," in Tintinalli, J. E. et al. *Emergency Medicine: A Comprehensive Study Guide, 4th Edition*. New York: McGraw-Hill, 1995.

ADMINISTERING ACTIVATED CHARCOAL TO AN INGESTED POISONING PATIENT

Obtain an order from medical direction either on-line or off-line (by standing orders).

↓

Confirm that the patient is alert, without an altered mental status, and is able to swallow.

↓

Shake the container thoroughly.

↓

Place the contents in a covered opaque container with a straw so that the patient cannot see what he is drinking. If the patient takes a long time to drink the solution, shake or stir it again.

↓

Record the name, dose, route, and time of administration.

↓

Transport the patient, monitoring his condition carefully and performing an ongoing assessment en route to the receiving facility. If the patient vomits soon after administration of the initial dose, one additional dose may generally be administered. (Check with medical direction or follow local protocols.)

↓

Bring all pill containers, bottles, and labels of the ingested substance to the receiving facility.

ADMINISTERING EPINEPHRINE TO A PATIENT WITH SEVERE ALLERGIC REACTION

Contact medical direction and obtain an order either on-line or off-line as per local protocol.

↓

If permission for use of epinephrine is obtained, then ensure the following:
• That the prescription is written for the patient having the allergic reaction
• That the medication is clear and not discolored (if you are able to see into the syringe)

↓

Remove the safety cap from the injector.

↓

Place the tip of the injector against the patient's bare lateral thigh midway between the waist and knee.

↓

Push the injector firmly against the thigh until the spring-loaded needle is activated.

↓

Hold the injector in place until all the medication is injected.

↓

Record the time of injection on the patient care report.

↓

Dispose of the empty auto-injector in an appropriate biohazard sharps container.

↓

Transport the patient to a receiving facility.

↓

Reassess the patient 2 minutes after the epinephrine injection and document all changes in the patient's condition.

↓

If patient's condition worsens:
• Contact medical control
• Consider an additional epinephrine dose if approved by medical direction
• Request an ALS intercept, if available
• Treat the patient for shock (hypoperfusion).
• Prepare to initiate life support measures:
  —Ventilation with 100 percent oxygen
  —CPR
  —Application of an AED if the patient suffers cardiac arrest

↓

If patient's condition improves, do the following:
• Provide supportive care
  —High flow oxygen
  —Treatment for shock (hypoperfusion)

↓

Continue to perform the ongoing assessment en route to the receiving facility.

Environmental Emergencies

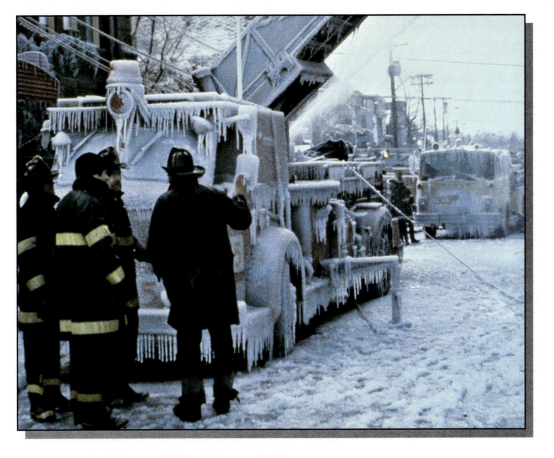

*A*s human beings, we constantly interact with the environment of the world that surrounds us. Yet some of those interactions—exposure to extremes of temperature, contact with water, or the bites or stings of animals or insects—may result in environmental medical emergencies. Children and the elderly as well as people with pre-existing medical conditions are at special risk to hazards posed by environmental conditions. In addition, firefighters are especially likely to encounter heat- and cold-related illnesses and injuries as part of fire suppression duties.

At the completion of this chapter, the EMT-Basic student should be able to meet the following objectives:

Knowledge and Understanding

1. Describe the various ways the body loses heat. (pp. 387–388)
2. List the signs and symptoms of emergencies arising from exposure to the cold. (pp. 390–391, 393–394)
3. Explain the steps in providing emergency medical care to patients suffering from cold-related emergencies. (pp. 391–392, 394–395)
4. List the signs and symptoms of emergencies arising from exposure to heat. (pp. 396–397)
5. Explain the steps in providing emergency medical care to patients suffering from heat-related emergencies. (pp. 397–398)
6. Recognize the signs and symptoms of water-related emergencies. (pp. 398–399)

7. Describe the complications of near drowning. (pp. 398–400)
8. Discuss the emergency medical care of bites and stings. (pp. 403–406)

Skills

1. Demonstrate the assessment and emergency medical care of a patient with exposure to the cold.
2. Demonstrate the assessment and emergency medical care of a patient with exposure to heat.
3. Demonstrate the assessment and emergency medical care of a near-drowning patient.
4. Demonstrate completing a prehospital care report for patients with environmental emergencies.

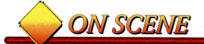

ON SCENE

DISPATCH: *ENGINE 31, ENGINE 2, TRUCK 1, SQUAD 2, BATTALION 8. RESPOND TO A REPORTED WORKING STRUCTURE FIRE. THE ADDRESS IS 1018 FURSTON STREET. CROSS STREET IS WARDS LANE. TIME OUT IS 0210.*

You are assigned to Truck 1 for this call on a bitterly cold January night. The scene proves to be a fire at an apartment building. About a dozen of the building's occupants have been driven to the street in the subfreezing temperatures. Two hours into the call, as you are conducting overhaul operations, you and the other EMT on the ladder company are ordered by the battalion chief to proceed to an alley beside the building. You are told to evaluate for possible cold exposure a patient who has been discovered there.

The fire is now out, and you know that the alley is safe from hazards of fire or collapse. As you walk up the alley, you see an elderly man sitting propped up against the wall and wearing only his underwear and a pair of shoes. You

approach him and begin your initial assessment, saying, "Hello. How are you doing? I'm with the fire department."

The patient does not respond to your greeting. You note that he appears to be very sleepy. As you touch his arm to get his attention, you can feel that his T-shirt is wet and frozen to his skin. As your partner places him on high flow oxygen, you continue your initial assessment and find that the patient only grunts in response to questions. You note his airway to be clear, but his respirations are slow and his pulse is also slow and weak. You assess the patient to be suffering from severe generalized hypothermia and radio for an ambulance to respond.

The ambulance is on scene within 2 minutes. You and your partner assist the ambulance EMTs in carefully loading the patient onto the stretcher. Once in the back of the ambulance, you make sure the cabin heat has been turned up to the maximum. You then remove the patient's wet and frozen clothing and wrap him in warm blankets. You quickly give a report to the ambulance crew, advising them that it is likely the patient has been outdoors in wet clothing for over 2 hours. You note that he displays an altered mental status and slowed respirations and pulse. The ambulance EMTs thank you for your help and begin transport. You later learn that the patient suffered a cardiac arrest in the emergency department and died despite an hour of attempted resuscitation by the hospital staff.

TEMPERATURE REGULATION AND THE BODY

The human body usually maintains a constant core body temperature of 98.6° Fahrenheit (37° Celsius). The body's own temperature regulation system helps to maintain this temperature. The regulation system is aided by the fact that people try to keep themselves in environments that are neither too hot nor too cold. Cold- and heat-related emergencies most often arise when patients find themselves in extreme environments without proper protection from the temperatures that surround them.

Mechanisms of Temperature Regulation (Thermoregulation)

The body's temperature regulation system works by preserving a balance between heat production and heat loss. This system is so well developed that, during a normal day, there is only about 1° Celsius of variation in body temperature.

The body generates heat through internal chemical reactions. A variety of events cause these heat-producing reactions, including food intake and activity. Even exposure of the body to cold can trigger heat production when the body reacts by shivering.

When the body's heat production and retention exceeds its heat loss, the resulting rise in body temperature above the normal level is called **hyperthermia.** When the body's heat loss exceeds its ability to produce and retain heat, then the resulting drop in body temperature below the normal level is called **hypothermia.**

Several mechanisms can work separately or together to produce a loss of body heat (Figure 16-1). It is important for you as an EMT to understand these mechanisms of heat loss and to recognize when they may be at work. If you do, you can act to prevent further heat loss in patients who are already too cold (hypothermic patients) and to cool down patients who are too hot (hyperthermic). Working with these mechanisms is the basis for treatment in many environmental emergencies.

- ◆ *Radiation* **Radiation** is the process by which energy, in the form of heat, is emitted from the body in waves or rays. This type of heat loss generally occurs when uncovered or non-insulated body parts are exposed to a cooler environment. The direct loss of body heat from an uncovered head is perhaps the most common source of radiation heat loss.

- ◆ *Conduction* Heat loss by **conduction** occurs when the body comes in direct contact with a colder object. Conductive heat loss can easily take place when a patient is lying on cold ground. Even more rapid and severe conductive heat loss occurs when a patient is immersed in cold water, a situation common in many water-related emergencies.

- ◆ *Convection* Heat loss by **convection** occurs when cooler air moves across the body and the body's heat is transferred to the moving air. This type of heat loss is common in windy conditions, as the wind sweeps away the thin layer of warmed air that normally surrounds the body. Convective heat loss is a particular problem for outdoor enthusiasts.

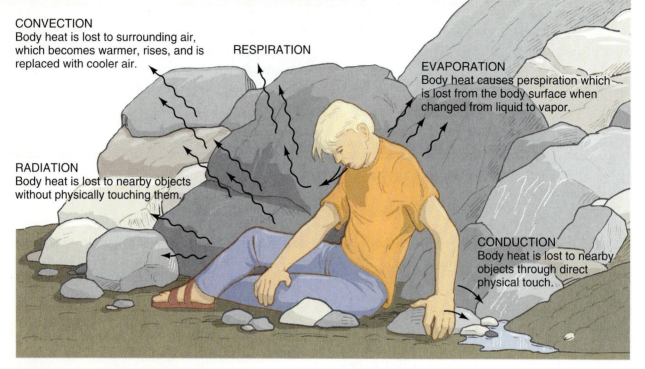

MECHANISMS OF HEAT LOSS

CONVECTION
Body heat is lost to surrounding air, which becomes warmer, rises, and is replaced with cooler air.

RESPIRATION

EVAPORATION
Body heat causes perspiration which is lost from the body surface when changed from liquid to vapor.

RADIATION
Body heat is lost to nearby objects without physically touching them.

CONDUCTION
Body heat is lost to nearby objects through direct physical touch.

Figure 16-1   This illustration shows various ways in which a person in an outdoor setting can lose body heat

◆ *Evaporation* Heat loss by **evaporation** occurs when a liquid is transformed into a vapor. Breathing is a common form of evaporative heat loss, during which warm, moist air is exhaled. Evaporative heat loss is the mechanism that allows the body to cool itself by producing perspiration.

Patients often lose heat through a combination of the mechanisms described above. The type of heat loss experienced by a patient will be affected by factors such the environment in which the patient is found, his length of exposure to it, and how he is clothed.

PEDIATRIC NOTE

Newborns are at particular risk for radiation heat loss from their uncovered heads and evaporative heat loss from amniotic and other fluids on the skin. All newborns should be carefully but thoroughly dried after birth, and their heads covered. (See Chapter 17, "Obstetrics and Gynecological Emergencies" for other ways to prevent heat loss.)

GERIATRIC NOTE

If you are treating an elderly patient who has fallen, be alert to the possibility of excessive conductive heat loss from contact with a cold floor, especially if there has been a delay between the fall and discovery of the patient.

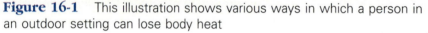

COLD-RELATED EMERGENCIES

A variety of factors—including pre-existing medical conditions, the age of the patient, and the type and length of cold exposure—influence the kind of cold-related emergency a patient will experience. Usually, these emergencies are divided into two major types. One type is generalized cold emergency or generalized hypothermia, which affects the patient's entire body. The other type is local cold injury, in which the cold causes damage to a particular part or parts of the body.

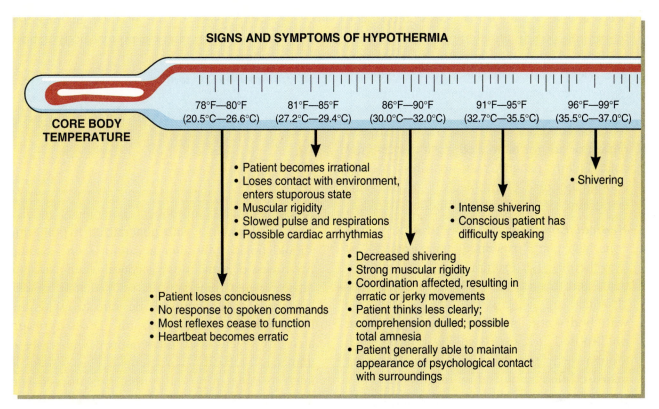

SIGNS AND SYMPTOMS OF HYPOTHERMIA

CORE BODY TEMPERATURE

| 78°F—80°F (20.5°C—26.6°C) | 81°F—85°F (27.2°C—29.4°C) | 86°F—90°F (30.0°C—32.0°C) | 91°F—95°F (32.7°C—35.5°C) | 96°F—99°F (35.5°C—37.0°C) |

• Shivering

• Patient becomes irrational
• Loses contact with environment, enters stuporous state
• Muscular rigidity
• Slowed pulse and respirations
• Possible cardiac arrhythmias

• Intense shivering
• Conscious patient has difficulty speaking

• Decreased shivering
• Strong muscular rigidity
• Coordination affected, resulting in erratic or jerky movements
• Patient thinks less clearly; comprehension dulled; possible total amnesia
• Patient generally able to maintain appearance of psychological contact with surroundings

• Patient loses conciousness
• No response to spoken commands
• Most reflexes cease to function
• Heartbeat becomes erratic

Figure 16-2   Signs and symptoms of hypothermia change as the body's core temperature drops.

Generalized Hypothermia

Generalized hypothermia is usually defined as the lowering of body temperature below 95°F (35°C). Generalized hypothermia may be mild or severe. The signs and symptoms displayed by a patient depend on the severity of the hypothermia (Figure 16-2). Generalized hypothermia can occur in a variety of settings and to a variety of patients. The belief that hypothermia can happen only in extreme winter conditions is false. For example, an elderly patient who is trying to save money in the winter by keeping her home thermostat at 50 to 55°F may develop generalized hypothermia over a period of hours or days.

Several factors predispose certain patients to the development of hypothermia. These include the following:

◆ **Cold or cool environment** Normally, the colder the environment is, the greater the risk that a person exposed to it will develop hypothermia. However, bitterly cold temperatures are not necessary to produce hypothermia. Patients who are exposed to relatively cool environments for extended periods of time may also develop hypothermia. Remem-

ber, for example, the case of the elderly woman cited above.

◆ **Age** As already mentioned, the very young and the very old are at particular risk of developing hypothermia.

Infants and children are at risk for several reasons. First, they have a large body surface area—especially the head—in comparison to their size. This means that they generally lose more heat via convection than do adults. Also, infants and children are less "bulky" (i.e., they have less body fat and muscle mass) than adults. Less body fat means that they have less insulation against the cold. A smaller muscle mass means they have a decreased ability to generate heat through shivering.

Various factors also leave the elderly more likely to develop hypothermia. Often they have pre-existing medical conditions that leave them more susceptible to the effects of the cold. Medications that they take for chronic medical conditions may interfere with temperature regulation (see next page). Also, elderly people living on fixed incomes may eat an inadequate diet, which can hinder the body's heat production; they may also keep their homes too cool in an attempt to save money.

Both children and geriatric patients may also wear inadequate clothing for environmental conditions. Infants and young children rely on others to dress them appropriately for weather conditions and may not be able to put on or ask for more clothing if they are too cold. Elderly patients may not dress warmly enough because of problems with dementia or because of impaired recognition of cold.

◆ **Medical Conditions** Certain medical conditions also place patients at increased risk of hypothermia. For example, patients with diabetes and those with low blood sugar (hypoglycemia) are at increased risk. Also, patients with body-wide infection (called sepsis) are predisposed to excessive heat loss even though such patients may initially have an increased body temperature from fever.

◆ **Drugs and poisons** Certain medications, particularly those prescribed for hypertension or psychiatric conditions, interfere with the body's normal thermoregulation system. In addition, substances like alcoholic beverages cause blood vessels in the skin that would normally constrict on exposure to cold to dilate inappropriately, accelerating heat loss.

◆ **Injuries** Several types of injuries place patients at increased risk of hypothermia. These include the following:

Burns—because the loss of skin results in loss of body fluids (evaporative loss), loss of insulation, and loss of the ability of blood vessels in the skin to constrict in response to the cold.

Head trauma—because damage to the parts of the brain that control temperature regulation may worsen hypothermia.

Spinal cord injury—because damage to nerves that control the body's ability to constrict blood vessels and to the nerves that allow muscles to shiver affects the body's ability to conserve or generate heat.

Shock (hypoperfusion)—because patients who are in shock and are hypothermic are more likely to die of their injuries than patients who have a normal body temperature are.

◆ **Immersion in water** Because heat transfer by conduction is 30 times greater in water than in air, immersion in water greatly accelerates the development of hypothermia.

Assessment of the Hypothermic Patient

Assessment and subsequent emergency medical care of the patient with generalized hypothermia should begin only after a careful scene size-up. Awareness of scene safety is critical when managing environmental emergencies or you may quickly become a victim yourself. Be sure to assess and be prepared for scene hazards. Dress appropriately for severe cold temperatures. With cases of immersion-related hypothermia, be especially keen to dangers posed by thin ice; proceed with a rescue only if you are trained and equipped to do so.

The patient with generalized hypothermia may present with obvious signs and symptoms of hypothermia, or may have a much more subtle presentation. You must look for environmental considerations and pre-existing conditions that place patients at increased risk of hypothermia. At the outset of the assessment, try to obtain a history of the patient's exposure either from the patient or from bystanders. Key questions to answer during the initial patient assessment might include the following:

◆ What was the length of exposure to the environment?

◆ Was there a loss of consciousness?

◆ Are there any preexisting conditions that may have contributed to hypothermia, such as alcohol intake or an underlying illness or injury?

Some signs and symptoms of generalized hypothermia may be detected during the initial assessment. Be alert to the following:

◆ **General impression** It is likely that you will detect an environment that may have rendered the patient hypothermic. Remember, however, that exposure to cool, as well as cold, temperatures can lead to hypothermia. Also, be alert to any potential mechanisms of injury if trauma is suspected in addition to hypothermia.

- ◆ *Mental status* As hypothermia progresses, a patient's mental status declines. Early in hypothermia, the patient may exhibit subtle mood changes. Poor coordination, problems with memory, speech difficulties, dizziness, and reduction in or loss of sensation may also be present. Poor judgment may actually cause the patient to remove his clothing. Eventually, as hypothermia becomes more and more severe, the patient may become difficult to arouse or even unconscious.

COMPANY OFFICER'S NOTES

During lengthy extrications in cool, cold, and/or wet conditions, patients are at particular risk of developing generalized hypothermia. A patient who starts out with a normal body temperature may become hypothermic if he remains pinned motionless in vehicle wreckage for an extended period. Other factors can also contribute to loss of body heat. For example, aggressive use of trauma scissors to expose injured body parts can contribute to radiant heat loss; contact with cold steel wreckage can result in conductive heat loss; and cool winds blowing through wreckage can produce convective heat loss.

Take steps during extrication to reduce the possibility that a victim may develop hypothermia. Remember, a hypothermic trauma patient is more likely to die from his injuries than one who maintains a normal body temperature.

Consider the following measures to protect an entrapped patient. Use salvage tarps to block the wind. Cover the exposed patient with either thermal or warmed blankets. Place blankets between the patient and metal contacts. Rotate blankets in and out of the warmed cab of on-scene emergency apparatus.

Utility companies and confined space rescue units may be able to provide additional resources for keeping patients and fire crews warm. Know your local resources.

- ◆ *Breathing* Breathing may be abnormally rapid early on but become abnormally slow as the patient's body temperature drops.

- ◆ *Circulation* The pulse is often rapid early in hypothermia, but becomes abnormally slow as the patient's body temperature falls. The pulse rate may be less than 30 beats per minute in advanced hypothermia. The pulse may be difficult to palpate because of decreased circulation to the extremities. Using the skin to assess circulation is very unreliable in generalized hypothermia; often the skin is pale or blue-gray in color due to the effects of the cold.

The final step in the initial assessment is to identify high priority patients. Anyone who is identified as a priority patient needs expedited transport and consideration of advanced life support (ALS) back-up. It is likely that patients with generalized hypothermia will meet criteria for immediate transport either because of a poor general impression, altered mental status, or inadequate breathing and circulation.

When obtaining vital signs and conducting the focused physical exam, you may note the following about patients with generalized hypothermia:

- ◆ Low or absent blood pressure
- ◆ Slowly responding pupils
- ◆ Shivering may be present or absent
- ◆ Muscle rigidity or a stiff posture

Determining the precise temperature of the patient in the field may be difficult. Some EMS agencies carry traditional mercury, electronic, or tympanic thermometers. These devices may be unreliable or impractical during assessment of the hypothermic patient. Rather than using a thermometer, place the back of your hand between the clothing and the patient's abdomen during the assessment. If the abdomen feels cold, then you should presume that the patient is hypothermic.

◆ Emergency Care—Generalized Hypothermia

Most hypothermic patients have suffered prolonged exposure to cool or cold temperatures. It is neither practical nor safe to attempt complete rewarming of such patients in the field. Instead, the goals of the out-of-hospital care for a hypothermic patient are these:

◆ To remove the patient from the cold environment

◆ To protect the patient from further heat loss

◆ To assure an open airway

◆ To support patient's breathing and circulation

In all aspects of emergency care, be extremely gentle when handling a hypothermic patient. Gentle handling is essential because the heart can easily become irritable in a hypothermic patient. Rough handling can result in cardiac arrest, often from dysrhythmias such as ventricular fibrillation. Ventricular fibrillation in patients with severe hypothermia is less likely to respond to defibrillation by an AED than in patients with normal body temperature. Follow local protocols on AED use in hypothermic patients.

Hypothermic patients who are found in cardiac arrest or who go into cardiac arrest after EMS arrival require immediate CPR. Even a patient who is stiff and rigid and has no apparent pulse requires CPR and immediate transport to a hospital. Because the heart does not function normally at low temperatures, resuscitation efforts may continue for hours at the hospital until the patient is rewarmed. Because body mechanisms act to protect the brain during conditions of generalized hypothermia, even patients in prolonged cardiac arrest may recover fully once circulation and breathing are restored. The saying "You're not dead until you're warm and dead" means that a physician cannot consider resuscitation to have failed until the heart has been given a chance to restart at a near normal temperature.

Provide the following treatment for all patients suspected of having generalized hypothermia:

1. **Perform the scene size-up.** Detect any hazards; call for specialized units as needed.

2. **Take BSI precautions.**

3. **Remove the patient from the cold environment.**

4. **Handle the patient as gently as possible.**

5. **Prevent further heat loss to the patient.**

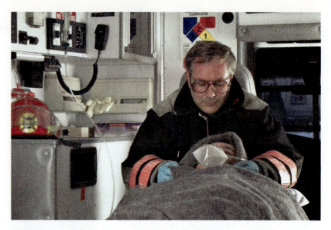

Figure 16-3 When wet clothes are removed and the body covered, the technique of passive rewarming allows the body to rewarm itself.

6. **Rewarm the patient.** If the patient is unresponsive and/or not responding appropriately, use techniques of *passive rewarming* (Figure 16-3). These include the following:

◆ Remove any cold, wet, or restrictive clothing.

◆ Apply blankets.

◆ Turn the heat up high in the patient compartment of the ambulance.

If the patient is alert and responding appropriately, you may use techniques of *active rewarming* (Figure 16-4). Active rewarming involves the application of external heat sources to the patient's body. By warming the blood in major arteries as they pass closely to the body's surface, this technique produces a

Figure 16-4 In active rewarming, an external heat source is applied to the body.

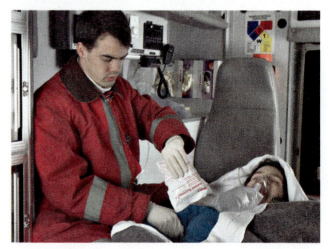

more rapid rise in body temperature than passive rewarming does. However, the technique also produces greater risk to the patient than passive rewarming. Use it only if your local protocols permit. To perform active rewarming, do the following:

◆ Follow all steps for the general management of the hypothermic patients as outlined above but use warmed blankets.

◆ Assure that the patient is alert and responding appropriately.

◆ Apply heat packs or warm water bottles to the patient's groin, armpits, chest, and cervical regions.

7. **Maintain an open airway.** Suction as needed.

8. **Support breathing and circulation.** Because respirations and pulse may be very slow, assess the patient for the presence of pulse and breathing for 30 to 45 seconds before starting CPR.

9. **Administer high flow oxygen if it has not already been provided during the initial assessment.** The oxygen should be warmed and humidified if possible.

10. **Do not allow the patient to try to walk or exert himself.**

11. **Do not allow the patient to eat or drink stimulants.**

12. **Do not massage the extremities.**

13. **Transport the patient as soon as possible.**

14. **Perform the ongoing assessment en route.**

Local Cold Injuries

Patients can suffer from exposure to the cold without developing generalized hypothermia. Inadequate protection of body parts from the cold often results in **local cold injuries.** (These are sometimes referred to as *localized cold injuries*.) The parts of the body farthest from its core are at the greatest risk of developing such injuries. The ears, nose, and other parts of the face are most commonly injured. The extremities, especially the toes, are also prime targets for local cold injuries.

Many of the factors that place certain patients at increased risk for generalized hypothermia also increase the risk of local cold injuries. Any condition, such as diabetes or alcohol intoxication, that decreases a person's ability to sense the cold increases the risk of local cold injury. Patients with poor circulation are also at increased risk. Children and geriatric patients are also likely to suffer from local cold injuries because their clothing is often inadequate for protection from the cold.

Local cold injury typically produces well-defined areas of tissue damage (Figure 16-5). Much as is the case with a burn, the depth of tissue injury depends upon length of exposure to the temperature extreme—the longer the exposure, the deeper and more severe the tissue injury.

Early or superficial local cold injury (sometimes called *frostnip*) results in a blanching, or pale discoloration, of the skin. If you palpate the

Figure 16-5 Deep local cold injuries (frostbite): **(A)** immediately after injury; **(B)** five days after injury.

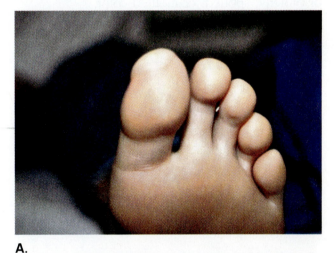

A.

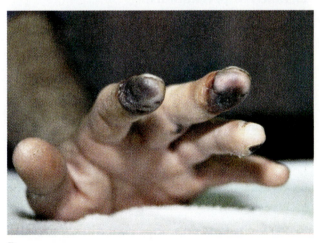

B.

affected area, the skin remains pale; normal capillary refill is absent. Despite the color change, the skin remains soft to the touch. In such cases, the patient will usually complain of a loss of feeling and sensation in the area. If proper rewarming procedures are followed at this early stage, most patients recover fully without permanent tissue loss. During rewarming, patients frequently complain of "tingling" sensations. These sensations usually indicate the return of normal blood circulation to the area.

Late or deep local cold injury is commonly known as *frostbite*. With this type of injury, the skin is often pale white and waxy-looking. On palpation, the skin feels hard, like wood. Blisters and/or local swelling may also be seen. In the most severe cases, as might be encountered with mountaineers, tissue as deep as the muscles and bones may be frozen. As deep injuries begin to thaw, the affected skin may show a purple-blue or blotchy, spotted, or mottled color.

◆ Emergency Care—Local Cold Injuries

The specific treatment of local cold injury will depend on the severity of the tissue damage. As with other cold-related emergencies, the following general steps should be taken for all local cold injury patients:

1. **Perform a thorough scene size-up.** Detect any hazards and call for additional specialized units as needed.

2. **Take BSI precautions.**

3. **As soon as possible, remove the patient from the cold environment.**

4. **Prevent further heat loss and remove any cold, wet, or restrictive clothing.**

5. **Administer high flow oxygen if not already provided in the initial assessment.** The oxygen should be warmed and humidified if possible.

6. **Protect the cold-injured area from further trauma.**

7. **Perform an ongoing assessment of the patient.**

The goal of treatment with local cold injury is to prevent further injury to or freezing of tissue. For this reason, rewarming of a local cold injury should usually take place in the controlled conditions of a hospital emergency department, not in the field. The greatest risk of thawing an affected body part in the field is the possibility that the part might refreeze. Refreezing of partially thawed areas of the body drastically increases tissue injury and subsequent tissue loss.

The specific steps for emergency care of *early or superficial local cold injury* are as follows:

1. **Splint the affected extremity.**

2. **Cover the cold-injured area with sterile dressings.**

3. **Remove any rings or jewelry from the affected area.**

4. **Do not rub or massage the area.**

5. **Do not re-expose the area to a cold environment.**

   Note: Some EMS systems allow EMTs to rewarm superficially injured areas by placing their hands (or the patient's) on the affected area without rubbing it; by breathing (or having the patient breathe) on the affected area through cupped hands; or by placing injured fingers in the patient's armpit. Follow your local protocols.

The specific steps for emergency care of *late or deep local cold injury* are as follows:

1. **Splint the affected extremity.** Do not allow the patient to walk on an affected extremity.

2. **Cover the cold-injured area with dry clothing or dressings.**

3. **Remove any rings or jewelry from the affected area.**

4. **Do not rub or massage the area.**

5. **Do not break blisters.**

6. **Do not apply heat or attempt to rewarm the affected area.**

7. **Do not re-expose the area to a cold environment.**

In wilderness areas or in certain rural settings where a delayed or extremely long transport is

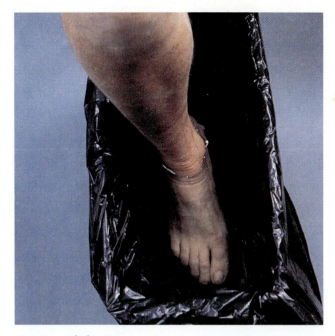

Figure 16-6 For rapid, active rewarming of a frozen body part, submerge the part in warm, not hot, water.

expected, rapid, active rewarming of the local cold injury should be initiated (Figure 16-6). Check with medical direction or follow local protocol in such cases. Remember, however, that rewarming should be started only if it is possible to protect the affected area from refreezing.

To actively rewarm a frozen body part, immerse the part in a warm (not hot!) water bath. Stir the water constantly. The ideal water temperature for rewarming is 108°F (42°C). The frozen body part will quickly cool the water, so monitor water temperature closely. Add warm water as necessary to keep the bath as close to 108°F as possible. Continue with the procedure until the body part softens and color and sensation begin to return. (This will usually take 20 or 30 minutes.) Once the affected part is thawed, apply dry sterile dressings to the area. If the hands or feet have been frozen, place sterile dressings between the fingers or toes. As thawing occurs and blood flow returns to the affected part, the patient may experience severe pain. Be prepared to comfort and reassure the patient.

Finally, even in wilderness settings, never attempt to rewarm a frozen extremity using dry heat such as that from a campfire. Because sensation is absent in the frozen skin, thermal burns from

radiant heat can further damage injured tissue without the patient being aware of what is happening.

HEAT-RELATED EMERGENCIES

As you read above, the body has various mechanisms by which it loses heat (Figure 16-1). In cold environments, such loss of body heat can have dire consequences. In a hot environment, however, the mechanisms that permit loss of body heat are essential for survival. If the body becomes unable to lose excess heat, death can be the result.

In a hot environment, the two major mechanisms by which the body loses heat are radiation and evaporation. As the temperature of the air surrounding the body rises, the amount of heat the body can lose by radiation is reduced. When the ambient air temperature is greater than the body's temperature, radiant heat loss is no longer possible. In fact, the body may begin to take on heat from the air.

At higher temperatures, the body relies more on evaporation for heat loss. Sweating accounts for most of this evaporative heat loss. The sweat contains not only water but also electrolytes of sodium and chloride that make up salt. The body can lose more than 1 liter (34 ounces) of sweat per hour. However, this cooling process does have limits. The body can sweat at the 1 liter per hour rate for only a few hours at a time. Also, environmental conditions can reduce evaporative heat loss. If the relative humidity of the air is high—that is, if the air surrounding the patient contains a lot of moisture—the evaporation of sweat slows and cooling is reduced (Figure 16-7).

If the mechanisms of heat loss are reduced, body temperature will continue to rise. As body temperature rises, the likelihood of a heat-related emergency increases. A variety of risk factors can add to the possibility of a heat-related emergency. These factors include the following:

◆ Age
—Infants (poor themoregulation, greater sweat losses, cannot remove their own clothing)

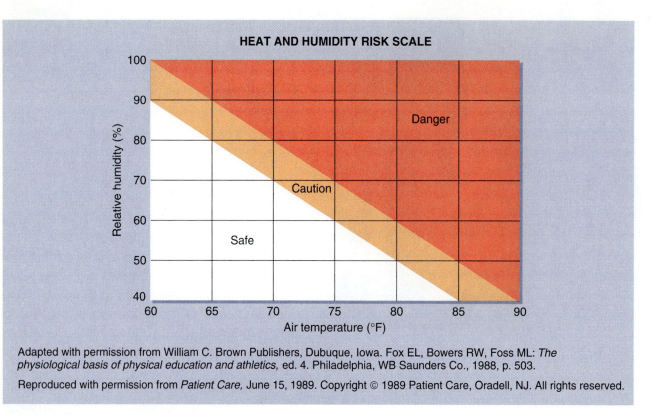

HEAT AND HUMIDITY RISK SCALE

Danger

Caution

Safe

Relative humidity (%)

Air temperature (°F)

Figure 16-7 As both the temperature and the humidity rise, the risk of heat-related emergencies increases.

—Elderly (poor thermoregulation, medications, cardiovascular disease, lack of adequate home cooling systems)

◆ Occupation

—Athletes

—Firefighters

—Laborers

—Military personnel

◆ Medications

—Especially medicines commonly prescribed for psychiatric illness

◆ Medical conditions

—Diabetes mellitus

—Heart disease

—Fever

—Dehydration

—Obesity

The three most common heat-related emergencies you are likely to encounter as an EMT are heat cramps, heat exhaustion, and heat stroke. Of these, heat stroke is the most serious. Failure to recognize the signs and symptoms of heat stroke and initiate aggressive care may result in the patient's death.

Heat Cramps

Heat cramps usually develop during strenuous activity in a hot environment. Excessive sweating results in loss of electrolytes (especially sodium). This leads to the cramping of muscles. Heat cramps are usually not serious. Most patients with them respond well to rest in a cool environment and replacement of fluids by mouth. Follow local protocols or check with medical direction before giving a patient fluids by mouth. If a person with heat cramps remains untreated and continues to lose fluid because of sweating, heat exhaustion may develop.

Heat Exhaustion

Heat exhaustion develops when the body's fluid volume is depleted. This can occur as a result of excessive sweating and the patient's failure to drink enough fluids, thus depleting the body's fluid volume. The end result is hypoperfusion of body organs. The signs and symptoms a patient displays may vary depending on the amount of fluid lost. Early signs may include fatigue, light-headedness, nausea, vomiting, and headache. The patient's skin is usually moist and pale, with a normal-to-cool temperature. If the condition is un-recognized and untreated, patients may develop more classic signs of shock (hypoperfusion) in-cluding increased heat rate, increased respiratory rate, and reduced blood pressure (hypotension).

Heat exhaustion is common among firefight-ers engaged in structural and wildland fire sup-pression without adequate rehabilitation. It can also occur during hazardous materials operations in which encapsulating suits are worn.

Heat Stroke

The most serious form of heat emergency occurs when the body's temperature regulating mecha-nism breaks down. This is the condition com-monly called *heat stroke*. Heat stroke usually develops over several days and most often affects the very young and the elderly. It is most com-monly encountered during summer heat waves. Unlike the patient with heat exhaustion whose temperature is normal or only slightly elevated, the patient with heat stroke will have a high tem-perature, up to 106° or 107°F (41° or 42°C). The patient's skin is likely to feel hot and either dry or moist. The patient with heat stroke will have an altered mental status, ranging from mild confusion to complete unresponsiveness.

Any patient found in a hot environment with altered mental status, elevated temperature, and hot dry or moist skin should be presumed to have a life-threatening heat-related emergency. You must provide aggressive cooling (see below) for such a patient.

◆ Emergency Care—Heat-Related Emergencies

Patients found in a hot environment with any of the following signs or symptoms should be treated for a heat-related emergency:

◆ Muscle cramps

◆ Weakness or exhaustion

◆ Dizziness or faintness

◆ Rapid heart beat

◆ Rapid, shallow breathing

◆ Skin that is

> Normal-to-cool temperature, pale, moist
>
> > or
>
> Hot temperature, dry or moist (a life-threatening sign)

◆ Headache

◆ Seizures

◆ Altered mental status ranging from mild con-fusion to unresponsiveness (a life-threatening sign)

All patients with suspected heat-related emer-gencies should receive the following treatment:

1. **Remove the patient from the hot environ-ment and place in a cool environment.** The air-conditioned patient compartment of an ambulance is ideal.

2. **Administer high flow oxygen if this has not already been done during the initial assessment.**

When a patient's skin is ***normal-to-cool tem-perature,*** *moist to the touch, and pale,* treat as follows:

1. **Loosen or remove the patient's clothing to allow cooling.**

2. **Cool the patient by fanning to enhance evaporation.**

3. **Place the patient in a supine position with his legs elevated.**

4. **If the patient is responsive and not nause-ated, you may have him sit up and drink water or other fluids as specified by local protocol.**

5. **If the patient is not responsive or is nau-seated or vomiting, transport him to the hospital on his left side, monitoring and maintaining the airway during transport.**

6. **Perform the ongoing assessment en route to the hospital.**

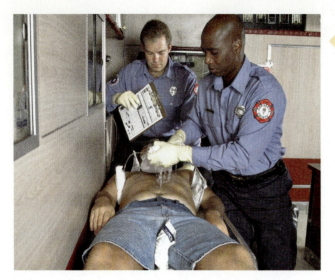

Figure 16-8 In cases where the patient's skin is hot in temperature and dry or moist, cool aggressively by applying cool packs to neck, armpits, and groin and by applying cool water with sponges or towels. At the same time, fan the patient aggressively.

In cases where the patient's skin is **hot in temperature** *and dry or moist to the touch,* treat the patient as follows (Figure 16-8):

1. **Remove the patient's clothing to allow cooling.**

2. **Apply cold packs to the patient's neck, groin, and armpits.**

3. **Keep the skin wet by applying cool water with sponges or wet towels or by wrapping the patient in sheets soaked in cool water.**

4. **Fan aggressively.**

5. **Use the maximum setting on the air conditioner in the patient compartment.**

6. **Give the patient nothing by mouth.**

7. **Transport immediately.**

8. **Perform the ongoing assessment en route to the hospital.**

A patient's survival and recovery from heat related emergencies will hinge on your recognizing the heat-related emergency, quickly removing the patient from the hot environment, and initiating the proper treatment for the patient in the out-of-hospital setting.

WATER-RELATED EMERGENCIES

Drowning is defined as death from suffocation due to submersion. *Near-drowning* is defined as survival, at least temporarily, after suffocation due to submersion. With the exception of occasional agricultural or industrial accidents, most drownings and near-drownings occur as a result of submersion in water. Each year there are more than 4,000 deaths in the United States from submersions. Drownings in fresh water are much more common than saltwater drownings, even in coastal areas.

PEDIATRIC NOTE

Most pediatric drownings and near-drownings occur in pools. However, unattended children may also drown in toilets, bathtubs, and even buckets. Drowning deaths in children are most common among those 4 years of age and under and then again in teenagers. Most pediatric deaths by submersion are preventable. Lack of supervision and inadequate or absent pool fencing are contributing factors in these deaths. Use of alcoholic beverages by adults supervising children is also a factor. Use of alcohol by teenagers is a major factor in drowning deaths among this age group as are drug use and peer pressure.

GERIATRIC NOTE

Elderly patients are at particular risk for drowning and near-drowning in bathtubs. Such cases may also be complicated when the patient suffers extensive burns from hot water because of a reduced ability to sense extreme heat (or cold).

A patient's survival after suffocation from submersion depends on several factors including the following:

◆ The length of time submerged prior to rescue

◆ Associated injuries, especially spinal injuries

◆ Water temperature

result of the so-called mammalian diving reflex. Full recovery has been reported in children who were submerged for more than one hour. Therefore, any pulseless, nonbreathing patient submerged in cold water should receive aggressive resuscitation including CPR and advanced life support.

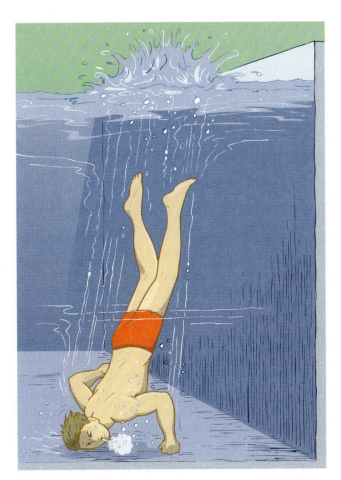

Figure 16-9 Spinal injuries are common in near-drowning cases in which diving was involved.

The shorter the time the patient has been under the water, the greater the chances of survival. Because the patient cannot breathe underwater, the brain will develop injury from lack of oxygen within several minutes unless the patient is rescued and either breathing is restored or the rescuer provides positive pressure ventilations.

Boating and diving accidents that lead to submersion frequently cause associated injuries. Injuries to the spine, especially the cervical spine, are common with drowning accidents in which patients dive into shallow water (Figure 16-9). Always assume that a spinal injury exists when you encounter any diving-related submersion or when the exact mechanism of the submersion is unknown.

Medical research and field experience have shown that the chances of survival for patients submerged in cold water are better than those for patients submerged in warmer water. This is a

---

COMPANY OFFICER'S NOTES

The exact period of time after which a rescue operation becomes a body recovery operation has not been well defined. The decision whether or not to initiate resuscitation should be based upon water temperature, the duration of submersion, and local medical protocol. When in doubt, initiate full CPR, consult medical control, and call for ALS back-up where available.

◆ Emergency Medical Care—Drowning/Near-Drowning Patients

The submerged patient's survival depends, to a large degree, on the speed with which a rescue can be made. If, however, the rescuers themselves become victims, then multiple lives may be lost to drowning. For this reason, the proper technique for assisting a submerged patient has been described as a "rapid, cautious rescue" (Figure 16-10). If you lack proper training, equipment, or sufficient personnel for a water rescue, then you must wait until the necessary resources are on the scene before initiating the rescue attempt.

The following steps should be taken when providing emergency care to a near-drowning victim:

1. **Ensure the safety of rescue personnel.**

2. **Assume that a spinal injury exists if a diving mechanism is involved or if the mechanism is unknown.** All medical and rescue procedures must assure spinal stabilization (Figure 16-11).

3. **If the patient is not breathing, then begin rescue breathing as soon as you reach the patient and are able.** In general, effective

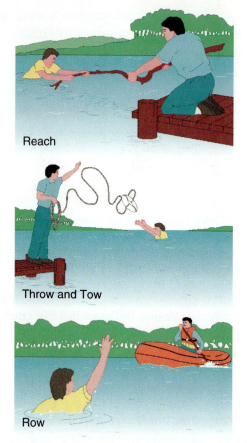

Figure 16-10 In a water rescue, first try to *reach* the patient by holding out an object from shore. If the patient cannot reach the object, *throw* him a floating object attached to a line and try to *tow* him to shore. If that fails, *row* to the patient in a boat. Only if none of these methods work and only if you are trained in water rescue should you attempt to *go* to the patient by swimming.

rescue breathing cannot begin until either the rescuer can stand in the water or the patient is on a firm surface. If the patient is pulseless, begin chest compressions as soon as the patient is on the shore or onboard a rescue craft.

4. **If there is no evidence of potential spinal injury, place the patient on his left side to allow drainage of water, vomitus, and other secretions.**

5. **Suction as needed.**

6. **Administer high flow oxygen via nonrebreather mask if it has not already been provided during the initial assessment.**

7. **If distention of the patient's abdomen keeps you from providing adequate posi-**

tive pressure ventilations, decompress the stomach. Use the following technique:

◆ Prepare a suction unit with large bore tip and tubing.

◆ Roll the patient on his left side to reduce the risk of possible aspiration.

◆ Place an open hand over the epigastric area of the abdomen and press firmly to relieve the distention.

◆ Clear the upper airway with suction prior to resuming ventilations.

8. **Transport immediately.**

9. **Perform the ongoing assessment en route.**

Special Water-Related Emergencies

Because submersion injuries occur in virtually every part of the world, all EMTs must be familiar with the emergency medical care of near-drowning patients. Depending on where you live and work, there are other types of water-related emergencies with which you may have to become familiar. Two such special situations are ice rescues and emergencies associated with SCUBA diving. It is not the intent of this text to present these topics in depth, only to familiarize you with them. If such special situations are common in your area, you are strongly encouraged to seek additional training in dealing with them through your fire department or rescue service.

Ice Rescue

As mentioned above, patients submerged in cold water generally have a better chance of survival than those found in warm water. Yet to complete the successful rescue of such patients, the rescue team may have to cross dangerous thin ice. In these circumstances, team members may be at high risk for submersion if proper rescue techniques are not used. The general guidelines for ice rescue include the following (Figure 16-12):

◆ Only properly trained personnel should attempt such rescues.

◆ Personal floatation devices (PFD) must be used by all rescuers.

◆ Immersion suits should be worn.

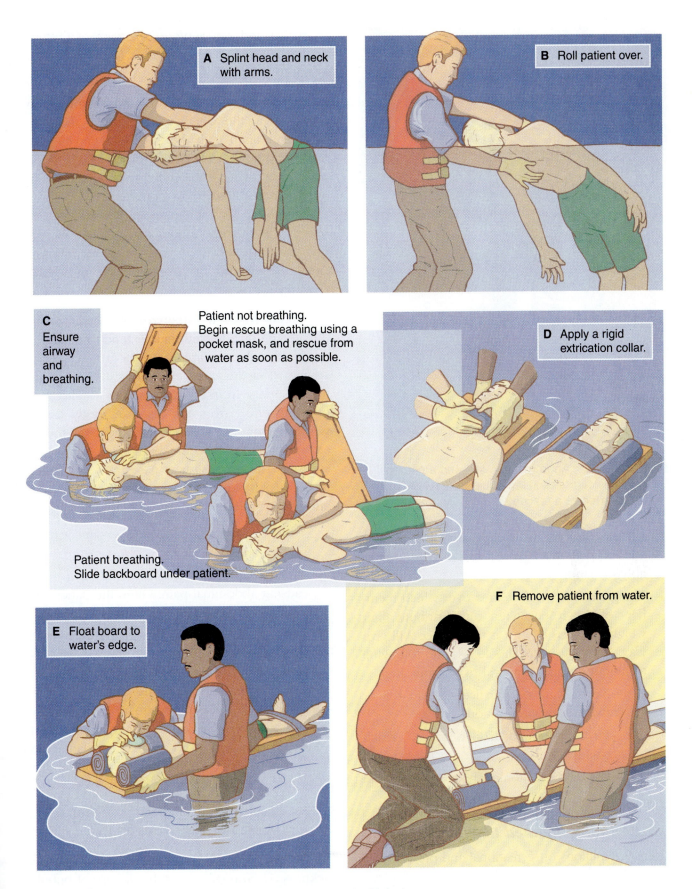

A Splint head and neck with arms.

B Roll patient over.

C Ensure airway and breathing.

Patient not breathing. Begin rescue breathing using a pocket mask, and rescue from water as soon as possible.

D Apply a rigid extrication collar.

Patient breathing. Slide backboard under patient.

E Float board to water's edge.

F Remove patient from water.

Figure 16-11 If a near-drowning patient may have spinal injuries, secure him to a long spine board before removing him from the water.

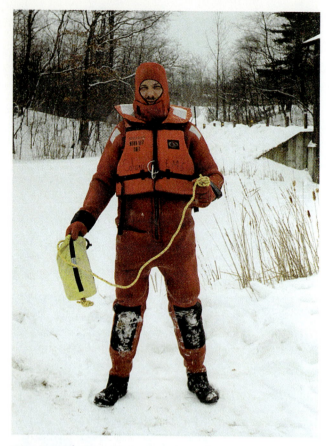

Figure 16-12 An immersion suit and a personal flotation device are required equipment when crossing ice to attempt a rescue.

◆ Lifelines should be attached to all ice rescuers and belayed from a secure position, preferably on land.

◆ The greater the surface area over which members of the rescue team can distribute their weight, the less likely it is that the ice will give way. Thus, rescuers should use the following techniques where practical or appropriate:

—Never walk on thin ice, instead roll or crawl in a prone position.

—Push a ground ladder out to reach across the ice.

—Use a flat-bottomed boat to reach the patient.

SCUBA Diving Related Emergencies

There are millions of recreational and professional divers in the United States. Most dives take place without complications. However, because of the pressure changes associated with going to depth

(descent) and returning to the surface (ascent), certain pressure-related injuries (barotrauma) do, at times, occur.

Descent-Related Barotrauma During a diving descent, the weight of the water above the diver combined with the effects of gravity place increasing pressure on the diver's body. Body cavities, especially those filled with air such as the inner ear and sinuses, are compressed. Divers call this compression "the squeeze." Patients with the squeeze frequently report ear fullness or pain and/or facial pain from sinus pressure. In severe cases, the eardrum may rupture, causing bleeding from the ear.

Ascent-Related Barotrauma The most life-threatening dive-related injuries tend to occur as a result of improper ascent to the surface. Gases contained in the body expand as a diver returns to the surface from the depths. This results in the opposite effect from the squeeze. Body tissues, which contain air, will become larger. As the gas expands during ascent, body tissues become stressed. The expansion of gases may even cause rupture of tissues. Areas of the body often affected include:

◆ *Teeth:* Air pockets in cavities expand causing severe pain.

◆ *Stomach and bowels:* Air expands in them causing abdominal pain. Often the patient will loudly and repeatedly belch or pass gas.

◆ *Lungs:* As air in the lungs expands, it can cause parts of the lungs to rupture. Air can also escape into the subcutaneous tissue of the skin resulting in subcutaneous emphysema. Air escaping into the bloodstream as bubbles or clusters of bubbles can cause an air embolism, which interferes with normal circulation and perfusion. The effects of air embolism can include cardiac arrest, seizures, or paralysis.

Ascent-related barotrauma can usually be avoided by gradual, staged ascents to the surface.

Decompression Sickness Decompression sickness (DCS) results from the deposit of bubbles of nitrogen gas in body tissue and the bloodstream. DCS is usually caused by too rapid an ascent from a dive. The classic form of DCS is the "bends," where the diver's joints become painful because of the presence of nitrogen bubbles within them. More severe cases of DCS can involve the lungs, spinal cord, and the brain.

◆ Emergency Care—Diving-Related Illness/Injury

In general, diving-related injuries should be managed as follows:

1. **Rescue the patient following appropriate precautions for rescuer safety.**

2. **Keep the patient in a supine position.**

3. **Administer high flow oxygen via nonrebreather mask.**

4. **Transport immediately.** Consider ALS backup if available.

5. **Contact medical direction.** Many serious diving-related conditions require treatment in specialized hyperbaric (recompression) chambers. Medical direction should be able to begin arrangements for hyperbaric treatment. The Diving Alert Network (DAN) is an organization that maintains a 24-hour hot line at (919)-684-8111 and can assist in finding the nearest hyperbaric center.

BITES AND STINGS

EMTs frequently encounter patients with bites from humans and other mammals. These bites can result in punctures and/or perforations of soft tissue. These injuries should be assessed and managed following procedures that will be discussed in Chapter 20, "Soft Tissue Injuries."

People also suffer from the bites and stings of snakes and insects in settings as varied as wilderness campgrounds, farm fields, suburban housing developments, and city parks. A large number of creatures are capable of delivering a bite or a sting. Bites and stings usually produce only minor irritation and discomfort in victims. But the effects of bites and stings vary with the creature doing the biting or stinging and the person who is bit-

ten or stung. In some cases, bites or stings can lead to life-threatening complications from venom or anaphylaxis. (You may wish to review the discussion of the assessment and treatment of anaphylaxis in Chapter 15, "Poisonings and Allergic Reactions," after completing this section.) As is the case in many environmental emergencies, the very young and the very old tend to be more severely affected by bites and stings.

You should become familiar with the animals and insects in your region that are likely to bite or sting people. Keep in mind, however, that ours is a highly mobile society; potentially dangerous creatures can easily be transported far from their normal habitats either accidentally or intentionally. While this chapter cannot describe in detail all the types of bites and stings you might encounter, it can give you a general approach to follow in assessing and treating bites and stings.

Insect Stings

Calls for EMS to assist people stung by bees, yellow jackets, hornets, and wasps are common. These insects inject **venom,** a substance poisonous to humans, through their stingers. Frequently, the stinger with the venom sac attached is left behind by the insect at the sting site. Reactions to a sting can include the following: localized pain, redness, and swelling at the sting site, generalized illness as a result of multiple simultaneous stings or systemic, life-threatening allergic reaction like anaphylaxis.

◆ Emergency Care—Insect Stings

General emergency care of insect stings is as follows:

1. **Perform a thorough, careful scene sizeup.** Remember that the insect(s) that stung the patient may still be present, even caught in the patient's clothing. Protect yourself from being stung.

2. **If stinger is still present, remove it.** Use the edge of a credit card to scrape it away (Figure 16-13). Do not use tweezers or forceps to remove the stinger; doing so may squeeze more venom into the wound.

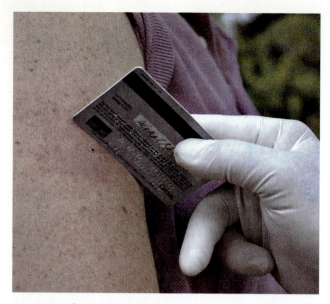

Figure 16-13 Use the edge of a credit card to scrape off a stinger.

3. **Gently wash the area of the sting.**

4. **Remove any jewelry from an injured area before swelling begins.** Failure to do so may result in loss of fingers or other tissue if swelling becomes severe.

5. **Place the injection site slightly below the level of the patient's heart.**

6. **Be alert for signs of generalized allergic reaction or anaphylaxis.** Be prepared to treat accordingly (see Chapter 15).

7. **Perform an ongoing assessment on the patient.**

Spider Bites

Spider bites are most common when webs are disturbed in areas such as barns or cabins. The venom delivered in most spider bites causes local reactions including swelling and itching at the site of the bite. However, two species of spiders—the brown recluse and the black widow—warrant special mention.

The brown recluse spider (Figure 16-14) has been reported in over 20 states. This spider prefers the warm, dry areas often found in abandoned buildings and basements. The spider's venom causes local tissue destruction that takes longer to heal than other spider bites. In some cases the bite may result in extensive tissue loss

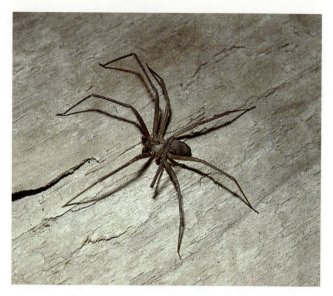

Figure 16-14 A brown recluse spider.

over days after the bite. Systemic symptoms of fever, chills, nausea, and vomiting may occur. The bites have been reported as fatal in some cases.

The black widow spider is found throughout the United States but is most common in the southern states. There are several species of black widow spiders, but only one has the classic orange hourglass pattern as shown in Figure 16-15. Black widow venom frequently causes systemic symptoms including muscle cramps of the extremities and abdomen.

The treatment for spider bites is similar to that for insect stings. Patients with any systemic symptoms such as shortness of breath, chest pain, or abdominal pain should be placed on high flow oxygen as well.

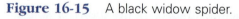

Figure 16-15 A black widow spider.

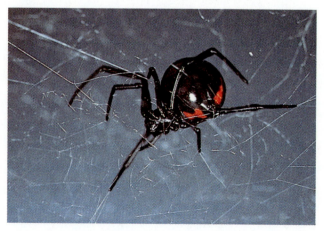

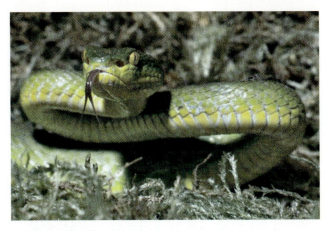

Figure 16-16 A pit viper. Note the elliptical eyes and pits below the eyes.

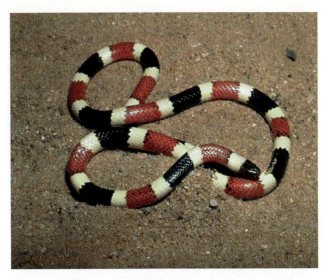

Figure 16-17 A coral snake.

Scorpion Stings

Scorpions are common in the southwestern United States. The stings of most species of scorpions cause only local reactions of redness, pain, and swelling at the sting site. One species, the bark scorpion, can cause serious systemic effects including increased heart rate, excessive salivation, roving eye movements, and difficulty in swallowing. Care includes normal management of stings, as well as high flow oxygen, and monitoring and maintaining an open airway clear of secretions.

Snake Bites

About 45,000 people a year are victims of snakebites in the United States. Some 8,000 of those bites are delivered by poisonous snakes. Most of those poisonous bites are from the group of snakes called *pit vipers*. This group includes rattlesnakes, copperheads, and water moccasins. These snakes can usually be identified by "pits" between and below the level of the eye and nostril and by elliptical or "cat-like" eyes (Figure 16-16). The other type of poisonous snake native to the U.S. is the *coral snake*. The coral snake can be identified by its colorful black, yellow, and red bands (Figure 16-17). Remembering the following rhyme can help you distinguish the coral snake from other colorful, non-poisonous snakes: "Red on black, venom lack/Red on yellow, kill a fellow."

The signs and symptoms of a venomous snakebite may take several hours to fully develop. Signs and symptoms vary with the species of

snake and the amount of venom injected in the bite. It is estimated that 25 percent of pit viper bites are "dry," with no venom injected. In these cases, only local skin damage may be present. If only small amounts of venom are injected, then swelling, redness, and some bruising may be seen at the site of the bite. When larger amounts of venom are injected, the following signs and symptoms are common:

◆ Swelling of an entire extremity

◆ Nausea and vomiting

◆ Numbness in the mouth

◆ Weakness and dizziness

◆ Increased pulse and respirations

◆ Shock

◆ Abnormal bleeding

◆ Emergency Care—Snakebite

Emergency care of snakebites includes the following steps:

1. **Assure your own safety.** Contact animal control or police officers for assistance if needed.

2. **Wash the area gently.**

3. **Remove any jewelry from an injured area before swelling begins.** Failure to do so may result in loss of fingers or other tissue if swelling becomes severe.

4. **Keep the site of the bite slightly below the level of the patient's heart.**

5. **Minimize patient movement.** Splint bitten extremities.

6. **Contact medical control or follow local protocols as to whether a constricting band should be placed proximal to the bite.**

7. **Administer high flow oxygen via nonrebreather mask if signs of systemic effects are seen.**

8. **Provide rapid transport.**

9. **Perform the ongoing assessment en route.**

Your out-of-hospital treatment should not delay getting the patient as rapidly as possible to the hospital where antivenin is available. The use of antivenin and intensive care interventions has decreased mortality among snakebite victims from over 20 percent of those bitten to less than 1 percent.

Chapter Review

SUMMARY

Environmental emergencies arise in many settings. They include cold- and heat-related emergencies, water-related emergencies, and bites and stings. You must develop a broad general knowledge of these emergencies—the situations in which they are likely to develop, their signs and symptoms, and their treatments. Remember that the frequency and type of these emergencies will vary with the natural features and conditions of a region. It is especially important for you to learn to recognize the environmental emergencies common in the region where you live and work.

REVIEWING KEY CONCEPTS

1. List the mechanisms by which the body loses heat.

2. List the signs and symptoms of generalized hypothermia.

3. Explain when it is appropriate to treat a cold emergency with active rewarming and when passive rewarming is appropriate.

4. Name the signs of a late or deep local cold injury.

5. Explain the steps in caring for a heat emergency patient who has skin that is moist, pale, and cool.

6. Explain the steps in caring for a heat emergency patient whose skin is hot and dry or moist.

7. Explain the steps in caring for a drowning or near-drowning patient.

8. Describe the proper care of a patient suffering from an insect bite or sting.

9. Describe the proper care of a patient suffering from snakebite.

RESOURCES TO LEARN MORE

Auerbach, Paul S., ed. *Management of Wilderness and Environmental Emergencies, 3rd Edition*. St. Louis: C. V. Mosby Co., 1996.

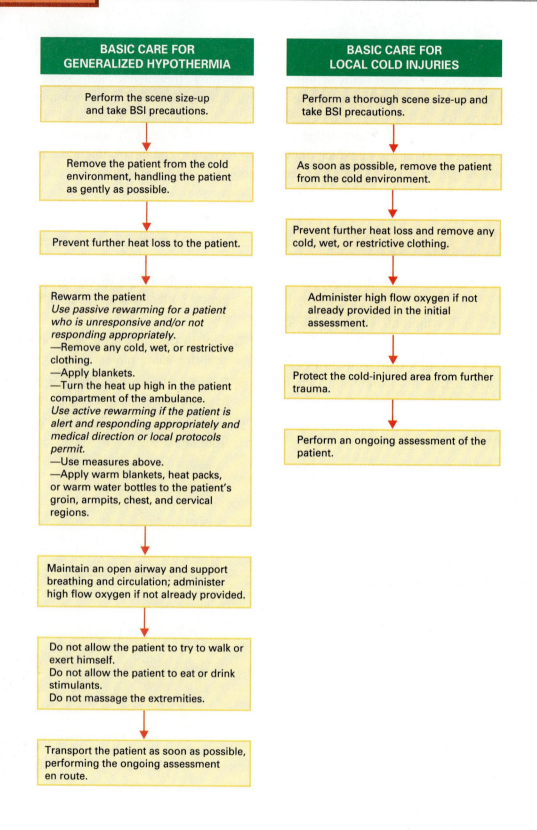

BASIC CARE FOR GENERALIZED HYPOTHERMIA

Perform the scene size-up and take BSI precautions.

Remove the patient from the cold environment, handling the patient as gently as possible.

Prevent further heat loss to the patient.

Rewarm the patient
Use passive rewarming for a patient who is unresponsive and/or not responding appropriately.
—Remove any cold, wet, or restrictive clothing.
—Apply blankets.
—Turn the heat up high in the patient compartment of the ambulance.
Use active rewarming if the patient is alert and responding appropriately and medical direction or local protocols permit.
—Use measures above.
—Apply warm blankets, heat packs, or warm water bottles to the patient's groin, armpits, chest, and cervical regions.

Maintain an open airway and support breathing and circulation; administer high flow oxygen if not already provided.

Do not allow the patient to try to walk or exert himself.
Do not allow the patient to eat or drink stimulants.
Do not massage the extremities.

Transport the patient as soon as possible, performing the ongoing assessment en route.

BASIC CARE FOR LOCAL COLD INJURIES

Perform a thorough scene size-up and take BSI precautions.

As soon as possible, remove the patient from the cold environment.

Prevent further heat loss and remove any cold, wet, or restrictive clothing.

Administer high flow oxygen if not already provided in the initial assessment.

Protect the cold-injured area from further trauma.

Perform an ongoing assessment of the patient.

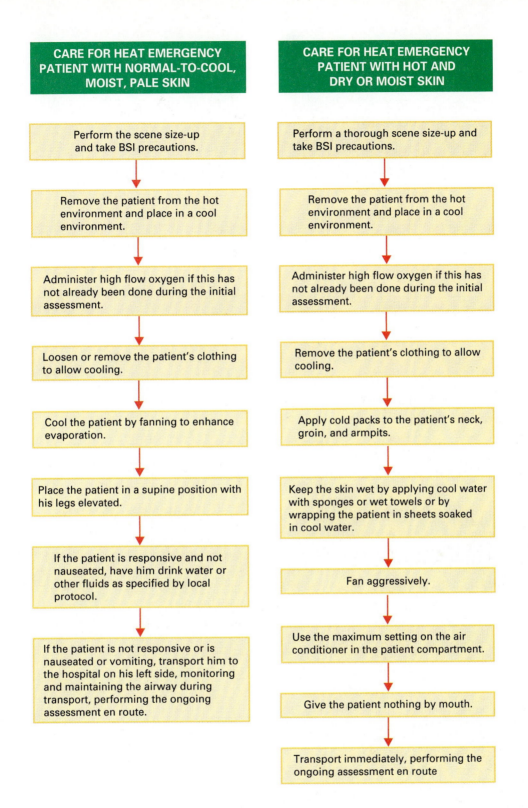

CARE FOR HEAT EMERGENCY PATIENT WITH NORMAL-TO-COOL, MOIST, PALE SKIN

Perform the scene size-up and take BSI precautions.

↓

Remove the patient from the hot environment and place in a cool environment.

↓

Administer high flow oxygen if this has not already been done during the initial assessment.

↓

Loosen or remove the patient's clothing to allow cooling.

↓

Cool the patient by fanning to enhance evaporation.

↓

Place the patient in a supine position with his legs elevated.

↓

If the patient is responsive and not nauseated, have him drink water or other fluids as specified by local protocol.

↓

If the patient is not responsive or is nauseated or vomiting, transport him to the hospital on his left side, monitoring and maintaining the airway during transport, performing the ongoing assessment en route.

CARE FOR HEAT EMERGENCY PATIENT WITH HOT AND DRY OR MOIST SKIN

Perform a thorough scene size-up and take BSI precautions.

↓

Remove the patient from the hot environment and place in a cool environment.

↓

Administer high flow oxygen if this has not already been done during the initial assessment.

↓

Remove the patient's clothing to allow cooling.

↓

Apply cold packs to the patient's neck, groin, and armpits.

↓

Keep the skin wet by applying cool water with sponges or wet towels or by wrapping the patient in sheets soaked in cool water.

↓

Fan aggressively.

↓

Use the maximum setting on the air conditioner in the patient compartment.

↓

Give the patient nothing by mouth.

↓

Transport immediately, performing the ongoing assessment en route

Obstetrics and Gynecology

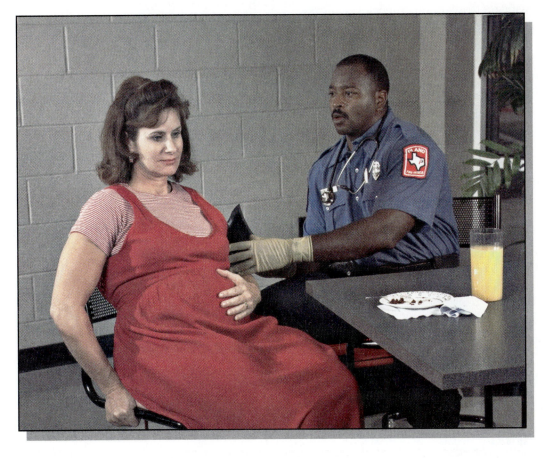

*A*s an EMT, you may be called upon to assist with out-of-hospital childbirths or attend to women with emergencies related to their reproductive systems. As a new EMT, you may initially feel nervous about approaching these situations.

   You should be reassured that childbirth is a natural process that has gone on for many thousands of years before there were EMTs or physicians available to assist the mother. In addition, the assessment skills and approaches to patient care you have learned throughout your EMT course will allow you to properly treat female patients with gynecological emergencies.

At the completion of this chapter, the EMT-Basic student should be able to meet the following objectives:

Knowledge and Understanding

1. Identify the following structures: uterus, vagina, fetus, placenta, umbilical cord, amniotic sac, perineum. (pp. 413–414)
2. Identify and explain the use of the contents of an obstetrics kit. (pp. 417–418)
3. Identify predelivery emergencies. (pp. 434–437)
4. State indications of an imminent delivery. (pp. 418–419)
5. Differentiate the emergency medical care provided to a patient with predelivery emergencies from a normal delivery. (pp. 434–437)
6. State the steps in the predelivery preparation of the mother. (pp. 417–420)
7. Establish the relationship between body substance isolation and childbirth. (p. 420)
8. State the steps to assist in delivery. (pp. 420–422)
9. Describe the care of the baby as the head appears. (p. 421)
10. Describe how and when to cut the umbilical cord. (pp. 425–427)
11. Discuss the steps in the delivery of the placenta. (pp. 427–428)
12. List the steps in the emergency medical care of the mother post-delivery. (pp. 427–428)
13. Summarize neonatal resuscitation procedures. (pp. 424–425)
14. Describe the procedures for the following abnormal deliveries: breech birth, prolapsed cord, and limb presentation. (pp. 429–434)
15. Differentiate the special considerations for multiple births. (pp. 431–432)
16. Describe special considerations of meconium. (pp. 433–434)
17. Describe the special considerations of a premature baby. (pp. 432–433)
18. Discuss the emergency medical care of a patient with a gynecological emergency. (pp. 437–438)
19. Explain the rationale for understanding the implications of treating two patients (mother and baby). (pp. 413, 434, 436)

Skills

1. Demonstrate the steps to assist in a normal cephalic delivery.
2. Demonstrate necessary care procedures of the fetus as the head appears.
3. Demonstrate infant neonatal procedures.
4. Demonstrate post-delivery care of the infant.
5. Demonstrate how and when to cut the umbilical cord.
6. Attend to the steps in the delivery of the placenta.
7. Demonstrate the post-delivery care of the mother.
8. Demonstrate the procedures for the following abnormal deliveries: breech birth, prolapsed cord, and limb presentation.
9. Demonstrate the steps in the emergency medical care of the mother with excessive bleeding.
10. Demonstrate completing a prehospital care report for patients with obstetrical/gynecological emergencies.

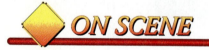

ON SCENE

DISPATCH: *ENGINE 6, RESPOND PRIORITY ONE TO THE WESTSHIRE MALL, FIRST FLOOR BATHROOM FOR A WOMAN IN LABOR. AMBULANCE IS EN ROUTE. TIME OUT IS 1328.*

On arrival at the mall, you size up the scene. You note the usual mid-day traffic problems, but detect no other scene hazards. You grab your usual first-in equipment. Because of the information provided by dispatch, you also bring the emergency obstetrical kit. A mall security guard meets your crew and guides you to the women's bathroom. There, several people are gathered around a woman lying on the floor. The security guard tells you the women's name is Helen Weaver.

As you approach Ms. Weaver, you begin your initial assessment. You see a woman who appears to be in her late 20s and is obviously pregnant. She is conscious, crying, and uncomfortable. She appears to have an adequate airway and breathing. You don your gloves as you introduce yourself, saying that you're an EMT with the fire department.

The woman replies, "I'm Helen, I've never done this before, but I think I'm about to have this baby right here."

You say, "Helen, we're here to help you. How far along are you in your pregnancy?"

"I'm four days past my due date."

You ask, "Are you having any contractions?"

"Yes, I had one about 5 minutes ago. That's when I felt this gush of fluid down there."

You then say, "Helen, I need to quickly look at your vaginal area to see if the baby is coming right now, or if we have time to get you to the hospital."

"OK, but I'm scared."

You reassure her, saying, "We're going to take good care of you and the baby."

You open your body substance isolation kit and put on your mask and goggles. As your lieutenant and mall security clear bystanders from the bathroom, the ambulance EMTs, both of whom are women, arrive. They continue to reassure Helen as you check for crowning. Your inspection reveals no signs of crowning.

Recognizing that delivery is not imminent, your crew and the ambulance EMTs load Helen onto the stretcher positioning her on her left side. You accompany the patient in the ambulance. During transport to the hospital, Helen has two more contractions about 4 minutes apart. At the hospital you take your patient directly to the Labor and Delivery suite. You later learn that Helen gave birth to a healthy girl 3 hours after her arrival at the hospital. Your knowledge of emergency childbirth assessment and procedures enabled Helen to give birth to her baby under the safest possible conditions—at the hospital.

Childbirth is a natural process. Most deliveries occur without complications because the anatomy and physiology of the female reproductive system and the anatomy and physiology of the baby allow the event to occur without significant risks to either the mother or the newborn. When an EMT is involved in an emergency childbirth in an out-of-hospital setting, it is usually only to perform procedures that *assist* the mother in giving birth and that ensure the well-being of the baby. However, it is crucial to remember that you are treating not one, but *two* patients during emergency childbirth. You must also be prepared to manage abnormal delivery situations where both the mother's and baby's lives may depend upon your assessment skills and your knowledge of emergency childbirth procedures.

A NATOMY AND PHYSIOLOGY OF PREGNANCY

Understanding the structure (anatomy) and function (physiology) of the female reproductive system is a vital basis for learning the emergency medical care of obstetric and gynecologic emergencies. Most of the human female's reproductive system is located within the pelvis in the lower abdomen (Figure 17-1). Major structures in the system include the two **ovaries** and two **fallopian tubes.** The fallopian tubes connect to the **uterus,** which connects to the **vagina** through the **cervix.** It is the lower part of the uterus, the cervix, and the vagina that form the **birth canal.** The area of

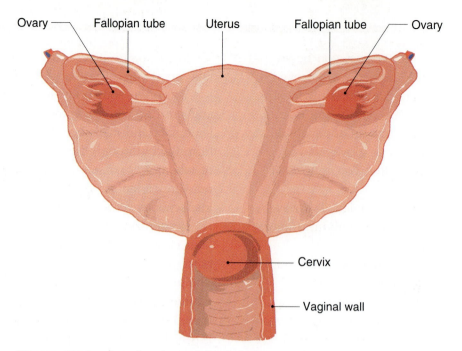

Figure 17-1 Anterior view of the female reproductive organs.

skin between the external vaginal opening and the anus is called the **perineum.** All of these structures have a very rich blood supply, which helps account for the severe bleeding often found with female reproductive system emergencies.

In a normal pregnancy, one of the ovaries produces a single egg that travels through a fallopian tube and, once fertilized by a sperm, implants itself in the uterus. Figure 17-2 illustrates the process after this point. The growing fertilized egg is called an embryo, which after several weeks grows into the **fetus.** A protective fluid-filled **amniotic sac** soon forms around the developing embryo and protects the fetus right up to the time of delivery. At the time of delivery, the sac will contain several quarts of amniotic fluid.

As the fetus grows, the **placenta,** a specialized structure that supplies nutrients from the mother to the fetus, develops within the uterus. The placenta provides a rich source of blood flow from the mother to the fetus through the **umbilical cord.** The placenta and umbilical cord supply oxygen to and remove waste products from the fetus right up until the moment the baby is born.

A normal human pregnancy lasts 9 months from fertilization until childbirth. The pregnancy is divided into three 3-month **trimesters.** During the first trimester, there is remarkable development from two cells at the time of conception to a complex fetus. In the second trimester, the fetus grows rapidly. By the fifth month, the uterus can be palpated at the level of the umbilicus. In the third and final trimester, the uterus can be palpated in the upper abdomen as the fetus grows to its full-term size, ready for birth to occur.

As pregnancy progresses, the mother's body undergoes many physiologic changes. Some of these changes are especially important for the EMT to be aware of (Table 17-1). Compared to a non-pregnant woman, a pregnant woman has an increased blood volume and an increased heart rate. This means that a pregnant woman's heart pumps a greater volume of blood, or has a higher cardiac output per minute, than that of a non-pregnant woman. Pregnant women also have a large increase in the number and size of blood vessels supplying their reproductive organs. This increased vascularity results in a somewhat decreased blood pressure as compared to normal.

The massive increase in the size of the uterus in the third trimester causes several anatomic and physiologic changes within the woman's abdomen. For example, the uterus compresses the digestive system, which results in delayed digestion and in increased risk of vomiting.

ANATOMY OF PREGNANCY

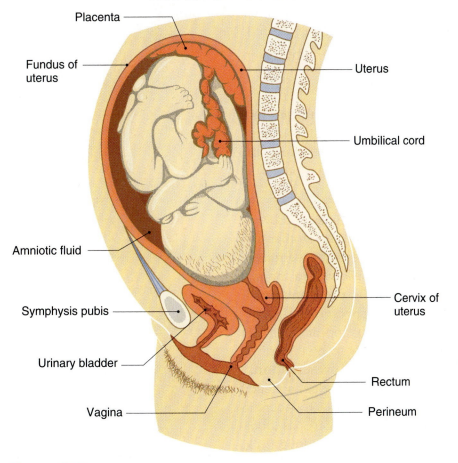

Figure 17-2 The structures of pregnancy.

The uterus may also compress the major vein in the abdomen, the inferior vena cava, when a pregnant women is in a supine position. This can decrease blood flow to the heart and result in falling blood pressure. This condition is known as **supine hypotensive syndrome.** The lowered blood pressure is potentially dangerous for the mother. It is also dangerous to the fetus because it decreases blood flow to the placenta, which can result in fetal distress. The condition is easily treated either by positioning the mother on her left side or by placing a rolled towel under her right hip. Both maneuvers move the uterus to the left side of the abdomen, away from the inferior vena cava.

Labor

Labor is the process by which a baby is born. This process is divided into three well-defined steps or **stages of labor** (Figure 17-3):

Table 17-1

Physiologic Changes During Pregnancy

Change	Significance to EMT
Increased blood volume and vascularity	Causes changes in the woman's vital signs: ◆ Increased pulse rate ◆ Decreased blood pressure
Increased size of the uterus results in pressure on digestive organs and delayed digestion	Increased risk of vomiting
Pressure on the inferior vena cava results in decreased blood flow to heart	Supine hypotensive syndrome with dangerously low blood pressure and fetal distress

- *First stage*—starts with regular contractions and thinning and gradual dilation of the cervix and continues until the cervix is fully dilated.

- *Second stage*—begins when the baby enters the birth canal and continues until the baby is born.

- *Third stage*—begins when the baby is born and continues until the afterbirth (placenta, umbilical cord, and some tissues from the amniotic sac and the lining of the uterus) is delivered.

By the end of the third trimester, several anatomic changes have prepared the mother and fetus for labor. The fetus will usually have rotated into a head-down position, allowing a normal head-first delivery, or **cephalic presentation.** If the fetus has not rotated, the **presenting part**—the first part of the baby to appear from the vagina during delivery—is likely to be the baby's buttocks. This is called a **breech presentation.**

Another change is that the cervix has softened to allow the process of dilation, which occurs in the first stage of labor. Picture the uterus as a bottle with the cervix forming the bottle's long neck. In order for the baby and then the placenta to pass out of the uterus, the neck of the bottle must be stretched to the size of a wide-mouth jar. (This process is called *effacement.*) Well before the onset of actual labor—sometimes as much as several days—uterine muscles begin mild contractions. Slight dilation occurs as the cervix begins to thin. When actual labor begins, the contractions of the uterus during the first stage of labor continue the thinning and dilation process, and the infant's head begins to move downward. As the cervix gradually shortens and thins enough to become flush with the wall of vagina (full effacement), the opening of the cervix becomes dilated in preparation for the passage of the fetus down the birth canal.

When contractions begin, they are widely spaced. As birth approaches, the time between contractions becomes shorter. Typically, the time between these contractions ranges from every 30 minutes down to 3 minutes apart or less at the time of birth. **Labor pains,** which the patient may feel in the lower abdomen or back, may accom-

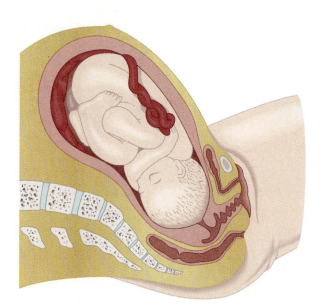

FIRST STAGE:
First uterine contraction to full dilation of cervix

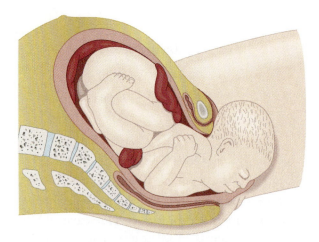

SECOND STAGE:
Birth of baby or expulsion

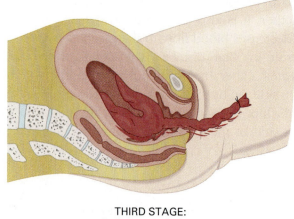

THIRD STAGE:
Delivery of placenta

Figure 17-3   The stages of labor.

pany the contractions. During a contraction, palpation of the mother's abdomen will reveal a "rock-hard" uterus in the center of the abdomen.

As the fetus moves downward and the cervix dilates, the amniotic sac usually breaks. The woman may describe this event as a "gush" of fluid or simply as a "trickle" of fluid. Normally, the amniotic fluid is clear. Fluid that is greenish or brownish-yellow in color may be an indication of maternal or fetal distress during labor. Such coloring is called **meconium** staining.

In addition to fluid from the breaking amniotic sac, there may be a watery, bloody discharge of mucus (not bleeding) in the first stage of labor. Part of this discharge will be from a mucus plug in the cervix that is displaced as the cervix dilates. This discharge is usually mixed with blood and is called the **"bloody show."** This event is not a cause for concern and it is not necessary to wipe the fluids away. Watery, bloody fluids discharging from the vagina are typical during all three stages of labor.

Full dilation of the cervix signals the end of the first stage of labor. Women giving birth for the first time remain in this first stage an average of 16 hours. However, some women may be in it for no more than 4 hours, especially if the birth is not a first child. As an EMT, you will not be able to determine when exactly the transition from the first to the second stage of labor occurs.

The second stage of labor begins after the full dilation of the cervix. During this time, contractions become increasingly frequent. Discomfort will become more severe. In the second stage of labor, the cramping and abdominal pains associated with the first stage of labor still may be present, but most women report a major new discomfort—they feel that they have to move their bowels. This sensation is produced as the baby's body moves downward and places pressure on the rectum.

Once the second stage of labor begins, childbirth may progress very rapidly. You must decide whether delivery is so imminent that it must be prepared for on the scene or whether the mother can be safely transported for an in-hospital delivery. It is always preferable that a baby be delivered in the controlled setting of the hospital. Therefore, the decision to stay and assist the mother with delivery on the scene must be based on careful assessment and physical examination of the mother. If assessment and examination reveal that delivery is likely in the next few minutes (as described below), you must then prepare to assist with an on-scene delivery.

NORMAL CHILDBIRTH

The Role of the EMT

Remember: *EMTs do not deliver babies—mothers do! Your primary roles will be determining whether the delivery will occur on the scene and, if it will, helping and assisting the mother as she delivers her child.*

Equipment and Supplies

Assisting the mother and providing care is much easier if a few basic items are standard supplies on the emergency vehicle. A sterile obstetric kit should contain the items needed for preparation of the mother, delivery, and initial care of the newborn (Figure 17-4). This kit should include:

◆ Several pairs of sterile surgical gloves to protect from infection

◆ Towels or sheets for draping the mother

◆ 1 dozen 2 × 10 (or 4 × 4) gauze pads (sponges) for wiping and drying the baby

◆ 1 rubber-bulb syringe (3 oz) to suction the baby's mouth and nostrils

◆ Cord clamps or hemostats to clamp the umbilical cord (plus extra clamps in case of a multiple birth)

Figure 17-4 The contents of an obstetrics kit.

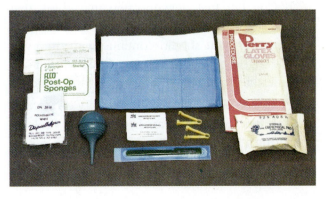

- Umbilical cord tape to tie the cord
- 1 pair of surgical scissors to cut the cord
- A baby blanket to dry and keep the baby warm
- Several individually wrapped sanitary napkins to absorb blood and other fluids
- Plastic bag.

Evaluating the Mother

A simple series of questions, an examination for crowning, and determination of vital signs will allow you to make the decision whether to transport. However, do not let the urgency of this decision upset the mother. Your patient needs emotional support at this time. Your calm, professional actions will help her feel more at ease and assure her that the required care will be provided for both her and her unborn child. *Remember: It is best to transport an expecting mother unless, based on your evaluation, you expect delivery within a few minutes.*

The process of evaluating the mother should include the following steps:

1. **Ask her name and age and expected due date.** Most women deliver close to their due dates. However, onset of labor may occur well before the due date.

2. **Ask if this is her first pregnancy.** The average time of labor for a woman having her first baby is about 16 to 17 hours. The time in labor is considerably shorter for each subsequent birth.

3. **Ask her how long she has been having labor pains, how often she is having pains, and if her "bag of waters" has broken. Ask if she has had any bleeding or bloody show.** At this point, with a woman having her first delivery, you may think that you can make a decision about transport. However, you should continue with the evaluation procedure. Also, you should begin to time the frequency and length of the patient's contractions.

4. **Ask her if she is straining or if she feels as though she needs to move her bowels.** If she says yes, this usually means that the baby has moved into the birth canal and is pressing the vaginal wall against the rectum. Birth will probably occur very soon. If a women in labor complains of having to move her bowels, do not allow her to use the bathroom because delivery of the baby directly into the toilet is a real possibility. The mother may tell you that she can feel the baby trying to move out through her vaginal opening. In this situation, cases, birth is probably very near.

5. **Examine the mother for crowning** (Figure 17-5). This is a visual inspection to see if there is bulging at the vaginal opening or if the presenting part of the baby is visible. *Crowning is the most reliable sign of an imminent delivery. If the head or presenting part is visible, immediately prepare for delivery.*

    In order to examine for crowning, you must expose the women's vaginal area. Examining for crowning may be embarrassing to the mother, the father, and any required bystanders. For this reason, fully explain what you are doing and why. It is essential that you maintain a professional attitude and take all reasonable steps to maintain the woman's privacy. Be certain that you protect the mother from the stares of bystanders. In a polite but firm manner, ask everyone who does not belong at the scene to leave. Carefully help the patient remove enough clothing to allow you an unobstructed view of the vaginal opening. Once the check for crowning is completed, be certain to immediately drape the abdomen and perineum with a sheet.

6. **Feel for uterine contractions.** You may have to delay this procedure until the patient

Figure 17-5 Crowning of the infant's head.

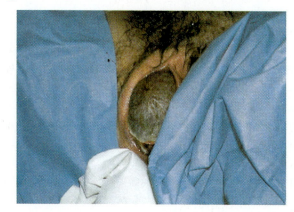

tells you she is having labor pains. Tell her what you are going to do, then place the palm of your gloved hand on her abdomen, above the navel. This can be done over the top of the patient's clothing. You should be able to feel her uterus and its contraction. All contractions should be timed. Keep track of their duration and frequency. The duration of the contraction is timed from the onset of the contraction until its relief. The frequency is timed from the onset of one contraction until the onset of the next contraction. As the delivery nears, the contractions will occur more frequently and with greater intensity.

7. **Take vital signs between contractions if you do not have a partner to do it.** Alert the hospital staff if the mother's vital signs are abnormal.

If this is the woman's first delivery, if she is not straining, and if there is no crowning, there is little reason why she cannot be transported to a medical facility for delivery. On the other hand, if this is not her first delivery, and she is straining, crying out, and complaining about having to go to the bathroom, birth will probably occur too soon for transport. If the mother is having labor pains from contractions about 2 minutes apart, birth is very near. If you determine that delivery is imminent based on the presence of crowning or other signs, you and your partner should prepare to assist the mother with delivery. Local protocol may require you to contact medical direction for the decision to commit to delivery on the site. If delivery does not occur in 10 minutes, contact medical direction for permission to initiate transport of the mother.

You may find a patient who is afraid of transport because she believes that birth will occur along the way. Assure her that you believe there is enough time before delivery. Let her know that you are trained to assist with the delivery and that the ambulance is well equipped to handle her needs and care for the newborn should she deliver en route. Intermittently assess for crowning during transport as part of the ongoing assessment. If crowning occurs, stop the ambulance and prepare for delivery.

Labor and delivery are emotionally charged events. As an EMT, you will need to provide constant emotional support to the mother throughout your care, from assessment through delivery. Some women may feel more comfortable if a female EMT is the primary provider of care and support; if this is possible, then see that it is done. In any case, once an EMT begins to provide the type of one-on-one support necessary for emergency childbirth, then that relationship should be maintained. It may be very stressful for the mother if EMS crew changes occur in the middle of labor. Even if normal operating procedures call for transition of care to another unit or agency, all efforts should be made to maintain continuity of care and support until arrival at the hospital.

Delivery Procedures

When your assessment reveals that on-scene delivery is imminent, you must prepare for delivery. *Remember at all times that you are providing care for two patients during delivery.* If necessary, and certainly if you are alone at the scene with

TRANSITION OF CARE

The first on-scene EMT should quickly obtain a history and baseline vital signs and assess the mother for crowning to determine whether it will be safe to initiate transport or if it will be necessary to assist with delivery on the scene. If working in a tiered response system, the EMT should advise incoming units of the result of this assessment and either prepare the patient for transport or open the emergency obstetrics kit and prepare for on-scene delivery.

If the first on-scene EMT has developed a particularly strong relationship with the mother—and certainly if the EMT has performed the on-scene delivery of the baby—it is appropriate for that EMT to accompany the mother to the hospital (even if patient care would usually be turned over to another crew for transport in your EMS system). This continuity of care is important not only for the emotional support of the mother, but also because the EMT's first-hand report of the delivery may provide important information to the hospital staff.

only a single partner, you should request additional personnel to respond. Having additional EMTs on the scene will be helpful especially after delivery, when you are assessing and caring for both the mother and the newborn.

COMPANY OFFICER'S NOTES

Maintaining patient privacy during an on-scene childbirth can present a significant challenge, especially in public gathering places. Maintaining control of on-scene crews and removing onlookers is essential. Makeshift protective screens can be improvised with salvage tarps, extra blankets, or sheets.

Preparing the Mother for Delivery

When preparing for an imminent delivery, you should follow these steps:

1. **Control the scene so that the mother will have privacy.** If you are not in a private room and transfer to the ambulance is not practical (crowning is present), ask bystanders to leave. (Her coach may remain.)

2. **In addition to surgical gloves, you and your partner should put on gowns, caps, face masks, and eye protection because there is a high probability of splashing blood and fluids during delivery.**

3. **Place the mother on a bed, sturdy table, or the ambulance stretcher. Elevate the buttocks with blankets or a pillow. Have the mother lie with knees drawn up and spread apart.** You will need about 2 feet of work space below the woman's buttocks to place and initially care for the newborn. Having the patient positioned on the stretcher may speed transport if complications arise.

4. **Remove any of the patient's clothing or underclothing that obstructs your view of the vaginal opening. Replace your initial non-sterile surgical gloves with sterile gloves from the obstetric kit.** Use sterile sheets or sterile towels to drape the mother's legs. Place a sterile towel or sheet below her buttocks and perineum. Clean sheets, clean cloths, towels, or materials such as tablecloths can be used if you do not have an obstetric kit.

5. **Position your assistant—your partner, the father, or someone the mother agrees to have assist you—at the mother's head.** This person should stay alert to help turn the mother's head should she vomit. This person should also provide emotional support to the mother, soothing and encouraging her.

6. **Position the obstetric pack on a table or chair.** All items must be within easy reach. ***Note:*** If delivery is to take place in an automobile, position the mother flat on the seat. Arrange her legs so that she has one foot resting on the seat and the other foot resting on the floor.

Delivering the Baby

Position yourself so that you have a constant view of the vaginal opening. Be prepared for the baby to come at any moment.

Be prepared for the patient to experience discomfort. Delivering a child is a natural process, but it will be accompanied by pain. Your patient may also have intense feelings of nausea. If this is her first child, she may be very frightened. All these factors may cause your patient to be uncooperative at times. You must remember that the patient is in pain and that she may feel ill. She will need emotional support and constant reassurance.

During delivery, talk to the mother. Encourage her to relax between contractions. Continue to time her contractions from the beginning of one contraction to the beginning of the next. Encourage her not to strain unless she feels she must. Remind her that her feeling of a pending bowel movement is usually just pressure caused by the baby moving into her birth canal. Encourage her to breathe deeply through her mouth. She may feel better if she pants, although she should be discouraged from breathing rapidly and deeply enough to bring on hyperventilation. If her "bag of waters" breaks, remind her that this is normal.

The steps for assisting the mother with a normal delivery include the following (Figure 17-6):

1. **Continue to keep someone at the mother's head to provide emotional support, moni-**

tor vital signs, and be alert for vomiting. If no one is on hand to help, be alert for vomiting and check vital signs between contractions.

2. **Position your gloved hands at the mother's vaginal opening when the baby's head starts to appear** (Figure 17-6A). Do not touch the area around the vagina except to assist with the delivery. For legal reasons, it is always preferable for both your protection and the patient's to have your partner present at all times when you are touching a woman's vaginal area.

3. **Support the baby's head as it is delivered.** Place one hand below the baby's head as it is delivered. Spread your fingers evenly around the baby's head, remembering that the skull contains "soft spots" or fontanelles. Support the baby's head, but avoid pressure to these soft areas at the top and sides of the skull. A slight, well-distributed pressure may help prevent an explosive delivery. Keeping one hand on the baby's head and using the other hand to hold a sterile towel to support the tissue between the mother's vagina and anus can help prevent tearing of this tissue during delivery of the head. *Do not pull on the baby!*

4. **If the amniotic sac has not broken by the time the baby's head is delivered, use your finger or a sterile clamp from the obstetric kit to puncture the membrane.** Pull the membranes away from the baby's mouth and nose. The amniotic fluid should be clear. Meconium-stained amniotic fluid is caused by fetal feces (wastes) released during labor, usually because of maternal or fetal stress. If the meconium is aspirated (breathed in) by the fetus, the baby can develop pneumonia or other complications.

5. **Once the head delivers, check to see if the umbilical cord is wrapped around the baby's neck.** Tell the mother not to push while you check. If she can "pant," or take short quick breaths for just a moment, it may help relieve the urge to push while you check, then gently loosen the cord if necessary. Even though the umbilical cord is very

tough, rough handling may cause it to tear. If the cord is wrapped around the baby's neck, try to place two fingers under the cord at the back of the baby's neck. Bring the cord forward, over the baby's upper shoulder and head.

If you cannot loosen and slip the cord over the baby's head, the baby cannot be delivered. Immediately clamp the cord in two places using the clamps provided in the obstetric kit. Be very careful not to injure the baby. With extreme care, cut the cord between the two clamps. Gently unwrap the ends of the cord from around the baby's neck, and then proceed with the delivery.

6. **Check the baby's airway.** Most babies are born face down and then rotate to the right or left. Support the baby's head so that it does not touch the mother's anal area. When the entire head of the baby is visible, continue to support the head with one hand and, with the other hand, wipe the mouth and nose with sterile gauze pads. Use the rubber bulb syringe to suction the baby's mouth, then the nose (Figure 17-6B). Compress the syringe *before* placing it in the baby's mouth. Suction the mouth first, then the nostrils. Carefully insert the tip of the syringe about 1 to 1½ inches (25 to 35 mm) into the baby's mouth and release the bulb to allow fluids to be drawn into the syringe. Control the release with your fingers. Withdraw the tip and discharge the syringe's contents onto a towel. Repeat this procedure two or three times in the baby's mouth and once or twice in each nostril. The tip of the syringe should not be inserted more than a ½ inch (12 mm) into the baby's nostril.

7. **Help deliver the shoulders** (Figure 17-6C). The upper shoulder (usually with some delay) will deliver after the head, followed quickly by the lower shoulder. You must support the baby throughout this entire process. Gently guide the baby's head downward, to assist the mother in delivering the baby's upper shoulder. After the upper shoulder has delivered, if the lower shoulder is slow to deliver, assist

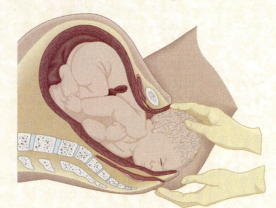

Figure 17-6A Support the infant's head.

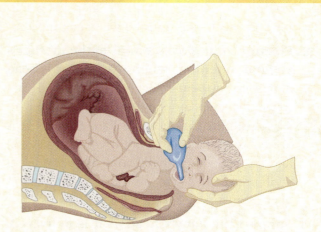

Figure 17-6B Suction the nose and mouth.

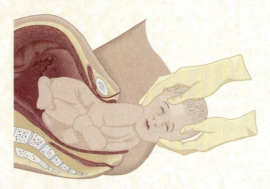

Figure 17-6C Support the head to prevent explosive delivery. Aid in the birth of the upper shoulder.

the mother by gently guiding the baby's head upward (Figure 17-6D).

8. **Support the baby throughout the entire birth process** (Figure 17-6E). Remember that newborns are very slippery. As the feet are born, grasp them to assure a good hold on the baby. Once the feet are delivered, lay the baby on its side with its head slightly lower than its body. This is done to allow blood, fluids, and mucus to drain from the mouth and nose. Suction the mouth and nose again with the bulb syringe. Keep the baby at the same level as the mother's vagina until the umbilical cord stops pulsating (Figure 17-6F). Wrap the infant in a warm, dry blanket.

9. **Note the exact time of birth for later documentation.**

10. **Once pulsation of the umbilical cord ceases, clamp and cut the cord as described below** (see "Cutting the Umbilical Cord").

11. **You or another EMT should initiate the care and assessment of the newborn as described below** (see "Assessment and Care of the Newborn").

12. **Prepare for delivery of the placenta and the remainder of the umbilical cord during the third stage of labor** (see " Delivering the Placenta").

13. **Continue ongoing emotional support and reassurance of the mother.**

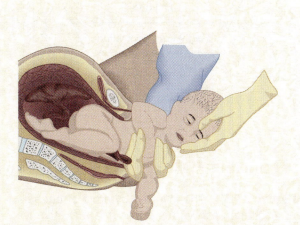

Figure 17-6D Support the trunk as the shoulders are delivered.

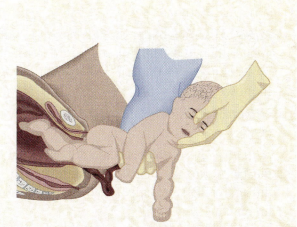

Figure 17-6E Use both hands to support the infant as the feet are delivered.

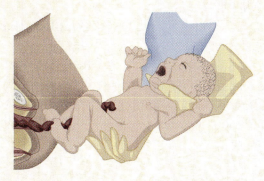

Figure 17-6F Keep the infant level with the vagina until the umbilical cord is cut.

Assessment and Care of the Newborn

Assessment

Once the baby is delivered, the EMT's attention must immediately turn toward assessing and caring for the newborn. All newborns should be initially positioned on a dry, warm surface, wiped dry, and placed in a dry newborn blanket with the head covered. The baby should receive additional suctioning of the mouth and nose. After the infant has been positioned, dried, wrapped, and suctioned, careful assessment should begin. The assessment of a normal newborn should reveal the following.

◆ *General appearance*—The baby's color should be pink in the trunk (the face, chest, and

COMPANY OFFICER'S NOTES

Because on-scene emergency childbirth involves the intensive care of two patients, the mother and the newborn, it is crucial that an adequate number of trained personnel be present to assist with patient care. Depending on your EMS system and department staffing, it may be necessary to order additional units to the scene to assist. Additional personnel may be life saving if either patient becomes unstable.

abdomen). Some cyanosis of the extremities is normal. Central cyanosis of the trunk is an abnormal finding.

◆ *Pulse*—The newborn should have a pulse greater than 100. The pulse is best determined by listening over the left nipple with a small stethoscope.

◆ *Grimace*—The baby should be vigorous and crying.

◆ *Activity*—The newborn should have good muscle tone as indicated by movement of the extremities. A limp baby is an abnormal finding.

◆ *Breathing effort*—The infant should cry and should be breathing spontaneously. Absent or gasping breathing requires that immediate steps be taken to improve breathing.

Newborn Resuscitation

Resuscitation of the newborn follows what has been depicted as an inverted pyramid (Figure 17-7). The pyramid is wider at the top because all newborns receive positioning, drying, warming, and suctioning, whereas only a few require advanced life support care.

Because resuscitation of the newborn is a procedure few EMTs have to perform on a regular basis, it is very important that you follow the procedures below carefully to insure proper treatment of the baby:

1. **Clear the baby's airway.** Use a bulb syringe, suctioning the mouth *first* and then the nostrils (Figure 17-8). It may be necessary to use a sterile gauze pad to clear mucus and blood from around the baby's nose and mouth. *Note:* When the nostrils are suctioned, the baby may gasp or begin breathing and aspirate any meconium, blood, fluids, or mucus from its mouth into its lungs. That is why it is imperative to suction the mouth before the nostrils.

2. **Keep the baby on its side and again suction the mouth, then the nose with a rubber bulb syringe.** If necessary, you can cradle the baby in your arms. However, it is best to keep the baby on the cot or table surface.

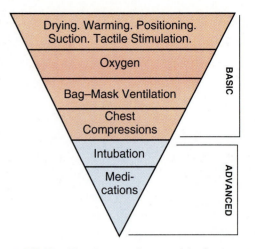

Figure 17-7 The inverted pyramid of neonatal resuscitation shows the approximate relative frequencies of neonatal care and resuscitative efforts. Note that a majority of infants respond to basic life support measures.

3. **Establish that the baby is breathing.** Usually the baby will be breathing on its own by the time you clear the airway. A newborn should begin breathing within 30 seconds. If it does not, then you must "encourage" the baby to breathe (Figure 17-9). Usually, a gentle but vigorous rubbing of the baby's back will promote spontaneous respiration. Should this method fail, snap one of your index fingers against the sole of the baby's foot. Do not hold the baby up by its feet and slap its bottom! Do not become alarmed if the hands and feet of a breathing newborn appear slightly blue. It is not uncommon for this blue color to remain for the first few minutes.

Figure 17-8 First suction the mouth, and then the nose of a newborn.

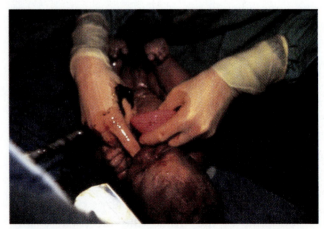

If assessment of the infant's breathing reveals shallow, slow, or absent respirations, provide artificial ventilations at a rate of 40 to 60 per minute (Figure 17-10). Remember: Provide only small puffs of air to the neonate if using mouth to mask, or small squeezes on the bag if using an infant-sized bag-valve-mask device. Reassess the infant's respiratory efforts after 30 seconds. If there is no change in the effort of breathing, continue with ventilations and reassessment.

4. **Assess the infant's heart rate.** A newborn's heart rate is best assessed by listening with a stethoscope over the left nipple. If the heart rate is less than 100 beats per minute, then provide artificial ventilations at a rate of 40 to 60 per minute. Reassess the heart rate after 30 seconds. If the heart rate is between 60 and 80 per minute and rising, continue to provide artificial ventilations and reassess again in 30 seconds. If the heart rate on reassessment is

less than 60 per minute, or between 60 and 80 per minute and not rising, continue ventilations and initiate chest compressions, as shown in Figure 17-10. Chest compressions in the neonate should be delivered at a rate of 120 compressions per minute, midsternum, with two thumbs, fingers supporting the back. Depth of compression is ½ to ¾ inch (12 to 18 mm). The ratio of compressions to breaths is 3 compressions to 1 breath.

5. **If the child has adequate respirations and a pulse rate greater than 100 per minute but exhibits cyanosis of the face and/or torso, provide supplemental oxygen.** Oxygen is best delivered at 10 to 15 liters per minute using oxygen tubing placed close to, but not directly into, the infant's face.

6. **The baby should be assessed repeatedly during transport to the hospital.** Should the baby cease breathing, begin gasping respirations, or develop a heart rate less than 100 beats per minute, repeat the above procedures. A neonate who requires intermittent or continuous ventilation should receive advanced life support care.

Cutting the Umbilical Cord

In a normal birth, the infant must be breathing on its own before you clamp and cut the cord. Before clamping and cutting the cord, palpate the cord with your fingers to make sure it is no longer pulsating. The general procedure for umbilical cord care is as follows (Figure 17-11).

1. **Keep the infant warm.** Dry the baby and wrap it in a baby blanket or infant swaddler, clean towel, or sheet prior to clamping the cord. Cover the top of the infant's head to prevent heat loss. Do not wash the infant. Sometimes the mother may request that you do so, but it is best to leave the protective coating (called the *vernix*) on the infant until it reaches the medical facility.

2. **Use the sterile clamps or umbilical tape found in the obstetric kit. Taking extreme care, form a knot slowly to avoid tearing the cord.** Ties should be made using a square knot (right over left, then left over right).

Figure 17-9 You can "encourage" a newborn to breathe by snapping an index finger against the sole of his foot or gently but vigorously rubbing his back.

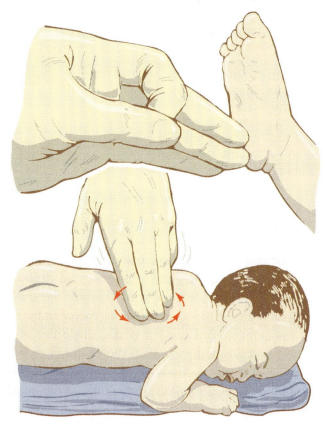

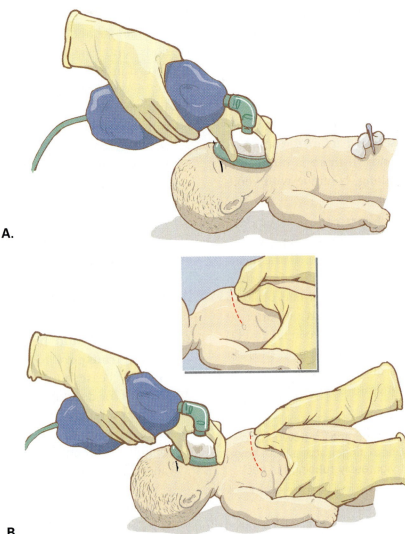

A.

B.

Figure 17-10 **A.** Use a bag-valve mask to provide positive pressure ventilations to a newborn. Maintain a good mask seal. Ventilate with just enough force to raise the infant's chest. **B.** To provide chest compressions, circle the torso with the fingers and place both thumbs on the lower third of the infant's sternum. If the infant is very small, you may need to overlap the thumbs. If the infant is very large, compress the sternum with the ring and middle fingers placed one finger's depth below the nipple line. Compress the chest from ½ to ¾ inch at the rate of 120 per minute.

3. **Apply one clamp to the cord or tie about 8 to 10 inches (200 to 250 mm) from the baby.** This leaves enough cord for intravenous lines to be used by paramedics or the staff at the hospital if they are needed.

4. **Place a second clamp or tie about 2 to 3 inches (50 to 75 mm) closer to the baby.** This second clamp should be about 4 fingers width from the neonate.

5. **Cut the cord between the clamps or knots using sterile surgical scissors.** Use caution and protect your eyes when cutting the cord as a spurt of blood is common. Never untie or unclamp a cord once it is cut. Place the placental end of the cord on the drape over the mother's legs to avoid contact with expelled blood, feces, and fluids. Examine the fetal end of the cord for bleeding. Don't attempt to

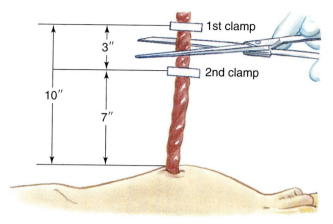

Figure 17-11 Cutting the umbilical cord.

adjust the clamp or retie the knot. If bleeding continues, apply another tie or clamp as close to the original as possible.

6. **Be careful when moving the baby so that no trauma is brought to the clamped cord.** If the cord does not remain closed off completely, the baby may bleed to death from seemingly little blood loss. In most cases, the cord vessels will collapse and seal themselves. **Warning:** *Do not tie, clamp, or cut the cord of a baby who is not breathing on its own unless you have to do so to remove the cord from around the baby's neck during birth, or unless you have to perform CPR on the infant. Do not cut or clamp a cord that is still pulsating.*

Keeping the Baby Warm

It is critical to keep the baby warm. Initially dry the newborn with a towel. Remove the initial drying towel and wrap the newborn in a fresh, dry infant swaddler or a warmed blanket or towel. Be sure to cover the infant's head (but not the face) to prevent heat loss. Bubble wrap can also be used to wrap the infant's torso. It provides padded protection, insulation, and allows visual monitoring of the infant. Let the mother hold the infant on her abdomen. During the delivery of the placenta, have your partner hold the baby unless the mother desires otherwise. Keep the ambulance warm.

Ongoing Care of the Mother

Remember that at the scene of a delivery you have two patients to care for: the mother as well as the baby. Care for the mother includes helping her deliver the placenta, controlling vaginal bleeding, and making her as comfortable as possible.

Delivering the Placenta

The third stage of labor is the delivery of the placenta with its umbilical cord section, membranes of the amniotic sac, and some of the tissues lining the uterus. (All of these together are known as the afterbirth.) Placental delivery begins with a brief return of the labor pains that stopped when the baby was born. You will notice a lengthening of the cord, which indicates the placenta has separated from the uterus. In most cases, the placenta will be expelled within a few minutes after the baby is born (Figure 17-12). Although the process may take 30 minutes or longer, avoid the urge to put pressure on the abdomen over the uterus or pull on the cord to hasten the delivery of the placenta. If mother and baby are doing well and there are no respiratory problems or significant uncontrolled bleeding, transportation to the hospital can be delayed up to 20 minutes while awaiting delivery of the placenta.

Save all afterbirth tissues. The attending physician will want to examine the placenta and other tissues for completeness since any afterbirth tissues remaining in the uterus pose a serious threat of infection and prolonged bleeding to the mother. Try to catch the afterbirth in a container. Place the container in a plastic bag, or wrap it in a towel, paper, or plastic. If no container is available, catch the afterbirth in a towel, paper, or a plastic bag. Label this material "placenta" and include the name of the mother and the time the

Figure 17-12 Delivery of the placenta.

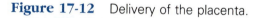

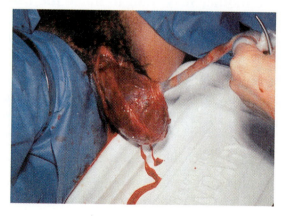

tissues were expelled. If the placenta does not deliver within 20 minutes of the baby's birth, transport the mother and baby to a medical facility without delay.

Note: Some EMS systems recommend transport without waiting for delivery of the placenta. There may be a condition in which the placenta does not separate from the uterine wall and it is important for mother and baby to get to the hospital. You can always stop the ambulance to deliver the placenta if necessary while en route.

Controlling Post-delivery Vaginal Bleeding

Delivery of the baby and placenta is *always* accompanied by some bleeding from the vagina. Although the blood loss is usually no more than 500 cc, it may be profuse, especially after delivery of the placenta. To control vaginal bleeding after delivery of the baby and placenta, you should do the following:

1. **Place a sanitary napkin over the mother's vaginal opening.** Do not place anything in the vagina.

2. **Have the mother lower her legs and keep them together.** Tell her that she does not have to "squeeze" her legs together. Elevate her feet.

3. **Massaging the uterus will help it contract.** This will help control bleeding. Feel the mother's abdomen until you note a "grapefruit-sized" object. This is her uterus. Rub this area lightly with a circular motion (Figure 17-13). It should contract and become firm, and bleeding should diminish.

4. **The mother may want to nurse the baby. This will aid in the contraction of the uterus.** Some pediatricians recommend the baby not nurse until a doctor has examined it.

5. **If vaginal bleeding continues despite uterine massage, the patient should be transported immediately.** Provide high flow oxygen, treat for shock, and perform an ongoing assessment during transport.

An additional source of post-delivery bleeding can arise from the skin between the vagina and

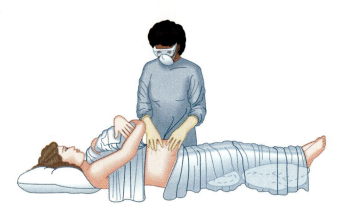

Figure 17-13 Massaging the uterus lightly in a circular motion can help control post-delivery bleeding.

the anus, known as the perineum. A tearing of tissue can occur in the perineum at the vaginal opening during the birth process. The mother may feel the discomfort from this torn tissue. Let her know that this is normal and that the problem will be quickly cared for at the medical facility. Treat the torn perineum as a wound. Dress by applying a sanitary napkin and applying some pressure.

Providing Comfort to the Mother

Keep contact with the mother throughout the entire birth process and after she has delivered. Your care for the mother does not end when you have delivered the placenta and controlled vaginal bleeding. Take her vital signs frequently. Be aware that she has just undergone a tremendous emotional experience and small acts of kindness will be appreciated and remembered. Childbirth is a rigorous task, and a woman is physically exhausted at the conclusion of delivery. Wiping her face and hands with a damp washcloth and then drying them with a towel will do wonders to refresh her and prepare her for the trip to the hospital. Replacement of blood-soaked sheets and blankets from under her buttocks will make that trip more comfortable. Make sure that both she and the baby are warm.

When delivery occurs at home, ask a member of the family or a trusted neighbor to help you clean up. You should clean up whatever disorder EMS care has caused in the house; however, you should not delay transport in order to complete these activities. Be sure to properly dispose of items that have been in contact with blood and other body fluids in a biohazard container.

Birth is supposed to be an exciting and joyous event. Talking to the mother and paying attention to her new baby are part of total patient care and good customer service. A good rule to follow is to treat your patient as you would wish a member of your family to be treated.

CHILDBIRTH COMPLICATIONS

Most women proceed through pregnancy, labor, and delivery without complications, and most neonates have a normal cephalic presentation. Although most babies are born without difficulty, complications may occur during delivery. We have already considered three such complications: the cord around the neck, an unbroken amniotic sac, and infants who need encouragement to breathe. These problems can be handled with simple procedures. However, there are other complications that can threaten the lives of both mother and newborn and for which definitive treatment is beyond an EMT's level of training. For emergencies that you detect during your physical exam such as a prolapsed umbilical cord, a breech presentation, and limb presentation, your treatment will be to provide high concentration oxygen and rapid transport to the hospital.

Prolapsed Umbilical Cord

Sometimes during delivery, the umbilical cord, rather than the baby, presents first. This occurrence is known as a **prolapsed umbilical cord.** With this condition, the cord can become compressed between the baby and the birth canal during delivery (Figure 17-14). The condition may be life threatening to the baby because the squeezing of the cord may cut off the baby's supply of oxygen. A prolapsed cord occurs most frequently when there is a breech or limb presentation. A prolapsed umbilical cord is detected during the assessment of the vaginal opening for crowning when the cord is seen protruding from the vagina.

The treatment goal with a prolapsed cord is to maximize oxygen delivery to the baby until it can be delivered at the hospital. The combination of increasing the mother's oxygen intake coupled with the manual prevention of the compression or squeezing of the cord against the birth canal is the mainstay of treatment. The emergency medical care of a prolapsed cord is the only time the EMT may insert a hand into the vagina.

◆ Emergency Care—Prolapsed Umbilical Cord

Upon recognition of a prolapsed cord, provide the following emergency care:

1. **Assure body substance isolation precautions including eye protection, mask, and gloves.**

Figure 17-14 Management of a prolapsed umbilical cord.

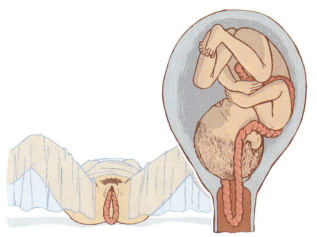

- Elevate hips, administer oxygen and keep warm
- Keep baby's head away from cord by placing fingers on the head
- Do not attempt to push cord back
- Wrap cord in sterile moist towel
- Transport mother to hospital, continuing pressure to baby's head

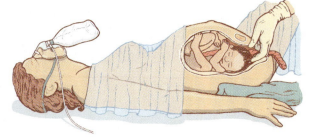

2. **Position the mother with her head down and buttocks raised with a blanket or pillow, using gravity to lessen pressure on the birth canal.**

3. **Administer high concentration oxygen to the mother via nonrebreather mask.**

4. **Don sterile gloves.**

5. **Carefully explain to the mother that you will have to insert your hand into her vagina to relieve the compression of the cord.** Provide emotional support throughout the procedure and subsequent transport.

6. **Insert several fingers of your sterile gloved hand into the vagina, gently pushing the baby's presenting part away from the umbilical cord.** Keep the gloved hand inside the mother's vagina and continue to push up on the baby until relieved by a physician at the hospital or directed otherwise by medical control.

7. **Initiate rapid transportation to the hospital.** Stay with the mother and continue to put pressure on the baby during the move to the transporting vehicle and during transport to the hospital. Notify the hospital of a prolapsed cord.

8. **Monitor the cord for palpations.** Palpations confirm blood flow through the cord.

9. **If possible, wrap the prolapsed cord in a moistened sterile towel to keep the cord warm and prevent drying.**

10. **Have your partner obtain frequent vital signs of the mother.**

Breech Presentation

Breech presentation is the most common abnormal delivery. It involves a buttocks-first or both-legs-first delivery. The risk of birth trauma to the baby is high in a breech presentation. In addition, there is an increased risk of a prolapsed cord with breech presentation.

If you evaluate a woman in labor and find the baby's buttocks or both legs presenting, rather than the head presenting, this is a breech presentation (Figure 17-15). Although breech presentations can spontaneously deliver successfully, the complication rate is high.

Figure 17-15   Management of a breech birth.

- Elevate hips, administer oxygen, and keep warm.
- Never attempt to deliver baby by pulling on its legs.
- Transport immediately.
- If baby delivers, support it and guide delivery of head.

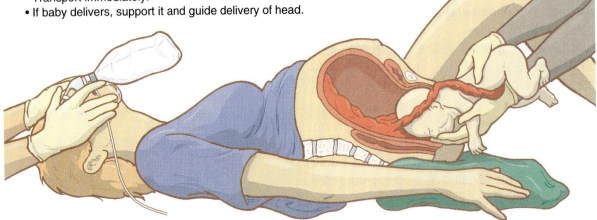

Emergency Care—Breech Presentation

Upon recognition of a breech presentation you should:

1. **Initiate rapid transport upon recognizing a breech presentation.**

2. **Never attempt to deliver the baby by pulling on its legs.**

3. **Provide high concentration oxygen to the mother**

4. **Place the mother in a head-down position with the pelvis elevated and provide her with emotional support.**

5. **Notify the receiving hospital of the breech presentation.**

6. **If the baby's buttocks and torso deliver, support the body with your hand until the head delivers.** Provide after-delivery care for the baby, cord, mother, and placenta as in a normal cephalic delivery.

Limb Presentation

A **limb presentation** occurs when a limb of an infant protrudes from the vagina as the presenting part. The presenting limb is commonly a foot when the baby is in the breech position. Limb presentations cannot be delivered in the prehospital setting. Rapid transport is essential to the baby's survival.

A limb presentation is detected when checking for crowning. You may see an arm, a single leg, or an arm and leg together, or a shoulder and an arm protruding from the vagina. A prolapsed cord may also be present. Never try to pull on the limb or replace the limb into the vagina. Instead, follow the procedures below.

Emergency Care—Limb Presentation

When you discover a limb presentation you should provide the following care (Figure 17-16):

1. **If there is a prolapsed cord, follow the same procedures as you would for any delivery involving a prolapsed cord.** Re-

member that you must keep pushing up on the baby until relieved by a physician.

2. **Place the mother in a head-down position with the pelvis elevated.**

3. **Administer high concentration oxygen via nonrebreather mask.**

4. **Provide rapid transport of the mother to the hospital.**

5. **Advise the hospital that you are inbound with a limb presentation.**

6. **Provide emotional support for the mother.**

Multiple Births

When more than one baby is born during a single delivery, it is called a **multiple birth.** A multiple birth, usually twins, is not considered to be a complication, provided that the deliveries are normal. Twins are generally delivered in the same manner as a single delivery, one birth following the other. However, if a multiple birth is encountered you should have enough personnel and equipment on scene to be prepared for multiple resuscitations. Call for additional personnel and ambulances to the scene as needed.

If the mother is under a physician's care, she will probably be aware that she is carrying twins. Without this information, you should consider a multiple birth to be a possibility if the mother's abdomen appears unusually large before delivery, or it remains very large after delivery of one baby. If the birth is multiple, labor contractions will continue after the first baby is delivered, and the second baby will be delivered shortly after the first. It is not unusual that the second baby presents in a breech position, usually within minutes of the first birth.

Emergency Care—Multiple Births

Special considerations for multiple births are as follows:

1. **Call for additional assistance to the scene once you determine that you have a multiple birth delivery situation.** Have several

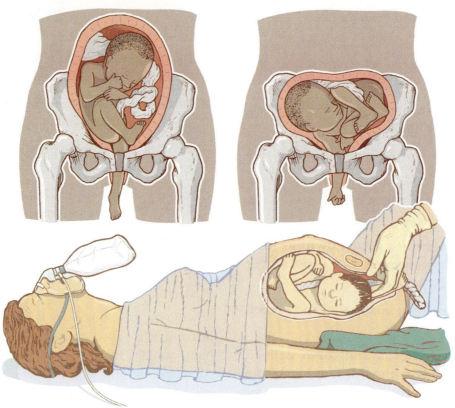

- Elevate hips, administer oxygen, and keep warm.
- If there is a prolapsed cord, gently push up on baby to keep it off cord.
- Transport immediately.

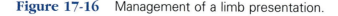

Figure 17-16 Management of a limb presentation.

emergency obstetrical kits available. Request enough personnel and ambulances to be prepared for multiple infant resuscitations. It is not practical to care for or resuscitate multiple infants in a single ambulance.

2. **Clamp or tie the umbilical cord of the first baby before the second is born.**

3. **Twins may share a single placenta or each have his own placenta. The placenta or placentas are delivered normally.** The second baby may be born either before or after the placenta is delivered. Care for infants, umbilical cords, and placentas just as you would in a single-birth delivery.

4. **Record the delivery time of each infant.** Identify them in the order they are born—for example, "baby boy A" and "baby boy B."

5. **Infants born as multiple births tend to be smaller than those born from a single delivery. Because of their smaller size**

these infants tend to deliver more swiftly; provide gentle support of the presenting part during delivery to prevent a rapid or explosive delivery. These infants also tend to lose heat more quickly; pay special attention to keeping the infants warm.

Premature Birth

By definition, a **premature infant** is one that weighs less than $5\frac{1}{2}$ pounds at birth, or one that is born before the 37th week of pregnancy. Since you will probably not be able to weigh the baby, you will have to make a determination as to whether the baby is full-term or premature based on the mother's information and the baby's appearance. By comparison with a normal full-term baby, the head of a premature infant is much larger in proportion to the small, thin, red body. You may encounter some infants whose delivery is so premature that they cannot survive outside the uterus, no matter what level of care is provided.

◆ Emergency Care—Premature Birth

Premature babies need special care from the moment of birth (Figure 17-17). The smaller the baby, the more important is the initial care. Special considerations in the care of the premature infant include the following:

1. **Keep the baby warm.** Premature babies lack fat deposits that would normally keep them warm. Premature infants are, therefore, at great risk of developing hypothermia. Once breathing, the baby should be dried and wrapped snugly in a warm blanket. Additional protection can be provided by an outer wrap of plastic bubble wrap (keep away from the face) or aluminum foil. The bubble wrap helps maintain warmth and allows for easier visual inspection of the clamped cord to check for bleeding. A stockinet cap should be placed on the baby's head to help reduce heat loss.

2. **Keep the airway clear.** Continue to suction fluids from the nose and mouth using a rub-

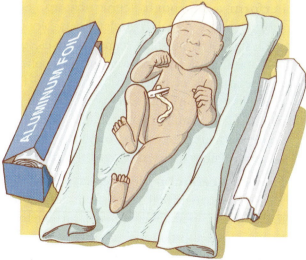

Figure 17-17 Premature infants need special care.

- Clear mouth and nose of fluid and mucus
- Prevent bleeding from cord
- Keep warm by wrapping in blanket and then in bubble wrap or aluminum foil. Cover head with stockinet cap.
- Administer oxygen if indicated

ber bulb syringe. Keep checking to see if additional suctioning is required.

3. **Provide ventilations and/or chest compressions as outlined earlier based upon the baby's pulse and respiratory effort.** In some cases resuscitation may not be possible if the baby is extremely premature. Contact the medical control physician immediately if you believe the infant is too premature to undergo resuscitative procedures.

4. **Provide oxygen.** Do not blow a stream of oxygen directly on the baby's face, but arrange for oxygen to flow past the baby's face.

5. **If the premature infant requires resuscitation, summon advanced life support backup either to the scene or to intercept the ambulance en route to the hospital.**

6. **Avoid contamination.** The premature infant is susceptible to infection. If the mother has defecated during the birth process, keep the infant away from such material. Keep the infant away from other people. Do not breathe directly onto the infant's face.

7. **Transport the infant in a warm ambulance.** The desired temperature is between 90°F and 100°F (32° and 38°C). Use the ambulance heater to warm the patient compartment prior to transport. In the summer months, the air conditioning should be turned off and all compartment windows should be closed or adjusted to keep the desired temperature.

8. **Notify the hospital emergency department of a premature delivery.** Early notification will allow the hospital to assemble the necessary equipment and medical staff to attend to the mother and infant.

Meconium

Meconium is a result of the fetus defecating (putting out wastes). It is a sign of fetal or maternal distress. Meconium stains amniotic fluid greenish or brownish-yellow in color. Infants born with meconium are at increased risk for respiratory problems, especially if aspiration of the meconium occurs at birth.

◆ Emergency Care—Meconium

Once you identify the presence of meconium at the vaginal opening you should:

1. **Avoid any stimulation of the infant before suctioning the mouth and oropharynx.** Many of the complications associated with meconium are the result of the baby aspirating meconium into his lungs. Therefore, it is very important not to stimulate the infant to breathe prior to suctioning as much meconium as possible out of the mouth and oropharynx. Remember to suction the mouth first and then the nose.

2. **Maintain an open airway and carefully monitor the baby.** Remember that meconium is a sign of fetal distress at the time of delivery. The newborn may require resuscitation. Provide artificial ventilations and/or chest compression, as indicated by effort of breathing and heart rate.

3. **Initiate transport as soon as possible.** Keep the infant warm during transport and advise the hospital of the presence of meconium during delivery.

EMERGENCIES IN PREGNANCY

Most women proceed through pregnancy without complications. However, pregnant women can have life-threatening predelivery emergencies that are a direct result of their pregnancies. In addition, pregnant women are susceptible to all the same medical and trauma emergencies as non-pregnant patients

As an EMT, you may be called upon to assess and provide emergency care for pregnant women with any of these emergencies. When assessing and providing care for any emergency where a pregnant woman is involved, remember that *"what's good for the mother is good for the fetus."* Assuring that the mother has an open airway and adequate breathing and circulation will in turn optimize the well being of the fetus during the emergency.

Spontaneous Abortion (Miscarriage)

The most common predelivery emergency EMTs are likely to encounter is a **miscarriage.** About 15 to 20 percent of pregnancies end in miscarriage. The medical term for miscarriage is **spontaneous abortion.** It is important to exercise caution when using the term "abortion" around the patient and family because of the ethical and religious implications of the word itself. A spontaneous abortion occurs when there is loss of the pregnancy prior to the 20th week of pregnancy. Indeed, if a miscarriage occurs very early in pregnancy, the woman may not even be aware that she is pregnant. During a spontaneous abortion the fetus and other contents of the uterus are passed through the cervix and out of the vagina. Because a fetus less than 20 weeks old cannot survive outside the uterus, a spontaneous abortion results in fetal death.

A woman who is having a spontaneous abortion will complain of vaginal bleeding, which may be associated with abdominal pain or cramping. The amount of vaginal bleeding experienced may be heavy and include clots and fetal tissue. The patient is also likely to be under great emotional stress because of the knowledge that vaginal bleeding during pregnancy is a serious symptom that may signal the loss of her pregnancy.

◆ Emergency Care—Spontaneous Abortion

The emergency care of a woman with a suspected spontaneous abortion includes the following:

1. **Perform a thorough scene size-up.** Body substance isolation is mandatory as blood is always present at such scenes. Gloves, goggles and a mask may be warranted depending on the amount of bleeding present. The EMT must also size-up the emotional state of the patient and family. Anger and frustration about the feared loss of the pregnancy may be inappropriately directed toward the EMT.

2. **Provide a careful patient assessment.** Your assessment may reveal a woman in distress due to abdominal pain. Women who are having a spontaneous abortion will usually present with an adequate airway and breathing status. Pro-

longed vaginal bleeding may result in signs of inadequate circulation such as pale and clammy skin and a rapid pulse. Immediate transportation and a request for advanced life support back-up should be the treatment priority for women with signs of inadequate circulation.

3. **Obtain a history.** This should include verification of the patient being pregnant and an estimate as to how far along the pregnancy is. Infants born at 24 or 25 weeks may survive with neonatal intensive care and are not considered miscarriages but rather premature infants and should be treated as described above.

4. **Conduct a physical exam, including baseline vitals.** If the patient is describing heavy vaginal bleeding or passing "clots" from her vagina, a brief inspection of the perineum is appropriate and allows placement of external vaginal pads. As always, examine the vaginal area in a professional manner, making every effort to respect the patient's privacy.

5. **Initiate treatment based on signs and symptoms.** Administer high flow oxygen if signs of inadequate breathing or perfusion are detected. Apply external vaginal pads to the vaginal area if bleeding is detected on examination.

6. **Provide on-going emotional support of the mother.**

7. **Bring any fetal tissue that has been passed to the hospital.** Doing so will allow it to be examined by the hospital staff.

Seizures During Pregnancy

Seizures during pregnancy are particularly serious because the mother's breathing is generally inadequate during a seizure. Because the mother is not receiving adequate oxygen while she is seizing, the fetus is also receiving inadequate amounts of oxygen.

Pregnant women who experience a seizure are likely either to have had a seizure history prior to pregnancy or to be having a seizure as a result of a pregnancy-related condition called **eclampsia** or **toxemia of pregnancy.** Patients

with eclampsia usually develop the condition in the third trimester of pregnancy. Signs and symptoms associated with eclampsia include a history of headache, high blood pressure, and swelling or edema of the ankles.

Take body substance isolation precautions when assessing the pregnant seizure patient. Determine the patient's mental status and whether the patient's airway and breathing are compromised by the seizure. During the focused history and physical exam, try to learn whether there is a previous history of seizures and what medications the patient may be taking. The detailed physical exam may reveal the presence of edema.

◆ Emergency Care—Seizures in Pregnancy

Regardless of the cause of a pregnant woman's seizure, the treatment is the same—protecting the patient from harm, maintaining an open airway, and assuring adequate breathing. Remember that any pregnant woman who is having or has had a seizure is a high priority patient who requires immediate transport to the hospital. Management steps for seizures during pregnancy include:

1. **Assess hazards around a seizing patient and move away objects that might injure the patient.**

2. **Ensure and maintain an open airway.**

3. **Administer high flow oxygen via nonrebreather mask.**

4. **Be prepared to assist ventilations with a bag-valve mask if necessary.**

5. **Have suctioning equipment ready to use if necessary.**

6. **Transport the patient positioned on her left side.**

7. **Consider requesting an ALS intercept if a prolonged transport is anticipated.**

Vaginal Bleeding Late in Pregnancy

Vaginal bleeding can occur during pregnancy at any time. As already discussed, vaginal bleeding early in pregnancy may signal a spontaneous abortion. Bleeding late in pregnancy, especially in the third trimester, can rapidly lead to the death of both the mother and fetus. The reason third trimester vaginal bleeding is so severe is that it frequently involves hemorrhage from the placenta. In some cases, the placenta separates from the wall of the uterus (*placental abruption*). In other cases, the placenta begins to bleed when it is positioned too close to the cervix (*placenta previa*). Vaginal bleeding late in pregnancy may or may not be associated with abdominal pain.

◆ *Emergency Care—Vaginal Bleeding Late in Pregnancy*

Management of pregnant women with vaginal bleeding should include the normal systematic approach to patient care.

1. **Be sure to take appropriate body substance isolation precautions as you perform the scene size-up.**

2. **During your initial assessment, pay careful attention for signs of inadequate circulation or shock (hypoperfusion).** Continue to assess for shock as you gather information during the focused history and physical exam.

3. **Consider any pregnant woman you treat who is having third trimester vaginal bleeding as a high priority patient who requires immediate transport to the hospital.**

4. **Base treatment on the woman's signs and symptoms.** Any pregnant patient with vaginal bleeding should receive high flow oxygen. Sanitary napkins can be placed over the vaginal opening to absorb the bleeding, but *do not place anything in the vagina*. Position the woman on her left side during transport.

5. **Advise the hospital that you are transporting a pregnant woman with vaginal bleeding.** This will allow the emergency department to notify the appropriate personnel.

Trauma During Pregnancy

Nowhere is the saying that *"what's good for the mother is good for the baby"* more true than in cases of trauma during pregnancy. Heeding that saying simplifies the care of the pregnant trauma patient because out-of-hospital care for pregnant trauma patients is virtually the same as for non-pregnant trauma patients. By assuring that the mother has an open airway and adequate breathing and circulation, you will be maximizing the fetus's chances for survival.

During these cases, you must be aware of the profound emotional stress the mother is experiencing because of her concerns for her baby. Reassure the mother that your care is designed not only to help her but also to help her baby as well.

◆ *Emergency Care—Trauma in Pregnancy*

Care of the pregnant trauma patient should include the following steps.

1. **Perform a thorough scene size-up.** Take appropriate body substance isolation precautions and assure scene safety. Be sure to assess the scene to determine, if possible, the mechanism of injury.

2. **Perform the initial assessment.** Carefully determine the patient's mental status, assure that she has an open and secure airway, and look for signs of inadequate breathing or circulation. A pregnant woman who has sustained significant injuries requires immediate transport to the hospital, preferably a trauma center.

3. **Perform the focused history and physical exam and take baseline vital signs.** Keep in mind that a pregnant woman's baseline vital signs will differ from those of a woman who is not pregnant; the pulse rate is usually higher and the blood pressure usually lower. Despite this normal variation in vital signs, always assume that a woman who has sustained trauma and has an increased heart rate and/or a decreased blood pressure is in shock and treat appropriately.

4. **Base your treatment on the patient's signs and symptoms.** Provide normal trauma care including cervical spine immobilization. However, any pregnant woman with trauma should receive high flow oxygen and be positioned on her left side during transport. For the pregnant

patient immobilized on a long backboard, the entire board can be tipped slightly with the left side down or a towel can be placed under the patient's right hip. Advanced life support should be summoned if the patient is unstable; assure that arrival at the hospital is not delayed by waiting for ALS treatment.

5. **Provide emotional support.** Reassure the patient that your emergency medical care is intended for baby's well-being as well as hers.

6. **Advise the hospital that you are transporting a pregnant trauma patient.** This will allow the emergency department to notify the appropriate personnel and resources.

GYNECOLOGICAL EMERGENCIES

There are several emergencies unique to the reproductive systems of non-pregnant women with which you as an EMT must be familiar.

Vaginal Bleeding

Vaginal bleeding that is not a result of direct trauma or a woman's normal menstrual cycle may indicate a serious gynecologic emergency. Since it will be impossible for you to determine a specific cause of the bleeding, it is important that all women who have vaginal bleeding be treated as though they have a potentially life-threatening condition. This is especially true if the bleeding is associated with abdominal pain. The most serious complication of vaginal bleeding is hypovolemic shock due to blood loss.

◆ Emergency Care—Vaginal Bleeding

Steps in the assessment and management of vaginal bleeding include the following:

1. **Perform a thorough scene size-up.** Take appropriate body substance isolation precautions. Wear gloves, mask, eye wear, and gown as indicated.

2. **Perform the initial assessment.** Carefully determine the patient's mental status, assure

that she has an open and secure airway, and look for signs of inadequate breathing or circulation. A pregnant woman who has sustained significant injuries requires immediate transport to the hospital, preferably a trauma center.

3. **Provide treatment based on the patient's signs and symptoms.** Administer high flow oxygen if signs of shock (hypoperfusion) are present. The use of the pneumatic anti-shock garment (PASG) may be indicated if the patient is hypotensive with other signs of hypoperfusion. Follow local protocols for PASG use.

4. **Provide rapid transport** Request an ALS intercept if signs of shock are present.

Trauma to External Genitalia

Trauma to a woman's external genitalia can be difficult to care for because of the patient's modesty and the severe pain often involved with such injuries. Injuries in this area tend to bleed profusely because of its rich blood supply. Injuries to the female external genitalia are frequently the result of straddle-type injuries such as one leg falling into a swimming pool while the other leg remains on the deck surface.

◆ Emergency Care—Trauma to the External Genitalia

Steps in the assessment and management of trauma to the external genitalia include the following:

1. **Perform a thorough scene size-up.** Assure appropriate body substance isolation. Observe for mechanism of injury.

2. **Perform the initial assessment.** Carefully observe for signs and symptoms of inadequate circulation.

3. **Provide treatment based on signs and symptoms.** Treat as you would other soft tissue injuries. Control bleeding with direct pressure applied to a bulky dressing or sanitary pad over the bleeding site. Do not pack or place any gauze within the vagina. Application of cold compresses in addition to sterile

dressings may aid in reducing pain. Remove unneeded bystanders and expose the patient's body only to the extent necessary to provide appropriate care. Administer high flow oxygen if signs of compromise of breathing or circulation are evident.

Sexual Assault

Situations where a sexual assault has occurred are always a challenge to the EMT. Care of the patient must include both medical and psychological considerations. In addition, law enforcement agencies are also frequently involved.

There is no question that the victim of sexual assault is under tremendous stress. You must be prepared to deal with the wide range of emotions that the patient may exhibit. The best approach is to be nonjudgmental and to maintain a professional but compassionate attitude. *It is generally preferable that an EMT of the same sex as the patient establish rapport and be the primary provider of emergency care whenever possible.*

◆ *Emergency Care—Sexual Assault*

Steps in the assessment and care of victims of sexual assault include the following:

1. **Perform a thorough scene size-up.** Since you may be entering a potential crime scene, assure that the scene is safe prior to entering. It may be necessary to stage your unit near the scene until it is rendered safe by police.

2. **During the initial assessment identify both the medical and the psychological needs of the patient.**

3. **Be alert to other injuries that the patient may have sustained during the assault while you are performing the focused history and physical exam.** Examine the genitals only if severe bleeding is present.

4. **Provide treatment based on the patient's signs and symptoms.** Be careful not to disturb potential criminal evidence unless it is absolutely necessary for patient care. Discourage the patient from bathing, voiding, or cleaning any wounds as doing so may result in the loss of important evidence.

5. **Fulfill any reporting requirements that are locally mandated.** Maintain patient confidentiality by not discussing the case with anyone who is not directly involved in the patient's care.

Chapter Review

SUMMARY

As an EMT, you may be called upon to assist with out-of-hospital childbirth or attend to women with emergencies related to their reproductive systems. You should possess the knowledge to assess and assist a mother with her delivery and assess and, if necessary, resuscitate the newborn baby. You must also be prepared to treat other injuries associated with women's reproductive systems.

REVIEWING KEY CONCEPTS

1. Name and describe the anatomical structures of a woman's body associated with pregnancy.

2. Describe physiological changes that take place in a woman's body during pregnancy and the implications of those changes for the EMT who is assessing a pregnant patient.

3. Describe the three stages of labor.

4. Explain how to evaluate a pregnant woman to determine whether delivery is imminent.

5. Explain the circumstances in which assisting with an on-scene delivery would be appropriate.

6. List the steps in assisting a patient in active labor with a normal delivery.

7. List the elements that should be considered in assessing a newborn infant.

8. Describe the indications and procedures for resuscitation of the newborn infant.

9. Describe the procedure for cutting the umbilical cord.

10. Explain how to help control post-delivery bleeding in the mother.

11. Describe the specific steps you would take to provide emergency care for the following conditions: (a) breech birth, (b) prolapsed cord, (c) multiple births, (d) meconium staining, (e) premature birth.

12. Describe the emergency care of a woman with a suspected spontaneous abortion.

13. Describe the basic emergency care for trauma to the external genitalia.

14. Describe the special considerations associated with the care of a victim of sexual assault.

RESOURCES TO LEARN MORE

"Emergency Aspects of Obstetrics" in Harwood-Nuss, A. L. et al., *The Clinical Practice of Emergency Medicine, 2nd Edition*. Philadelphia: Lippincott-Raven, 1995.

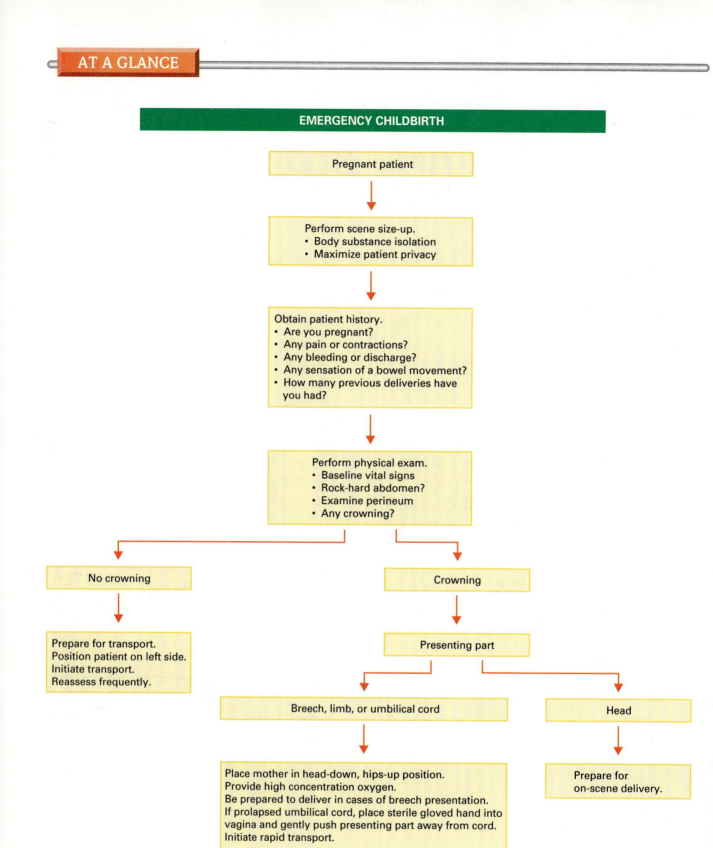

EMERGENCY CHILDBIRTH

Pregnant patient

Perform scene size-up.
• Body substance isolation
• Maximize patient privacy

Obtain patient history.
• Are you pregnant?
• Any pain or contractions?
• Any bleeding or discharge?
• Any sensation of a bowel movement?
• How many previous deliveries have you had?

Perform physical exam.
• Baseline vital signs
• Rock-hard abdomen?
• Examine perineum
• Any crowning?

No crowning

Prepare for transport.
Position patient on left side.
Initiate transport.
Reassess frequently.

Crowning

Presenting part

Breech, limb, or umbilical cord

Place mother in head-down, hips-up position.
Provide high concentration oxygen.
Be prepared to deliver in cases of breech presentation.
If prolapsed umbilical cord, place sterile gloved hand into vagina and gently push presenting part away from cord.
Initiate rapid transport.

Head

Prepare for
on-scene delivery.

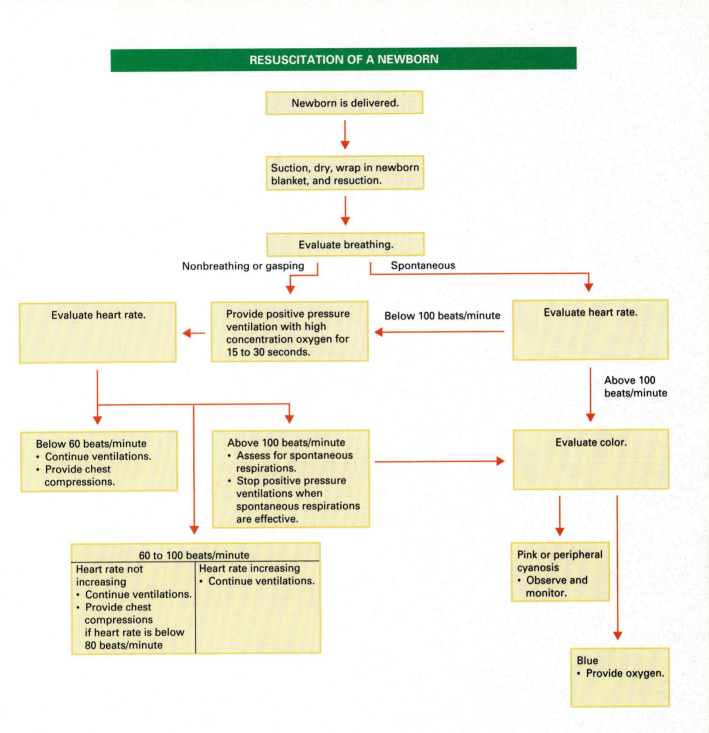

Behavioral Emergencies

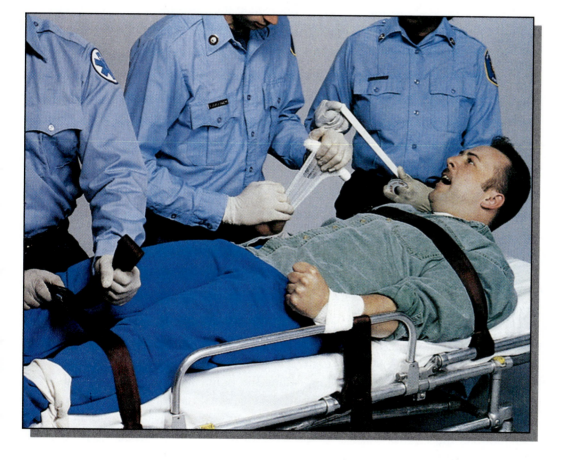

*S*ome of the most difficult—and dangerous—situations you will face as an EMT involve patients who are behaving in unexpected ways. Their behaviors may arise from a variety of causes—stress, alcohol or drugs, injuries, physical or mental illness. Because the behaviors of these patients are often unpredictable, you may feel it necessary to request law enforcement assistance before beginning assessment and treatment.

At the completion of this chapter, the EMT-Basic student should be able to meet the following objectives:

Knowledge and Understanding

1. Define behavioral emergencies. (p. 445)
2. Discuss the general factors that may cause an alteration in a patient's behavior. (pp. 445–446, 448–449)
3. State the various reasons for psychological crises. (pp. 446, 448–449)
4. Discuss the characteristics of an individual's behavior that suggest the patient is at risk for suicide. (pp. 448–449
5. Discuss special medical/legal considerations for managing behavioral emergencies. (pp. 450, 452–453)
6. Discuss the special considerations for assessing a patient with behavioral problems. (pp. 446–450)

7. Discuss the general principles of an individual's behavior that suggest he is at risk for violence. (p. 449)
8. Discuss methods to calm behavioral emergency patients. (pp. 446–447, 449–450)
9. Explain the rationale for learning how to modify your behavior toward the patient with a behavioral emergency. (pp. 446–447)

Skills

1. Demonstrate the assessment and emergency medical care of the patient experiencing a behavioral emergency.
2. Demonstrate various techniques to safely restrain a patient with a behavioral problem.

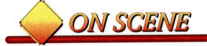

ON SCENE

DISPATCH: *ENGINE 4, RESPOND TO THE CORNER OF FIFTH AND ADDISON FOR A PSYCHIATRIC EMERGENCY. POLICE ARE ALSO EN ROUTE.*

When the engine company arrives at the scene, two police units are already there. Two police officers are talking to a naked man who is standing in front of a church. The lieutenant hears the man shouting to the police officers, "I am the arm of the Lord Almighty!" The man paces in a tight circle, waving his arms. He is angry that he can't go inside the church.

As one police officer motions the engine lieutenant over, an additional police car pulls up. The other firefighters stay on the engine. A police office and the lieutenant both try to calm the man and convince him to be transported for treatment. The man does not reply directly, but shouts, "I am the arm of the Lord who will strike down the wicked who oppose him." He stops pacing and turns, glowering, his fists clenched.

The police officer and the lieutenant back off several paces. Then they try to convince him again. Several similar attempts at communicating with the man fail. The police then decide to restrain him. The officers plan their moves carefully. At the agreed signal, four of them move in and quickly restrain the patient.

Once the restraint is complete, the lieutenant calls the other firefighters over to examine the patient. The man is fighting the restraint and screaming, calling the police and firefighters "devils." It is impossible to obtain a history. One of the police officers advises that he has seen the patient before and knows he has a psychiatric history.

The patient is not wearing a medical alert bracelet; he shows no signs of any other medical condition. The patient has an open airway and is breathing adequately. His pulse is 104. His continuing struggles don't allow the firefighters to determine blood pressure or respirations.

The firefighters monitor the patient carefully, paying special attention to his ABCs, until the ambulance arrives.

BEHAVIORAL EMERGENCIES

Behavior is the manner in which a person acts or performs. It includes both a person's physical and mental activities. All people exhibit behavior. However, behavior may differ from person to person and from situation to situation.

A **behavioral emergency** is defined as a situation where the patient exhibits abnormal behavior within a given situation that is unacceptable or intolerable to the patient, family, or the community.

Note that this definition of behavioral emergency says "within a given situation." What behavior is "acceptable" depends on the situation in which it is performed. For example, unexpected news of the death of a loved one may produce reactions in people that range from sobbing to screaming to a silent, shock-like state. In the circumstances, those behaviors would be considered acceptable. However, if a person walking through a shopping mall began sobbing or screaming for no apparent reason, such actions might be signs of a behavioral emergency.

Also remember that "acceptable behavior" is shaped by the culture in which a person lives. The United States is a huge nation. Many of its residents came from other lands and cultures. In certain circumstances, they may behave in ways that seem unusual to you but might be quite normal in their native cultures.

If you are called to a behavioral emergency, you must perform a careful, thorough patient assessment just as you would at the scene of a medical or trauma emergency. As you perform that assessment, remain objective. Do not judge patients solely on the way they look or act.

Behavioral Changes

There are many medical and traumatic conditions that can alter a patient's behavior. When dealing with a person who appears to be having a behavioral emergency, always first consider the possibility that the unusual behavior is caused by something other than a psychological problem. These causes might include the following:

◆ *Low blood sugar* This can cause the rapid onset of erratic or hostile behavior (similar to alcohol intoxication), dizziness and headache, fainting, seizures, sometimes coma, profuse perspiration, hunger, drooling, and rapid pulse but normal blood pressure.

◆ *Lack of oxygen* This can cause restlessness and confusion, cyanosis (blue or gray skin), and altered mental status.

◆ *Inadequate blood flow to the brain or stroke* These can cause confusion or dizziness, impaired speech, headache, loss of function or paralysis of extremities on one side of the body, nausea and vomiting, and rapid full pulse.

◆ *Head trauma* This can cause personality changes ranging from irritability to violent, irrational behavior, altered mental status, amnesia or confusion, irregular respirations, elevated blood pressure, and decreasing pulse.

◆ *Mind-altering substances (both prescription and illegal drugs)* These may cause highly variable signs and symptoms depending on the substance ingested.

◆ *Excessive cold* This can cause shivering, feelings of numbness, altered mental status, drowsiness, staggering walk, slow breathing, and slow pulse.

◆ *Excessive heat* This can cause decreased or complete loss of consciousness.

When at the scene of what seems to be a behavioral emergency, always consider the possibility that there may be a physiological rather than a psychological reason for the way the person is acting. Some signs that the problem might have a physiological cause include the following:

◆ Unusual odors on the patient's breath

◆ Dilated, constricted, or unequally reactive pupils

◆ Rapid rather than gradual onset of symptoms

◆ Excessive salivation

◆ Loss of bladder or bowel control

◆ Visual rather than auditory hallucinations

Situational Stress Reactions

At many of the incidents you will be called to as an EMT, you will find patients—and sometimes family members or bystanders—exhibiting fear, grief, and anger. These are typical reactions to the stress of an accident or a fire as well as common reactions to serious illness and death. In most cases, as you take control of the situation and treat the patient as an individual, personal interaction will inspire confidence in your ability to help. People will begin to calm down and feel cable of coping with the emergency.

Be as unhurried as you can in these stressful situations. Rushing the survey and the interview may leave the patient feeling that the situation is out of control. The patient also may believe that you are more concerned with the problem than with him. Let the patient know that you are there to help.

Whenever you care for a patient who is displaying typical stress reactions, do the following:

◆ Act in a calm manner.

◆ Give the patient time to gain control of emotions.

◆ Quietly and carefully evaluate the situation.

◆ Keep your own emotions under control.

◆ Honestly explain things to the patient.

◆ Let the patient know that you are listening to what he is saying.

◆ Stay alert for sudden changes in behavior.

By following these guidelines, you are applying crisis management techniques to help the patient deal with stress. If the patient does not begin to interact with you or to calm down, you must assume that there is a problem of a more serious nature, such as an emotional or psychiatric problem. You should then proceed according to the recommendations for dealing with behavioral emergencies described below.

Psychiatric Emergencies

There are many types of psychiatric problems. Some patients with psychiatric conditions may be withdrawn and not wish to communicate, while others are agitated, or talk ceaselessly, or exhibit bizarre or threatening behavior. Some patients may act as if they wish to harm themselves or others.

There are a number of different psychiatric conditions that can cause behavioral emergencies. These conditions include anxiety, phobia, depression, bipolar disorder, paranoia, and schizophrenia. It is not important that you be able to identify each of these conditions. Rather, you should recognize that a patient is having a behavioral emergency and treat him according to the steps below.

Whenever you are called to a scene where a patient is experiencing a psychiatric—or any behavioral—emergency, there are some general rules to follow that can make dealing with the patient easier (Figure 18-1). These include the following:

◆ Identify yourself and your role.

◆ Speak slowly and clearly. Use a calm and reassuring tone.

◆ Listen to the patient. You can show you are listening by repeating part of what the patient said back to him.

◆ Do not be judgmental. Show compassion, not pity.

◆ Use positive body language. Avoid crossing your arms or looking uninterested.

Figure 18-1 Be calm and reassuring when talking to a behavioral emergency patient. Do not enter the patient's personal space and remain alert to changes in his emotional status.

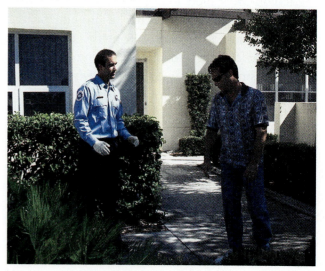

- Acknowledge the patient's feelings.

- Do not enter the patient's personal space. Stay at least 3 feet (1 m) from the patient. Making the patient feel closed in can cause an emotional outburst.

- Be alert for changes in the patient's emotional status. Watch for increasingly aggressive behavior and take appropriate actions for safety.

Assessment of Behavioral Emergency Patients

When performing the assessment of a behavioral emergency patient, begin with a careful scene size-up. If for any reason you suspect violence or the possibility of violence, do not enter a scene or, if you have already entered the scene, retreat from it. Do not hesitate to call for law enforcement assistance in such cases. The police can provide protection. Also, if a patient must be transported, the police can be valuable witnesses. Finally, if a patient must be restrained, their presence will be vital (see below).

Once you have assured that the scene is safe and you have entered it, identify yourself and your role. It may not be obvious to the patient who you are and what you intend to do.

Complete an initial assessment of the patient. Be certain to include an assessment of the patient's mental status (level of responsiveness and orientation to person, place, and time).

Perform as much of the focused and detailed examinations as possible. Be alert for medical and traumatic conditions that could be causing the patient's behavior.

Gather as thorough a patient history as possible. This will alert you to past psychiatric problems, psychiatric medications the patient may be taking, or not taking—causing the outburst. (See Table 18-1 on page 453 for a list of common psychiatric medications.) This may also alert you to other conditions, such as diabetes, that can closely mimic a psychiatric condition. Be aware, however, that with behavioral emergency patients, you sometimes may not get much information. Some patients will ignore you. Others will respond inappropriately to your questions. Do the best you can, and be sure to document how the patient responds.

When you are assessing behavioral emergency patients, you may encounter some of the following common signs and symptoms:

- Panic or anxiety

- Fear

- Agitated or unusual activity, such as repetitive motions or threatening movements

- Unusual appearance, disordered clothing, poor hygiene

- Unusual speech patterns, such as too-rapid speech, repetitions, or inability to carry on a coherent conversation

- Depression

- Withdrawal

- Confusion

- Anger, often inappropriately directed and often brief but intense

- Bizarre behavior or thought patterns

- Loss of contact with reality, hallucinations

- Suicidal or self-destructive behavior

- Violent or aggressive behavior with threats or intent to harm others

◆ Emergency Care—Behavioral Emergencies

Follow these general guidelines when treating a patient with a behavioral emergency.

1. **Be alert for personal or scene safety problems during scene size-up and throughout the call.** Consider requesting police back up.

2. **Treat any life-threatening problems during the initial assessment.**

3. **Be alert for medical or traumatic conditions that could mimic a behavioral emergency.**

4. **Be prepared to spend time talking to the patient and stay with the patient.** Use the skills listed earlier when dealing with the patient. Remember to talk in a calm reassuring voice. Use positive body language and good eye contact. Avoid unnecessary physical contact and quick movements. Never turn your

back on or drop your guard with a violent or potentially violent patient.

5. **Encourage the patient to discuss what is troubling him.**

6. **Never play along with any visual or auditory hallucinations that patient may be experiencing. Do not lie to the patient.**

7. **If it appears it will help, involve family members or friends in the conversation.** Evaluate the response of the patient to the presence of others. If it agitates the patient, ask the others to leave.

8. **As possible, perform a focused history and physical exam and provide any necessary emergency care.**

9. **Perform a detailed physical exam only if it is safe and you suspect the patient may have an injury.**

10. **Consider using restraints if it is necessary to keep the patient from harming himself or others.** Request assistance from law-enforcement personnel. See the discussion below of factors to be considered when using restraints.

11. **If necessary, transport the patient to a facility where he can get appropriate physical and psychological treatment.**

12. **Perform the ongoing assessment.** Stay alert for any sudden changes in the patient's behavior.

13. **Contact the receiving hospital and report on current mental status and other important information.** Your medical protocols or procedures should direct you to the most appropriate medical facility within your community. Not all hospitals are prepared to treat behavioral emergencies.

SPECIAL CONSIDERATIONS

Two types of behavioral emergencies can be especially challenging—and dangerous—for EMTs. These are calls that involve attempted suicide or that involve a hostile or aggressive patient.

Suicide

Each year in this country, thousands of people commit suicide. Many more suffer both physical and emotional injuries in suicide attempts. Anyone may become suicidal if emotional distress is severe, regardless of gender, age, or ethnic, social, or economic background.

People attempt suicide for many reasons. These include depression caused by chemical imbalance, the death of a loved one, financial problems, the end to a love affair, poor health, loss of esteem, divorce, fear of failure, and alcohol and/or drug abuse. People use a variety of methods in attempts to end their lives. You may observe suicides or attempted suicides by drug overdose, hanging, jumping from high places, ingesting poisons, inhaling gas, wrist-cutting, self-mutilation, stabbing, or shooting.

Whenever you are called to care for a patient who has attempted or is about to attempt suicide, *your first concern must be your own safety*. Not all patients will wish to harm you, but the mechanism used to attempt suicide will be capable of causing death. It could intentionally or accidentally be turned on you.

The following factors can help you assess the patient's risk for suicide.

◆ *Depression*. Take seriously a patient's feelings and expressions of despair or suicidal thoughts.

◆ *High current or recent stress levels*. If these are present, take the threat of suicide seriously.

◆ *Recent emotional trauma*. This might include job loss, loss of a significant relationship, serious illness, arrest, imprisonment.

◆ *Age*. High suicide rates occur at ages 15–25 and over age 40. The elderly are a population in which suicide is increasing.

◆ *Alcohol and drug abuse*.

◆ *Threats of suicide*. The patient may have told others that he is considering suicide.

◆ *Suicide plan*. A patient who has a detailed suicide plan is more likely to commit suicide. Look for a plan that includes a method to carry out the suicide as well as notes and other arrangements, such as giving away personal possessions and getting affairs in order.

◆ *Previous attempts or suicide threats*. Does the patient have a history of self-destructive behavior? Too often, patients who have attempted suicide before are considered to be "looking for attention" and are not taken seriously. Statistics reveal that persons with a prior suicide attempt are more likely to commit suicide than those without an attempt. Take all threats of suicide seriously.

◆ *Sudden improvement from depression*. Patients who have made the decision to commit suicide may actually appear to improve from a recent depression. The fact that the decision has been made and an end is in sight can cause this apparent "improvement." You may find family members and friends of suicidal patients who will report that the patient had seemed "better" in the past few days.

In cases of threatened or attempted suicide, remember that you are the first professional to begin both the physical and mental health care of the patient. The more reassurance you can provide for the patient, the easier it will be for the hospital emergency department staff to continue care.

Your care for the patient who has threatened or attempted suicide is basically similar to that for other patients with emotional or psychiatric emergencies. Your personal interaction with the patient is key. Try to establish visual and verbal contact with the patient as soon as possible. Avoid arguing. Make no threats, and show no indication of using force.

The importance of safety at the scene of such emergencies cannot be emphasized too strongly. Make sure the scene is safe and make sure it is safe to approach the patient. If the scene is not safe, request assistance from the police and wait until they have secured the scene. Do not leave the patient alone unless you are at risk of physical harm. Try to talk with the patient from a safe distance until the police arrive.

When the scene is secure, look for and treat life-threatening problems to the extent that the patient will permit. Seek police assistance in restraining the patient if necessary for care of life-threatening problems.

Throughout your interaction with the patient, speak slowly—and patiently await answers to your questions. As you gain the patient's confidence, explain what questions must be answered and what must be done as part of the physical exam and vital sign assessment. Let the patient know that you think it would be best if he goes to the hospital and that you need his cooperation and help. Back off if necessary. If the patient's fear or aggression increases, do not push the issues of the examination or transport. Instead, try to re-establish the conversation and give the patient more time before you again say that going to the hospital is a good idea.

Note that you should *transport all suicidal patients*. Seek police assistance if necessary. Report any attempted suicide or expression of suicidal thoughts to the medical facility, police, or government agency designated by your state law and local protocols.

Hostile or Aggressive Patients

Aggressive or disruptive behavior may be caused by trauma to the brain and nervous system, metabolic disorders, stress, alcohol and other drugs, or psychological disorders. Sometimes you will know that your patient is aggressive from the information you receive from dispatch. At other times, the scene may provide quick clues (e.g., drugs, yelling, unclean conditions, broken furniture). Neighbors, family members, or bystanders may tell you that the patient is dangerous or angry or has a history of aggression or combativeness. The patient's stance (tense muscles, clenched fists, or quick irregular movements, for example) or position in the room may give you an early warning of possible violence (Figure 18-2). On rare occasions, you may start with an apparently calm patient who suddenly turns aggressive. Additional signs that you may be dealing with a hostile or aggressive patient are that the patient:

◆ Responds to people inappropriately

◆ Tries to hurt himself or others

◆ May have a rapid pulse and breathing

◆ Usually displays rapid speech and rapid physical movements

◆ May appear anxious, nervous, "panicky"

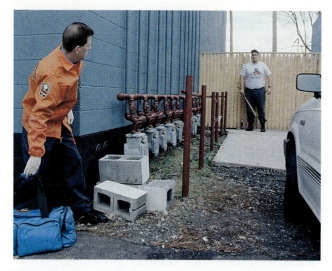

Figure 18-2 A patient's stance and position can indicate a potential for violence. If you determine that there is a potential for violence, request police assistance.

As with other behavioral emergencies, safety is the key concern. When a patient acts as if he may hurt himself or others, *your first concern must be your own safety*. Take the following precautions.

◆ *Do not isolate yourself from your partner or other sources of help.* Make certain that you have an escape route. Do not let the patient come between you and the door. Should a patient become violent, retreat and wait for police assistance.

◆ *Do not take any action that may be considered threatening by the patient.* To do so may bring about hostile behavior directed against you or others.

◆ *Always be on the watch for weapons.* Stay out of kitchens; they are filled with dangerous weapons. Stay in a safe area until the police can control the scene.

◆ *Be alert for sudden changes in the patient's behavior.*

◆ *Always carry a portable radio to maintain contact with other units or the dispatcher.*

Your assessment of the aggressive or hostile patient may never go beyond the initial assessment phase. Most of your time may be spent trying to calm the patient and ensuring everyone's safety. Otherwise, treatment steps follow those cited above for a patient in a behavioral emergency. Remain ready at all times to retreat from the scene if you suspect danger. Request assistance from law enforcement, before approaching the patient if necessary or if you feel the use of restraints is necessary.

Reasonable Force and Restraint

As noted above, patients in behavioral emergencies sometimes threaten or attempt to hurt themselves or others. **Reasonable force** is the force necessary to keep such a patient from injuring himself or others. Reasonableness is determined by looking at all circumstances involved. These include the patient's strength and size, type of abnormal behavior, mental status, and available methods of restraint. Understand that you may protect yourself from attack, but otherwise you must avoid actions that can cause injury to the patient.

Note that in most localities an EMT cannot legally restrain a patient, move a patient against his or her will, or force a patient to accept emergency care—even at the family's request. The restraint and forcible moving of patients is within the jurisdiction of law enforcement. The police (and in some jurisdictions a physician) can order you to restrain and transport a patient to the appropriate medical facility. However, the physician is not empowered to order you to take action that could place you in danger. If the police order restraint and transport, they must assist with these procedures as necessary. Remember to follow local protocols.

Never try to assist in restraining a patient unless there are sufficient personnel to do the job. You must be able to ensure your safety and the safety of the patient. If you help the police or a physician to restrain a patient, make certain that the restraints are humane. Handcuffs and "throwaway" plastic criminal restraints should not be used because of the soft-tissue damage they can inflict. Initially, the police may have to use such restraints. However, in some states they can be replaced with soft restraints such as leather cuffs and belts. If authorized in your state and by local protocol, an ambulance should carry leather cuffs, a waist-size belt, and at least three short belts. Restraints for the wrists and ankles can be made from gauze roller bandages.

Restraining a Patient

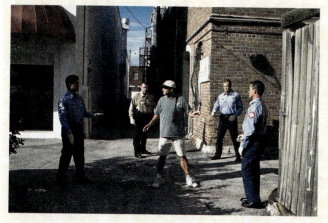

Figure 18-3A Plan your approach to the patient in advance and remain outside the range of his arms and legs until you are ready to act.

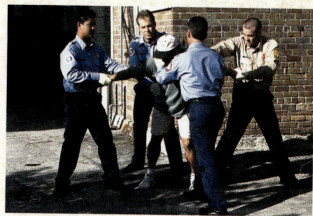

Figure 18-3B Assign one person to each limb and approach the patient at the same time.

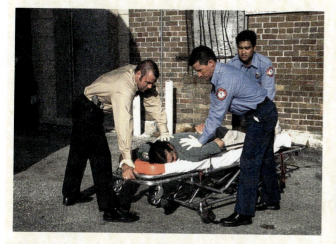

Figure 18-3C Place the patient on the stretcher as his condition and local protocols indicate. Do not let go until he is properly secured.

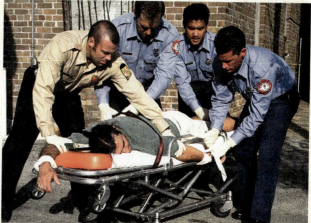

Figure 18-3D Use multiple straps or other soft restraints to secure the patient to the stretcher.

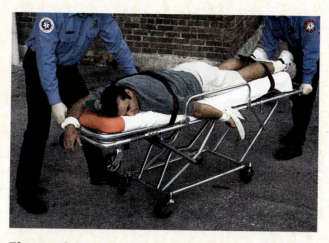

Figure 18-3E Once the patient is secured to the stretcher, be sure to reassess his distal circulation and monitor his airway and breathing continually.

Do not remove police restraints until you and the police are certain that soft restraints will hold the patient. To ensure everyone's safety, once they are on, *do not* remove soft restraints, even if the patient appears to be acting rationally.

Follow these guidelines when a patient must be restrained (Figure 18-3A-E):

♦ *Be sure to have adequate help.*

♦ *Plan your activities.*

♦ *Estimate the range of motion of the patient's arms and legs and stay beyond that range until ready.*

♦ *Once the decision to restrain the patient has been reached, act quickly.*

♦ *Have one EMT or crew member talk to and reassure the patient throughout the restraining procedure.*

♦ *Approach with a minimum of four persons,* one assigned to each limb, all to act at the same time.

♦ *Secure all four limbs with restraints approved by medical direction.*

♦ *Position the patient face up or face down.* The position will be dictated by what the restraining process itself permits, by the patient's condition (e.g., injuries, breathing problems), and by local protocols. Monitor the patient's airway. Never "hog tie" the patient or restrain the patient in any manner that will impair breathing. Patients who have been improperly

restrained have died as a result of a condition called **positional asphyxia.** Monitor all restrained patients carefully.

♦ *Use multiple straps or other restraints to ensure that the patient is adequately secured.* Anticipate that the patient's behavior may turn more violent and be sure that restraint is adequate for this possibility.

♦ *If he is spitting on rescuers, place a surgical mask on the patient if he has no breathing difficulty or likelihood of vomiting and if local protocols permit,* or have rescuers wear protective masks, eye wear, and clothing.

♦ *Reassess the patient's distal circulation frequently* and adjust restraints as safe and necessary if distal circulation is diminished.

♦ *Use sufficient force, but avoid unnecessary force.*

♦ *Document the reasons why the patient was restrained and the technique of restraint* and provide a hand-off report to the transporting EMS crew.

DOCUMENTING BEHAVIORAL EMERGENCIES

It is highly important to document your observations and actions when writing your report for a behavioral emergency call. Document your observations of the patient objectively and professionally. Do not interject opinions or unprofessional comments (i.e., "The patient was acting nuts.") Describe behavior in exact terms ("The patient was pacing with clenched fists. He was shouting at all times. He referred to himself as 'the arm of the lord' and referred to police and fire department personnel as 'the wicked who defile the earth.'")

Document the scene thoroughly. If a behavioral emergency patient demolished his own apartment and possessed a knife, document this on your report. Hospital and mental health personnel will not be able to see the scene, making your accurate documentation vital for continuing care.

When documenting, include statements supporting your belief that the patient might have harmed himself or others had you not provided

COMPANY OFFICER'S NOTES

Positional asphyxia is a condition in which breathing is restricted during the restraint process. This can ultimately lead to death. As company officer, you must personally verify that restraint is used properly and humanely and does not restrict breathing. Monitor the patient's respirations carefully. Note both the rate *and* depth of respirations to be sure breathing is adequate. You will obviously expose yourself and your department to tremendous liability if a patient dies from positional asphyxia while in your care.

Table 18-1

Commonly Prescribed Psychiatric Medications

Generic Name	Trade Name®
sertraline	Zoloft
thiothixene	Navane
haloperidol	Haldol
thioridazine	Mellaril
risperidone	Risperdal
alprazolam	Xanax
lithium carbonate	Lithotabs
clozapine	Clozaril
amitriptyline	Elavil
paroxetine hydrochloride	Paxil
fluoxetine hydrochloride	Prozac

care. If you suspect use of alcohol or other drugs by the patient, this too should be documented. (See Table 18-1 for a list of common psychiatric medications.) Finally, if you suspect that illness or injury may have caused a behavioral emergency, record the facts that support your belief.

Be sure to include in your report the names of law enforcement personnel or other witnesses.

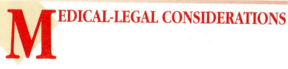

MEDICAL-LEGAL CONSIDERATIONS

A patient who refuses emergency care or transport is a significant medical/legal risk for EMTs. What should you do when a behavioral emergency patient refuses or resists your efforts to provide care?

Most states have provisions in their laws that allow a patient to be transported against his will if he is a danger to himself or others. This is the exception to the rule that patients must provide consent for their care and transportation. *Know your state laws on treating patients without consent.* Many states give this authority to law-enforcement personnel. It will always be beneficial to have the police present if the patient must be restrained as a matter of safety.

You may also be required to contact medical direction about a psychiatric patient who refuses care. Many communities have mental health teams that will respond to the scene to help with the care of a patient with behavioral problems. Such teams will also help evaluate the need for transporting the patient against his will.

Emotionally disturbed patients sometimes accuse EMTs of sexual misconduct. If possible, EMTs of the same sex as the patient should attend to emergency care of disturbed patients. For the same reason, two EMTs should remain with such a patient at all times if possible. With aggressive or violent patients, make sure law-enforcement officers accompany you to the hospital to protect both you and the patient. In the event of a legal problem, they can serve as third party witnesses.

Chapter Review

SUMMARY

As an EMT, you will respond to many behavioral emergencies. Because treatment for these patients usually requires long-term management, little medical intervention can be done in the prehospital situation. However, your interactions with the patient during an emergency can make a difference—to the patient and to the medical professionals who take over his treatment. On these calls, remember that you must assure your own safety, consider the legal ramifications of your actions, and transport the patient in a safe and effective manner to an appropriate facility. Know your local protocols.

REVIEWING KEY CONCEPTS

1. Describe several physical conditions that can cause behavioral emergencies.

2. List signs and symptoms that may indicate the cause of a behavioral emergency is physical.

3. Describe methods you may follow to help calm the behavioral emergency patient during assessment and treatment.

4. List presentations that are common in patients with behavioral emergencies.

5. Describe the steps in the emergency care of the behavioral emergency patient.

6. List factors that may indicate that a patient is at risk for suicide.

7. Describe steps to follow when restraint of a violent/aggressive patient is necessary.

8. List some of the considerations you should keep in mind when preparing a prehospital care report on a behavioral emergency patient.

RESOURCES TO LEARN MORE

Hafen, Brent Q. and Frandsen, Kathryn J. *Psychological Emergencies and Crisis Intervention.* Upper Saddle River, NJ: Brady/Prentice Hall, 1985.

CARE OF THE BEHAVIORAL EMERGENCY PATIENT

Be alert for personal or scene safety problems during scene size-up and throughout the call.

Treat any life-threatening problems during the initial assessment.

Be alert for medical or traumatic conditions that could mimic a behavioral emergency.

Be prepared to spend time talking to the patient and stay with the patient.
- Encourage the patient to discuss what is troubling him.
- Never play along with any visual or auditory hallucinations that patient may be experiencing.
- Do not lie to the patient.
- If it appears it will help, involve family members or friends in the conversation.

As possible, perform a focused history and physical exam and provide any necessary emergency care.

Perform a detailed physical exam only if it is safe and you suspect the patient may have an injury.

Consider using restraints if it is necessary to keep the patient from harming himself or others.

If necessary, transport the patient to a facility where he can get appropriate physical and psychological treatment.

Perform the ongoing assessment en route and contact the receiving hospital to report on current mental status and other important information.

Bleeding and Shock

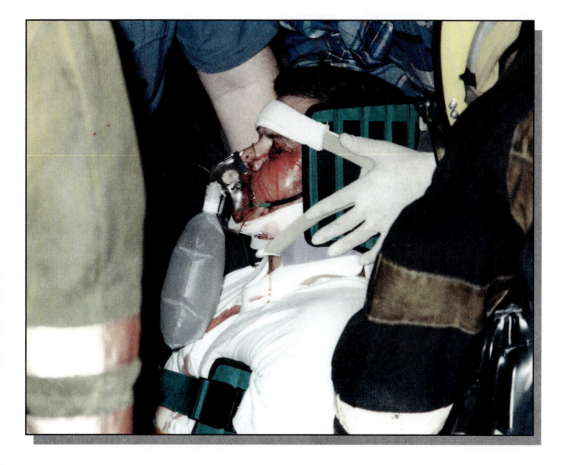

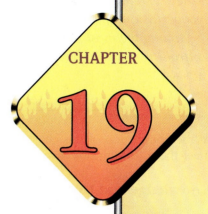

*A*s an EMT, you will often treat patients who are bleeding. At times, the bleeding will be obvious. For example, a patient may have a cut on the scalp from which large amounts of blood are flowing. At other times, the bleeding may not be as obvious. For example, you may see no blood on a patient who has been in a motor vehicle crash. Yet if that patient has a bruised and swollen abdomen, there is a strong likelihood that he is bleeding internally.

Uncontrolled and untreated bleeding, internal or external, is a grave emergency. If it progresses, the patient will deteriorate. The loss of ▶

blood means its flow to vital organs such as the brain, heart, and kidneys is reduced. This leads to a condition called shock, or hypoperfusion. If shock is left untreated, the patient will die.

Among the most important things you will do as an EMT are controlling external bleeding and recognizing and treating shock.

OBJECTIVES

At the completion of this chapter, the EMT-Basic student should be able to meet the following objectives:

Knowledge and Understanding

1. List the structures and functions of the circulatory system. (pp. 459–461)
2. Differentiate between arterial, venous, and capillary bleeding. (pp. 462–463)
3. State methods of emergency medical care of external bleeding. (pp. 464–469)
4. Establish the relationship between body substance isolation and bleeding. (p. 462)
5. Establish the relationship between airway management and the trauma patient. (pp. 464, 471, 473)
6. Establish the relationship between mechanism of injury and internal bleeding. (pp. 469–470)
7. List the signs and symptoms of internal bleeding. (p. 470)
8. List the steps in the emergency medical care of patients with signs and symptoms of internal bleeding. (p. 471)
9. List the signs and symptoms of shock (hypoperfusion). (pp. 470, 471–472)
10. State the steps in the emergency medical care of the patient with signs and symptoms of shock (hypoperfusion). (pp. 472–473)

11. Understand the urgency of transporting patients who are bleeding and show signs of shock (hypoperfusion). (pp. 464, 471, 473)

Skills

1. Demonstrate the use of direct pressure as a method of emergency medical care of external bleeding.
2. Demonstrate the use of diffuse pressure as a method of emergency medical care of external bleeding.
3. Demonstrate the use of pressure points and tourniquets as a method of emergency medical care of external bleeding.
4. Demonstrate the care of the patient exhibiting signs and symptoms of internal bleeding.
5. Demonstrate the care of the patient exhibiting signs and symptoms of shock (hypoperfusion).
6. Demonstrate completing a prehospital care report for a patient with bleeding and/or shock (hypoperfusion).

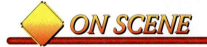 ON SCENE

DISPATCH: *PARAMEDIC RESCUE 2 AND ENGINE 1, A REPORTED STABBING. THE ADDRESS IS 214 FIRST STREET. POLICE ARE ON THE SCENE AND THE SCENE IS SECURED. YOU MAY PROCEED DIRECTLY INTO THE SCENE. TIME OUT IS 0214.*

As your engine company turns the corner onto First Street, you note several police units already on the scene. A police sergeant comes to the dri-

ver's-side window and advises that the scene is secure. She also says that your crew will be treating a single stabbing patient.

One firefighter off-loads your trauma and airway kits, while you don your gloves and eye protection. Stepping from the vehicle onto the sidewalk, you see a trail of blood on the sidewalk. The trail leads to a young man lying on the ground surrounded by police officers. As you and your crew approach the group, a police officer turns to you and says, "It looks like he was stabbed about a block a way and made it this far before he collapsed."

The young man lying on the ground looks up at you and pleads, "Please help me, man. I'm bleedin' bad."

You kneel down beside him and say, "My name is Kevin. I'm an EMT with the fire department. We're here to help you. What's your name?"

"Bobby."

You have begun your initial assessment, noting that Bobby has an open airway and is able to speak. His respirations are shallow and rapid. When you check for bleeding, you find a wound in the front of his left thigh that is bleeding profusely. Another EMT on the crew immediately applies direct pressure over the wound with gauze pads and a gloved hand. You cannot find a pulse at Bobby's wrist, but do find a carotid pulse that is weak and rapid at 120 beats per minute. You assess that Bobby is unstable and in shock from blood loss and inform your captain and the crew of your findings.

Based on this assessment, you provide Bobby with high flow oxygen via a nonrebreather mask. Your crew log-rolls him onto a long spine board and immobilizes him there.

During your initial assessment, a commercial ambulance staffed by other EMT-Basics arrives on the scene. Your captain informs you that Paramedic Rescue 2 is still 10 minutes away. Given the seriousness of Bobby's condition and the fact that you are only 5 minutes from the trauma center, you decide to begin transport immediately. You and another firefighter EMT go with the ambulance, backing up its EMTs.

En route to the hospital, you cut off the rest of Bobby's clothes to check for other wounds and find none. The other firefighter continues to hold direct pressure on the leg wound, while the ambulance EMT elevates the leg. You reassess Bobby's carotid pulse just prior to arrival at the hospital and find that his heart rate is now 140.

In the emergency department, the staff starts two IVs and initiates a blood transfusion. Bobby is in the operating room even before you complete your prehospital care report.

THE CIRCULATORY SYSTEM

To understand how to assess and treat for bleeding and shock, you must understand some basic facts about the circulatory system, which is also called the cardiovascular system. (This would be a good time to review the information about the circulatory system in Chapters 5 and 13.)

Simply stated, the circulatory system has three major components—the pump (the heart), the pipes (the blood vessels), and the fluid in the system (blood). The system delivers oxygen and other nutrients to the cells of the body's organs and removes waste products from those same cells.

This delivery-and-removal process is called **perfusion.** In order for the system to work effectively, all three components (the heart, the blood vessels, and the blood) must function correctly.

The Heart

The heart is the center of the circulatory system (Figure 19-1). The heart is a muscular organ about the size of a fist located just to the left of the sternum within the lower chest. The heart is comprised of four chambers, the two upper atria (which receive blood) and the two lower ventricles (which pump blood out of the heart).

Functionally, the heart is divided into a right-side pump and a left-side pump. The right atrium and ventricle form a low-pressure pump. This

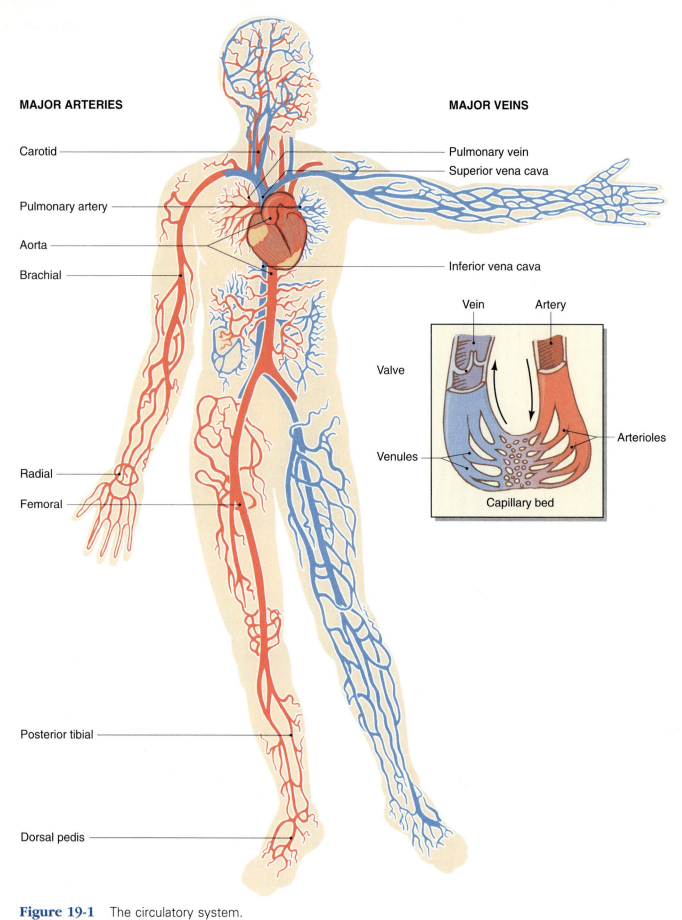

MAJOR ARTERIES

Carotid

Pulmonary artery

Aorta

Brachial

Radial

Femoral

Posterior tibial

Dorsal pedis

MAJOR VEINS

Pulmonary vein

Superior vena cava

Inferior vena cava

Vein

Artery

Valve

Venules

Arterioles

Capillary bed

Figure 19-1 The circulatory system.

pump takes oxygen-depleted blood in from the major veins and sends it to the lungs to be reoxygenated. The left atrium then receives the blood back from the lungs, and the left ventricle pumps it out of the heart under high pressure into the body's arteries. It is the force created by the pumping action of the left ventricle that produces the pulse of an artery. Such pulses can be felt (palpated) where the artery crosses a bone, as with the radial pulse at the wrist.

The Blood Vessels

There are three major types of blood vessels. Together, they carry blood from the heart to all parts of the body and then back to the heart.

The *arteries* carry blood away from the heart. The major artery of the body is the aorta. Blood is pumped directly from the left ventricle into the aorta. The aorta then branches into smaller arteries. Because arteries carry blood under pressure, they have thick, muscular walls. The arteries, in turn, branch into smaller vessels called arterioles.

Eventually, the arterioles branch down in the organs into the tiny, thin-walled structures called *capillaries*. The walls of capillaries are usually only one cell thick. Through the capillaries' thin walls, the bloodstream and the body's cells exchange oxygen and other nutrients the cells need for carbon dioxide and other waste products of the cells.

Veins then carry the oxygen-depleted blood back to the right side of the heart. Small venules carry blood from the capillaries to larger veins and eventually to the superior and inferior vena cavae, which empty into the heart. Compared to the arteries, the veins are thin walled and under low pressure.

Upon return to the right side of the heart, blood is pumped by the right ventricle to the lungs, where carbon dioxide is exchanged for inhaled oxygen. The newly oxygenated blood then returns to the left side of the heart to be pumped through arteries to the body's organs.

The Blood

An average adult weighing 150 pounds (6.8 kg) has a blood volume of about 10 to 12 pints (9.5 to 11.4 L). That blood, which is pumped by the heart through the blood vessels, is made up of several components.

Red blood cells carry oxygen to the body's cells and carry carbon dioxide away from them. The red blood cells also give the blood its color.

White blood cells are part of the body's immune system. They help fight infection.

Platelets are specialized parts of cells. When they become activated, they release materials to form clots that help stop bleeding.

Plasma makes up about over half the volume of the blood. This watery, salty fluid carries the red and white blood cells and the platelets to all parts of the body.

BLEEDING

The circulatory system functions constantly, delivering oxygen to the body's organs and removing carbon dioxide and wastes from them. Problems with any component of the system—for example, heavy bleeding from a damaged blood vessel—can lead to inadequate perfusion of the body's organs. When organs don't receive enough blood flow and nutrients, waste products build up within them. Eventually, the body's cells begin to die. This situation is called **hypoperfusion** (from *hypo-* meaning "under"), or shock. It is a life-threatening situation. Bleeding is a common cause of hypoperfusion encountered by EMTs.

Blood loss can range from minor to severe. The patient's size has a great effect on the seriousness of blood loss. The sudden loss of 100 cc (a little over a third of a cup) of blood would not be a problem for most adults. An infant, on the other hand, may have a total blood volume of only 500 to 800 cc. For such an infant, a 100 cc blood loss would be very serious. In general, sudden blood loss of 1 liter (1000 cc or a little over 4 cups) in an adult, one-half liter (500 cc or a little over 2 cups) in a child, and 100 cc in an infant should be considered serious.

You must be able to recognize severe blood loss and realize the impact that loss can have on a patient. With external bleeding, such as from a scalp wound, the fact that blood is being lost may be obvious. However, it is often difficult or impossible to determine how much blood has been lost since clothing, upholstery, rugs, or the ground can absorb blood. The problem of determining blood loss is even greater with internal bleeding, where a massive loss of several liters of blood can occur unseen by the EMT.

Your assessment of the severity of blood loss, therefore, should be based on the patient's signs and symptoms, not only on the quantity of visible blood. If the bleeding patient exhibits *any* of the signs and symptoms of shock (hypoperfusion) listed on page 472, then you should presume the patient's blood loss is severe.

Severe bleeding may be further complicated by the failure of the body's mechanisms to control bleeding. Under normal circumstances, injured blood vessels constrict, or clamp down, to reduce blood loss. The blood also contains clotting factors and platelets, which form clots. Both normal blood vessel constriction and clotting may be lost as shock (hypoperfusion) progresses.

A patient's medications can also affect bleeding. Some patients take prescription medications that inhibit the blood's ability to clot. The most common of these is Coumadin® (wafarin). It is often taken by patients who have received artificial heart valves and by elderly patients with chronic irregular heart rhythms (i.e., atrial fibrillation). Patients on such blood-thinning medications may suffer abnormally severe bleeding as a result of trauma. Determine whether a patient is using such medications during your scene size-up. Also, a patient's mentioning that he takes such medications when you are gathering the SAMPLE history should alert you to the possibility of increased severity of bleeding.

Body Substance Isolation

Bleeding can pose serious danger not only to the patient but also to the EMT. In general, blood is the most infectious type of body fluid. HIV and various forms of hepatitis are most commonly acquired through contact with an infected person's blood.

When treating patients with bleeding, take all necessary body substance isolation (BSI) precau-

tions to prevent coming into contact with the patient's blood. At a minimum, gloves must be worn. If there is severe bleeding or bleeding from the airway, then wear eye protection, a face mask, and a gown or another type of garment impervious to blood.

After every contact with body fluids, wash your hands with soapy water when you remove your gloves. In addition, decontaminate equipment such as the interior of an ambulance or a backboard that comes in contact with a patient's blood. Whenever decontaminating equipment, follow the same BSI precautions, including masks and eye protection, used in direct patient care because splashing is common. (Review Chapter 3, "Infection Control and Body Substance Isolation.")

EXTERNAL BLEEDING

External bleeding is bleeding through a break in the skin. Contact between the skin and an object or objects outside it, such as a knife, car wreckage, or a road surface, most commonly causes external bleeding. Sometimes, the break in the skin results from something inside the body moving outward, as when a broken bone erupts through the skin in an open fracture. Because the site of bleeding can be seen, you can assess and take the steps necessary to control the bleeding.

Types of Bleeding

The type of blood vessel damaged will affect the characteristics of the bleeding. There are three basic types of bleeding (Figure 19-2):

◆ ***Arterial bleeding*** This occurs when an artery or arteriole is cut. Blood within arteries is oxygen rich and under high pressure. Thus, the blood from such a wound is bright red (oxygen rich). It usually spurts (high pressure) with each heartbeat. Arterial bleeding is often profuse and difficult to control because of its high pressure. Left uncontrolled, the spurting of arterial bleeding would begin to subside as shock worsened and the patient's blood pres-

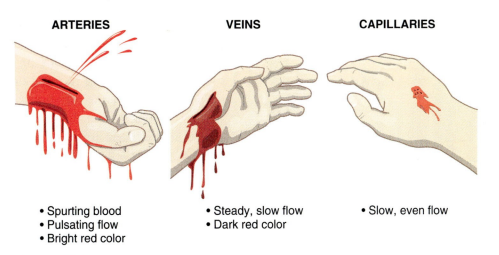

ARTERIES	VEINS	CAPILLARIES
• Spurting blood • Pulsating flow • Bright red color	• Steady, slow flow • Dark red color	• Slow, even flow

Figure 19-2 Types of bleeding.

sure began to fall. Arterial bleeding is most often seen in lacerations.

◆ ***Venous bleeding*** This occurs when a vein or venule is cut. Veins contain oxygen-poor blood under low pressure. Blood from such a wound, then, is usually dark red. Bleeding tends to be in a steady (low-pressure) flow. Bleeding from veins (especially larger veins) can be life threatening. Fortunately, because of its low-pressure flow, venous bleeding is easier to control than arterial bleeding. This type of bleeding is also common in lacerations.

◆ ***Capillary bleeding*** Because the capillaries are tiny, bleeding from them is slow and oozing. The color of the blood is dark red. Capillary bleeding is routinely seen in areas of abrasion. Although abrasions may cover large surface areas (as in a motorcyclist's "road rash" from a fall and slide on pavement), bleeding is easily controlled. Many abrasions clot spontaneously, resulting in very little blood loss.

You should also consider several other factors when assessing a patient with external bleeding. For example, the type of a wound and its location affect the severity of bleeding. Lacerations and abrasions are the most common types of wounds causing external bleeding (Figure 19-3A and B). (A more in-depth discussion of specific wound types can be found in Chapter 20, "Soft Tissue Injuries.") Because blood vessels become smaller as they branch out, the closer (more proximal) a

Figure 19-3 Among the most common causes of external bleeding are **(A)** lacerations and **(B)** abrasions.

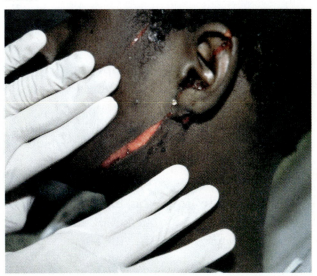

A.

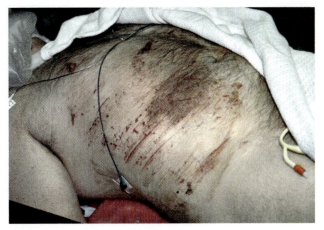

B.

wound is to the center of the body, the greater the likelihood that a wound will cause severe bleeding.

◆ Emergency Care—External Bleeding

"All bleeding stops eventually" is a truism of emergency care. However, the bleeding may stop either as a result of good patient care or because the patient bleeds to death, dying from shock (hypoperfusion). As an EMT, it is your job to stop external bleeding by assuring the proper steps are taken to control blood loss. These steps are as follows:

1. **Take appropriate body substance isolation (BSI) precautions.** You can begin to don basic BSI gear while en route to the scene. Be prepared to add additional gear if your scene size-up reveals the need for it.

2. **Perform the scene size-up upon arrival.** Determine that the scene is safe to enter. Note if more BSI gear should be worn. Determine if additional resources will be needed because of the number of patients or because of problems in reaching the patient(s).

3. **Perform the initial assessment** Form a general impression of the patient and his mental status. Ensure the ABCs by

   ◆ Maintaining an open airway

   ◆ Providing artificial ventilations if breathing is inadequate

   ◆ Administering oxygen if signs and symptoms of shock (hypoperfusion) are present (Table 19-1)

4. **Control the bleeding.** Once the steps above have been taken, management of external bleeding can begin. Remember that serious bleeding is a life-threatening emergency and must be addressed as part of the initial assessment. Controlling such bleeding has priority over other emergency care except airway and breathing.

   There are three standard methods for controlling external bleeding: *direct pressure, ele-*

vation, and *pressure points.* If these methods fail, consider the use of a *tourniquet* for uncontrolled bleeding from an amputated extremity. If bleeding remains uncontrolled or if signs or symptoms of shock (hypoperfusion) are present, assign the patient a high priority for immediate transport and treat for shock (see page 472).

5. **Monitor the patient carefully for renewed bleeding throughout the focused history and physical exam, the detailed exam, and the ongoing assessment.** Remain prepared to treat for shock if its signs and symptoms develop.

Control of Bleeding

Follow this sequence of methods when trying to control external bleeding (Figure 19-4, pages 466–467).

◆ **Direct pressure** Press on the site of the bleeding with a gloved hand. The initial application of direct pressure to the wound should be made with a gloved finger for small points of bleeding or a gloved hand for larger wounds. Sterile dressings should be placed over the wound as soon as possible while continuing direct pressure. With large, gaping wounds, it may be necessary to pack the wound with sterile dressings and then apply direct pressure with a gloved hand to control bleeding.

If direct pressure alone does not stop the bleeding, continue to apply pressure and use—

◆ **Elevation** Raise the wound above the level of the heart, if possible. For example, you might elevate the arm of a patient with a wrist wound above his heart or have a patient with a head wound sit up rather than lie supine. Remember, however, that external wounds are the result of trauma and often occur with other musculoskeletal or spinal injuries. *Do not* use elevation if you suspect musculoskeletal injury in a bleeding extremity. For example, it would not be safe to raise the wrist of a patient with a possible upper arm fracture or to have a patient with a head wound and a neck or spine injury sit up. However, if the patient is immobilized to a backboard, you could raise one end of the backboard.

If the combination of direct pressure and elevation fails to stop bleeding on an extremity, you should use—

◆ ***Pressure points*** Pressure points are places where large arteries pass over bones and can be compressed to reduce blood flow to a wounded extremity (Figure 19-5, page 468). The most frequently used pressure points are the brachial artery in the upper arm and the femoral artery in the groin, which supplies blood to the leg. (The temporal artery's pressure point on the lateral face can be used to control bleeding there.) Pressure points can be used to control bleeding with patients in a variety of positions. They can also be used with patients who have other associated injuries.

Most external bleeding can be controlled using these general steps in the sequence described above (Figure 19-4). Once bleeding is controlled, use a bandage to secure the wound dressing in place.

The 1994 U.S. DOT EMT-Basic Curriculum states that if external bleeding does not stop, it may be necessary to remove the dressing and reassess the wound. If a specific point of bleeding is seen during reassessment, reapply direct finger pressure to the site. If the area of bleeding is larger than originally appreciated, apply additional pressure with gloved hands to the site. Elevation and pressure points may again be used to assist in bleeding control. Note, however, that some EMS systems strongly discourage the removal of original wound dressings because doing so may disrupt blood clotting that has begun at the wound site. Follow your local EMS system protocols.

Devices Used in Controlling Bleeding

Several devices can be used to assist in the control of external bleeding, especially wounds on the extremities. The devices include rigid splints, pneumatic (air) splint devices, and tourniquets.

Rigid Splints

Rigid or fixation splints, such as ladder and corrugated box splints, are especially helpful in controlling external bleeding on extremities. By reducing movement of the limb, these devices also reduce the blood loss associated with any fractures of the same extremity.

Pneumatic Splints

Pneumatic splints include air splints, vacuum splints, and the pneumatic anti-shock garment (PASG). These devices stabilize an extremity while also providing pressure over the wound. They are particularly useful in controlling bleeding from large wounds with extensive tissue damage.

An air splint should be inflated by mouth not beyond the point at which a thumb pressed to the outside surface can just indent the splint material. Inspect the inflation stem before you begin to inflate the device to assure that there is no blood or body fluid contamination of it.

When using the PASG to control bleeding in a lower extremity, inflate only the section of the garment that covers the wounded extremity. If there is injury to the pelvis, inflate all sections of the garment. The PASG is usually inflated to approximately 30 mm Hg for splinting. Use of the PASG is controversial. Follow local protocols concerning the device. (See Figure 19-9, page 476.)

Tourniquets

A tourniquet is your *last* resort when attempting to control life-threatening bleeding from an amputated or near-amputated extremity. Use of a tourniquet can result in extensive damage to muscles, blood vessels, and nerves. This may worsen the patient's condition and make reattachment of the severed limb impossible. A tourniquet is rarely necessary to control bleeding and, because of the associated risks, should only be used when all the other methods of bleeding control have failed. If a tourniquet must be used, keep these general precautions in mind:

◆ Always use a wide bandage and secure it tightly.

Control of External Bleeding

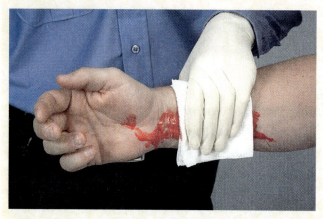

Figure 19-4A Using a gauze pad, apply direct pressure to the wound. If bleeding is heavy, apply direct pressure with your gloved hand rather than allowing more blood to be lost while you search for a dressing.

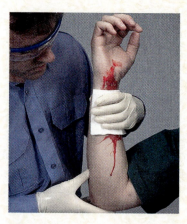

Figure 19-4B Elevate the extremity above the level of the heart.

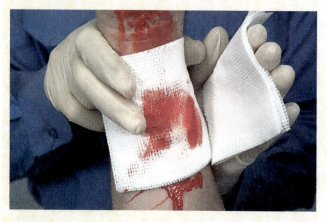

Figure 19-4C If the wound continues to bleed apply more dressings over it: *do not* remove earlier dressings.

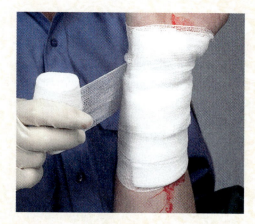

Figure 19-4D Bandage the dressing in place.

◆ Always leave an applied tourniquet in open view.

◆ Never use wire, rope, or a belt that may cut into the tissue underneath.

◆ Do not loosen a tourniquet once it is applied unless ordered to do so by medical direction.

◆ Do not apply the tourniquet over a joint.

When applying a tourniquet, follow these steps (Figure 19-6, page 468):

1. Use a bandage material 4 inches (100 mm) wide and 6 to 8 layers thick.

2. Wrap the bandage twice around the extremity just above or proximal to the bleeding, but as distal as possible on the injured limb.

3. Tie one knot in the bandage and place a stick or rod on top of the knot. Then tie the ends of the bandage over the top of the stick with a square knot.

4. Twist the stick until the bleeding stops.

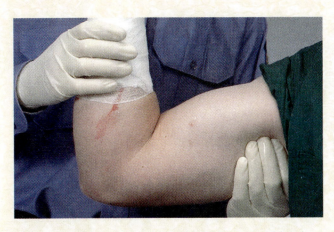

Figure 19-4E If the wound continues to bleed, apply pressure to the brachial artery to control bleeding from an arm wound.

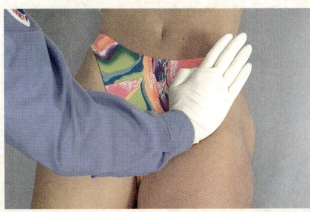

Figure 19-4F Apply pressure to the femoral artery to control continued bleeding from a leg wound.

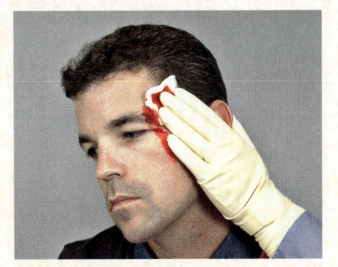

Figure 19-4G Apply pressure on the temporal artery to control bleeding from a face wound.

5. Once the bleeding has stopped, secure the stick or rod in position to prevent it from loosening.

6. Notify any other EMS personnel who are to take over the care of the patient (such as paramedics, the transporting ambulance crew, or the emergency department staff) that a tourniquet has been applied and at what time the device was put in place. Document the fact that you applied a tourniquet and the time you did so on your written patient care report.

7. Apply sterile dressings over the wounds distal to the tourniquet to reduce the risk of infection.

8. Monitor the area distal to the tourniquet for any additional bleeding.

9. *Do not loosen the tourniquet unless ordered to do so by medical direction.*

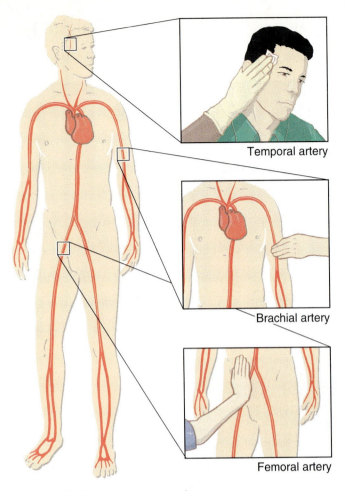

Temporal artery

Brachial artery

Femoral artery

Figure 19-5   Pressure points.

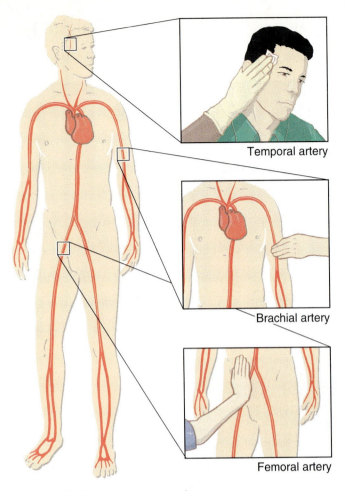

Figure 19-6   To apply a tourniquet, (1) place bandage material just above the bleeding, but as distal as possible on the injured limb. (2) Tie one knot in the bandage and place a stick on top of the knot. Then tie the ends of the bandage over the top of the stick with a square knot. (3) Twist stick until the bleeding stops and secure the stick in position. (4) Document tourniquet use and time of application on the PCR and on patient's forehead.

A continuously inflated blood pressure cuff can also be used as a tourniquet. This is the preferred method of tourniquet application in many EMS systems. If a blood pressure cuff is used, inflate the cuff only to the pressure necessary to control the life-threatening external bleeding. Once the bleeding is controlled, make a note of the pressure reading on the sphygmomanometer. Be alert to gradual air loss from the cuff. Maintain the cuff at the pressure necessary to control bleeding, reinflating from time to time if necessary. To prevent a pressure loss, some experts recommend clamping the hose to the inflation bulb with a surgical clamp after an adequate pressure is obtained. As with any tourniquet device, document use of the blood pressure cuff and the time of its application on your care report and pass this information along to any other emergency personnel who assume care of the patient.

Special Situations

Bleeding from the ears, mouth, or nose can result from a wide variety of causes and requires special mention. This kind of bleeding is most commonly due to direct trauma to these areas. Bleeding from the nose and/or ears when significant head trauma has occurred may also be the result of a skull fracture. Non-traumatic causes of bleeding from the mouth and nose include sinus and respiratory infections, high blood pressure, and bleeding disorders that prevent the proper clotting of blood.

In general, manage bleeding from the ears by applying a loose dressing to collect the blood and to prevent infection. Bleeding from the mouth requires careful attention in order to assure that the airway remains open; provide suctioning as needed.

Nosebleeds

Nosebleeds (also called epistaxis) are common and can result in significant blood loss. Common causes of nosebleeds include nose picking, excessive drying of the nasal lining, high blood pressure, sinus or respiratory infections, and bleeding disorders. Nosebleeds can be very frightening to patients. Treatment of nosebleeds should include the following steps:

1. Place the patient in a sitting position and have him lean forward.

2. Apply direct pressure to the bleeding by pinching the fleshy part of the nose. Maintain this pressure for at least 10 to 15 minutes before reassessing the bleeding.

3. Assist the patient in removing any clotted blood that may collect in the mouth. Do not attempt to remove clotted blood from the nostrils.

4. Keep the patient at rest.

5. Provide calm reassurance to the patient.

INTERNAL BLEEDING

Internal bleeding is bleeding from organs and blood vessels unseen by the EMT. It can result from blunt trauma, the rupture of a blood vessel, or a variety of other causes. Such bleeding can be massive and can quickly lead to shock (hypoperfusion) and death. Internal bleeding in the chest, abdomen, and pelvis can be especially life threatening. Even the internal bleeding from injuries to the extremities can lead to blood loss of several liters.

Because internal bleeding cannot be seen, you must base your assessment of internal bleeding on the mechanism of injury and the patient's signs and symptoms.

Mechanisms of Injury Associated with Internal Bleeding

There are several mechanisms of injury associated with an increased risk of serious internal bleeding. This is because the greater the force involved in the injury (for example, the greater the height of the fall or the speed of the crash), the more energy the body must absorb. This means a greater likelihood of internal injury. You should maintain a high index of suspicion for internal injuries and bleeding when you are called to accidents involving the following mechanisms.

Blunt injury mechanisms that can cause internal injuries and bleeding include:

◆ **Falls from height** Falls from heights of greater than 15 feet (5 m) or more than 3 times the patient's height are especially serious.

◆ **Motorcycle crashes** These provide increased risk of serious injury because riders are relatively unprotected and are frequently ejected from their vehicles.

◆ **Pedestrians struck by autos** These patients may have three separate impacts—the initial bumper impact, a second impact on the hood or windshield, and often a third impact when the pedestrian is run over by the same or another car or impacts the pavement.

◆ **Automobile collisions** High speed impacts, rollovers, and crashes in which an occupant is ejected are particularly likely to produce serious internal injuries.

Penetrating injury mechanisms that can cause internal injuries and bleeding include:

◆ **Gunshot wounds** All gunshot wounds except those isolated to the hands and feet may result in serious internal bleeding.

◆ **Stab wounds** All stab wounds to the head, neck, chest, abdomen, pelvis, and proximal extremities can result in serious internal bleeding.

◆ **Impalements** Impalements of the head, neck, chest, abdomen, pelvis, upper legs, and arms can result in serious bleeding.

Combination blunt and penetrating injury mechanisms that can cause internal injuries and bleeding include:

◆ **Blasts** Blasts may produce blunt injuries from the pressure wave and/or the impact of a patient thrown by the blast against a station-

TRANSITION OF CARE

A quick and accurate determination of details about the mechanism of injury should be a part of the scene size-up. Information about the mechanism of injury should be carefully documented and a verbal report made to the transporting EMT or ALS crew. As a first arriving EMT, you may be in a unique position to determine the mechanism of injury from scene conditions or the reports of bystanders. Documenting such mechanisms is critical because many EMS systems use mechanism of injury as a factor in determining which patients to transport to a trauma center. The emergency surgery that can treat the internal bleeding likely to be caused by certain mechanisms of injury is usually most readily available at a trauma center.

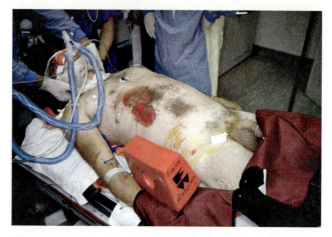

Figure 19-7 A bruised and rigid or distended abdomen is one of the signs of possible internal bleeding.

ary object. Penetrating injuries may result from flying shrapnel.

Signs and Symptoms Associated with Internal Bleeding

Patients with internal bleeding may present with a wide variety of signs and symptoms. Often, early signs and symptoms of internal bleeding are detected only after a careful history and physical examination. Later, patients with serious internal bleeding may present with extensive signs and symptoms of shock (hypoperfusion). Specific signs and symptoms of internal bleeding include:

◆ Increased pulse rate
◆ Areas of abrasions, contusions, deformity, impact marks, and swelling on the head, neck, chest, abdomen, and/or pelvis at suspected sites of injury
◆ Painful, swollen, and deformed extremities
◆ Bleeding from the mouth, rectum, vagina, or other orifice
◆ Vomiting of bright red blood or material the color of coffee grounds
◆ Dark, tarry stools or red, bloody stools
◆ Tender, rigid and/or distended abdomen (Figure 19-7)

If internal bleeding is severe, the signs and symptoms of shock (hypoperfusion) may be present:

◆ Altered mental status, including anxiety, confusion, restlessness, or combativeness
◆ Weakness, faintness, or dizziness
◆ Marked thirst
◆ Nausea or vomiting
◆ Dilated pupils that are sluggish to respond to light
◆ Increased breathing rate
◆ Shallow, labored, or irregular breathing
◆ Rapid, weak pulse
◆ Pale, cool, clammy skin
◆ Pallor (pale or gray skin)
◆ Cyanosis (bluish discoloration) of the lips or conjunctiva of eyes
◆ Capillary refill of greater than 2 seconds in infants and children
◆ A low or falling blood pressure (a late sign)

 COMPANY OFFICER'S NOTES

There is particular risk of internal bleeding within the chest or abdomen when painful, swollen deformities that may represent fractures are present in both upper and lower extremities of the same patient. Assign such trauma patients a high priority. Assume that they have internal bleeding in addition to their extremity injuries and treat them accordingly.

◆ Emergency Care—Internal Bleeding

Unlike cases of external bleeding, there is little an EMT can actually do to stop internal bleeding. The goals of the emergency care are to identify a patient with potentially serious internal bleeding and to provide supportive care until arrival at the emergency department. Emergency care of the patient with possible internal bleeding includes the following steps:

1. **Take appropriate body substance isolation (BSI) precautions.**

2. **Perform the scene size-up upon arrival.** Pay particular attention to potential mechanisms of injury in cases of trauma.

3. **Perform the initial assessment.** Form a general impression of the patient and his mental status. Ensure the ABCs by maintaining an open airway, suctioning if needed. Provide positive pressure ventilation if breathing is inadequate. *If serious external bleeding is present, control it. Assign a high priority for immediate transport to patients with inadequate airway, inadequate breathing, and/or uncontrolled bleeding.* Remember also that a patient with external bleeding may also be bleeding internally. Pay attention to signs and symptoms.

4. **Monitor the patient carefully during the focused history and physical exam, especially if your general impression of the patient and the mechanism of injury suggest internal bleeding.** If there are painful, swollen, or deformed extremities and/or if the patient shows signs and symptoms of shock, assume that internal bleeding is present.

5. **Provide high flow oxygen if not already provided during the initial assessment.**

6. **Splint any painful, swollen, or deformed extremities.**

7. **Provide immediate transport for patients with signs and symptoms of shock.** Consider requesting an Advanced Life Support (ALS) intercept.

8. **Perform an ongoing assessment every 5 minutes during transport.**

SHOCK (HYPOPERFUSION)

Throughout this chapter, you have read that both internal and external bleeding, if uncontrolled, will eventually lead to shock. Shock is also referred to as hypoperfusion or hypoperfusion syndrome. Understanding shock is important, because it makes more clear how specific signs and symptoms develop in patients with shock and why to be on the lookout for them.

In its normal state, the cardiovascular system provides an adequate supply of oxygenated blood to the body's organs and removes the waste products of the cells (especially carbon dioxide) from those same organs. This is the process known as perfusion. When the cardiovascular system fails to supply adequate amounts of oxygen and to remove adequate amounts of wastes from the body's organs, the condition known as hypoperfusion results. If left uncorrected, hypoperfusion will lead to cell and organ damage and dysfunction. When enough cells and organs are damaged, the patient will die. There are three major causes of hypoperfusion: failure of the heart to pump correctly; failure of the blood vessels to constrict normally; and loss of blood or other body fluids. In this chapter, we are most concerned with the third cause.

Shock (hypoperfusion) that results from blood loss is termed **hemorrhagic** or **hypovolemic shock.** When blood loss occurs, the cardiovascular system attempts to maintain organ perfusion by increasing the heart rate and, to some extent, constricting blood vessels. This response explains why an increased heart rate is a frequent early sign of shock. This compensation mechanism allows perfusion to continue for a time. If bleeding continues, however, hypoperfusion will develop. Peripheral (skin and extremity) perfusion is markedly reduced. This produces the characteristic signs of a weak, thready pulse and pale, clammy skin. As blood flow to organs further decreases, those organs no longer function correctly and signs and symptoms specific to those organ systems develop (Table 19-1).

Table 19-1

The Body's Responses to Significant Blood Loss

Organ	Response to Blood Loss	Resulting Signs and Symptoms
Brain	Decrease of perfusion in higher centers of thinking in order to maintain cardiac and respiratory control centers	Altered mental status —Confusion —Restlessness —Anxiety
Cardiovascular system	Heart pumps faster; blood vessels constrict	Increased pulse rate Increased breathing rate Rapid, weak pulse Low or falling blood pressure Delayed capillary refill time (pediatric patients)
Gastrointestinal organs	Decrease of perfusion in the digestive tract	Nausea and vomiting
Kidneys	Reduction in function to conserve the body's salt and water	Decreased urine production Increased thirst
Skin	Marked loss of perfusion as blood vessels to the skin constrict	Cool, clammy, pale skin Pallor Cyanosis
Extremities	Marked loss of perfusion	Weak or absent peripheral pulses Decreased blood pressure

◆ Altered mental status, including anxiety, confusion, restlessness, or combativeness

◆ Weakness, faintness, or dizziness

◆ Marked thirst

◆ Nausea or vomiting

◆ Dilated pupils that are sluggish to respond to light

◆ Increased breathing rate

◆ Shallow, labored, or irregular breathing

◆ Rapid, weak pulse

◆ Pale, cool, clammy skin

◆ Pallor (pale or gray skin)

◆ Cyanosis (bluish discoloration) of the lips or conjunctiva of eyes

◆ Capillary refill of greater than 2 seconds in infants and children

◆ A low or falling blood pressure (a late sign)

PEDIATRIC NOTE

Infants and children have different physiologic responses to hypovolemic shock than adults. Children with serious blood loss will usually maintain a compensated heart rate and blood pressure longer than adults. A child can lose up to half his blood volume before blood pressure begins to fall. However, when blood pressure does fall, cardiac arrest may rapidly follow since the child has much less cardiovascular reserve than does an adult. For this reason, *do not* wait for signs and symptoms of shock to appear. Provide treatment based on mechanism of injury or suspicion of trauma.

◆ Emergency Care—Hypovolemic Shock

Shock (hypoperfusion) from blood loss may quickly lead to death if aggressive care is not provided. Ideally, you will treat external blood loss so quickly that shock (hypoperfusion) does not develop. However, there are times you will arrive on the scene after significant external or internal bleeding has occurred. You must be alert and prepared to recognize the early signs of shock from both internal and external bleeding and provide appropriate care and rapid transport.

Treatment of patients with signs and symptoms of shock should include the following steps: (Figure 19-8).

1. **Assure scene safety.**

2. **Take appropriate BSI precautions.**

3. **Maintain an open airway.** Provide artificial ventilations if breathing is inadequate.

4. **Administer high flow oxygen.**

5. **Control any external bleeding.**

6. **Use the PASG, if appropriate conditions apply.** If no chest injuries are present, if the patient has signs and symptoms of shock, and if the pelvis or lower abdomen is tender to examination, apply and inflate the PASG if permitted to do so by your local protocol or medical director (Figure 19-9, pages 476–477).

7. **Elevate the lower extremities approximately 8 to 12 inches (200 to 300 mm).** If the patient has signs or symptoms of injuries to the spine, head, chest, abdomen, or lower extremities, keep the patient supine. Alternatively, place the patient on a long backboard and then elevate the lower end of the backboard as a unit.

8. **Splint any suspected bone or joint injuries.**

9. **Prevent additional heat loss from the patient.** Cover the patient with a blanket or thermal rescue tarp.

10. **Provide immediate transportation to the emergency department.**

11. **Continue to monitor the patient.** Look for changes in mental status and vital signs during the focused history and physical exam, detailed physical exam, and ongoing assessment. Do not delay transport of the patient; remember that you can perform these operations during transport.

Care for a Patient in Shock

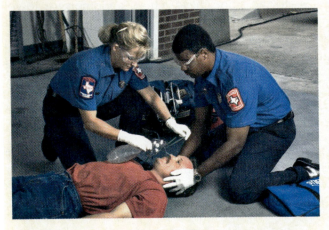

Figure 19-8A Maintain an open airway and provide high concentration oxygen via nonrebreather mask. Provide positive pressure ventilations and CPR if necessary.

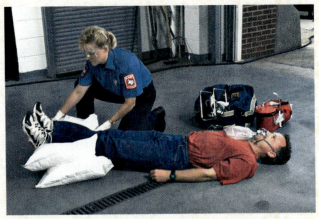

Figure 19-8B Elevate the patient's legs 8 to 10 inches if there are no signs of serious injuries to the spine, head, chest, abdomen, or lower extremities.

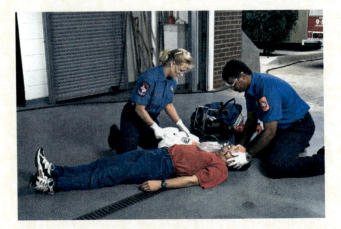

Figure 19-8C If there are signs of serious injury to the spine, head, chest, abdomen, or lower extremities, leave the patient supine.

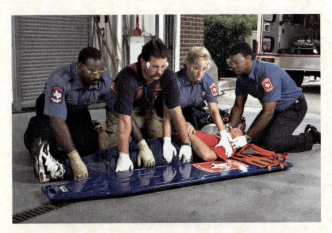

Figure 19-8D   Positioning the patient on a long spine board will have the effect of splinting his entire body. Splint injuries to individual bones or joints en route to the hospital.

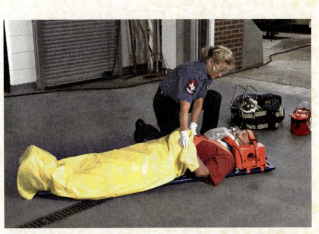

Figure 19-8E   Cover the patient with a blanket or thermal rescue tarp to prevent heat loss.

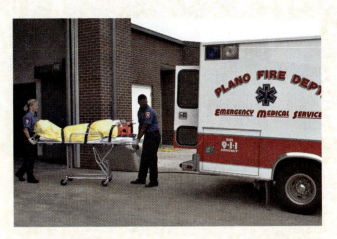

Figure 19-8F   Transport the patient immediately.

Using the Pneumatic Anti-Shock Garment

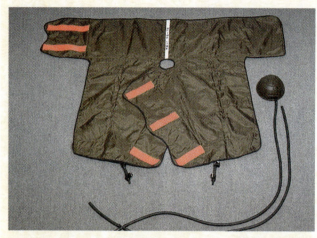

Figure 19-9A   The pneumatic anti-shock garment (PASG) and inflation pump.

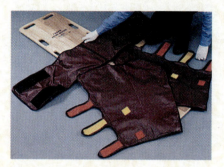

Figure 19-9B   Unfold the PASG and lay it out flat on a long spine board.

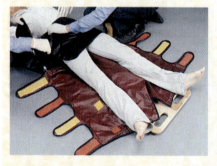

Figure 19-9C   Log roll the patient onto the PASG or slide it under him so that the upper edge of the PASG is just below the patient's bottom rib. (In actual practice, remove the patient's clothing before applying the PASG.)

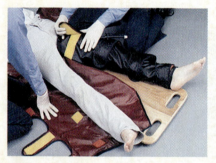

Figure 19-9D   Enclose the left leg and secure the straps.

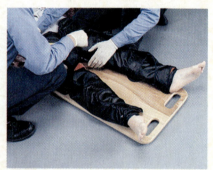

Figure 19-9E   Enclose the right leg and secure the straps.

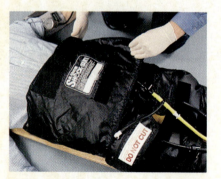

Figure 19-9F   Enclose the abdomen and pelvis and secure the straps.

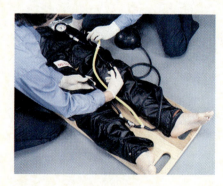

Figure 19-9G   Check the inflation tubes leading from the pump to the compartments.

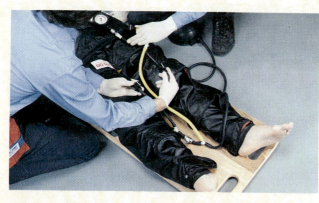

Figure 19-9H Open the stopcocks to the legs and close the stopcock to the abdominal compartment.

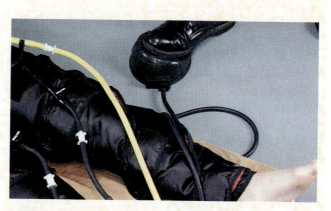

Figure 19-9I Inflate the leg compartments simultaneously using the pump. Inflate until the Velcro on the straps makes a crackling noise.

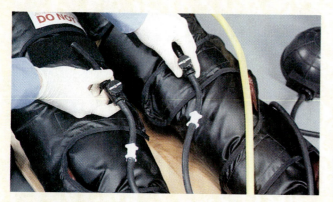

Figure 19-9J Close the stopcocks of the leg compartments.

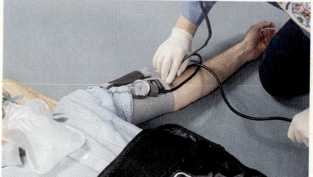

Figure 19-9K Check the patient's blood pressure.

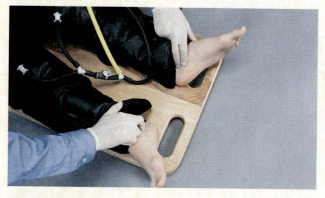

Figure 19-9L Check both extremities for distal pulses.

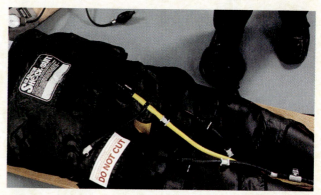

Figure 19-9M If systolic blood pressure is below 90 mmHg, open the abdominal compartment stopcock, inflate the compartment, and close the stopcock.

Monitor and record vital signs every 5 minutes. Add air if compartments lose pressure. Follow your local protocols when using the PASG.

Chapter Review

SUMMARY

As an EMT, you will often be called to assist patients who are bleeding. If uncontrolled and untreated, bleeding will eventually lead to death from hypoperfusion of the body's organs and hypovolemic shock. You must be prepared to control external bleeding and to recognize the signs and symptoms of internal bleeding and hypoperfusion from blood loss.

REVIEWING KEY CONCEPTS

1. Define *perfusion* and *hypoperfusion*.
2. Describe the amount of blood loss that would constitute severe bleeding in adult and child patients.
3. Name the three major types of bleeding and describe the characteristics of each.
4. Describe the sequence of steps to follow in controlling external bleeding.
5. List precautions to follow whenever a tourniquet is used.
6. List common mechanisms of injury associated with internal bleeding.
7. List the early and late signs and symptoms of internal bleeding.
8. Describe steps in the emergency care of a patient with internal bleeding.
9. Explain how a child's physiologic response to shock differs from that of an adult.
10. List the signs and symptoms of shock.
11. Describe the steps in the emergency care of a patient in shock.

RESOURCES TO LEARN MORE

"Management of Shock" in Moore, E. E. et al., eds. *Trauma, 2nd Edition*. Norwalk, CT: Appleton and Lang/Prentice Hall, 1991.

CARE FOR EXTERNAL BLEEDING

Take appropriate body substance isolation (BSI) precautions.

↓

Perform the scene size-up upon arrival.

↓

Perform the initial assessment and assure ABCs:
- Maintain an open airway.
- Provide artificial ventilations if breathing is inadequate.
- Administer oxygen if signs and symptoms of shock (hypoperfusion) are present

↓

Control the bleeding using techniques in the following order:
- Direct pressure
- Elevation
- Pressure points
- Tourniquet (only as a last resort)

↓

Monitor the patient carefully for renewed bleeding throughout the focused history and physical exam, the detailed exam, and the ongoing assessment.

CARE FOR INTERNAL BLEEDING

Take appropriate body substance isolation (BSI) precautions.

↓

Perform the scene size-up upon arrival, paying particular attention to potential mechanisms of injury.

↓

Perform the initial assessment.
- Ensure the ABCs
- If serious external bleeding is present, control it.
- Assign a high priority for immediate transport to patients with airway problems, inadequate breathing, and/or uncontrolled bleeding.

↓

Monitor the patient carefully during the focused history and physical exam, especially if your general impression of the patient and the mechanism of injury suggest internal bleeding.

↓

Provide high flow oxygen if you have not already done so during the initial assessment.

↓

(continued) ▶

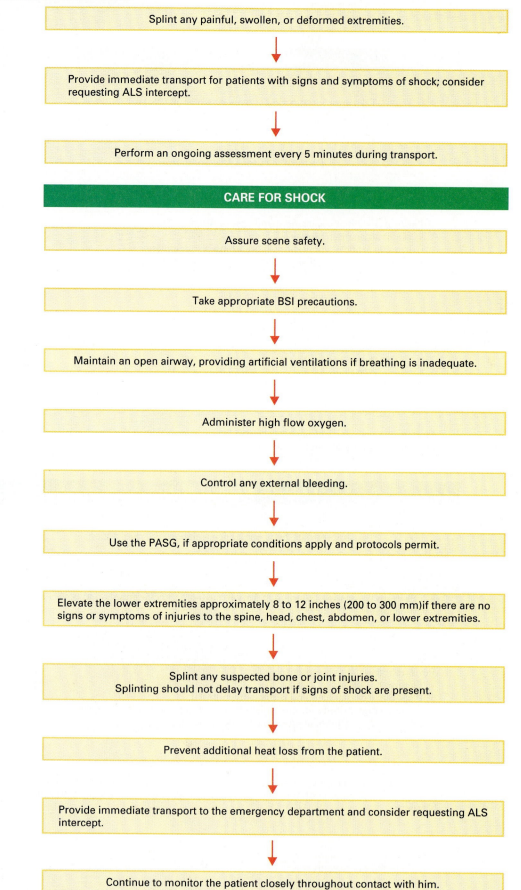

Splint any painful, swollen, or deformed extremities.

Provide immediate transport for patients with signs and symptoms of shock; consider requesting ALS intercept.

Perform an ongoing assessment every 5 minutes during transport.

CARE FOR SHOCK

Assure scene safety.

Take appropriate BSI precautions.

Maintain an open airway, providing artificial ventilations if breathing is inadequate.

Administer high flow oxygen.

Control any external bleeding.

Use the PASG, if appropriate conditions apply and protocols permit.

Elevate the lower extremities approximately 8 to 12 inches (200 to 300 mm) if there are no signs or symptoms of injuries to the spine, head, chest, abdomen, or lower extremities.

Splint any suspected bone or joint injuries.
Splinting should not delay transport if signs of shock are present.

Prevent additional heat loss from the patient.

Provide immediate transport to the emergency department and consider requesting ALS intercept.

Continue to monitor the patient closely throughout contact with him.

Soft Tissue Injuries

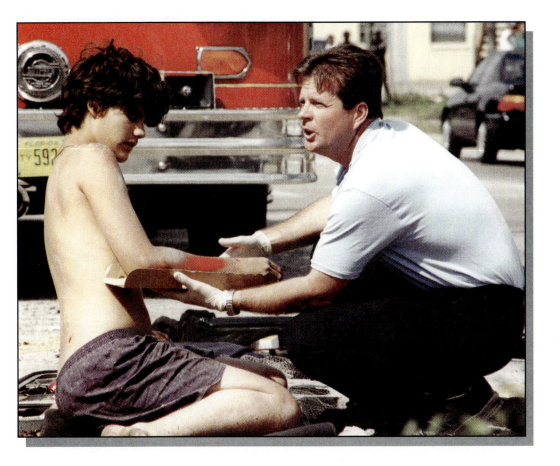

*I*njuries to the soft tissues of the body are perhaps the most common type of injuries that you will encounter as an EMT. Injuries to the skin are seen with even the most minor of traumas. More significant soft tissue injuries, including burns and injuries involving the chest and abdomen, may be life threatening because of associated blood loss, shock, and compromise of the airway and breathing.

As an EMT, you will need to recognize and to treat effectively a wide variety of soft tissue injuries. In addition, because soft tissue injuries ▶

often cause heavy external bleeding, you must be sure to take all appropriate body substance isolation precautions when assessing and treating patients.

OBJECTIVES

At the completion of this chapter, the EMT-Basic student should be able to meet the following objectives.

Knowledge and Understanding

1. State the major functions of the skin. (p. 484)
2. List the layers of the skin. (p. 484)
3. Establish the relationship between body substance isolation and soft tissue injuries. (p. 489)
4. List types of closed soft tissue injuries. (pp. 485–486)
5. Describe the emergency medical care of the patient with a closed soft tissue injury. (pp. 486–487)
6. State the types of open soft tissue injuries. (pp. 487–489)
7. Describe the emergency medical care of the patient with an open soft tissue injury. (pp. 489–502)
8. Discuss the emergency medical care considerations for a patient with a penetrating chest injury. (pp. 495–496)
9. State the emergency medical care considerations for a patient with an open wound to the abdomen. (pp. 496–497, 498)
10. Differentiate the care of an open wound to the chest from an open wound to the abdomen. (pp. 495–497)
11. List classifications of burns. (p. 503)
12. Define superficial burn. (pp. 503–504)
13. List characteristics of superficial burns. (pp. 503–504)
14. Define partial thickness burn. (pp. 504–505)
15. List characteristics of partial thickness burns. (pp. 504–505)
16. Define full thickness burn. (p. 505)
17. List characteristics of full thickness burns. (p. 505)
18. Describe the emergency medical care of the patient with a superficial burn. (pp. 508–509)
19. Describe the emergency care of the patient with a partial thickness burn. (pp. 508–510)
20. Describe the emergency care of the patient with a full thickness burn. (pp. 508–510)
21. List the functions of dressing and bandaging. (p. 490)
22. Describe the purpose of a bandage. (p. 490)
23. Describe the steps in applying a pressure dressing. (p. 492)
24. Establish the relationship between airway management and the patient with chest injury, burns, and blunt and penetrating injuries. (pp. 487, 490, 495–496, 507–509, 512)
25. Describe the effects of improperly applied dressings, splints, and tourniquets. (p. 500)
26. Describe the emergency medical care of a patient with an impaled object. (pp. 497, 500)
27. Describe the emergency medical care of a patient with an amputation. (pp. 500–501)
28. Describe the emergency care for a chemical burn. (pp. 510–511)
29. Describe the emergency care for an electrical burn. (p. 512)

Skills

1. Demonstrate the steps in the emergency medical care of closed soft tissue injuries.
2. Demonstrate the steps in the emergency medical care of open soft tissue injuries.
3. Demonstrate the steps in the emergency medical care of a patient with an open chest wound.
4. Demonstrate steps in the emergency care of a patient with open abdominal wounds.
5. Demonstrate the steps in the emergency medical care of a patient with an impaled object.
6. Demonstrate the steps in the emergency medical care of a patient with an amputation.
7. Demonstrate the steps in the emergency medical care of an amputated part.
8. Demonstrate the steps in the emergency medical care of a patient with superficial burns.
9. Demonstrate the steps in the emergency care of a patient with partial thickness burns.
10. Demonstrate the steps in the emergency care of a patient with full thickness burns.
11. Demonstrate the steps in the emergency medical care of a patient with a chemical burn.
12. Demonstrate completing a prehospital care report for patients with soft tissue injuries.

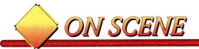

DISPATCH: *FIRE BOARD TO ALL UNIVERSITY HEIGHTS FIREFIGHTERS. A REPORTED STRUCTURE FIRE AT THE BAXT PHYSICS CENTER OF THE STATE UNIVERSITY. TIME IS 2314.*

You respond to the main station from your home and make the jump seat of the first engine out. Upon arrival on scene, you are met by a campus security officer who advises you that there is a fire condition in the first floor lab area.

As your captain calls in a second alarm, you and your partner stretch a 2½ inch (65 mm) preconnect down the entry hall of the building. As you crawl under the banking smoke, you hear a faint moaning for help just before the hoseline is charged.

Suddenly, you come across a person lying in the hall. Your helmet light reveals a young man, whose chest is bare and charred and whose jeans are still burning. You crack the nozzle of your hoseline and immediately extinguish the burning clothing. Your partner transmits a message indicating that you've located a civilian casualty, and then the two of you begin to drag the patient back out of the hall. As you do, members of the second due engine arrive and take over your hoseline, continuing fire suppression.

Once outside and clear of the building, you and your partner take off your SCBA and attend to the patient. Your initial assessment reveals that the man's eyes are open. You note that his airway is open, but he speaks in a hoarse, soft voice and coughs up black sputum frequently. He tells you, "It feels tight to breathe." The movement of the patient's chest wall as he breathes is shallow, and his entire chest is blackish-brown in color and leather-like to the touch.

Your partner applies high flow oxygen via a nonrebreather mask just as the crew from Ambulance 249 arrives with their stretcher. You give the crew a quick report on the patient while he is packaged and loaded into the ambulance. The ambulance EMT radios the hospital with your assessment of a patient with major burns and difficulty breathing. Riding along with the patient, you continually reassess his airway and breathing status during the 4-minute ride to the emergency department while speaking to him and comforting him.

At the community hospital emergency department, a physician assistant intubates the patient while the physician on duty makes surgical incisions on both sides of the patient's chest to permit better ventilations by relieving the constriction caused by the patient's burns. Within 25 minutes of arrival at the hospital, the patient is loaded onto a Mercy Flight helicopter and flown to the regional burn center 110 miles (177 k) away. You learn the next day that your patient died at the burn center as a result of full thickness burns over 95 percent of his body.

Your engine crew, the Ambulance 249 crew, and the emergency department staff participate in a critical incident stress debriefing (CISD) the next day. It is agreed that, despite the excellent care given by both fire department and emergency department personnel, the patient's fate was determined by the severity of his burns before you even stepped off the apparatus at the fire scene.

Injuries that involve or pass through the skin to involve muscles, nerves, blood vessels, and organs are termed **soft tissue injuries** (Figure 20-1). Soft tissue injuries are extremely common. Some, such as abrasions, are relatively minor in nature. Others, such as major burns and penetrating injuries to the chest, can quickly result in a patient's death.

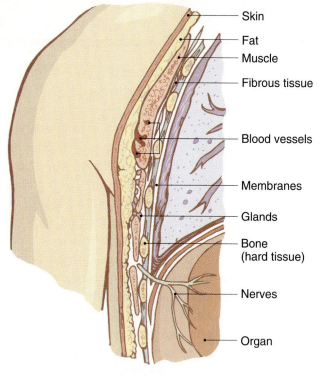

Labels (top to bottom):
- Skin
- Fat
- Muscle
- Fibrous tissue
- Blood vessels
- Membranes
- Glands
- Bone (hard tissue)
- Nerves
- Organ

Figure 20-1   The soft tissues.

SKIN FUNCTIONS AND STRUCTURES

The skin is the human body's largest organ. The skin has several major functions, including the following:

◆ It serves as a barrier to prevent infections and other materials from entering the body.

◆ It helps hold water and other fluids in the body.

◆ It helps regulate the body's temperature.

◆ It and its underlying layers of fat act as a shock absorber to protect underlying organs from blunt trauma.

Injuries to the skin, especially open injuries, can disrupt any or all of these functions. For example, full thickness burns like those received by the patient in On Scene can destroy the body's ability to regulate its temperature, permit major losses of body fluids, and allow the free entry of

microorganisms carrying life-threatening infections into the body.

There are three major layers of the skin (Figure 20-2). From the outside in, these are the epidermis, the dermis, and the subcutaneous layers. Each layer has specific functions and structures.

The various layers of the skin cover deeper structures of the body such as muscles, bones, and internal organs. Always remember that injuries that seem to involve only the skin may in fact have caused serious injuries to deeper structures as well.

◆ **The epidermis** The epidermis is the outermost layer of the skin. The surface of the epidermis is actually composed of dead skin cells that are gradually rubbed off and replaced from cells from layers deeper within the skin. The epidermis is the layer that makes skin water resistant and that forms the initial barrier to the entry of infection. The epidermis contains no blood vessels or nerve cells. However, hair shafts and the drainage of sweat glands pass through this layer.

◆ **The dermis** The dermis is the skin layer below the epidermis. This layer is filled with many different structures including blood vessels, nerve fibers, sweat glands, sebaceous (oil) glands, and hair follicles.

Injuries to the dermis can cause significant bleeding because of the many blood vessels present in that skin layer. Injuries can also be very painful because of the number of nerve fibers in this layer. If the dermis is destroyed by injury or burns, then the risk of infection passing from the outside the body into its deeper structures is profound.

◆ **The subcutaneous layers** Below the dermis are fatty layers called the subcutaneous tissue. The fat and connective tissue in these layers give the skin its insulating and shock absorbing qualities. Larger blood vessels pass through the subcutaneous layers as do nerve fibers. This means that bleeding and pain are likely to accompany injuries that affect the subcutaneous layers.

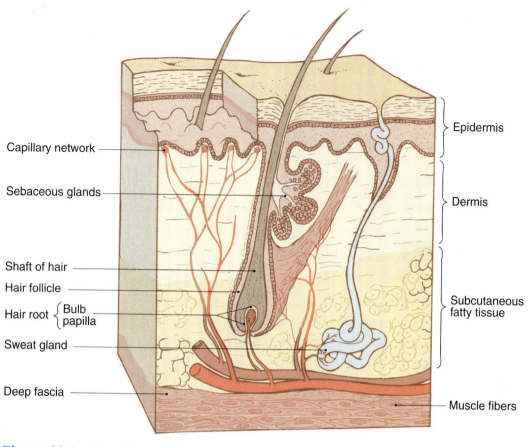

Figure 20-2 The skin.

Labels on figure:
- Capillary network
- Sebaceous glands
- Shaft of hair
- Hair follicle
- Hair root { Bulb / papilla
- Sweat gland
- Deep fascia
- Epidermis
- Dermis
- Subcutaneous fatty tissue
- Muscle fibers

S OFT TISSUE INJURIES

Soft tissue injuries are usually broadly categorized as either "closed" or "open." A **closed injury** is one in which the trauma does not break the surface of the skin, although structures in and beneath the skin's surface are injured. An **open injury** is one in which the surface of the skin is broken. In addition to harming the skin, an open injury may also damage body structures beneath the skin.

Closed Soft Tissue Injuries

Closed soft tissue injuries usually result when a blunt force is applied to the body. Examples of blunt trauma that might cause closed injuries include a patient struck by a fist or a patient, driving without a seat belt, whose chest impacted his vehicle's steering wheel during a collision.

The basic types of closed soft tissue injuries include contusions, hematomas, and closed crush injuries.

Contusions

Contusions, or bruises, are the most minor of closed soft tissue injuries (Figure 20-3). With a contusion, the epidermis remains intact, while cells and blood vessels in the dermis are damaged. Blood from the damaged structures usually accumulates in the dermis, giving a contusion a typical bluish-purple color. There is also usually swelling, pain, and tenderness at the site of the injury.

Hematomas

Hematomas, like contusions, result from damage to blood vessels beneath the epidermis. However,

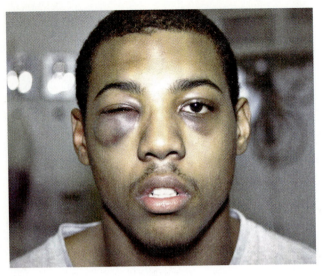

Figure 20-3 A contusion.

hematomas tend to involve larger blood vessels and larger amounts of tissue damage in the dermis and the subcutaneous layers. With a hematoma, a liter or more of blood can pool beneath the skin. Hematomas can produce large swollen, discolored areas on the body's surface. Hematomas can also occur deep within the body—for example, in the brain or the abdomen—where they may not be detected during patient assessment. Depending on its location and size, a hematoma may cause shock (hypoperfusion) in the patient.

Crush Injuries

Crush injuries are those in which damaging forces are passed from the exterior of the body to internal structures because the body or some part of it has been compressed between two or more surfaces. These compression injuries can cause massive tissue damage without breaking the skin's surface. A patient who strikes his thumb with a hammer, one whose arm is caught in the gears of an industrial machine, or one who is buried in a structural collapse may all experience crush injuries. Depending of the weight of the object and the region of the body involved, crush injuries may result in massive tissue damage and sufficient blood loss to cause shock (hypoperfusion). Damage to the skeletal system is also common with crush injuries. This damage can result in painful, swollen, and deformed extremities that may indicate underlying bone fractures.

One specific type of crush injury is called *traumatic asphyxia*. This can occur when the chest is suddenly compressed, producing severe pressure on the heart and lungs and forcing blood out of the chest and into the veins of the head, neck, and shoulders (Figure 20-4).

Assessment of Closed Soft Tissue Injuries

When dealing with any soft tissue injury, assure appropriate BSI precautions including wearing gloves. Be sure to wash your hands thoroughly after patient care is completed.

During the scene size-up, study the area for possible mechanisms of injury to the patient. If you note a mechanism of injury that may have caused spinal injury or your general impression of the patient suggests the possibility of spinal injury, establish in-line stabilization of the spine during your initial assessment.

During the focused history and physical exam, reconsider the mechanism of injury. If the mechanism of injury is significant, perform a rapid trauma assessment. If you continue to suspect spinal injury, apply a cervical spine immobilization collar as soon as you have examined the patient's neck. Maintain manual stabilization. If the mechanism of injury is not significant, perform a focused trauma assessment.

◆ Emergency Care—Closed Soft Tissue Injuries

The specific treatment of closed soft tissue injuries will vary depending on the magnitude of the

Figure 20-4 A patient suffering from traumatic asphyxia.

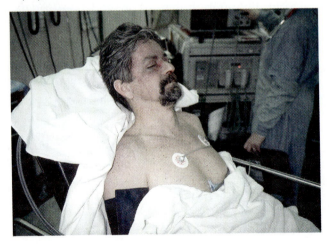

injury. Simple contusions may only require the application of a cold compress or ice pack to reduce the swelling and pain. Patients with major crush injuries may require aggressive management of airway and breathing problems as well as emergency care for shock (hypoperfusion).

Steps in the care of closed soft tissue injuries may include the following:

1. **Assure that appropriate BSI precautions are taken.**

2. **Assure an open airway.** If a patient suffering from a closed soft tissue injury requires manual maneuvers to open his airway, use a jaw thrust because the amount of force that produced the trauma is likely to have been sufficient to cause cervical spine injury.

3. **Provide supplemental high flow oxygen if signs or symptoms of respiratory distress or shock are present.**

4. **Provide artificial ventilations if the patient's respiratory effort is inadequate or if the patient is in respiratory arrest.**

5. **Treat for shock (hypoperfusion) as needed.** (See Chapter 19, "Bleeding and Shock.")

6. **Splint any painful, swollen, or deformed extremities.** This will reduce the patient's pain, lessen blood loss, and reduce the risk of further injuries.

7. **Apply cool compresses or ice packs to contusions and hematomas when possible to reduce swelling and pain.**

8. **Transport.** Provide an ongoing assessment en route.

Open Soft Tissue Injuries

Injuries in which the surface of a patient's skin is broken are classified as open injuries. These injuries can be caused by either blunt trauma or penetrating trauma, such as gunshot or stab wounds. Common types of open soft tissue injuries include abrasions, lacerations, avulsions, amputations, penetrations/punctures, and open crush injuries.

Abrasions

Abrasions are the most superficial of soft tissue injuries. Abrasions are caused by scraping, rub-

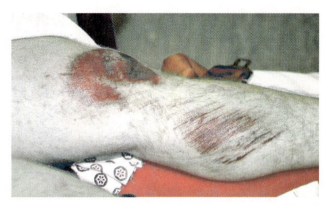

Figure 20-5   Abrasions.

bing, or shearing forces applied to the epidermis (Figure 20-5). Abrasions usually penetrate into the dermis as a result of shearing forces. Abrasions can be very painful but usually result in relatively minor bleeding. In certain mechanisms of injury, large areas of abrasions may be present. For example, large areas of the skin of a patient thrown from a motorcycle may come into prolonged contact with the abrasive surface of the road as the patient slides along it.

Lacerations

Lacerations are breaks in the skin of various lengths and depths (Figure 20-6). They usually result from forceful impact with sharp objects. There are various types of lacerations: straight-line lacerations are called *linear* or *regular;* jagged lacerations are called *stellate* or *irregular.* Lacerations may occur in isolation or in combination with other soft tissue injuries, including hematomas, abrasions, avulsions, and crush injuries.

Figure 20-6   Lacerations.

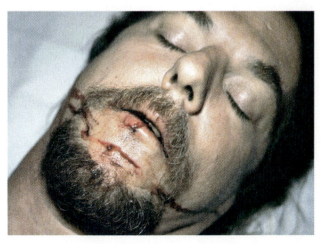

Bleeding from lacerations can range from relatively minor to severe. Deeper lacerations that injure large blood vessels may result in immediately life-threatening bleeding that must be controlled during the initial assessment. In addition, lacerations to parts of the body with rich blood supplies such as the face, scalp, and genital areas may cause significant external blood loss.

Avulsions

Avulsions occur when flaps of skin or tissue are torn loose from or pulled completely off the body surface (Figure 20-7). Bleeding is often severe with avulsions because multiple veins, capillaries, and arteries may have been ripped. A specific kind of avulsion injury frequently encountered in industrial accidents is called a *degloving injury*. In degloving injuries, the skin is pulled or peeled off circumferentially from a limb (Figure 20-8).

Amputations

Amputations occur when parts of extremities or other body parts are severed from the body (Figure 20-9). When a body part is completely separated from the body, it is termed a *complete amputation*. When the separation of a part from the body is not entirely complete, it is termed a *partial amputation*. The blood loss associated with amputations can range from minor to massive. The amount of blood loss will depend on the site of the amputation and the amount of damage done to major blood vessels.

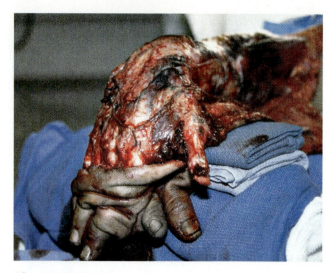

Figure 20-8 An avulsion injury that caused a degloving.

Figure 20-9 Amputations. **A.** Partial amputation. **B.** Partial amputation on right leg, complete amputation on left.

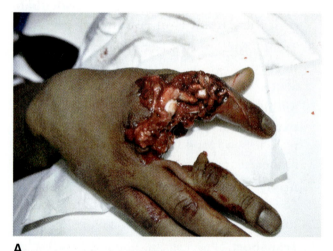

A.

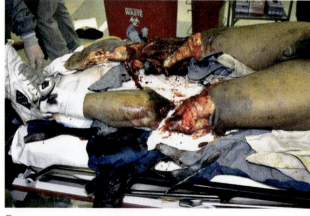

B.

Figure 20-7 An avulsion.

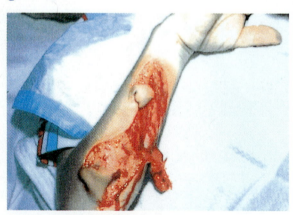

Penetrations/Punctures

The forceful contact of sharp, pointed objects or high-velocity objects, such as bullets, with the body produces **penetrations** and **punctures** (Figure 20-10). With these injuries, the amount of damage seen on the skin's surface may have little bearing on the amount of damage that has occurred to deeper structures. Wounds that show little or no bleeding at the skin's surface may have caused liters of internal blood loss. In some cases, especially with gunshot wounds, both an entry wound, where the object entered the body, and an exit wound, where it left the body, may be present. Often there is little or no external bleeding seen at the site of the entry wound. Any penetrations or punctures on the head, neck, torso, or proximal extremities should be considered potentially serious injuries because of the risk of severe internal bleeding.

Open Crush Injuries

If sufficient force is applied during a crush injury, the skin may rupture open (Figure 20-11). The skin may also be ripped open because of shearing force. These injuries often result in extensive injuries to the soft tissues, internal organs, and bones. With these injuries also, external bleeding may be minimal while internal bleeding is enough to lead to shock (hypoperfusion).

Assessment of Open Soft Tissue Injuries

With all open injuries, you will be exposed to blood and, possibly, other body fluids. *You must take all appropriate BSI precautions when caring for patients with open soft tissue injuries.* At a minimum, gloves should be worn at all times during patient contact. In cases of more severe bleeding, it may be appropriate to wear eye protection, impervious gowns, and masks during your efforts to control bleeding.

During the scene size-up, study the area for possible mechanisms of injury to the patient. If you note a mechanism of injury that may have caused

Figure 20-10 Penetrations and punctures. **A.** Penetration with an impaled nail. **B.** Gunshot wound to thigh—entry wound on left, exit on right.

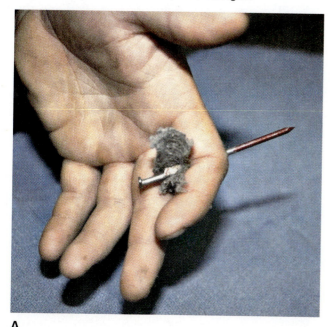

A.

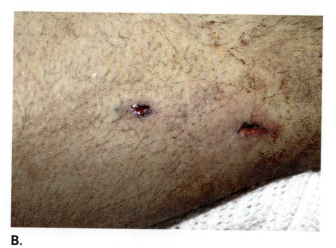

B.

Figure 20-11 An open crush injury.

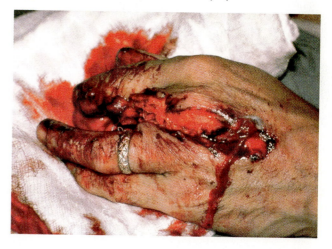

spinal injury or your general impression of the patient suggests the possibility of spinal injury, establish in-line stabilization of the spine during your initial assessment. Your priorities during the initial assessment of a patient with open soft tissue injuries will be assuring an open airway, adequate breathing, and rapid control of life-threatening external bleeding.

During the focused history and physical exam, reconsider the mechanism of injury. If the mechanism of injury is significant, perform a rapid trauma assessment. If you continue to suspect spinal injury, apply a cervical spine immobilization collar as soon as you have examined the patient's neck and maintain manual stabilization. If the mechanism of injury is not significant, perform a focused trauma assessment.

Dressings and Bandages

A basic in the care of any open wound is the proper use of wound dressings and bandages. The functions of dressings and bandages are to stop bleeding, to protect wounds from further damage, and to prevent further contamination, thereby reducing the risk of infection (Figure 20-12).

A **dressing** is applied directly to the wound to control bleeding. Dressings used by EMTs are

Figure 20-12   A dressing is applied to a wound to control bleeding. A bandage is used to hold a dressing in place.

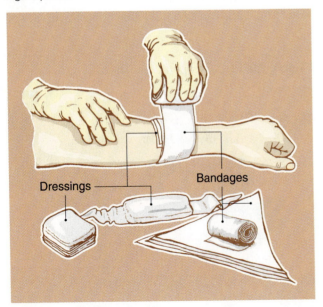

sterile, which means they are free of contamination and infectious organisms up to the time their packages are opened. When you handle a sterile dressing, take care to handle it by the edges, avoiding contact with the part of the dressing that will come in contact with the wound itself. Doing this will reduce the risk of introducing contamination from your non-sterile gloves into the patient's wound.

As an EMT, you will become familiar with the use of several common types of dressings including the following (Figure 20-13):

◆ *Universal dressings* These are large, bulky dressings used to cover large areas such as abdominal wounds.

◆ *Gauze pads* These are made of layered gauze and come in a variety of sizes. Perhaps the most commonly used are the 4" x 4" dressings. This size will cover most wounds that you will encounter. Because they are thinner than the universal dressings, it is likely that you will use multiple 4" x 4" pads to control bleeding from open soft tissue injuries.

◆ *Occlusive dressings* These are dressings that are impregnated with petroleum jelly or other substances that will prevent the passage of air or fluids through the dressings. In prehospital care, occlusive dressings are used almost exclusively for the care of chest and neck wounds. The dressings keep air from passing in or out of the wounds and can prevent development of some serious complications common with such wounds (see below).

◆ *Self-adhesive dressings* These dressings include plastic strips that adhere to themselves when overlapped. They are most often used to cover minor soft tissue injuries. Larger adhesive dressings are relatively expensive and, because they are usually removed at the receiving facility staff so wounds can be evaluated, are not routinely used by most EMTs.

A **bandage** is used to hold dressings in place (Figure 20-14). Because bandages usually are in direct contact with the dressing and not the wound itself, they may be sterile or non-sterile. Common types of bandages include the following:

Dressings

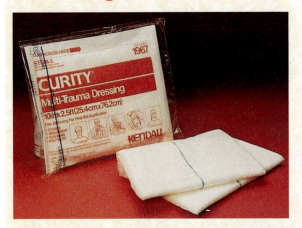

Figure 20-13A Universal, or multi-trauma, dressings.

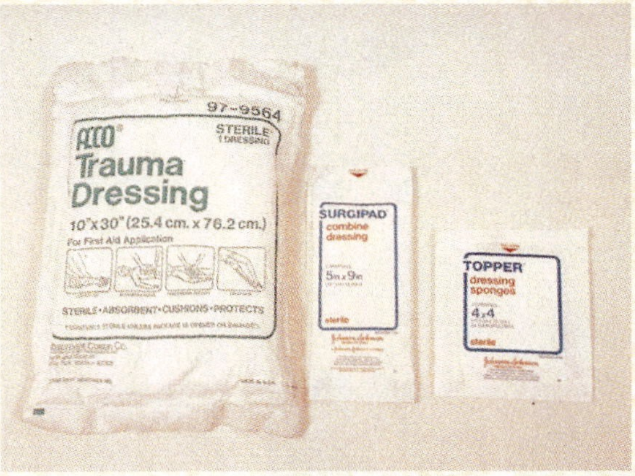

Figure 20-13B Sterile gauze pads.

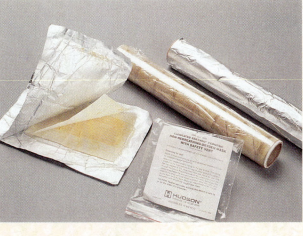

Figure 20-13C Occlusive dressings.

◆ *Gauze rolls* These are the most commonly used bandaging materials. Gauze rolls come in various widths usually ranging from 2 to 6 inches (51 to 152 mm). After being applied, the end or "tail" of the bandage is usually secured in place with adhesive tape.

◆ *Triangular bandages* These bandages are usually made from 40-inch (1,016-mm)-square pieces of cloth. They can be used for scalp wounds and extremity injuries.

◆ *Air splints* Air splints are used for secure dressings that cover multiple lacerations or large areas of abrasion on extremities. You should inflate the air splint by mouth to a pressure at which you can still readily dent the outside of the splint with your fingertip.

◆ *Adhesive tape* Adhesive tape is useful when securing dressings to a small wound such as one covered with a single 4" x 4" dressing. Blood and other material around the wound may make the tape less likely to adhere.

◆ *Self-adhering bandages* These usually come in rolls. The bandage material adheres to itself when overlapped (Figure 20-15, page 494).

Examples of Bandaging

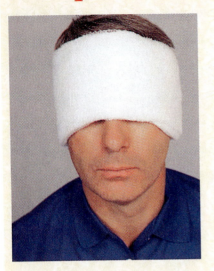

Figure 20-14A   Head and/or eye bandage.

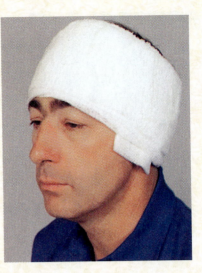

Figure 20-14B   Head and/or ear bandage.

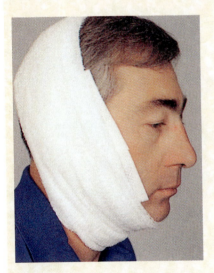

Figure 20-14C   Cheek bandage. (If you use this, make sure that the patient's mouth can open.)

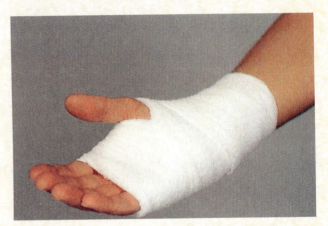

Figure 20-14D   Hand bandage.

A combination of dressings and bandages are applied to create a **pressure dressing,** used to control bleeding. The steps in applying a pressure dressing are as follows:

1. Cover the wound with a universal dressing or several gauze pads.
2. Put pressure on the dressing with your hand until bleeding stops.

3. Apply a bandage over the dressing tightly enough to maintain the pressure controlling the bleeding, but not so tightly that circulation is cut off. Check distal pulses to assure circulation.
4. If blood soaks through the original dressing and bandage, do not remove them. Instead, apply additional dressing over the original and bandage in place.

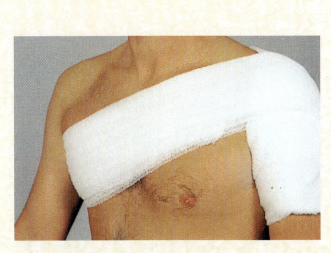

Figure 20-14E   Shoulder bandage.

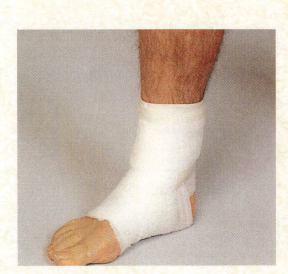

Figure 20-14F   Foot and/or ankle bandage.

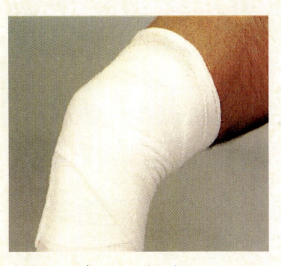

Figure 20-14G   Knee bandage.

◆ *Emergency Care—Open Soft Tissue Injuries*

The basic steps in management of open soft tissue injuries include the following (Figure 20-16):

1. **Assure BSI precautions.**

2. **Expose the wound.** Identify the edges of the wounds to assure that adequate dressings can be applied. In cases of penetrating injuries, check for exit wounds.

3. **Control the bleeding, taking whatever steps are necessary to control blood loss.** Use the techniques taught in Chapter 19, "Bleeding and Shock. These include direct pressure, elevation, pressure points, and—if necessary—tourniquets.

Applying a Self-Adhering Bandage

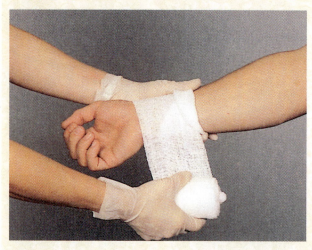

Figure 20-15A Secure the self-adhering roller bandage with several overlapping wraps.

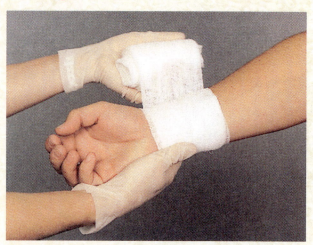

Figure 20-15B Overlap the bandage, keeping it snug.

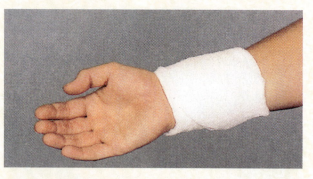

Figure 20-15C Cut the bandage and use adhesive tape or tie the bandage to secure it in place.

4. **Prevent further contamination of the wound.** Do not probe the wound, but if you can see large pieces of foreign material on the surface of the wound remove them with a gloved hand.

5. **Apply a sterile dressing and secure it in place with appropriate bandaging material.**

6. **Keep the patient calm and quiet.** Remember that keeping the patient informed and providing continuous reassurance are important components of patient care. Doing this can help to lower the patient's blood pressure and heart rate, thereby assisting with control of the bleeding.

7. **Treat the patient for shock (hypoperfusion) if signs and symptoms are present.** See Chapter 19, "Bleeding and Shock."

8. **Provide ongoing patient assessment.** Be sure to check the wounds to assure that bleeding remains controlled.

Emergency Care Considerations for Specific Injuries

Certain types of soft tissue injuries carry with them risks of additional complications. The basic care steps described above still apply with these injuries; however, they also require that some special care measures be taken.

General Procedures for Open Wound Care

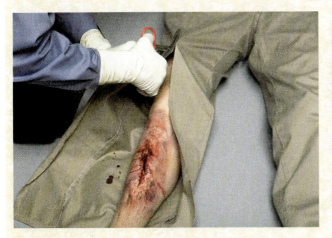

Figure 20-16A Having taken appropriate BSI precautions, expose the wound.

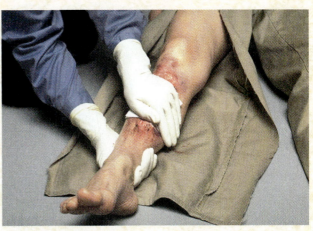

Figure 20-16B Control the bleeding. Try direct pressure first. If that fails, try elevating the wound, using pressure points, or—as a last resort—a tourniquet.

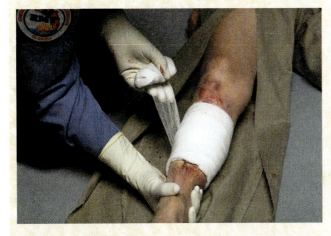

Figure 20-16C Apply a dressing and secure it with a bandage.

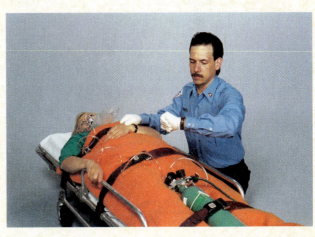

Figure 20-16D Keep the patient calm and quiet.

Open Chest Injuries

Penetration or perforation of the chest wall produces what is known as an **open chest injury.** The penetration/puncture allows direct communication between the inside of the chest cavity and the outside air. This type of injury can produce what is called a *sucking chest wound* because you can sometimes hear sucking sounds or see bubbling around the wound as the patient breathes. An open chest injury is a life-threatening condition. In this situation, air can accumulate between the inside of the chest wall and the lung, leading to collapse of the lung and impairing adequate breathing (Figure 20-17). This condition is known as a *pneumothorax.*

Emergency medical care of open chest injuries includes the following steps:

1. **Assure that BSI precautions are adequate.** The accumulation of pressure within the chest can cause blood to spray from an open wound during respirations. Use of eye protection, a mask, and a gown may be indicated.

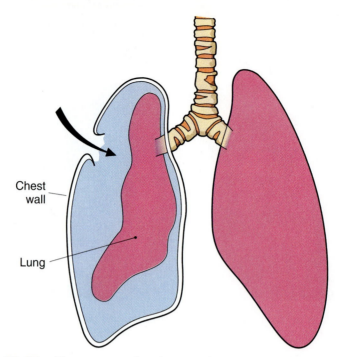

Figure 20-17 Air can enter the chest cavity through a puncture in the chest wall. This can cause a collapse of a lung and impaired breathing, a condition known as pneumothorax.

Chest wall

Lung

2. **Administer high concentration oxygen.**

3. **Secure an occlusive dressing in place over the wound with tape to seal it.** This will prevent the movement of air through the wound. The dressing should be at least 2 inches (50 mm) wider than the wound. Secure it on all four sides, or follow local protocols (see below). Remember to seal both entry and exit wounds if an object has perforated the chest (gone through the chest wall twice).

4. **Place the patient in a position of comfort if no spinal injury is suspected.**

5. **Transport the patient immediately and provide ongoing assessment en route.**

In some cases, securing an occlusive dressing over the wound may trap air in the chest, causing excessive pressure to build up within the chest cavity, a condition called a *tension pneumothorax*. If the patient's condition deteriorates during transport with signs of decreased mental status, worsening respiratory distress, or a falling blood pressure, then the occlusive dressing should be briefly removed to allow escape of the air under tension in the chest. Some EMS systems direct that

the occlusive dressing be secured with tape on only three sides with an open chest injury (Figure 20-18). This creates a "blow-off" or "flutter" valve, allowing air to escape through the untaped fourth side if a tension pneumothorax develops.

Abdominal Open Injuries

On rare occasions you may encounter open abdominal injuries where internal organs such as the bowel protrude out of the abdominal cavity. These injuries are termed **eviscerations**. The emergency care of patients with eviscerations includes the following (Figure 20-19, page 498):

1. **Assure appropriate BSI precautions.**

2. **Administer high concentration oxygen.**

3. **Expose the wound but do not touch or try to push the protruding abdominal contents back into the wound.**

4. **Cover the exposed organs and wound with a sterile dressing moistened with sterile saline and secure the dressing in place.**

5. **Flex the patient's knees and hips if they are not also injured.** This maneuver

On inspiration, dressing seals wound, preventing air entry

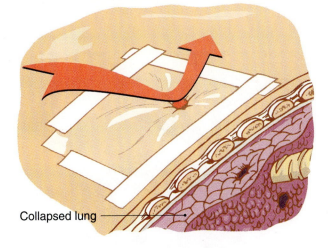

Collapsed lung

Expiration allows trapped air to escape through untaped section of dressing

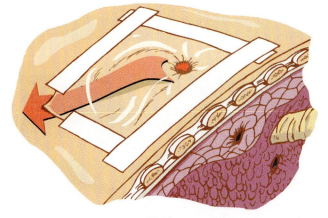

Figure 20-18 Some EMS systems recommend use of a "flutter" valve dressing with open chest wounds. This type of dressing allows air to escape from the chest cavity.

reduces the amount of stress on the abdominal wall.

6. **Transport the patient immediately and provide ongoing assessment en route.**

Impaled Objects

Objects such as knives, fence posts, and shards of glass that caused penetrations or punctures may still be imbedded in the patient when you arrive on the scene. You must handle these impaled objects in a way that minimizes further injury to the patient through additional movement of the object. When you encounter a patient with an impaled object, follow these steps (Figures 20-20 and 20-21, pages 499 and 500):

1. **Assure BSI precautions.**
2. **In general, do not remove an impaled object unless it does any of the following:**
   —The object prevents transport of the patient and all reasonable efforts to trim or to make the object of manageable size have failed.
   —The object interferes with the performance of chest compressions.
   —The object is solely through the cheek and doesn't involve deeper structures in the mouth or pharynx (Figure 20-22, page 500).
3. **Manually secure the object.** Often a single rescuer is assigned this single task for the duration of the call.
4. **Expose the wound area.** Cut away clothing, but be careful not to move the object.
5. **Control bleeding.** Use direct pressure on the wound edges, not on the impaled object. Treat the patient for shock (hypoperfusion) if signs and symptoms are present.
6. **Use bulky dressings to help stabilize the object.** Surround the object with layers of dressings, then tape the dressings in place.
7. **Transport the patient carefully, providing ongoing assessment en route.**

Large Open Neck Injury

Large open neck wounds often involve massive bleeding from the large arteries and veins in the neck. With such injuries, the danger exists that air may be sucked into a large neck vein as blood flows back to the heart. The resulting **air embolus,** or air bubble, may then travel into the heart and lungs and may cause the patient's death.

Another danger associated with open neck wounds is that of putting too much pressure on the carotid artery during attempts to control bleeding. Doing so may reduce blood flow to the brain enough to cause a stroke.

To avoid the problems, follow the steps below when caring for a patient with a large open neck injury (Figure 20-23, page 501):

1. **Assure adequate BSI precautions.**
2. **Place a gloved hand over the open wound to control bleeding.**

Care for an Open Abdominal Wound

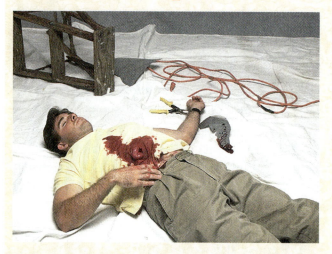

Figure 20-19A A patient with an open abdominal wound with evisceration.

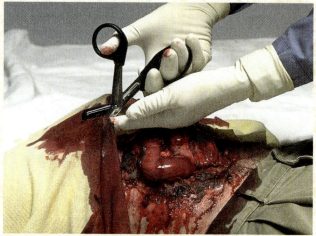

Figure 20-19B Having taken appropriate BSI precautions, cut away clothing and expose the wound.

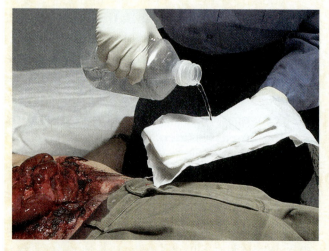

Figure 20-19C Use sterile saline to soak a sterile dressing.

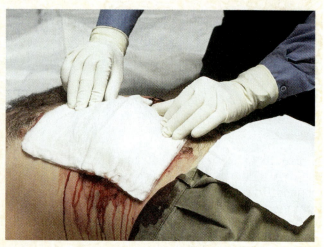

Figure 20-19D Place the moist dressing over the wound.

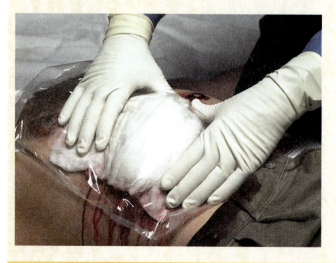

Figure 20-19E Some EMS systems call for placing an occlusive dressing over the moist dressing to keep it moist. Secure the dressing(s) loosely in place with bandages tied above and below the wound.

General Care for a Patient with an Impaled Object

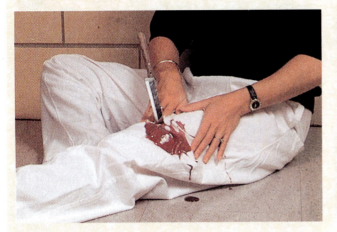

Figure 20-20A A patient with an impaled kitchen knife.

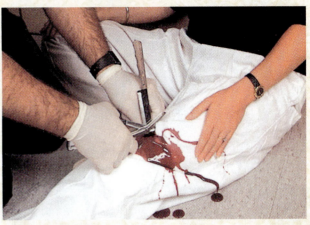

Figure 20-20B Manually stabilize the impaled object while cutting away clothing to expose the wound.

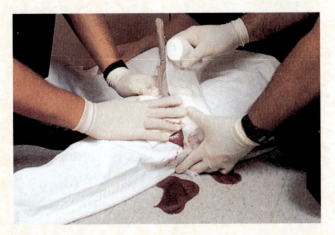

Figure 20-20C When bleeding is controlled, use bulky dressings to stabilize the object and bandage the dressings in place.

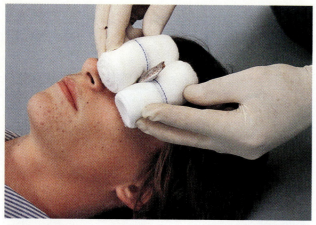

A.

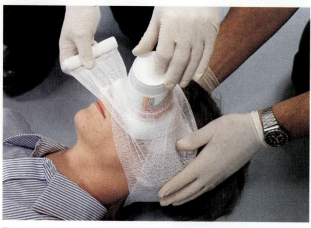

B.

Figure 20-21 When an object is impaled in the eye, **(A)** stabilize it in place with rolls of gauze bandage on either side of the object. **(B)** Place a disposable paper cup over the bandage rolls and the object (not allowing it to touch the object) and secure the cup in place with a roller bandage or gauze wrapping. Dress and bandage the uninjured eye to reduce sympathetic eye movements.

3. **Cover the open neck wound with an occlusive dressing, and then place a sterile dressing over the occlusive dressing.**

4. **Apply only enough pressure to control the bleeding.** Compress the carotid artery only if necessary to control bleeding. If you must compress the carotid artery, never compress both carotid arteries at the same time.

3. **Bandage the dressing in place when the bleeding stops.**

4. **Transport the patient immediately, and provide ongoing assessment en route.**

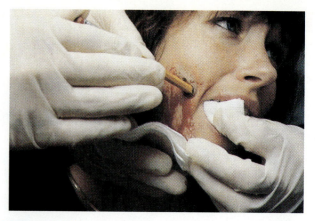

Figure 20-22 An object impaled solely through the cheek may be removed if no deeper structures in the mouth or pharynx are involved or if the airway cannot be managed with the object in place. Dress the outside of the wound and inside between the cheek and the teeth.

Amputations

When managing a patient with an amputation, control of bleeding and proper care of the amputated part are both essential. Reattachment of the part may be possible at the hospital. Even when the part cannot be reattached, tissue from the part may be used for some reconstruction at the amputation site.

Emergency care of patients with amputations should include the following:

1. **Assure adequate BSI precautions.**

2. **Control bleeding.** Use pressure dressings over the stump. Use a tourniquet only as an absolute last resort.

3. **Do not complete partial amputations.** Even the smallest link between the body and the amputated part may significantly improve the likelihood of successful reattachment.

   Splint or immobilize partially amputated parts in anatomical position to stabilize them and to prevent further injury.

   There are rare situations in which completion of a partial amputation might be considered. For example, if a patient in shock is hopelessly entrapped in machinery by a partially amputated body part, completing the partial amputation may help save the patient's life. In situations like these, contact medical direction immediately for advice.

Care for a Patient with a Large Open Neck Wound

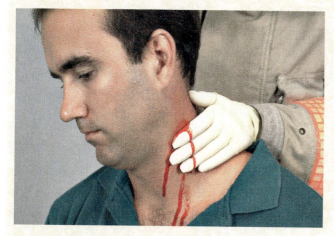

Figure 20-23A Place a gloved hand over the open wound to control bleeding.

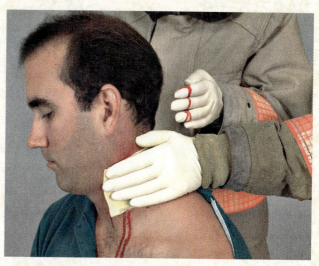

Figure 20-23B Place an occlusive dressing over the wound.

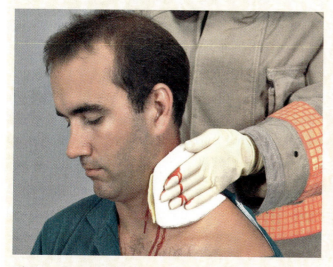

Figure 20-23C Place a sterile gauze dressing over the occlusive dressing. Use only enough pressure as is needed to control the bleeding.

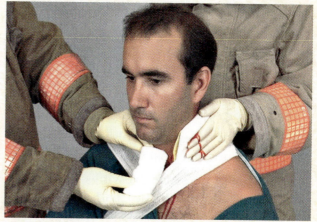

Figure 20-23D Bandage the dressings in place. Use a figure 8 configuration when applying the bandage, winding it under the arm opposite the wound. Never wrap it circumferentially around the neck.

4. If a complete amputation has occurred, follow these steps: (Figure 20-24, page 502):

◆ Wrap the amputated part in sterile dressing. Many systems recommend moistening the dressing with sterile saline. Follow local protocols.

◆ Seal the amputated part in a plastic bag and keep it cool. Place it in a cooler or other suitable container, but do not allow direct contact between the amputated part and ice or an ice pack. Do not use dried ice.

◆ Transport the amputated part along with the patient. Label the part with the patient's name, the date, and the name of the amputated body part.

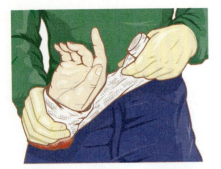
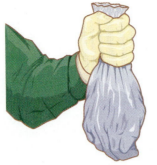
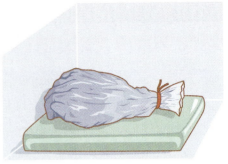

(1) Wrap completely in sterile dressings.

(2) Place in plastic bag and seal shut.

(3) Place sealed bag on top of a cold pack. Do not allow the tissue to freeze.

Figure 20-24   One procedure for caring for an amputated or completely avulsed body part. Follow your local procedures.

Avulsions

If you encounter a patient with an avulsion where the avulsed tissue is still attached, try to prevent it from becoming separated from the wound. If a large flap of skin or tissue has been torn off, treat it as any amputated part (see above) and transport it with the patient. It may be possible to use the tissue for wound repair at the hospital.

Emergency care of the patient with an avulsion that is still attached includes the following:

1. **Protect the avulsed tissue from further damage or separation from the wound.**

2. **Replace any attached avulsed skin or tissue to its normal position if possible.**

3. **Apply bulky pressure dressings to control bleeding and hold the avulsed part in place.**

4. **Transport the patient.**

Emergency care of the patient with an avulsion that has been torn completely free of the body includes the following steps:

1. **Apply bulky pressure dressings to control bleeding.**

2. **Save the avulsed part.**

   ◆ Wrap the avulsed part in a sterile dressing. Many EMS systems recommend that the dressing be moistened with sterile saline if possible. Follow your local protocol.

   ◆ Seal the avulsed part in a plastic bag and keep it cool. Place it in a cooler or other suitable container, but do not allow direct

contact between the amputated part and ice or an ice pack. Do not use dried ice.

   ◆ Transport the avulsed part along with the patient. Label the part with the patient's name, the date, and the part of the body from which the avulsed skin came.

BURNS

Burns are a significant cause of injuries for firefighters. Minor and moderate burns have always been looked upon as an occupational hazard of the profession. Fortunately, advances in protective clothing, including protective hoods and better gloves, have made these injuries somewhat less common among firefighters.

Among civilians, burns are also a frequent cause of soft tissue injuries. Most burns occur in the home, with about half of these being from

PEDIATRIC NOTE

Some 50 percent of all burns occur in patients younger than 20 years of age, and 30 percent of all burn patients are younger than 10 years of age. Scalding injuries from hot household liquids such as soup, tea, and coffee are especially common among these younger patients.

GERIATRIC NOTE

Burns are a common cause of death in the elderly. Burns that would be considered less serious in younger adults represent significant life threats in older patients. Several factors explain why burns affect the elderly more severely than they do younger patients:

◆ The skin thins as people age, and it also heals more slowly.

◆ Reaction time slows as people age so that older patients tend to remain in contact with sources of heat longer, resulting in more extensive burns.

◆ Geriatric patients frequently have underlying medical conditions, such as lung diseases, that can complicate recovery from burns.

direct contact with flame. Over 2 million thermal burns occur each year in the United States, accounting for about 100,000 hospitalizations and 10,000 deaths.

Burns can cause the death of patients in various ways, some immediate and some delayed. Immediate causes of burn-related deaths are highly relevant to prehospital care and include airway compromise and inadequate respirations. Delayed causes of burn-related deaths are largely related to the loss of normal skin coverage and include profound fluid loss resulting in hypoperfusion—so-called "burn shock"—and overwhelming infections.

As an EMT, you will need to learn how to properly assess the extent and severity of burns and to provide appropriate emergency care for patients with burns.

Classification of Burns

Classification of burns is based on three major elements:

◆ **Mechanism of burn injury** (see Table 20-1)

—Thermal

—Chemical

—Electrical

—Radiation

◆ **Depth of the burn**

—Superficial

—Partial thickness

—Full thickness

◆ **Percentage of body surface area (BSA) burned**

When you describe a burn, your description should include each of these elements. For example, you might say, "The patient has a partial thickness chemical burn covering 18 percent of his body surface area."

Depth of Burn

Burns that involve the skin are classified based on the depth of tissue damage. Current terminology for burn depths, proceeding from the shallowest to the deepest, is *superficial, partial thickness,* and *full thickness* (Figure 20-25). These terms correspond to the older terminology of *first degree, second degree,* and *third degree burns,* respectively. A single patient may have burns of different depths. This is common when the duration or intensity of exposure to the burn mechanism varies in different body areas.

Superficial Thickness Burns These are the least serious of burns. They affect only the epidermis (Figure 20-26). The most common superficial thickness burn is a sunburn that results from

Table 20-1

Mechanisms of Burn Injury

Mechanism	Possible Sources
Thermal	Flames; excessive heat from fire, steam, hot liquids, hot objects; radiation
Chemical	Various acids, bases, caustics
Electricity	Alternating current, direct current, lightning
Radiation	Nuclear sources; ultraviolet light is also considered a source of radiation burns, as in sunburn

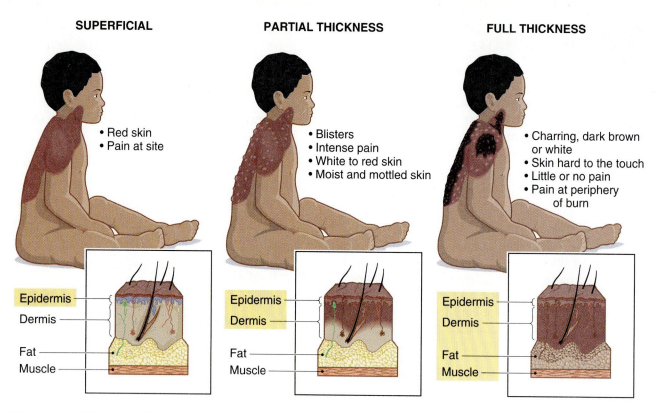

SUPERFICIAL	PARTIAL THICKNESS	FULL THICKNESS

SUPERFICIAL
- Red skin
- Pain at site

Epidermis
Dermis
Fat
Muscle

PARTIAL THICKNESS
- Blisters
- Intense pain
- White to red skin
- Moist and mottled skin

Epidermis
Dermis
Fat
Muscle

FULL THICKNESS
- Charring, dark brown or white
- Skin hard to the touch
- Little or no pain
- Pain at periphery of burn

Epidermis
Dermis
Fat
Muscle

Figure 20-25   Classification of burns by depth.

overexposure to the sun's ultraviolet radiation. Other common causes of superficial burns include thermal burns from hot liquids, like coffee or soup, and chemical burns.

Superficial burns are identified by reddened skin and pain and tenderness at the burn site. The pain of these burns may be intense. If there is extensive body surface area involvement, patients may summon the assistance of EMS solely because of the pain of these injuries.

Partial Thickness Burns These burns are more extensive than superficial burns. They involve both the epidermis and the dermis (Figure 20-27). Thermal agents are the most common causes of these burns. Because deeper layers of tissues are involved, partial thickness burns carry risks of serious complications such as fluid loss and subsequent infection.

Partial thickness burns are characterized by red, white, or blotchy skin and blisters at the burn

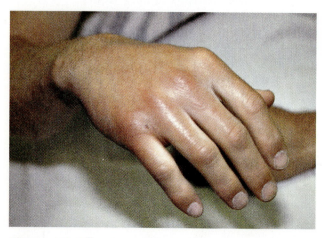

Figure 20-26   A superficial burn.

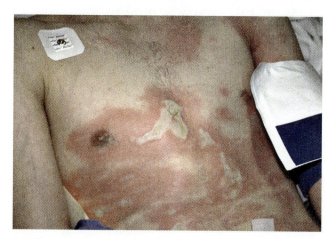

Figure 20-27   A partial thickness burn (note blistering).

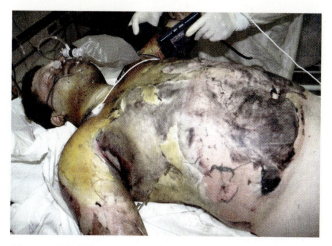

Figure 20-28 A full thickness burn.

site. The burned skin is moist because body fluids seep out through the damaged area. Because there are many nerve fibers in the dermis, these injuries are very painful.

Full Thickness Burns Full thickness burns cause the most extensive tissue damage. All skin layers—epidermis, dermis, and subcutaneous layers—are damaged (Figure 20-28). The damage from these burns may extend even deeper to the muscles, bones, or the internal organs.

Full thickness burns have a typically dry or leather-like appearance. The burned area can be a white, brown, or charred color. Because parts of the dermis and subcutaneous layers containing nerve fibers are destroyed, these most serious of burns often cause little or no pain for patients. However, areas of full thickness burns are commonly surrounded by partial thickness burns, which are very painful.

Body Surface Area and Burns

The amount of a patient's body surface area (BSA) that is burned also affects how severe the burn is. You must be able to estimate rapidly the extent of the BSA burned so that you can set correct priorities for treatment and transport.

The most widely used system for estimating the extent of BSA burned in adults is called the **rule of nines** (Figure 20-29). With this system, the body is divided into areas each of which represents 9 percent of the BSA. These areas are as follows:

◆ The head and neck
◆ Each upper extremity
◆ The chest

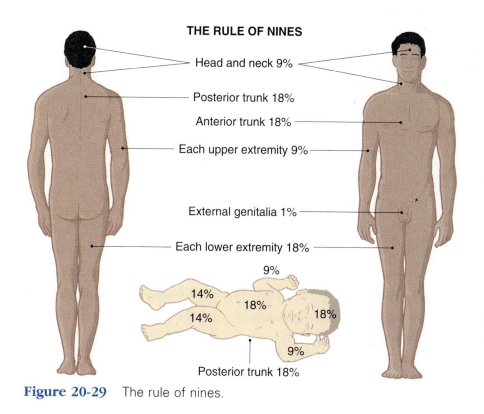

THE RULE OF NINES

Head and neck 9%

Posterior trunk 18%

Anterior trunk 18%

Each upper extremity 9%

External genitalia 1%

Each lower extremity 18%

9%

14%   18%   18%

14%

9%

Posterior trunk 18%

Figure 20-29 The rule of nines.

- The abdomen
- The upper back
- The lower back
- The front of each lower extremity
- The back of each lower extremity

These areas represent 99 percent of the total BSA. The genital area makes up the remaining 1 percent.

The rule of nines is most helpful when determining the extent of large burns. With smaller burns, you can use a method based on the size of the palm of the patient's hand. The palm of the hand equals approximately 1 percent of the total BSA. Thus, a burn about the size of 4 of the patient's palm surface areas would represent about 4 percent of the BSA.

PEDIATRIC NOTE

You must modify the rule of nines when estimating the extent of burns in young children and infants. This is necessary because the heads of infants and young children are proportionally larger in relationship to the rest of the body than are those of adults.

In the modified system, the various areas and the percentages of BSA they represent are:

- The head and neck—18 percent
- Each lower extremity—14 percent
- The chest and abdomen combined—18 percent
- The entire back—18 percent
- Each upper extremity—9 percent
- The genital area—1 percent

This adds up to a BSA of 101 percent, but still provides for a reasonable estimate of the burned area.

Burn Severity

There are three levels of burn severity—minor burns, moderate burns, and critical burns (see Table 20-2). Many EMS systems use the level of severity in determining the hospital to which a burn patient should be transported—for example, a burn center rather than the hospital to which

emergency patients are usually taken. Hospital staff also use the level of severity when deciding which patients can be treated and discharged from the emergency department, which patients will be admitted to the hospital, and which patients will require transfer to a burn center.

The depth of the burn and the percentage of BSA burned are basic elements in determining the severity of a burn. There are several additional factors that can affect how to classify the severity of a burn. These include the following:

- *The age of the patient* Children less than 5 years old and adults older than 55 are more prone to suffer complications as a result of burn injuries. *Indeed, burns that normally be classified as moderate for most other patients are classified as critical for these two age groups.*

- *Airway involvement* Patients showing evidence of respiratory injury such as burns around the mouth, singed nasal hairs, or complaints of shortness of breath are likely to have suffered a burn injury to the respiratory system (Figure 20-30). Such injuries are more common when the patient has received burns in a confined space, such as when trapped in a room by a blaze.

  Patients whose burns involve the airway are at greater risk for developing immediate problems—for example, acute airway obstruction and respiratory failure—as well as long-term complications of their burn injuries.

- *Preexisting medical conditions* Patients with underlying medical conditions such as diabetes, lung disease, and heart disease will generally not tolerate burn injuries as well as patients who do not suffer from these illnesses.

- *Associated injuries* When patients have experienced other injuries such as internal bleeding or injuries to the bones, they will require more careful management.

- *Location of the burn* Burns to certain regions of the body increase the risk of long-term complications and may require more specialized care. These areas include the face, the hands, the feet, and the genitalia.

Table 20-2

Classification of Burn Severity: Adults

Severity	Burn Depth	BSA percentage/Complicating Factor
Minor	Full	Less than 2% BSA, excluding face, hands, feet, genitalia, or respiratory tract
Minor	Partial	Less than 15% BSA
Minor	Superficial	Less than 50% BSA
Moderate	Full	2–10% BSA, excluding face, hands, feet, genitalia, or respiratory tract
Moderate	Partial	15–20% BSA
Moderate	Superficial	More than 50% BSA
Critical	Partial or full	Complicated by injury to respiratory tract, other soft tissue injury, bone injury
Critical	Partial or full	Any burns involving face, hands, feet, genitalia, or respiratory tract
Critical	Full	More than 10% BSA
Critical	Partial	More than 30% BSA
Critical	Partial or full	Complicated by musculoskeletal injury
Critical	Partial or full	Involving circumferential burns

◆ *Circumferential burns* These are burns that completely encircle an extremity or any other part of the body. They can cause the skin to constrict or tissues to swell, interfering with circulation and/or breathing.

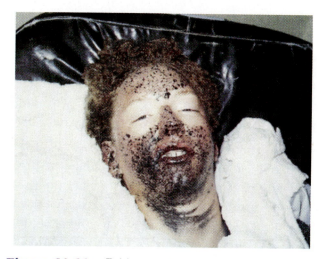

Figure 20-30 Evidence of burns to the face should suggest the possibility of airway involvement.

Assessment of the Patient with Burns

You must conduct a proper scene size-up before you can begin to provide proper emergency medical care for a burn patient. Determine the mechanism of the burn and take steps to assure that it will no longer pose a threat to you, other rescuers, or the patient. These steps may range from fire suppression activities, to the shutting down of electrical power sources, to simply securing hot liquids on a stovetop.

With a burn patient, the first task in the initial assessment may be to stop the burning process. Flames and smoldering materials must be extinguished and the patient cooled down. Use water or saline to accomplish this. Do not, however, keep the burn area immersed in water, as this may lead to hypothermia.

Once the burning material is out, proceed to evaluate the ABCs. Remember that the airway and breathing of patients can be easily compromised by burns. Provide high flow oxygen by nonrebreather mask. Provide positive pressure ventilations if breathing is inadequate. Electrical burns

General Care for Patients with Burns

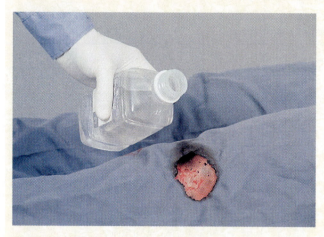

Figure 20-31A Stop the burning process.

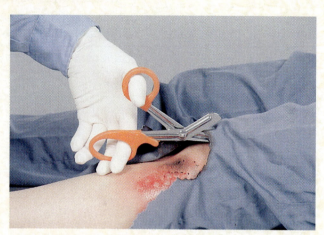

Figure 20-31B Remove smoldering clothing and expose the burned area.

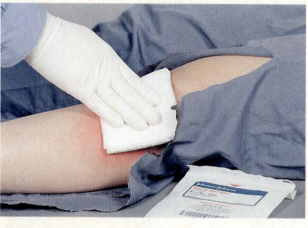

Figure 20-31C Cover the burned area with dry sterile dressings.

can often disrupt a patient's heartbeat, so be prepared to perform CPR and use an AED. Complete the initial assessment by determining the severity of the patient's burns to determine priority for transport. Treat any other life-threatening conditions you may have detected.

Perform a focused history and physical exam. Patients with burns often have other injuries; be alert for these as you perform the rapid trauma assessment. If you have the opportunity, gather a SAMPLE history from the patient, family members, or bystanders. Do not, however, delay transport of a patient with critical burns to do this.

◆ Emergency Care—Patient with Burns

General steps for the emergency care of patients with burns include the following (Figure 20-31):

1. **Stop the burning process.** If flames or smoldering clothing are present, extinguish them with water or saline. If there is burning semisolid material like grease, wax, or tar on the patient's skin, cool it with water or saline, but do not attempt to remove the material. Always check the patient over completely to be sure no areas still burning escape detection.

Care for Burned Fingers or Toes

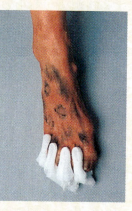

Figure 20-32A Separate burned toes with dry sterile gauze.

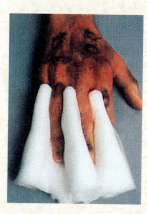

Figure 20-32B Separate burned fingers with dry sterile gauze.

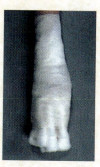

Figure 20-32C Cover burned fingers or toes completely with dry sterile dressings.

2. **Take appropriate BSI precautions.**

3. **Assess and continually monitor the airway for evidence of burns or airway obstruction.** Any patient who shows signs of airway burns or respiratory distress or who has been exposed to fire in a confined space should receive high concentration oxygen.

4. **Remove any surrounding clothing to expose the burned area completely.** Also remove any jewelry such as earrings, necklaces, or rings from burned areas. If synthetic materials have melted and bonded to the skin, do not attempt to rip them free.

5. **Evaluate the severity of the burn.** If the burn is critical, transport the patient immediately. If it is not critical, continue with the steps below.

6. **To prevent further contamination of the burned area, cover it with dry sterile dressings.*** If hands or feet are burned, separate fingers and toes with sterile gauze pads (Figure 20-32). *Do not* attempt to break any blisters. *Do not* apply any type of ointment, lotion, or antiseptic to the burn.

7. **Keep the patient warm.** Remember that serious burns can upset the body's thermoregulating mechanisms.

8. **Treat any other injuries that the patient may have.**

9. **Transport the patient to appropriate local facility, following your local protocols.** Perform an ongoing assessment en route, remaining alert for signs of airway compromise, breathing difficulty, or shock (hypoperfusion).

*Note: The 1994 U.S. DOT EMT-Basic National Standard Curriculum states that only dry dressings should be applied to burns. Your local medical director or the protocols of your EMS system may direct that saline-moistened sterile dressings be used for certain smaller burns (usually those involving less than 10 percent BSA). Follow your local protocols. Wet dressings should never be used on large burns because of the risk that their use may induce hypothermia.

Special Considerations with Infants and Children

The general principles of burn care remain the same when you are treating infants and children. However, there are some special considerations you should keep in mind when providing that care for pediatric patients.

Remember that infants and children have a greater skin surface area in relationship to their total body size than do older patients. For this reason, children are more prone to increased fluid loss and to the possibility of developing hypothermia. In addition, other differences in the anatomy and physiology of infants and children mean that burn severity is determined differently in these patients (see Table 20-3). Indeed, any burn in a child less than 5 years of age that would be classified as "moderate" severity in an adult is automatically upgraded to the "critical" category.

Finally, as you assess and manage burns with a pediatric patient, be alert for signs that the burns are the result of physical abuse. Burns are a common form of physical child abuse seen in emergency departments. During your assessment, make sure that the mechanism of the burn described by parents or caregivers matches the pattern of injury that you see in the child. Consider the possibility of child abuse when you discover the following:

◆ Multiple burns from point contacts such as cigarettes, hot irons, etc.

◆ Bilateral burns

◆ Indications of similar past burns

◆ Burns from scalding hot water in a "immersion pattern." This pattern is marked by circumferential burns to the lower extremities, but with the knees and anterior thighs usually spared because the child tries to draw up his legs to escape further burns.

Chemical and Electrical Burns

Burns that result from contact with chemicals or with electricity warrant special discussion. In both these mechanisms, it is especially crucial that the firefighter-EMT take extensive safety precautions so as not to also become injured.

Chemical Burns

Chemicals can burn patients in several ways (Figure 20-33). Some chemicals are strong acids or bases that directly erode through the layers of the skin. Other chemicals can burn both by chemical action and by generating heat as they react with human tissue.

Unless the chemical burn is the result of a very small spill onto the skin, act on all calls involving chemical burns as you would at a hazardous materials incident. Take all precautions to assure that you are not exposed to chemicals that

Table 20-3

Classification of Burn Severity: Children Less Than 5 Years Old

Severity	Burn Depth	BSA percentage
Minor	Partial	Less than 10% BSA
Moderate	Partial	10–20% BSA
Critical	Partial or full	More than 20% BSA

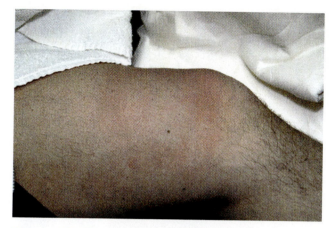

Figure 20-33   A patient with chemical burns.

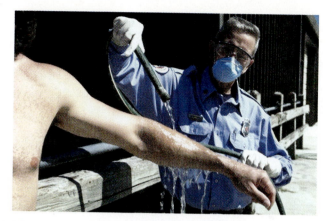

Figure 20-34   Flushing with large amounts of water is the suggested emergency treatment for many chemical burns.

burned the patient. At the minimum, wear gloves and eye protection when caring for these patients. Higher levels of protection, including SCBA and encapsulating suits, may be indicated based on the substance(s) present on the scene.

Emergency care of chemical burns should include the steps of general burn care described above. Additional care measures include the following:

◆ Flushing with large amounts of water is a key step in the management of most chemical burns. Large amounts of water will dilute the chemical, weakening its actions or stopping them entirely. Before you begin to flush away the chemical, find a description of it in the *North American Emergency Response Guidebook* or some other publication or check with medical direction or your poison control center to assure that it is safe to use water with that specific chemical. Combustion may occur when some chemicals come into contact with water.

When you have established that the use of water is safe, immediately flush the area of the burn with large amounts of water (Figure 20-34). Be careful with the runoff as you flush. Position the patient or the water source so that runoff does not flow onto uninjured areas. This is especially crucial when flushing eye injuries or facial burns that have not yet involved the eyes (Figure 20-35). If contamination of the patient(s) is heavy, contain the runoff using procedures that would apply in a hazardous materials

incident. Continue to flush affected areas during transport if possible.

◆ With dry chemicals such as dry lime, brush as much of the substance as possible off the patient before flushing with water. (Again, check to be sure it is safe to use water with the dry chemical.) Be aware that brushing may make particles of the chemical airborne, posing threats of respiratory burns and secondary contamination to the patient and rescuers. Use respiratory precautions, including SCBA, as indicated.

Electrical Burns

Electrical burns can result from lightning strikes or from contact with electrical current from a wide variety of sources. In general, the higher the voltage and amperage of the electrical source, the more severe the burn. Sources of alternating current (AC) tend to produce more serious burns and related injuries than sources of direct current (DC).

Frequently electrical injuries will have an "entry" burn where the patient contacted the electrical source and an "exit" burn where the current exited the patient going to ground. In a patient struck by lightning, a characteristic fern leaf-like burn pattern is often seen.

Electrical burns can be very deceptive (Figure 20-36). Often they can produce relatively minor external burns while causing extensive internal burns as current passes through the body. The electrical current can also cause sudden contractions of the patient's muscles. Some of these

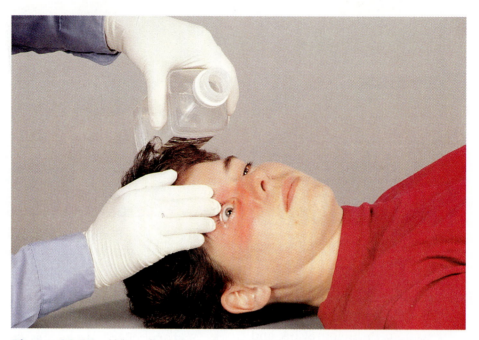

Figure 20-35 When flushing a chemical burn to a patient's eye, be sure the water that runs off does not flow into the unaffected eye.

may be so strong as to fracture or dislocate the patient's bones. The electricity can also disrupt the body's cardiac conduction system, producing an irregular heart rhythm or even cardiac arrest.

The management of electrical burns includes a careful scene size-up. Be aware that the source of the electricity that injured the patient may still be present and "live." Look for downed wires or some other source of electricity. Approach the patient slowly. If you feel a sensation of tingling in your feet or lower legs, you may be experiencing a *ground gradient,* which indicates that you are entering an energized area. Stop at once. Turn around and retreat immediately.

Do not attempt to shut down or remove the patient from an electrical source unless you are trained to do so. Otherwise, request the assistance of power company personnel or a specialty rescue team. *If you are unsure whether or not an electrical source is still energized, assume that it is and act accordingly.*

Steps in the emergency care of patients with electrical burns include the following:

1. **Assure scene safety and take appropriate BSI precautions.**

2. **Administer high flow oxygen via nonrebreather mask.** Provide artificial ventilations if the patient experiences respiratory failure or arrest.

3. **Carefully monitor for cardiac arrest.** Apply an AED if the patient goes into cardiac arrest.

4. **Treat external burns following the general guidelines for treatment of burns described above.** Always assess for entry and exit burns.

5. **Treat any other injuries the patient may have sustained as a result of contact with the electrical current.**

6. **Make note of the energy involved (voltage, amperage, etc.) and document this information on your patient care report.**

7. **Transport the patient as soon as possible.** Perform an ongoing assessment en route to the hospital.

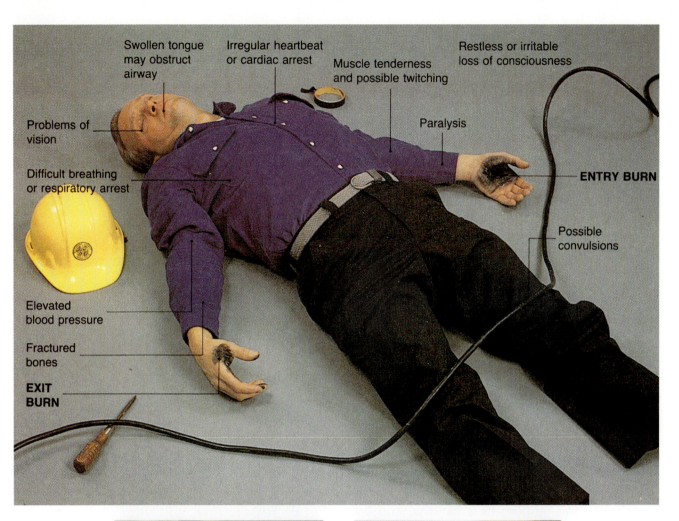

Swollen tongue may obstruct airway

Irregular heartbeat or cardiac arrest

Muscle tenderness and possible twitching

Restless or irritable loss of consciousness

Problems of vision

Paralysis

Difficult breathing or respiratory arrest

ENTRY BURN

Possible convulsions

Elevated blood pressure

Fractured bones

EXIT BURN

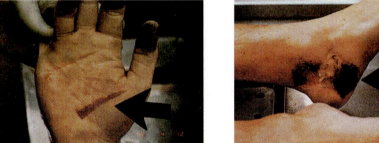

Entrance wound

Exit wound

Figure 20-36   Possible injuries resulting from an electrical shock.

Chapter Review

SUMMARY

Injuries to the soft tissues of the body are perhaps the most common types of trauma you will encounter as an EMT. These injuries include open and closed wounds as well as burns. Some of these injuries can be life threatening. Knowing how to assess and knowing how to provide the appropriate emergency care for these soft tissue injuries are essential parts of your responsibilities as an EMT.

REVIEWING KEY CONCEPTS

1. Describe the major functions of the skin.

2. Identify the three layers of the skin.

3. Define a closed soft tissue injury and list three types of such injuries.

4. Describe the general steps in the care of a closed soft tissue injury.

5. Define an open soft tissue injury and list six types of such injuries.

6. Describe the purpose of a dressing and list several common types that EMTs use.

7. Describe the purpose of a bandage and list several common types that EMTs use.

8. Describe the steps in applying a pressure bandage.

9. Describe the steps in the general care of a patient with an open soft tissue injury.

10. Explain the possible complications of an open chest injury.

11. Describe the steps in the care of an open chest injury.

12. Describe the steps in the care of a patient with an evisceration.

13. Describe the steps in the care of a patient with an impaled object.

14. Explain how a fully amputated body part should be treated.

15. List the basic mechanisms that cause burn injuries and give an example of each.

16. Define the three different burn depths.

17. Describe the rule of nines as it applies to adult patients and to pediatric patients.

18 Explain how the severity of a burn is determined.

19. Describe the steps in the general care of a patient with burns.

20. Explain the additional considerations to follow in providing emergency care for a patient with chemical burns.

21. Describe the steps in the care of the patient with electrical burns.

RESOURCES TO LEARN MORE

Moore, E.E. et al., eds. *Trauma, 2nd Edition*. Norwalk, CT: Appleton and Lange/Prentice Hall, 1991.

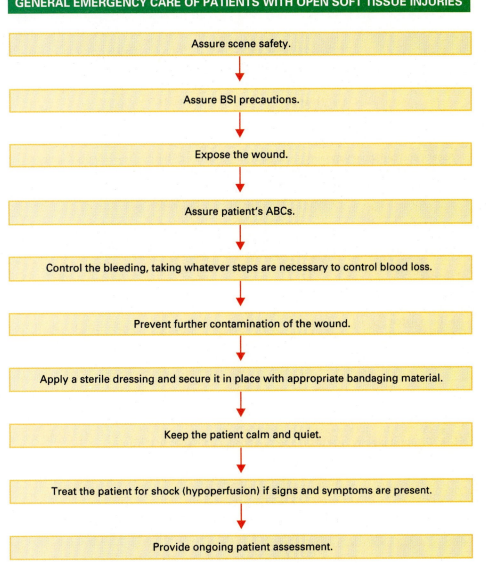

GENERAL EMERGENCY CARE OF PATIENTS WITH OPEN SOFT TISSUE INJURIES

Assure scene safety.

↓

Assure BSI precautions.

↓

Expose the wound.

↓

Assure patient's ABCs.

↓

Control the bleeding, taking whatever steps are necessary to control blood loss.

↓

Prevent further contamination of the wound.

↓

Apply a sterile dressing and secure it in place with appropriate bandaging material.

↓

Keep the patient calm and quiet.

↓

Treat the patient for shock (hypoperfusion) if signs and symptoms are present.

↓

Provide ongoing patient assessment.

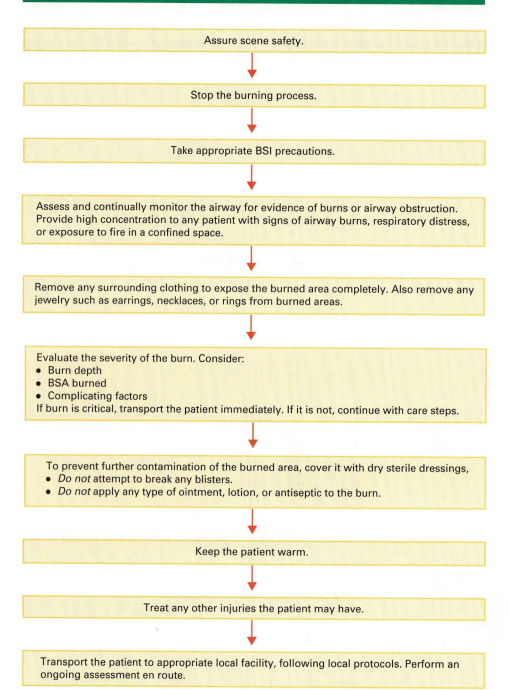

Assure scene safety.

↓

Stop the burning process.

↓

Take appropriate BSI precautions.

↓

Assess and continually monitor the airway for evidence of burns or airway obstruction. Provide high concentration to any patient with signs of airway burns, respiratory distress, or exposure to fire in a confined space.

↓

Remove any surrounding clothing to expose the burned area completely. Also remove any jewelry such as earrings, necklaces, or rings from burned areas.

↓

Evaluate the severity of the burn. Consider:
• Burn depth
• BSA burned
• Complicating factors
If burn is critical, transport the patient immediately. If it is not, continue with care steps.

↓

To prevent further contamination of the burned area, cover it with dry sterile dressings,
• *Do not* attempt to break any blisters.
• *Do not* apply any type of ointment, lotion, or antiseptic to the burn.

↓

Keep the patient warm.

↓

Treat any other injuries the patient may have.

↓

Transport the patient to appropriate local facility, following local protocols. Perform an ongoing assessment en route.

Musculoskeletal Injuries

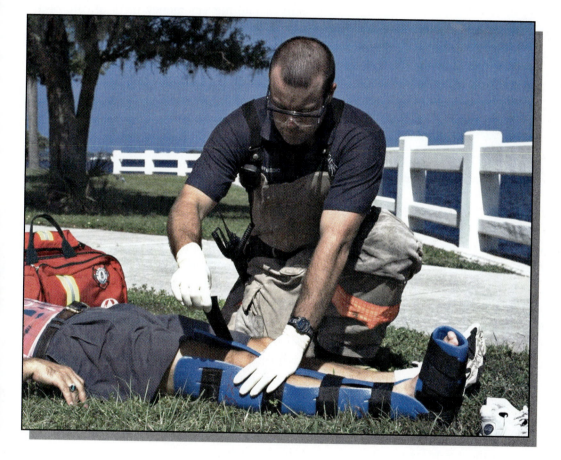

*E*MTs commonly encounter injuries to the musculoskeletal system. Injuries to bones and associated structures can occur as isolated injuries or in the setting of multiple traumas. Most musculoskeletal injuries that do not involve the spine are not immediately life threatening. The appropriate prehospital emergency care of these injuries can reduce the risks of both short- and long-term complications affecting the bones and associated structures.

At the completion of this chapter, the EMT-Basic student should be able to meet the following objectives:

Knowledge and Understanding

1. Describe the functions of the muscular system. (p. 519)
2. Describe the functions of the skeletal system. (p. 521)
3. List the major bones or bone groupings of the spinal column; the thorax; the upper extremities; the lower extremities. (pp. 519–521)
4. Differentiate between an open and a closed painful, swollen, deformed extremity. (pp. 524–525)
5. State the reasons for splinting. (p. 527)
6. List the general rules for splinting. (pp. 528–532)
7. List the complications of splinting. (p. 527)
8. List the emergency medical care for patients with a painful, swollen, deformed extremity. (pp. 526–527)
9. Explain the rational for splinting at the scene versus "load and go" management. (pp. 526–527)
10. Explain the rationale for immobilization of the painful, swollen, deformed extremity. (p. 527)

Skills

1. Demonstrate the emergency medical care of a patient with a painful, swollen, deformed extremity.
2. Demonstrate completing a prehospital care report for patients with musculoskeletal injuries.

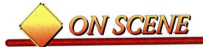

ON SCENE

DISPATCH: *LADDER 11 AND AMBULANCE 2, RESPOND TO 17 BROADWAY, THE GYMNASIUM OF ST. MATTHEW'S ACADEMY FOR A REPORTED LEG INJURY. TIME OUT IS 1524.*

You are the acting captain on Ladder 11. As your truck leaves the station, you notify the dispatcher via the mobile data terminal that you are en route to the call. You are aware that the response of the paramedics on Ambulance 2 is likely to be delayed because they are at the hospital restocking supplies after transport and care of a cardiac arrest patient.

As your unit approaches the scene, you note that it is close to dismissal time. Many school buses are lined up in the parking lot. Large numbers of children crowd the steps and walks at the front of the school. Your driver maneuvers Ladder 11 through the lot slowly and carefully toward the wing of the building that contains the gym. A man in sweat clothes is standing by an open door there, waving you in. You radio your arrival to the dispatcher and request that Ambu-

lance 2 be advised of the congestion present at the scene. You make sure that one of the crew members brings the splint bag from the EMS supply compartment as you get off the truck.

As you enter the gym, you note a crowd of children and adults surrounding a boy lying on the floor at the far end of the basketball court. As you walk toward the apparent patient, the man who had been waving from the door says, "I'm Coach Davis and the boy who's down is Kevin Wallace. Kevin came down from a rebound and heard something snap in his ankle."

When you reach the patient's side, you observe that he is a boy of about 12, lying supine and grimacing in pain. You introduce yourself and add, "Kevin, we're here to help you. How are you feeling now?"

"I hurt my leg real bad," he replies. You can tell from this response that his airway and breathing are adequate.

"Did you hurt yourself anywhere else, Kevin?"

He shakes his head and says, "No."

Two crew members move to Kevin's leg to begin an assessment. Because Kevin is wearing shorts, the swelling and deformity of his right lower leg just above the ankle is immediately evident. While the two crew members stabilize Kevin's leg and continue assessment of the injury, you carefully explain to the patient that the other EMTs will be asking him questions and splinting his leg.

After assessing and determining that both a strong pulse and sensation are present in Kevin's foot distal to the injury site, your crew applies a rigid lower leg splint that covers not only the injury site but immobilizes the knee joint and ankle as well. After the splint is applied, they reassess and find that normal pulse and sensation are still present below the injury site. The crew has just obtained a set of baseline vital signs when the paramedics of Ambulance 2 arrive with their stretcher. Your crew members gently move Kevin onto the ambulance stretcher, being careful to support his splinted leg.

While you provide an oral report and a copy of the patient's baseline vital signs to the paramedics, the patient's father arrives. He climbs into the ambulance to accompany Kevin to the hospital. Your crew prepares to put your unit back in service. As they do, you briefly talk about fire safety to the students who are now hanging out around the truck.

To properly assess and care for musculoskeletal injuries, you should understand some basics of the anatomy and physiology of the musculoskeletal system. You should also be aware of the common mechanisms that cause injuries to the bones and associated structures.

ANATOMY AND PHYSIOLOGY OF THE MUSCULOSKELETAL SYSTEM

The musculoskeletal system has three major functions:

◆ It gives the body shape.

◆ It protects vital internal organs.

◆ It provides for body movement.

Bones of the Pelvis and Extremities

The bones of the musculoskeletal system provide the body's physical structure and serve to protect the internal organs. The bones of the body make up the human skeleton and are thus considered the "skeletal" system (Figure 21-1). This chapter will discuss injuries to the musculoskeletal structures of the pelvis and the extremities. Injuries to the bones of the head and spine will be covered in Chapter 22.

The pelvis is made up of two sets of paired bones, the ilium and the ischium. The pelvis is joined anteriorly at the **pubis** and posteriorly on both sides at the sacral spine. The **iliac crest** of the pelvis can be palpated laterally and the **ischium** can be palpated inferiorly.

The lower extremities extend from the pelvis, where the head of the femur forms a ball that sits in the indentation or socket of the pelvis called the **acetabulum** to form the hip joint (Figure 21-2). The femur angles downward at the greater trochanter to form the thigh bone. Three bones form the knee joint—the distal femur, the **patella** or knee cap, and the proximal **tibia.** The lower leg is formed by the tibia (shin bone) and the **fibula** laterally. The distal lateral portion of the fibula is the **lateral malleolus** and the distal medial portion of the tibia is the **medial malleolus.** These two structures are the surface landmarks of the ankle joint, which is formed by the connection of the lower leg bones to the **tarsal bones** of the foot. A tarsal bone called the **calcaneus,** or heel bone, is the most posterior portion of the foot. In the mid-

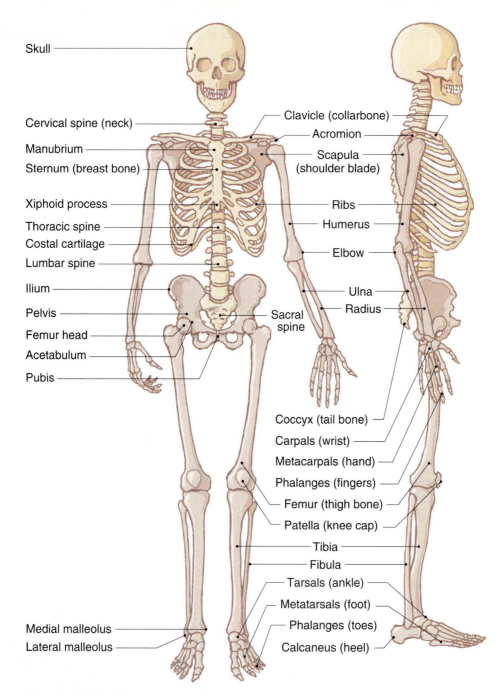

Skull

Cervical spine (neck)

Manubrium

Sternum (breast bone)

Xiphoid process

Thoracic spine

Costal cartilage

Lumbar spine

Ilium

Pelvis

Femur head

Acetabulum

Pubis

Clavicle (collarbone)

Acromion

Scapula (shoulder blade)

Ribs

Humerus

Elbow

Ulna

Radius

Sacral spine

Coccyx (tail bone)

Carpals (wrist)

Metacarpals (hand)

Phalanges (fingers)

Femur (thigh bone)

Patella (knee cap)

Tibia

Fibula

Tarsals (ankle)

Metatarsals (foot)

Phalanges (toes)

Calcaneus (heel)

Medial malleolus

Lateral malleolus

Figure 21-1   The human skeleton.

foot are the **metatarsal bones,** which connect to the toes **(phalanges).** The toes are clinically identified by numbers, with the great toe being the first toe and the small toe being the fifth.

The upper extremities extend from the shoulder (Figure 21-3). Each shoulder is made up of a **scapula** (shoulder blade), **clavicle** (collar bone), and **acromion** (which forms the lateral tip of the shoulder). The head of the **humerus** rests in the shoulder joint. The humerus forms the proximal portion of the upper extremity commonly called the "arm." The elbow joint is the connection between the distal humerus and the two bones of the forearm, the **radius** (lateral and aligning with the thumb) and the **ulna** (medial and aligning with the fifth finger). The bony prominence easily palpated on the posterior aspect of the elbow is the **olecranon** process of the ulna.

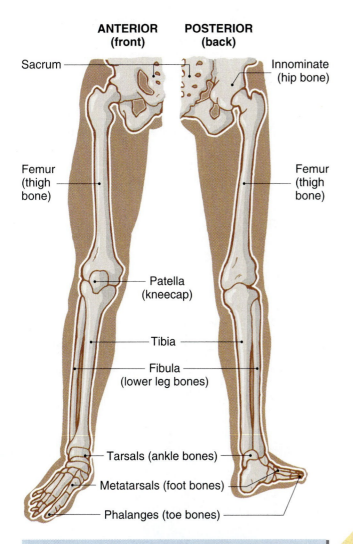

ANTERIOR (front)   **POSTERIOR** (back)

Sacrum

Innominate (hip bone)

Femur (thigh bone)

Femur (thigh bone)

Patella (kneecap)

Tibia

Fibula (lower leg bones)

Tarsals (ankle bones)

Metatarsals (foot bones)

Phalanges (toe bones)

THE LOWER EXTREMITIES

COMMON NAME	ANATOMICAL NAME
Pelvic girdle (pelvis or hips)	Ilium and ischium joined anteriorly at pubis and posteriorly at sacral spine
Thigh bone (1/limb)	Femur (FE-mer)
Kneecap (1/limb)	Patella (pah-TEL-lah)
Shin bone (1/limb)	Tibia (TIB-e-ah) – medial
	Fibula (FIB-yo-lah) – lateral
Ankle bones (7/foot)	Tarsals (TAR-sals)
Foot bones (5/foot)	Metatarsals (meta-TAR-sals)
Toe bones (14/foot. Some people have two bones in their little toe, others may have three.)	Phalanges (fah-LAN-jez)

Figure 21-2   The bones of the lower extremities.

The wrist is made up of the distal radius and ulna and the proximal bones of the hand called the **carpals.** The carpals connect to the **metacarpals,** which form the bones of the palm of the hand. The fingers or **phalanges** are also clinically identified by number, with the thumb being the first finger, and the little finger being the fifth.

Connective Tissue, Joints, and Muscles

The human skeleton can move as it does because the body has many joints. **Joints** are the places where bones connect to other bones. Joints are held together and kept stable by strong band-like connective tissue called **ligaments.** The two most common types of joints are **ball-and-socket joints** like the hip and **hinge joints** like the finger joints. **Muscles** are attached to bones by **tendons** and with them allow movement across joints (Figure 21-4, page 523). The muscles that move the body are called **skeletal** or **voluntary muscles** because they can be purposefully, or voluntarily, controlled by the brain to move many of the bones that make up the human skeleton (Figure 21-5, page 523). These muscles are different from the smooth muscles found in many internal organs and the cardiac muscles found only in the heart.

TRAUMA AND THE MUSCULOSKELETAL SYSTEM

One of the most serious types of trauma the musculoskeletal system can sustain is a break or fracture to a bone. When a bone is broken, the normal structure and contour of the part of the body supported by the bone can become greatly deformed.

A break or fracture of a bone can also cause serious bleeding. Some of this bleeding can come from the bone itself. Although very hard, bones are made of living tissue with a rich blood supply. Other bleeding can come from vessels near the bone. The body's major arteries often run alongside long bones like the femur or humerus. When a bone breaks, its jagged edges can damage surrounding blood vessels and other tissue such as muscles. The bleeding from the bone and from damaged blood vessels and tissue can lead to substantial swelling at the site of injury.

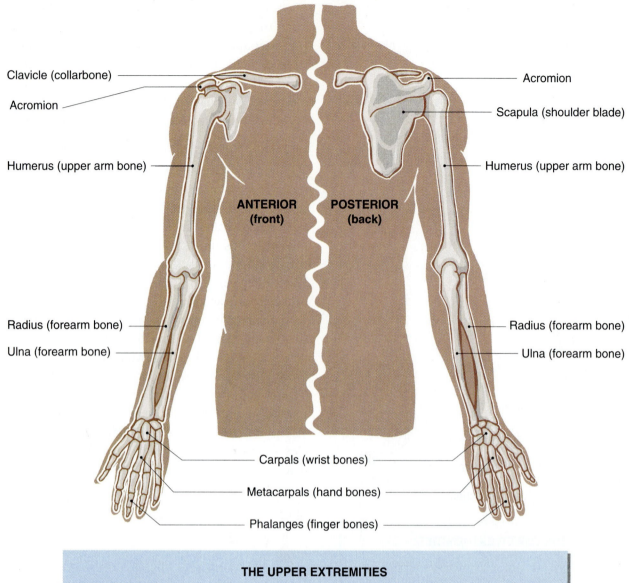

Clavicle (collarbone)

Acromion

Humerus (upper arm bone)

ANTERIOR (front)

POSTERIOR (back)

Acromion

Scapula (shoulder blade)

Humerus (upper arm bone)

Radius (forearm bone)

Ulna (forearm bone)

Radius (forearm bone)

Ulna (forearm bone)

Carpals (wrist bones)

Metacarpals (hand bones)

Phalanges (finger bones)

THE UPPER EXTREMITIES

COMMON NAME	ANATOMICAL NAME
Shoulder girdle	Pectoral girdle (pek-TOR-al): clavicle, scapula, and head of humerus
Collarbone (1/side)	Clavicle (KLAV-i-kul)
Shoulder blade (1/side)	Scapula (SKAP-u-lah)
Arm bone (1/limb, from shoulder to elbow)	Humerus (HU-mer-us)
Forearm bones (2/limb, from elbow to wrist: 1/medial, 1/lateral)	Ulna (UL-nah)–medial Radius (RAY-de-us)–lateral
Wrist bones (8/wrist)	Carpals (KAR-pals)
Hand bones (5/palm, palm bones)	Metacarpals (meta-KAR-pals)
Finger bones (14/hand)	Phalanges (fah-LAN-jez)

Figure 21-3   The bones of the upper extremities.

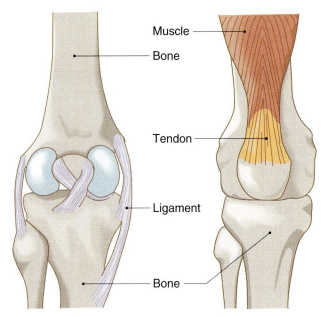

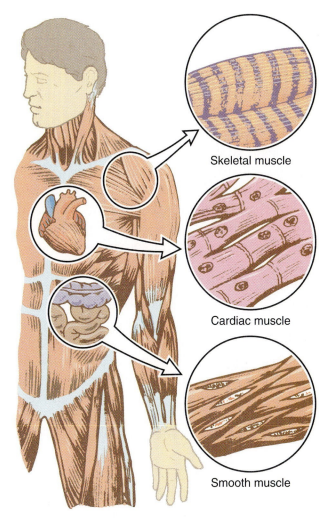

Figure 21-4   The knee joint. Ligaments attach bone to bone. Tendons attach muscle to bone.

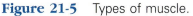

Breaks or fractures in bones can also affect nearby nerves. The nerves may be damaged or compressed as a result of the trauma. Nerve involvement can produce the symptom of pain and the sign of tenderness at the injury site.

The combination of loss of structure, internal bleeding, and involvement of nerves leads to the classic finding associated with musculoskeletal injuries—a painful, swollen, and deformed area. *All injuries that result in a painful, swollen, and deformed area are presumed to be serious and to require appropriate immobilization with splinting.*

Mechanisms of Musculoskeletal Injury

Injuries to the bones, muscles, and connective tissues result when excessive or abnormal force is applied to the musculoskeletal system. There are three basic mechanisms by which this force can be applied (Figure 21-6).

Direct Force

The easiest-to-understand mechanism that produces musculoskeletal injury is **direct force.** With this mechanism, force is applied directly to the bone or other structure. Injury occurs where the force is applied. Examples of direct force injuries would include the ulna of the forearm that is broken when a person is struck by a pipe during an assault or the painful, swollen, and deformed fin-

Figure 21-5   Types of muscle.

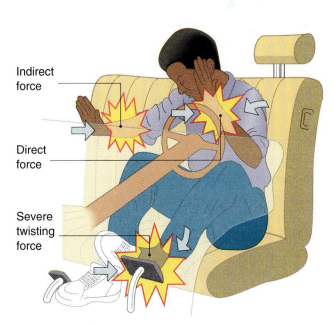

Figure 21-6   Mechanisms of musculoskeletal injury.

gers that result when a brick falls onto a construction worker's hand.

Indirect Force

Indirect force can also cause musculoskeletal injury. In this case, energy is applied to the body in one area and transmitted through the bones to cause injury at another site. A typical example of this type of injury occurs during a head-on collision. Energy that enters the body when a passenger jams his knees against the car dashboard is then transmitted up his legs, resulting in a fracture of the midshaft femur or a posterior dislocation of the hip.

Twisting Force

Twisting force is a variation of indirect force. In twisting force injuries, the weight and motion of the body itself contributes to the application of abnormal strain on the bones and joints of the body. These types of injuries are common in sports activities. An example is when a skier falls on a slope, twisting his torso in opposition to his lower extremities, causing an injury to his lower leg.

Types of Musculoskeletal Injuries

It will not be your responsibility as an EMT to try to decide exactly what type of injury to the musculoskeletal system has occurred. The fact is that *any* painful, swollen, and deformed extremity will receive the same emergency medical care. That care is based on preventing further injury and reducing pain by stabilizing the injury through use of an appropriate splinting technique.

It is helpful, however, for you to understand the medical terminology used to describe common musculoskeletal injuries:

◆ *Fracture* When a bone is broken or is simply cracked, the condition is termed a **fracture.** Fractures can produce severe bleeding, great pain for the patient, and the potential for long-term disability from the injury. The risk of disability is greatest when the fracture occurs at the end of a bone where it forms a joint or in the growing areas of children's bones called *growth plates.*

◆ *Dislocation* Disruption of the normal structure of a joint where one bone connects (artic-

ulates) with another is called a **dislocation.** The extreme flexion or extension of a joint is what usually renders a joint "dislocated." Finger joints, the shoulder, and the hip are the most common sites of dislocations that you will encounter.

◆ *Sprain* A stretching or tearing of the ligaments that surround or support a joint is called a **sprain.** Sprains commonly result from the application of twisting force to a body part. For example, a patient might miss a step off a curb and twist his ankle medially under his lower leg resulting in damage to ligaments surrounding the ankle joint.

◆ *Strain* The injury that results from the abnormal stretching of the tendons that connect muscles to bones and of the muscles themselves is called a **strain.**

COMPANY OFFICER'S NOTES

One of the crucial tasks of the fire officer is maintaining a broad perspective of the emergency scene that confronts the crew. To accomplish this, an officer should try to be "less hands on, and more heads up" than the firefighters under his or her command. During an EMS call, this need for maintaining a view of the big picture still applies.

When firefighter EMTs are providing emergency medical care for a patient with both musculoskeletal injuries and other serious trauma, it is the officer in charge of the EMS operation who should be sure that the crew works toward the goal of moving the patient off the scene as rapidly as possible. The officer should assure that valuable time in the "Golden Hour" is focused on packaging and transporting the patient rather than squandered in splinting minor fractures. It is often difficult for EMTs heavily involved in patient care to maintain this officer-level objectivity.

Open and Closed Musculoskeletal Injuries

As was the case with soft tissue injuries, injuries to the musculoskeletal system are also classified as either open or closed. When the skin overlying a painful, swollen, and deformed extremity is bro-

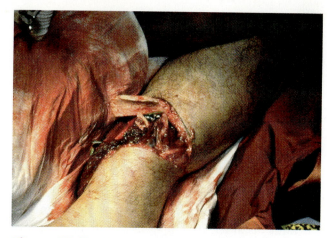

Figure 21-7 An open musculoskeletal injury of the lower leg with bone fragments protruding.

ken, then the condition is termed an **open musculoskeletal injury** (Figure 21-7). If there is no break in the continuity of the skin, then the condition is termed a **closed musculoskeletal**

Figure 21-8 Photographs showing visible swelling and deformity with closed musculoskeletal injuries and corresponding x-rays revealing underlying damage. **A.** Dislocation of the knee. **B.** Fracture and dislocation of the wrist.

A.

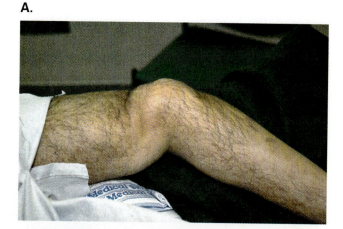

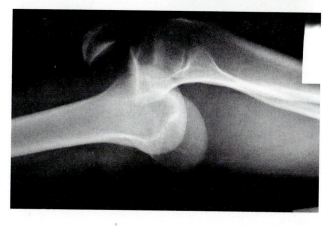

injury (Figure 21-8). Prehospital personnel usually assume that an injury is closed unless otherwise informed; therefore, during a transition of care be sure to report the fact when you have a patient with an open injury.

Open, painful, swollen, and deformed extremity injuries are of particular concern because they may have resulted from fractured bone puncturing the skin from within rather than from an external object breaking the skin. Open fractures are an orthopedic emergency because they carry a high risk for development of limb-threatening infection in the exposed bone.

B.

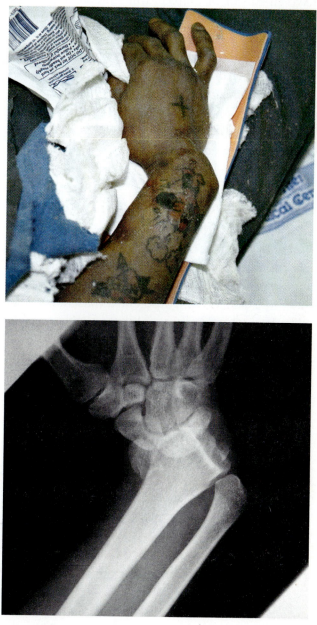

Assessment of Musculoskeletal Injuries

The scene size-up is a critical part of any call for suspected musculoskeletal injuries. During it, you will of course take appropriate BSI precautions and assure the safety of yourself and the patient. However, you should also pay particular attention to any potential mechanisms of injury that may have caused the patient's problem.

Remember to follow the steps of the patient assessment process. Musculoskeletal injuries can often be gory and grotesque. They can easily distract you from properly checking for and treating potential life-threatening conditions. Once you have ruled out or corrected life-threatening problems with the ABCs, you can turn your attention to the musculoskeletal injuries.

Perform a focused history and physical exam. If the patient is unresponsive or the mechanism of injury is significant, start with a rapid trauma assessment. If the patient is responsive or the mechanism of injury is not significant, perform a focused trauma assessment. Remember to record baseline vital signs and obtain a SAMPLE history if possible.

Signs and Symptoms of a Musculoskeletal Injury

When bones, tendons, muscles, or ligaments are injured, you can expect to observe certain signs and symptoms (Figure 21-9). During the assessment of a patient with a potential musculoskeletal injury, you should assess carefully to determine if any of the following are present:

◆ Deformity or abnormal angulation (difference in shape or position) of an extremity

◆ Pain and tenderness at the site of the injury

◆ Swelling

◆ Bruising or discoloration at the site

◆ The sensation or sound of grating of bones **(crepitus)** if the limb is moved

◆ Open wounds or exposed bone at the site of injury

◆ A joint that no longer moves normally or is locked into position

◆ Paleness, coolness, or lack of pulse in the limb distal to the injury (a sign that the artery that supplies the distal limb has been disrupted within the injury site)

Of these signs and symptoms, those most commonly encountered with musculoskeletal injuries are pain, swelling, and deformity of the extremity.

◆ Emergency Care— Musculoskeletal Injuries

Whenever you encounter a patient with a painful, swollen, or deformed extremity, assume a musculoskeletal injury is present. Treat the injury as if a fracture has occurred. Even if a fracture has not occurred, the basic prehospital emergency care is the same.

Although the splinting of painful, swollen, deformed extremities is a key part of the emergency medical care of musculoskeletal injuries, you must keep the "big picture" of the patient's condition in mind as you treat him. Although it is ideal to splint all the painful, swollen, and deformed injuries you encounter, splinting should never take priority over assessing and assuring that the patient has an open airway and adequate

Figure 21-9 Signs and symptoms of musculoskeletal injury.

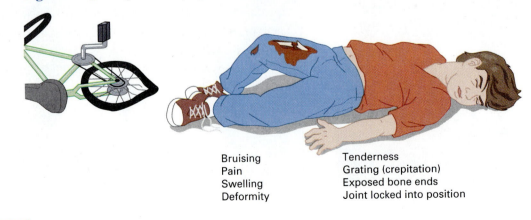

Bruising
Pain
Swelling
Deformity

Tenderness
Grating (crepitation)
Exposed bone ends
Joint locked into position

breathing and circulation. This is especially true in cases where the patient has sustained multiple serious injuries. In such a setting, avoid the error of "splinting a patient to death." You do a patient no good by applying five splints in the field when the patient is in life-threatening shock and your focus should be on providing rapid transport to a facility where definitive care could be provided.

The general emergency medical care of patients with injuries to the musculoskeletal system includes the following steps:

1. **Perform a thorough scene size-up.** Take appropriate BSI precautions and ensure scene safety. Study the area to detect any possible mechanisms of injury.

2. **Perform an initial assessment to assure that the patient has an open airway and adequate breathing and circulation.** If the airway, breathing, or circulation is compromised, attempt to correct the problem(s). When the ABCs are compromised, correcting the problems and initiating transport become the patient care priorities, not managing the musculoskeletal injuries. If a priority patient requires rapid transport, provide "whole body splinting" by securing him to a long backboard.

3. **Administer high flow oxygen if indicated by shortness of breath, inadequate breathing, or signs of shock (hypoperfusion).**

4. **Control any bleeding from open wounds.**

5. **After you have controlled any immediate life-threats, splint painful, swollen, or deformed extremities in preparation for transport.** (Follow the "General Guidelines for Splinting" below.)

6. **Once you have applied a splint, elevate the limb if possible and apply a cold pack to reduce swelling and pain at the site of injury.**

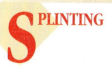

SPLINTING

The goal in caring for musculoskeletal injuries is stabilization of the injury site to reduce the likeli-

hood of further injury and reduce pain. The most common means of stabilizing these injuries is by splinting. Remember, however, that you will begin to splint the injuries only after other life-threatening conditions have been corrected or stabilized. In situations where a patient has a life-threatening condition and painful, swollen deformities are present, splint the patient as a unit by immobilizing him to a long backboard while you try to manage the airway, breathing, and circulation.

Splinting stabilizes the skeleton where stability has been lost due to injury. Splinting prevents or minimizes further movement of fractured bones and bone fragments. Without splinting, fractures of the bones can result in the following:

◆ Further damage to nerves, muscles, and blood vessels caused by the sharp bone ends created by a fracture

◆ Increased internal bleeding as bone edges injure additional soft tissue during movement

◆ Increased suffering for the patient due to the pain of fractured bone movement

◆ Conversion of a closed injury to a more serious open injury as edges of fractured bones push through the skin from underneath

Splinting must be done carefully and correctly. Splinting that is performed incorrectly or that is performed without proper regard for the patient's overall condition can result in the following:

◆ Any of the complications associated with fractured bones that are listed above can occur when a splint is too loose.

◆ Compression of the blood vessels, nerves, muscles, or other soft tissues can occur when the splint is too tight.

◆ A patient's death can result when patient priorities are ignored or incorrectly assigned—for example, when time is spent splinting extremity injuries rather than transporting a patient with other life-threatening injuries.

Types of Splints

Splinting is a skill that takes repeated practice to master. Once you learn basic splinting techniques, be aware that you may have to exercise consider-

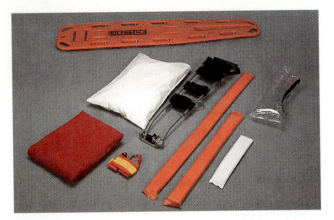

Figure 21-10 An array of different splints and accessories.

able ingenuity in adapting those techniques to certain types of extremity injuries. As you splint a patient's injury, always remember that the goal of splinting is to stabilize a part of the body that has been rendered potentially unstable due to injury.

A wide variety of splinting devices is available to stabilize the many different types of musculoskeletal injuries you may encounter (Figure 21-10). Some of these devices are only appropriate with certain types of injuries and are less useful or even contraindicated with other injuries and conditions. Become familiar with these devices and the ways they can best be used.

◆ **Rigid splints** These splints are ideal for stabilizing extremity injuries that involve the shafts of long bones such as those of the forearm and lower leg. Examples of rigid splints include padded board splints, preformed

Figure 21-11 An example of a commercially produced rigid splint system.

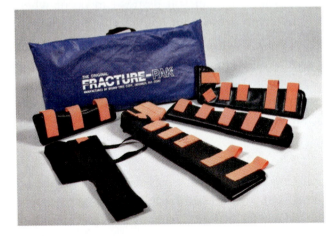

splints, ladder splints, and box splints (Figure 21-11).

◆ **Traction splints** Traction splints are specifically designed to stabilize injuries that result in pain, swelling, or deformity in the mid-thigh (Figure 21-12). Examples of traction splints include the Thomas half-ring, Hare™, and Sager™ splints.

◆ **Pneumatic splints** Pneumatic splints use either air pressure (inflatable air splint) or a vacuum to immobilize injuries (Figure 21-13). These splints are very useful when immobilizing injuries to joints such as the elbow or ankle.

◆ **Pneumatic anti-shock garment (PASG)** The PASG can be used as a splint for the patient with a pelvic injury or one with multiple lower extremity injuries that require rapid immobilization. When used as a splint, the PASG is usually inflated to a pressure of about 30 mm Hg. Be sure to follow local protocols regarding use of the PASG.

◆ **Sling and swathe** The sling and swathe, which can be formed from triangular bandages, are often used for shoulder, upper arm, elbow, and forearm injuries. The sling cradles the elbow and forearm, while the swathe splints the injured extremity against the body to further reduce potential movement.

◆ **Improvised splints** In emergency situations when actual splints are not available, many readily available objects can be used to splint painful, swollen, and deformed extremities. For example, a pillow might be wrapped around an ankle and secured with cravats to stabilize an ankle injury (Figure 21-14). Or a rolled-up newspaper might substitute for a rigid splint when stabilizing a forearm injury.

General Guidelines for Splinting

No matter what type of splint you use, there are some general guidelines that you should keep in mind when applying the device (Figure 21-15, page 530). These include the following:

◆ Keep splinting simple.

◆ Use the device that is best suited for the injured area.

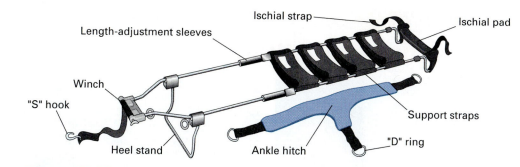

Figure 21-12   A bipolar traction splint.

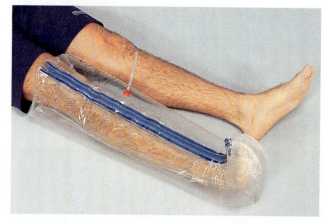

Figure 21-13   An air splint.

If you have any doubts about whether or not an injury involves the bones and/or related structures, assume that it does and splint the injury.

If the patient with musculoskeletal injuries has signs of shock (hypoperfusion) or any other condition that make transport a priority, then

Figure 21-14   An improvised pillow splint.

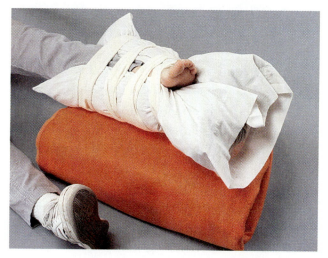

align the injuries in normal anatomic position and secure the patient to a long backboard. This will provide adequate immobilization in this situation where rapid transport is a higher priority than splinting.

Never delay transport of a seriously injured patient in order to splint every painful, swollen, or deformed extremity.

Before splinting, assign one rescuer to manually stabilize the injury site by placing one hand proximal to and one hand distal to the injury. Stabilization should be held until the splint is applied and secured.

Before splinting, assess the pulse, motor function, and sensation in the extremity distal to the injury. When you have completed splinting, reassess distal pulse, motor function, and sensation. Always document your findings on the patient care report both before and after splinting.

Remove or cut away any clothing around a painful, swollen, or deformed area of injury. Carefully assess the area for any open wounds.

Cover any open wounds with sterile dressings and secure them in place with tape or bandages before splinting.

If there is severe deformity to the extremity or if the distal extremity is cyanotic (bluish-gray) or lacks a pulse, realign the limb in its normal anatomic orientation by applying gentle manual traction (pulling) before splinting.

If you see bone edges coming through an open injury, do not try to push them back into the wound.

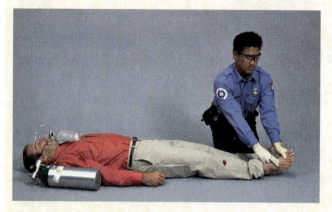

Figure 21-15A Assess pulse, motor function, and sensation function distal to the injury.

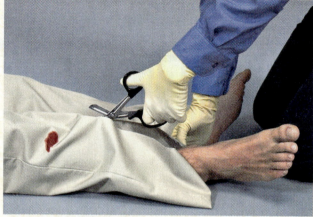

Figure 21-15B Cut away clothing, if necessary, to expose the injury site.

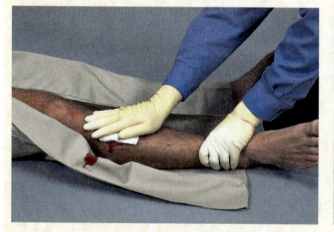

Figure 21-15C Cover an open wound with a sterile dressing and secure it in place.

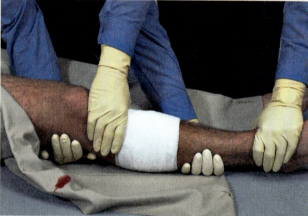

Figure 21-15D Use gentle manual traction to realign the extremity if there is severe deformity, cyanosis, or absence of a pulse distal to the injury.

◆ Pad each splint to prevent pressure and discomfort to the patient.

◆ Pad open or hollow spaces (voids) between the splint and the patient whenever possible.

◆ Splint the patient before moving him whenever possible, unless there are potentially life-threatening conditions that mandate more rapid transport.

◆ Immobilize the joints above and below the injury site. For example, with an injury to the mid-forearm immobilize both the wrist and elbow in addition to the injury site.

◆ Immobilize the bones above and below the site of a joint injury. For example, with an elbow injury immobilize both the upper arm and the forearm.

◆ When splinting distal extremities including the hands and feet, always leave the tips of fingers and toes exposed so that you can assess distal circulation during transport.

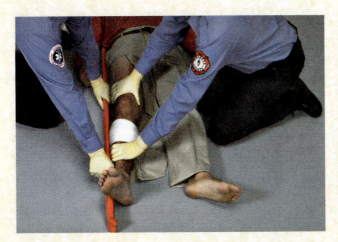

Figure 21-15E Select a splint that will immobilize the extremity above and below the injury.

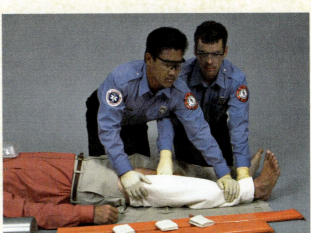

Figure 21-15F Pad the splint to prevent discomfort for the patient.

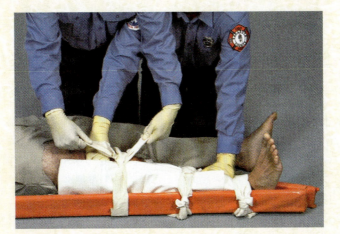

Figure 21-15G Maintain manual traction until the splint has been secured in place. Then reassess pulse and motor and sensory function distal to the injury.

◆ When splinting the arm, forearm, wrist, hand, or fingers, remove any bracelets, wrist watches, or rings that may cut off circulation as distal swelling develops. Bag the items and give them to a family member or be sure they are transported along with the patient.

Realigning Injured Extremities

If a musculoskeletal injury has decreased or completely stopped the flow of blood to a distal extremity, you should try to realign the extremity before you splint it. The distal extremity in these cases will be cyanotic (bluish-gray) or pale and lack a pulse.

Realigning an injured extremity can be an intimidating experience for many EMTs. There is a natural worry that realignment will cause the patient further pain. Also, there may be a fear of doing further damage to the extremity. If you are faced with the need to realign an extremity, remember that the maneuver may save the patient's limb, which is threatened by the compromised blood flow.

Begin a realignment by first supporting the limb above and below the site of the injury. Then apply gentle traction (pulling) along the long axis of the bone. In some cases, it may be necessary to rotate the limb to return it to its normal position. In these cases, apply traction and rotate simultaneously in one smooth action.

Some pain and grating of bone ends is inevitable when realigning a limb. Keep in mind that the only reason you are performing the maneuver is to save an endangered limb. However, if you encounter a lot of resistance as you attempt to realign the limb or if it appears that bone ends will come through the skin, stop attempts at realignment and splint the extremity in the position in which you found it.

Splinting Long Bone Injuries

The long bones of the body include the upper extremity long bones (humerus, radius, ulna, metacarpals, and phalanges) and lower extremity long bones (femur, tibia, fibula, metatarsals, and phalanges). Long bone injuries are injuries that occur along the shafts of the bone(s) of the extremity. Remember that long bone injuries may also involve injuries to adjacent joints.

In addition to following the general guidelines for splinting above, perform these steps when splinting a long bone injury:

1. **Perform a scene size-up and assure scene safety.** Determine the mechanism of injury and that there is no continued risk to you or the patient from it.

2. **Take appropriate BSI precautions.**

3. **Stabilize the injury site manually.**

4. **Assess pulse, motor function, and sensation distal to the injury site before splinting.** Document your findings.

5. **If there is severe deformity present or if the distal limb is cyanotic or pulseless, gently realign the limb into normal anatomic position by using manual traction.** If you feel significant resistance, stop

attempts at realignment and splint the limb in the position you found it.

6. **Select and measure an appropriate splint.**

7. **Assure that not only the injury site but also the joints above and below it are also immobilized.**

8. **Reassess distal pulse, motor function, and sensation after splinting.** Document your findings.

9. **Protect the splinted extremity during all subsequent movement of the patient.** Assign one person to manually stabilize the splinted long bone injury to assure this protection. Make sure that the entire injured extremity is adequately secured and protected.

10. **Elevate the splinted injured limb and apply cold packs if possible.**

Special Techniques for Long Bone Injuries

Because of differences in the structure, location, and functions of the various long bones and the joints they comprise, there are some special splinting techniques that you should use when splinting injuries in these areas. Skill Summaries depicting these techniques are collected on pages 537–544 at the end of this chapter.

Injuries to the Arms

Injuries that involve the humerus are best splinted with a sling and swathe. (See Figure 21-21, pages 537–538.) A rigid splint can also be used in conjunction with the sling and swathe.

With injuries to the forearm bones, the best choices for immobilization are a padded board splint secured with a rolled bandage, a commercially produced forearm splint, or a pneumatic splint. Once the splint is applied, place the forearm in a sling and swathe to immobilize the elbow and wrist joints and to further protect the injured site. (Other splinting techniques involving the arms are shown in Figure 21-22, page 539.)

Injuries to the Hand

When there are injuries to the hand and also when you are splinting injuries to the wrist and forearm, you should immobilize the hand in a **position of function.** This is the position of the hand in which the fingers are slightly curled, as if they are holding a ball.

Put the hand into a position of function by placing a rolled bulky dressing in the palm of the patient's hand. Then, when treating a hand injury, immobilize the forearm with a padded board splint so that the distal portion of the splint supports the wrist and the proximal part of the hand. This procedure places the hand in slight flexion. The entire forearm, wrist, and hand can be wrapped in a rolled gauze bandage. You can then place the splinted extremity in a sling. (Several ways of splinting injuries to the forearm, wrist, and hand are shown in Figure 21-22, page 539.)

Injuries to the Feet

When there are injuries to the long bones of the feet (and also when you are splinting injuries to the ankle and lower leg), the foot should also be immobilized in a position of function. In this position, the foot is at its normal 90° angle to the leg. To accomplish this, splint the entire lower extremity in a preformed or ladder splint that supports the sole of the foot at the proper angle to the lower leg.

There is a strong association between heel (calcaneus) fractures and spinal injuries when patients fall from height. Because of this, patients who have received head injuries in such falls should have both their feet and lower legs splinted and receive spinal immobilization on a long backboard.

Injuries to the Lower Legs

Immobilize painful, swollen, and deformed injuries to the lower legs with rigid splints. If you use a rigid splint, select one long enough to immobilize both the knee and the ankle of the injured leg. Alternatively, you can place padding such as a folded or rolled blanket between the patient's legs, bind the legs together with folded triangular bandages or wide straps, and place the patient on a backboard.

Injuries to the Thighs

Always assume that a painful, swollen, and deformed injury to the thigh region is the result of

a fractured femur. This is a serious injury and may result in blood loss totaling several liters. In fact, a fractured femur poses the greatest risk of causing significant blood loss and shock (hypoperfusion) of all the long bone fractures. The large muscles of the thigh are extremely strong; when they contract after an injury they can pull the ends of a fractured femur and cause them to overlap. The jagged ends of the femur can then severely damage the tissues and large arteries found in the thigh.

Before development of the prehospital traction splint during World War I, a fractured femur was often a fatal injury. Development of the traction splint provided a better way of stabilizing the fractured femur. This meant a great reduction in blood loss from these injuries and in other complications associated with them.

> ### COMPANY OFFICER'S NOTES
> When some types of traction splints are applied to tall patients, the splint can extend well beyond the end of the ambulance stretcher. If this happens, be certain that the end of the splint is supported by a backboard. Sometimes, the "package" of a tall patient with a traction splint who is immobilized on a stretcher may be too long to allow the back doors of the ambulance to close. It may be necessary to load the patient onto the stretcher so that his head is near the back doors and the leg with the splint is pointed toward the front of the ambulance.
>
> If a patient is being packaged for helicopter evacuation, be aware that certain brands of traction splints may not fit onto the helicopter. You should learn whether the helicopter(s) that service your jurisdiction can accommodate the type of traction splint carried on your unit.

A traction splint immobilizes an injured femur by first establishing two fixed points surrounding the injury—at the ring of the pelvis (proximal to the injury) and at the ankle (distal to the injury). Tension is created between the two points with a ratchet device at the distal part of the splint. As tension is increased, the broken ends of the femur are realigned, lessening the likelihood of damage to tissues, nerves, and blood vessels.

The traction splint is the splinting device of choice when stabilizing a painful, swollen deformity of the thigh. However, there are several situations in which the device should *not* be used. In these cases, the device might worsen other injuries that are present. Contraindications to the use of the traction splint include the following:

◆ Injury to the hip or pelvis

◆ Injury to the knee

◆ Injury close to the knee

◆ Injury to the ankle

◆ Injury to the lower leg

◆ Any partial amputation or any avulsion of the limb where application of the traction device might complete the amputation or separation of the tissue

The application of a traction splint is shown in Figures 21-23 and 21-24 on pages 540–543. Note, however, that there are several types of traction splints with differences in the application of each. You must become familiar with the specific type of traction splint used by your department and practice its application.

Injuries to the Joints

Injuries to the joints are managed in much the same manner as injuries to the long bones. Joint injuries often result in loss of function of the limb distal to the joint injury. They often cause marked deformities either at the site of the dislocation or distally, where the normal orientation of the limb is altered by the injury. For example, with a fracture of the hip, the foot on the injured side rotates outward and the leg on the injured side appears shorter than that on the uninjured side. With a dislocation of the proximal femur from the hip joint, the leg may be rotated outward or inward depending on whether the dislocation is anterior or posterior.

When you encounter a patient with a joint injury, follow these general rules for splinting shown in Figure 21-25 on page 544.

1. **Perform a scene size-up and assure scene safety.** Determine the mechanism of injury and that there is no continued risk to you or the patient from it.

2. **Take appropriate BSI precautions.**

3. **Stabilize the injury site manually.**

4. **Assess the pulse, motor function, and sensation in the extremity distal to the joint before splinting.** Document your findings.

5. **In general, splint a joint injury in the position in which it was found.** However, if the distal extremity is cyanotic or lacks a pulse, align the injured joint with gentle manual traction. If pain or a grating sound or sensation increases, stop your efforts to realign the joint and splint it in the position in which it was found.

6. **Immobilize not only the injury site but also, if possible, the joints above it and below it.** This is not usually possible when managing shoulder or hip injuries.

7. **After the splint is applied, reassess distal pulse, motor function, and sensation.** Document your findings.

8. **Protect the splinted joint during all subsequent movement of the patient.** To assure this protection, assign one person to manually stabilize the splinted joint. Make sure that the entire injured extremity is adequately secured and protected.

9. **Apply ice to the injured joint if possible.**

Injuries to the Hips and Pelvis

The hip is the joint formed by the proximal femur and the pelvic acetabulum. Injuries to the hip are extremely common among the elderly as a result of falls. The most common hip injury is a fracture of the proximal femur at the hip joint. This injury produces pain and tenderness of the hip and deformity of the leg in which the entire leg appears outwardly rotated and shortened. This rotation and shortening can be most readily observed at the ankle. Because of the amount of soft tissue overlying the hip, it is often difficult to detect swelling there.

In patients other than the elderly, pelvic injuries are usually caused by forces greater than those involved in a simple fall. Such pelvic injuries are commonly seen in patients involved in motor vehicle crashes and in pedestrians struck by cars. You can detect the tenderness characteristic of these injuries by *gently* compressing and then releasing pressure on the wings of the pelvis or by applying downward pressure to the pelvis anteriorly.

Pelvic fractures may result in life-threatening internal blood loss of several liters. The management of pelvic injuries should include treatment for shock (hypoperfusion) if indicated and immobilization of the patient on a long backboard (Figure 21-16). The PASG can also be used to immobilize patients with pelvic injuries (Figure 21-17).

Figure 21-16 A patient with a hip or pelvic injury can be immobilized by **(A)** binding the legs together or **(B)** using padded long-board splinting.

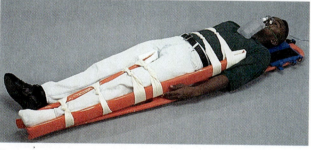

A.

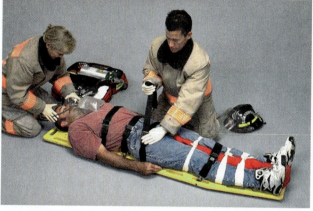

B.

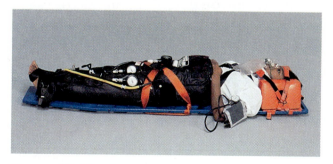

Figure 21-17 The PASG can be used to splint a suspected pelvic injury.

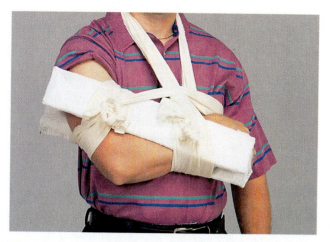

Figure 21-18 Use a sling and swathe when immobilizing a patient's elbow in a bent position.

Injuries to the Shoulders

Injuries to the shoulders are common. These injuries frequently occur in the course of athletic activities. Shoulder injuries will typically display the usual signs of tenderness, swelling, and deformity over the affected joint. Often these patients will be found sitting with the affected shoulder slumped forward and the uninjured arm being used to protect it. Shoulder injuries are best splinted with a sling and swathe.

Injuries to the Elbow

Elbow injuries carry a high risk of associated nerve and blood vessel damage because these structures run very close to the joint. Always carefully assess distal pulses, motor function, and sensation with these injuries. The sling and swathe is usually ideal for immobilizing this injury when you encounter a patient whose elbow is in a bent position (Figure 21-18). If the patient's elbow is in a straight or extended position, immobilize the joint with a long padded board splint (Figure 21-19).

Injuries to the Ankle

Ankle injuries are very common. One of the most common types is the "step-down" injury in which the foot turns under the lower leg when the patient misses a step. When this mechanism has produced the injury, you will often detect the most severe tenderness, swelling, and deformity over the lateral malleolus.

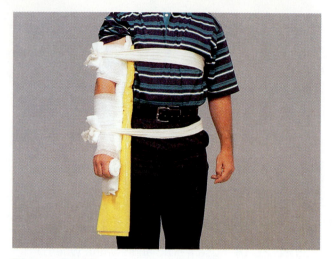

Figure 21-19 A long padded splint can be used to immobilize an elbow injury in a straight position.

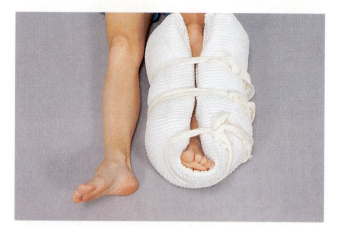

Figure 21-20 You can immobilize a patient's ankle and foot with a splint improvised from a blanket roll and bandages.

To immobilize these injuries, always place the foot and ankle in a position of function. You can use a padded long splint that extends from above the knee to at least 4 inches (100 mm) below the foot to secure the ankle and foot in proper alignment. Commercially available rigid splints that immobilize the foot, ankle, and lower leg can also be used. Finally, an improvised soft splint made of a pillow or a blanket roll secured with cravats can also be effective with this type of injury (Figure 21-20).

Applying a Sling and Swathe

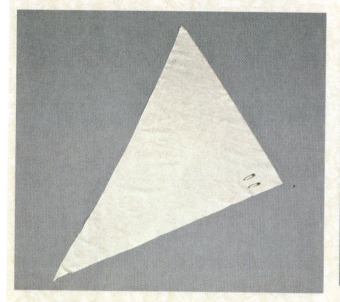

Figure 21-21A The sling should be made from a triangular bandage measuring about 36″ by 36″ by 50-60″. Assess pulse, motor function, and sensation before applying the sling.

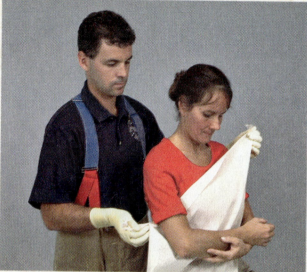

Figure 21-21B Position the sling over the top of the patient's chest. One point of the triangle should extend well below the elbow on the injured side. Position the patient's injured arm across the chest. Allow the patient to assist in stabilizing the arm.

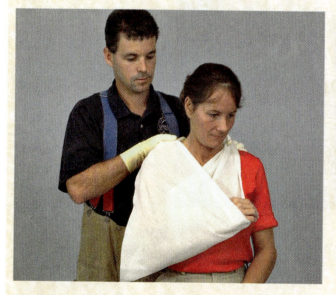

Figure 21-21C Bring the bottommost point of the sling up over the patient's arm and over the top of the shoulder. Draw up on the two ends of the sling so that the patient's hand is about four inches above the elbow.

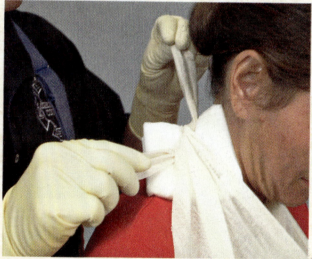

Figure 21-21D Tie the two ends of the sling together behind the patient's neck. To ensure that the knot doesn't press against the neck use bulky dressings or sanitary napkins as padding.

(continued)

Applying a Sling and Swathe (continued)

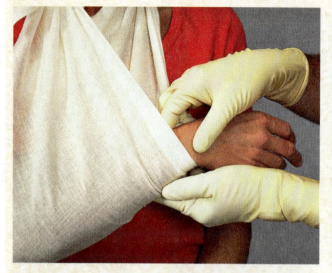

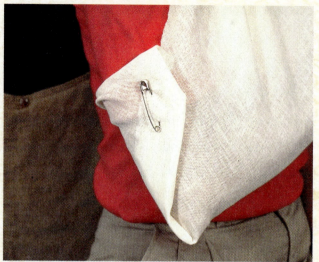

Figure 21-21E Leave the patient's fingertips exposed so you can check distal circulation, motor function, and sensation.

Figure 21-21F Take the material at the patient's elbow, fold it forward, and pin it to the front of the sling. This makes a pocket for the elbow.

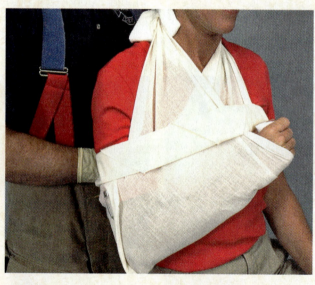

Figure 21-21G Fasten a swathe around the chest and over the sling. You can use bandages or Velcro straps for the swathe. Do not place the sling over the uninjured arm.

Splinting Arm, Forearm, Wrist, and Hand Injuries

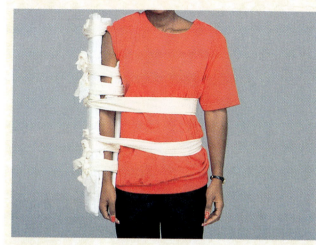

Figure 21-22A A rigid splint used with an arm injury.

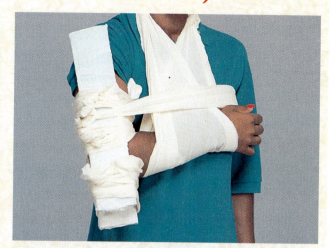

Figure 21-22B A rigid splint with a sling and swathe for an upper arm injury.

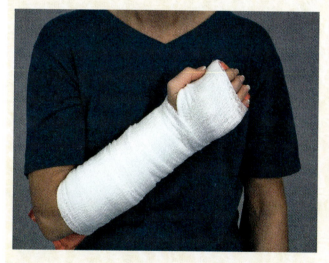

Figure 21-22C When there are injuries to the hand, immobilize it in a position of function.

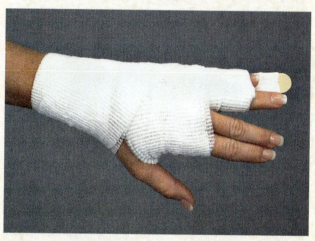

Figure 21-22D When there are injuries to individual fingers, you can use a tongue depressor as a splint.

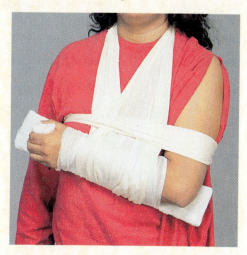

Figure 21-22E You can use a sling and swathe together with a rigid splint for injuries to the forearm, wrist, and hand.

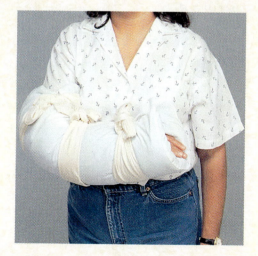

Figure 21-22F You should be prepared to improvise and create splints from items like blankets or pillows.

Applying a Bi-Polar Traction Splint

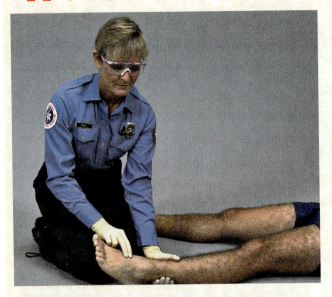

Figure 21-23A Assess distal pulse, motor function, and sensation.

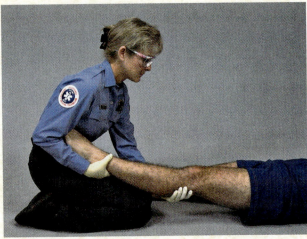

Figure 21-23B Stabilize the leg by applying gentle manual traction.

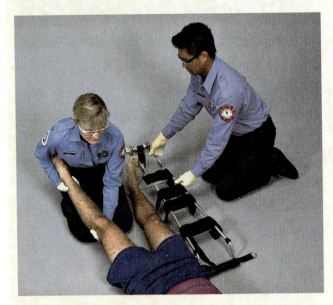

Figure 21-23C Adjust the splint to the proper length.

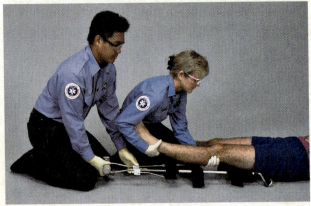

Figure 21-23D Position the splint under the injured leg so that the ischial pad rests against the bony prominence of the buttocks. Once the splint is positioned, raise the heel stand.

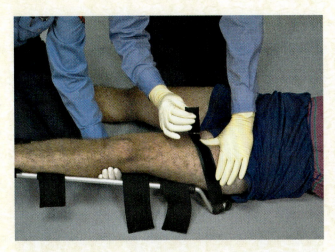

Figure 21-23E Attach the ischial strap over the groin and thigh.

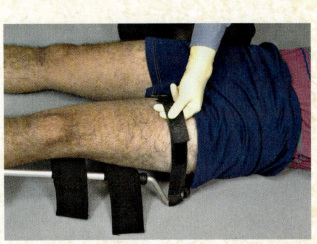

Figure 21-23F Be sure that the strap is snug, but not tight enough to cut off circulation.

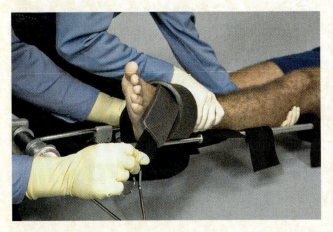

Figure 21-23G With the patient's foot upright, secure the ankle hitch.

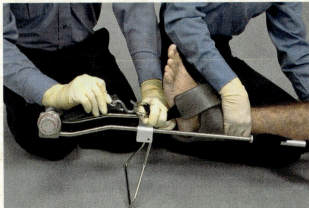

Figure 21-23H Attach the "S" hook to the "D" ring of the ankle hitch and apply mechanical traction. Full traction is applied when mechanical traction equals the manual traction and pain and muscle spasms are reduced. In an unresponsive patient, adjust traction until the injured leg is approximately the same length as the uninjured leg.

(*continued*)

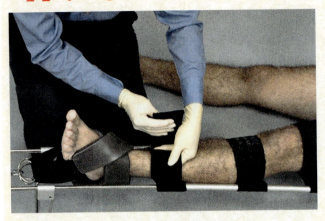

Figure 21-23I Fasten the leg support straps.

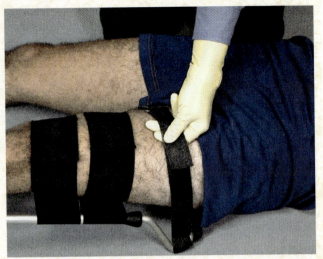

Figure 21-23J Recheck both the ischial strap and the ankle hitch to ensure that they are securely fastened.

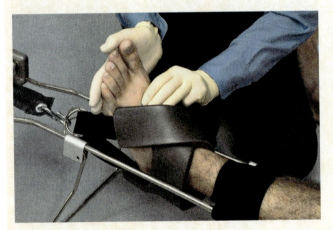

Figure 21-23K Reassess distal pulses, motor function, and sensation after splinting.

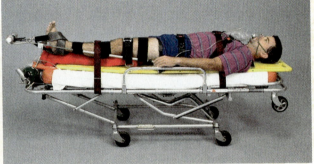

Figure 21-23L Place the patient on a long spine board and secure with straps. Pad between the splint and the uninjured leg. Secure the splint to the board.

Applying a Unipolar Traction Splint

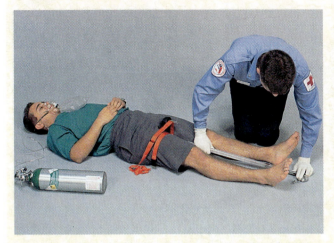

Figure 21-24A Place the splint along the medial aspect of the injured leg. Adjust it so that it extends about 4″ beyond the heel.

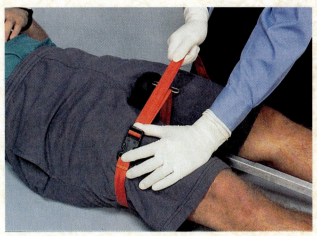

Figure 21-24B Secure the strap to the thigh.

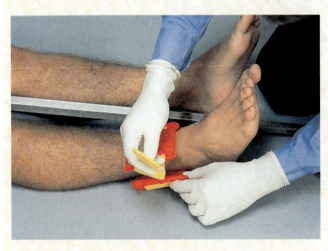

Figure 21-24C Apply the ankle hitch and attach it to the splint.

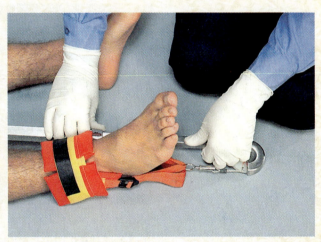

Figure 21-24D Apply traction by extending the splint. Adjust the splint to 10% of the patient's body weight.

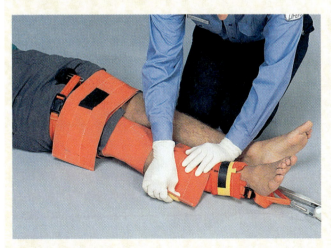

Figure 21-24E Apply the straps to secure the leg to the splint. Reassess distal pulses, motor function, and sensation.

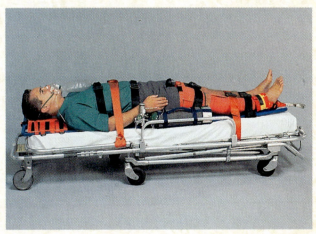

Figure 21-24F Place the patient on a long spine board. Strap the ankles together and secure to the board.

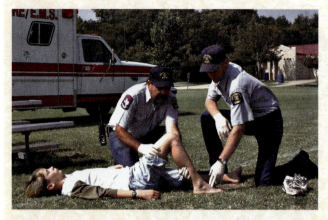

Figure 21-25A Manually stabilize the joint in the position in which you find it. Assess pulse, motor function, and sensation distal to the joint.

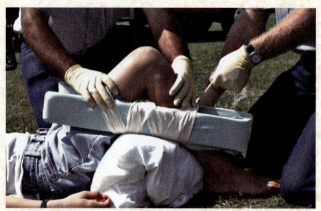

Figure 21-25B Apply the splint to immobilize the bones above and below the injured joint.

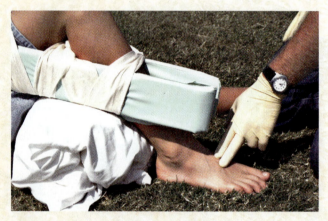

Figure 21-25C After the splint is applied, reassess distal pulse, motor function, and sensation.

Chapter Review

SUMMARY

Knowing how and when to apply splints is the key to emergency care of musculoskeletal injuries. Splinting, properly done, will stabilize an injured extremity. This reduces the patient's pain and decreases the possibility that broken bone ends will cause further damage to nerves, muscles, blood vessels, and other soft tissue. Ideally, splinting should be done before a patient is transported. However, if a patient has a life-threatening condition, do not waste time splinting—immobilize the whole patient to a long backboard and transport him rapidly.

REVIEWING KEY CONCEPTS

1. Describe the major functions of the musculoskeletal system.

2. List the indications that would lead you to suspect injury to the musculoskeletal system.

3. Identify common mechanisms of injury responsible for damage to bones, muscles, and associated structures.

4. Describe common musculoskeletal injuries.

5. Explain the difference between an open and a closed painful, swollen, and deformed extremity injury.

6. Describe the steps in the general emergency care of a patient with a musculoskeletal injury.

7. Explain the reasons for splinting a musculoskeletal injury and the possible consequences of not splinting or improperly splinting the injury.

8. Describe the basic types of splints.

9. List general guidelines to keep in mind when splinting.

10. Explain the reason for realigning a swollen, painful, deformed extremity before splinting. Describe how to carry out the realignment.

11. List contraindications for use of a traction splint on a swollen, painful, deformed extremity.

RESOURCES TO LEARN MORE

Simon, R. R. and Koenigsknecht, S. J. *Emergency Orthopedics: The Extremities, 3rd Edition*. Norwalk, CT: Appleton & Lange, 1995.

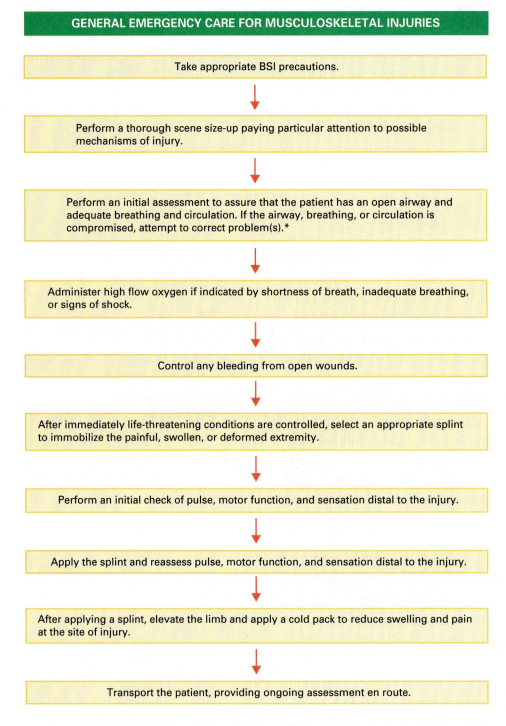

GENERAL EMERGENCY CARE FOR MUSCULOSKELETAL INJURIES

Take appropriate BSI precautions.

↓

Perform a thorough scene size-up paying particular attention to possible mechanisms of injury.

↓

Perform an initial assessment to assure that the patient has an open airway and adequate breathing and circulation. If the airway, breathing, or circulation is compromised, attempt to correct problem(s).*

↓

Administer high flow oxygen if indicated by shortness of breath, inadequate breathing, or signs of shock.

↓

Control any bleeding from open wounds.

↓

After immediately life-threatening conditions are controlled, select an appropriate splint to immobilize the painful, swollen, or deformed extremity.

↓

Perform an initial check of pulse, motor function, and sensation distal to the injury.

↓

Apply the splint and reassess pulse, motor function, and sensation distal to the injury.

↓

After applying a splint, elevate the limb and apply a cold pack to reduce swelling and pain at the site of injury.

↓

Transport the patient, providing ongoing assessment en route.

* *Note:* If patient is unstable or ABCs are compromised, treatment priority is rapid transport rather than splinting. A long backboard can be used to provide whole body splinting.

Injuries to the Head and Spine

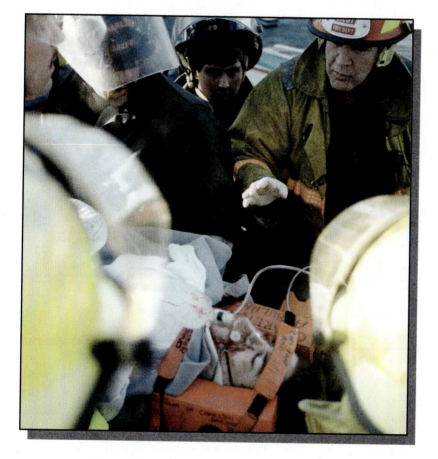

*I*njuries to the head and spine are among the most potentially
devastating you will encounter as an EMT. Injuries to the head can
be life-threatening or result in permanent disruption of the patient's
life due to disability. Injuries to the spine and spinal cord can also be
fatal or result in lifelong paralysis. The emergency medical care that you
provide patients with these injuries is essential both for their survival
and for reducing the risks of permanent disability. For these reasons,
assessment and care of head and spine injuries will be among your most
important responsibilities as an EMT.

At the completion of this chapter, the EMT-Basic student should be able to meet the following objectives:

Knowledge and Understanding

1. State the components of the central nervous system. (p. 551)
2. List the functions of the central nervous system. (p. 551)
3. Define the structure of the skeletal system as it relates to the nervous system. (pp. 550–551)
4. List the major bones and bone groupings of the spinal column. (pp. 550–551)
5. Relate mechanism of injury to potential injuries of the head and spine. (pp. 552–553)
6. Describe the implications of not properly caring for potential spine injury. (pp. 552, 553, 557–558)
7. State the signs and symptoms of a potential spine injury. (pp. 556–557)
8. Describe the method of determining if a responsive patient may have a spine injury. (pp. 555, 556–557)
9. Relate the airway emergency medical care techniques to the patient with a suspected spine injury. (p. 553)
10. Describe how to stabilize the cervical spine. (pp. 558, 560, 562–563)
11. Discuss indications for sizing and using a cervical spine immobilization device. (pp. 560, 562, 563)
12. Establish the relationship between airway management and the patient with head and spine injuries. (pp. 553, 565)
13. Describe a method for sizing a cervical spine immobilization device. (pp. 560, 562)
14. Describe how to log roll a patient with a suspected spine injury. (pp. 566, 570–572)
15. Describe how to secure a patient to a long spine board. (p. 569)
16. List instances when a short spine board should be used. (p. 560)
17. Describe how to immobilize a patient using a short spine board. (pp. 561, 567–568)
18. Describe the indications for the use of rapid extrication. (p. 566)
19. List the steps in performing rapid extrication. (pp. 575–576)
20. State the circumstances when a helmet should be left on the patient. (p. 585)
21. Discuss the circumstances when a helmet should be removed. (p. 585)
22. Identify different types of helmets. (p. 585)

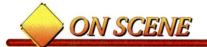

ON SCENE

DISPATCH: *COLDEN AMBULANCE 1, RESPOND MUTUAL AID TO WEST FALLS WITH ENGINE 82 TO THE CORNER OF WEST GROVE AND MARKET STREETS FOR A MOTOR VEHICLE CRASH WITH PERSONAL INJURIES. TIME OUT IS 0254.*

You respond to the call with two other EMTs on your department's ambulance. En route, you monitor the radio traffic from the scene and learn that one patient has already been airlifted from the scene to the county trauma center. Approaching the scene, you radio for instructions: "West Falls Command, this is Ambulance 1."

"West Falls Command."

"We are 2 minutes out. Request instructions."

"Ambulance 1, you will have a male patient with neck pain who is currently with the sheriff's deputy at the sheriff's car. Park directly behind the sheriff's car in the westbound lane."

"Ambulance 1. Received."

On your arrival, the fire police direct you in. Traffic has been diverted and there are no downed power lines visible. You note that the crew from Engine 82 has a charged hoseline stretched to the vicinity of the two cars involved in the crash. It is obvious from the damage to the vehicles that this was a high-speed collision with a significant mechanism of injury. One of

23. Describe the unique characteristics of sports helmets. (p. 585)

24. Explain the preferred methods to remove a helmet. (pp. 586–587)

25. Discuss alternative methods for removal of a helmet. (p. 588)

26. Describe how the patient's head is stabilized to remove the helmet. (pp. 586, 588)

27. Differentiate how the head is stabilized with a helmet compared to without a helmet. (p. 585)

28. Explain the rationale for immobilization of the entire spine when a cervical spine injury is suspected. (pp. 552, 557–558)

29. Explain the rationale for utilizing immobilization methods apart from the straps on the cots. (pp. 557–558, 560)

30. Explain the rationale for utilizing a short spine immobilization device when moving a patient from the sitting to the supine position. (pp. 560–561)

31. Explain the rationale for utilizing rapid extrication approaches only when they indeed will make the difference between life and death. (p. 566)

32. Defend the reasons for leaving a helmet in place for transport of a patient. (p. 585)

33. Defend the reasons for removal of a helmet prior to transport of a patient. (p. 585)

Skills

1. Demonstrate opening the airway in a patient with suspected spinal cord injury.

2. Demonstrate evaluating a responsive patient with a suspected spinal cord injury.

3. Demonstrate stabilization of the cervical spine.

4. Demonstrate the four person log roll for a patient with a suspected spinal cord injury.

5. Demonstrate how to log roll a patient with a suspected spinal cord injury using two people.

6. Demonstrate securing a patient to a long spine board.

7. Demonstrate using the short board immobilization technique.

8. Demonstrate procedure for rapid extrication.

9. Demonstrate preferred methods for stabilization of a helmet.

10. Demonstrate helmet removal techniques.

11. Demonstrate alternative methods for stabilization of a helmet.

12. Demonstrate completing a prehospital care report for patients with head and spinal injuries.

---

the fire police directs you to your patient, who is standing next to a sheriff's deputy and talking to the officer. Your initial impression is of a male patient in his 30s with no apparent airway or breathing problems, because he is talking easily.

You approach directly to the front of the patient and introduce yourself, adding, "Sir, I'm an EMT with the fire department. What seems to be the problem?"

"My neck is killing me."

"Sir, I'd like you to hold your head still. My partner is going to move behind you and gently support your neck." As you say this, your partner gets into position and manually stabilizes the patient's neck. You then ask the patient if he has any pain elsewhere or if he has any numbness or weakness in his arms or legs.

He replies, "Not pain, exactly. It feels more like electric shocks going down my arms." He denies any other pains, abnormal sensations, or injuries. You palpate his neck and note that the patient says it is tender to your touch over the area of the mid-cervical spine.

Because of the patient information you received from Command, the other crew members have brought from the ambulance a rigid cervical collar, a long backboard, and a head immobilizing device. As one of the EMTs applies the cervical collar, you explain to the patient that you and your crew will be immobilizing him onto the backboard as a precaution in case he has sustained a spinal injury. You decide to use a standing takedown technique. You explain to the patient that you'll be placing the board behind him as he is standing and then lowering both him and the board to the ground as a unit.

Before the takedown, you check the patient's grip by having him squeeze your hands. You note that the strength of his grip seems normal and equal in both hands. You and your crew then lower the patient to the ground.

During the takedown and after its completion, one EMT continues to manually stabilize the patient's head. Once the board is on the ground, you and the other EMT strap the patient to it and then apply and secure the head immobilization device. When the patient is fully immobilized, you check his grip again and note that it

has remained normal and equal. You also check motor function and sensation in his feet and determine them to be normal and equal as well.

Your crew loads the patient into the ambulance, where you obtain a set of baseline vital signs. En route to the hospital, you perform an ongoing assessment, checking the patient's ABCs and obtaining additional sets of vital signs. You also repeat a focused assessment of the extremities and note that sensation, strength, and motor function appear to remain normal in all of them. You document all your findings and pass them on to the hospital staff in both your oral report and your written PCR.

Later in the day, you learn that the patient sustained a fracture of the fourth cervical vertebra. He was transferred to the trauma center that afternoon.

ANATOMY OF THE SKULL, SPINE, AND CENTRAL NERVOUS SYSTEM

Injuries to the head, neck, and spine can have serious consequences because they may involve the brain and central nervous system. To understand how to deal with these injuries, you should first review the anatomy of the skull, spine, and the central nervous system.

The Skull

The bones of the skull protect the brain. The skull is made up of several bones joined together at seam-like sutures (Figure 22-1). In infancy and childhood, these sutures are expandable and allow the brain and skull to grow. By adulthood, the sutures become fused, making the skull a rigid capsule enclosing the brain. The names of the regions of the scalp, which you should know, are based on the underlying bones of the skull. They include the *frontal, occipital, parietal,* and *temporal* regions.

The bones of the face have several functions. All the facial bones help to protect the brain from frontal impacts. The *orbits* (eye sockets) are made up of several bones that surround and protect the eye. The *mandible* (lower jaw) and the *maxillae* (upper jaw) provide support for the teeth. The *nasal bones* support the nose, which allows for the sense of smell. The *zygomatic bones* (cheek bones) contribute to facial structure by forming the cheeks.

The Spine

The head is supported by the bony *spinal column.* The spinal column extends from the base of the brain into the pelvis and contains and protects the spinal cord (Figure 22-2). The spinal column or "spine" is the most crucial support structure of the body. The spine is made up of 33 stacked bones called *vertebrae.* The spinal column is separated into five sections: the seven neck or *cervical* vertebrae, the twelve chest or *thoracic* vertebrae, the five lower back or *lumbar* verte-

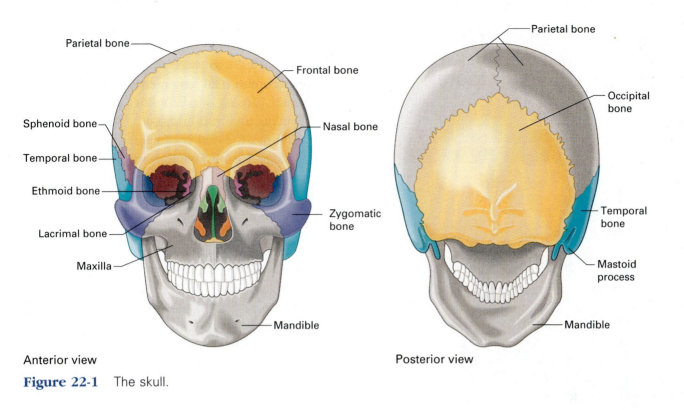

Anterior view

Figure 22-1 The skull.

Posterior view

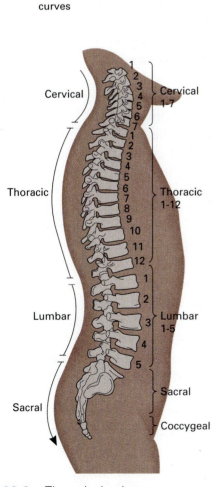

Figure 22-2 The spinal column.

brae, the five fused *sacral* vertebrae that make up the posterior wall of the pelvis, and the four fused tailbone or *coccyx* vertebrae. Because the thoracic spine is supported by the ribs and the sacral and coccyx vertebrae are supported by the pelvis, they are less prone to injury than the unsupported cervical and lumbar vertebrae.

The Central Nervous System

The central nervous system is made up of the brain and the spinal cord. The brain is located within the skull, or cranium. The brain is responsible for control of both higher functions, such as thought and memory, as well as the more basic functions, such as breathing. The spinal cord extends from the base of the brain and descends down the back, protected by the vertebrae of the spinal column. The spinal cord carries messages from the brain to the body (Figure 22-3). Such messages might include directions for the peripheral nervous system to cause movement of voluntary muscles. The spinal cord also carries messages back to the brain from the body. Such messages might include information gathered by the peripheral nervous system about the body's functions and environment.

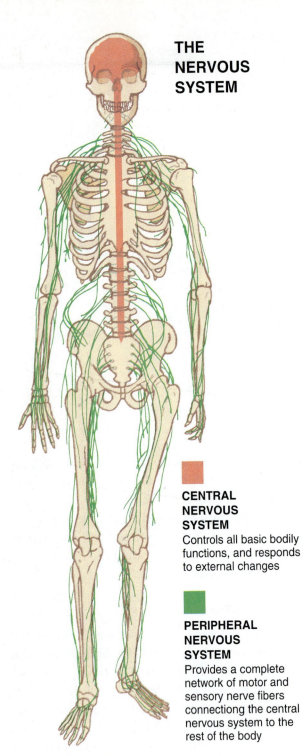

THE NERVOUS SYSTEM

CENTRAL NERVOUS SYSTEM
Controls all basic bodily functions, and responds to external changes

PERIPHERAL NERVOUS SYSTEM
Provides a complete network of motor and sensory nerve fibers connectiong the central nervous system to the rest of the body

Figure 22-3   The nervous system.

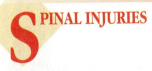

SPINAL INJURIES

Spinal injuries are serious, and failure to handle them properly can have long-term, even fatal, consequences for patients. In fact, one of the chief reasons that formal EMT training was begun over two decades ago was the realization that untrained prehospital emergency responders were routinely causing or worsening spinal cord injuries of patients involved in motor vehicle crashes.

The most feared consequence of spinal injury is damage to the spinal cord. This damage can result in the loss of control of voluntary muscles. This loss of control, or paralysis, is often permanent. Spinal cord injuries can affect not only the muscles of the arms and legs but also the muscles responsible for breathing. Be aware that patients with cervical spinal cord injuries may present with or rapidly develop inadequate breathing.

The vertebrae of the spinal column surround, support, and protect the spinal cord. Damage to the bones of the spinal column does not by itself cause paralysis or the other signs and symptoms of spinal cord injury. However, spinal column instability and/or the fractures in the bones themselves can produce the injuries to the spinal cord that lead to paralysis.

When damage to the spinal cord does occur, nervous system function distal to the injury is generally lost. For example, if a spinal cord injury occurs at the level of the 1st or 2nd cervical vertebrae, then the patient is likely to lose the ability to move both his arms and his legs. In addition, an injury high on the cervical spine is likely to affect the nerves that control the muscles of breathing, meaning that the patient may well suffer respiratory arrest.

Throughout this book, you have read that you must provide immediate manual in-line stabilization and, later, full immobilization whenever you suspect that a patient has sustained serious head, neck, or spine injury. The purpose of these maneuvers is to stabilize the bones of the spinal column in the hopes of preventing them from further damaging the spinal cord. You will learn much more about methods of stabilizing and immobilizing patients with suspected spinal injuries later in this chapter.

Mechanisms of Injury

Certain mechanisms of injury carry an increased risk of damage to the spinal column and spinal cord for patients. Any mechanism that causes excessive or abnormal motion of the spine can produce this damage (Figure 22-4). These mechanisms include the following:

- **Flexion** This is the bending forward, or anteriorly, of the spine. It is a common mechanism in head-on crashes and in diving injuries.
- **Extension** This is the bending backward, or posteriorly, of the spine. It is a common mechanism in rear-end crashes.
- **Lateral bending** This is the bending of the spine to one side or the other. It often occurs in side-impact collisions.
- **Rotation** This is the twisting of the spine. It is common in many types of falls and motor vehicle crashes.
- **Compression** This is the application of force directly onto the spine from either a superior or inferior direction. This is a common mechanism in motor vehicle crashes, falls from height, and diving accidents.
- **Distraction** This is the application of force that results in the spinal cord and vertebrae being stretched or pulled apart. It is common in hangings and motor vehicle crashes.
- **Penetration** This occurs when some object enters the spinal cord or spinal column. It is common in shootings and stabbings.

Because the cervical spine and the lumbar spine are not supported by other bones as the thoracic and sacral spine are, these areas will be of special concern when you are assessing and managing injuries that result from the mechanisms described above.

Assessment of Spinal Injury Patients

The scene size-up can be critical to your care of the patient with suspected spinal injury. A careful survey of the scene can reveal whether mechanisms likely to have caused spinal injury were involved. Emergency scenes that commonly involve those mechanisms include the following:

- Motor vehicle crashes
- Motorcycle crashes
- Pedestrian vs. automobile collisions
- Falls

- Blunt trauma
- Sporting injuries, such as those from football, hockey, bicycling, or horseback riding
- Hangings
- Diving accidents and near drownings where diving may have been involved
- Penetrating trauma to the head, neck, or torso including gunshot wounds

Whenever there is any chance that the mechanism of injury could have produced a spinal injury, assume that it did. Immediately take steps to provide manual in-line stabilization and prevent any additional movement of the spine. Manual stabilization must be maintained until the patient is properly immobilized to a long backboard.

You may at times encounter a patient like the one in On Scene who is standing or walking at a scene where the mechanism of injury suggests spinal injury. The fact that he is standing or walking does not mean that spinal injury has not occurred. In such a case, tell the patient not to move and have someone provide manual in-line stabilization while you assess the patient for signs and symptoms of spinal injury.

As noted earlier, airway obstruction and inadequate breathing are often associated with serious spinal injuries. Pay careful attention to the patient's airway and breathing during the initial assessment. If you detect problems in these areas, correct them immediately while maintaining manual in-line stabilization. If necessary, open and control the airway using the jaw-thrust maneuver. Be prepared to provide positive pressure ventilations if necessary.

Conduct a focused history and physical exam. This includes the rapid trauma assessment and the gathering of vital signs and a SAMPLE history. As you carry out these tasks, continue to maintain manual in-line stabilization.

During the rapid trauma assessment, inspect for signs of deformities, contusions, abrasions, lacerations, punctures or penetrations, swelling, and other findings that suggest the possibility of injury to the spine (Figure 22-5). Gently palpate the spine for areas of tenderness or deformity. These injuries are best assessed while the patient is being log-rolled onto a long spine board for immobilization.

MECHANISMS OF SPINAL INJURIES

FLEXION INJURY

COMPRESSION INJURY

HYPEREXTENSION INJURY

DISTRACTION INJURY

FLEXION-ROTATION INJURY

PENETRATION INJURY

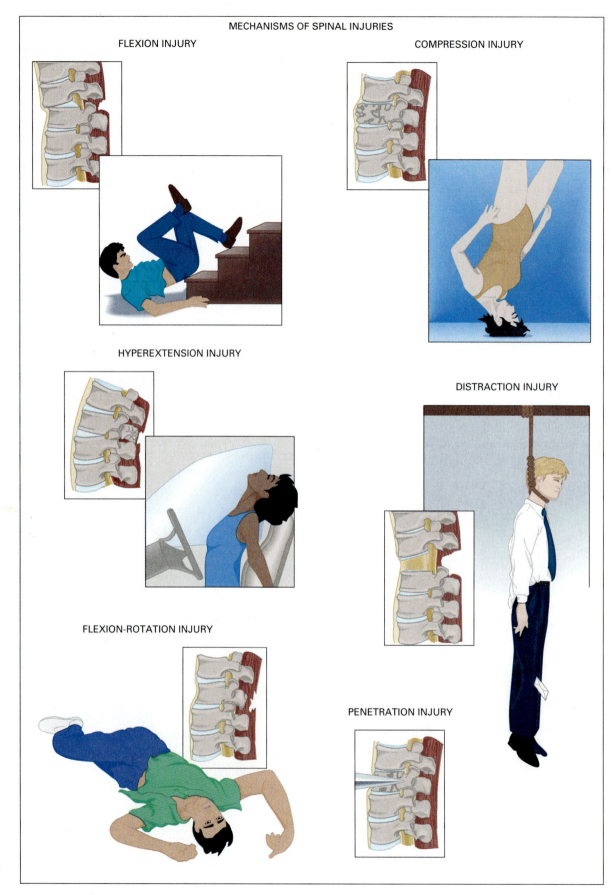

Figure 22-4 Mechanisms of spinal injury.

- **PAIN**   Unprovoked pain in area of injury, along spine, in lower legs.

- **TENDERNESS**   Gentle touch of area may increase pain.

- **DEFORMITY** (rare)   There may be abnormal bend or bony prominence.

- **SOFT TISSUE INJURY**   Injury to the head, neck, or face may indicate cervical-spine injury. Injury to shoulders, back, and abdomen may indicate thoracic- or lumbar-spine injury. Injury to extremities may indicate lumbar- or sacral-spine injury.

- **PARALYSIS**   Inability to move or inability to feel sensation in some part of body may indicate spinal fracture with cord injury.

- **PAINFUL MOVEMENT**   Movement may increase pain. Never try to move the injured area.

- **ABNORMAL SENSATION**   Tingling or "pins and needles" sensation in torso or extremities.

- **ALSO:**   Loss of bowel or bladder control, priapism, impaired breathing.

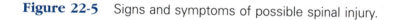

Figure 22-5   Signs and symptoms of possible spinal injury.

If the patient is responsive, perform a brief neurological exam to test for sensation and motor function in all four extremities (Figure 22-6):

◆ Ask the patient if he can move his fingers and toes.

◆ Ask the patient to grip your fingers with both his hands simultaneously and squeeze. Then compare the strength and equality of the response in each of his hands.

◆ Ask the patient to gently push his feet against your hands ("step on the gas"), and compare the strength and equality of the response in each of his feet.

◆ Ask the patient if he can feel it when you touch his fingers and toes.

When you are conducting the rapid assessment of a patient with a suspected spinal injury, keep the following points in mind:

◆ Assume that any unresponsive patient with a mechanism of injury that suggests the possibility of spinal injury has one.

◆ Remember that patients who deny having tenderness in the area of the spine may still have a spinal injury.

◆ *Never* ask a patient to move his spine in order to test for pain with motion.

Try to gain as much specific information as possible from the responsive patient during the SAMPLE history. Consider asking questions such as the following:

◆ What happened?

◆ Does your neck or your back hurt?

◆ Can you move your hands and feet?

◆ Do you have any pain or any numbness or tingling in your arms or legs?

Assessing Motor Function and Sensation in the Extremities

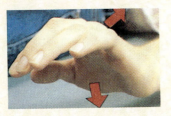

Figure 22-6A Assess the patient's ability to move the hands.

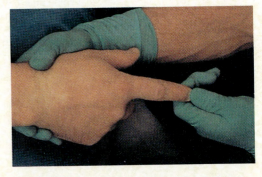

Figure 22-6B Assess sensation in the fingers and hands.

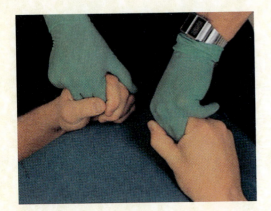

Figure 22-6C Check for equal strength in the upper extremities.

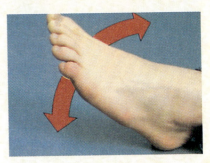

Figure 22-6D Assess the patient's ability to move the feet.

♦ Did you move or did anyone move you before the EMTs arrived?

If the patient is unresponsive, obtain as much of the SAMPLE history as you can from family members or bystanders. Question them about the possible mechanism of injury. Ask about the patient's condition before your arrival. Be sure to ask whether there was any change in the patient's mental status before you arrived.

The following are signs and symptoms of spinal injury that you may detect during the focused history and physical examination of the patient:

♦ Tenderness of the spine in the area of injury

♦ Deformity of the spine

♦ Soft tissue injuries associated with spinal injuries

—Injury to head and/or neck: consider possible cervical spine injury

—Injury to shoulders, back, or abdomen: consider thoracic or lumbar spine injury

—Injury to pelvis or lower extremities: consider possible lumbar or sacral spine injury

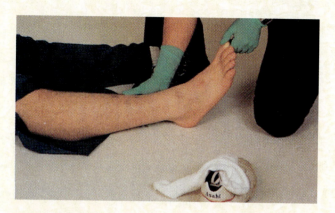

Figure 22-6E Check sensation in the feet by touching a toe and asking if the patient can identify which one it is.

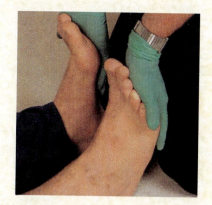

Figure 22-6F Check for equal strength in the lower extremities.

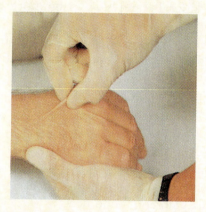

Figure 22-6G If a patient is unresponsive or does not feel a light touch, pinch the back of the hand and watch for a response.

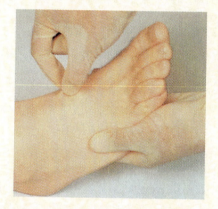

Figure 22-6H If a patient is unresponsive or does not feel a light touch, pinch the top of the foot and watch for a response.

- Loss of sensation or paralysis below the level of the suspected spinal injury
- Loss of sensation or abnormal sensation such as weakness or tingling in the upper or lower extremities
- Priapism, a persistent and emotionally unjustified erection of the penis
- Evidence of bowel or bladder incontinence
- Impaired breathing
- Pain, either with or without movement, along the spinal column
- Pain, either constant or intermittent, in the buttocks and legs

Immobilization and Spinal Injuries

Immobilization is the key element in emergency care of patients with suspected spinal injuries. Patients are immobilized in order to help stabilize spinal injuries that have already occurred and to prevent further injuries by limiting body movement. Spinal immobilization is, of course, performed in conjunction with other interventions that may be necessary such as maintaining an open airway, administering supplemental oxygen, providing positive pressure ventilations, and treating for shock.

There are many different types of spinal immobilization devices (Figure 22-7). As an EMT, you must become familiar with those used in your system and know when and how to apply them.

Manual In-Line Stabilization

Manual in-line stabilization is the first step in providing all types of spinal immobilization. To perform manual in-line stabilization, you hold the patient's head in a neutral position with your hands (Figure 22-8, page 560). This prevents motion of the cervical spine that would occur if the patient moved his head.

Manual in-line stabilization is maintained during the processes of applying a rigid cervical collar, of securing the patient to a short spine board or vest-type extrication device, and of placing the patient on a long spine board. Manual stabilization should only be released when the patient's head is fully immobilized on the long spine board with blanket rolls, head blocks, or some other commercial head-immobilization device. Even then, it may be necessary to provide continued manual stabilization if the patient has an altered mental status and is attempting to move or thrash about while secured to the long spine board.

You can provide manual in-line stabilization for a patient found in any position. When the patient's head and neck are in a position other than neutral—for example, flexed forward or turned to the side—bring the head and neck into a neutral position in line with the long axis of the

Immobilization Devices

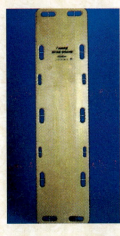

Figure 22-7A A long spine board.

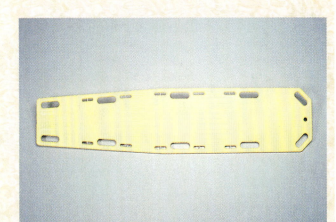

Figure 22-7B A fiberglass long board.

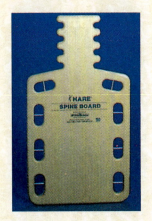

Figure 22-7C A short spine board.

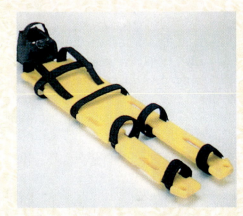

Figure 22-7D A full-body splint.

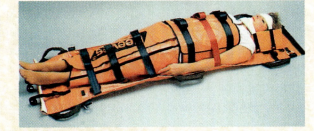

Figure 22-7E A full-body immobilizer.

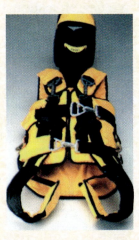

Figure 22-7F A vest-type, half-back immobilizer.

Establishing Manual In-Line Stabilization

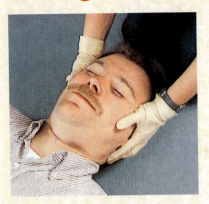

Figure 22-8A Properly position your hands. Spread your fingers around the sides of the head to hold it steady.

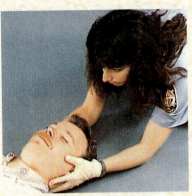

Figure 22-8B Keep the head in a neutral position and the patient's nose in line with his navel.

body. If the patient is lying on the ground, you would normally position yourself above the patient's head and then place one hand on each side of the head, maintaining it in or returning it to a neutral position. If the patient is sitting, you can place yourself in front of or behind him, depending on the position that gives you the best access for stabilization.

Remember that manual stabilization must be held until the patient is immobilized to a spine board. This can be a prolonged time in cases such as complicated rescues or extrications. In these circumstances, your hands and arms can begin to tire, which can make your stabilization less effective. Always try to make the task of holding stabilization less fatiguing by positioning yourself wisely. If the patient is supine, use the ground to support your hands and forearms. If the patient is sitting, use the back of the seat or the patient's shoulders for support.

Cervical Collars (Cervical Spine Immobilization Devices)

Whenever you provide emergency care to a patient with a suspected spinal injury, you should use a rigid cervical collar, or cervical spine immobilization device (Figure 22-9). The cervical collar must be used in conjunction with manual in-line stabilization and subsequent immobilization to a

spine board. Note that use of the collar by itself *does not* provide adequate stabilization or immobilization for the patient.

To be effective, the cervical collar must be rigid. Avoid using the soft collars sometimes worn by people with chronic neck problems. They have no value in the prehospital setting.

To be effective, the cervical collar must also be the proper size. Various manufacturers produce cervical collars in a range of sizes. You must learn how to size and apply the type(s) of collar used by your department (Figures 22-10, 22-11, and 22-12 on pages 562, 563, and 564). An improperly sized collar can do more harm than good for a patient. Improperly sized collars can allow too much motion or hyperextend the neck, worsening spinal injuries, or they can position the jaw so as to cause airway obstruction.

Short Spinal Immobilization Devices

Short spinal immobilization devices include the short, rigid spine board and vest-type extrication devices. These devices are used to immobilize non-critical patients with suspected spinal injuries who are found in a sitting position, as in a car after a crash. These devices immobilize the head, neck, and torso. Once the patient is immobilized to the short device, he is moved to a supine position on a long spine board and immobilized to that device.

Identifying Cervical Collars (Cervical Spine Immobilization Devices)

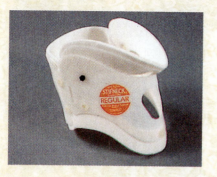

Figure 22-9A A Stifneck® cervical collar.

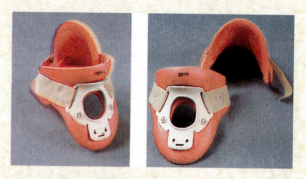

Figure 22-9B A Philadelphia® Cervical Collar assembled and disassembled.

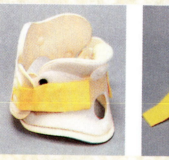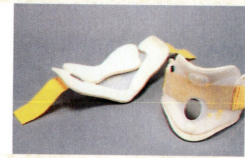

Figure 22-9C A Nec-Loc® cervical collar assembled and disassembled.

The general procedure for applying a short spinal immobilization device to a sitting patient is as follows (Figure 22-13 on page 567):

1. **Provide and maintain manual in-line stabilization throughout the procedure.**

2. **Assess pulses, motor function, and sensation in all extremities.**

3. **Assess the cervical area.**

4. **Size and apply a rigid cervical immobilization device.**

5. **Position the short spinal immobilization device behind the patient.**

6. **Secure the patient's torso to the device with chest and leg (groin) straps.**

7. **Evaluate how well the patient's torso is secured to the device.** Adjust securing straps as necessary, moving the patient as little as possible while you do.

8. **Evaluate the positioning of the patient's head against the device and pad as necessary to maintain a neutral, in-line position.**

9. **Secure the patient's head to the device.** You may release manual stabilization of the head at this point, but if extensive extrication is still required, it is advisable to maintain manual stabilization until the patient is secured to a long board.

10. **Pivot and lower the patient to a supine position on a long spine board.**

11. **Immobilize the patient to the long board.**

12. **Reassess pulses, motor function, and sensation in all extremities.**

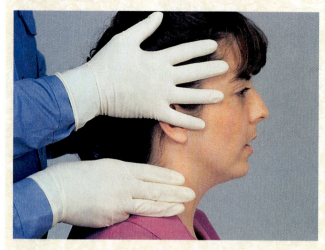

Figure 22-10A First, draw an imaginary line across the top of the shoulders and the bottom of the chin. Use your fingers to measure the distance from the shoulder to the chin.

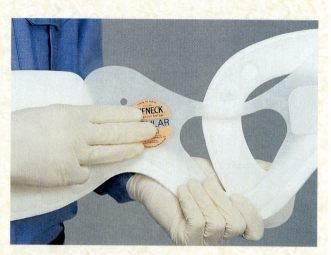

Figure 22-10B Check the collar you select. The distance between the sizing post (black fastener) and lower edge of the rigid plastic should match that of the number of fingers you measured from the patient's shoulder to chin.

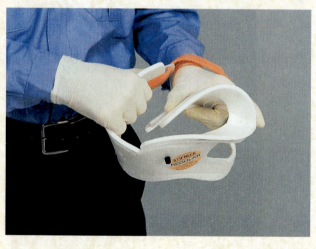

Figure 22-10C Assemble and preform the collar.

Be aware that different types of short spinal immobilization devices use different strapping systems to secure the patient to the device. You must become thoroughly familiar with the device(s) used by your department.

Full Body Spinal Immobilization Devices

Full body spinal immobilization devices are also known as long spine boards or long backboards. When a patient is properly secured to one of

these devices, his head, neck, torso, pelvis, and extremities are immobilized. The devices can be used to immobilize patients with suspected spinal injuries who are found lying, sitting, or standing. As noted above, long spine boards are often used in conjunction with short spinal immobilization devices.

There are several types of full body spinal immobilization devices available. You must become familiar with both the type of device used by your department as well as the strap and head

Applying a Cervical Collar, Seated Patient

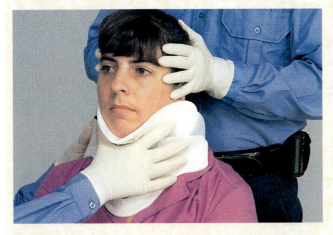

Figure 22-11A When you have chosen a proper size collar, slide the cervical collar up the patient's chest wall. The chin must cover the central fastener in the chin piece.

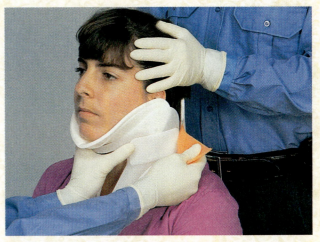

Figure 22-11B Bring the collar around the neck and secure the Velcro. Check the patient's head and collar for proper alignment. Again, be sure the patient's chin covers the central fastener of the chin piece.

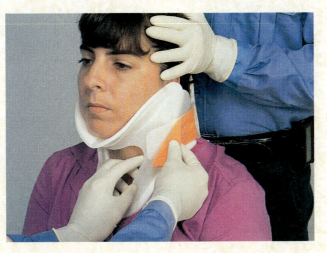

Figure 22-11C If the chin is not covering the fastener of the chin piece, readjust by tightening on the Velcro until you get a proper sizing. If tightening will cause hyperextension of the patient's neck, use the next smaller size of collar.

immobilization system that secures the patient to the device.

The general procedure for immobilizing a patient to a full body spinal immobilization device is described below. Procedures for immobilization of patients in a variety of different circumstances are illustrated in Figures 22-14, 22-15, and 22-16 on pages 568, 570, and 572.

1. **Provide and maintain manual in-line stabilization throughout the procedure.**

2. **Assess pulses, motor function, and sensation in all extremities.**

3. **Assess the cervical area.**

4. **Size and apply a rigid cervical immobilization collar.**

Applying a Cervical Collar, Supine Patient

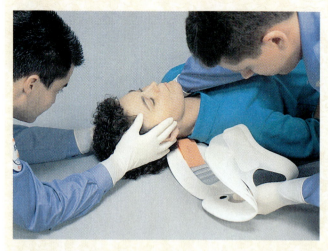

Figure 22-12A Slide the back part of the cervical collar behind the patient's neck. Fold the loop part of the Velcro strap inward on the foam padding.

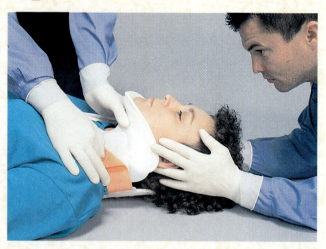

Figure 22-12B Position the collar so that the chin fits properly. Secure the Velcro.

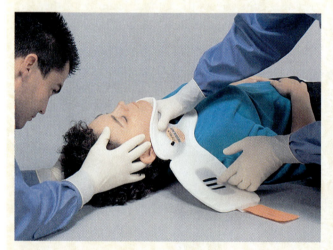

Figure 22-12C Alternatively, you can start by positioning the chin piece and then sliding the back part of the collar behind the patient's neck.

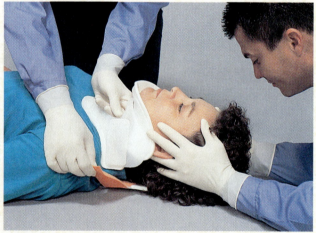

Figure 22-12D Hold the collar in place by grasping the trachea hold. Align the loop part of the Velcro with the hook part and attach the parts.

5. **Position the full body spinal immobilization device beside the patient.**

6. **Move the patient onto the device using the log-roll technique, a suitable lift or carry, or a scoop stretcher.**

    If you use a log roll, proceed as follows:

    —Position one EMT at the patient's head to maintain manual in-line stabilization of the head and neck.

    —The EMT at the patient's head will coordinate and direct all movements of the patient.

    —From one to three additional rescuers kneel along one side of the patient and reach across him, positioning their hands on his other side as they prepare to log roll the patient toward them.

—At the direction of the EMT at the patient's head, the rescuers roll the patient as a unit toward them. Rescuers must maintain full control of movement of the patient's hips and shoulders during the entire log roll. They must not allow any twisting of the patient's spine.

—One rescuer should quickly inspect and palpate the patient's neck and back, assessing for tenderness and DCAP-BTLS injuries.

—One rescuer should slide the immobilization device into place against the patient.

—At the direction of the EMT at the patient's head, the rescuers roll the patient back down onto the board as a unit, being careful to avoid any twisting of his spine.

7. **Pad any voids between the patient and the board.** With adults, pay careful attention to spaces under the torso and under the head. With infants and children, it may be necessary to pad from the shoulders down to the heels to keep the spine in a neutral position. (See the Pediatric Note on page 566.)

8. **Immobilize the patient's torso to the device by applying straps across the pelvis and superior chest.** Adjust the straps as snugly as necessary.

9. **Immobilize the patient's head to the device using head blocks and straps, a rolled blanket and tape, or some other commercial head immobilization system.**

10. **Immobilize the patient's legs to the device by applying straps above and below the knees.**

11. **Release manual in-line stabilization of the head.**

12. **Advise a responsive patient to keep his hands across his abdomen.** With an unresponsive patient, loosely tie his hands across his abdomen or at his sides with either a cravat or bandage material.

13. **Reassess pulses, motor function, and sensation in all the patient's extremities.**

Note that you should immobilize the patient's head to the long spine board only after the torso has been secured with chest and pelvis straps. If the head were immobilized first, the body's weight could still allow side-to-side motion of the cervical spine. For this same reason, it is never adequate to secure only the patient's head to the long spine board without also securing the torso.

◆ General Emergency Care— Patients with Suspected Spinal Injuries

Immobilization is only part of the comprehensive emergency care of patients with suspected spinal injuries. The general steps in this comprehensive emergency care include the following:

1. **Perform a good scene size-up with special attention to the mechanism of injury.**

2. **Assure scene safety, including appropriate BSI precautions.**

3. **Establish and maintain manual in-line stabilization.**

   —Place the patient's head in a neutral position in line with the axis of his spine unless the patient complains of pain or his head does not move easily into position.

   —Maintain manual in-line stabilization until the patient's head is fully immobilized to a long spine board.

4. **Perform an initial assessment.**

   —If the assessment reveals that airway control measures or ventilations are necessary, be sure to maintain manual stabilization while ventilations are provided. Use a jaw-thrust maneuver to maintain an open airway if necessary.

5. **Assess pulses, motor function, and sensation in all extremities.**

6. **Assess the cervical spine region and the anterior neck for signs of injury such as wounds, deformities, or tenderness.**

7. **Size and apply a rigid cervical immobilization collar.**

8. **Select an appropriate method and device for spinal immobilization based on the patient's position and condition:**

—If the patient is found lying on the ground, immobilize him directly to a long spine board as shown in Figures 22-15 and 22-16 on pages 570 and 572.

—If the patient is found in a sitting position and is stable and in no immediate danger, immobilize him to a short spinal immobilization device as shown in Figure 22-13 on page 567.

—If the patient is found standing (as in the On Scene at the beginning of this chapter), immobilize him using the standing takedown technique shown in Figures 22-17 and 22-18 on pages 573 and 574.

—If the patient is found in a sitting position and is either in unstable condition or in immediate danger, as in a burning car, transfer him directly to a long spine board using the rapid extrication technique shown in Figure 22-19 on page 575.

9. **Once the patient is fully immobilized to a long spine board, reassess pulses, motor function, and sensation in all extremities.**

10. **Transport the patient rapidly, performing an ongoing assessment en route. Provide high concentration oxygen and positive pressure ventilations if the patient's breathing is or becomes inadequate.**

PEDIATRIC NOTE

Spinal immobilization with infants and children can present special challenges:

◆ Children do not readily tolerate being strapped down in an immobilization device for any length of time. Provide constant reassurance. When possible, allow a parent or caregiver to stay with the child to provide reassurance and explanations.

◆ Finding a cervical collar of the proper size for your pediatric patient may be difficult. Remember that an improperly sized collar can do more harm than good. If you cannot find a collar that fits properly, use rolled towels on both sides of the head and neck and secure them with tape to the head and spine board.

◆ Because the occiput, or back of the head, is very prominent in infants and children, it may be difficult to get the pediatric patient's head into a neutral position on a standard spine board. You may have to pad the length of the pediatric patient's body, from the shoulders to the heels, to achieve a neutral body position in relation to the cervical spine.

◆ If you encounter an infant or toddler who is already strapped into a child safety seat, use can use the safety seat itself to immobilize the child by applying rolled towels or padding in the spaces between the seat and the child's head and neck and then securing them to the child and the seat with tape (Figure 22-20, page 577). (At other times, it may be necessary to perform a rapid extrication from the safety seat. See Figure 22-21, page 578 for this procedure.)

Immobilizing a Patient with a Short Spinal Immobilization Device

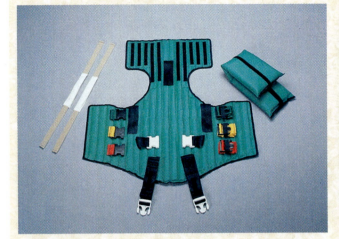

Figure 22-13A A Ferno (K.E.D.) Extrication Device.

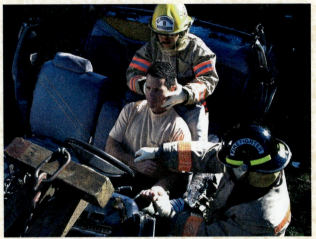

Figure 22-13B Provide manual in-line stabilization. Maintain manual stabilization until the patient is fully immobilized to a long spine board.

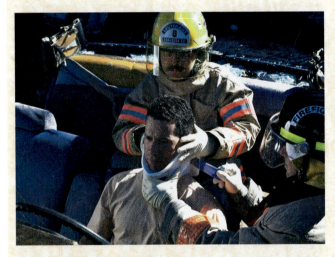

Figure 22-13C Apply a cervical collar.

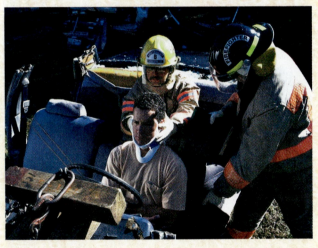

Figure 22-13D Slip the K.E.D. behind the patient and center it.

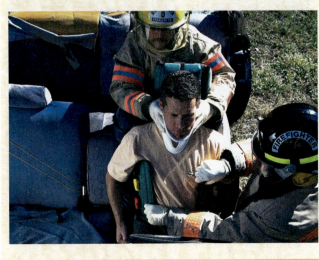

Figure 22-13E Align the device and wrap it around the patient's torso.

(*continued*)

Immobilizing a Patient with a Short Spinal Immobilization Device (continued)

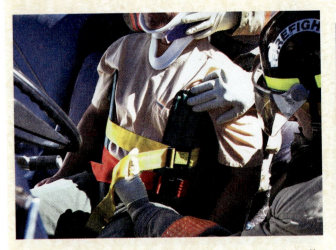

Figure 22-13F Be sure the device is tucked well up into the patient's armpits and then secure the chest straps.

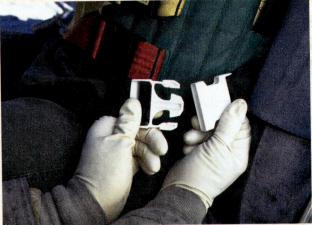

Figure 22-13G Secure the leg straps.

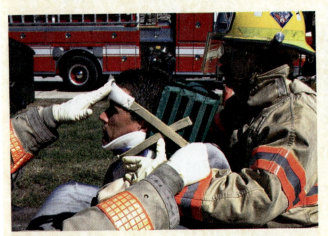

Figure 22-13H Secure the head with the Velcro head straps.

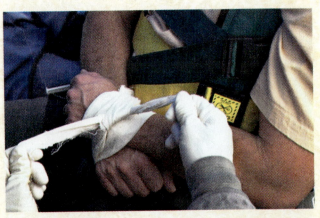

Figure 22-13I Tie the patient's hands together.

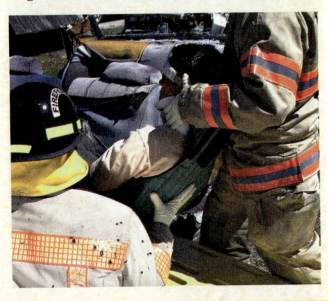

Figure 22-13J Pivot the patient onto a long spine board while maintaining in-line stabilization.

Immobilizing a Patient to a Long Spine Board

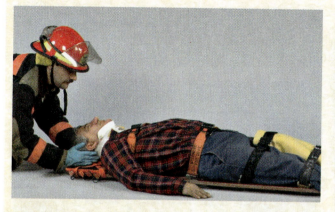

Figure 22-14A The patient can be secured with straps placed across the chest, the hips, above the knee, and below the knee. Pad between the knees.

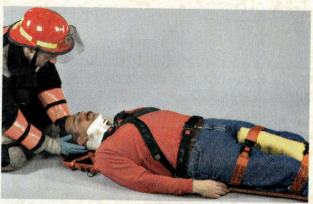

Figure 22-14B Alternatively, use the straps in an "X" configuration to secure the torso. Apply the other straps at the hip and above and below the knee.

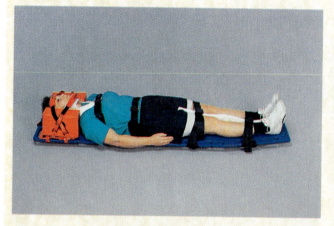

Figure 22-14C Use a head immobilization device to secure the patient's head to the long board.

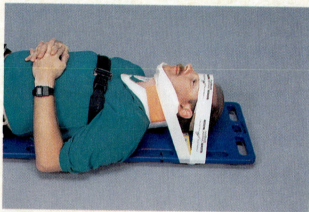

Figure 22-14D A disposable commercial head immobilization device.

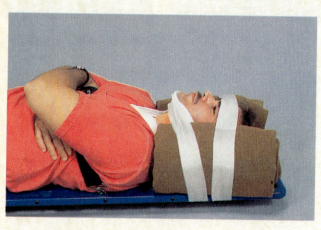

Figure 22-14E Blanket rolls and tape can be used to improvise a head immobilization device.

Four-Rescuer Log Roll and Long Spine Board Immobilization

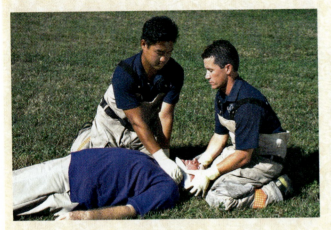

Figure 22-15A Establish in-line manual stabilization and maintain it until the patient is immobilized to the long spine board. Apply a cervical collar.

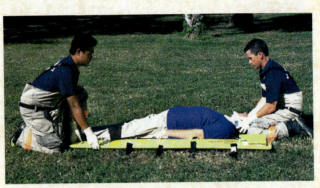

Figure 22-15B Position the long spine board next to and parallel to the patient. Be prepared to pad voids under the head and torso.

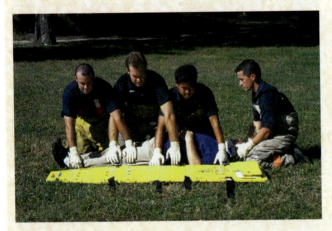

Figure 22-15C Three rescuers kneel on the side of the body opposite the patient, leaving room to roll the patient toward them.

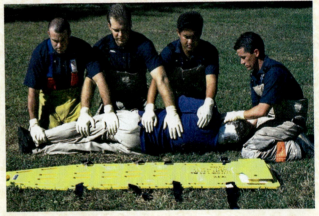

Figure 22-15D On command of the EMT at the patient's head, the three rescuers roll the patient toward them as a unit. While the patient is held up on his side, his back should be assessed.

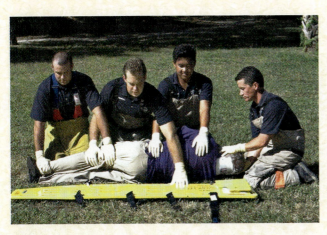

Figure 22-15E The rescuer at the patient's waist pulls the spine board into position against the patient. (This can be done by a fifth rescuer, if available.)

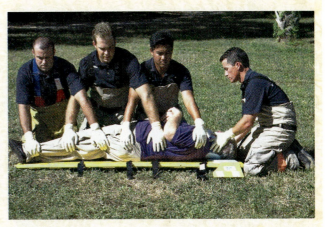

Figure 22-15F The EMT at the patient's head directs the rescuers to roll the patient back down onto the board.

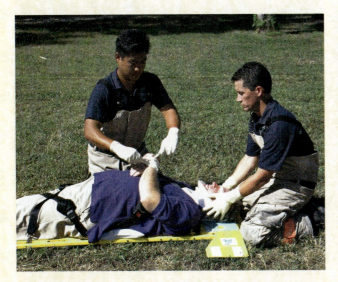

Figure 22-15G Pad voids under head and torso as needed. The patient is then secured to the board with straps. His wrists should be loosely tied.

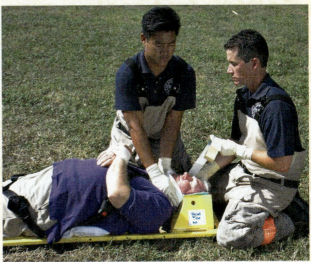

Figure 22-15H The patient's head is secured to the board with a head immobilizer device.

Figure 22-15I Transfer the patient and long board to the cot as a unit. Secure them to the cot.

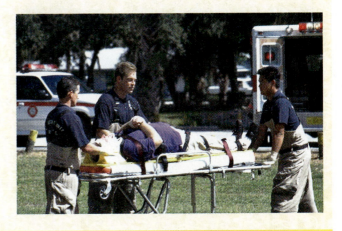

SKILL SUMMARY

Two-Rescuer Log Roll

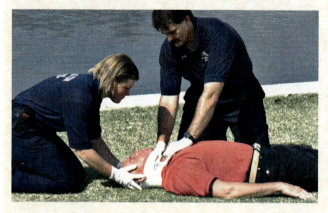

Figure 22-16A Establish in-line manual stabilization and apply a cervical collar.

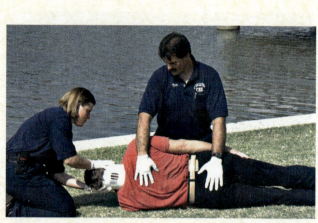

Figure 22-16B Maintain stabilization while moving the patient onto his side.

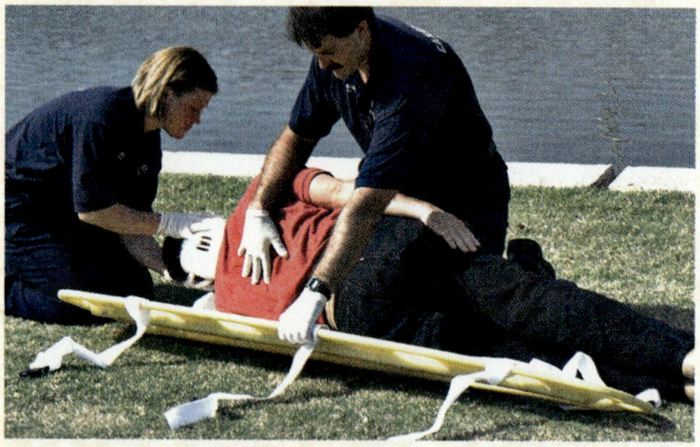

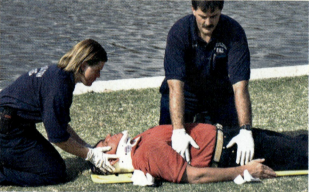

Figure 22-16C Pull the long spine board against the patient.

Figure 22-16D Gently roll the patient down onto the long board and immobilize him to it.

Standing Takedown—Three Rescuers

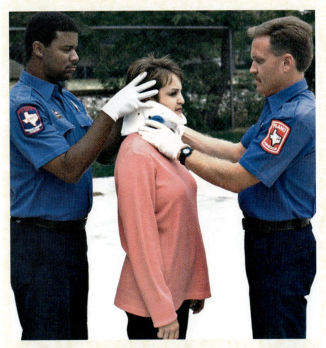

Figure 22-17A One rescuer should hold manual in-line stabilization while another applies a cervical collar.

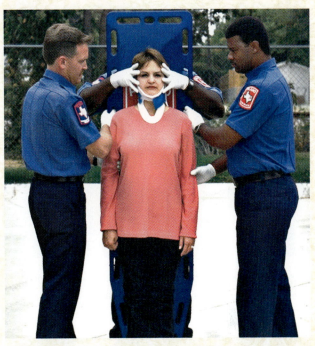

Figure 22-17B With a rescuer continuing to hold in-line stabilization, position a long spine board behind the patient.

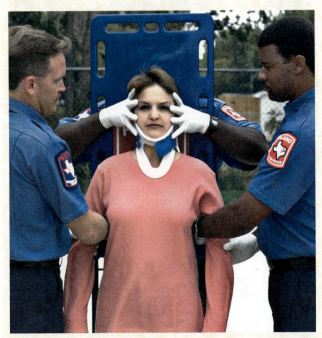

Figure 22-17C Rescuers at the patient's sides each place a hand under a patient's arm and grasp the next highest handhold on the board. Their other hands grasp the patient's elbows.

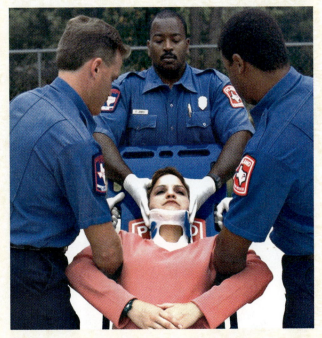

Figure 22-17-D Working together, the rescuers proceed to slowly and smoothly lower the patient to the ground. The rescuer at the head should continue to hold stabilization until the patient is fully immobilized to the long board.

Standing Takedown—Two Rescuers

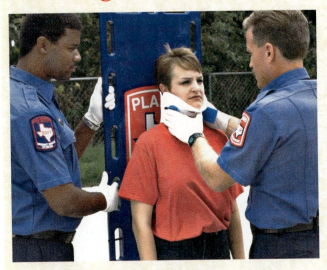

Figure 22-18A Apply a cervical collar and position a long spine board behind the patient.

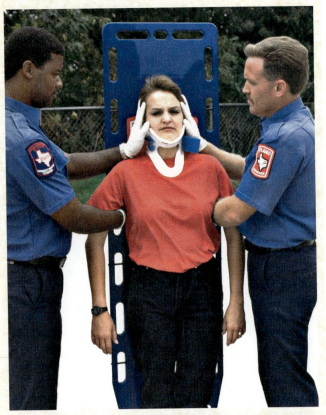

Figure 22-18B Each rescuer should reach one hand under the patient's arm and grasp the next highest handhold. The rescuers' other hands should be used to maintain the patient's head in a neutral in-line position.

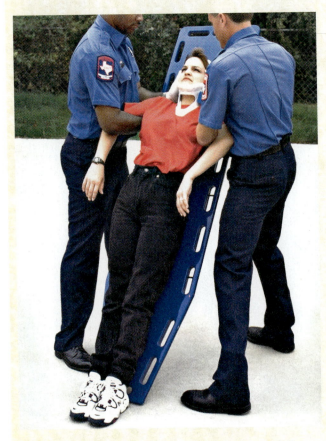

Figure 22-18C Rescuers should then carefully lower the board to the ground.

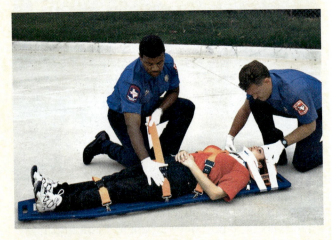

Figure 22-18D One rescuer should then take over and maintain manual in-line stabilization until the patient is completely immobilized to the board.

Rapid Extrication Procedure—For High-Priority Patients Only

Note: In this skill summary, the roof has been removed to better illustrate the procedure. In most cases, the roof of the vehicle will be in place when the procedure is performed, and the skill should be practiced under those conditions.

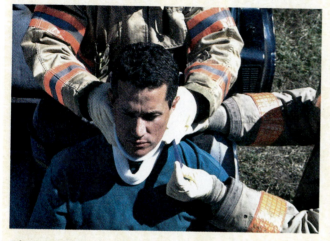

Figure 22-19A Provide manual in-line stabilization and apply a cervical collar.

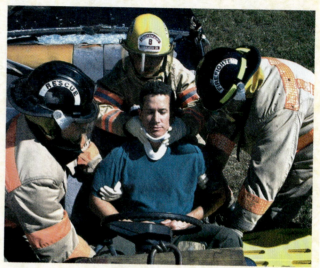

Figure 22-19B At the direction of the rescuer holding stabilization, two rescuers lift the patient by his armpits and buttocks just enough to slide a long spine board onto the seat under the patient and lower him onto it.

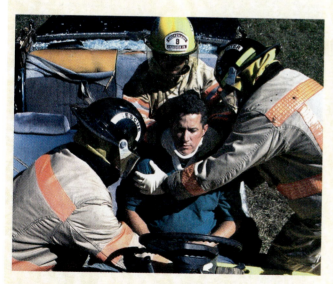

Figure 22-19C The rescuer inside the vehicle then holds the patient's legs and pelvis. The rescuer outside the vehicle holds the upper chest and arms. The rescuer at the head continues to maintain stabilization.

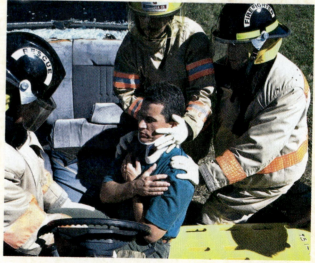

Figure 22-19D At the direction of the rescuer holding stabilization, the patient is carefully moved a quarter turn, so that his back is facing the side door of the vehicle. If another rescuer is available, he may help to hold the board steady during the procedure.

(continued)

Rapid Extrication Procedure—For High-Priority Patients Only (continued)

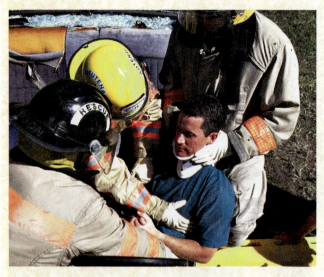

Figure 22-19E The rescuer who was holding the pelvis temporarily holds the chest. The rescuer who was holding the chest takes over in-line stabilization. The rescuer in the back seat then reaches over and holds the chest, allowing the rescuer who had been holding the pelvis to return to it.

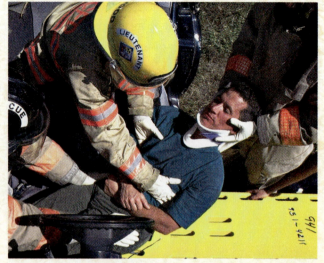

Figure 22-19F The rescuer now holding stabilization directs the other rescuers to lower the patient gently to the long board.

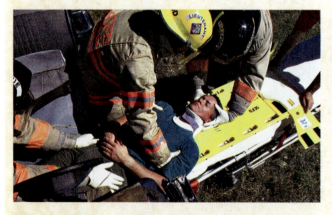

Figure 22-19G As an additional rescuer or bystander holds the end of the board, the rescuers gently slide the patient to its head.

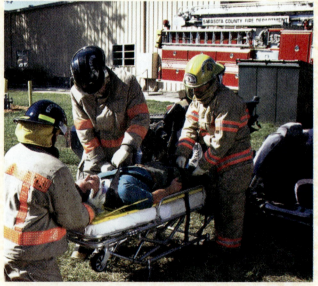

Figure 22-19H Rescuers quickly attach straps across the patient's chest, hips, and legs. At the direction of the rescuer holding stabilization, they move the patient to a stretcher or the ground. Full immobilization should then be completed.

Immobilizing a Patient in a Child Safety Seat

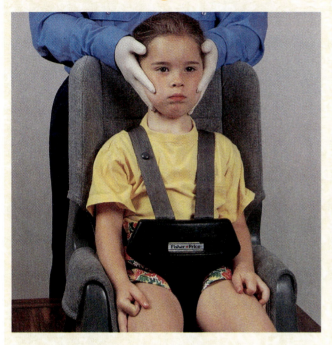

Figure 22-20A One EMT stabilizes the car seat in an upright position and applies and maintains manual in-line stabilization throughout the immobilization process.

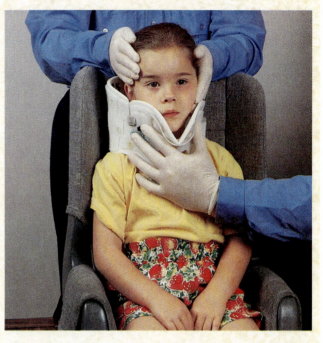

Figure 22-20B A second EMT applies an appropriately sized cervical collar. If one is not available, improvise using a rolled hand towel.

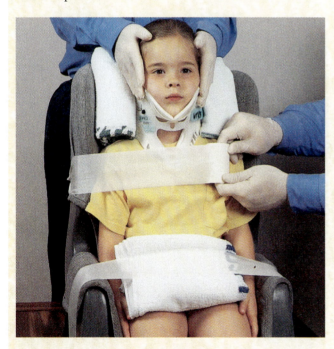

Figure 22-20C The second EMT places a small blanket or towel on the child's lap, then uses straps or wide tape to secure the chest and pelvis areas to the seat.

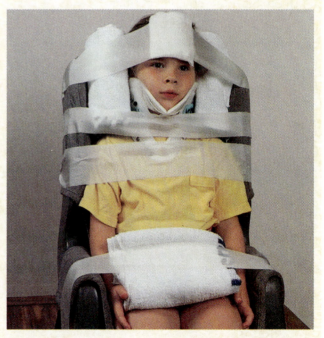

Figure 22-20D The second EMT places towel rolls on both sides of the child's head to fill voids between the head and seat. He then tapes the head into place, taping across the forehead and the collar, but avoiding taping over the chin, which would put pressure on the neck. The patient and seat can be carried to the ambulance and strapped to the stretcher, with the stretcher head raised.

Rapid Extrication from a Child Safety Seat

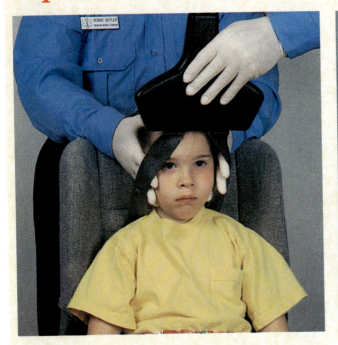

Figure 22-21A One EMT stabilizes the car seat in the upright position and provides manual in-line stabilization throughout the process. The second EMT prepares the equipment, then loosens or cuts the seat straps and raises the front guard.

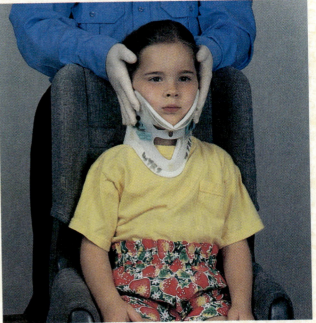

Figure 22-21B The second EMT applies a cervical collar.

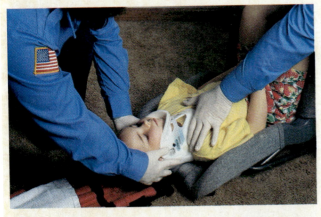

Figure 22-21C While the first EMT continues to hold stabilization, the second EMT centers the safety seat on a back board and slowly tilts it into a supine position. During this maneuver, exercise care that the child does not slip out of the chair. For a child with a large head, place a towel under the area where the shoulders will eventually be placed on the board to prevent the head from sliding forward.

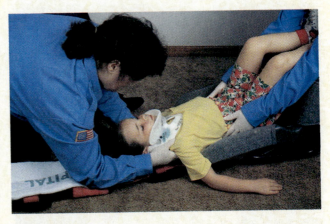

Figure 22-21D The EMT holding stabilization directs a coordinated long axis move of the child from the seat onto the board.

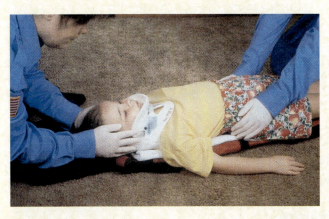

Figure 22-21E Stabilization is maintained as the move is completed. The child's shoulders are now over the folded towel.

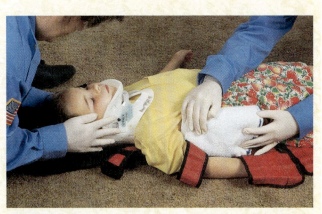

Figure 22-21F The second EMT places rolled towels or blankets on both sides of the patient.

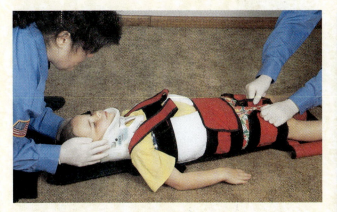

Figure 22-21G The second EMT secures the patient to the board with tape or straps across the upper chest, pelvis, and lower legs. *DO NOT* strap across the abdomen.

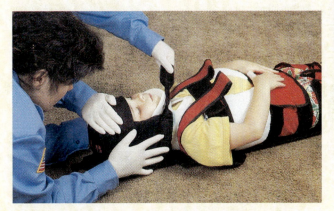

Figure 22-21H The second EMT places rolled towels on both sides of the head and tapes the head securely in place across the forehead and maxilla or cervical collar. In order to avoid putting pressure on the neck, *DO NOT* tape across the chin.

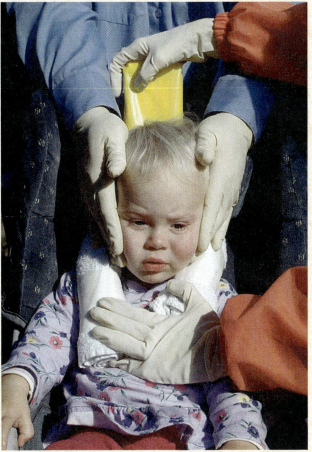

Figure 22-21I The procedure is the same with newborns and infants, except an armboard is inserted behind the patient when the cervical collar is applied. If the patient is very small, the armboard can actually be used as a spine board.

INJURIES TO THE HEAD

Injuries to the head fall into two general categories: injuries to the brain and injuries to the other soft tissues and the bony structures of the head, including the scalp, facial bones, and skull.

The skull and the facial bones provide reasonably good protection for the brain. In cases of head trauma, these bones frequently act as "shock absorbers." The skull and facial bones sustain fractures and other injuries while reducing the amount of energy that affects the brain itself. In cases of severe trauma, however, both the brain and the other structures of the head may be damaged (Figure 22-22).

Figure 22-22   Trauma can produce injuries to the head and brain.

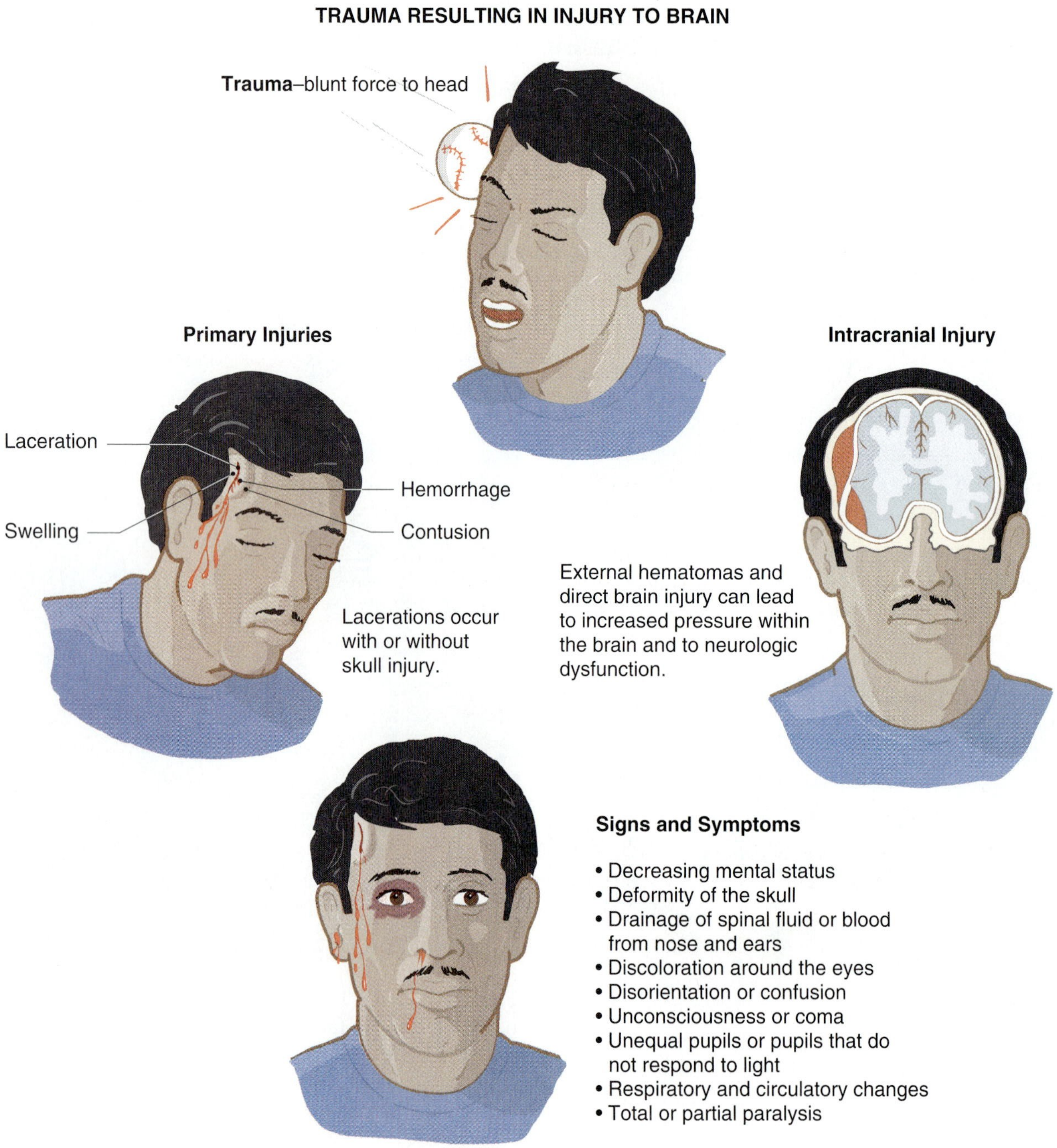

TRAUMA RESULTING IN INJURY TO BRAIN

Trauma–blunt force to head

Primary Injuries

Laceration

Swelling

Hemorrhage

Contusion

Lacerations occur with or without skull injury.

Intracranial Injury

External hematomas and direct brain injury can lead to increased pressure within the brain and to neurologic dysfunction.

Signs and Symptoms

- Decreasing mental status
- Deformity of the skull
- Drainage of spinal fluid or blood from nose and ears
- Discoloration around the eyes
- Disorientation or confusion
- Unconsciousness or coma
- Unequal pupils or pupils that do not respond to light
- Respiratory and circulatory changes
- Total or partial paralysis

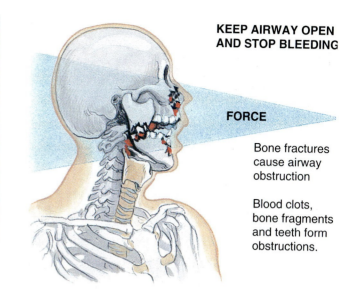

**KEEP AIRWAY OPEN
AND STOP BLEEDING**

FORCE

Bone fractures
cause airway
obstruction

Blood clots,
bone fragments
and teeth form
obstructions.

Figure 22-23   Injuries to the face can have serious complications.

GERIATRIC NOTE

As part of the aging process, the brain shrinks, creating more space between the skull and the brain. This means that, in cases of serious injury such as bleeding in the tissue surrounding the brain, it will take a longer time for the blood to accumulate to the point where it begins to compress the brain. Because it is often compression of the brain by hematomas that causes changes in patients' mental status, it may take longer for geriatric patients to develop signs and symptoms of brain injury. In addition, older patients have more fragile blood vessels and may be using blood-thinning medications like Coumadin®. These factors can contribute to bleeding within the brain and skull.

For these reasons, always consider elderly patients with serious mechanisms of injury to be at high risk for brain injury even if they initially have a normal mental status.

Scalp and Facial Injuries

Injuries to the soft tissues and bones of the skull and face are generally less serious than injuries to the brain itself. However, these injuries can cause serious problems. Scalp lacerations, for example, may bleed excessively because of the rich blood supply in the scalp. Also, injuries to the facial structures can produce partial or complete obstruction of the upper airway as the normal structures are distorted by injuries and swelling and by blood filling the nose and mouth (Figure 22-23).

Skull Injuries

Like all bones, the skull can be fractured if sufficient force is applied. Because the skull is in such close proximity to the brain tissue, fractures of the skull are often associated with injuries to the brain itself (Figure 22-24). Because of this close relationship between skull and brain and because it takes significant force to fracture the skull, when you assess that a skull injury has occurred you should always assume that there is a potential brain injury as well. Signs of a skull injury include the following:

- A mechanism of injury that generates substantial force
- Severe contusions, deep lacerations, or hematomas (swellings due to pooled blood) of the scalp
- Deformities of the skull such as depressions or sudden "step-offs" on the surface of the skull
- Blood or clear (cerebrospinal) fluid leaking from the nose or ears
- Bruising around the eyes ("raccoon eyes")
- Bruising behind the ears over the mastoid process (Battle's sign)

Brain Injuries

The severity of traumatic injuries to the brain can vary widely. Sometimes the brain tissue itself can be damaged by lacerations or contusions. At other times, trauma can cause hematomas, or pools of blood, to collect on the outer surface of the brain or between the thin layers of tissue between the brain and the skull. Because the skull is rigid and doesn't permit outward swelling, these hematomas can quickly compress the brain. The brain tissue itself may swell when injured, increasing pressure within the skull and causing further injury to the brain. Finally, trauma can cause damage to brain tissues at the level of the cells.

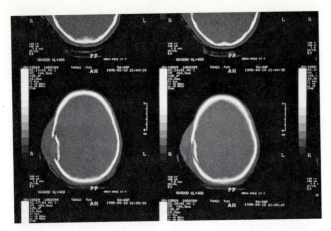

A.

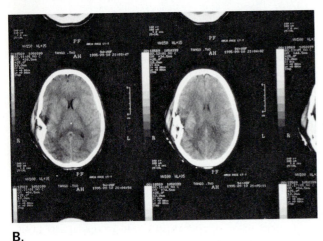

B.

Figure 22-24 CAT scans of a head injury, **(A)** one showing just the deformity of the skull fracture and **(B)** the other revealing how fragments of the skull impinge on the brain.

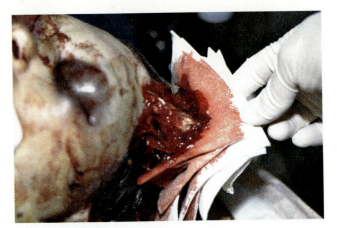

Figure 22-25 An open head injury from a gunshot wound with visible brain tissue.

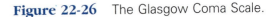

GLASGOW COMA SCALE		
Eye Opening	Spontaneous	4
	To Voice	3
	To Pain	2
	None	1
Verbal Response	Oriented	5
	Confused	4
	Inappropriate Words	3
	Incomprehensible Sounds	2
	None	1
Motor Response	Obeys Command	6
	Localizes Pain	5
	Withdraw (pain)	4
	Flexion (pain)	3
	Extension (pain)	2
	None	1
Glasgow Coma Score Total		

TOTAL GLASGOW COMA SCALE POINTS	
14-15=5	CONVERSION = APPROXIMATELY ONE-THIRD TOTAL VALUE
11-13=4	
8-10=3	
5-7=2	
3-4=1	

Neurologic Assessment	

Figure 22-26 The Glasgow Coma Scale.

An open soft tissue injury that reaches down through the skull to the level of the brain, is termed an *open head injury*. In some severe cases, brain tissue may be visible in the wound (Figure 22-25). Various objects can be impaled in the head causing open head injuries. Such objects should be stabilized and left in place while you assess, treat, and transport the patient.

The hallmark of brain injury is an alteration in a patient's mental status. An initial loss of consciousness at the time of injury is common; if one has occurred, be sure to document it when caring for a patient with head injuries. The extent of the altered mental status can vary widely. It can range from a brief loss of consciousness, to confusion, to complete unresponsiveness. With cases of severe brain injury, there is often a progressive deterioration in mental status. In such a case, a patient may be initially awake but confused, repeating a question or statement over and over. As time passes, he becomes less and less responsive and, finally, completely unresponsive.

Some EMS systems use an objective measure called the Glasgow Coma Scale to assist in determining the extent of the alteration in mental status. This scale assigns number values to the various ways a patient displays eye opening, motor, and verbal responses during an examination (Figure 22-26).

In addition to an altered mental status, you should be alert to several other signs and symptoms when evaluating patients with possible brain injury. These include the following:

◆ Any of the signs of skull injury described earlier
◆ Nausea and/or vomiting
◆ Irregular breathing patterns
◆ Loss of normal neurologic function. This may include loss or decrease of motor function on only one side of the body and/or other loss of motor function or sensation.
◆ Seizures
◆ Unequal pupils associated with altered mental status

Assessment of Head Injuries

Perform a thorough scene size up. Study the scene to determine the mechanism of injury. Specifically look for evidence that significant force was applied to the patient's head. For example, in a motor vehicle collision you should check to see if the windshield was "starred" by contact with the patient's head (Figure 22-27). In incidents involving motorcycles or bikes, check to see if the operator's helmet was damaged (Figure 22-28).

Take appropriate BSI precautions. Be aware that head wounds tend to bleed extensively. In addition, head injury patients often have blood in their airways and may vomit. For this reason, eye and face protection should be considered in addition to gloves.

During the initial assessment, be alert for the possibility of injury to the cervical spine. *Remember that any mechanism that could produce a significant injury to the soft tissue and/or bones of*

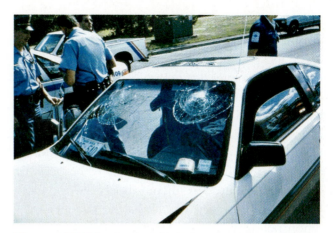

Figure 22-27   A windshield "starred" by contact with a patient's head in a crash.

the head likely had sufficient energy to injure the cervical spine as well. Presume that any patient with a significant injury above the level of the clavicles has a spinal injury. Provide initial manual in-line stabilization and appropriate immobilization for that patient.

Determine the patient's mental status using the AVPU scale. Protect the patient's airway and breathing. If it is necessary to open the airway, use the jaw-thrust maneuver. Provide supplemental oxygen and positive pressure ventilations as necessary, maintaining manual in-line stabilization.

Conduct a focused history and physical exam. This includes the rapid trauma assessment and the gathering of vital signs and a SAMPLE history. Look for the signs and symptoms of head and brain injury described above. As you carry out

Figure 22-28   A motorcyclist's helmet that was damaged in a crash.

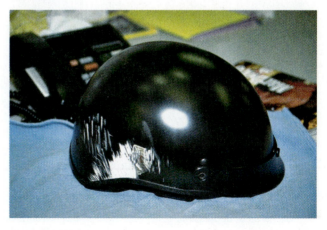

these tasks, continue to maintain manual in-line stabilization.

If the patient is responsive, be aware that his mental status may deteriorate because of the head injury. If another EMT is present, one of you may gather the SAMPLE history while the other performs the rapid trauma assessment. If the patient is unresponsive, obtain as much of the SAMPLE history as you can from family members or bystanders. Question them about the possible mechanism of injury. Ask about the patient's condition before your arrival. Be sure to ask whether there was any change in the patient's mental status before you arrived.

Use extreme care when you perform a rapid trauma assessment on a patient with a head injury. Palpate for deformities, depressions, lacerations, and impaled objects (Figure 22-29). Do not, however, jab at the skull or apply excessive pressure.

◆ *Emergency Care—Patient with Head Injuries*

1. **Assure scene safety and personal safety, including appropriate BSI precautions.**
2. **Assume that a spinal injury exists and provide manual in-line stabilization.**
3. **Maintain an open airway.** Use a jaw-thrust maneuver to open the airway if necessary.
4. **Assure that the patient receives adequate oxygen.** If the patient's breathing is adequate, provide high flow oxygen via nonrebreather mask. If breathing is inadequate, provide positive pressure ventilations with supplemental oxygen.
5. **Complete spinal immobilization as determined by the patient's position and priority.** Be prepared to use the rapid extrication technique if necessary.
6. **Closely monitor the patient's airway, breathing, pulse, and mental status for signs of deterioration.** Be prepared to suction blood, secretions, and vomitus from the patient's airway.
7. **Control bleeding from head wounds as you would for any soft tissue injury.** Be sure, however, to avoid applying excessive pressure over an open head wound or a depression in the skull. Stabilize impaled objects in place. If clear (cerebrospinal) fluid is flowing from the patient's ears or nose, do not attempt to stop it. Instead, use a loose gauze dressing to absorb the fluid.
8. **Transport the patient immediately.** Provide an ongoing assessment en route, continually monitoring airway, breathing, pulse, and mental status.

Figure 22-29 Types of deformities, depressions, lacerations, and impaled objects possibly encountered during the rapid trauma assessment.

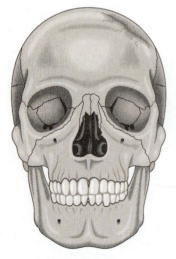

Soft area or depression.

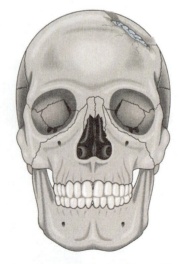

Open wound with bleeding and/or exposed brain tissue.

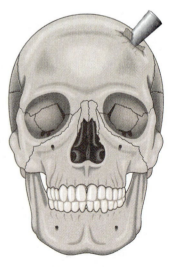

Impaled object in skull.

HELMET REMOVAL

The assessment and care of a patient with a possible head or spine injury can become more complicated when the patient is wearing a helmet. Helmets have become standard head protection in many sports and occupations. A helmet does provide the wearer with some protection. However, an activity that calls for a helmet to be worn is by its nature hazardous, and a person who engages in that activity remains at increased risk for head and spine injury even when he wears a helmet. Some of the people who commonly wear helmets whom you may encounter as patients include the following:

◆ Motorcycle drivers and passengers
◆ Bicycle riders
◆ Football players
◆ Ice hockey players
◆ Skiers
◆ Construction workers
◆ Firefighters

Helmet designs can vary greatly. The helmets that present the greatest challenges for EMTs attempting patient care are those with full face shields, such as football helmets and certain types of motorcycle helmets. These helmets can prevent immediate access to the patient's airway.

When you encounter a patient still wearing a helmet, you must make several decisions before you can properly assess and care for that patient. The most basic decision is whether or not to remove the helmet in order to assess, care for, and immobilize the patient.

Indications that a helmet can be left in place include the following:

◆ The helmet does not interfere with assessment and monitoring of the patient's airway and breathing.
◆ There are no current or impending airway or breathing problems.
◆ Removal of the helmet would risk further injury to the patient.
◆ The patient can be adequately immobilized with the helmet in place.
◆ The patient's head rests snugly within the helmet, assuring that there will be little or no movement of the patient's head once the helmet is secured to the long spine board.

Indications that a helmet should be removed include the following:

◆ The helmet prevents assessment and monitoring of the airway and breathing.
◆ The helmet interferes with efforts to manage the patient's airway or provide ventilations.
◆ The design of the helmet prevents adequate spinal immobilization. For example, the wide brim on a fire helmet makes it almost impossible to adequately stabilize the head and neck of a patient who is wearing one.
◆ The patient's head moves too freely within the helmet to allow adequate stabilization.
◆ The patient is in respiratory or cardiac arrest.

If you decide that it is necessary to remove a helmet, follow the basic procedures shown in Figures 22-30 and 22-31. Remember, however, that procedures for removal will vary depending on the design of the helmet a patient is wearing.

COMPANY OFFICER'S NOTES

Accomplishing a safe helmet removal, especially when there is an urgent need to manage airway and breathing problems, can be a tense undertaking. When you are facing a helmet whose design you have not encountered before, don't forget to use the expertise of civilians on the scene who may be familiar with techniques for removing such a helmet. For example, sports trainers usually have the knowledge and equipment that will allow them to quickly remove face guards from football, hockey, and lacrosse helmets. Also, think ahead! If there is a good possibility that airway or breathing problems will develop en route to the hospital, either remove the helmet before you begin transport or bring the trainer and any necessary equipment for removal along with the patient in the ambulance.

Helmet Removal

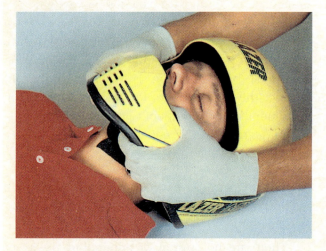

Figure 22-30A One EMT applies stabilization by placing hands on each side of the helmet with fingers on the patient's mandible. This prevents slippage if the strap is loose.

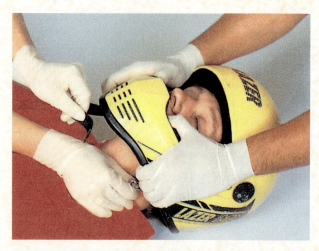

Figure 22-30B While the first EMT maintains stabilization, a second EMT loosens the strap at the D rings.

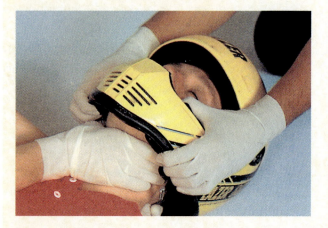

Figure 22-30C The second EMT places one hand on the mandible at the angle, the thumb on one side, the long and index fingers on the other.

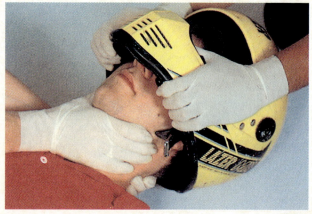

Figure 22-30D With his other hand, the second EMT holds the patient's occipital region and thus takes over stabilization from the first EMT. The first EMT then removes the helmet in two steps, allowing the second EMT to adjust his hand at the occipital region. Keep these factors in mind when removing the helmet: (a) the helmet is egg-shaped and must be expanded laterally to clear the ears; (b) if the helmet provides full facial coverage, the patient's glasses must be removed first; (c) if the helmet provides full facial coverage, it must be tilted backwards to clear the nose.

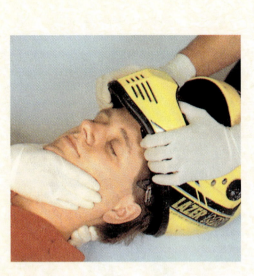

Figure 22-30E The second EMT maintains stabilization to prevent head tilt during removal.

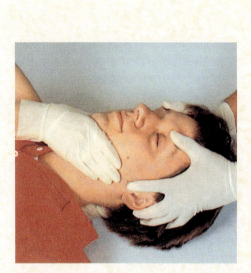

Figure 22-30F When the helmet is off, the first EMT resumes stabilization.

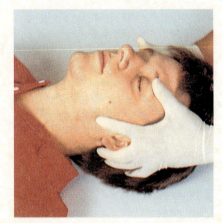

Figure 22-30G The first EMT maintains stabilization while a cervical collar is applied and until the patient is fully immobilized to a spine board.

Alternative Helmet Removal

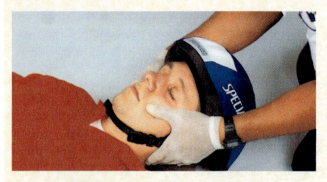

Figure 22-31A The first EMT should apply manual in-line stabilization.

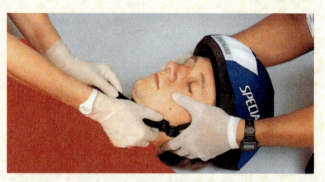

Figure 22-31B A second EMT should remove the chin strap.

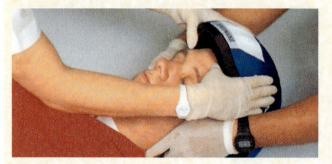

Figure 22-31C The second EMT should remove the helmet by pulling out laterally on each side.

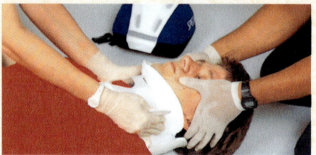

Figure 22-31D The second EMT should then apply a cervical collar. The first EMT should maintain in-line stabilization until the patient is fully immobilized to a long spine board.

Chapter Review

SUMMARY

It is common to encounter patients with both head and spine injuries. These injuries are among the most potentially devastating you will encounter as an EMT. The emergency medical care you provide for patients with these injuries can save their lives and reduce the risk that they will suffer permanent disability.

REVIEWING KEY CONCEPTS

1. List the components of the central nervous system and describe their functions.

2. Explain why providing spinal stabilization is important in cases of suspected spinal injury.

3. List and describe mechanisms of injury that carry increased risk of causing spinal injuries.

4. Explain how you can test for motor function and sensation in a patient with suspected spinal injury.

5. List common signs and symptoms of spinal injury.

6. List the circumstances in which you should apply a cervical collar to a patient.

7. Explain how to provide manual in-line stabilization for a patient in a standing position and one in a supine position.

8. Describe the basic procedure for immobilizing a patient to a full body spinal immobilization device.

9. Describe the steps in the emergency care of a patient with a suspected spinal injury.

10. List common signs of skull injury.

11. List common signs of brain injury.

12. Describe the steps in the emergency care of the patient with a head injury.

13. Identify circumstances in which it is acceptable to leave a helmet on a patient. Identify circumstances in which the helmet should be removed.

RESOURCES TO LEARN MORE

Article

Brown, L. H., Gough, J. F., and Simonds, W. B. "Can EMS Providers Adequately Assess Trauma Patients for Cervical Spinal Injury?" in *Prehospital Emergency Care*. 1998; 2:33–36.

Book

"Injuries of the Cranium" and "Injuries of the Vertebrae and Spinal Cord" in Moore, E. E., Mattox, K. L., and Feliciano, D. V. *Trauma, 3rd Edition*. Philadelphia: Appleton-Lange, 1996.

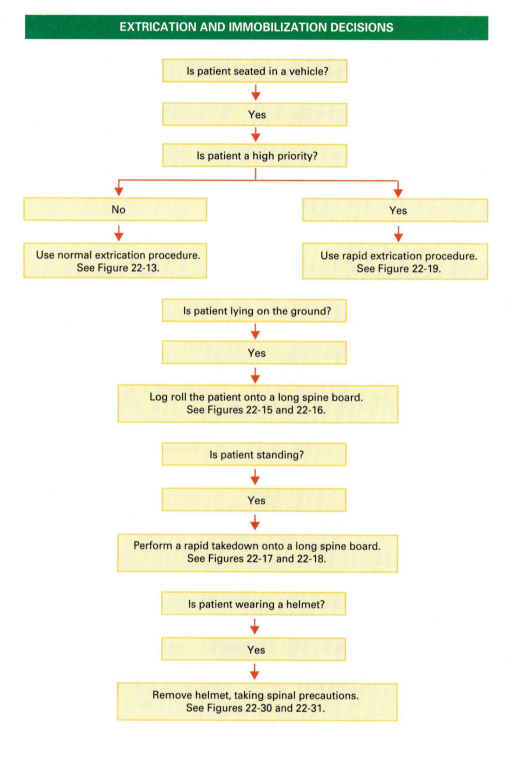

EXTRICATION AND IMMOBILIZATION DECISIONS

Is patient seated in a vehicle?

Yes

Is patient a high priority?

No

Use normal extrication procedure.
See Figure 22-13.

Yes

Use rapid extrication procedure.
See Figure 22-19.

Is patient lying on the ground?

Yes

Log roll the patient onto a long spine board.
See Figures 22-15 and 22-16.

Is patient standing?

Yes

Perform a rapid takedown onto a long spine board.
See Figures 22-17 and 22-18.

Is patient wearing a helmet?

Yes

Remove helmet, taking spinal precautions.
See Figures 22-30 and 22-31.

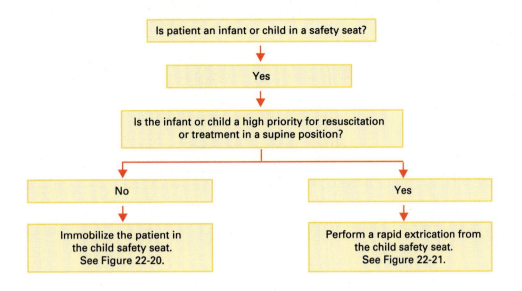

Infants and Children

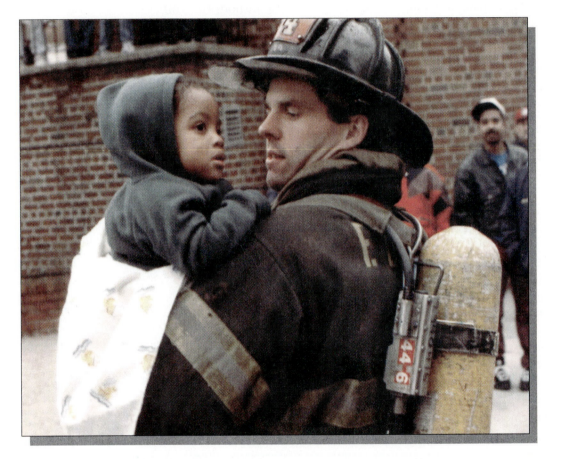

*A*s a firefighter EMT, you will sometimes be called upon to provide emergency medical care for infants and children. Although the assessment and treatment priorities are largely the same as for adults, there are also many differences in their anatomy, physiology, and responses to illness that make pediatric patients unique. Because infants and children are not simply small adults, it is vitally important that you acquire the knowledge and learn the skills that go into providing the best possible care for them.

At the completion of this chapter, the EMT-Basic student should be able to meet the following objectives:

Knowledge and Understanding

1. Identify the developmental considerations for the following age groups: (pp. 598, 599)
   —infants
   —toddlers
   —preschool
   —school age
   —adolescent

2. Describe the differences in the anatomy and physiology of the infant, child, and adult patient. (pp. 595–597)

3. Differentiate the response of the ill or injured infant or child (age specific) from that of an adult. (pp. 595–599)

4. Indicate various causes of respiratory emergencies. (pp. 611, 613–614)

5. Differentiate between respiratory distress and respiratory failure. (pp. 613–614)

6. List the steps in the management of foreign body airway obstruction. (pp. 602–604, 611–612)

7. Summarize emergency medical care strategies for respiratory distress and respiratory failure. (pp. 613–614)

8. Identify the signs and symptoms of shock (hypoperfusion) in infants and children. (p. 616)

9. Describe the methods of determining end organ perfusion in infants and children. (pp. 609–610)

10. State the usual causes of cardiac arrest in infants and children versus adults. (p. 598)

11. List the common causes of seizures in infants and children. (p. 614)

12. Describe the management of seizures in infants and children. (pp. 614–615)

13. Differentiate between the injury patterns in adults, infants, and children. (pp. 618–622)

14. Discuss the field management of the infant and child trauma patient. (pp. 618–622)

15. Summarize the indicators of possible child abuse and neglect. (p. 623)

16. Describe the medical legal responsibilities in suspected child abuse. (pp. 623–624)

17. Recognize the need for EMT-Basic debriefing following a difficult call involving an infant or child transport. (p. 628)

18. Explain the rationale for having knowledge and skills appropriate for dealing with the infant or child patient. (pp. 593, 595)

19. Attend to the feelings and needs of the family when dealing with an ill or injured infant or child. (pp. 598, 618, 627–628)

20. Understand the provider's own emotional responses to caring for infants and children.

Skills

1. Demonstrate the techniques of foreign body airway obstruction removal in the infant.

2. Demonstrate the techniques of foreign body airway obstruction removal in the child.

3. Demonstrate assessment of infants and children.

4. Demonstrate bag-valve-mask artificial ventilations technique for the infant.

5. Demonstrate bag-valve-mask artificial ventilations technique for the child.

6. Demonstrate oxygen delivery for infants and children.

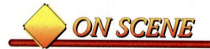

ON SCENE

You are an EMT assigned to Ladder 11. Engine 11 is out doing inspections, and your crew is cleaning up the station and getting dinner ready. Suddenly there is a loud pounding at the bay doors. You raise the doors and see a teenage girl holding a limp toddler in her arms. She screams, "Help! Mickey's not breathing!"

You quickly move to assess the child as the other members of your crew grab a pediatric jump kit and transmit an alarm. You note that the patient is a toddler about 2 years old who is unresponsive and cyanotic around the mouth and nose. You take the child from the girl's arms as she explains to you that she is Mickey's babysitter. She says that he suddenly stopped breathing while she was sharing a hot dog with him at the food stand next to your station.

As you lay the child on the bay floor, you open the airway with a modified head-tilt, chin-lift maneuver and note that there is no air exchange. The other EMT from Ladder 11 begins to ventilate the toddler with a pediatric BVM, but there is no chest rise. Even after you reposition Mickey's head, a second ventilation also fails to expand the chest.

You then immediately deliver four abdominal thrusts and inspect Mickey's mouth. You see a large chunk of a hot dog, which you remove. The other EMT again attempts to ventilate the patient, and this time the chest rises easily. You

check for a pulse while your partner continues ventilations. Mickey's brachial pulse is initially slow, but it rises almost immediately to about 130 beats per minute. The child's color quickly becomes pink, and he begins to cry and cough. He then opens his eyes and tries to push the mask away from his face.

Your reassessment reveals that Mickey is now breathing normally. To calm the child, you hand him a stuffed animal from the pediatric jump kit. You have switched over to providing oxygen using the blow-by method instead of a mask by the time the paramedic ambulance arrives. You give the ambulance crew an account of your initial assessment of respiratory arrest due to airway obstruction and report Mickey's response to your treatment.

The ambulance crew transports Mickey to the hospital. He's admitted to the pediatric intensive care unit overnight, but is released the next day.

INTRODUCTION TO PEDIATRIC EMERGENCY CARE

Pediatrics is the medical specialty of caring for infants and children. Infants and children are commonly referred to as *pediatric patients.* In most EMS systems, compared to adult patients, pediatric patients make up a relatively small percentage of calls. Although life-threatening illnesses and injuries are not commonly encountered, such conditions can and do occur in infants and children.

Because most EMS personnel care for pediatric patients less frequently than adults and because there are always heightened emotions when caring for a seriously ill or injured child, calls involving pediatric patients are often more stressful than adult calls. You can reduce some of this stress by learning the characteristics that distinguish infants and children from adults. Knowing the anatomical and physiological differences will help you better understand the differences in emergency medical care between the two groups.

Because calls for infants and children are relatively infrequent, you may find that you will want or need to review from time to time the material in this chapter and the skills associated with assessing and treating pediatric patients even after you have completed your EMT course.

ANATOMY AND PHYSIOLOGY CONSIDERATIONS

The differences between the anatomy and physiology of infants and children and that of adults are the basis for the differences in the emergency medical care of the two groups (Figure 23-1). As an infant grows, its anatomy and physiology both change. Since an infant must grow, many of its tissues are designed to accommodate this growth. This is especially true of rigid or bony structures such as the skull, ribs, and long bones, which are softer than in older children and adults. The rings and cricoid cartilage of the trachea are also softer.

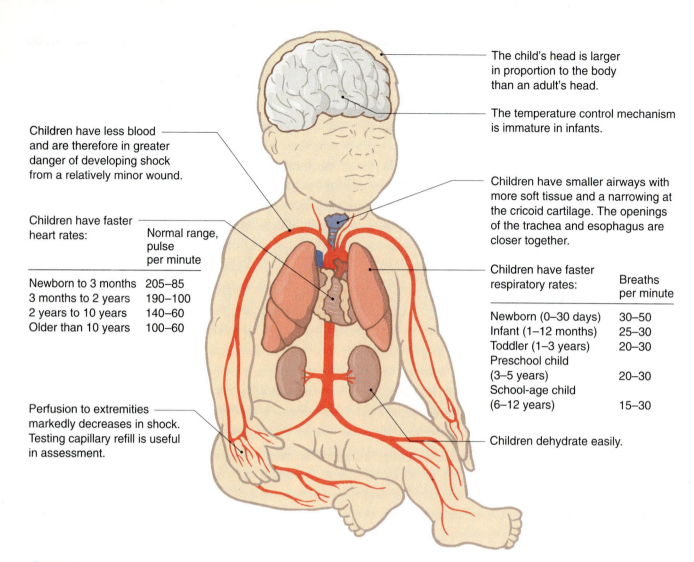

Children have less blood and are therefore in greater danger of developing shock from a relatively minor wound.

Children have faster heart rates:

Normal range, pulse per minute	
Newborn to 3 months	205–85
3 months to 2 years	190–100
2 years to 10 years	140–60
Older than 10 years	100–60

Perfusion to extremities markedly decreases in shock. Testing capillary refill is useful in assessment.

The child's head is larger in proportion to the body than an adult's head.

The temperature control mechanism is immature in infants.

Children have smaller airways with more soft tissue and a narrowing at the cricoid cartilage. The openings of the trachea and esophagus are closer together.

Children have faster respiratory rates:

	Breaths per minute
Newborn (0–30 days)	30–50
Infant (1–12 months)	25–30
Toddler (1–3 years)	20–30
Preschool child (3–5 years)	20–30
School-age child (6–12 years)	15–30

Children dehydrate easily.

Figure 23-1   Anatomic and physiologic considerations in infants and children.

These softer bones and cartilage have an important influence on trauma and airway considerations in pediatric patients. Some of the major anatomical and physiological differences and what those differences may mean for assessment and care are summed up in Table 23-1.

The organ systems of pediatric patients are much less likely to be diseased than those of adults. For example, coronary artery disease, which is responsible for angina, myocardial infarctions, and sudden cardiac death in adults, is very rare in children. Similarly, breathing problems in infants and children tend to be the result of reversible causes, such as infection or asthma, as compared to breathing problems in adults, which are often caused by more chronic or irre-

versible diseases like emphysema. Their healthier organ systems allow infants and children to have a greater "physiologic reserve" in many cases; that is, infants and children can generally withstand or compensate for many illnesses better than adults. This is especially true of diseases affecting the respiratory and cardiovascular systems.

Although children can compensate well for short periods of time, when they do begin to succumb to an illness or injury the change is much more rapid than it usually is for adults. For instance, a toddler who has been in respiratory distress may have a sudden drop in pulse and immediately go into cardiac arrest, whereas this type of decompensating event tends to occur more gradually in an adult.

Table 23-1

Anatomical and Physiological Characteristics of Infants and Children

Differences in Infants and Children as Compared to Adults	Potential Effects That May Impact Assessment and Care
Tongue proportionally larger	More likely to block airway
Smaller airway structures	More easily blocked
Abundant secretions	Can block the airway
Deciduous (baby) teeth	Easily dislodged; can block the airway
Flat nose and face	Difficult to obtain good face mask seal
Head heavier relative to body and less-developed neck structures and muscles	Head may be propelled more forcefully than body producing a higher incidence of head injury in trauma
Fontanelle and open sutures (soft spots) palpable on top of young infant's head	Bulging fontanelle can be a sign of intracranial pressure (but may be normal if infant is crying); shrunken fontanelle may indicate dehydration
Thinner, softer brain tissue	Susceptible to serious brain injury
Head larger in proportion to body	Tips forward when supine causing flexion of neck, which makes neutral alignment of airway difficult
Shorter, narrower, more elastic (flexible) trachea	Can close off trachea with hyperextension of neck
Short neck	Difficult to stabilize or immobilize
Abdominal breathers	Difficult to evaluate breathing
Faster respiratory rate	Muscles easily fatigue, causing respiratory distress
Newborns breathe primarily through the nose (obligate nose breathers)	May not automatically open mouth to breathe if nose is blocked; airway more easily blocked
Larger body surface relative to body mass	Prone to hypothermia
Softer bones	More flexible, less easily fractured; traumatic forces may be transmitted to and injure internal organs without fracturing ribs; lungs easily damaged with trauma
Spleen and liver more exposed	Organ injury likely with significant force to abdomen

TRANSITION OF CARE

Putting a child (and sometimes a parent as well) at ease with the personnel providing emergency care can be very difficult. Developing trust between an EMT and a pediatric patient in the brief period of time of an average EMS call is a skill that is both taught and learned with time and the experience of caring for children. When it is obvious that a bond has developed between a crew member and a patient, it may be very damaging to overall care to sever that bond too suddenly. A terrified child who has been calmed by a specific provider is likely to become terrified again if that provider suddenly disappears. This is especially true when the child's environment suddenly changes as well, as in the move from the home to the back of an ambulance. If a particular provider has developed a bond with the patient, it may very beneficial to have that provider accompany the patient all the way to the hospital, even if, as in the case of a first-responding engine company member, that provider would not normally do so.

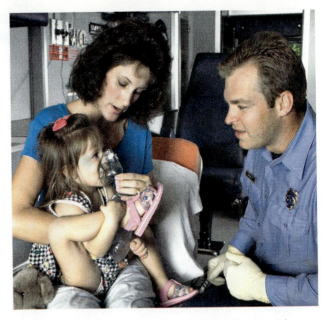

Figure 23-2 It is characteristic of infants and young children to be suspicious of strangers and to fear separation from parents. If possible, have a parent hold the child during assessment and care.

DEVELOPMENTAL CONSIDERATIONS

Infants and children develop and grow throughout childhood, not only physically but emotionally as well. The emotional development of infants and children is important to prehospital care because it influences how infants and children respond to illness and injury and how they will react to you, the EMT (Figure 23-2). Developmental considerations relevant to the prehospital care for infants and children are presented in Table 23-2.

MANAGEMENT OF THE PEDIATRIC AIRWAY AND BREATHING

Airway and breathing problems that may be immediately life threatening are often encountered in seriously ill infants and children.

Obstructed airways and respiratory failure are the most common causes of cardiac arrest in infants and young children. Management of the pediatric patient's airway and breathing problems is, therefore, one of the most crucial and life-saving skills you will learn as an EMT.

The immediate management of problems detected with the airway and breathing is an important part of the initial assessment of infants and children just as it is for adults. For this reason, issues of airway and breathing management will be discussed here, before a specific discussion of pediatric assessment.

There are several special anatomic and physiologic and considerations that influence the way you manage the airway of an infant or child as compared to an adult (Figure 23-3):

◆ *The face, mouth, and nose of the pediatric patient are smaller than the adult's.* The smaller diameters of the mouth and nose are more easily blocked by secretions.

◆ *The tongue takes up more space proportionately in a child's mouth.* It can more easily obstruct the airway in an unconscious infant or child.

Table 23-2

Psychological and Social Characteristics of Infants and Children

Infant Birth to 1 year	Toddler 1 to 3 years	Preschool 3 to 6 years	School Age 6 to 12 years	Adolescent 12 to 18 years
Has minimal stranger anxiety				
Needs to be kept warm (so warm hands and stethoscope before use)				
Fears being touched by strangers (so examine heart and lungs first, head last to build confidence)				
Doesn't like being separated from parents (so have patient sit on parent's lap when possible)				
Feels suffocated by oxygen mask (so try blow-by method)				
	Fears needles and instruments (so explain what you are doing; reassure)			
	Thinks injury or illness is punishment for being bad (so assure this is not true)			
	Fears pain (so do not lie to patient, but reassure)			
		Fears blood (so explain and reassure)		
		Fears permanent injury (so do not lie to patient, but reassure)		
		Is modest (so protect privacy)		
			Fears disfigurement (so do not lie to patient, but reassure)	
				Sensitive to violations of dignity (so talk as if to an adult; assess away from parents or guardians; have same-sex EMT examine if possible)

Airway structures are smaller and more easily obstructed.

Cricoid cartilage is less rigid and less developed.

Tongue takes up more space in pharynx.

Trachea is narrower.

Nose and mouth are smaller.

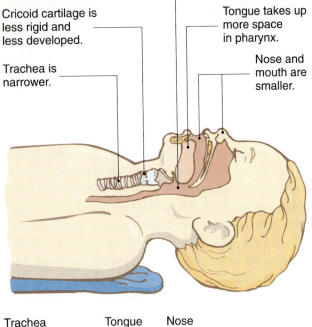

Trachea Cricoid cartilage Tongue Nose

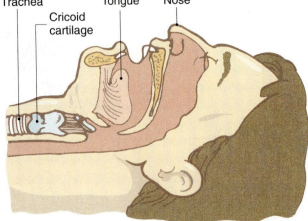

Figure 23-3 Child and adult airways compared.

- *The trachea (windpipe) is softer and more flexible in a child.* The trachea can collapse if the neck and head are hyperextended during maneuvers for opening the airway. It can also collapse if the head is allowed to fall into a position of hyperflexion.

- *The trachea is narrower.* It is easily obstructed by swelling.

- *Stimulation of the pharynx during suctioning may result in a sudden drop in the heart rate.* This is especially dangerous when the child is hypoxic (oxygen starved), as that condition may also contribute to a slowed heart rate (bradycardia).

- *Infants breathe predominantly through their noses (obligate nose breathers) rather than through their mouths.* If the nose is blocked, for example by mucus, the infant may not "know" to open its mouth to breathe.

- *The chest wall is softer, and infants and children tend to depend more on the diaphragm rather than their chest or intercostal (between-the-rib) muscles for breathing.*

- *Children can compensate well for problems with the airway and breathing for short periods of time by increasing the rate of breathing and the effort of breathing.* They may accomplish this through the use of accessory muscles, including the abdominal muscles. Compensation can be followed by a rapid decompensation to respiratory failure and arrest as normal respiratory and accessory muscles become fatigued.

- *Hypoxia (insufficient oxygen in the bloodstream) in an infant or child will frequently result in a slow (bradycardic) heart rate, which may rapidly progress to cardiac arrest.*

Take account of these anatomic and physiologic differences in the following ways when you manage the pediatric airway:

- Use properly sized face masks to assure a good seal when providing pocket mask or BVM ventilations. All first response and transporting vehicles should be equipped with assorted pediatric sizes of pocket masks and BVMs.

- Use pediatric-sized nonrebreather masks and nasal cannulas when administering supplemental oxygen.

- Open the airway gently. Infants can be placed in a neutral neck position and children may require only slight extension of the neck (Figure 23-4). Do not overextend the neck, because doing so may collapse the trachea. Placing a folded towel under the shoulders of an infant can help compensate for the infant's larger head and help you to maintain the proper extension.

- Obstruction by the proportionally larger tongue may require that one EMT be assigned

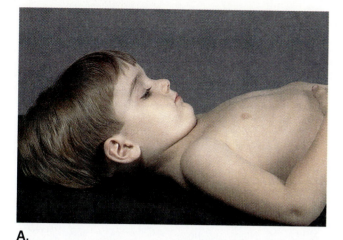

A.

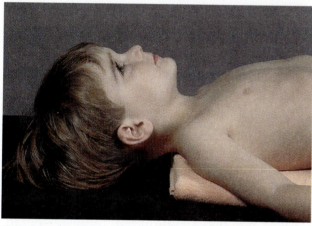

B.

Figure 23-4 **A.** In the supine position, an infant's or child's larger head will tip forward, causing airway obstruction. **B.** Placing padding under the patient's shoulders will bring the airway to a neutral or slightly extended position.

to constantly maintain the airway-opening maneuver.

◆ Because any device placed in the infant's or child's airway further narrows the passage's diameter and may result in localized swelling, consider use of an oral or nasal airway only after other manual maneuvers have failed to keep the airway open.

◆ When suctioning infants and children, use a rigid-tip catheter, but be careful not to cause trauma to the surfaces of the mouth and not to touch the back of the airway. Trauma in the mouth can cause local swelling that may obstruct the airway. Also, prolonged stimulation of the back of the throat may suddenly and dangerously slow the patient's heart rate.

◆ Suctioning secretions from the nose and nasopharynx may significantly improve airway and breathing problems in an infant.

◆ If any infant or child demonstrates an increased respiratory rate or signs of increased effort of breathing—such as nasal flaring, retractions, or use of accessory muscles—place him on high concentration oxygen and conduct a continuous ongoing assessment so you can immediately detect signs of decompensation into respiratory failure.

◆ If any infant or child has a slow heart rate, assume that he is hypoxic. Immediately provide high flow oxygen, plus assisted ventilations with a pocket mask or BVM if necessary.

Airway Skills

Opening the Airway

As with all patients, the first pediatric care priority is to assure an open airway. Use the head-tilt, chin-lift maneuver without hyperextending the child's neck (Figure 23-5). In cases of suspected trauma, use the jaw thrust (Figure 23-6). When performing either maneuver, keep your fingertips on the bony part of the lower jaw, avoiding any excess pressure on the soft tissue under the mandible. Pressure in this area may accidentally compress the trachea.

Figure 23-5 When using the head-tilt, chin-lift maneuver to open an infant or child's airway, avoid hyperextending the neck.

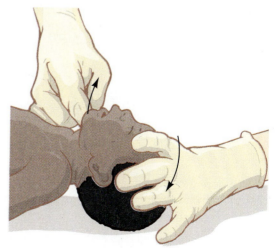

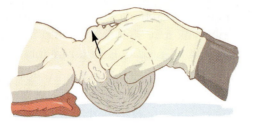

Figure 23-6 Use the jaw-thrust maneuver to open the airway if trauma is suspected.

Suctioning

Careful but effective suctioning is an essential skill in pediatric airway management. Suction whenever there are heavy secretions or other fluids in the patient's mouth or nose. Suctioning is especially important when the patient has an altered mental status or is unresponsive, because his ability to protect his own airway may be diminished or absent. A bulb syringe, a flexible suction catheter, or a rigid-tip suction catheter can be used, depending on the situation and the patient's age (Figure 23-7). When a flexible catheter is used it should be appropriately sized (Table 23-3).

Suctioning can potentially cause the same dangerous complications in infants and children as in adults. Be especially alert for hypoxia, which can develop when supplemental oxygen is removed from the patient for an overly long period of suctioning. You can generally prevent hypoxia by providing the patient with high flow

Figure 23-7 Pediatric suction catheters. **Top:** a soft suction catheter. **Bottom:** a rigid or hard suction catheter.

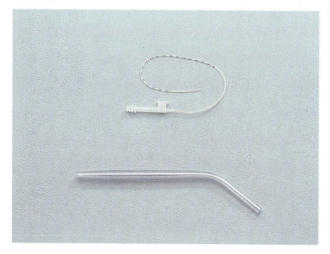

Table 23-3

Suction Catheter Sizes for Infants and Children

Age	Suction Catheter Size (French)
up to 1 year	8
2 to 6 years	10
7 to 15 years	12
16 years	12 to 14

oxygen or ventilations with 100 percent oxygen before suctioning. Also be sure to limit suctioning to less than 15 seconds per attempt.

Deep suctioning into the pharynx may also stimulate the vagus nerve. In a pediatric patient, this can cause a dangerously slow heart rate or even cardiac arrest. To avoid this complication, suction no deeper than you can see and avoid suctioning for an excessive period of time.

As already mentioned, newborns and young infants are obligate nose breathers. They depend greatly on the unobstructed passage of air through the nose. Keep the infant's nose clear of obstruction by suctioning with either a bulb syringe or a flexible suction catheter appropriately sized for the infant's age. To avoid soft tissue trauma and nosebleeds, be careful not to place the tip of the suction bulb or catheter too deeply into the nostril. Remember, don't place the tip any deeper than you can see.

Clearing Complete Airway Obstructions

In your basic life support (CPR) course, you learned the steps for clearing an obstructed airway in an infant or child. Upper airway obstruction by such objects as hot dogs, peanuts, marbles, and balloon pieces remains a major cause of accidental death among young children. Because of its importance, airway obstruction clearance will be discussed again, in more depth, later in this chapter.

It is important to determine immediately if an airway obstruction is partial or complete. Infants and children with a partial airway obstruction can have a hoarse cry or voice, a cough, or an audible high-pitched sound during inhalation (stridor). Any of these sounds indicates that at least some air is passing through the airway. Avoid performing a maneuver that risks making a complete obstruction out of one that is only partial. Instead, place the patient in the position of greatest comfort, carefully monitor the patient for developing signs of complete airway obstruction, and transport immediately.

In cases of complete airway obstruction, the patient may be either responsive or unresponsive. The unresponsive pediatric patient will likely be cyanotic (gray or blue in color). The responsive patient with a complete airway obstruction may also be cyanotic and will not be able to cry or speak.

In an infant less than 1 year of age who has a complete airway obstruction, perform a series of 5 back blows followed by 5 chest thrusts (Figure 23-8). At the completion of each series of back blows and abdominal thrusts, quickly but carefully look into the infant's mouth for a dislodged foreign body that you can then remove with a gloved finger. In a child older than 1 year of age with complete airway obstruction, perform a

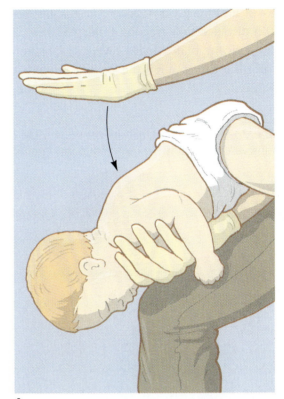

A.

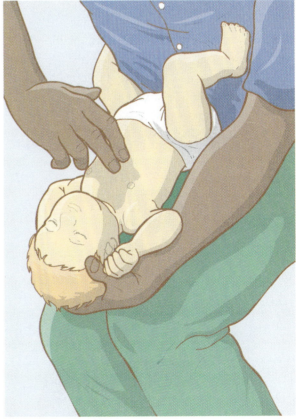

B.

Figure 23-8 Positioning the infant with a foreign body airway obstruction to deliver **(A)** back blows and **(B)** chest thrusts.

series of abdominal thrusts and check the mouth for the displaced obstructing object (Figure 23-9). *Never* perform blind finger sweeps. Continue to perform the thrusts until the patient becomes unresponsive.

Figure 23-9 Delivering abdominal thrusts **(A)** on a responsive child and **(B)** on an unresponsive child.

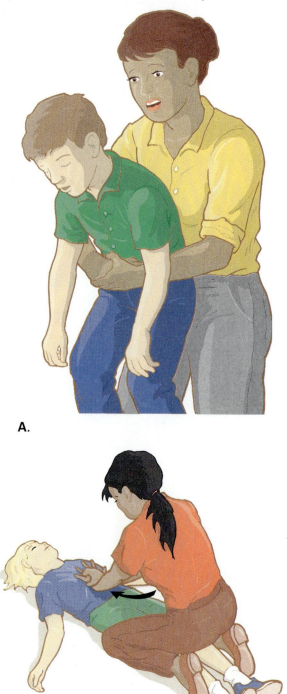

A.

B.

Use of Airway Adjuncts

Oropharyngeal and nasopharyngeal airways are used in infants and children who require *prolonged* artificial ventilations. Unlike adults, in whom these devices are usually placed as soon as artificial ventilation begins, with children they should *not* be used for initial artificial ventilations. Because the breathing efforts and oxygenation of infants and children will often improve quickly as a result of artificial ventilations with 100 percent oxygen, it is often not necessary to place these devices at all. Avoiding the immediate use of an airway adjunct in a pediatric patient also avoids the complications these devices often cause that can worsen the patient's airway and breathing status. These complications include soft tissue damage resulting in bleeding in or swelling of the airway, vomiting, and stimulation of the vagus nerve, which may result in a sudden and dangerous drop in heart rate.

Oral Airways Oropharyngeal airways come in a variety of pediatric sizes. Use a properly sized airway with a pediatric patient. Too small an airway can become an airway obstruction; too large an airway can both block the airway and result in trauma to the mouth and pharynx. Measure a pediatric oral airway by sizing from the corner of the mouth to the front of the earlobe. Again, these devices are not generally used for initial artificial ventilation. They should only be used in patients who have no gag reflex, because stimulation of the gag reflex can cause vomiting and a decreased heart rate.

Insertion of the oropharyngeal airway in children is done as follows (Figure 23-10):

1. **Insert a tongue blade to the base of the tongue.** *If the patient begins to gag or cough, a gag reflex is present and the procedure should be stopped.* If a gag reflex is present, continue to maintain an open airway with a head-tilt, chin-lift or jaw-thrust maneuver, and consider the use of a nasal airway.
2. **If there is no gag reflex, push down against the tongue while lifting it slightly forward.** This maneuver will create the largest possible passageway through the mouth and will enable smooth insertion of the airway.

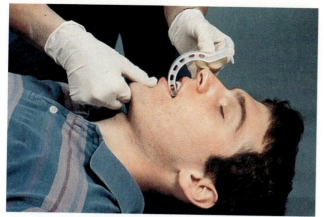

A.

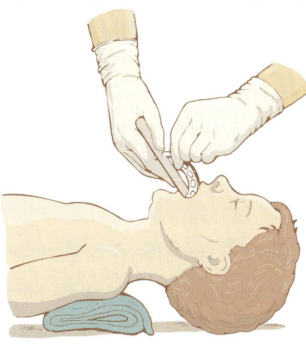

B.

Figure 23-10 **A.** In an adult patient, the airway is inserted with the tip pointing to the roof of the mouth, then rotated into position. **B.** With a pediatric patient, insert the airway with the tip pointing toward the tongue and pharynx, in the same position it will be when insertion is completed.

3. Insert the airway directly into the mouth until the flange rests against the lips. Insert the airway following its curvature *without rotation*.

If the patient begins to cough or gag at any time after airway insertion, remove the airway and be prepared to suction as needed.

Nasal Airways Although pediatric nasopharyngeal airways are not as commonly used as oral pharyngeal airways, they can be an effective airway adjunct for the patient who requires prolonged artificial ventilation but cannot tolerate an oral airway because of the presence of a gag reflex. Nasopharyngeal airways come in a variety of children's sizes but are not routinely available for infants less than 1 year of age. Select a nasal airway of a diameter that will comfortably fit in the child's nostril. The outside diameter of the patient's little finger is approximately the airway diameter that can be used.

Insertion of a nasal airway in a pediatric patient is done in the same fashion as in adults:

1. **Select an appropriately sized airway.**

2. **Lubricate the tip and shaft of the airway with a water-soluble lubricant.**

3. **Insert the airway with the beveled opening toward the nasal septum.** If resistance is met, attempt to insert the airway in the other nostril.

4. **Gradually but steadily insert the airway into the nostril and advance it into the nasopharynx.** If the child gags or coughs with the insertion of the airway, remove it immediately and continue to maintain an open airway with a head-tilt, chin-lift or jaw-thrust maneuver.

The most frequent complication of inserting a nasal airway is nose bleeding. You can usually control this by pinching the patient's nostrils together. Be aware that bleeding from the nostrils may cause bleeding into the nasopharynx and pharynx. Be prepared to suction the airway of blood. However, since children who require nasal airways are likely to be on oxygen or receiving artificial ventilations, attempts at controlling minor bleeding from the nose should not take priority over keeping the airway clear and providing ventilations and supplemental oxygen.

Another serious complication can occur in cases of head or midface trauma where any tube passed through the nostrils may inadvertently be passed through facial or skull fractures into the sinuses or the brain. For this reason, never use a nasal airway when children have sustained trauma to the nose, midface, or head.

Supplemental Oxygen Therapy

All infants and children with signs or symptoms of inadequate breathing or shock (hypoperfusion) should receive supplemental oxygen of the highest possible concentration that can be delivered and that the child will tolerate. Methods used to deliver supplemental oxygen to infants and children include pediatric-sized nonrebreather masks and "blow-by" techniques. Nonrebreather masks deliver the highest concentration of supplemental oxygen.

Often infants and children, because of fear or anxiety, will not allow a nonrebreather be applied to the face. To overcome resistance to the mask, you might place it first over your own face or have the parents place it over their faces to show the child that it's "OK" to wear the mask (Figure 23-11). In systems that use stuffed animals like bears as comforting objects for kids, applying the mask to the bear's face may also ease the child's fears (Figure 23-12).

When the child will not tolerate application of the mask, then use the blow-by technique to deliver supplemental oxygen (Figure 23-13). You can deliver blow-by oxygen by holding a nonrebreather mask or oxygen tubing as close as the

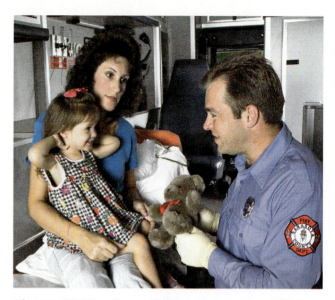

Figure 23-12 Some EMS systems use stuffed animals to help put children at ease during assessment and care.

patient will tolerate—hopefully within a few inches of the face. Alternatively, you can place oxygen tubing into the bottom of a colorful paper cup, possibly covered with familiar cartoon characters, and hold the cup close to the patient. Often the child will not react with the same fear to such an alternative blow-by device as he would to a piece of strange-looking medical equipment like a nonrebreather mask. Although blow-by oxygen does not deliver as a high a concentration of oxy-

Figure 23-11 To overcome the child's fear of the nonrebreather mask, try it on yourself or have the parent try it on before attempting to place it on the child.

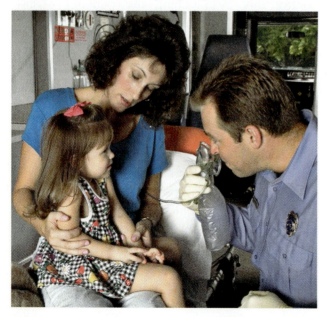

Figure 23-13 Blow-by administration of oxygen. **A.** Using a paper cup and oxygen tubing. **B.** Using oxygen tubing held about 2 inches (50 mm) from the child's face.

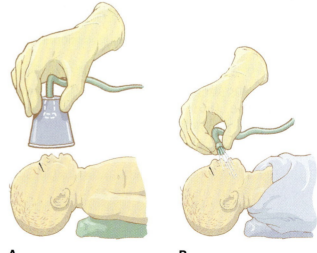

A.   B.

Table 23-4

Artificial Ventilations in Children

	Over 8 Years	1 to 8 Years	Birth to 1 Year
Ventilation Duration	1½ to 2 seconds	1 to 1½ seconds	1 to 1½ seconds
Ventilation Rate	12 breaths/minute (1 breath every 5 seconds)	20 breaths/minute (1 breath every 3 seconds)	20 to 30 breaths/minute (1 breath every 3 seconds)

gen as a nonrebreather mask, it can be an important technique for providing supplemental oxygen.

Some EMS systems also carry pediatric-sized nasal cannulas for oxygen delivery. Although cannulas are effective as a source of supplemental oxygen, infants and children often fear them as they do nonrebreather masks. High-flow blow-by oxygen can provide similar or even higher concentrations of supplemental oxygen than nasal cannulas in children.

Artificial Ventilation

Pediatric patients in respiratory arrest or respiratory failure should receive immediate artificial ventilations with high concentration oxygen. (See Table 23-4 for rates and durations of artificial ventilations.) Similarly, patients with signs of inadequate breathing associated with an abnormally slow heart rate should also receive artificial ventilations, as these patients are at risk for cardiac arrest due to hypoxia. When a patient is breathing inadequately, deliver artificial ventilations by "assisting" the ventilations that are present; if the patient is breathing too slowly, deliver additional ventilations between the patient's own breaths. When assisting with ventilations, carefully watch the beginning of the child's chest rise and deliver the artificial breath at the same time he begins inhalation.

Methods of artificial ventilation in children include mouth-to-mask and BVM ventilation. With either technique, a good mask seal is essential for adequate ventilations. A properly sized mask should fit snugly over the mouth and nose of the patient (Figure 23-14). Use one hand or two hands to assure an adequate mask seal so that no oxygen escapes around the edges of the mask

(Figure 23-15). Important points to remember when providing artificial ventilations to infants and children include the following:

◆ Avoid excessive bag pressure and volume. Use only enough to make the chest rise. Squeeze the bag slowly and steadily.

◆ Use properly sized face masks to assure a good mask seal.

◆ Flow-restricted, oxygen-powered ventilation devices are contraindicated (should not be used) in infants and children.

◆ Infants and children are prone to gastric distention during ventilations or respiratory distress. This may impair adequate ventilations as the distended abdomen pushes up on the diaphragm, limiting expansion of the lungs. In

Figure 23-14 A mask should fit on the bridge of the nose and the cleft above the chin.

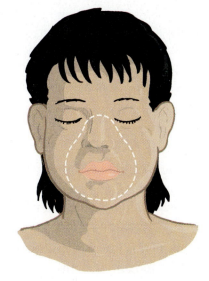

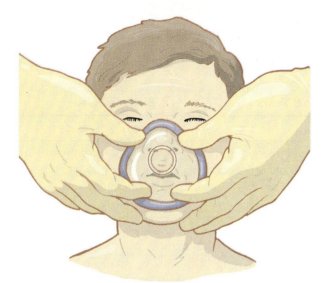

A.

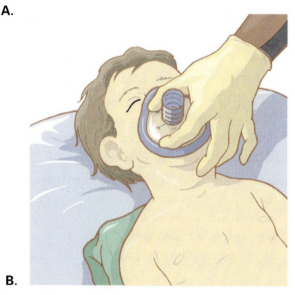

B.

Figure 23-15   A. Holding a mask seal with two hands. **B.** Holding a mask seal with one hand.

such cases it may be necessary to insert a nasogastric tube to decompress the abdomen. (See nasogastric tube insertion in Chapter 29, "Advanced Airway Management.")

◆ An oral or nasal airway may be considered when other measures fail to keep the airway open and artificial ventilations are prolonged.

◆ When suctioning infants and children during artificial ventilations, use a rigid-tip catheter but be careful not to touch the back of the airway.

◆ Avoid overextending the neck during artificial ventilations as this may collapse the trachea in infants and younger children.

◆ The jaw-thrust maneuver should be used when ventilating patients with possible head or spinal injuries.

◆ Provide 100 percent oxygen by using a reservoir attached to a BVM.

◆ Do not use BVMs with "pop-off" valves. These devices may reduce the effectiveness of ventilations by not allowing adequate volumes of oxygen to be delivered to the lungs.

◆ If a pocket mask with an oxygen inlet is used, attach high concentration oxygen to the inlet when delivering ventilations.

ASSESSMENT OF THE PEDIATRIC PATIENT

As with all patients, assessment of the pediatric patient is a systematic process that begins with scene size-up and progresses through initial assessment and an appropriate detailed history and physical examination.

Initial Assessment

Initial assessment begins upon arrival at the scene or from across the room. The assessment should include observations about any mechanism of injury, the surroundings, and a general impression that the patient is a "sick" child or a "well" child.

General Impression

In pediatrics, the general impression you form is designed to place the patient in one of two categories: a "well"-appearing child versus a "sick"-appearing child. Observations of several things, when put together, will form your overall impression of the infant or child. A "sick" child will have a high priority for transport. Observations that go into forming the general impression of the patient include:

◆ *Skin color* Well children should have a pink hue to their skin. Gray, pale, mottled, or cyanotic skin indicates a sick infant or child.

◆ *Quality of cry or speech* An infant who is crying loudly or a child who is able to speak normally is likely to have an adequate airway and breathing. If the infant has a weak cry or does not cry at all in circumstances that would normally cause crying, this indicates a potentially sick child.

- *Interaction with surroundings* A well child should demonstrate normal attentive interactions with his environment, such as playing, moving about, making eye contact, and recognizing and responding to his parents. The child who lies listlessly still, does not react to significant changes in the environment such as the arrival of the fire department crew, and fails to react to or recognize his parents is likely to be a sick child.

- *Emotional state* A well pediatric patient should show emotions appropriate for the child's age and the situation. A sick child will display limited or inappropriate emotional response.

- *Response to the EMT* A well child is likely to have some fear of the EMT especially when it comes to being touched or having procedures performed, such as obtaining a blood pressure or applying oxygen. The child who allows himself to be poked and prodded by the EMT with little or no response is most likely sick.

- *Body tone and positioning* A well child should have good muscular tone and be positioned as one would expect for a child of that age. The infant who is limp or the child who assumes abnormal body positions, such as leaning forward on his hands (tripod position) or lying on his side with his knees drawn up (fetal position), is more likely to be a sick pediatric patient.

Mental Status

Quickly determine the patient's mental status, using the AVPU method described in Chapter 7, "Patient Assessment." If the child is not awake and alert, shout at the child to determine a reaction to verbal stimulus. (Asking "Are you OK?" is obviously not appropriate when assessing an infant.) If there is no response to verbal stimulus, use a pinch or a brisk rub on the sole of the foot to determine response to painful stimulus. (Never shake a baby or a young child.) Be alert to the fact

that altered mental status is often a result of inadequate circulation (hypoperfusion) of the brain.

Airway, Breathing, and Circulation

The respiratory assessment of a child is designed to immediately detect any airway or breathing problems. It is accomplished by careful observation and listening.

- *Observe the respiratory rate.* Breathing at a rate that is faster or slower than normal for the child's age is a sign of respiratory distress (Table 23-5).

- *Observe for full and symmetrical chest rise with inspiration.* Shallow breathing or asymmetric chest movements are signs of inadequate breathing.

- *Note the effort or work of breathing.* Retractions of the skin above the sternal notch and clavicles and between and below the ribs are a sign of increased work of breathing. Nasal flaring (where the nostrils "flare" open and closed with respirations) and "seesaw" breathing (where the work of inhaling draws the chest in and pushes the abdomen out) are also signs of increased effort.

- *Listen for abnormal breathing sounds.* Grunting, stridor, crowing, and other noisy breathing are signs of airway and breathing compromise.

- *Listen with a stethoscope to both sides of the chest.* Normal breath sounds should be present and equal on both sides of the chest. High-pitched sounds on exhalation (wheezes) or on inhalation (stridor or, sometimes, wheezes) or the absence of breath sounds are abnormal findings that indicate breathing problems.

Circulation is another crucial component of pediatric assessment.

- *Assess peripheral perfusion* (how well blood is circulating to all parts of the body). Feel for brachial, femoral, or peripheral pulses (see Table 23-5 and Figure 23-16). Capillary refill time is also an excellent means of determining the adequacy of circulation in children 5 years of age or younger. (In older patients, other factors make capillary refill a less reliable measure of perfusion.) Use your thumb to compress the

Table 23-5

Normal Vital Sign Ranges: Infants and Children

Normal Pulse Rates (Beats per Minute, at Rest)

Newborn	120 to 160
Infant 0–5 months	90 to 140
Infant 6–12 months	80 to 140
Toddler 1–3 years	80 to 130
Preschooler 3–5 years	80 to 120
School age 6–10 years	70 to 110
Adolescent 11–14 years	60 to 105

Normal Respiration Rates (Breaths per Minute, at Rest)

Newborn	30 to 50
Infant 0–5 months	25 to 40
Infant 6–12 months	20 to 30
Toddler 1–3 years	20 to 30
Preschooler 3–5 years	20 to 30
School age 6–10 years	15 to 30
Adolescent 11–14 years	12 to 20

Normal Blood Pressure Ranges

	Systolic	Diastolic
	Approx. 80 plus 2 X age	Approx. 2/3 systolic
Preschooler 3–5 years	average 99 (78 to 116)	average 65
School age 6–10 years	average 105 (80 to 122)	average 69
Adolescent 11–14 years	average 114 (88 to 140)	average 76

Note: A high pulse in an infant or child is not as great a concern as a low pulse. A low pulse may indicate imminent cardiac arrest. Blood pressure is usually not taken in a child under 3 years of age. In cases of blood loss or shock, a child's blood pressure will remain within normal limits until near the end, then fall swiftly.

back of the infant's or child's hand or the top of the foot for several seconds. When you release your thumb, the skin beneath will be blanched but should return to its normal color within 2 seconds. If the return of normal skin color takes more than 2 seconds, then capillary refill is delayed, which likely indicates inadequate circulation or shock.

- *Assess the skin for color, moisture, and temperature.* Pale or mottled skin, or skin that is cool and moist, are other signs of hypoperfusion in pediatric patients.
- *Take a blood pressure reading in children older than 3 years.* Be sure to use an appropriately sized blood pressure cuff. (See Table 23-5 for normal blood pressure ranges.)

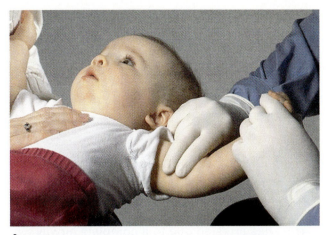

A.

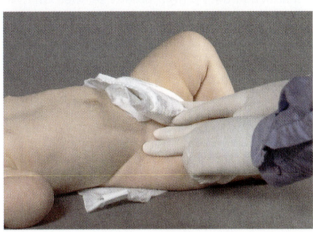

B.

Figure 23-16 **A.** Checking the brachial pulse in an infant. **B.** Checking the femoral pulse in an infant.

Some pediatric experts recommend the "Pediatric Assessment Triangle" as a rapid conceptual way of condensing the pediatric initial assessment and determining the level of severity and need for immediate treatment intervention. The three sides of the triangle are formed by the *general appearance* of the patient, the *work of breathing* that is present, and the *circulation to the skin* as determined by capillary refill. It is a rapid "eyes-open, hands-on" approach that does not require you to use a stethoscope, blood pressure cuff, pulse oximeter, or any other medical device in determining how ill your pediatric patient is.

History and Physical Examination

Most children have a limited past medical history. But if there is a past medical history, it can be critically important and should be obtained and documented. You should obtain the history of the

present illness—the duration of symptoms and associated problems (fever, rash, cough, and so on)—from the patient, a parent, or a caregiver.

The patient's age and situation will determine the need for and extent of a physical examination. When you perform a physical exam, start with the extremities, then work inward toward the trunk, leaving the head for last. Infants and children will become more at ease with you if you first touch them in areas away from the torso and face. If you first touch and play with the child's feet or abdomen, this should reduce anxiety.

See Table 23-5 for normal pediatric vital signs, which you will measure during the physical examination.

COMMON MEDICAL PROBLEMS IN INFANTS AND CHILDREN

There are several common reasons why EMS is summoned to care for pediatric patients. Because these are emergencies you are likely encounter, it is important to recognize and understand the special considerations and emergency medical treatment of the following conditions:

◆ Airway obstruction

◆ Respiratory emergencies

◆ Seizures

◆ Altered mental status

◆ Fever

◆ Poisonings

◆ Shock

◆ Near drowning

◆ Sudden infant death syndrome (SIDS)

Airway Obstruction

Infants and children frequently put objects into their mouths to teethe and suck on. Any object placed in the mouth is a potential choking and obstruction hazard. The risk for choking is especially high in infants and children under 5 years of age. Objects that often cause pediatric airway obstruction include peanuts, balloon fragments, coins, hot dog pieces, raw carrots, marbles, and small toy pieces.

When faced with a pediatric airway obstruction, you must quickly determine whether the obstruction is partial or complete.

Partial Obstruction

In a partial airway obstruction, the pediatric patient is still able to exchange some air past the obstruction. The patient with a partial airway obstruction is generally found alert and sitting up. These children often instinctively assume positions on their own that allow for the best possible air exchange around the obstruction. However, they will often appear panicked.

Signs of a partial airway obstruction that is allowing an adequate air exchange include:

◆ Stridor on inspiration

◆ Noisy breathing or crowing

◆ Retractions present on inspiration

◆ Strong cough

◆ Normal mental status

◆ Pink skin color

◆ Good circulation with normal capillary refill

◆ Emergency Care—Partial Airway Obstruction

Emergency medical care of partial airway obstruction in children includes the following:

1. **Allow the child to remain in a position of comfort.** Younger infants should usually be placed in a sitting position in their parent's arms.

2. *DO NOT* **forcibly lay the patient down, as this may worsen the obstruction.**

3. *DO NOT* **agitate the child.**

4. **Perform only a limited examination.** Do not assess blood pressure.

5. **Initiate transport as soon as possible.**

6. **Offer blow-by oxygen but do not agitate the patient.**

7. **Consider a request for ALS (paramedic) assistance or intercept if not already dispatched.** Paramedic units have specialized equipment to clear the airway obstruction should it become complete.

8. **Carefully monitor the patient at all times.** It is crucial to remember that a partial airway obstruction can instantaneously become a complete airway obstruction.

COMPANY OFFICER'S NOTES

You must presume that any previously healthy infant, toddler, or young child who is suddenly found in respiratory or cardiac arrest has arrested due to a complete airway obstruction until proven otherwise. (See On Scene for this chapter.) Since airway obstruction is a potentially reversible cause of arrest, quickly evaluate for it and treat for it if found. Carefully assess the scene for evidence of choking hazards such as small toy pieces. Remember that paramedic units carry specialized equipment that will allow removal of upper airway obstructions that basic life support procedures have failed to dislodge. Request paramedic back-up to the scene of all such calls or as an intercept en route to the hospital.

Complete Obstruction or Partial Obstruction with Cyanosis or Altered Mental Status

Patients with complete airway obstruction must be immediately recognized and treated during the initial assessment. The same holds true for a patient who has a partial airway obstruction without air exchange adequate to sustain life as indicated by cyanosis or altered mental status.

Signs of complete airway obstruction or partial airway obstruction that is *NOT* allowing adequate air exchange include:

◆ Cyanosis

◆ No crying or speaking

◆ Ineffective, weak cough

◆ Altered mental status

◆ Increasing respiratory difficulty accompanied by stridor

◆ Loss of consciousness

◆ Emergency Care—Complete Obstruction or Partial Obstruction with Cyanosis or Altered Mental Status

Emergency medical care for complete obstruction or partial airway obstruction with inadequate air exchange in children includes the following:

1. **Clear the airway.** For infants less than 1 year old, use back blows and chest thrusts, followed by checking the mouth for dislodged objects. For children older than 1 year of age, use abdominal thrusts followed by checking of the mouth for dislodged objects. (See "Clearing Complete Airway Obstructions" earlier in the chapter.)

2. **Attempt artificial ventilations with a BVM.** Assure a good mask seal.

3. **Call for ALS (paramedic) assistance or intercept if not already dispatched.**

Respiratory Emergencies

Infants and children may present with a wide variety of respiratory emergencies. Since respiratory failure is the leading cause of cardiac arrest in pediatric patients, all calls involving respiratory complaints must be carefully evaluated and the appropriate emergency medical care quickly provided.

Upper Airway Obstruction vs. Lower Airway Disease

One of the important skills you must learn is recognizing the difference between upper airway obstruction (complete or partial) and lower airway disease. This recognition is important because the specific emergency medical care is different for each condition. For example, placing a gloved finger into the mouth to remove a visible foreign object may be appropriate in caring for airway obstruction. Placing a finger into the mouth of patient with lower airway disease, however, can cause spasms that will close the airway.

As already discussed, partial upper airway obstruction is indicated by stridor (high-pitched sounds heard loudest over the neck and trachea) on inspiration. Increased work of breathing may

also be noted during inhalation as the patient tries to force air past the partial obstruction. Complete airway obstruction is indicated by an inability to cry or speak, cyanosis, altered mental status, and an inability to cough. Lower airway disease is likely when stridor is absent but wheezing (high-pitched sounds best heard over the chest) during exhalation and increased work of breathing are present.

Recognition of Early Respiratory Distress, Severe Respiratory Distress/Failure, and Respiratory Arrest

Respiratory emergencies may quickly progress from respiratory distress to respiratory failure to respiratory arrest. You must learn to recognize where, in this range of conditions, your pediatric patient with a respiratory emergency falls. Prompt recognition and immediate appropriate treatment can be life saving.

Early Respiratory Distress Early respiratory distress is indicated by signs of moderately increased work of breathing (Figure 23-17). This takes place as the infant or child tries to increase oxygen delivery and expel carbon dioxide to compensate for a respiratory problem such as

Figure 23-17   Early signs of respiratory distress.

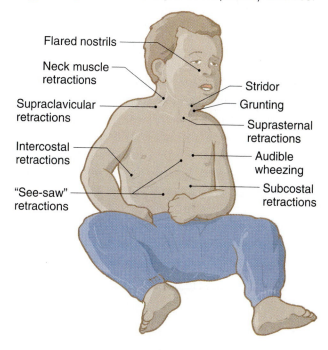

Flared nostrils
Neck muscle retractions
Supraclavicular retractions
Intercostal retractions
"See-saw" retractions
Stridor
Grunting
Suprasternal retractions
Audible wheezing
Subcostal retractions

asthma or infection. Early respiratory distress is indicated by *any* of the following:

◆ Nasal flaring. The nostrils will collapse with inhalation and "flare" open with exhalation as a sign of the patient's increased respiratory effort.

◆ Retractions of the skin and muscles above the sternal notch (suprasternal), between the ribs (intercostal), and under the ribs (subcostal) with inhalation

◆ Stridor

◆ Grunting sounds at the beginning of exhalation

◆ Audible wheezing

◆ Use of neck and abdominal muscles in breathing

◆ *Emergency Medical Care—Early Respiratory Distress*

Any infant or child with signs of respiratory distress should be placed on the highest possible concentration of oxygen that the patient will tolerate. High flow delivery with a nonrebreather mask is ideal, but blow-by oxygen may also be used if the child will not tolerate the mask. Carefully monitor the patient for progression to respiratory failure or arrest that will require the delivery of artificial ventilations. If the patient has a history of asthma and has a home medication nebulizer or metered dose inhaler, you should consult with medical direction about assisting with the use of these prescribed medications.

Severe Respiratory Distress/Failure Pediatric patients with serious respiratory conditions may progress to or present with signs of respiratory failure. Severe respiratory distress and respiratory failure are indicated when the signs and symptoms of early respiratory distress are present and *any* of the following are also observed:

◆ Respiratory rate greater than 60 or less than 10 breaths per minute

◆ Cyanosis

◆ Decreased muscle tone

◆ Heavy use of accessory muscles

◆ Poor peripheral perfusion

◆ Altered mental status

◆ Severe and constant grunting

◆ *Emergency Care—Severe Respiratory Distress/Failure*

Patients with signs of respiratory failure and severe respiratory distress should have their ventilations assisted with 100 percent oxygen delivered via BVM.

Respiratory Arrest The signs of pediatric respiratory arrest are as follows:

◆ Absent breathing

◆ Limp muscle tone

◆ Unresponsiveness

◆ Slow pulse rate (bradycardia)

◆ Weak or absent distal pulses

◆ *Emergency Medical Care— Respiratory Arrest*

All patients in respiratory arrest should receive artificial ventilations with 100 percent oxygen via a bag-valve mask. If the patient requires prolonged ventilations, consider the use of a properly sized oropharyngeal airway as an adjunct to ventilation.

Seizures

A seizure in an infant or child is a common reason for a call to EMS. The most common reason for seizures in pediatric patients is a fever that rises rapidly. Children with a pre-existing seizure disorder also commonly have seizures despite being on prescription anti-seizure medications. Less common causes include infections such as meningitis, head injuries, hypoglycemia, poisonings, or hypoxia. Although most pediatric seizures are relatively brief and not life threatening, as an EMT you should consider all seizures as serious.

Begin assessment of a patient with a seizure by assuring an open airway and adequate breathing. Airway problems due to secretions, as well as diminished respiratory efforts, are common during and after seizures. It is also common for patients to have an altered mental status after a seizure (called a "postictal period"). Assess the patient for injuries that may have occurred as a result of the seizure. Ask parents or caregivers these specific questions:

♦ Has the child had a recent illness or fever?

♦ Does the child have a past history of seizures? If yes:

—Is this a normal pattern of the seizures?

—Is the patient on any anti-seizure medications?

Prolonged seizures or seizures that are not typical for a patient with a past history of seizures are more likely to be potentially life threatening than brief or typical seizures.

◆ Emergency Care—Seizures

Emergency care for seizures should include the following:

1. **Assure an open airway.**
2. **Position the patient on his side if no cervical injury is suspected.**
3. **Suction the airway as needed.**
4. **Provide supplemental oxygen.**
5. **If there are signs of respiratory failure, assist ventilations with 100 percent oxygen via BVM. If respiratory arrest is present, provide artificial ventilations.**
6. **Transport.** Although the seizure itself may not be immediately life threatening, there may be a serious underlying condition that triggered the seizure.
7. **Call for ALS assistance or intercept** if not already dispatched in cases of prolonged (greater that 10 or 15 minutes) seizures.

Altered Mental Status

Altered mental status is another reason that you may be called to care for a pediatric patient. A parent or caregiver will often simply report that the infant or child is "just not acting right." On further questioning, you may discover that the child is less responsive to his environment than usual.

Altered mental status in children may be caused by many conditions including:

♦ Low blood sugar (hypoglycemia)

♦ High blood sugar (hyperglycemia)

♦ Poisoning

♦ Aftermath of a seizure (postictal)

♦ Infection

♦ Head trauma

♦ Hypoxia

♦ Shock (hypoperfusion)

While on scene, you should quickly search for clues to the reason for the altered mental status. Open medication bottles or disrupted house plants may be signs of poisoning. A history of recent illness may indicate that infection is a cause of the change in mental status. A mechanism of injury may be apparent that indicates trauma as the cause of the altered mental status.

◆ Emergency Care—Altered Mental Status

When your patient presents with altered mental status, provide the following care:

1. **Assure an open airway by manual maneuvers and suctioning as needed.**
2. **Administer supplemental oxygen.**
3. **Be prepared to assist or provide artificial ventilations.**
4. **Transport.**

Fever

Fever is a common reason that you will be called by parents to care for an infant or child. Almost all children develop fevers at some point. Most fevers are not life threatening. Perhaps the most feared cause of fever in children is meningitis, an infection of the tissue surrounding the brain and spinal cord. These patients may present with fever associated with stiff neck, seizures, or a body-wide rash. Conditions and circumstances that are more likely to indicate a potentially life-threatening cause of the fever include the following:

♦ Fever with an associated seizure or altered mental status

♦ Any fever in an infant less than 1 month of age

♦ High fever (greater than 102.5°F or 39.2°C) in a child less than 3 years of age

♦ Fever with an associated rash

◆ Emergency Care—Fever

Provide the following emergency care for the pediatric patient with fever:

1. **Lightly bundle the patient.** (Heavy bundling will cause retention of heat.)

2. **Transport.**

3. **Be alert for changes in the patient's condition such as respiratory distress or seizures.**

Some EMS systems will allow EMTs to initiate treatment to begin cooling children with high fevers prior to arrival at the emergency department. Follow your local protocol.

Poisonings

Poisonings, especially those due to oral ingestion, are very common in pediatric patients. As part of your scene size-up and assessment, attempt to identify the exact substance that was ingested. Medications, household plants, and substances that look pretty and taste good, such as mouthwashes containing alcohol, are common sources of poisoning in infants and children. If the ingested poison is identified, bring it to the emergency department along with its container. (You may also wish to review Chapter 15, "Poisonings and Allergic Reactions," at this time.)

◆ Emergency Care—Poisoning

Care should be based on whether the patient is responsive or unresponsive.

Responsive poisoning patient

1. **Administer oxygen.**

2. **Contact medical direction to discuss the need for activated charcoal.**

3. **Transport.**

4. **Ongoing assessment is essential because the patient may suddenly become unresponsive.**

Unresponsive poisoning patient

1. **Assure an open airway, including suctioning as needed.**

2. **Administer oxygen.**

3. **Provide artificial ventilations if signs of respiratory failure or arrest are present.**

4. **Transport.**

5. **Contact medical direction.**

6. **Be sure to exclude trauma as a cause of the altered mental status.**

Shock (Hypoperfusion)

Critically ill infants and children may present with signs and symptoms of shock (Figure 23-18). Commonly encountered causes of hypoperfusion in pediatric patients include dehydration from vomiting and/or diarrhea, trauma, infection, and blood loss from abdominal injuries. Less commonly encountered causes of shock in this age group include allergic reactions, poisonings, and cardiac illness. As an EMT, you should attempt to identify, if possible, the likely cause of the patient's hypoperfusion based on your assessment and findings at the scene and report your findings to the emergency department staff.

Signs and symptoms of shock include:

◆ Rapid respiratory rate with or without signs or respiratory distress

◆ Pale, cool and clammy skin

◆ Weak or absent peripheral pulses

◆ Capillary refill time of more than 2 seconds

◆ Mental status changes

◆ Absence of tears even when crying (a sign of dehydration)

◆ Decreased urine output. (Determine this by asking the parents whether a diapered baby has had a normal number of wet diapers or whether an older child has been to the bathroom as much as usual.)

◆ Sunken fontanelle (soft spot) on an infant's head

◆ Emergency Care—Shock (Hypoperfusion)

Provide the following emergency care for the patient with signs or symptoms of shock (hypoperfusion):

1. **Maintain an open airway.**

2. **Administer high concentration oxygen.**

SIGNS OF SHOCK (HYPOPERFUSION) IN A CHILD

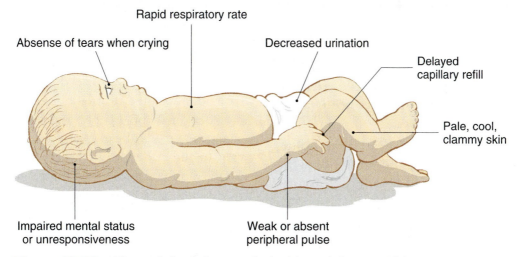

Rapid respiratory rate

Absense of tears when crying

Decreased urination

Delayed capillary refill

Pale, cool, clammy skin

Impaired mental status or unresponsiveness

Weak or absent peripheral pulse

Figure 23-18 Signs of shock (hypoperfusion) in an infant or child.

3. **Control bleeding if present.**

4. **Elevate legs if no spinal injury is suspected.** If spinal injury is suspected, secure the patient to a backboard and then elevate the foot section of the board.

5. **Keep the patient warm.**

6. **Initiate rapid transport.** Complete the focused examination en route to the hospital, as permitted by the situation.

Near Drowning

As already described in Chapter 16, "Environmental Emergencies," near drownings are a tragically frequent reason why EMS units are called to care for children. Infants left unattended in baths, toddlers inadequately supervised near pools and other bodies of water, and teenagers involved in alcohol- or diving-related water accidents are common scenarios in which pediatric patients become submerged. If these patients are rescued and either have or regain a pulse, then they are considered "near drownings." Patients who die as a result of submersion—that is, who suffer cardiac arrest from which they never regain a pulse despite CPR—are called "drowning" patients.

Special considerations when treating near-drowning patients must include the following:

◆ Always assure your own safety. Personal flotation devices should always be worn in water

rescue situations. (See Chapter 28, "EMS Special Operations.")

◆ Presume a spinal injury has occurred in any diving-related situation or fall from a height into a body of water.

◆ Consider the possibility of generalized hypothermia with prolonged submersion.

◆ In adolescents, consider the possibility that alcohol ingestion may have been a factor. That ingestion can cause altered mental status and increased risk of vomiting.

There is a medical phenomenon called *secondary drowning syndrome*. In these cases, submersion patients have normal, adequate breathing immediately after a submersion but develop respiratory distress, failure, and even arrest minutes to hours later. For this reason, *all* near-drowning patients must be transported to the hospital for careful evaluation and monitoring.

◆ Emergency Medical Care—Near Drownings

Emergency medical care for the near-drowning patient should include the following:

1. **Assure an open airway.** Use a head-tilt, chin-lift maneuver or a jaw-thrust maneuver if a spinal injury is suspected.

2. **Suction the airway as needed.**

3. **Provide high concentration oxygen if the patient has adequate spontaneous breathing.**

4. **If signs of respiratory distress, failure, or arrest are present, provide immediate artificial ventilations with 100 percent oxygen via BVM or high concentration oxygen via pocket mask.**

5. **Manually stabilize the head and spine, apply a cervical collar, and immobilize the patient to a backboard if indicated by the mechanism of injury.**

6. **Keep the patient warm by removing wet clothing and applying dry blankets.**

COMPANY OFFICER'S NOTES

Most cases of pediatric near drowning result from inadequate adult supervision of infants and children while they are close to water. On occasion, you may be called to assist a near-drowning victim who appears to be in no acute distress. His parents or caregivers may refuse further assistance or transportation for further evaluation because the child currently looks "OK." Parents or caregivers may refuse transport in such cases for several reasons. The adults may feel guilty about having allowed the event to occur. They may fear that they will get into trouble because of their lack of supervision. They may also not understand the potential problems or their judgment may be clouded by alcohol or other drugs. You must persuade these adults to allow treatment and transport because of the risk posed to the patient by secondary drowning syndrome. If you cannot persuade the adults to permit transport, have the police respond to the scene to assist in assuring that the child receives proper treatment and evaluation at the hospital.

Sudden Infant Death Syndrome

Sudden infant death syndrome (SIDS) is the most common reason that EMS is called for infant cardiac arrests. SIDS is the sudden death of an infant less than 1 year of age. The exact cause of SIDS is unknown, and the syndrome likely results from several factors. Recent studies have indicated that positioning the infant in a face-up rather than a prone position in the crib may reduce the incidence of SIDS deaths. SIDS patients are most often discovered in the early morning, but SIDS can occur at other times, such as during afternoon naps.

SIDS is devastating. The aftermath for the family often includes misplaced guilt, obvious despair, and even the divorce of parents. Prehospital providers may be deeply affected as well. The emergency medical care that you, as an EMT, provide to the patient and the professionalism and compassion you show the family can have a profound impact on a tragic situation.

◆ *Emergency Medical Care—SIDS*

In a case of suspected SIDS, provide the following care:

1. **Initiate full resuscitative measures unless there is obvious stiffening of the body (rigor mortis).**

2. **Transport immediately.**

3. **Consider ALS back-up or intercept.**

4. **Avoid any comments that might suggest blame, such as "If only they had called sooner. . . ."**

TRAUMA IN INFANTS AND CHILDREN

Trauma is the leading cause of death in infants and children in North America. Although in some urban areas penetrating trauma from stabbings and shootings is a common mechanism of injury, the vast majority of injuries sustained by pediatric patients result from blunt trauma.

Trauma Considerations by Mechanism of Injury

Although pediatric patients can be injured in the same ways as adult patients, there are several patterns of injury that are more common in children than in adults.

Seat Belt Injuries

Because children in the back seats of automobiles are often restrained with only lap belts, they are prone to "lap-belt complex" injuries. This injury pattern, which includes lumbar spine fractures and associated internal abdominal injuries, is the result of severe flexion of the patient's torso over the lap belt. Assume that any child found with the line of a seat belt mark across the lower abdomen has suffered serious internal injuries. This patient should receive full spinal immobilization and should be a high priority for transport to an appropriate hospital, ideally a trauma center.

Bicycle-Related Injuries

Children are frequently injured while riding their bicycles. Simple falls from bikes may result in injuries ranging from abrasions and broken bones to life-threatening injuries. Children who are struck in the upper abdomen by the end of a handlebar as they fall may sustain serious abdominal injuries that include hematomas of the small bowel and injuries to the spleen and liver. When children are struck by automobiles while riding their bicycles, they can have head, spinal, and abdominal injuries.

Many states have laws requiring children to wear helmets when riding bicycles. These laws have helped reduce the incidence of head injuries.

Car vs. Pedestrian Injuries

This mechanism of injury is frequently encountered in cities where children play in or near narrow streets. Adults hit by cars often sustain only injuries to the lower leg from impact with bumpers. Children, however, tend to be much more seriously injured. They are physically smaller and shorter than adults and are more apt to be stuck higher on their bodies by car bumpers. Children struck by autos frequently sustain serious femur and pelvic fractures, neck injuries, head injuries, as well as internal bleeding in the abdomen.

Head and Neck Injuries

Children sustain head and neck injuries by various mechanisms. Sports activities, falls from heights, diving into shallow water, and physical abuse are common causes of these injuries in infants and children. Always consider such mechanisms dur-

ing scene size-up. Manually stabilize the head and spine, apply a cervical collar, and immobilize the patient to a backboard if you suspect a neck or head injury. Children with suspected head and neck injuries frequently develop airway problems, including obstruction of the airway by the tongue. Monitor these patients carefully, administer high concentration oxygen, and maintain an open airway, using the jaw-thrust maneuver.

Burns

Burns are common injuries in childhood. They are the second leading cause of death in children in the United States, resulting in some 2,000 to 3,000 deaths per year. Certain types of burns, such as scalding injuries from liquids, are seen more commonly in infants and children than in adults.

Remember that the body surface area of burns in children is calculated differently than in adults. This means that the traditional rule of nines for determining burn area must be modified. (You may wish to review material on burns in Chapter 20, "Soft Tissue Injuries.") In general, any child with a full thickness or partial thickness burn covering more than 20 percent of body surface area or burns involving the hands, face, airway, or genitalia is considered to have critical burns that require care at a burn center.

All burns should be covered with sterile, nonadhering dressings. Some EMS systems allow moistening of burn dressings. Follow your local protocol. Assess all infants and children with burns carefully for the presence of airway injury and the development of signs of respiratory distress. Treat with high flow oxygen or artificial ventilations.

Trauma Considerations by Body Regions

Head Injuries

When assessing and providing emergency medical care for infants and children, the number one priority is the management of airway and breathing.

In cases of head injury, airway obstruction is most commonly caused by the tongue in an unresponsive patient. Airway obstruction will quickly lead to hypoxia and then to respiratory and cardiac

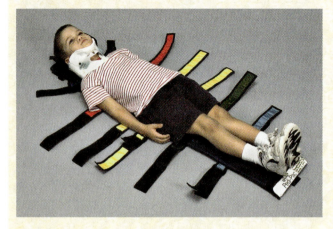

Figure 23-19A Position the patient on the immobilization system.

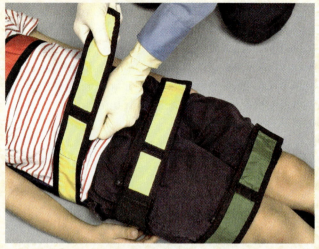

Figure 23-19B Adjust the color-coded straps to fit the child.

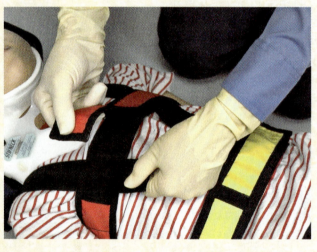

Figure 23-19C Attach the four-point safety harness.

arrest without immediate and continual management. Always open the airway of a trauma patient using the jaw-thrust maneuver. Children with even minor head injuries often have nausea and vomiting, so you must always be prepared to suction the airway as needed.

Respiratory failure and arrest are common in children with serious head injuries. Assist the ven-tilations of any child with a head injury and signs of respiratory failure, using a pocket mask or a BVM. If the child is in respiratory arrest, immediately provide artificial ventilations with 100 percent oxygen.

Spinal injuries are commonly associated with head injuries. All patients with a significant mechanism of injury, major injuries to the face and

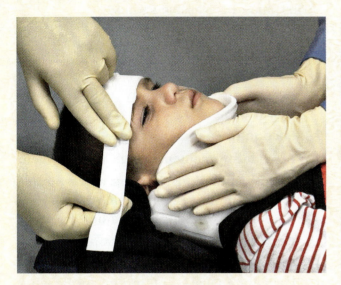

Figure 23-19D Fasten the adjustable head-support system.

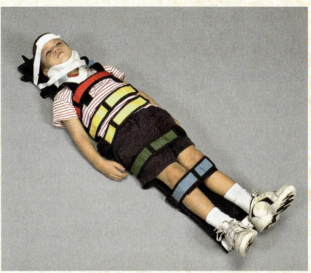

Figure 23-19E The patient fully immobilized to the system.

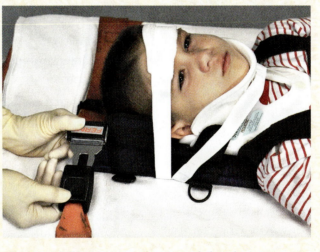

Figure 23-19F Move the immobilized patient onto the stretcher and fasten the loops at both ends to connect to the stretcher straps.

head, or altered mental status as a result of a head injury must receive full spinal immobilization (Figure 23-19). You can use commercial pediatric immobilization devices or foam head blocks to stabilize the head and neck once the patient is secured to the backboard. (If a pediatric patient is found in a car seat, you can also use the seat to immobilize the child. See Figure 22-20 in Chapter 22, "Head and Spine Injuries.") Never use sand bags when immobilizing a pediatric patient's head, because the weight of the bag may worsen a head injury if the backboard is turned on its side to help manage the patient's vomiting.

Medical research and experience have shown that infants and children who sustain serious head injuries often have associated internal injuries.

This is because a mechanism of injury forceful enough to cause serious head injury is also forceful enough to cause chest and abdominal injuries. When assessing a trauma patient with a head injury and associated signs of shock (hypoperfusion), assume that the patient has sustained more than just a head injury and is likely losing blood either internally or externally from a site of injury other than the head.

Chest Injuries

The most crucial aspect of assessing chest injuries in infants and children is to remember that children's ribs are relatively soft compared to those of adults. For this reason, pediatric patients may suffer significant chest injuries with little sign of external injury. In adults, a rigid rib cage absorbs a lot of traumatic energy, protecting the internal organs by allowing ribs to fracture. In children, soft and pliable ribs allow such energy to pass through the chest wall without rib fractures. This results in more serious injuries to the lungs and even the heart. If the mechanism of injury is consistent with a serious chest injury, proceed accordingly, even if there is little sign of chest trauma on the chest wall such as crepitus, bruising, or tenderness.

Abdominal Injuries

Injuries to the abdomen are commonly encountered in children. Serious abdominal injuries may not be immediately evident when you assess the pediatric trauma patient. However, injuries to internal organs such as the liver and spleen can result in life-threatening blood loss. Always consider the possibility of abdominal injuries in trauma patients who show signs of hypoperfusion without obvious external blood loss.

Extremity Injuries

The in-hospital and long-term care of skeletal injuries in infants is often more complicated than in adults. Issues involving the healing of bones and other structures that are rapidly growing are the reason for this. The prehospital care of extremity injuries, however, is generally the same for adults and pediatric patients. To assure proper prehospital care for extremity injuries in children, properly sized splinting equipment, such as pediatric-sized traction splints and prefabricated rigid splints, must be available and used.

◆ Emergency Care—Pediatric Trauma Patients

1. **Assure an open airway using the jaw-thrust maneuver.**
2. **Suction the airway as needed.**
3. **Provide supplemental high flow oxygen.**
4. **Assist ventilations if signs of respiratory failure are present. Provide artificial ventilations in cases of respiratory arrest.**
5. **Provide spinal immobilization.**
6. **Consider use of the pneumatic anti-shock garment in cases of trauma only where signs of severe hypoperfusion or pelvic instability are present.** Use only properly sized garments. Do not try to put a child or infant in the single leg of an adult PASG. Do not inflate the abdominal compartment, as this may interfere with adequate breathing. Follow local protocols.
7. **Transport immediately.**

CHILD ABUSE AND NEGLECT

An unavoidable reality of our society is that some people cause physical and psychological harm to children. **Abuse** is defined as performing an improper or excessive action so as to injure or cause harm. **Neglect** is defined as giving insufficient attention or respect to someone who has a claim to that attention or respect. As an EMT, you may encounter infants and children who have been the victims of abuse and neglect. Physical abuse and neglect are the two most common forms of child abuse you are likely to encounter. You must learn how to recognize signs and symptoms of child abuse (Figure 23-20).

Common signs of and symptoms of injuries that may be consistent with physical abuse and include the following:

- *Multiple bruises in various stages of healing*—Bruises go through color changes as they heal. They are initially red in color but will soon turn to a typical black and blue-purple color. Finally, just before fading, bruises will exhibit a yellow color.

- *Injury inconsistent with the mechanism of injury*—As you have already learned, certain mechanisms of injury produce predictable patterns of injury. Whenever the injuries you encounter appear far more serious than those that you might expect from the mechanism described to you, consider the possibility of abuse. For example, you might be called to treat a child who has multiple linear belt-width abrasions across his back. Yet his parents report that he was clawed by the family dog. In this case, the mechanism of injury described is obviously inconsistent with your physical findings and should suggest the possibility of abuse.

- *Fresh burns*—Fresh burns, especially those for which parents or caregivers report mechanisms of injury that are unlikely for the child to have caused himself, are highly suspicious. Examples would include a toddler with cigarette burns to his back or an infant with hot water burns only to the palms and soles of the hands and feet.

- *Children found in the home with severe head injuries*—Head injuries are the most lethal of child abuse injuries. "Shaken baby syndrome" results in severe head injuries with little external sign of injury.

- *Repeated calls to the same address for children with injuries*

- *Parents or caregivers who seem inappropriately unconcerned with a child's injuries*

- *Conflicting stories as to how injuries occurred*

- *Fear on the part of the child to discuss how the injury occurred*

Common conditions that may be consistent with neglect include the following:

- *Lack of parental supervision in potentially dangerous settings*—for example, a child playing on the street at 2 A.M., or a toddler left alone at home while the parent goes to the gym to work out

- *Unsafe living environment*—for example, a child living in a home with crack cocaine on the table

- *Untreated chronic illness*—for example, a child with medical conditions such as asthma whose prescriptions are never filled despite multiple trips to the emergency department

- *Appearance of malnourishment*

Approaches to Suspected Abuse or Neglect Situations

It is rarely productive or in the patient's best interest to accuse or confront suspected perpetrators of child abuse in the field. Such actions usually serve only to delay transportation and further upset the child. The one exception is when parents or caregivers refuse to allow the EMT to assess, treat, or transport infants or chil-

COMPANY OFFICER'S NOTES

There are over a million confirmed cases of child abuse each year in the United States. About a quarter of these cases are identified by emergency medical personnel, including prehospital care providers and emergency department staff. There are approximately 2,000 abuse-related deaths of children each year.

As the person in charge of an emergency medical scene, you must be familiar with the signs of child abuse. You must also be familiar with the obligations you have as an emergency medical worker to make formal reports of suspected child abuse to personnel of child protective or law enforcement agencies. Laws on reporting suspected child abuse vary from jurisdiction to jurisdiction; know the specifics of those laws in your area. Even if you are not specifically required under local law to make a report yourself, you must inform the staff of the receiving emergency department of your concerns.

Looking the other way and not reporting witnessed or suspected abuse of a child may result in that child's eventual death at the hands of the abuser.

Child Abuse

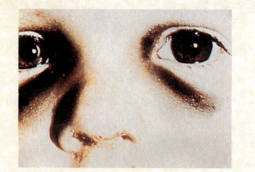

Figure 23-20A Injuries resulting from physical abuse.

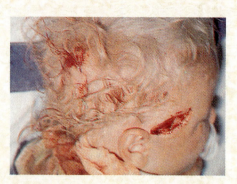

Figure 23-20B Multiple lacerations from physical abuse.

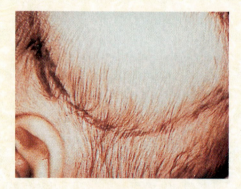

Figure 23-20C Evidence of physical abuse.

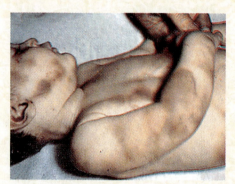

Figure 23-20D Child abuse death from multiple injuries.

dren whose injuries are serious and are likely the result of physical abuse. In this case, a police agency should be summoned to the scene for assistance.

When you suspect that abuse or neglect has occurred, you should report your findings to the emergency department staff upon arrival at the facility. Remember that such reports of possible abuse should be based upon objective information about what you saw and heard, not what you think. In some areas you may be required by law to formally report your findings to child protective services. Your instructor will be able to tell you about any such regulations that are in effect in your jurisdiction.

INFANTS AND CHILDREN WITH SPECIAL NEEDS

Medical advances have allowed infants and children to live at home who would not previously have survived or been able to leave the hospital because of devastating congenital conditions and diseases. Many of these children are now able to live at home only because of advanced medical devices. Some of the devices, and special considerations relating to them, will be discussed here. These patients and their devices can be very intimidating for EMTs to encounter. Remember, however, that parents and caregivers of children

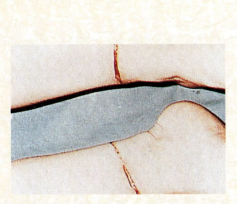

Figure 23-20E Child physical abuse—child restrained by tying.

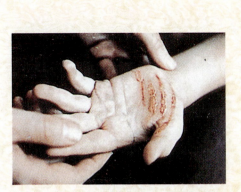

Figure 23-20F Child physical abuse—burns on a hand held to an electric stove.

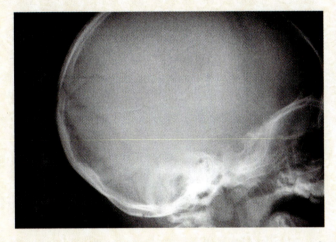

Figure 23-20G Evidence of child abuse—x-ray of a fractured skull.

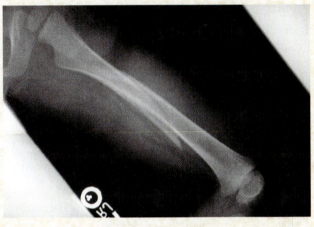

Figure 23-20H Evidence of child abuse—x-ray of a spiral femur fracture.

with special needs are very knowledgeable about their children and their medical equipment. Always listen to them, because they know their children better than anyone else.

Tracheostomy Tubes

Tracheostomy tubes are airways that are surgically placed into the anterior portion of the lower trachea. There are various types of these tubes, but all provide an airway from the outside directly into the trachea (Figure 23-21). Pediatric patients with tracheostomy tubes in place usually suffer from chronic respiratory problems and may even be on home ventilators.

Common complications encountered in patients with tracheostomy tubes include obstruction by mucus plugs, bleeding around the tube site, leaking of air around the tubes, and the tubes falling out. In addition, these infants and children often develop respiratory distress when infections worsen their already impaired breathing.

The emergency medical care of pediatric patient with tracheostomy tubes includes the following:

1. **Maintain an open airway.**
2. **Suction the tube as needed.**
3. **Allow the patient to maintain a position of comfort.**

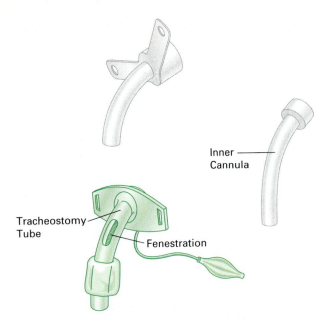

Figure 23-21 Tracheostomy tubes. **Top:** Plastic tube. **Bottom:** Metal tube with inner cannula.

4. **Administer oxygen if the patient is in respiratory distress.**

5. **Assist ventilations via the tube in cases of respiratory failure.**

6. **Provide artificial ventilations via the tube in cases of respiratory arrest.**

7. **Transport.**

Home Ventilators

A pediatric patient with chronic respiratory insufficiency may be on a home ventilator. This device provides the patient with mechanical artificial ventilations. There are several types of these devices, and patients may receive ventilations at all times or only at certain times, such as while they sleep.

The most common complications with these devices are mechanical failure and the need for energy during an electrical failure. The emergency medical care of patients on ventilators requires keeping the airway open and providing artificial ventilations via an appropriately sized BVM with supplemental oxygen. It is safest to transport these patients so that they can be placed on ventilators in the emergency department while repairs are made to their home units.

Central Intravenous Lines

Children who require long-term IV therapy, such as intravenous nutrition, antibiotics, or chemotherapy for cancer, will often have specialized IV catheters called *central lines* placed into the superior vena cava near the heart. Often these lines are placed in the upper chest just below the clavicles. In cases where IV access is only necessary for a few weeks, PIC (percutaneous intravenous catheter) lines may be placed in the arm and threaded into the superior vena cava.

Common complications of central and PIC lines include cracking of the exposed catheter, bleeding at the insertion site, and clotting of the lumen of the catheter so fluids can no longer flow through it. In addition, children with central or PIC lines are at risk for severe infections caused by bacteria introduced through the catheter.

Emergency medical care of central line complications includes controlling any bleeding with direct pressure and transporting the patient.

Gastric Feeding Tubes and Gastrostomy Tubes

There are many chronic disorders in children that prevent them from eating and swallowing food normally. Many of these patients either have *gastric feeding tubes* placed through the nostril into their stomach, or have *gastrostomy tubes* placed directly through the abdominal wall into the stomach. Specially formulated liquids provide nutrition for these patients. The patients also receive routine medications through these tubes.

Complications with these devices include bleeding at the site of gastrostomy tube insertion and tubes falling out. More serious complications may occur in diabetic patients who require constant feedings to maintain adequate glucose levels and who may develop an altered mental status if tube feedings are stopped. Finally, patients with tube feeding devices commonly develop respiratory problems as a result of tube feeds backing up through their esophagus and being aspirated into their trachea and lungs.

Emergency medical care includes management of the airway and breathing, as for any patient, including suctioning and supplemental oxygen administration. These patients should be transported either sitting or lying on their right side with the head elevated to reduce the risk of aspiration.

Shunts

A *shunt* is a surgical connection from the brain to the abdominal cavity. It is used to drain excessive cerebrospinal fluid (CSF) from the brain. There is usually a reservoir that can be felt on one side of the skull. The reservoir is used by physicians to test that the system is working properly. These devices are often placed early in childhood and need to be revised from time to time as the child grows.

The most common shunt-related problem that you will encounter as an EMT is "shunt failure." This occurs when the shunt's connections separate (usually as a result of the child's growth) and CSF begins to back up into the brain. The back-up of fluid causes changes in mental status, often reported by the parents simply as the child being more sleepy than usual. Some children develop respiratory arrest as a result of shunt failure. Shunt failure requires surgical repair of the drain system in the operating room.

Emergency medical care of patients with shunt-related problems includes the following:

1. **Maintain an open airway.**
2. **Assure adequate ventilations.**
3. **Transport to an appropriate facility.**

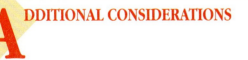

ADDITIONAL CONSIDERATIONS

Advance Directives

Although the situation is rarely encountered, the EMT must be aware that children with terminal illnesses such as untreatable cancer or certain genetic diseases may suffer cardiac and respiratory arrests out of the hospital. In some cases the parents may have already decided that they do not want any heroic measures, such as CPR, performed on their child. When faced with this situation, you must quickly obtain the necessary information and, if any questions arise, contact medical direction. Although such situations are difficult, it is important to comply with the parents' wishes if legally recognized directives are in place.

The Family

A child cannot be cared for in isolation from his family. Therefore, you will find yourself having to develop a relationship with both your patient and his parents or caregivers. A good interaction with the parents is essential to a good interaction with the patient. If a parent is upset, it is likely that the child will be upset as well. A calm parent helps calm the child.

Parents will respond in a variety of ways to the illness or injury of their child. They are likely to be very anxious over his well being. These anxieties are heightened by conditions such as the child being in pain or bleeding externally. Parents may show this anxiety by reacting toward the EMT with a variety of emotions including anger or hysteria. Again, try to remain calm and supportive in your interactions with the family despite such displays of emotion.

Most parents are not medically trained. They often feel a sense of helplessness at being unable to help their child directly. So it is important to allow the parents to participate in the child's care whenever possible.

When a child is critically ill, such as in cardiac or respiratory arrest, it is not appropriate for the parents to assist in patient care. However, it is still important to keep the parents as informed as possible. Explain what is being done and why.

In non-critical situations, ask parents to help calm the child by holding his hand or stroking his head. A parent can hold the child in a position of comfort and also hold blow-by oxygen. Allowing parents to participate in care in this way makes them feel more in control of the situation. This will likely help to reassure them and, as a result, reassure their child as well.

Again remember that, although they are not trained emergency medical personnel, parents are experts on their own children. They know when something abnormal is going on with their child, and they know what actions will help calm their child. All calls involving pediatric patients will go more smoothly when you develop a positive interaction with the parents by listening carefully to them and enlisting their help as much as possible.

The EMT's Response to Pediatric Patients

Few EMTs are as comfortable caring for infants and children as for adults. This is largely because pediatric calls are less common than calls involving adults, and calls involving critically ill infants and children are even less common. In addition, EMTs with their own children may identify aspects of their own children in the patients they are caring for. For these reasons, calls involving infants and children are likely to trigger a certain amount of anxiety for you as an EMT.

Tactics to minimize your anxiety over caring for infants and children include the following:

- Remember that much of what you've learned about adult patients also applies to children. Remember that *A*irway, *B*reathing, and *C*irculation remain the top priorities of patient care.

- Remember, however, that children are not simply small adults and that their developmental stage, anatomy, and physiology do alter some of the ways they are cared for.

- Drill and practice with pediatric equipment. Maintain pediatric assessment skills through training. Frequently inspect the pediatric jump kit to maintain familiarity with its contents.

- If you have your own children, use your personal experience and skills in interacting with children to your advantage.

- If an incident involving a child has been particularly stressful or emotional, consider contacting your department's critical incident stress debriefing (CISD) team.

Chapter Review

SUMMARY

As an EMT, you will be called upon to provide emergency medical care for infants and children. Although the assessment and treatment priorities are largely the same for these patients as for adults, there are also many differences in their anatomy, physiology, and response to illness that make pediatric patients unique. Because infants and children are not simply small adults, it is vitally important that you acquire the knowledge and learn the skills that go into providing their optimal care.

REVIEWING KEY CONCEPTS

1. Describe at least five ways in which the anatomy and physiology of infants and children differ from those of adults. Explain how the differences you described might affect the assessment and care of pediatric patients.

2. Explain the considerations to be alert to when suctioning the airway of an infant or child.

3. Describe strategies to use when a pediatric patient will not accept supplemental oxygen via nonrebreather mask or nasal cannula.

4. List observations during the initial assessment that might support the general impression of a "sick" child.

5. List the signs and symptoms of partial airway obstruction and complete airway obstruction.

6. Explain how to distinguish between upper airway obstruction and lower airway disease.

7. List common causes of seizures in pediatric patients. Describe steps in the emergency care of pediatric seizure patients.

8. List indications that a fever in a pediatric patient may be potentially life threatening. Describe steps in the emergency care of the pediatric fever patient.

9. List signs and symptoms of shock (hypoperfusion) in pediatric patients.

10. Define secondary drowning syndrome and explain its implications for your treatment of pediatric near-drowning patients.

11. Describe some of the patterns of injury common in pediatric trauma patients.

12. Describe steps in the care of a pediatric trauma patient.

13. Define *abuse* and *neglect*. List common signs, symptoms, and conditions that may indicate abuse and neglect in pediatric patients.

14. Describe ways EMTs might deal with the special stresses that accompany the emergency care of pediatric patients.

RESOURCES TO LEARN MORE

American Heart Association and American Academy of Pediatrics. *Textbook of Pediatric Advanced Life Support.* Dallas: American Heart Association, 1998.

Eichelberger, M. R. et al. *Pediatric Emergencies: A Manual for Prehospital Care Providers, 2nd Edition.* Upper Saddle River, NJ: Brady/Prentice Hall, 1998.

Fleisher, G. R. and Ludwig, S. *Textbook of Pediatric Emergency Medicine, 3rd Edition.* Baltimore: Williams & Wilkins, 1993.

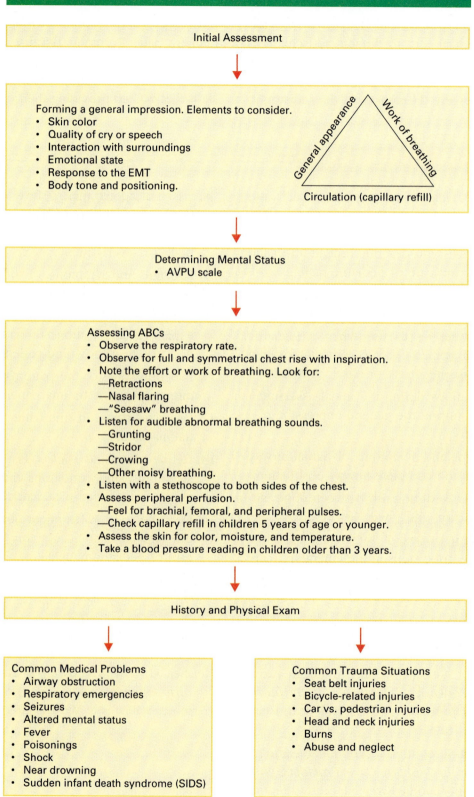

BASICS OF PEDIATRIC ASSESSMENT

Initial Assessment

Forming a general impression. Elements to consider.
- Skin color
- Quality of cry or speech
- Interaction with surroundings
- Emotional state
- Response to the EMT
- Body tone and positioning.

General appearance   Work of breathing

Circulation (capillary refill)

Determining Mental Status
- AVPU scale

Assessing ABCs
- Observe the respiratory rate.
- Observe for full and symmetrical chest rise with inspiration.
- Note the effort or work of breathing. Look for:
  —Retractions
  —Nasal flaring
  —"Seesaw" breathing
- Listen for audible abnormal breathing sounds.
  —Grunting
  —Stridor
  —Crowing
  —Other noisy breathing.
- Listen with a stethoscope to both sides of the chest.
- Assess peripheral perfusion.
  —Feel for brachial, femoral, and peripheral pulses.
  —Check capillary refill in children 5 years of age or younger.
- Assess the skin for color, moisture, and temperature.
- Take a blood pressure reading in children older than 3 years.

History and Physical Exam

Common Medical Problems
- Airway obstruction
- Respiratory emergencies
- Seizures
- Altered mental status
- Fever
- Poisonings
- Shock
- Near drowning
- Sudden infant death syndrome (SIDS)

Common Trauma Situations
- Seat belt injuries
- Bicycle-related injuries
- Car vs. pedestrian injuries
- Head and neck injuries
- Burns
- Abuse and neglect

Geriatrics

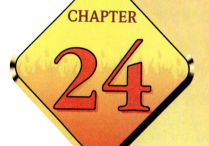

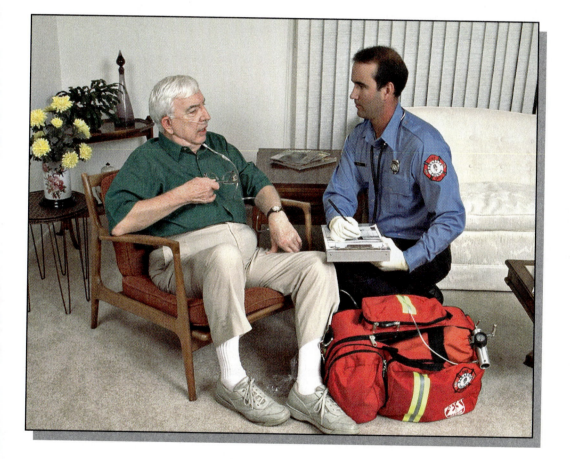

*G*eriatrics *is the medical specialty involving care of the elderly. In most EMS systems today, people older than 65 years of age make up about 40 percent of the patients transported by ambulance. By the year 2030, as the population ages, it is estimated that some 70 percent of EMS calls will be for geriatric patients.*

In these patients, the aging process has produced distinctive physiological and anatomical changes. In addition, these older patients often have special medical, emotional, and social needs. As an EMT, you will be encountering growing numbers of older patients. Therefore, ▶

it is vital that you acquire a good understanding of the special considerations involved in the assessment and care of these geriatric patients.

OBJECTIVES

At the completion of this chapter, the EMT-Basic student should be able to meet the following objectives. These objectives are supplemental to the U.S. DOT 1994 EMT-Basic curriculum.

Knowledge and Understanding

1. Understand the major changes in anatomy and physiology that occur with aging. (pp. 633–634)
2. Describe how the changes in physiology that occur with aging impact upon the assessment of geriatric patients. (pp. 634–635)
3. Identify other factors such as mental status impairment, patient fear and pride, and communication problems that impact upon assessment and treatment of geriatric patients. (pp. 635–636)
4. Describe the importance of determining the baseline mental status of geriatric patients from family or care facility staff members. (p. 636)
5. Identify trauma emergencies, such as falls, motor vehicle crashes, head injuries and physical abuse, that are common among geriatric patients. (pp. 636–639)
6. Discuss how the assessment and the treatment of geriatric trauma patients differ from those processes with younger adult patients. (pp. 636–639)
7. Identify medical emergencies, such as syncope, acutely altered mental status, chest pain, shortness of breath, and abdominal pain, that are common among geriatric patients. (pp. 639–640)
8. Discuss how the assessment and the treatment of geriatric medical patients differ from those processes with younger adult patients. (pp. 639–640)
9. Discuss the impact of advanced directives, including living wills and Do Not Resuscitate orders, on the care of geriatric patients. (p. 639)

Skills

1. Demonstrate how to modify backboard immobilization to accommodate anatomical changes in an elderly patient's cervical spine.

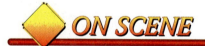

ON SCENE

DISPATCH: *ENGINE 15, MEDIC SQUAD 1. RESPOND TO A LIFELINE® MEDICAL ALARM. THE ADDRESS IS 113 NINTH STREET. TIME OUT IS 1756.*

You are the firefighter-EMT assigned to Engine 15. As you arrive on-scene, the emergency medical dispatcher advises that he has been unable to contact the residence using the phone number provided by the Lifeline service company. The company did advise the dispatcher that the patient is Mrs. Ada Schwartz, an 84-year-old woman. The company also stated that the

woman's son has been contacted and that he is en route from his office.

The address to which you've been dispatched is a single-story ranch-style house. Your scene size-up reveals no obvious hazards, so you approach the house. There is no response when you ring the front doorbell. Your officer then directs you to look for other access into the house. As you check the back door, you see through the window a woman lying on the kitchen floor. Determining that there is a potential immediate threat to life, your officer orders forcible entry into the residence.

Once inside, you find an elderly women lying on the floor. She has an obvious bleeding laceration and a large bruised area above her left eye. As another firefighter puts on gloves and applies a dressing to her laceration, you introduce yourself while applying a cervical collar "Hello, my name is Peter. I'm an Emergency Medical Technician with the fire department. We're here to help you. Can you tell me your name?"

The woman replies, "Who are you people? Who broke my door?"

"I'm sorry about the door, ma'am. We had to break it to get to you because all the doors were locked. We're with the fire department, and we'd like to help you. Do you remember falling?"

Mrs. Schwartz's only response is to repeat, "Who are you people?"

You now begin to assess the patient as being confused. In addition to her head injuries, you note that her right leg appears shorter than the left and that her right foot is outwardly rotated. As you begin to obtain baseline vital signs, the paramedic unit arrives, as does the patient's son.

You tell the paramedics, "We found the patient here on the floor. She appears to be confused. It's not clear whether she slipped and fell or whether she passed out and fell. We noted a laceration and contusion above her eye; that bleeding is controlled. She also appears to have a right hip injury."

As the medics place the patient on a cardiac monitor, you question the patient's son, asking, "Is your mother normally confused like this?"

He answers, "No, normally she's sharp as a tack."

The paramedics report that the patient has an unstable heart rhythm. After an IV is started and intravenous medications given, Mrs. Schwartz appears somewhat less confused. Your crew assists in carefully immobilizing the patient to a backboard just prior to transport.

You later learn from the Squad 1 paramedics that Mrs. Schwartz had fractured her right hip and that she was admitted to the Intensive Care Unit because of her cardiac condition. The paramedics report that her unstable cardiac rhythm most likely caused her to lose consciousness, resulting in her fall.

ANATOMY AND PHYSIOLOGY IN AGING

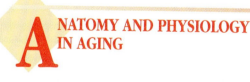

The aging process produces many changes in the structure (anatomy) and function (physiology) of the body (Figure 24-1). In general, as the body ages, body systems begin to function less well. They become more prone to disease and more prone to injury as a result of trauma. The changes can also make assessment and treatment of geriatric patients more difficult and time-consuming. Table 24-1 shows some of the common effects of the aging process.

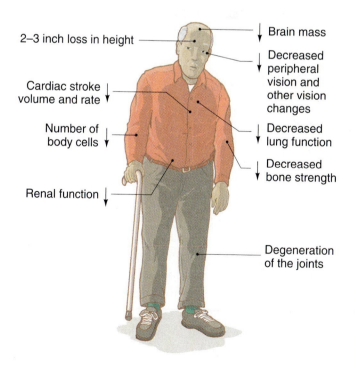

- 2–3 inch loss in height
- Cardiac stroke volume and rate ↓
- Number of body cells ↓
- Renal function ↓
- Brain mass ↓
- Decreased peripheral vision and other vision changes ↓
- Decreased lung function ↓
- Decreased bone strength ↓
- Degeneration of the joints

Figure 24-1   Age-related changes in the body.

Table 24-1

Anatomical and Physiological Changes with Aging

Body System	Changes With Aging	Clinical Importance
Neurological	Brain tissue shrinks Loss of memory Clinical depression common Altered mental status common Impaired balance	Delay in appearance of symptoms with head injury Difficulty in patient assessment Increased likelihood of falls
Cardiovascular	Loss of elasticity and hardening of arteries Changes in heart rate, rhythm, efficiency	Hypertension common Greater likelihood of strokes, heart attacks Greater likelihood of bleeding from minor trauma
Respiratory	Loss of strength and coordination in respiratory muscles Cough and gag reflexes reduced	Increased likelihood of respiratory infection
Musculoskeletal	Loss of bone strength (osteoporosis) Loss of joint flexibility and strength (osteoarthritis)	Greater likelihood of fractures Slower healing Increased likelihood of falls
Gastrointestinal	Diminished digestive functions	Constipation common Greater likelihood of malnutrition
Renal	Loss of kidney size and function	Increased problems with drug toxicity
Skin	Thins and becomes more fragile Perspires less	More subject to tears and sores Bruising more common Heals more slowly Heat-related emergencies more common

APPROACHES TO THE GERIATRIC PATIENT

It is important to understand that a variety of physical, emotional, psychological, and social factors affect how a geriatric patient reacts in a medical emergency. For example, if the patient lives in his or her own home, then a trip to the hospital may cause the patient to become very fearful. The patient might fear that he will loose the ability to live independently and perhaps have to go into a nursing home. In addition, fears may arise from the knowledge that geriatric patients are more likely to die during hospitalization than younger patients with the same illness or injury. Many elders have known friends who have died after going to an emergency department. They may view hospitalization not as a step in healing but as a potential death sentence.

Another factor that can influence the responses of older patients in medical emergencies is pride. Geriatric patients often take a rightful pride in their achievements and the fact that they have out-lived many of their peers. Such patients may view their injury or illness as embarrassing.

Approach the geriatric patient with respect. Don't automatically begin using the patient's first name in an attempt to put him or her at ease. Instead, address the patient as "Mr.," "Mrs.," or "Miss" unless the patient requests otherwise.

Avoid being curt and rushed with geriatric patients. Never assume that, because a patient's responses to you seem slow, the patient's mental capacities are diminished. Give the patient the chance to hear you, think about what you have asked, and reply appropriately (Figure 24-2).

Talk to the patient about the problem, even though it might seem faster or easier to *talk about* the patient with a family member or care facility staff member. Of course, there are times when an elderly patient will not be able to respond appropriately and you will have to speak to others. But, when possible, show the patient the courtesy of directing your attention to him.

Remember, showing simple politeness with geriatric patients can go a long way toward easing those patients' concerns and fears about dealing with EMS services. Easing those concerns and fears will aid you in your assessment and treatment of geriatric patients.

Scene Size-Up

You should take appropriate body substance isolation precautions with elderly patients just as you would with younger ones. Be aware, however, that there is an increased risk of tuberculosis in patients who live in nursing homes. Consider

Figure 24-2 Use good communications techniques during assessment of the geriatric patient. Position yourself at the patient's level, make good eye contact, and speak slowly and clearly.

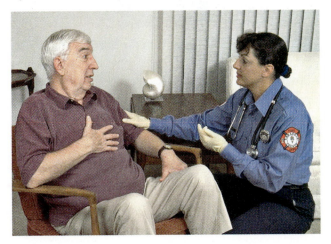

using a HEPA or N-95 respirator if you are called to assist a patient with respiratory problems in such a facility.

Be alert to the temperature of the surroundings in which you find a geriatric patient. The body's ability to adapt to heat or cold is often impaired in the elderly. This impairment leaves them more apt to suffer from heat- or cold-related emergencies than younger adults. In addition, economic factors can contribute to such problems. Many elderly people live on fixed incomes. To save on fuel costs, they may keep temperatures too low in winter or too hot in summer.

Remember also that geriatric patients may not be able to communicate clearly with you about their medications. Check the scene for prescription or nonprescription medications and home oxygen equipment that might give clues to the nature of an emergency.

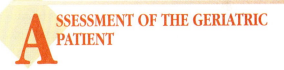

ASSESSMENT OF THE GERIATRIC PATIENT

The priorities of patient assessment—airway, breathing, circulation, determining mental status, and determining patient priority—are the same for all patients regardless of age. However, geriatric patients commonly require more detailed and lengthy assessments than younger patients. There are several reasons why geriatric assessment is more complicated and time-consuming than that of most other patients:

◆ *The presence of multiple diseases* Older patients often have one or more long-standing or chronic illnesses. When an acute injury or illness occurs, the presence of these other diseases may make assessment of the acute problem much more complicated. For example, if a patient with chronic breathing problems sustains a chest injury in a motor vehicle crash, it may be more difficult to assess the adequacy of respirations since he or she may commonly have some degree of shortness of breath.

◆ *The use of multiple prescription medications* Elderly patients often take one or more prescription medications for chronic illnesses.

Figuring out when, why, and how much of the medications have been taken may be confusing for both the EMT and the patient. In some cases, the patient may not know or understand exactly what the medication was for. In other cases, the patient may have all his medications deposited in a "pill minder," making them hard to identify. Further confusion can result when a patient has prescribed medications from more than one physician. If you are to assist a patient with additional doses of inhalers or nitroglycerine, it is important to take the time to determine when and how much of the medications were taken (see Chapter 12, "Respiratory Emergencies," and Chapter 13, "Cardiac Emergencies").

◆ **Communication difficulties** Many elderly patients have visual or hearing impairments. If the patient has eyeglasses and/or a hearing aid, make sure he uses them. In addition, some patients may not completely understand the medical questions you ask. Always speak at an appropriate volume and speed to the geriatric patient. Remember that not all geriatric patients are hard of hearing; some may be offended if you assume they are and shout at them. Always make good eye contact to confirm that the patient is hearing you properly. Try to explain any actions or procedures you will be performing on the patient in clear, simple language; avoid excessive medical jargon.

◆ **Alteration of mental status** You may note that some geriatric patients are confused during their assessment. Some elderly people suffer from conditions such as Alzheimer's disease and normally experience some confusion. It is very important to determine whether the patient's confusion is a chronic problem or whether it is a new development brought on by or contributing to the current emergency. Ask family members or nursing home staff whether the altered mental status of the patient is chronic or newly developed. In addition, ask the family and/or staff for any information about the current problem they can provide.

Geriatric Trauma Emergencies

Trauma is a leading cause of death among the elderly. Geriatric patients who sustain moderate to severe trauma are much more likely to die from the injuries than younger patients with similar injuries.

Falls

Falls are the most common type of trauma among geriatric patients. Approximately one of every three falls in geriatric patients results in at least one fractured bone. The most common fall-related fracture in the elderly is a proximal femur or "hip" fracture. Other common fall-related fractures in elderly patients are listed in Table 24-2. When assessing elderly patients who have fallen, it is important to palpate and inspect the hips, pelvis, chest, forearms, and proximal arms for injuries. In addition to fractures, falls produce serious brain or abdominal injuries in about 10 percent of geriatric patients.

Although some geriatric patients simply trip and fall, with others medical conditions play a part in causing the fall. For example, an irregular heart rhythm (dysrhythmia) might cause a patient to "black out" and subsequently fall and injure himself. During assessment of a geriatric fall victim, you should ask the patient if he remembers falling or "blacking out." You must also evaluate such patients for signs of cardiac or other medical emergencies. When obtaining baseline vital signs, carefully evaluate the blood pressure and pulse. Be especially alert to an irregular pulse, which may indicate a heart dysrhythmia.

Table 24-2

Fractures Common in Geriatric Falls

Proximal femur / hip (most common)
Pelvis
Distal forearm
Proximal humerus
Ribs
Cervical spine

Remember, the evaluation of a geriatric patient who has fallen must include both careful consideration of the events preceding the fall as well as assessment of the injuries the fall may have caused.

Motor Vehicle Crashes

Although the number of miles a person drives per year declines with age, the risk of being involved in a motor vehicle crash (MVC) increases. Several factors contribute to this increase. One key factor is the decrease in side or peripheral vision that occurs with age. This decline in peripheral vision, combined with a decrease in reaction time to hazards, may contribute to the increased number of side-impact collisions involving elderly patients. In side-impact or "T-bone" crashes, the elderly driver's car is usually struck on the side by another vehicle that the older driver failed to see in time.

The injuries sustained by geriatric patients in MVCs will largely depend on the mechanism of injury of the crash. When assessing and treating the geriatric patient who has been involved in a MVC, remember that such patients are many times more likely to die of injuries that younger patients would survive.

Survival of geriatric patients injured in MVCs depends upon high-quality prehospital care that is alert to the anatomic and physiologic differences between elder and younger patients. The geriatric patient must be carefully assessed to detect injuries and signs of shock (hypoperfusion). Cervical spine injuries are more common in geriatric MVC patients because, with age, the neck tends to become less flexible (due to arthritis) and weaker (due to osteoporosis). Therefore, it is important to provide all older patients involved in MVCs with immediate manual cervical spinal stabilization at the time of initial assessment.

Recognizing signs of shock may be difficult in geriatric patients. Common signs of shock can be misleading in the elderly. For example, an elevated pulse rate, a common early sign of hypoperfusion, is sometimes absent in elders. This sign may be missing either because of chronic heart disease or because the patient is taking prescription medications that keep the heart from beating too rapidly. These "blocker" medications are frequently prescribed to treat patients who have high blood pressure or who have had heart attacks (myocardial infarctions) in the past. Patients on these medications may show a normal or slow heart rate even with advanced shock.

Blood pressure readings in older patients can also be deceptive. Those readings are normally higher in older patients than in younger ones. Thus, a blood pressure reading of 110/70 that might be considered normal in a 20-year-old may, in fact, represent a very low blood pressure and a sign of late shock in a 78-year-old MVC patient whose normal blood pressure is 160/90.

Because older patients may not show the normal signs of shock and hypoperfusion, it is important to treat all older patients injured in severe MVCs as though they are in shock. This is especially true if the patient has an altered mental status, such as confusion or agitation. Altered mental status is one of the most common signs of shock in the elderly. Such geriatric patients should be rapidly transported to the hospital, and ideally a trauma center, as soon as possible. Remember that the "golden hour" of trauma care (from the time of injury until the patient's transfer to a surgeon's care) is especially critical in the survival of geriatric trauma patients.

Head Injuries

Head injuries are common among the elderly. They may result from falls, motor vehicle crashes, or assaults. Because of frail blood vessels and thinning of the skin, even minor head injuries in geriatric patients may produce severe bruising (Figure 24-3). Serious head injuries that produce bleeding inside the skull and brain are also more common in older patients. Frequently, signs and symptoms of these more serious head injuries do not show up as quickly in geriatric patients as in younger ones. Loss of consciousness or confusion after head trauma should alert you to the possibility of serious head injury in a geriatric patient. Older patients who are on "blood thinner" medications such as Coumadin® are at especially high risk of life-threatening bleeding with even minor head trauma.

Because the risk of cervical spinal fracture during trauma is increased for geriatric patients, you should always perform spinal immobilization on older patients with head injuries. However, changes in the spine that occur with aging can make immobilization difficult. Some elderly

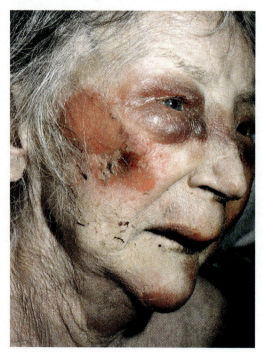

Figure 24-3 Even minor head injuries can produce serious bruising in elderly patients.

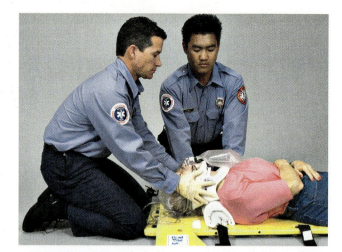

Figure 24-4A In an elderly patient with curvature of the spine, place padding behind the neck when immobilizing a patient to a long spine board.

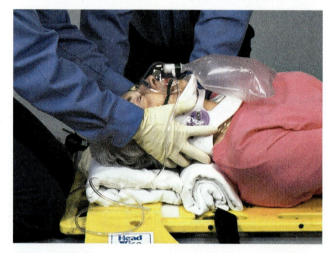

Figure 24-4B Additional padding, such as rolled blankets or towels behind the head may be needed to keep the head in a neutral, in-line position.

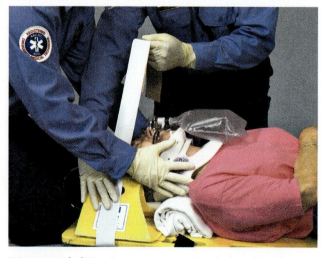

Figure 24-4C Secure the patient's head with a head immoblizer device. Maintain manual stablization until the head is secured.

patients develop such severe curving of the spine (kyphosis) that their head will not touch the backboards when they are placed in supine positions on them. Be prepared to modify normal techniques when immobilizing such a patient to a backboard (Figure 24-4). You may have to use blankets or other padding beneath the head to obtain proper immobilization and to prevent further injury.

Abuse of Geriatric Patients

When assessing and treating geriatric patients, be alert to the possibility that they may be victims of physical and/or mental abuse. An abuser might be a family member, a nursing home staff member, or another elderly person. As with cases of child abuse, you should suspect physical abuse whenever the injuries seem unusually severe for the mechanism of injury that has been reported by the patient, bystanders, nursing home staff, or family members.

Some states require EMTs to report suspected cases of elder abuse. Often, the patients themselves are afraid to report abuse because they are dependent upon the abuser(s) for their daily care. Even if your state does not require you to make a direct report in suspected cases of elder abuse, you should advise the transporting crew or the emergency room staff of your concerns.

Medical Emergencies

In general, geriatric patients face the same types of medical emergencies as younger adults. With geriatric patients, however, illnesses may be more severe than in younger patients. Also, the signs and symptoms of illnesses may be different.

When assessing geriatric patients, always consider these chief complaints as symptoms of a serious or life-threatening illness:

◆ Syncope (passing out) or near-syncope (dizziness)

◆ Acute confusion

◆ Chest pain

◆ Shortness of breath

◆ Abdominal pain

Syncope

Syncope (sin-co-pee) is a temporary loss of consciousness. Syncope results from a reduced flow of blood to the brain. In the elderly, it is often caused by an irregular heart rhythm. The patient will often have a low blood pressure associated with syncope. Treatment of syncope includes administration of high flow oxygen, treatment for shock, and management of injuries resulting from related falls. A request for an Advanced Life Support (ALS) unit should also be considered if one is not normally dispatched.

Acute Confusion

Geriatric patients suffering from a variety of different illnesses may present to the EMT with an altered mental state or sudden confusion. Among the many medical conditions common in the elderly that can produce altered mental status are stroke, heart attack, severe infection, abnormal blood sugar levels, and shock. In such cases, it is important that you determine if the patient's presenting mental status is normal or if it represents a change for the patient. Question family members, friends, or the nursing home staff to learn what the patient's normal mental status is and how it differs from what is now present.

Chest Pain and Shortness of Breath

Many elderly patients suffer heart attacks with little or no chest discomfort. In fact, shortness of

TRANSITION OF CARE

An altered mental status such as confusion or agitation may be a sign of life-threatening illness in a geriatric patient. Because many geriatric patients normally have some degree of confusion, you must determine from the family or care facility staff whether the current altered mental status represents a change for that patient. It is essential that you document whether the alteration in mental status is chronic or new and pass this information along to the transporting crew along with other assessment and treatment information.

breath may be the only symptom of a cardiac emergency in the elderly patient. Any geriatric patient with chest pain and/or shortness of breath should be considered potentially unstable. Provide high flow oxygen and careful ongoing assessment. Patients who suffer chronic chest pain may take nitroglycerin. If the patient's chest pain/shortness of breath are typical of his angina symptoms and the patient has nitroglycerin, follow local protocols for assisting with its administration. If an ALS unit is not routinely dispatched, request that one respond to the scene or intercept the ambulance en route to the hospital.

Abdominal Pain

Abdominal pain is a symptom in a variety of illnesses. In the elderly, abdominal pain can be very serious because geriatric patients are almost ten times more likely to die of abdominal conditions such as appendicitis than younger patients. In addition, certain life-threatening conditions that cause abdominal pain, such as a ruptured abdominal aorta, are seen almost exclusively in older patients. Elderly patients with abdominal pain should be considered to have a life-threatening condition. Assign them a high priority.

Advanced Directives

Advanced directives are documents such as "living wills" or Do Not Resuscitate orders. These documents are usually signed by the patient and a physician prior to a medical emergency. Most advanced directives detail the patient's wishes if he or she becomes unresponsive and suffers respiratory or cardiac arrest. Usually, the directive limits the care that is to be provided the patient, stating that CPR or other resuscitation should not be initiated. Many geriatric patients suffering from chronic or terminal diseases will have advanced directives.

Advanced directives may be confusing to emergency care providers. You should follow state laws and local EMS system protocols whenever you are presented with an advanced directive document by the patient's family or by members of the care facility staff. Some states have standard legal forms for DNR orders to prevent confusion (Figure 24-5). Cases in which you encounter patients with advanced directives are truly "life or death" situations. If there is any doubt about what an advanced directive says or that the document is valid, begin treatment and contact medical direction immediately.

Department of Health

Nonhospital Order Not to Resuscitate (DNR order)

Person's Name (Print) _____

Date of Birth ____/____/____

Do not resuscitate the person named above.

Person's Signature_____

Date____/____/____

Physician's Signature_____

Print Name_____

License Number _____

Date____/____/____

It is the responsibility of the physician to determine, at least every 90 days, whether this order continues to be appropriate, and to indicate this by a note in the person's medical chart. The issuance of a new form is **NOT** required, and under the law this order should be considered valid unless it is known that it has been revoked. This order remains valid and must be followed, even if it has not been reviewed within the 90 day period.

Figure 24-5   A Do Not Resuscitate order.

Chapter Review

SUMMARY

Geriatric patients represent a large number of those served by EMS systems. Because of the aging process, geriatric patients are more prone to injury and illness. The aging process and greater use of medications may also make assessment of these patients more difficult for EMTs. It is crucial that you understand these special considerations when caring for the geriatric patient.

REVIEWING KEY CONCEPTS

1. Describe some changes associated with aging in the following body systems: neurological, cardiovascular, respiratory, musculoskeletal, gastrointestinal, renal, skin.

2. Explain some of the emotional, psychological, or social factors that might cause a geriatric patient who needs EMS care to be fearful.

3. Describe basic approaches to follow to improve communications during assessment of the geriatric patient.

4. List things to be on the lookout for during scene size-up on calls involving geriatric patients.

5. List four factors that can complicate the assessment of geriatric patients.

6. Explain factors that you should consider when evaluating the geriatric patient who is the victim of a fall.

7. Explain why recognizing signs of stroke can be difficult with geriatric patients.

8. Describe the special considerations that may be involved in the immobilization of a geriatric patient with suspected head, neck, or spine injury.

9. List chief complaints that should be considered symptoms of life-threatening illness in geriatric patients.

RESOURCES TO LEARN MORE

Dickinson, E. T. et al., "Geriatric Utilization of Emergency Medical Services," *Annals of Emergency Medicine,* Volume 27, Number 2, pp. 199-203.

"Geriatric Considerations" in Harwood-Nuss, A. L. et al., eds., *Clinical Practice of Emergency Medicine, 2nd Edition.* Philadelphia: Lippincott-Raven, 1996.

"Geriatric Trauma" and "Abuse in the Elderly and Impaired" in Tintinalli, J. E. et al., eds., *Emergency Medicine: A Comprehensive Study Guide, 4th Edition.* New York: McGraw-Hill, 1995.

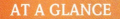
SPECIAL CONSIDERATIONS IN THE ASSESSMENT OF GERIATRIC PATIENTS

SCENE SIZE-UP CONSIDERATIONS
- Consider additional BSI protection because of possibility of TB in patients with respiratory problems in nursing facilities.
- Note whether the environment of the patient's home is too hot or too cold.
- Check scene for presence of prescription or non-prescription medications and home oxygen equipment.

ASSESSMENT CONSIDERATIONS
- Consider presence of multiple diseases.
- Consider that the patient may be using multiple prescription drugs.
- Be prepared for difficulties communicating with the patient.
- If the patient's mental status is altered, determine whether this status is a chronic condition or a new problem.

TRAUMA EMERGENCIES
- Falls
  —Consider events, such as syncope, that preceded the fall as well as fall itself.
- Motor Vehicle Crashes
  —Provide immediate manual cervical stabilization; pad as necessary behind neck and head when immobilizing patient to long spine board.
  —Treat all geriatric patients in severe MVCs as though they are in shock.
- Head Injuries
  —Provide immediate manual cervical stabilization; pad as necessary behind neck and head when immobilizing patient to long spine board.
- Elder Abuse
  —Be aware of reporting requirements.

MEDICAL EMERGENCIES
With geriatric patients, always consider these chief complaints as symptoms of a serious or life-threatening illness:
- Syncope (passing out) or near-syncope (dizziness)
- Acute confusion
- Chest pain
- Shortness of breath
- Abdominal pain

Follow department protocols when providing care to a patient who has an advanced directive such as a living will or a Do Not Resuscitate order.

PART

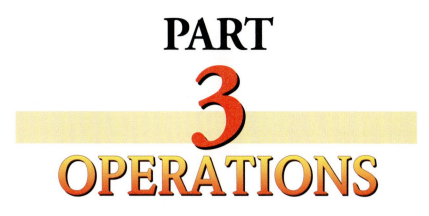

3

OPERATIONS

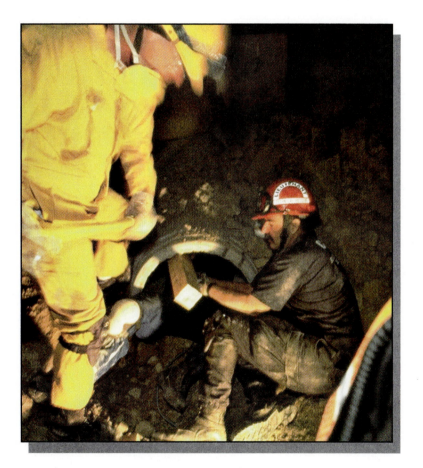

*T*he chapters on EMS Operations that follow are designed to give you a broad overview of many of the technical aspects of working as a firefighter-EMT. Although some medical information is presented, the greatest part of the material in these chapters relates to the non-medical aspects of good patient care.

The information presented here is not meant as a substitute for formal departmental training and drills on the crucial topics of emergency vehicle operations, extrication, rehabilitation, and other special rescue situations and operations. The material is, however, ▶

intended to highlight steps to assure that a well-trained firefighter-EMT can function most effectively in these situations. These steps are detailed in the chapters of Part 3.

Chapter 25   Emergency Vehicle Operations
Chapter 26   Gaining Access and Basics of Extrication
Chapter 27   Emergency Incident Rehabilitation
Chapter 28   EMS Special Operations

Emergency Vehicle Operations

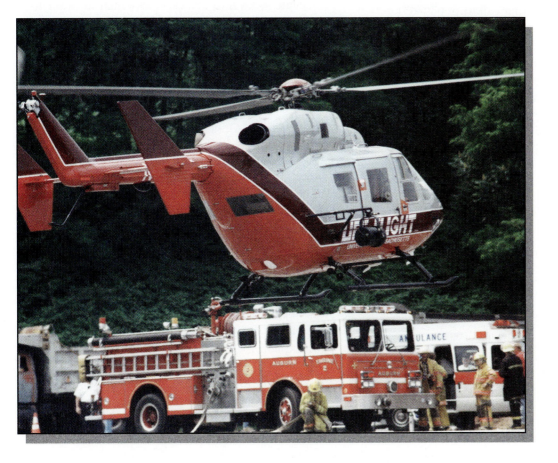

*A*s a firefighter-EMT, you may be called upon to provide patient care in a variety of settings and system configurations. You may carry out your duties as a part of a BLS or ALS engine company or as a crew member on a dedicated, transport-capable ambulance. You will be working with a number of different types of vehicles when responding to emergencies.

Although it is likely you will work with a variety of emergency vehicles on your job, some guidelines for safety and procedures apply with all of them. Being sure that a vehicle is operated safely is the highest ▶

concern. Emergency vehicles exist for the well-being of patients who need their services. Any practices that cause additional risk to patients— or to the personnel caring for them—must be avoided.

This chapter deals with the basics of emergency vehicle operation— stocking the vehicle, driving it safely, and using it to respond to a call. It also provides an overview of air medical evacuations.

OBJECTIVES

At the completion of this chapter, the EMT-Basic student should be able to meet the following objectives:

Knowledge and Understanding

1. Discuss the medical and non-medical equipment needed to respond to a call. (pp. 650–651, 653–654)
2. List the phases of an emergency medical response. (p. 649)
3. Describe the general provisions of state laws relating to the operation of emergency vehicles and privileges in any or all of the following categories: (pp. 655–657)
   —Speed
   —Warning lights
   —Sirens
   —Right-of-way
   —Parking
   —Turning
4. List contributing factors to unsafe driving conditions. (pp. 655, 657–658)
5. Describe the considerations that should be given to: (pp. 657–658)
   —Requests for escorts
   —Following an escort vehicle
   —Intersections

6. Discuss "Due Regard for Safety of Others" while operating an emergency vehicle. (p. 656)
7. State what information is essential in order to respond to a call. (pp. 651, 654)
8. Discuss various situations that may affect response to a call. (pp. 651, 654, 658, 660)
9. Differentiate between the various methods of moving a patient to the unit based upon injury or illness. (p. 660)
10. Apply the components of the essential patient information in a written report. (p. 662)
11. Summarize the importance of preparing the unit for the next response. (pp. 662–665)
12. Identify what is essential for completion of a call. (pp. 662–665)
13. Distinguish among the terms cleaning, disinfection, high-level disinfection, and sterilization. (p. 663)
14. Describe how to clean or disinfect items following patient care. (p. 663)
15. Explain the rationale for appropriate report of patient information. (pp. 658, 660–662, 666)
16. Explain the rationale for having the unit prepared to respond. (pp. 647–648, 649–651)
17. Describe basic procedures for safe air medical evacuation. (pp. 665–666)

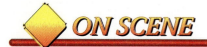

ON SCENE

DISPATCH: *STATION 25, MEDIC AMBULANCE 11. SUBJECT FALLEN AND REPORTED UNCONSCIOUS. 103 COLORADO AVENUE, COUNTRY HILLS. SHE IS A 65-YEAR-OLD FEMALE REPORTED BREATHING BUT UNRESPONSIVE. TIME OUT, 1706 HOURS.*

You are a firefighter EMT assigned to Engine 25, which is responding to this incident. The company officer indicates that your engine will be the first unit on the scene. As the driver navigates the streets, you and your paramedic partner don latex gloves and mentally review which equipment you'll be responsible for taking into the residence.

Once you arrive and determine that the scene is secure, you take the oxygen administration equipment and medical bag, while your partner takes the drug bag, suction unit, and cardiac monitor/defibrillator. A woman who meets at the curb gives her name as Glenda Kincaid and says that it is her mother, Eileen Tyrell, who has fallen. She directs you into the house and to a door to the basement. At the bottom of the basement stairs, you see the patient lying on her side.

You descend to her and find that Mrs. Tyrell is now awake, but somewhat disoriented. She complains of pain in her hip and cannot recall the events leading to her fall. You and your EMT partner provide manual stabilization, apply a cervical collar, and administer supplemental oxygen.

You then obtain a set of baseline vital signs. The company officer records your observations and obtains additional information from the family.

Ambulance 11 arrives a few minutes after your unit. You give an oral report on Mrs. Tyrell's condition and your interventions and transfer her care to its paramedics. They establish cardiac monitoring and start an intravenous line. You help the paramedics complete the immobilization of the patient and remove her from the basement. Mrs. Tyrell is then loaded into the ambulance for the trip to the hospital. You return to the basement for a last check to make sure no equipment has been left behind. You make a mental note to contact the crew of Ambulance 11 for additional information about Mrs. Tyrell's condition later that evening.

The scenario presented in On Scene above is a fairly typical one for firefighter-EMTs. It illustrates how the firefighter-EMT can work with a variety of emergency vehicles and equipment during the course of a single call. The numbers of emergency care personnel and emergency vehicles will vary from call to call. Nevertheless, every call can be broken down into distinct phases. For each of those phases, there are procedures and practices you should follow.

PHASES OF AN EMERGENCY RESPONSE

The basic phases of an emergency medical call are as follows:

◆ Preparing for the call

◆ Dispatch and response

◆ En route to the scene

◆ At the scene

◆ En route to the receiving facility

◆ At the receiving facility

◆ Returning to service

Preparing for the Call

It is essential that you, your vehicle, and its equipment are prepared at all times for an emergency response. This preparation involves routinely checking not only the required equipment and supplies but also the readiness of the crew.

Emergency Vehicles

Like other EMTs, firefighter-EMTs will learn to be familiar with a variety of ambulances. The U.S. Department of Transportation has issued specifications for ambulances outlining possible configurations of the vehicles and requirements for such things as cot-retention systems, hand-held spotlights, and venting systems. The U.S. DOT specifications define Type I, Type II, and Type III ambulances (Figure 25-1A to C). In recent years, the extra weight and space requirements of

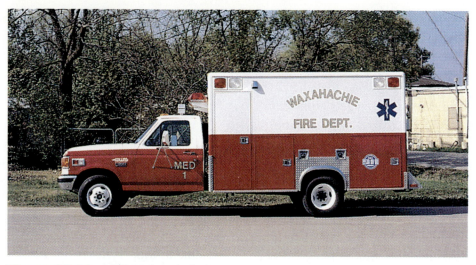

Figure 25-1A   A Type I ambulance.

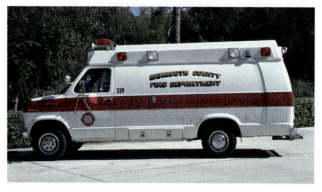

Figure 25-1B   A Type II ambulance.

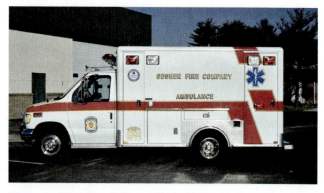

Figure 25-1C   A Type III ambulance.

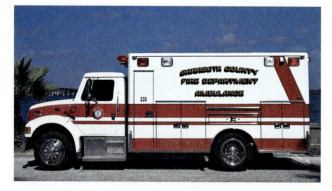

Figure 25-1D   A medium-duty-chassis ambulance.

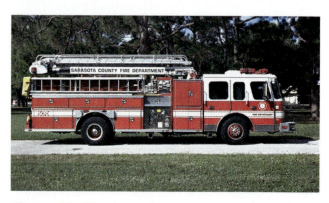

Figure 25-1E   An engine company equipped for EMS duty.

equipment now available for advanced life support and hazardous materials operations have led to the use of a medium-duty truck chassis for some ambulances (Figure 25-1D). In addition, as fire-service-based EMS systems have evolved, more pumpers, rescue units, and ladder trucks are carrying emergency medical equipment and can

thus be considered EMS vehicles (Figure 25-1E). Indeed, some pumpers are now equipped to transport patients.

Equipment Check

Whether you are assigned to an engine company with specific first-response medical supplies or to

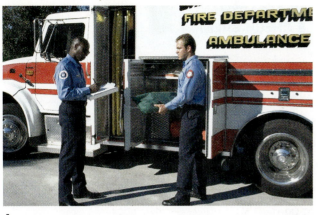

A.

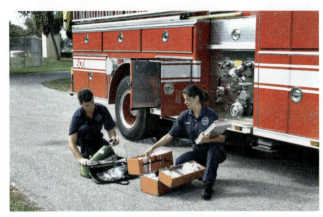

B.

Figure 25-2 At the beginning of each shift, check the equipment required on board the emergency vehicle whether it is **(A)** an ambulance or **(B)** an engine company.

an ambulance with the entire range of emergency medical equipment and supplies, you must verify that all required equipment is on board and in working order at the beginning of your shift (Figure 25-2). Be certain to check that the batteries of any equipment that uses them—for example, the portable suction device or the AED—are fully charged. Your agency should have a checklist of required equipment for the vehicle (Figure 25-3). Use it!

Equipment requirements vary from state to state and jurisdiction to jurisdiction. Table 25-1 shows the different types of equipment required on ambulances in one state.

At the end of each run, you should restock any equipment that has been used and disposed of. Clean, maintain, or repair other gear that has been used.

Vehicle Check

The daily check of your assigned equipment should also include a comprehensive inspection of the vehicle and vehicle systems. Regardless of the type of vehicle (engine, ladder, ambulance, squad), an inspection should be performed at the beginning of each shift. Table 25-2 provides a list of items to be inspected.

Dispatch and Response

An emergency vehicle's run begins with a call from dispatch. Most major metropolitan areas in the nation use a centralized 9-1-1 emergency telephone number for police, fire, and emergency medical services. These central communications centers have personnel available 24 hours a day who obtain information about emergencies from callers and dispatch appropriate units to the situation (Fig. 25-4, page 655).

Emergency Medical Dispatchers

Many dispatch centers have trained and certified their personnel as Emergency Medical Dispatchers (EMDs). These EMDs receive specialized training in the processing, prioritization, and coordination of medical incidents and resources. They are trained to perform the following functions:

◆ Obtain information from the caller regarding the location, nature, and priority of the incident

◆ Dispatch and coordinate EMS resources, and relay all information to responding crews

◆ Provide pre-arrival medical instructions to callers

◆ Coordinate the response with other public safety agencies as required

Required Dispatch Information

Personnel responding to an emergency incident should receive this information from dispatch:

◆ The nature of the incident

◆ The location of the incident

◆ The location of the patient

◆ The number of patients and the severity of the problem

(*text continues, page 654*)

SARASOTA COUNTY FIRE DEPARTMENT
DAILY RESCUE VEHICLE CHECK SHEET

GENERAL		MECHANICAL		AUDIO/VISUAL		DRIVERS COMPARTMENT	
UNIT/ID #	_____	ENGINE OIL:	_____	SIREN/PA	_____	HAND LIGHTS	_____
PIC NAME/ID #	___/___	STEERING FLUID	_____	AIR HORN	_____	RAINCOATS	_____
EMT NAME/ID #	___/___	BRAKE FLUID	_____	ELECTRIC HORN	_____	KEYS & CARDS	_____
DATE	_____	BATTERIES	_____	BEACONS	_____	MAPS/BOOKLETS	_____
HOURS	_____	COOLANT	_____	FLASHERS	_____	GAS KEY	_____
P.M. DUE	_____	**START VEHICLE**		SPOT LIGHT	_____	GRID BOOK	_____
HOURS TILL P.M.	_____	TRANS. FLUID	_____	LOAD LIGHTS	_____	LOG BOOK	_____
RADIOS		FUEL MAIN	_____	FRONT INT. LIGHTS	_____	CLIPBOARD	_____
MOBILE:	_____	FUEL RESERVE	_____	REAR INT. LIGHTS	_____	EMS COMM. VOL II	_____
PORTABLE:	_____	BRAKES	_____	STANDARD LIGHTS	_____	BAYFLIGHT INFO	_____
MEDICAL:	_____	TIRES	_____	MIRRORS	_____	ACCOUNTABILITY TAGS	_____
		WIPERS/WASHERS	_____				

SPLINT EQUIPMENT				ON BOARD EQUIPMENT			
LONG BOARDS	_____	JUMPER CABLES	_____	TRAUMA BAG	_____	STRAPS	_____
SHORT BOARDS	_____	EXTINGUISHER	_____	ADULT M.A.S.T.	_____	RESTRAINTS	_____
K.E.D.	_____	S.C.B.A.	_____	PEDS M.A.S.T.	_____	NITROUS	_____
SCOOP	_____	SAFETY GEAR	_____	AIRWAY SUPPLIES	_____	VENTILATOR	_____
"C" COLLARS	_____	TRAUMA BOX	_____	IV SUPPLIES	_____		
FERNO DEVICE	_____	DRUG BOX	_____	O2 ADJUNCTS	_____	**OXYGEN PSI**	
SANDBAGS	_____	MONITOR/DEFIB	_____	EKG SUPPLIES	_____	ON BOARD	_____
TRACTION SPLINTS	_____	PORTABLE SUCTION	_____	TRAUMA SUPPLIES	_____	PORTABLE	_____
BOARD SPLINTS	_____	O.B. SUCTION	_____	LINENS	_____		
TOOL BOX	_____	PEDS KIT	_____	GLOVES	_____	SPARE	_____
		EXTRA DRUGS	_____	INFECTION CONTROL KIT	_____	NITROUS #	_____

LIST ALL DEFICIENCIES

_____

_____

_____

_____

Figure 25-3 Most departments have lists of equipment that should be checked at the start of the shift.

Table 25-1

Typical Ambulance Equipment

Patient Transfer Equipment

◆ Wheeled ambulance cot capable of carrying a patient in Fowler's position

◆ A stair chair or other stretcher capable of moving a patient through narrow spaces and down stairways

◆ Crash-resistant fasteners capable of securing two patient carrying devices

Airway, Ventilation, Oxygen, and Suction Equipment

◆ A bag-valve-mask device

◆ 4 oropharyngeal airways in adult sizes

◆ D-size portable oxygen cylinder with pressure gauge and flowmeter

◆ Spare oxygen cylinder (D-size or larger)

◆ On-board oxygen system with two E-size or larger cylinders, yoke(s) or CDC fitting, pressure gauges, regulators, and flowmeters

◆ 4 nonrebreather masks

◆ 4 nasal cannulas

◆ Portable suction equipment that can generate a vacuum of 300 mmHg

◆ On-board suction equipment that can generate a vacuum of 300 mmHg

◆ 2 rigid-tip-type wide-bore suction tips

Immobilization Equipment

◆ 1 full-size backboard with straps

◆ 1 short backboard with straps

◆ 1 traction splinting device for the lower extremity

◆ 2 each of the following size padded boards

    4½ by 3 inches

    3 feet by 3 inches

    15 inches by 3 inches

◆ 1 set of rigid extrication collars, sized large, medium, and small

◆ Head immobilizing device

Bandages and Dressings

◆ 24 sterile gauze pads, 4 inches by 4 inches

◆ 3 rolls of adhesive tape in 2 or more sizes

◆ 10 rolls of conforming gauze bandages in 2 or more sizes

◆ 2 sterile universal dressings, 10 inches by 30 inches

◆ 10 large sterile dressings, 5 inches by 9 inches minimum

◆ 1 pair bandage shears

◆ 2 sterile bed-size burn sheets

◆ 6 triangular bandages

◆ 1 liter of sterile normal saline

◆ 1 roll of plastic or aluminum foil or equivalent occlusive dressing

Emergency Childbirth Supplies

◆ Disposable gloves

◆ Scissors or scalpel

◆ Umbilical clamps or tape

◆ Bulb syringe

◆ Drapes

◆ 1 individually wrapped sanitary napkin

Miscellaneous Equipment

◆ Linen and pillow on wheeled cot

◆ Spare pillow

◆ 2 sheets, pillow cases, and blankets

◆ 4 cloth towels

◆ 1 box facial tissues

◆ 2 emesis containers

◆ 1 adult-size blood pressure cuff with gauge

◆ Stethoscope

◆ Carrying case for essential emergency equipment and supplies

◆ 4 chemical cold packs

◆ 1 male urinal

◆ 1 bed pan

(continued)

Table 25-1

Typical Ambulance Equipment (continued)

- 2 sets masks and goggles or equivalent
- 2 pairs of disposable rubber or plastic gloves
- 1 container liquid glucose or equivalent
- 6 sanitary napkins individually wrapped
- 1 penlight or flashlight

Safety Equipment

- 6 flares or 3 U.S. DOT-approved reflective road triangles
- 1 battery lantern
- 1 chemical fire extinguisher

Pediatric Equipment

- Pediatric bag-valve-mask device
- Face masks in newborn, infant, and child sizes

- 2 nasal cannulas
- 2 oxygen masks including nonrebreather
- Oropharyngeal airways, 2 each in newborn, infant, and child sizes
- Sterile DeLee-type suction catheters, 2 each in sizes 5, 8, and 10 French
- 1 sterile single-use oxygen humidification setup
- Child- and infant-size blood pressure cuffs with gauges
- 1 pediatric-size rigid extrication collar
- 1 pediatric stethoscope
- 1 commercially prepared infant swaddler

Table 25-2

Vehicle Inspection

- Fuel levels
- Oil and all other fluid levels
- Engine cooling system
- Battery
- Brakes
- Wheels and tires
- Headlights
- Stoplights
- Turn signals
- Emergency warning lights
- Wipers
- Horn
- Siren
- Function of all doors (closing and latching)
- Communications system
- Air conditioning/heating system
- Ventilation system

- Any special problems or circumstances
- Whether additional units have been dispatched to the scene

All information should be considered "reported" until confirmed by a public safety official (law enforcement officer, other fire apparatus personnel, etc.) who is on the scene. Additional information, such as a past history of the premises to which the unit is dispatched or ongoing situational changes, may also be provided while a unit is responding to the scene. Some communications centers have the ability to provide a complete view of the computer incident file to all responding units, either through printers in the station or through mobile data terminals (MDTs) mounted in each vehicle.

Write down information that you receive from dispatch. Refer to it as you think of the resources you may need on the call. If anything in the dispatch information is unclear, ask the dispatcher to repeat or clarify it. If yours is the first responding unit to reach the scene, remember to contact dispatch and provide a clear and concise size-up report once you have assessed the incident.

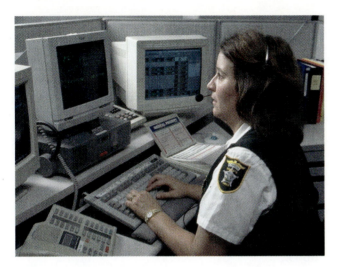

Figure 25-4 Dispatchers try to obtain from callers as much information as possible about the nature of an emergency and pass what they learn on to responding EMS personnel.

En Route to the Scene

The response to the scene can be one of the most dangerous phases of an emergency response (Figure 25-5). In fact, emergency vehicle operations represent one of the largest sources of liability for any public safety agency.

Basic Safety Measures

Each crew member on an emergency vehicle responding to an incident is responsible for taking steps to assure personal safety—for example, by wearing a seat belt. Additionally, all persons on the vehicle share the responsibility of being alert

Figure 25-5 The risk of collision with other vehicles can be high during responses to emergency calls.

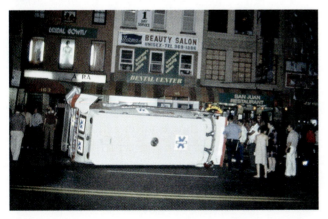

for hazards, such as inattentive operators of other vehicles, other responding apparatus, etc. The safety of the responding unit thus becomes a team responsibility. Basic safety practices that should be followed while driving an emergency vehicle include the following:

- All occupants of the emergency vehicle should wear safety belts. Many departments have a mandatory use policy for all employees, regardless of the type of vehicle.

- Emergency vehicle operators should be familiar with the unique characteristics of each vehicle they are required to operate in the performance of their duties. All employees must complete an emergency vehicle operator's course before driving under emergency conditions.

- Emergency vehicle operators should be alert for changes in weather and road conditions, particularly in geographic areas susceptible to changeable road conditions, such as fog, snow, or ice.

- Exercise caution in use of red lights and siren (RLS). Studies show that emergency vehicle operators have a tendency to accelerate with continuous use of audible and visual warning devices. Follow local and state regulations when using RLS. Be aware of the limitations of the warning devices installed on the particular vehicle you are driving.

- Select an appropriate route, and consider that other emergency vehicles may be responding to the same location. Be prepared to use an alternate route in the event of unforeseen problems with the primary route.

- Maintain a safe following distance from all vehicles. Be prepared for the possibility that other motorists may take sudden or unexpected actions when they encounter an emergency vehicle.

- Drive with due regard for the safety of your crew and other motorists on the road. This is particularly important because emergency vehicles may place themselves in areas or positions that would not be used by "normal" traffic.

The headlights are the most visible warning devices on an emergency vehicle. It is good practice for drivers of emergency vehicles to turn on their headlights whenever they are on the road—day or night—to increase visibility to other motorists.

Be familiar with any hazards associated with the design and style of your vehicle.

All emergency vehicle operators should be familiar with their department's policies and procedures in cases of collisions involving the vehicle. Procedures should include provisions for reporting, investigating, and reviewing all collisions involving departmental personnel and equipment. The provisions should also incorporate a review of operational practices to discover ways of preventing similar incidents in the future.

Laws Governing Emergency Vehicle Operations

Traffic laws in most states grant drivers of emergency vehicles exemptions from many of the provisions that govern civilian drivers. However, these exemptions require that the operator of the emergency vehicle demonstrate *due regard for the safety of others* on the roads. To drive with due regard involves operating a vehicle in a fashion that is reasonable and careful, with consideration for other motorists. Thus, despite the special exemptions, emergency vehicle operators can, and have, been found criminally and civilly liable for their actions if they are involved in or cause collisions. In fact, many traffic laws contain specific clauses stating that *"emergency vehicle exemptions shall not be a defense to the emergency vehicle operator in a action brought forth for criminal negligence or reckless conduct."*

Drivers of authorized emergency vehicles are normally granted some or all of the following exemptions. Note, however, that the exemptions often apply only in cases of true emergency, which are defined as those in which life or limb are endangered. Be familiar with and obey the laws in effect in your jurisdiction.

Speed Emergency vehicle operators may exceed the posted speed limits, provided they do not endanger persons or property.

COMPANY OFFICER'S NOTES

All officers should be familiar with the traffic laws specifying the requirements that must be met by emergency vehicle operators in their jurisdiction. Additionally, company officers should be familiar with their department's standard operating procedure(s) for initial qualification and training of emergency vehicle operators, and with ongoing proficiency requirements. Company officers should stay alert and be prepared to upgrade or downgrade response to a call based on changes in patient conditions or field conditions.

Warning lights Emergency vehicle operators may use visual warning signals in conformance with local laws to request the right of way from operators of other vehicles.

Sirens Emergency vehicle operators may use audible warning devices to request the right of way from operators of other vehicles.

Right of way Emergency vehicle operators may proceed against the right of way at uncontrolled intersections and may disregard the proper traffic lanes. They may also drive the wrong way down a one-way street.

Traffic signals Emergency vehicle operators may proceed through red stop lights or red flashing lights. Some states require the emergency vehicle to come to a full stop before proceeding; all states require the operator to use caution when going through such signals. Note that IFSTA and NFPA recommend that all emergency vehicles come to a full stop at all red lights, stop signs, and active rail crossing signals. These guidelines are based on the fact that a large proportion of accidents occur at intersections and could be prevented if vehicles came to a full stop before entering them.

Turning Emergency vehicle operator may operate against signs or traffic control devices that govern the direction of traffic flow or that indicate the directions in which turns can be made.

Parking An emergency vehicle may park or stand in areas designated as "no-parking" zones, regardless of ordinance or statute. An operator may basically park anywhere, as long as doing so does not endanger lives or property.

◆ *Passing* Emergency vehicle operators may pass other vehicles in no-passing zones.

The privileges granted to the operator of an emergency vehicle do not provide immunity from the responsibility to drive with due regard for the safety of others. As stated earlier, an emergency vehicle operator who was involved in a collision and failed to exercise due regard for others may be found criminally and civilly responsible for his or her actions.

Multiple-Vehicle Hazards

It is common for more than one emergency vehicle to be dispatched to the same incident. For example, a police car may be dispatched with a fire department engine and an ambulance to a reported cardiac arrest. Such a situation presents an increased potential for collisions involving the emergency vehicles. Motorists, having seen one emergency vehicle, often do not expect another and pull from the curbside or into an intersection without looking. Also, the sirens of two vehicles converging on a scene from different areas can cause confusion for motorists. In addition, the sound of your vehicle's siren may prevent you from hearing the siren of another emergency vehicle, increasing the possibility of an accident.

Emergency Vehicle Escorts

The use of escort vehicles can pose dangers similar to those found in multiple-vehicle responses. Escort vehicles, usually police cars, are assigned in the belief that additional emergency vehicles can facilitate faster travel for the ambulance. Fortunately, this practice has fallen out of favor for a variety of reasons. First, as noted above, motorists often do not expect more than one emergency vehicle and may pull directly into the path of the vehicle receiving the escort. Additionally, the driver of the escorting vehicle will most likely travel much faster than the driver of the vehicle transporting the patient, who is trying to provide a smooth ride for the patient and crew. As a result,

the driver of the emergency vehicle may speed up unnecessarily or lose the escort. It is more desirable to have police control traffic at busy or dangerous intersections than to have them provide an escort.

Under rare circumstances, use of an escort may be indicated. If, for example, the driver and crew of a responding unit are unfamiliar with the location of either the patient or the receiving facility, use of an escort would be appropriate. When an escort is used, all vehicles involved must be sure to maintain safe following distances. Also, there should be direct communications between vehicles so that the escort can be properly coordinated while on the road.

Intersections

Intersections present a special hazard for emergency vehicles. In fact, a majority of the collisions involving emergency vehicles occur at intersections. An emergency vehicle traveling against the traffic flow or against the pattern established by the intersection's traffic-control devices can confuse other motorists. Frequently, other drivers are not looking for an approaching vehicle in an oncoming lane, or may not have heard the audible warning devices. Table 25-3 lists some additional hazards found at intersections.

Table 25-3

Factors Contributing to Intersection Collisions

◆ Motorists' failure to anticipate vehicles approaching from an unexpected direction

◆ Motorists' inability to hear or to correctly detect the direction of sirens or horns

◆ Motorists entering an intersection despite a change in traffic light

◆ Failure of motorists to anticipate more than one emergency vehicle responding to the same incident

◆ Limited visibility due to other vehicles either parked or waiting at the intersection

Emergency vehicle operators must exercise extreme caution when entering intersections. Many departments require responding apparatus to go no faster than the posted speed limit when entering an intersection *with the traffic-control devices*. IFSTA and many departments require the apparatus operator to come to a complete stop when entering an intersection *against the traffic-control device*. An intersection presents another opportunity for all crew members to assist the emergency vehicle operator by remaining alert for hazards during a response. Do not proceed through any intersection until all lanes of traffic can be accounted for.

Factors Affecting Emergency Response

Many factors can affect the response to an emergency incident. Weather, traffic patterns, and road conditions are just a few of the things that can delay or prevent responders from reaching a scene. Be ready for the possibility that your route to the scene of the emergency may be blocked. As you set out, have an alternate route in mind. If it looks like you will face a significant delay in reaching the scene for any reason, contact dispatch and report your delay, also giving the reason for it. Doing so will permit the incident commander to dispatch other units that may be able to reach the scene before yours.

At the Scene

Once you reach the scene, your goals should be to assure scene safety and then get to, assess, provide emergency care for, and transport the patient as safely and efficiently as possible.

Positioning Units at the Scene of an Emergency

When you reach the scene, inform dispatch of your arrival. After that, your primary concern, as it should be during any emergency response, is the safety of all responding personnel. The members of the first crew on the scene should position their vehicle to shield them from immediate hazards, such as traffic flow. Park out of the traffic flow if possible, for example, in a parking lot or

driveway. If the vehicle must be left in the street, be sure to leave its warning lights on.

Be alert for potential hazards and maintain a safe distance from them (Figure 25-6). For instance, park the unit uphill, upwind, and at least 2,000 feet (610 meters) from a potential hazardous materials leak. All crew members should be on the lookout for other potential hazards such as unruly crowds, downed power lines, leaking fuel, unstable terrain, etc.

It is important for all vehicles at an emergency scene to be positioned so that the transporting ambulance can gain access to the patient and then exit the scene (Figure 25-7). Blocking the route of the transporting ambulance with engines, rescue units, or command vehicles increases on-scene time for the patient. It also adds to the chance of a vehicle collision as apparatus is hurriedly moved to make a path for the ambulance.

Reporting to Dispatch

The first-in unit should provide an initial progress report to dispatch that includes the following:

◆ A brief summary of the situation

◆ Any changes in your unit's location from that to which it was originally dispatched

◆ Number of patients with initial assessment of severity

◆ Additional resources required, recommended travel route, staging location

◆ Weather, landmark, and landing zone information if helicopter evacuation is requested.

Once the unit is safely positioned, determine if the patient requires immediate movement to protect him from hazards. First-responding apparatus should divide up patient care tasks among the crew to assure fast and efficient assessment and treatment of the patient. The first-response unit should strive to have the patient prepared for transport by the time the ambulance or paramedic unit arrives on scene.

Multiple-Casualty Incidents

The multiple-casualty incident (MCI), or mass-casualty situation (MCS), presents some unique

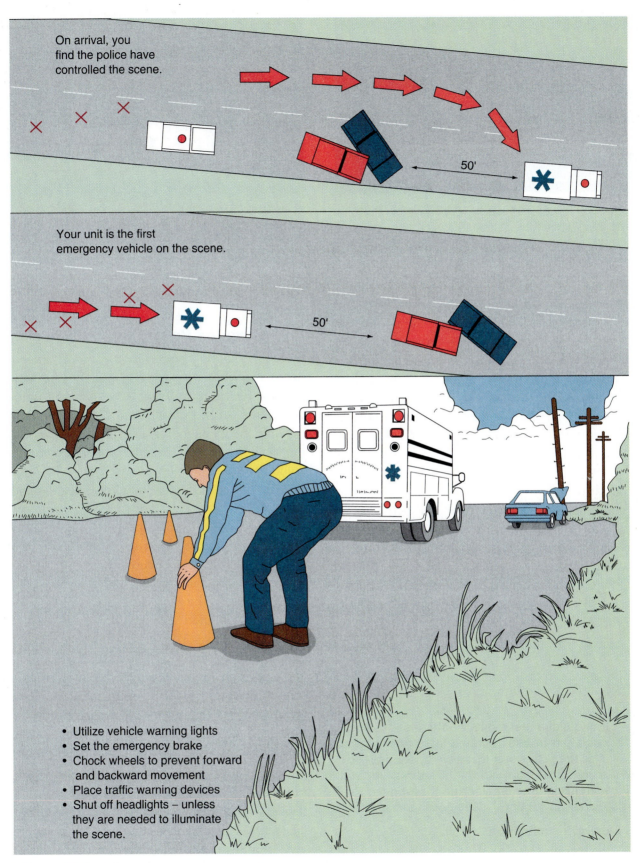

On arrival, you find the police have controlled the scene.

50'

Your unit is the first emergency vehicle on the scene.

50'

- Utilize vehicle warning lights
- Set the emergency brake
- Chock wheels to prevent forward and backward movement
- Place traffic warning devices
- Shut off headlights – unless they are needed to illuminate the scene.

Figure 25-6 Positioning the first-responding apparatus at the emergency scene.

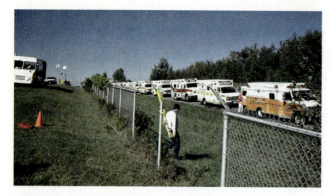

Figure 25-7 When multiple vehicles respond to a scene, they should be staged in a way that permits safe and easy access and departure from the scene.

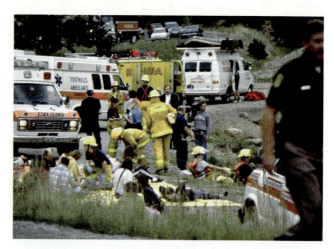

Figure 25-8 The first-arriving unit at a multiple-casualty incident should recognize the need for additional resources and request them promptly.

challenges to firefighter-EMTs (Figure 25-8). The first-arriving unit should determine the number of patients, request additional resources, and begin patient triage. The organization and structure for the entire incident will be determined in the first 5 minutes of the first-arriving unit's activities on the scene. The unit's actions can thus "make" or "break" the incident. It is imperative that the first-in unit at an MCI provide an overview of the situation to the communications center that will allow dispatchers to anticipate the needs of the on-scene units or to initiate the jurisdiction's disaster plan. During the early stages of the incident is the time to request additional resources; waiting can lead to unnecessary delays in moving patients to area receiving facilities. (Multiple-casualty incidents will be discussed in greater detail in Chapter 28, "EMS Special Operations.")

COMPANY OFFICER'S NOTES

Individual personnel on the first-arriving unit can be pre-assigned tasks prior to arrival at the scene. For instance, a response to an "unconscious subject" might prompt the officer to assign the crew to the following areas of responsibility:

◆ Airway management

◆ Chest compressions

◆ Semi-automatic external defibrillator operation

Preparing the Patient for Transport

Once you have completed all critical interventions, you must package and prepare the patient for transfer to an ambulance, paramedic unit, or helicopter for transport to the hospital. Before moving the patient, recheck all interventions. If immobilized, is the patient properly secured to spine board? Is he properly covered? Are all devices (oxygen, cardiac monitor, pulse oximeter, intravenous lines, etc.) prepared for the transfer? Are bandages and splints properly applied? Is the patient properly strapped to the stretcher? Is the stretcher locked and secured in the ambulance? Remember that all lifting and moving of the patient should be accomplished following the guidelines outlined in Chapter 10, "Lifting and Moving Patients." You may wish to review that chapter at this time.

Too often, unnecessary problems disrupt this stage of the process. Hasty, unplanned movement of the patient can result in disconnection from oxygen devices, pulled intravenous lines, or disconnection from patient monitoring equipment.

Transition of Care

If you are transferring care of the patient to ambulance EMTs or a paramedic unit, be prepared to give a brief oral or written report of the patient's condition. Include pertinent findings from your assessment, any interventions you have performed, and the patient's response to them.

Remember that your initial on-scene observations, as well as information provided by bystanders, can be valuable to the transporting EMS personnel, as well as to the hospital staff who will ultimately receive the patient. Review the procedures for turning over care of a patient in Chapter 9, "Transition of Prehospital Care."

Patients involved in accidents often have various types of personal property with them. Be alert for any of the patient's personal effects at the scene. Secure such items with the patient and transfer them to the custody of the staff at the receiving facility. You should be familiar with your agency's policies or procedures for dealing with patient property.

En Route to the Receiving Facility

The communications center should be notified when the emergency vehicle departs from the scene of the call and told of its intended destination. In fact, some agencies require the unit to provide the vehicle's mileage at the beginning and end of patient transport. During transport, at least one certified EMT should—and in many states, must—accompany the patient in the patient compartment. In some situations, additional personnel may be required to assist with a critical patient, such as one in cardiac arrest.

Your mode of response from the scene to the hospital should be determined by your patient's condition. A high-priority patient should generally get RLS transport. This level of response usually is not appropriate for non-critical patients. Consult and follow your local protocols.

During transport to the receiving facility, conduct an ongoing assessment to ensure the effectiveness of any interventions and that the patient's condition is not deteriorating (Figure 25-9). Be sure to explain to the patient any assessments or procedures that you undertake. Doing so will help ease the patient's fears and uneasiness. It will also reduce the possibility of the patient becoming resistant as you attempt to provide care.

Always be prepared for the possibility of complications and deterioration of the patient during transport. Anticipating problems will enable you to have the resources ready to manage any situation that may arise during transport.

The transport phase is also an opportunity to obtain additional information regarding the patient's history and the circumstances of the current incident. You might also begin to complete the prehospital patient care report at this time.

Some EMS systems require all ambulances to contact the receiving facility by radio or phone before arrival with a patient. Other systems only require contact if the patient will need special services or resources. At the very minimum, an EMT should request that the dispatcher notify the receiving facility when a priority patient is being transported. This notification will permit the receiving facility to prepare for the patient's arrival by clearing a room, gathering specialized staff, or summoning assistance for lifting and transfer of the patient. You should be familiar with and follow all local policies regarding contact with receiving facilities.

Figure 25-9 Provide ongoing assessment of the patient during transport to the receiving facility.

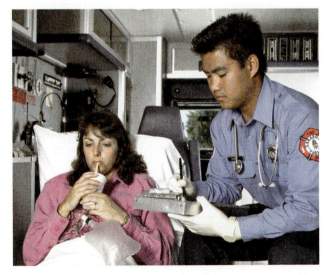

At the Receiving Facility

As you arrive at the receiving facility, contact dispatch and provide an update of your status. Then check with emergency department personnel to see where the patient should be placed. Many hospitals require arriving ambulance crews to report to triage areas, where a brief summary of the patient's condition is presented. The triage area staff may also wish to ask the patient direct questions to assist in determining the proper destination in the emergency department. Continue to care for the patient until he is actually transferred to the emergency department staff.

The transfer of patient responsibility from the prehospital EMS crew to the hospital staff takes place at the patient's bedside. There, you should provide a detailed oral report on the patient's condition to the emergency room personnel (Figure 25-10). *NEVER leave a patient in a room without notifying the hospital staff and providing a bedside oral report.* Assist emergency department staff with the patient until your services are no longer required.

Many fire departments require EMTs to assure that a stretcher's side rails are in the up position before leaving the patient in the emergency department. This reduces the risks both of patient injury and of subsequent lawsuits.

Leave a written report documenting all observations and treatment you have provided with the patient's hospital chart before the unit returns to

Figure 25-10 An oral report of the patient's condition is an essential part of the transfer of patient care to the receiving facility staff.

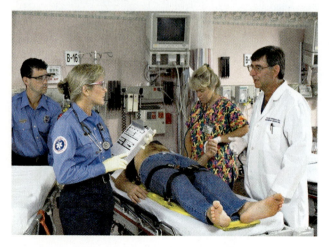

service (see Chapter 8, "Communication and Documentation"). Also be sure that the patient's personal effects are transferred to responsible hospital personnel per your department's policy.

Before leaving the hospital, confirm with the emergency department physician or nurse that your services are no longer needed. Often, emergency department staff may have additional questions about the patient's history or prehospital assessment. In some cases, you might be required to perform further transport duties. For example, if the patient's condition is not serious enough to warrant admission, you may have to return him home.

Returning to Service

The transfer of the patient to the receiving facility is not the end of the EMT's responsibilities during a run. The unit must be prepared for return to available status. You can begin this process while still at the receiving facility.

Clean-up at the Receiving Facility

Begin to prepare the ambulance by giving it a quick cleaning while at the receiving facility. Use heavy-duty, dishwashing style gloves while you clean up blood, vomitus, and other body substances that may have soiled the ambulance floor, walls, and other surfaces. Dispose of contaminated wastes by following approved procedures. Bag dirty clothing and linens for later laundering.

Make up the ambulance cot so that it will be ready for the next patient. Likewise, clean and disinfect other reusable equipment so that it will be ready for service.

Whenever you are cleaning equipment, always be sure to take appropriate BSI precautions. When you are through, wash your hands (Figure 25-11).

Obtain replacements for equipment, such as spine boards and linens, that you have had to leave at the hospital. If you have an agreement with the facility, you may also be able to replace expendable items that you have used, such as dressings, bandages, gloves, etc.

En Route to the Station

When you leave the receiving facility, radio in to inform dispatch that you are returning to the sta-

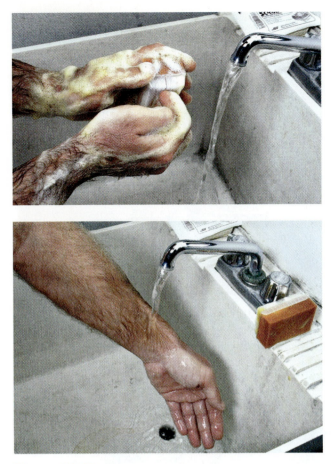

Figure 25-11 Proper handwashing is an important part of the post-run cleanup.

tion. Indicate whether you are or are not available for service.

All crew members should wear seat belts while returning to base. However, a crew member can still continue to clean the patient compartment while belted in.

You may refuel the vehicle at this time. Follow department policy on when to refuel.

At the Station

Once you have returned to the station, complete any unfinished report forms. Do not postpone this task.

Cleaning and Disinfection Procedures If you were unable to do so at the receiving facility, clean and disinfect the ambulance and its equipment or complete whatever cleaning and disinfection you were unable to do there (Fig. 25-12A to D). Remember that failure to properly clean devices or to wash your hands frequently can result in cross-contamination of co-workers and future patients, in addition to increasing risk to your own health.

Cleaning of equipment or a vehicle involves the removal of any obvious debris from an object. Although a device or vehicle will no longer have any visual signs of contamination, it is still possible for bacteria or other pathogens to remain on a device that has been cleaned.

Disinfection refers to the physical or chemical removal or inactivation of bloodborne pathogens on a surface or item to the point that they are no longer capable of transmitting infectious particles. The surface or item is then considered safe for handling, use, or disposal.

Standard disinfection involves wiping equipment or surfaces with an EPA-registered hospital disinfectant or use of a 1:100 chlorine bleach to water solution. Standard disinfection would be utilized for routine cleaning of ambulance floors, walls, and countertops. If these surfaces have been contaminated with blood or higher levels of organic matter, use intermediate-level disinfection.

Intermediate-level disinfection is used for items that have been contaminated with greater levels of organic matter. These items might include splints, stethoscopes, or blood pressure cuffs. Use a 1:10 bleach to water solution or an EPA-registered disinfectant that is tuberculocidal.

High-level disinfection would normally be used for reusable equipment that has been in contact with mucous membranes. This would include laryngoscopes, blades, handles, etc. For this process, use hot water pasteurization, soaking equipment for 30 minutes at 176° to 212°F (80° to 100°C). Equipment can also be immersed in an EPA-approved chemical sterilizing agent for 10 to 45 minutes following the manufacturer's instructions.

Sterilization refers to the use of physical or chemical procedures to destroy all microbial life including highly resistant bacterial spores. Sterilization is normally used for instruments that penetrate the skin during invasive procedures. Sterilization can be accomplished with steam autoclaving, gas autoclaving, or immersion in an EPA-approved chemical sterilization agent for 6 to 10 hours.

Launder linens or clothing soiled during the call or the post-run clean-up. Dispose of all wastes according to department policy.

Cleaning and Disinfecting Equipment

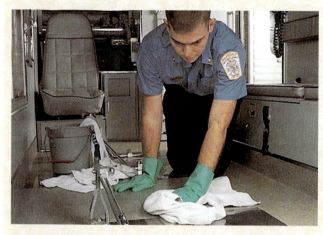

Figure 25-12A Use a low-level disinfectant approved by the U.S. Environmental Protection Agency—for example, a cleanser like Lysol—to clean and to kill germs on ambulance floors and walls.

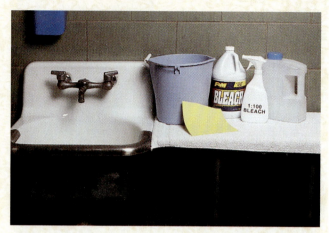

Figure 25-12B Use an intermediate-level disinfectant—for example, a 1:10 mix of bleach to water—to clean and to kill germs on equipment surfaces.

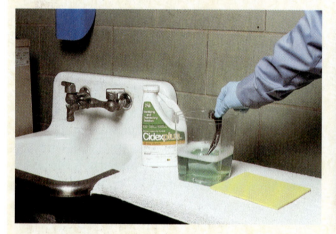

Figure 25-12C Use a high-level disinfectant—for example, Cidex Plus—to destroy all forms of microbial life except high numbers of bacterial spores.

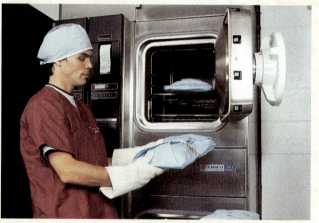

Figure 25-12D Use techniques of sterilization to destroy all possible sources of infection on equipment that is used invasively.

Always take appropriate BSI precautions when cleaning and disinfecting equipment. Always wash your hands thoroughly when done.

Preparing the Vehicle Once the vehicle is cleaned, make sure that it is ready for service again. Some examples of tasks required for returning a unit to "available" status include:

◆ Checking the vehicle's fuel and fluid levels

◆ Replacing or changing linens

◆ Replacing or refilling oxygen cylinders

◆ Replacing patient care equipment so that the vehicle is fully stocked

◆ Performing any post-run vehicle maintenance required by agency protocols

◆ Cleaning the exterior of the unit

- Completing any remaining report forms if you have not already done so
- Contacting dispatch and reporting that the unit is ready for service

AIR MEDICAL TRANSPORT

Air medical transportation via helicopter has become an increasingly important component of EMS systems throughout the country. Fire departments routinely interact with helicopter medical teams. Such interactions include the transfer of patients from ground personnel to air medical personnel (Figure 25-13). Engine companies might also provide stand-by fire suppression services at helicopter landing zones.

Helicopter services can help patients—and EMTs—in several ways:

- The helicopter will usually bring advanced life support personnel and equipment. These assets are particularly useful during MCIs or in jurisdictions without ground-based ALS capabilities.
- Helicopter transport is usually faster than ground transport, especially when ground transport routes are impeded.
- The helicopter can provide rapid, direct transport of patients from the scene to specialty care centers (i.e., trauma centers, pediatric centers, hyperbaric facilities, etc.)

Figure 25-13 Helicopters can provide rapid transport of patients to regional trauma centers.

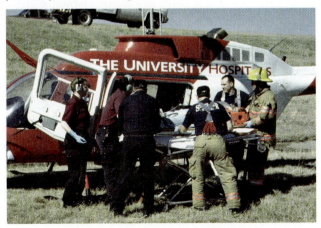

- The helicopter can provide a platform for rescue or access to remote locations inaccessible to regular vehicles, as in a wilderness rescue situation.

Requesting Air Medical Support

A request for air transport should be considered under the following circumstances:

- *Operational considerations:* The patient needs the services of a distant specialty care facility. The patient is in a remote region difficult to access by ground transportation. Normal ground routes to a receiving facility are blocked. An extended extrication has delayed transport of a high-priority patient.
- *Medical considerations:* The patient is considered high-priority for transport. This might include patients in shock; those with extensive burns; those with chest trauma and respiratory distress; those with penetrating injuries to the body cavity; those with head injuries and altered mental status who are less than alert; those with serious mechanisms of injury. Follow local protocols when determining priority.

If you determine air transport is necessary, follow your department's protocols for contacting a service. The communications center will usually have contact information about air transport services on file. You should be prepared to provide some specific information to the service whenever a helicopter is requested. This information includes:

- Your name and department
- The nature of the incident and its exact location, including crossroads and major landmarks
- Radio frequencies or channels so that the helicopter can communicate directly with units at the scene
- Specific hazards at the scene, such as power lines, trees, traffic, etc.
- The exact location of the landing zone
- Number and condition of patients

Selecting a Landing Zone

Select the site of the landing zone (LZ) for a helicopter carefully. Depending on where the LZ is located, you may need to request additional units for security or for assistance in transferring the patient from the scene of the incident to the LZ.

The size of the LZ will be determined by the type of aircraft being used and by department protocols. A 60-foot by 60-foot (19-meter by 19-meter) square area is usually adequate for daytime use by small helicopters. For nighttime operations, however, a 100-foot by 100-foot (30-meter by 30-meter) square area is usually required. For medium-sized or larger helicopters, an even larger area is needed. Mark the corners of the LZ with traffic cones, flares, or light sticks.

The area for the LZ should be level and free of overhead wires, towers, and trees. If possible, choose a site that can be secured to prevent bystanders from wandering into it. In some jurisdictions, an engine company stand-by is required when a helicopter transport is requested to provide security, rescue, and fire-suppression capabilities in the event of a crash. Note that the aircraft pilot has the ultimate authority to accept the LZ or choose an alternative landing site.

Ground Safety Procedures

Most air medical services present safety orientation programs to EMS agencies that they serve. These programs lay out safety procedures to be followed with the specific types of aircraft used by the air medical service. However, there are basic ground safety procedures that should be followed whenever a helicopter transport is requested (Figure 25-14). These include the following:

◆ Do not approach a helicopter unless directed or escorted by the flight crew.

◆ Always follow the flight crew's instructions exactly.

◆ Approach and leave the helicopter from the front of the aircraft when possible.

◆ Never walk around the tail rotor area.

◆ Do not smoke in or around the LZ.

◆ Do not shine spotlights up at an approaching helicopter at night.

◆ Do not use headlights to illuminate the LZ because the white lights can interfere with the air crew's night vision.

◆ Keep patient and ground crew clear of or protected from the "rotor wash" produced by the helicopter's rotors on landing or take-off. The sand, gravel, dirt, and other items blown about by the rotor wash can be hazardous.

◆ Provide a person to monitor the helicopter's tail rotor until the aircraft leaves the scene.

COMPANY OFFICER'S NOTES

Company officers should ensure that all personnel under their command have completed an aircraft safety program offered by their local air medical service. These programs offer an opportunity to discuss preferred and prohibited actions when a helicopter is used in an emergency response.

It is also important for incident commanders to coordinate the use of a helicopter with the primary medical care providers on the scene. The decision to use, not use, or cancel a helicopter should be made jointly with the persons providing medical care to the patients.

Transition of Care

The transfer of patient treatment from ground EMS personnel to the air medical crew should include the same information that would normally be provided to a ground-based transport provider (see Chapter 9, "Transition of Prehospital Care"). Make every effort to provide a *written* report outlining your observations and treatment. The noise of the helicopter can interfere with a spoken report. Also, the helicopter crew may be transporting the patient to a distant location and may not have access to the on-scene units for follow-up questions.

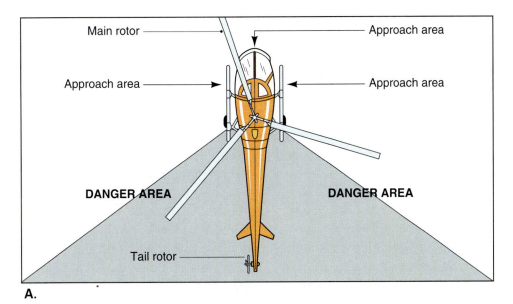

A.

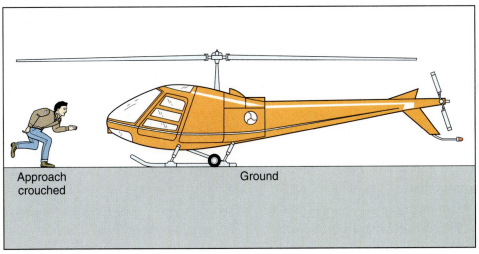

B.

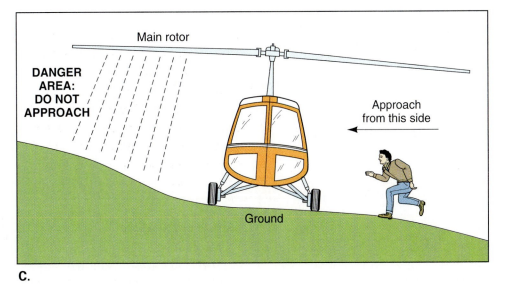

C.

Figure 25-14 Danger areas around helicopters. **A.** The area around the tail rotor is extremely dangerous even in rear-loading aircraft. **B.** Sudden wind gusts can cause the main rotor of a helicopter to dip. Always approach a helicopter in a crouch when the rotor is moving. **C.** When the helicopter has landed on a hillside, approach it from the downhill side.

Chapter Review

SUMMARY

Firefighter-EMTs may provide patient care on a variety of vehicles, including engine companies, ambulances, heavy rescue units, and paramedic units. Whatever type of apparatus you ride on, you must be familiar with its operation and its equipment. You must also be aware of agency policies and procedures setting out your responsibilities during a call. Although you have responsibilities to the patient, remember that you are also responsible for your own safety and the safety of your co-workers. These responsibilities include the safe operation of the emergency vehicle both on the way to the scene and during transport of the patient to the receiving facility.

Your responsibilities do not end at the door of the receiving facility. Be ready to ensure a proper transition of patient care to the staff of the receiving facility. Provide the staff with an oral report on the patient's condition and provide written documentation of your interventions and pertinent observations as well. Finally, you must ensure that the emergency vehicle is cleaned, restocked, and ready to go back into service to assist other patients.

REVIEWING KEY CONCEPTS

1. List the basic phases of an emergency medical call.

2. List the items that should be checked during a daily vehicle inspection.

3. Explain what information responders to an emergency call should receive from dispatch.

4. Describe basic safety procedures that should be followed when you are driving an emergency vehicle.

5. Explain what the driver of an emergency vehicle must do to qualify for exemptions to traffic laws.

6. Explain why the following are particularly dangerous situations for operators of emergency vehicles: multiple-vehicle responses to a call; intersections; escorting vehicles.

7. List some basic guidelines for safe parking at an emergency scene.

8. Describe procedures to follow when transferring a patient to an ambulance; when en route with the patient to a receiving facility; when transferring care of the patient to receiving facility staff.

9. Explain steps that should be followed in preparing to return the emergency vehicle to service.

10. Describe basic ground safety procedures to follow around medical transport helicopters.

RESOURCES TO LEARN MORE

Book

Peto, Gloriajean and Medve, William. *EMS Driving: The Safe Way.* Upper Saddle River, NJ: Brady/Prentice Hall, 1992.

Wieder, M., ed. *Fire Department Pumping Apparatus.* Stillwater, OK: IFSTA, 1989.

Slide Presentation

Air-Medical Dispatch Guidelines for Trauma Scene Response. National Association of EMS Physicians, PO Box 15945-281, Lenexa, KS 66285.

PHASES OF AN EMERGENCY CALL

PREPARING FOR THE CALL
- Equipment check
- Vehicle check

DISPATCH AND RESPONSE
- The nature of the incident
- The location of the incident
- The location of the patient
- The number of patients and the severity of the problem
- Any special problems or circumstances
- Whether additional units have been dispatched to the scene

EN ROUTE TO THE SCENE
Follow basic safe driving procedures
- All occupants of the emergency vehicle should wear safety belts.
- Be familiar with the characteristics of the emergency vehicle.
- Be alert for changes in weather and road conditions.
- Exercise appropriate caution when using red lights and siren (RLS).
- Select an appropriate route; have an alternate route in case of unforeseen problems.
- Maintain a safe following distance from all vehicles.
- Drive with due regard for the safety of your crew and other motorists on the road.
- Use headlights—day or night—to increase visibility to other motorists.
- Be familiar with any hazards associated with the design and style of your vehicle.

AT THE SCENE
- Position unit properly.
- Report to dispatch.
- Request additional resources if necessary.
- Provide patient assessment and care.
- Prepare patient for transport.
- Provide for proper transition of care.

EN ROUTE TO THE RECEIVING FACILITY
- Provide appropriate mode of transport (RLS vs. no RLS).
- Provide ongoing assessment.
- Communicate with dispatch and receiving facility.

AT THE RECEIVING FACILITY
- Communicate with dispatch.
- Provide oral and written reports to receiving facility staff.
- Transfer patient care to receiving facility staff.

RETURNING TO SERVICE
- Restock supplies.
- Clean and disinfect vehicle and equipment.
- Check and prepare vehicle.
- Inform dispatch the unit is back in service.

Gaining Access and Basics of Extrication

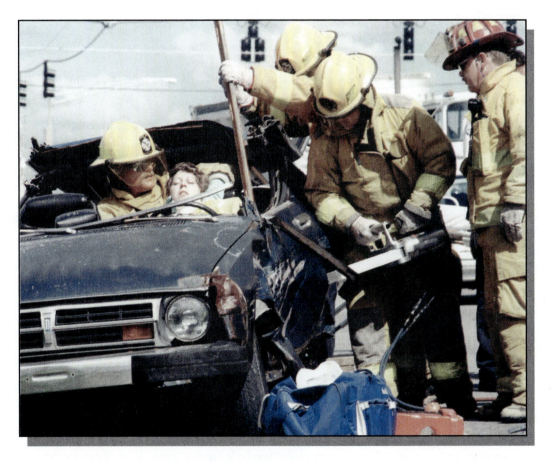

*A*s a firefighter-EMT, you will respond on many types of calls. On most of them, access to the patient will not be a problem. The patient may be in chair, on a bed, or on the floor—someplace you can easily walk to. The exceptions will be when the patient is in a hard-to-reach location or is entrapped and a special rescue or extrication is required to get the patient safely removed, treated, and transported.

The most common rescues are at vehicle crash scenes, where you may have one or many patients trapped in one or several vehicles in a ▶

variety of conditions. As an EMT, your assignment may be patient care, not actual extrication or rescue, but it is important to understand how the extrication or rescue process is carried out. You need to know how extrication may affect the patient and when and how you can provide patient care during the process.

At the completion of this chapter, the EMT-Basic student should be able to meet the following objectives:

Knowledge and Understanding

1. Describe the purpose of extrication. (pp. 673–674)
2. Discuss the role of the EMT-Basic in extrication. (pp. 674–678, 680–685, 686. 692–694, 695)
3. Identify what equipment for personal safety is required of the EMT-Basic. (pp. 677–678)
4. Define the fundamental components of extrication. (pp. 674, 686–691, 694–695)
5. State the steps that should be taken to protect the patient during extrication. (pp. 678, 683, 693–694)
6. Evaluate the various methods of gaining access to the patient. (pp. 686–691)
7. Distinguish between simple and complex access. (pp. 686–687)

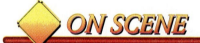

ON SCENE

DISPATCH: *ENGINE 1, LADDER 5, AND MEDIC 1, RESPOND TO A TWO-VEHICLE CRASH AT THE INTERSECTION OF BROADWAY AND STATE STREET. THIS IS REPORTED AS A SIDE-IMPACT COLLISION, MULTIPLE PATIENTS, EXTRICATION REQUIRED. PD EN ROUTE WITH EXTENDED ETA. TIME OUT IS 1701.*

You are the captain on Engine 1 (E1), which is dispatched as part of a multi-company (engine, ladder, and ambulance) response to a two-vehicle "T-bone" crash with possible extrication. The information you are given by the dispatcher includes the location, cross street, and the fact that several patients are involved. An update from dispatch tells you that there are four patients still in the two vehicles. Bystander information relayed to you indicates there are serious injuries and that the victims can't get out on their own. You know this is an intersection where high-speed crashes are common. As com-

pany officer, you consider the location and number of patients, then decide to call for an additional engine and two additional ambulances. You ask dispatch if they have any reports of power lines or hazards on the scene and are told there is no other information available.

Arriving near the intersection, you have the engineer slow down so you can view the scene from a distance. Your initial visual assessment confirms that only two vehicles are involved, and that there are no downed power lines or other obvious hazards in the area. You radio to dispatch that you are on scene at a two-vehicle crash, both vehicles are on the roadway, on their wheels, and that Engine 1 will be establishing Broadway Command.

Staging the engine so as to provide a safe working area between it and the crash scene, you instruct the engineer and a firefighter-EMT to pull and stage a charged, pre-connected line for hazard and fire control in case it is needed.

As the hose is being set up, you walk around both vehicles, looking inside, underneath, and into the crowd of bystanders for hidden hazards, ambulatory injured, and a confirmation of patient conditions. Your crew meets you at the vehicles with the charged line and a jump kit.

Your scene survey reveals the four patients in the two vehicles. The two people in vehicle 1 that broadsided the other car (vehicle 2) complain of leg injuries and minor pain in their chests, probably resulting from deployment of the front air bags in their vehicle. They were wearing seat belts and feel they are not badly hurt, but the doors won't open. You identify these patients as not needing immediate assistance but requiring minor extrication.

Your evaluation of vehicle 2, which was broadsided, is different. The driver is unresponsive. The passenger is responsive and complaining of shortness of breath and pain in her side. The bucket seats are leaning toward each other, the floor of the car is severely buckled down, and there is at least a 24-inch (600 mm) intrusion into the driver's side door. You try the passenger-side door handle but are not able to open the door. You assess that both patients have serious injuries and need rapid extrication, treatment, and transport. You radio to the now-arriving ladder company to set up extrication tools on the broadsided car. You assign the just-arriving para-

medics of Medic 1 to vehicle 2. You also assign the second-due engine to care for the patients in vehicle 1.

The Engine 1 engineer and firefighter-EMT break out some window glass to reach the patients in vehicle 2. The EMT performs an initial assessment and rapid trauma assessment and provides high flow oxygen via nonrebreather masks to both patients. The engineer covers the patients with an aluminized blanket and removes the remaining window glass in the doors. You assist with stabilization by applying step chocks under the vehicle. The ladder company then removes the front doors from their hinges.

Engine 2 crew members have by now reached the patients in the vehicle 1, applied cervical collars and vest-type extrication devices to the patients, immobilized them to backboards, and loaded them into an ambulance for transport. The Engine 2 crew is now available to work with the ladder company to remove the roof and doors of vehicle 2 and assist the Medic 1 crew with extrication and packaging of the two severely injured patients for rapid transport. Your firefighter-EMT is asked to go along with Medic 1 to assist the crew.

You call dispatch to report that extrication is complete and that you will be en route to the hospital to pick up your personnel after Engine 1 is put back in service. On-scene time was 16 minutes.

There are at least a dozen types of specialty rescue teams that may be available in various communities or regions. They include swift water rescue, dive rescue, ice rescue, technical-rope high angle/low angle rescue, back country/wilderness rescue, trench rescue, hazardous materials rescue, confined space rescue, farm rescue, heavy-vehicle rescue, aircraft rescue, and building collapse. Participation in any of these teams requires special equipment and training that are not discussed in this chapter. You may or may not be part of one of these teams, but the most

important thing to know as a firefighter-EMT is how or where to get them if needed. Usually the teams are located in an area based on need. For example, if there are lakes or rivers in an area, then there will probably be some sort of water-related rescue team in place. In this chapter, the emphasis is on vehicle rescue, since it is the most common type of rescue (Figure 26-1).

The extent to which you, as a firefighter-EMT, will participate in vehicle rescue depends on the roles your particular unit and department play in the local area. Remember that the main reason for

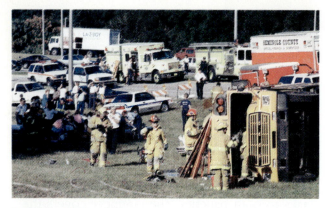

Figure 26-1 The number of patients and the complexity of vehicle rescue operations you take part in can vary significantly.

the EMT to know extrication procedures is to be able to incorporate them into the patient care plan.

VEHICLE RESCUE

There are ten phases or processes of vehicle rescue that you, as an EMT, should understand.

1. Preparing for the rescue
2. Sizing up the scene
3. Recognizing and managing the hazards
4. Stabilizing the vehicle prior to entering
5. Gaining access to the patient
6. Providing initial patient assessment and a rapid trauma exam
7. Immobilizing the patient
8. Extricating the patient
9. Providing transport to the most appropriate health care facility with a detailed physical exam and ongoing assessment en route
10. Terminating the rescue/extrication

Some of these phases, such as patient assessment, the rapid trauma exam, and immobilization, have been discussed at length in earlier chapters. This chapter will focus less on the phases that involve patient care and more on those that involve operations.

Preparing for the Rescue

Vehicle rescue has changed tremendously since its organized inception during the 1950s and 1960s. Many units still have some of the same tools that were first adapted from auto body shop equipment, but most units have converted to better, higher tech, more powerful tools. The vehicles that patients are rescued from have also changed from very large, heavy, mechanically simple cars to smaller, lighter-weight, more technically complex cars.

One thing has not changed since the early days of rescue: The most important part of preparing for the rescue is having proper tools and the training to use them properly.

- *Tools*—No matter what kind of tools your department or company uses, they *must* be in good working order. You should inspect the rescue tools according to your department's and the manufacturer's guidelines, making sure that they operate, that fluids are topped off, that hoses and cords are attached and in working order, and that all necessary attachments and components are accounted for. You should be thoroughly familiar with where the tools are and with how to use them.

- *Training*—Training is without a doubt one of the most important ways we prepare for the rescue. Showing up at a rescue scene and confidently knowing what to do exhibits professionalism. Everyone expects you to be well trained when you arrive—so be prepared, train often, train hard, and train smart.

Sizing-up the Scene

Size-up begins before you get to the emergency scene. Most often, you can form a good mental picture of the incident while you are en route. Information collected from dispatch, what you know of the area, the time of day, the terrain, and the weather, will help you start to build a mental image of what you might see at the scene. Don't be afraid to ask questions en route, because many times the dispatcher does not anticipate exactly what information you may need.

The next phase of size-up takes place when you arrive on scene. The things you see and do will set the stage for rescue operations, so a good, thoughtful on-scene survey will help you make the right decisions from the beginning. If you rush in, neglecting to take a careful look at the scene, the hazards, the vehicles, and the patients involved, you may well take less desirable actions during the extrication that can slow the process to a standstill. This wastes the patient's time. *Never waste the patient's time; doing so can result in unnecessary suffering—even death!*

Some of the things to look for during the initial on-scene survey include the following:

◆ *Location*—Is the crash scene safe or are there hazards associated with it as, for example, the middle of a busy intersection with traffic running through it?

◆ *Stability*—Are the vehicles stable? On a hillside? In water?

◆ *Electrical hazards*—Are there downed power lines?

◆ *Fire*—Do you have potential fire problems?

◆ *Hazmats*—Could hazardous materials be involved?

◆ *Special rescue*—Is there a need for specialty rescue teams?

◆ *How many patients can be seen?*

　　—Are they all in the vehicle(s)?

　　—Are there patients who are out of the vehicle(s)?

　　—What is each person's medical status?

　　—Who is critical, serious, moderate, or "walking wounded"?

The survey also includes making an initial plan for how to rescue the occupants. You should assess resources at hand and decide if there is a need for more than those already on scene or en route. By walking around the crash site, you can see if airbags are deployed or fuel lines are leaking, gauge the condition of the patients, and note other factors that you may not have caught during the initial size up.

All of the factors and information obtained during the size-up should tell you which patients have time and which ones don't. Those patients who do not have life-threatening injuries can wait while you take care of the ones who do. The seriously injured priority patients have very little time to make it to the hospital before their survival rates start diminishing rapidly—about an hour from the moment of the crash to surgery. This time period is called the "golden hour." Extrication can take up much of that "golden hour," leaving precious few minutes to get the patient to the hospital and definitive care.

Recognizing and Managing Hazards

Scene Safety

Vehicle rescue scenes are inherently dangerous. There are dangers present both from the vehicles involved and from the environment. Scene safety and personal safety are your highest considerations. If a safety hazard is present, take care of it or at least identify it and/or post guards so rescue personnel can avoid the hazard. Possible hazards include:

◆ *Broken glass and debris*—with potential for loss of footing and injury

◆ *Downed wires and power poles*—with the possibility of electrocution

◆ *Spilled fuel*—posing risks both for fire and for health problems

◆ *Barriers, holes, ditches, trenches, uneven terrain*—raising possibilities of falls or trips

◆ *Traffic*—with the risk that drivers will be watching the scene instead of the road . . . or you

◆ *Bystanders*—who can get unruly, over-helpful, or in the way

◆ *Animals*—with the possibility of bites

◆ *Poor lighting*—complicating all of the above

There are a number of things you can do to deal with these hazards before beginning extrication. You may need to cover, sweep, or avoid debris; avoid or cordon off power equipment; use foam and place sand or an absorbent on the spilled fuels and oil; set up scene lighting; post guards; and charge protective hoselines.

There are also vehicular hazards that can affect the way you perform the extrication and rescue.

- *Bumpers*—The shock-absorbing, or "loaded," bumpers that have been compressed in a collision can spring out from the vehicle and injure rescuers who are standing too close to the front of a car or truck. There are ways of chaining up or securing loaded bumpers, all of which should be decided by the unit you work with. Everyone needs to understand that if a loaded bumper "unloads" and a rescuer is standing in front of it, the injury he receives will probably be career ending.

- *Charged fuel systems*—Vehicles with modern electronic fuel systems can be pressurized to 90 psi (630 kPa) or better. It is important to *at least turn off the ignition* to ensure that power to the fuel pump is cut off. Cutting into a pressurized fuel line during the extrication could spray the rescuers, patients, and the scene with gasoline and create a risk of serious burns.

- *Active suspensions*—Many vehicles now have computer-controlled suspensions that inflate and deflate to provide a smooth ride in various road conditions. The systems employ small air bags located around the running gear to adjust the ride. Cutting or puncturing these bags can cause a vehicle to immediately drop up to 6 inches (150 mm). This sudden drop can aggravate a patient's head, neck, and spine injuries. Using devices such as "step chocks" under the vehicle will help reduce the chance of sudden drops.

- *Fuel tanks*—In newer cars, fuel tanks are constructed of plastic-type materials. The tanks are often relocated forward, to behind the rear passenger's seat or under it. This placement allows automobile manufacturers to provide more space in the smallest of trunks. Relocation also puts the tank nearer to the hot parts of the exhaust system, mainly the catalytic converter. In this more forward location, a fuel tank has a greater chance of melting or of being overheated or ignited by the hot exhaust system following a crash.

- *Seat belts*—There are many styles of seat belts in vehicles. There are variations of the combination lap/shoulder belt, and there are separate lap and shoulder belts. The separate lap and shoulder belts can pose special problems. If an occupant of a vehicle wears only the shoulder portion (which is automatically driven into place when the door is closed), there is a great chance he will still strike the windshield. If the occupant wears both lap and shoulder belts, you must remember to disconnect the lap belt after you've disconnected the shoulder belt before you try to remove the patient. Some seat belts in foreign vehicles are "active"; they retract and tighten up against an occupant, keeping him from sliding forward. If the vehicle is struck from the side, the belt may not activate, and cutting into the mechanism during extrication could present a hazard. Rule of thumb: *Never cut into a seat belt retractor or mechanism!*

- *Hardened metals*—There are several parts of the vehicle that are constructed of harder steel than others. Latches, hinges, seat belt retractors and mounts, some seat components, and some steering shafts are among the parts commonly made of hardened steel. In a few makes (mostly European models, such as Mercedes, Volvo, and Saab), you can find tougher door-collision beams. Parts made of hardened metals pose a problem because they have about the same hardness as the steel of the cutting blades on hydraulic rescue tools. This means that during a rescue you may either cut or break the hardened component or you may break your cutting blades. Either result can send steel parts and pieces flying at high speed, posing risk of injury to patients or rescuers. In addition, the tool may be placed out of service for the rest of that rescue and will be expensive to repair or replace.

- *Airbags*—Vehicle airbags are safety features that can be hazards for rescuers. There are three types of airbags: frontal-impact, side-impact, and head-protection bags. The frontal-impact bags have been around for some time. While they have saved many lives, they have also created some problems. The bags deploy from the center of the steering wheel or from a mount in the passenger side of the dash.

They deploy fast, generally within 1/25 of a second, or a little less than it takes to show *one* of the 24 frames-per-second of a movie. Potential problems come when an airbag has not deployed. If one is accidentally activated during rescue, it could injure a rescuer or aggravate a patient's injuries. Be aware of the locations of wiring and control units for the airbags. *Never cut into the steering column, never push against the center dash console, and do not work between an occupant and an undeployed air bag.* There are commercially available wheel cover devices that can contain an airbag if it deploys; they might provide an added margin of safety.

The side-impact airbags are located either in the side of the seat back or in the door. The seat-mounted bags are activated when the seat base is pressed in from the side as occurs in side-impact collisions. The door-mounted bags are activated by a sensor in the door or B-post (the post to which the door latches) when an intrusion into the car is made. If these bags have not deployed, pushing against the seat base from the side during a prying operation or "popping" the door at the latch may activate them. Hinge-side door removal is therefore recommended. Learning what makes of cars have side-impact bags can be of assistance in rescue operations.

Some cars also use head-protection airbags. These tube-like bags come out of the headliner above the doors, also during side impacts. They stay inflated a little longer than other airbags and may be in the way during rescue and treatment. These head-protection bags can be cut out with a sharp knife or heavy duty shears. Again, accidental activation of undeployed bags can cause injury to patients or rescuers.

Safeguarding Yourself from Hazards

When you, as a firefighter-EMT, arrive at the crash scene, your job is to rescue, extricate, treat, and transport the injured. Your first responsibility, though, is not to get hurt yourself. As noted above, many things can contribute to injury on the scene. However, you do have control over the things that are most likely to cause problems. These include the following:

◆ *A careless attitude toward personal safety*—not wearing all of the protective gear provided, not paying attention

◆ *Lack of skill in tool use*—not learning how to use the tools on hand, not training enough

◆ *Physical problems that impede strenuous effort*—not being in shape

Unsafe and improper acts and omissions also cause injuries.

◆ *Failure to eliminate or control hazards*

◆ *Failure to select the proper tool for the task*

◆ *Using unsafe tools*

◆ *Failure to recognize mechanisms of injury and unsafe surroundings*

◆ *Failure to use proper lifting technique with heavy objects*

◆ *Deactivating safety devices on rescue equipment designed to prevent injury*

◆ *Failure to wear highly visible outer clothing, especially when exposed to highway traffic*

Good protective clothing is a must at any crash scene (Figure 26-2). There are two basic kinds of attire used by responders: full protective clothing, such as the firefighter's structural gear; and lighter-weight clothing, such as nylon or cotton flame-resistant jackets, Nomex® jumpsuits, and work pants used by many agencies such as ambulance crews, search and rescue teams, and flight crews. The guidelines for selecting helmets, gloves, footwear, and turnout gear can be found in NFPA standard 1971. Guidelines for station/work uniforms are in NFPA standard 1975. Always be sure to wear the protective clothing specified by your department for rescue scenes.

Headgear/Helmets One of the most important things you should do before even starting to provide rescue is to put an approved helmet on your head. Baseball-style caps, watch caps, and "bump caps" are of little use. Either use a structural fire helmet with a face shield and chin strap or use a rescue-style helmet, which is usually a little

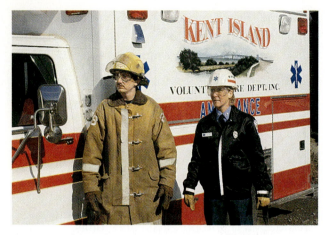

Figure 26-2 Two firefighter-EMTs dressed for vehicle operations.

lighter and more comfortable, especially in non-vehicle rescues such as trench, confined-space, and high-angle rescues. Helmets worn by rescue crews should be uniform, highly visible, and identifiable.

Eye Protection Putting on eye protection should be automatic. The shields provided on structural fire helmets, eyeglasses, and everyday sunglasses are not adequate. The most common thing people do when objects fly toward their face is to turn their heads. This exposes the unprotected area around the eyes, the area on the side of the face that the shield or glasses does not cover. It is best to purchase clear safety glasses with side protection. Even better, if available, are form-fitting goggles that are vented to prevent fogging.

Hand Protection Because firefighters and EMTs sometimes need to put their hands into places where there are sharp edges and where tools are being used, and because direct contact with patients is likely, optimal hand protection is mandatory. Remember that *any chance of contacting a patient's body fluids or allowing your body fluids to contact a patient must be eliminated.* If you are working on the scene and there is even a remote chance of contacting a patient, put on latex or vinyl gloves first, before you put on leather work or structural fire fighting gloves. Also keep in mind that the hydraulic fluid used in all rescue tools is an extreme hazard if injected into your skin; so cover up! Durable leather work gloves are acceptable if you want dexterity when

using rescue tools, but structural fire fighting gloves provide better protection, although at the expense of some dexterity.

Body Protection As noted earlier, it is important to protect your body, as well as your head, eyes, and hands. Always wear the appropriate layers of fluid- and flame-resistant clothing during rescue, especially in the action area of an extrication. Jagged metal, glass, hazardous fluids, flash fire, and adverse weather—either alone or in combination—may be present during almost any extrication. You should be prepared and be safe. Protective coats and pants will generally shield you from these hazards. Shoes or boots should be approved for industrial or fireground operations, and steel toes and shanks, high tops, and chemical resistance are recommended.

Safeguarding Your Patient from Hazards

The occupants of the vehicle that has been in a crash have already had a bad day. It is your job, as an EMT, to make sure that nothing more unpleasant happens to them while you care for them during and after the extrication and rescue. You can help to prevent injuries to occupants by providing a cover during extrication that will protect them from heat, cold, rain, snow, dust, glass, and flying particles of glass (Figure 26-3). Some of the coverings you can use, along with their benefits and drawbacks, are listed in Table 26-1.

Managing Traffic Hazards

Traffic hazards should be a big concern to you as a firefighter-EMT, and even more so if you are the company officer. Control of traffic is usually a law enforcement responsibility. However, fire department personnel are often the first to arrive at many rescue scenes. This means that the fire department personnel often have to handle and control the hazards posed by traffic. If you are assigned responsibility for traffic control, consider using the following methods:

◆ Assign personnel, if enough are available, to flag traffic through the scene.

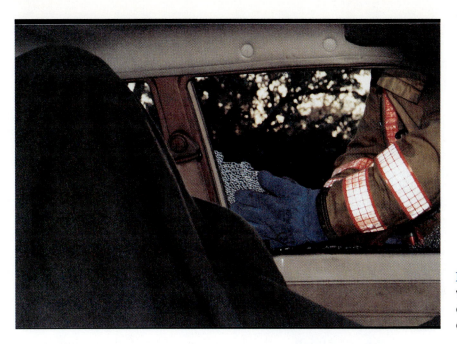

Figure 26-3 Cover the patient with a blanket, tarp, or salvage cover to provide protection from debris during rescue operations.

Table 26-1

Coverings for Patient Protection

Item	Benefits	Drawbacks	Rating
Aluminized rescue blanket	Good protection. Will reflect 95% of heat from a flash fire. Will not absorb glass, dirt, or water	Expensive	Excellent
Disposable foam blanket	Good protection. Water resistant, inexpensive	Not fire resistant	Good
Polytarp-style cover	Good protection. Water resistant, inexpensive	Not fire resistant	Good
Canvas	Good protection. Sturdy, readily available.	Large and awkward. Hard to clean.	Good
Disposable paper blanket	Protects from dust and glass particles	Not water resistant. Not fire resistant.	Poor
Wool blanket	Good protection from cold weather	Too warm in hot weather. Not water resistant. Not fire resistant. Attracts glass particles like a magnet.	Poor
Hard hats, safety goggles, masks	Good protection for head and face	Awkward. Can get in way of treatment.	Poor

- Use flares (fusees), chemical luminescent light sticks, or reflective traffic cones to create a visual barrier for night operations.

- Use apparatus with warning lights to create a protective wall between the scene and traffic. Position the apparatus between oncoming traffic and the scene where operations are being carried out.

- Be sure that all personnel are wearing clothing that is brightly colored and reflective or clothing that contains reflective material for high visibility.

Positioning Flares or Cones Flares and cones have both good points and drawbacks. Flares are bright in darkness and work well in fog and snow. Many can be stored in a small space, and they are relatively inexpensive. They can be a fire hazard, however, and must be replaced as they burn down. Traffic cones are highly visible and are not a fire hazard. They are more expensive than flares but are reusable.

When using and placing signal devices, consider the following points (Figure 26-4):

- Look for and avoid spilled fuel, dry vegetation, and other combustibles before you ignite and position flares, especially on roadsides. If not positioned properly, flares will roll and may not be where you need them to be.

- Do not throw flares or cones out of moving vehicles.

- Position a few signal devices behind the last vehicle after it's parked to help identify it to other drivers.

- When placing flares or cones, walk facing traffic and place them approximately 10 feet (3 m) apart.

- If the collision has occurred on a two-lane road, position signal devices in both directions.

- Never use a flare as a traffic wand. Molten phosphorus can splatter on you, causing severe burns.

Controlling Spectators

Spectators can cause many problems at a crash scene if they are not managed correctly. They may get into traffic and become victims themselves. They can become injured by falling in the fuel, oil, battery acid, and other fluids on the ground around wrecked vehicles. Sometimes they can cause problems by trying to remove patients who have not been stabilized or immobilized from wreckage because they fear the cars may "blow-up."

Use law enforcement personnel, highway crew members, or other firefighters to keep bystanders away from the wreckage. Use a roll of barricade tape or traffic cones to create a clear working space around the wreckage, then only permit authorized rescue workers into that space. Sometimes the best way of controlling bystanders is to enlist their aid in creating the clear working space with tape or cones. If you do, however, be careful that the bystanders do not themselves enter dangerous areas.

Coping with Electrical Hazards

Electricity poses many dangers at vehicle collision scenes. When there is an electrical hazard, establish a danger zone and a safe zone. Only individuals who are responsible for controlling the hazard, such as power company personnel or specialty rescue team members, should enter the danger zone. The safe zone should be sufficiently far away to assure that an arcing or moving wire could not possibly injure any of the rescue personnel or bystanders.

COMPANY OFFICER'S NOTES

There are different devices on the market designed to find downed, energized power lines. Never fully trust these items. Although they may work, remember that power can come back on at any time and injure or kill anyone too close to the conductor.

Keep in mind the safety points listed below when you are working in potential electrical hazard areas. Many of these points have to do with taking precautions around conductors. *Remember that a conductor is a wire or any other object or material that will carry electricity.*

Positioning Flares to Control Traffic

Posted speed (mph)	Stopping distance for that speed*		Posted speed (in feet)		Distance of the farthest warning device
20 mph	50 feet	+	20 feet	=	70 feet
30 mph	75 feet	+	30 feet	=	105 feet
40 mph	125 feet	+	40 feet	=	165 feet
50 mph	175 feet	+	50 feet	=	225 feet
60 mph	275 feet	+	60 feet	=	335 feet
70 mph	375 feet	+	70 feet	=	445 feet

Figure 26-4A Position flares according to a formula that includes the stopping distance for the posted speed plus a margin of safety. (*Distances given are for passenger cars.)

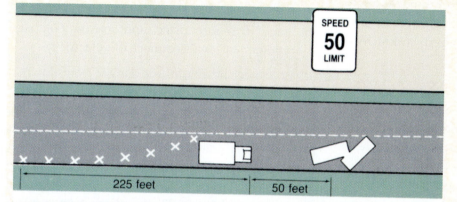

Figure 26-4B Positioning flares on a straight road. Approaching vehicles are moved into the correct lane before they reach the edge of the danger zone.

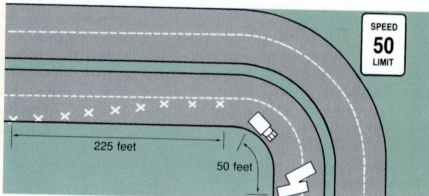

Figure 26-4C Position flares ahead of a curved section of road. The start of the curve should be considered the edge of the danger zone.

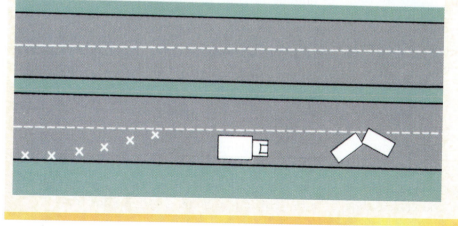

Figure 26-4D Positioning flares on a hill. The flares slow vehicles and make them turn into the correct lane before they reach the top of the hill.

- High voltages are not as uncommon on roadside utility poles as people often think. In some areas, wooden poles support conductors of as much as 500,000 volts.

- When you suspect an electrical hazard, assume that the entire area is extremely dangerous. Conductors may have touched and energized many things in the area. These include electrical, telephone, cable TV, and other wires supported by the utility pole; guy wires; ground wires; the pole itself; and nearby guard rails and fences. Assume that severed or displaced conductors may be touching and energizing every wire and conductor at the highest voltage present. Assume that dead wires may be re-energized at any moment. Assume that energized conductors may arc to the ground.

- Ordinary protective clothing does not protect against electrocution.

Remembering these points and the procedures discussed below may keep you and your crew members alive at the scene of a motor vehicle crash where unconfined and uncontrolled electricity is a hazard.

Broken Utility Pole with Wires Down A broken utility pole with downed wires is very dangerous. You probably cannot work safely in the immediate area until power company representatives assure you that the power is off or secured and the scene safe.

If you discover that a utility pole is broken and wires are down, do the following:

1. Stage your apparatus outside the identified danger zone, which IFSTA defines as the distance between utility poles.

2. Before you leave your vehicle, be sure that no portion of it, including the radio antenna, is in contact with any sagging wires or potential conductors.

3. Order spectators and nonessential emergency personnel out of the danger zone. Use perimeter tape to set up a large safety zone.

4. Discourage the occupants of vehicles involved in the collision from leaving the wreckage or from touching any portions of the vehicle they are not already in contact with, especially the outside of the vehicle.

5. Prohibit traffic flow through the danger zone.

6. Determine the pole number of the nearest power pole you can safely approach, and ask your dispatcher to advise the power company of the pole number and location.

7. Do not attempt to move downed wires. Unless you have certified and tested high voltage equipment and have the power company's training and approval, you shouldn't play the part of a power company helper. Fire department tools with even the smallest amount of carbon on them will conduct electricity, as will natural fiber ropes.

8. Stage in a safe place until power company workers cut or disconnect the electricity.

Be especially careful for danger from downed wires when you approach a collision in a dark area, such as a rural road side at night. As you walk from your fire apparatus, sweep the area in front of you, side to side and overhead, with a light. An energized conductor may be hanging just at head level. If you discover that a wire is down, report it immediately to the power company, and be especially careful of the area.

Sometimes, especially in wet weather, a phenomenon known as *ground gradient* may provide your first clue that a wire is down. Voltage is greatest at the point where the conductor touches the ground, then diminishes with distance from the point of contact. That distance may be a few inches or several feet. Being able to recognize and respond properly to energized ground can save your life.

Stop your approach immediately if you feel a tingling in your legs and lower torso. This sensation means you are on energized ground. Current is entering one foot, passing through your body, and exiting through your other foot. If you continuing walking in the direction you were heading, you risk electrocution! Turn 180 degrees and take one of two escape measures. Either hop away to a safe place on one foot or shuffle away from the danger area with both feet together, allowing no break in contact with the ground or the other foot. Either technique helps to keep you from creating a circuit through your body.

Broken Pole with Wires Intact Even if the wires are intact, a broken utility pole is still dangerous. Sometimes a vehicle will break right through the bottom of a pole and leave it hanging by the wires. The wires may break under the weight at any time. If you arrive and find such a situation:

1. Park the apparatus outside the danger zone.
2. Notify the dispatcher of the situation.
3. Stay outside the danger zone until the power company can de-energize the conductors and stabilize the pole.
4. Keep spectators and other emergency personnel out of the danger area.

Damaged Pad-Mounted Transformer When electrical cables are run underground, the transformer may be mounted on a pad above the ground (Figure 26-5). When one of these transformers is struck, it poses a serious threat. In such a situation:

1. Request immediate power company response.
2. Do not touch either the vehicle or the transformer case, and warn other emergency personnel and bystanders not to touch it.
3. Stage in a safe place until the power company arrives and de-energizes the equipment

Coping with Vehicle Fires

Extinguishing vehicle fires is best done by those equipped for it—firefighters! A vehicle fire can be simple and taken care of with a 5-pound (2.3 kg) dry chemical or CO_2 extinguisher, or it can be serious with victims trapped in the vehicle. The best bet against fire on the scene is to make sure a charged fire hose that discharges at least 100 gallons (400 L) per minute is on hand. Watch for the following when putting out a car fire:

◆ *Bumpers*—There are pistons under bumpers of many vehicles that are likely to go off under fire conditions. Start your attack from a distance and put the water onto the exterior first to cool the bumpers, McPherson struts, drive line, and tires.

◆ *Fire in the engine compartment*—Be careful when opening the hood (Figure 26-6). If you can extinguish the fire without opening the hood, the "frying pan lid effect" will keep the fire from getting the oxygen it needs to go into the free burning stage. Engine compartment fires may be extinguished without opening the hood by directing the fire stream through the front grill or openings into the wheel well. The resultant steam conversion under the hood will control the fire. After the victim is removed from the vehicle and as time allows, the hood should eventually be opened to assure that complete extinguishment has been made and the fire should be overhauled.

◆ *Fire in the passenger compartment*—This can be life threatening and should be handled quickly. If you are using an extinguisher, be careful not to asphyxiate the occupants with the powder cloud, but make sure the fire is out (Figure 26-7). Any fire involving a vehicle should be attacked wearing self-contained breathing apparatus (SCBA) because extremely toxic gases are created when plastics and other materials in a car burn. Also watch out for fuel, fuel cans, hazardous materials, aerosol cans, and propane bottles that may be carried in the vehicle's interior or trunk.

◆ *Fire under the vehicle*—Use the ground under the vehicle to help direct the water or powder up against the bottom of the car. Be wary of plastic fuel tanks, which may melt and create a pool of fuel. In a parking lot or near other

Figure 26-5 A pad-mounted electrical transformer.

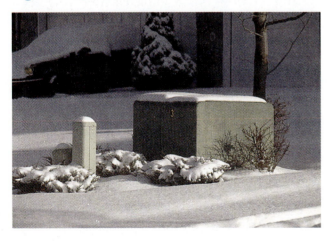

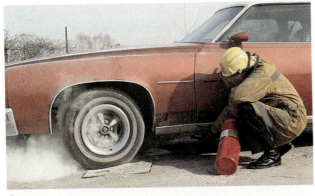

A.

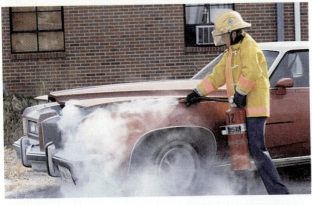

B.

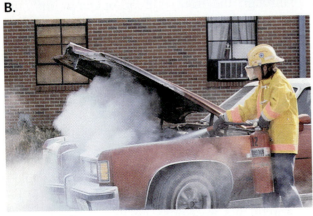

C.

Figure 26-6 Many engine compartment fires can be handled with a small chemical extinguisher. If possible, leave the hood **(A)** closed or only **(B)** partially open. This will keep the fire from getting oxygen. **(C)** If the hood is already open, approach cautiously.

vehicles, this pooled fuel can develop into a much larger fire.

◆ *Truck fire*—Trucks are not just large cars. They have entirely different systems that can be dangerous: larger fuel tanks and batteries, unknown loads or cargo, and split rims that can fly if the tires catch fire.

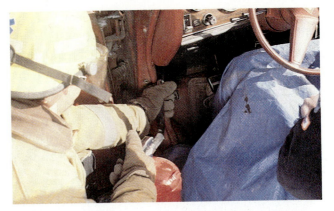

Figure 26-7 Try not to spread a cloud of chemicals over entrapped occupants when extinguishing a fire in the passenger compartment.

If you have a vehicle fuel leak, charge a hose line and stop the leak if at all possible. Fuel lines can be pinched over; holes can be plugged with a commercial sealing clay or wooden wedges. Other items like golf tees can also be used. On a hot day, the fuel on the pavement will turn to vapor much faster than on a cold day, and there is a greater chance of a vapor or fuel explosion. Also keep in mind that diesel fuel has a flash point of about 100°F (38°C). Therefore, the chances of igniting a pool of diesel fuel are smaller on a cold day than on a very hot day.

Coping with a Vehicle's Electrical System

Older motor vehicles were constructed differently than today's. They contained more combustible material and had more primitive fuel systems; fire after a crash in an older vehicle was more likely than in a newer vehicle. Disabling the electrical systems of those older vehicles was a standard part of rescue and extrication operations.

Today, disconnecting a vehicle's power can be more of a problem than a help and may also be needlessly time consuming. Many cars have electric locks and seats, so that cutting the vehicle's battery cables may disable the best method of moving the seats or unlocking the doors to gain access to the passengers. Unless there is an obvious hazard, you should simply switch off the vehicle's ignition and proceed with extrication efforts.

If you do need to shut down a vehicle's electrical system, getting to the battery may prove to

Stabilizing Vehicles

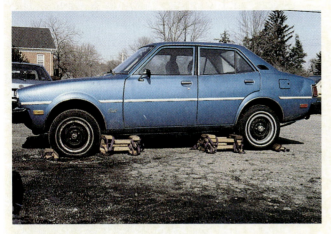

Figure 26-8A A vehicle on its wheels can be stabilized with standard wooden cribbing under the rocker panels.

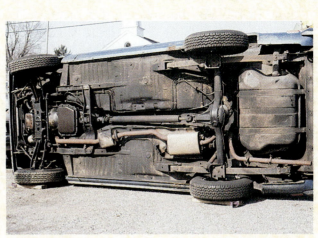

Figure 26-8B A vehicle on its side should be stabilized using at least four contact points. Here cribbing is positioned under the wheels . . .

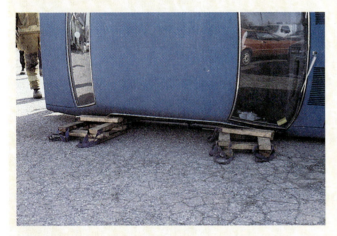

Figure 26-8C and under the A- and C-posts. With the car stabilized in this way, rescuers can pull the roof down to access the vehicle's interior.

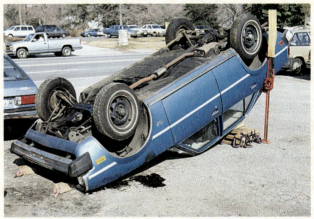

Figure 26-8D Overturned cars are often found in a nose-down position. Such a vehicle should be stabilized using at least four contact points. A combination of cribbing and jacks stabilize this vehicle.

be difficult. If you can reach the battery, disconnect or cut the ground cable. This reduces the chance of arcing and sparks and adds a measure of safety.

Stabilizing a Vehicle

Stabilization of vehicles involved in collisions is very important but something that is unfortunately often left undone. A vehicle may look stable because of its position, the terrain on which it sits, or an apparent lack of damage. However, stabilization means more than just keeping a vehicle from falling over or from lying on its side. It also means taking the "bounce" out of the radial tires and the "sway" out of the suspension.

If a rescuer or bystander shakes the car, moves it with hydraulic tools, or climbs on it to get in, these actions may well move the patient enough to cause additional injury. By stabilizing all vehicles, these types of injury can be avoided. Stabilization procedures for a variety of situations are described below (Figure 26-8).

- *A vehicle on its wheels*—Walk around the vehicle during the scene size-up. You may find that the car is stable because the axles are gone or broken, the tires are flat, or because positioning has "high centered" it. If none of these situations has stabilized the vehicle, you can build a box crib with standard wooden cribbing. Alternatively, you can place at least three step blocks under the vehicle and drive wedges between the vehicle and the blocks. You can also use wheel chocks from your engine, basic wooden cribbing, jacks, or a wrecker truck (if you have worked with them in preparation for this type of task). Set the parking brake of the vehicle and shift the transmission gear to Park. This should sufficiently reduce the instability of the vehicle.

- *A vehicle on its side*—A vehicle on its side can be found in one of two positions. It can be "halfway over," resting on its side, doors, and tire sidewalls, but not resting on its top at all. Or it may be found "more than halfway over," leaning against the roof and posts. This is the most unstable position, because the natural tendency of the car is to roll back to the halfway-over position. When approaching a vehicle on its side, *never shake the vehicle to see if it is stable.* Chock the vehicle in place with at least four points of contact so that it won't be knocked over as weight shifts in the interior with patient treatment or movement. Jacks, cribbing, anchors, and anchoring systems such as a come-along are all good methods of stabilization.

  Regardless of what you use to stabilize the vehicle, remember to make sure that you are not relying on something that will be removed during the extrication process. For example, if you will be removing the roof, then it is unwise to use the door posts as cribbing points. When the roof is removed, the side strength of the posts is severely reduced, and the vehicle may tip over.

- *A vehicle on its roof*—Upside-down vehicles pose problems in patient care and extrication. It is easy to run out of cribbing material rapidly when trying to stabilize a vehicle in this position. If the vehicle's roof is smashed flat and the vehicle is basically on the ground with no roof showing, it may be considered stable until a lifting operation is started. Then you will need four equally spaced points of contact on the ground for cribbing as well as rescue airbags or jacks. If the vehicle is resting on an intact roof (not flattened), the car will probably be situated in the "engine down" position. In this position, the points of contact with the ground are the vehicle's nose and the top at the windshield because most of the weight is at the front of the vehicle. This position may require jacks or rescue airbags to hold up one end of the vehicle while the other is rested against at least two fixed box-cribbing stacks. Be careful to not go over 24 inches (600 mm) high with standard 18-inch (450 mm) cribbing in this situation.

ACCESS

Simple vs. Complex Access

When making the decision to extricate, one of the easiest traps to fall into is wanting to "cut the vehicle up" in spite of the occupant's injuries or needs. It is normal for a trained firefighter-EMT to want to exercise both his skills and the tools and techniques he has been trained to use. Sometimes, however, using *all* the skills and tools available may not be in the best interest of the patient.

In serious crashes, the patients routinely need the definitive care provided only in hospitals. The most important thing you can do to help a patient is to get him to a hospital as quickly and safely as possible. The key in vehicle rescue operations is to consider the whole range of access and extrication options and then to choose ones that will provide the fastest way of make an opening from which the patients can be removed with the least manipulation. (See Access Evolutions, below.)

Always try *simple access* first. This means getting into the vehicle in an ordinary way, without tools, like simply opening a door. If a door won't open, decide if a passenger seems uninjured enough to unlock a door or lower a window from the inside.

If simple access isn't possible, consider your range of options for *complex access*. Complex access involves using tools and special equipment in a series of steps, or evolutions, to progressively open up the vehicle until the space is wide enough to remove the patient easily and safely.

COMPANY OFFICER'S NOTES

As the company officer, you will probably be the one who makes the determination about which access pathway to follow. Once you have selected a method, you should stick to it with reasonable determination. Changing plans mid-extrication can create additional delay at the scene.

Tool Staging

To save time on the scene, it is advisable to set up a tool staging area near the action area (within 20 feet or 6 meters) but not in it. With a tool staging area you will save time by eliminating the need to run back and forth to the rescue vehicle for tools and equipment. The area will also serve as a visual tool box where you can study the tools available and decide which ones you need.

Here is a small list of what you should have in your tool staging area (Figure 26-9). It isn't necessary to unload the entire truck for most crashes, but this list is a good start.

◆ Hydraulic spreader or spreader/cutter
◆ Rams or jacks
◆ Come-along and chain set(s)
◆ Reciprocating saw and blades
◆ Ram block
◆ Hand tools
◆ Air bags
◆ Standard wooden cribbing, step blocks, wedges

Glass Removal

After you have gained entrance into a vehicle and have covered the patient with an appropriate pro-

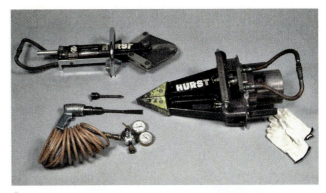

A.

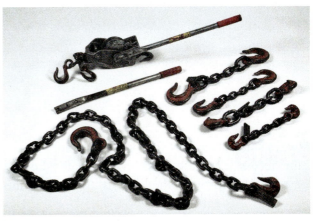

B.

Figure 26-9 A variety of tools should be available in extrication operations. These include **(A)** hydraulic cutters, hydraulic spreaders, and air chisels and **(B)** come-alongs and chains for pulling.

tection device, glass removal begins (Figure 26-10). Using tools such as a spring-loaded center punch or screwdriver, remove the side and rear glass, taking care to pull the glass to the outside instead of pushing it inside with the occupant. If you can, roll the windows down, then break the glass into the door by striking it on the top edge. If you need to remove the front windshield, use an ax and chop around the outer edge, or use a reciprocating saw with a wood- or metal-working blade in it. In addition, a commercial glass-removal device may also be used.

Access Evolutions

There are a variety of different procedures for gaining access to patients in vehicles. The aim of these procedures is to allow rescuers to reach patients in the quickest, safest way possible.

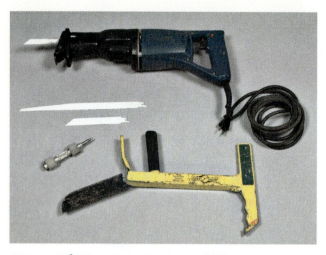

Figure 26-10 Tools for glass removal include a reciprocating saw and blades, a spring-loaded center punch, and a Glas-Master™ saw.

Always study a scene before you begin attempts to gain access. Pick the method that will take the least time and provide the least risk of moving the patient as it is carried out. Procedures for displacing parts of a vehicle to gain access are described below. Note that these procedures use the A-, B-, and C-posts of a car as standard reference points (Figure 26-11). Procedures for removing a roof and displacing doors and the front end of a car are also illustrated in Figures 26-12, 26-13, and 26-14.

1. Try the door first. If the door opens only partially, widen the opening by pulling the door with a come-along or force it forward manually. The come-along is preferred since it is designed to pull and hold.

2. If the door is jammed, then remove it completely by breaking the hinges and forcing the door off the latch. You can also force the door at the latch (beware of any side-impact airbags), pull the door around with a come-along, or manually bend the door forward.

3. If opening a front door of a four-door vehicle does not provide enough space to get the patient, then open or force the back door. Cut the top of the B-post (center) completely through. Manually pull and force the post and door out and down to the ground (perpendicular to the vehicle). The result should resemble a wing.

4. If the post and door won't fold out and down, cut completely through the bottom of the B-post and remove the post and door from the action area.

5. At times, the doors are not the first choice for access because of obstacles such as a wall, another vehicle, or some other type of barrier. Removing the roof may be the best route for extricating the patient. Don't waste time with door work if it appears that the chance of removing the patient that way is less than 80 percent. Instead, cut the roof to create a fold-back or "flap." (The flap can be laid back, to the side, or forward over the engine compartment). In some cases, completely removing and disposing of the roof may be the safest and fastest course of action. Base this decision on the patient's condition, the type of tools available, and special roof considerations, such as roof racks, sunroofs, and vehicle height.

Figure 26-11 The locations of the A-, B-, and C-posts on a car.

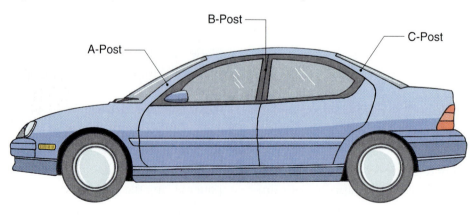

Disposing of the Roof of a Car

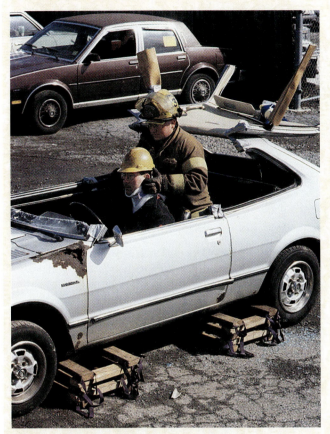

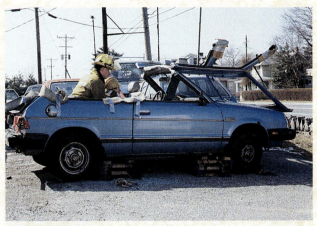

Figure 26-12B Alternatively, the roof can be folded forward by cutting the C-posts. Depending on how much working space is needed, the roof can be hinged forward at either the top or the bottom of the windshield.

Figure 26-12A Sever the A- and B-posts, cut through the roof rails just ahead of the C-posts, and fold the roof back like the roof of a convertible. The windshield should either be removed or cut depending on the amount of working space needed.

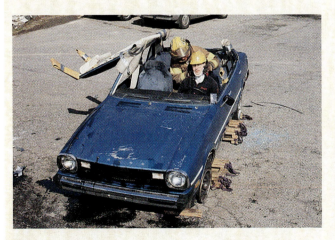

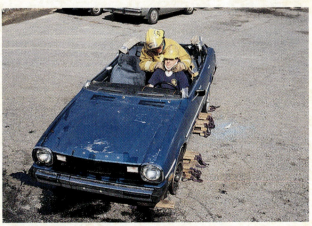

Figure 26-12C Another option is displacing the roof to one side by cutting the A-, B-, and C-posts on the other side.

Figure 26-12D If necessary, the roof can be removed entirely.

Displacing Car Doors

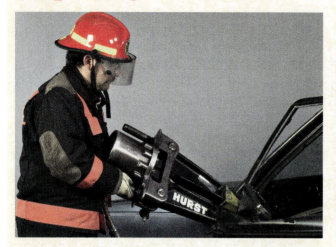

Figure 26-13A Work with the spreader against the A-post side door jamb above the top hinge to spread the door away from the patient and break the top hinge.

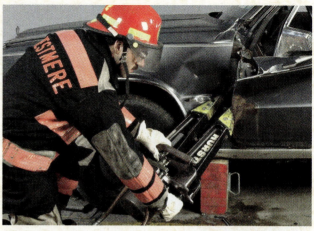

Figure 26-13B Work against the bottom hinge to spread the door farther and to break the bottom hinge. This will leave the door held by its latch.

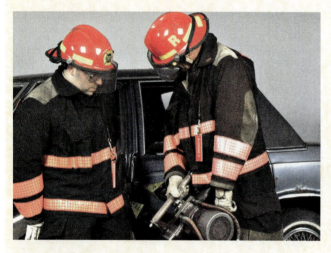

Figure 26-13C Position the spreader above the latch and force the door off the latch. Have an assistant hold or guide the door.

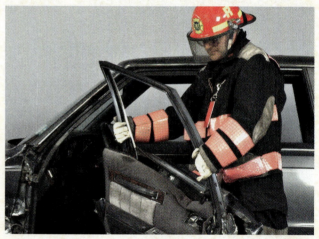

Figure 26-13D Move the door out of the action area.

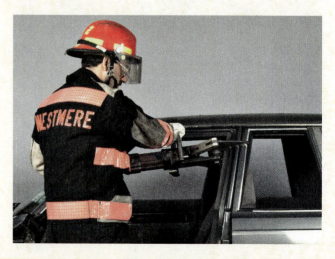

Figure 26-13E If the opening is not large enough, cut the top of the B-post.

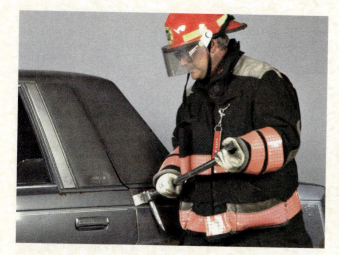

Figure 26-13F Force open the back door.

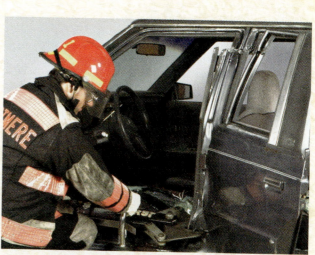

Figure 26-13G Try folding the door down. If it doesn't move easily, cut the bottom of the B-post.

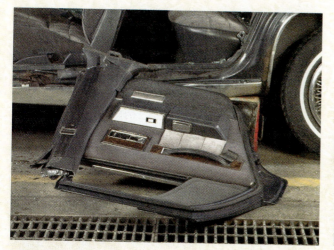

Figure 26-13H You can then fold the door down.

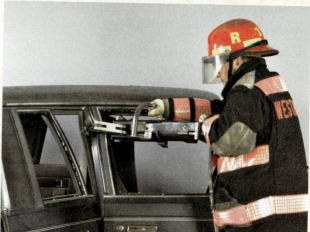

Figure 26-13I Using an alternative method, cut the top and bottom of the B-post.

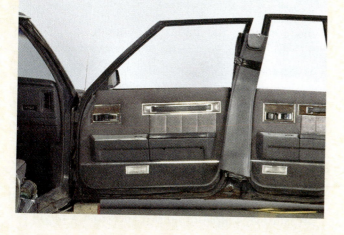

Figure 26-13J Then swing both doors forward as a unit.

Displacing the Front End of a Car

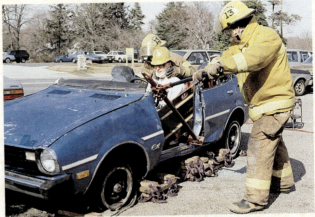

Figure 26-14B Use heavy duty jacks to pivot the front end away from the relief cuts.

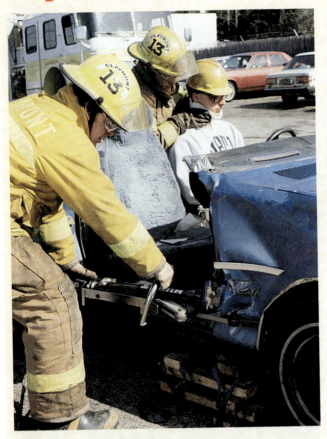

Figure 26-14A Make relief cuts at the junction of the A-post with the rocker panel and in the A-post between the door hinges.

INITIAL AND RAPID TRAUMA ASSESSMENT

You can begin to form a general impression of the patient's mental status and physical condition as soon as you can see the patient, even before gaining access. Once access has been gained and before the patient is extricated, have someone initiate manual stabilization of the head and spine as you complete the initial assessment and manage any life-saving problems with airway, breathing, or circulation. Also perform a head-to-toe rapid trauma assessment, apply a cervical collar, and provide high flow oxygen. These procedures can be going on while other crew members prepare for extrication.

Getting good vital signs and breath sounds can be difficult when power tools are running and saws are cutting. You may need to rely on blood pressure by palpation and realize that it might not

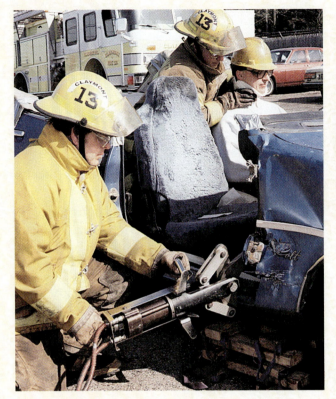

Figure 26-14C Use the combination hydraulic tool in the spreading mode to displace the front end.

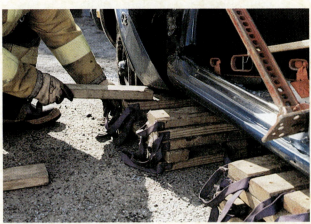

Figure 26-14D Displacing the front end will tend to lift the vehicle from the cribbing. Add cribbing to keep the vehicle stable.

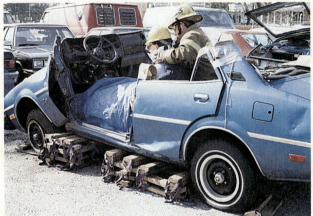

Figure 26-14E Displacing the front end will create working room by moving mechanisms of entrapment away from front-seat patients.

be possible to get an accurate assessment until you are into the back of the ambulance.

EXTRICATION

Normal vs. Rapid Extrication

The access pathway you choose will be closely related to another key decision: whether to use rapid or normal extrication techniques to remove the patient. As you learned earlier (see Chapter 22, "Head and Spine Injuries"), *normal extrication* of a patient seated in a vehicle involves applying a short spine board or a vest-type immobilization device along with manual stabilization of the head and neck and application of a cervical collar, before the patient is moved onto a long spine board for transfer to an ambulance. In *rapid extrication*, after manually stabilizing the head and neck and applying a cervical collar, you can save time by manually immobilizing the patient's torso instead of applying a short spine board or vest-type immobilizer. Maintain manual immobilization until the patient is fully secured to the long spine board.

Rapid extrication should be used *only* when the patient's condition or the environmental conditions in which he is found are serious enough that the need for speed in getting him out of the vehicle outweighs the need for the degree of spinal protection provided by normal extrication. Criteria for rapid extrication should be set by local protocols, but some obvious reasons for rapid extrication are a patient with difficulty breathing, uncontrolled bleeding, multi-system trauma, and signs of shock or an unsafe environment (e.g., a car on fire).

As you perform the initial and rapid trauma assessments, you should assign the patient a priority and decide which extrication procedure should be used.

Partial vs. Full Extrication

When you can get the patient out of a wrecked vehicle by removing the doors or the roof, that is defined as a *partial extrication*. A *full extrication* is required when the patient is trapped and part of the vehicle has to be lifted or removed in order to free the trapped body parts. In this case, you need to consider another set of evolutions that will gain room to free the trapped occupant.

Vehicle on Its Wheels

1. Create "purchase" areas around the front door hinges in order to gain a tool push-point above the hinge.

2. Cut the roof for a fold back, fold-to-the side, fold forward, or removal.

3. By using the A-post as a fulcrum for a spreader tip and pushing down on the top of the door with the other spreader tip, you can create a good starting point for pushing the hinge apart.

4. Then place the spreader on top of the bottom hinge, and push it apart. The door should be hanging by the latch. Force the door from the latch and remove it from the action area. You should end up with no roof and no door(s).

5. If this hasn't produced enough room to remove the patient, then you need to push the dash forward and up. Cut a relief point below the front hinge just above the floor boards.

6. Place a ram or jack against the base of the B-post and against the top hinge area of the front door and push. This should provide enough room to remove victims from a head-on type of collision.

Vehicle on Its Side

1. Stabilize the vehicle first, then gain access to the patient through the back window or the up-side doors in order to provide protective cover.

2. Cut the up-side posts.

3. Cut horizontally through the roof just above the down-side posts. Then create another cut or a fold-line to remove the roof or fold it forward or back.

4. Pull the seats or displace the dashboard as needed.

5. Pull the steering column if necessary. Exercise extreme caution when pulling the steering column on a front-wheel-drive vehicle.

Vehicle on Its Roof

1. Crib and stabilize the vehicle in position to keep it from falling onto patients or rescuers.

2. Force the doors with a hydraulic spreading tool.

3. Use a reciprocating saw to cut the windshield and any internal items that are in the way, such as the gearshift or steering wheel.

TRANSPORT, DETAILED PHYSICAL EXAM, AND ONGOING ASSESSMENT

Once the extrication has created a large-enough space, remove the patient(s), using normal or rapid extrication procedures as discussed earlier. Use a long backboard to help remove the patient though the doors. *Never take victims out through the window when you have a door that can be used.* When the patient is fully immobilized and secured to the long spine board, transfer him into the ambulance for transport to an appropriate facility.

En route in the ambulance if time and the patient's condition permit, perform a detailed physical exam to find and manage any problems that were overlooked during the initial and rapid trauma assessments. If the patient's condition is serious and unstable, you may need to omit the detailed physical exam and spend all the time en route performing ongoing assessment and managing life-threatening conditions. Always assess and reassess the patient as often as possible both during and after the extrication.

TERMINATING THE RESCUE

After you have completed the extrication and rescue and the patients have been transported, you need to close up your operation, get back to the station, and prepare to go back into service.

You will need to terminate your command post, if you used one, and collect your crew for a brief, informal critique, followed by a bigger one later, as needed. (Consider the need for a critical incident stress debriefing if the call has involved serious injuries.) Check in with law enforcement agencies and other EMS agencies to make sure you are free to go and to see if there are any other requests for your unit.

It goes without saying that rescue situations can be physically draining. Even if you are very tired, however, service any tools used in the rescue. Fueling, oiling, washing, lubrication, drying, and storing all come before completing reports or relaxing. Your unit must be ready to go back into service as quickly as possible.

Chapter Review

SUMMARY

As an EMT, you will not automatically be responsible for vehicle or other kinds of rescue and extrication unless you undertake special training. You should, however, understand how the process is done, how it may affect the patient, and how you can gain early access to the patient to begin care. Vehicle extrication or rescue includes 10 phases: Preparing for the rescue; sizing up the scene; recognizing and managing hazards; stabilizing the vehicle; gaining access to the patient; providing initial assessment and a rapid trauma exam; immobilizing the patient; extricating the patient; providing transport, a detailed physical exam, and ongoing assessment; and terminating the rescue.

REVIEWING KEY CONCEPTS

1. List the ten phases of a vehicle rescue operation.

2. Explain the role of the firefighter-EMT in the size-up of a motor vehicle collision.

3. Identify types of passenger restraints used in vehicles and the problems they may pose in rescue operations.

4. Describe what a firefighter-EMT should do upon arrival at a collision if a power pole is broken in half and the lines are down on the street.

5. Describe ways of stabilizing a vehicle that is: resting on its wheels; resting on its side; and resting on its roof.

6. Explain the difference between simple access and complex access.

7. Explain the difference between partial extrication and full extrication.

RESOURCES TO LEARN MORE

Grant, H. D. and Gargan, J. B. *Vehicle Rescue, 2nd Edition*. Upper Saddle River, NJ: Brady/Prentice Hall, 1997.

Wieder, M., ed. *Principles of Extrication*. Stillwater, OK: IFSTA, 1990.

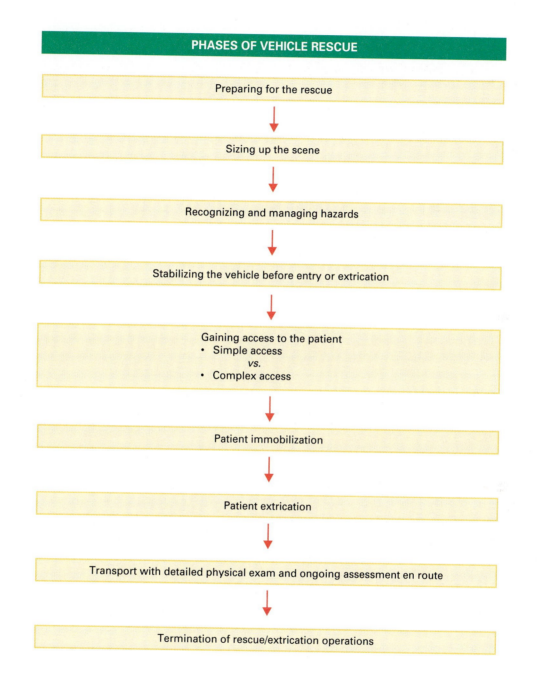

PHASES OF VEHICLE RESCUE

Preparing for the rescue

↓

Sizing up the scene

↓

Recognizing and managing hazards

↓

Stabilizing the vehicle before entry or extrication

↓

Gaining access to the patient
- Simple access
  vs.
- Complex access

↓

Patient immobilization

↓

Patient extrication

↓

Transport with detailed physical exam and ongoing assessment en route

↓

Termination of rescue/extrication operations

Emergency Incident Rehabilitation

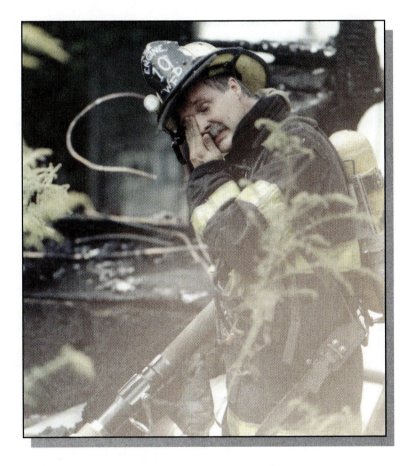

*F*irefighters die of stress- and heat-related illnesses far more often than they do of burns or injuries suffered in structural collapses. Although fire fighting is a hazardous, physically demanding occupation, appropriate emergency scene rehabilitation, or "rehab," can reduce the risks of stress- and heat-related illnesses and deaths associated with it.

As a firefighter, you must be alert to your own physical and mental limitations when on duty and also look out for the physical and

▶

emotional well being of your fellow firefighters. As an EMT, you may also be assigned to evaluate and care for fellow firefighters when you are assigned to the Rehabilitation Sector/Group at a fire or rescue scene.

OBJECTIVES

At the completion of this chapter, the EMT-Basic student should be able to meet the following objectives. These objectives are supplemental to the U.S. DOT 1994 EMT-Basic curriculum.

Knowledge and Understanding

1. Understand the principles of Emergency Incident Rehabilitation. (pp. 700–704)
2. Describe the set-up and components of a rehabilitation area. (pp. 704–711)
3. Describe the role of the EMT in the evaluation and care of firefighters in the rehabilitation area. (pp. 704–711)

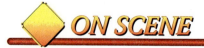

ON SCENE

DISPATCH: *COLUMBIA COUNTRY FIRE CONTROL TO ALL TRI-VILLAGE FIREFIGHTERS. YOU ARE REQUESTED MUTUAL AID TO RESPOND ONE ENGINE AND YOUR RESCUE UNIT FOR MANPOWER TO THE SCENE OF A WORKING STRUCTURE FIRE IN EAST CHATHAM ON ROUTE 295, ONE MILE SOUTH OF MILL ROAD. 1342. DISPATCHER 11-49.*

You respond from your home to the station and drive your department's rescue truck. It is a sunny July day. Temperatures are in the mid-90s and the relative humidity is high. As you near the scene, East Chatham Command orders your unit to establish a Rehab Group upon arrival.

Other fire crews are engaged with a heavily involved house fire as you approach. You drive about 50 yards past the fire scene and park your vehicle in front of a neighbor's home. You and the two other EMTs on your crew deploy the tarps and other rehabilitation supplies stored on the rescue unit. For the location of the Rehab Group, you have selected an area that is upwind of the fire and a safe distance from it. Because it is a hot day, you have also picked a spot well shaded by a large oak tree.

At your request, a neighbor provides you with a garden hose. Using water from the hose, which the neighbor assures you is drinkable, you mix two large coolers of electrolyte replacement solution. You then set up the hose to provide a cooling shower for firefighters who will be coming to the Rehab Group. You also set up electric-powered smoke ejectors to assist in cooling firefighters.

You then advise Command that the Rehab Group is operational and that you will be using the radio identifier "Rehab." As the Rehab Group supervisor, you assign the EMT crew members to their stations, one in the Medical Evaluation/ Treatment area and one in the Rest and Refreshment area.

Just as you and your crew complete final set-up of the Rehab Group, two firefighters arrive. They advanced the first hose line into the house and have now gone through two SCBA bottles each. They appear physically exhausted as they remove their Nomex® hoods, SCBAs, and turnout coats. You log the crew into the Rehab Group and obtain baseline blood pressures and pulse rates for both. Both firefighters have heart rates greater than 120, so you assign them to the Medical Evaluation/Treatment area for hydration and monitoring.

Soon more fire crews with potential stress- and heat-related illnesses arrive in the Rehab Group. You advise Command that you will need two or three additional EMTs assigned to Rehab to assist in evaluation and monitoring. You also request that two ambulances be dispatched to the scene and assigned to your group in case any firefighters require further evaluation and treatment at the local hospital's emergency department.

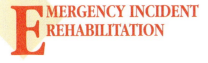

EMERGENCY INCIDENT REHABILITATION

The concept of on-scene Emergency Incident Rehabilitation (EIR) is relatively new in the fire service. The recognition that stress- and heat-related emergencies are the primary causes of on-duty firefighter death has made EIR an integral part of fire ground operations.

All fire departments should have formal standard operating procedures (SOPs) for Emergency Incident Rehabilitation. Such procedures will help to assure the well being of personnel subjected to periods of sustained physical exertion. At the scene of an incident, the incident commander should put the SOPs into action as soon as it becomes clear that conditions exist in which firefighters are likely to develop heat- or stress-related illnesses. The Rehabilitation Sector/Group is a recognized component of the Incident Management System (see Chapter 28, "Special Situations and Operations").

As an EMT, you may be assigned to the Rehab Sector/Group to evaluate and monitor fellow firefighters. Even when you are not specifically assigned to the Rehab Sector/Group, you should always be aware of your own physical and psychological limitations when performing fire fighting and rescue duties. As a firefighter-EMT, you should also be able to recognize signs of exhaustion and heat-related illness in other crew members as well (Figure 27-1). Remember that an exhausted firefighter risks not only his or her own life, but the lives of others as well. If you feel you are at your physical or psychological limits or see others who appear to be at theirs, your crew needs to report to the Rehab Sector/Group for rest and evaluation.

STRESS- AND HEAT-RELATED EMERGENCIES

As noted above, heat-related emergencies are a common danger for firefighters on the job. Chapter 16, "Environmental Emergencies," explores this subject in detail. You may wish to refer back to

Figure 27-1 Firefighter-EMTs must be alert for signs of heat- and stress-related emergencies in themselves and in other crew members as well.

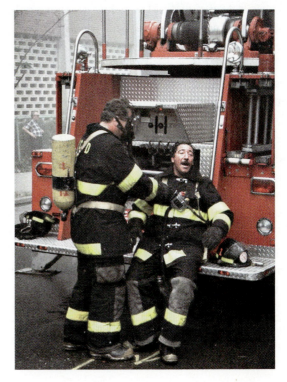

that chapter. In addition, the physical stress of fire fighting can result in cardiac emergencies such as acute myocardial infarction and sudden death. You may refer back to Chapter 13, "Cardiac Emergencies," for more on this subject. Because the goal of EIR is to prevent and/or treat stress- and heat-related emergencies, a review of concepts important to remember at an emergency scene is provided here.

Mechanisms of Heat Loss

The body generates increased heat during periods of increased physical activity. Under normal conditions, the body uses several mechanisms to dissipate this heat. Most of the heat is lost through convection and evaporation.

Heat loss through convection occurs when cooler air moves across the body and the body's heat is transferred to the moving air. The moving air sweeps away the thin layer of warmed air surrounding the body and permits the body to lose still more heat.

Heat loss through evaporation occurs when warmed body moisture is lost to the environment. Evaporative heat loss occurs with normal breathing as warm, moist air is exhaled. Most evaporative heat loss, however, occurs during the process of perspiration. As the body generates heat, it releases a warmed fluid—sweat. The sweat then evaporates into the air, cooling the body surface. The more the body sweats, the more heat is lost.

There are limits to the effectiveness of these mechanisms. Convection works as cooler air moves heat away from the body. As the environmental temperature approaches the body's temperature, convectional cooling becomes less effective. For sweat to evaporate and cool the body, the air surrounding the skin has to be relatively low in humidity. As humidity increases, heat loss through evaporation decreases.

Heat-related emergencies are common in fire fighting for several reasons. First, fires emit heat. In structural or wildland fires, heavy fire loads may produce extreme heat (Figure 27-2). Also, the intense physical activity associated with fire fighting causes firefighters' bodies to generate increased heat. Finally, the protective clothing worn by firefighters, although essential for safety, impairs heat

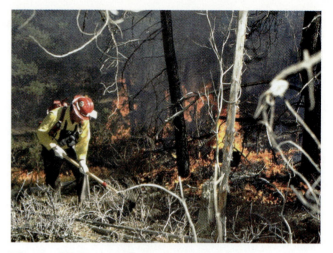

Figure 27-2 Heat-related emergencies are common among crews fighting wildland fires.

loss through evaporation and convection (Figure 27-3). The combination of high temperatures radiated by fires, increased heat produced by firefighters' bodies, and diminished heat loss because of protective gear places crews fighting fires at serious risk for heat-related emergencies.

Figure 27-3 Protective clothing worn by firefighters can limit cooling by convection and evaporation, increasing the risk of heat-related emergencies.

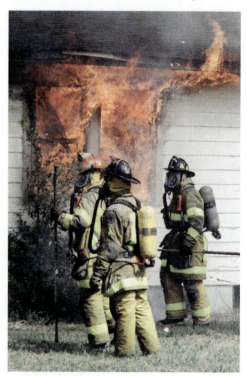

The three most important heat-related emergencies that the EMT will encounter in the Rehab Sector/Group are *heat cramps, heat exhaustion,* and *heat stroke.* Of these conditions, heat stroke is the most serious. Failure to recognize the signs and symptoms of heat stroke and to begin aggressive care may result in the patient's death.

Heat Cramps

Heat cramps usually develop during strenuous activity in a hot environment. Excessive sweating results in loss of electrolytes (especially sodium), which contributes to muscle cramping. Heat cramps are usually not a serious problem. They respond well to rest in a cool environment and replacement of fluids by mouth. If a person with heat cramps is untreated and continues to lose fluid because of sweating, heat exhaustion may develop.

Heat Exhaustion

Heat exhaustion occurs when excessive sweat loss and inadequate oral hydration cause depletion of the body's fluid volume. The end result is hypoperfusion of the body's organs. The signs and symptoms of heat exhaustion may vary with the amount of fluid lost. Early signs may include fatigue, light-headedness, nausea, vomiting, and headache. The firefighter's skin is usually pale and moist to the touch, with cool or normal temperature. If the condition is unrecognized and untreated, a patient with heat exhaustion may develop more classic signs of shock or hypoperfusion. These signs include increased heart rate, increased respiratory rate, and—eventually—reduced blood pressure.

Firefighters who engage in structural and wildland fire suppression without adequate rehabilitation often suffer from heat exhaustion. The condition is also common in hazardous materials operations in which firefighters wear encapsulating suits.

Heat Stroke

Heat stroke occurs when the body can no longer regulate its body temperature in hot conditions. Unlike emergency personnel with heat exhaustion whose temperatures are normal or only slightly elevated, those with heat stroke have very high temperatures (up to 106 or 107°F [41° to 41.7°C]). Because of the high temperature, the skin is likely to feel hot and either dry or moist. The firefighter with heat stroke will have an altered mental status. That mental status may range from mild confusion to complete unresponsiveness.

Any emergency personnel found in a hot environment with altered mental status and skin that is hot in temperature and dry or moist to touch should be presumed to have a life-threatening heat related emergency. Such a patient should be aggressively cooled (see below).

◆ *Emergency Care—Stress- and Heat-Related Emergencies*

Firefighters found at an emergency scene who exhibit any of the following symptoms should be treated for a heat-related emergency:

◆ Muscle cramps

◆ Weakness or exhaustion

◆ Dizziness or faintness

◆ Chest pain

◆ Shortness of breath

◆ Rapid heart beat

◆ Skin that is

—Normal-to-cool temperature, pale, moist

or

—Hot temperature, dry or moist (a life-threatening sign)

◆ Headache

◆ Seizures

◆ Altered mental status ranging from mild confusion to unresponsiveness (a life-threatening sign)

All firefighters with suspected heat-related emergencies should receive the following treatment:

1. **Remove the firefighter from the hot environment, remove his protective clothing, and place him in a cool environment.** The air-conditioned patient compartment of an ambulance is ideal.

2. **Administer high flow oxygen if not already done during initial assessment.**

In cases of apparent heat exhaustion, where the skin is normal-to-cool in temperature, moist to the touch, and pale in color, treat as follows:

1. **Remove the firefighter's protective clothing, including head gear, to allow cooling.**
2. **Cool him by fanning.** Use an electric-powered fan to assist in cooling.
3. **Place him in a supine position with legs elevated.**
4. **If he is responsive and not nauseated, have him drink water or other fluids as specified by local protocol.**
5. **If he is not responsive or is nauseated or vomiting, transport him to the hospital on his left side, monitoring and maintaining the airway during transport.**
6. **Perform the ongoing assessment en route to the hospital.**

In cases of apparent heat stroke, where the firefighter's skin is hot in temperature and dry or moist to the touch, treat the patient as follows:

1. **Remove the firefighter's protective clothing, including head gear, to allow cooling.**
2. **Apply cold packs to the firefighter's neck, groin, and armpits.**
3. **Keep his skin wet by applying cool water with sponges or wet towels or by wrapping him in sheets soaked in cool water.**
4. **Fan aggressively.**
5. **Use the maximum setting on the air conditioner in the patient compartment of the ambulance.**
6. **Give the firefighter nothing by mouth.**
7. **Transport immediately.**
8. **Perform the ongoing assessment en route to the hospital.**

Remember, the firefighter's survival and recovery from a heat-related emergency hinges on your recognizing the emergency, quickly removing him from the hot environment, and initiating the proper treatment in the out-of-hospital setting.

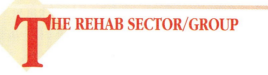

THE REHAB SECTOR/GROUP

Most of the tasks associated with EIR are carried out in the Rehab Sector/Group. EMTs usually play key roles in the staffing of that sector.

Functions in the Rehab Sector/Group

EMTs assigned to the Rehab Sector/Group perform several functions:

◆ EMTs must assure that the sector provides a safe area in which fire and rescue crews can rest and receive **rehydration,** or replacement of water and electrolytes lost in sweating. During prolonged incidents, food should also be supplied to crews in the rehabilitation area.

◆ EMTs must identify firefighters and rescue personnel entering Rehab who are at risk for heat- and stress-related illness.

◆ EMTs must medically monitor crews and determine whether they:
  —Are fit to return to active fire/rescue duty
  —Require additional hydration and rest
  —Require transport to an emergency department for further evaluation and treatment

◆ EMTs must assure accountability for firefighters and rescue personnel who enter and exit Rehab.

◆ EMTs must give regular reports/updates to the Safety Officer or the Incident Commander.

The Rehab Sector/Group must be equipped with materials and personnel adequate to accomplish these functions. The amount of materials and number of personnel in the Rehab Sector/Group will be determined by the magnitude of the incident and by the climatic conditions.

Staffing of the Rehab Sector/Group

The Rehab Sector/Group should be staffed with adequate personnel to provide medical evaluation and treatment and to assure that firefighters receive sufficient food and fluid replenishment.

The most highly trained and qualified EMS personnel on the scene should provide medical

COMPANY OFFICER'S NOTES

A fire officer must be aware of the conditions and circumstances that require establishment of a Rehab Sector/Group as part of the Incident Management System. The Rehab Sector/Group must be set up as early as possible to prevent unnecessary casualties. Conditions that require establishment of a Rehab Sector/Group include the following:

◆ Large, multi-jurisdiction incidents (Figure 27-4)

◆ All multiple-alarm fires

◆ Hazardous materials incidents

◆ All incidents of long duration (greater than one hour)

◆ Extremes of weather conditions including:
—High temperature
—Low temperature
—High humidity
—High winds

evaluation and treatment in the Rehab Sector/Group. At the minimum, the area should be staffed by EMTs. In large-scale incidents or in those where a trend toward serious heat- and stress-related illness is detected among firefighters, advance life support (ALS) units should be requested and assigned. Often, outside EMS agencies such as mutual aid companies or ambulance squads provide medical evaluation and treatment

Figure 27-4 Rehab Sector/Groups should be established at all large, multi-jurisdictional or multiple-alarm fires.

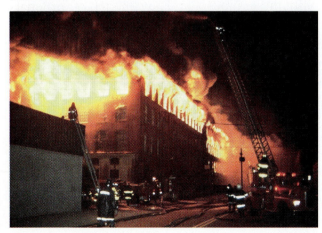

in the Rehab Sector/Group. If such agencies are used, it is essential that they have direct radio communication with Command.

Personnel without medical training can help provide food and fluid replenishment in the Rehab Sector/Group. In many volunteer fire departments, members of the department's Ladies' Auxiliary or an Explorer Post fill this function. In addition, agencies such as the American Red Cross or local food retailers may offer additional nutritional support. When such organizations are involved in EIR, they must follow the directions of Command or the Rehab Sector/Group officer. This is especially important in order to assure that proper types of fluids—non-carbonated and caffeine-free—are administered.

Design and Location of the Rehab Sector/Group

The EIR area should be set up in a location that truly allows firefighters and rescue personnel to get physical and psychological rest. A good rehabilitation site includes the following features (Figure 27-5):

◆ *The site should be outside and upwind of the operational hazard area or "hot zone." This*

Figure 27-5 Location of the Rehab Sector/Group relative to the hazard area.

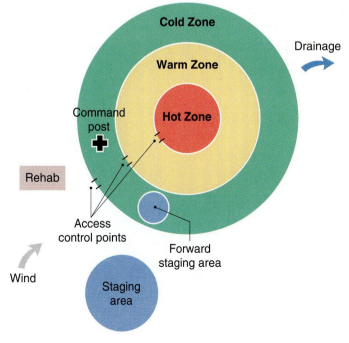

allows personnel to remove their turnout gear and SCBAs safely.

◆ *The site should permit prompt re-entry into emergency operations when personnel have completed rehabilitation.*

◆ *The site should provide protection from environmental extremes.* Locations such as a shaded, cool area in hot weather conditions and a warm, dry, protected area during cold weather operations are preferred.

◆ *The site should be large enough to accommodate all those who may need rehabilitation.* Remember when laying out the site that crews in rehabilitation will need room to sit or lie down.

◆ *The site should be free of vehicle exhaust.*

◆ *The site should not be immediately accessible to the media.*

◆ *The site should provide access to SCBA replenishment/refill.*

◆ *The site should be close to a potential ambulance staging area in case transport to the emergency department for further evaluation and treatment becomes necessary.*

◆ *The site should have a supply of running and drinkable water.* This simplifies ongoing rehydration operations. It also enables Rehab personnel to set up a cooling water spray in hot conditions.

◆ *If the incident involves the recovery of fatalities, the site should be out of view of the work area.*

Site selection is usually made either by Command or by the officer assigned to establish the Rehab Sector/Group. Site selection should always take into account the possibility that the emergency scene may expand, as with an uncontained fire. Making a good initial site selection for the Rehab Sector/Group is vital because trying to relocate the site in the middle of an emergency incident creates delays and confusion for both sector personnel and the crews who need its services. Once the site is selected, its location should be made known to all incident participants.

In large-scale incidents, more than one Rehab Sector/Group may be needed. If more than one area is established, Rehab personnel at each site must keep accurate logs of the entries and exits of crews in order to assure proper fireground accountability. If the departments involved use some sort of identification marker system (such as passports), make sure all standard procedures for collecting and returning them are followed.

The size of the Rehab Sector/Group will vary with the size of the incident it is set up to service. Local fire department SOPs should describe a general physical layout for Rehab Sector/Groups (Figure 27-6). The layout should provide for a single

Figure 27-6 Layout of a typical Rehab Sector/Group.

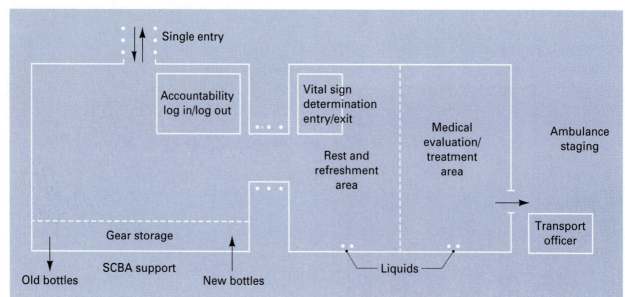

entry/exit point with adjacent areas for logging crews in and out and for performing medical evaluations upon entry.

Most of the space within the Rehab Sector/Group should be devoted to two large, clearly designated areas: the Rest and Refreshment area and the Medical Evaluation/Treatment area. Large tarps of different colors can be used to distinguish the two areas. Specifically assigning personnel who need assistance to these distinct areas makes monitoring and accountability during rehab easier.

Criteria for Entering the Rehab Sector/Group

Local SOPs detailing when crews must enter rehabilitation may vary. However, the following guidelines are among the most commonly accepted.

First, whenever a firefighter or emergency incident responder feels that he has reached the limit of his physical or psychological endurance, he should report to the Rehab Sector/Group. A fatigued firefighter places not only himself but also the other firefighters in that crew at risk. For this reason, the entire crew should report to Rehab when one crew member becomes fatigued. This "whole crew to Rehab" approach is a sound one. It assures better tracking and accountability of personnel on the scene. Further, it recognizes the reality that if one member of the crew is at the limits of endurance, then others in the crew may be also.

Another common indicator for mandatory rehabilitation is the "two-cylinder rule." Under this standard, firefighters must report to the Rehab Sector/Group after going through two 30-minute-capacity SCBA air cylinders.

Finally, some departments use a time limit. A common SOP sets the rule that, after 45 minutes of active fire suppression duty, rehabilitation is mandatory.

Accountability in the Rehab Sector/Group

Accountability refers to the process by which fire crews and individual firefighters are tracked and accounted for at the scene of an incident. Accurate accountability can be life saving during a fire or complex rescue situation. Too often, the lack of an efficient accountability system has led to delays in recognizing that firefighters were missing; these delays have been contributing factors in some firefighters' deaths. Accurate accountability is especially important when there is a sudden change in fire conditions. Those conditions might include the abandoning of interior attack operations for a defensive exterior attack or a catastrophic structural collapse.

Individual fire departments have various accountability systems (Figure 27-7). These include Velcro® name tags removed from firefighters' turnout coats or helmet shields and placed on the command post status board or magnetic name tags placed on pump panels.

Figure 27-7 A reliable system for assuring accountability must be in place in the Rehab Sector/Group. **A.** In one department, the Rehab officer collects clip-on tags as firefighters enter Rehab. **B.** In another department, Velcro name tags are attached to a board to show the whereabouts of fire personnel.

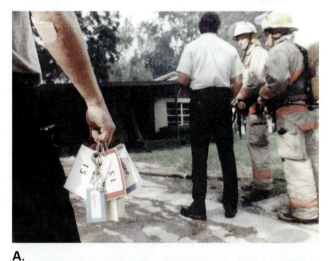

A.

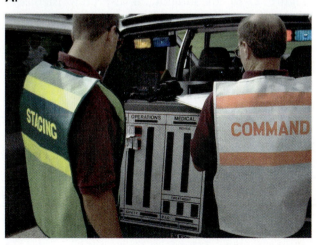

B.

CREWS OPERATING ON THE SCENE: _____ E8, E24, R1, L14, BAT6 _____

UNIT #	# PERSONS	TIME IN	TIME OUT		UNIT #	# PERSONS	TIME IN	TIME OUT
E8	4	1301	1335					

Figure 27-8 A sample company check-in/check-out log sheet.

In the Rehab Sector/Group, the following measures will assist in assuring accountability:

◆ *SOPs should direct that entire crews, not individuals, be assigned to the Rehab Sector/Group.*

◆ *Crews should enter and exit the Rehab Sector/Group as a unit.*

◆ *The Rehab Sector/Group staff should log crews in and out.*

◆ *All entry to and exit from the Rehab Sector/Group should be through a single access point.*

The Rehab Sector/Group officer must be able to instantly account for crews that have been or are currently assigned to rehabilitation. For this reason, a company check-in/check-out log sheet should be developed and used to track crews (Figure 27-8). In addition, if any crew members who have entered the Rehab Sector/Group require transport to the hospital, their names, their unit designations, and their destination hospitals must also be recorded and made immediately available to Command (Figure 27-9).

Entry and Triage

As noted, all crews must enter and exit Rehab through a single designated entry point and be time-logged in by the sector staff. Upon entering Rehab, fire crews should be allowed to remove their SCBAs, hoods, and turnout gear. Once gear is removed, each crew member should be evaluated for injuries and for heat- and stress-related illnesses.

The first step in evaluation is obtaining entry vital signs, including blood pressure and pulse. Rehab staff should rapidly question crew members, being alert to potentially life-threatening complaints such as the presence of chest pain or shortness of breath. Remember the goal of the entry medical evaluation is to identify personnel with potential heat- or stress-related illnesses or injuries, not to keep firefighters from rest and rehydration.

Figure 27-9 Information on crew members who have entered the Rehab Sector/Group must be instantly available to Command.

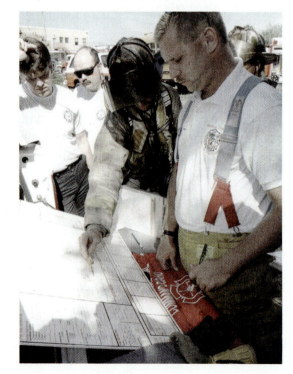

Table 27-1

Entry Evaluation Findings Mandating Triage to the Medical Evaluation/Treatment Area

Heart Rate	> 120
Blood Pressure	> 200 systolic
	< 90 systolic
	> 110 diastolic
Injuries	Any

When the entry evaluation is complete, Rehab staff should assign crew members either to the Rest and Refreshment area or to the Medical Treatment/Evaluation Area. Patients assigned to the Medical Treatment/Evaluation Area will receive more intensive evaluation and monitoring as well as rehydration and rest. The findings in the entry medical evaluation determine the area to which crew members are assigned. Local protocols vary, but firefighters with pulse rates greater than 120 per minute at entry, who have a markedly abnormal blood pressure, or who have sustained any injuries should be assigned to the Medical Evaluation/Treatment Area (Table 27-1).

Medical Evaluation/Treatment Area

Crew members are triaged to the Medical Evaluation/Treatment Area because their entry evalua-tions indicate a potential risk for having or devel-oping heat- or stress-related illnesses. They may also be triaged to this area because of injuries that they have sustained. Patients triaged with abnormal vital signs require ongoing assessment of their vital signs and conditions while they are resting and taking in oral rehydration and/or food. These patients should, at a minimum, have their vital signs reassessed 20 minutes after entering the Rehab Sector/Group. Each patient's sequential vital signs and assessments should be logged on a flow sheet (Figure 27-10). After 20 minutes of cool down with rest and rehydration, vital signs of most crew members will return to normal levels.

Some patients may still have elevated heart rates (greater than 100 beats per minute) after 20 minutes. These patients must generally remain in the Rehab Sector/Group for additional rehydra-tion. Some EIR SOPs prohibit such personnel from returning to duty for the remainder of the incident or shift.

The exact amount of time that crews should spend in the Rehab Sector/Group will depend on their level of exhaustion and need for rest, rehydration, and—during prolonged operations—nutrition. At a minimum, crews should remain in the Rehab Sector/Group for 20 minutes. Before returning to fire fighting or rescue duties, all crew members should have a repeat pulse and blood pressure check. If a crew member still has abnor-mal vital signs at this time, then the entire crew

Figure 27-10 In the Rehab Sector/Group, a firefighter's sequential vital signs and assessments should be logged on a flow sheet like this one.

EMERGENCY INCIDENT REHABILITATION REPORT   INCIDENT: Palmer Rd. structure fire

DATE: 6/18/99

NAME / UNIT #	TIMES(S)	TIME /# Bottles	BP	PULSE	RESP	TEMP	SKIN	TAKEN BY	COMPLAINTS/CONDITION	TRANSPORT?
John Skoda	0940	NA	140/70	78	16	NA	NL	ETD	Swollen, deformed ankle	Yes/St. Mary's Hospital

Table 27-2

Reevaluation Findings Mandating Continued Time in the Rehabilitation Sector

Heart Rate	> 100
Blood Pressure	> 160 systolic
	< 100 systolic
	> 90 diastolic

must remain in rehabilitation and receive additional rehabilitation and monitoring (Table 27-2).

All personnel who enter the Rehab Sector/Group with injuries should have those injuries promptly evaluated. Appropriate treatment should be given and transport to a medical facility provided if warranted. If a crew member is transported, other members of that crew can potentially go back on line. However, be sure that those crew members and Command are informed that a crew member has been transported.

Because a goal of EIR is detecting and preventing heat-related emergencies, many fire department SOPs call for monitoring of the patient's oral temperature. Some rehabilitation SOPs mandate obtaining oral temperatures on all patients with heart rates greater than 110 to 120 beats per minute at entry into Rehab. If the patient's temperature is greater than 100.6°F, then he is not permitted to put turnout gear or SCBA back on. For example, the Phoenix Fire Department Rehabilitation SOP states that any patient with a temperature higher than 101°F (38.3°C) must receive intravenous (IV) hydration and transport to the emergency department.

In winter months, generalized hypothermia and local cold injuries such as frostbite must be considerations during medical evaluation of fire and rescue crews. In these conditions, the Rehab Sector/Group must provide crews with warmth and protection from ice and snow hazards. Remember, however, that heat- and stress-related illnesses can also occur in cool and cold weather.

During rehabilitation and medical monitoring of crews, Rehab Sector/Group personnel may detect signs and symptoms of potentially life-threatening emergencies. These signs and symptoms include the following:

- Chest pain
- Shortness of breath
- Altered mental status (confusion, seizures, dizziness, etc.)
- Skin that is hot in temperature and either dry or moist
- Irregular pulse
- Oral temperature greater than 101°F.
- Pulse greater than 150 at any time
- Pulse greater than 140 after cool down
- Systolic blood pressure greater than 200 mm Hg after cooldown
- Diastolic blood pressure greater than 130 mm Hg at any time

If any of these conditions is detected, place the patient on high flow oxygen, initiate appropriate care, and transport the patient immediately to the emergency department for further evaluation and treatment. Use of an advanced life support (ALS) unit is indicated for all of these conditions. However, transport from the Rehab Sector/Group should not be delayed if ALS is unavailable.

One other thing that Rehab Sector/Group personnel must be on the lookout for when monitoring fire or rescue crews is a pattern of unusual complaints, illnesses, or injuries. Such patterns may indicate unexpected hazards involved in the incident. For example, if several patients at a fire scene complain of excessive salivation, runny noses, and diarrhea, it is a good indication that organophosphate pesticides are involved in the fire. Complaints of burning eyes could indicate the presence of metal gases. If unusual patterns such as these are noted, the EMT assigned to the Rehab Sector/Group must immediately report the finding to the Incident Commander so that appropriate actions can be taken.

Hydration and Nourishment in the Rehab Sector/Group

Oral rehydration is essential during periods of prolonged strenuous activity such as fire fighting (Figure 27-11). Both water and crucial electrolytes

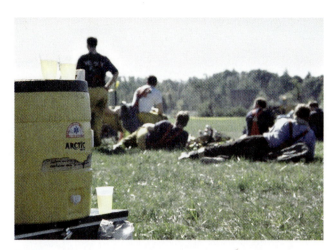

Figure 27-11 Liquids for rehydration must be available in the Rehab Sector/Group. In addition, the area selected for the site must be large enough to allow personnel to sit or lie down.

are lost from the body through sweating. Fluid replacement should, therefore, include both water and electrolytes.

Commercially available sports activity beverages are ideal for fluid replacement in EIR. Some agency SOPs recommend that these commercial rehydration preparations be diluted in a 50/50 mixture with water. Other agencies prefer to use the undiluted preparations. These fluids should be served either cool or at the ambient temperature, but not with ice or ice cold. Beverages that are too cold can cause problems such as spasm of the esophagus and a sudden drop in heart rate.

Beverages containing caffeine or alcohol should be excluded because they can alter cardiovascular performance and heat-regulation mechanisms. Carbonated beverages should also be avoided because they can cause digestive upset leading to nausea and vomiting.

Patients who are unable to tolerate oral rehydration due to nausea or vomiting should be assigned to the Medical Evaluation/Treatment area. These patients should be closely monitored. They will likely require intravenous (IV) hydration by ALS providers and transport to the emergency department.

During incidents that involve more than 2 to 3 hours of ongoing physical activity, fire and rescue crews should receive solid nourishment in the Rehab Sector/Group. Foods that are easily prepared and served and easily digested are ideal for EIR nourishment. Soups or stews are often appropriate food choices. In addition, fruits such as oranges and apples are good sources of fluids and sugars.

Chapter Review

SUMMARY

Although fire fighting is an inherently hazardous and physically demanding occupation, it is likely that good on-scene rehabilitation can reduce the risks of heat- and stress-related illness and death associated with the job. All fire departments should have formal SOPs for Emergency Incident Rehabilitation.

REVIEWING KEY CONCEPTS

1. Explain the factors that place firefighters at increased risk for heat- and stress-related illnesses.

2. List and describe the three most common heat-related illnesses an EMT will encounter in the Rehab Sector/Group.

3. List the symptoms that indicate that a firefighter should be treated for a heat-related emergency.

4. Describe the steps in the care of a firefighter with a heat-related emergency whose skin is normal-to-cool, moist to the touch, and pale in color.

5. Describe the steps in the care of a firefighter with a heat-related emergency whose skin is hot in temperature and dry or moist to the touch.

6. Explain the basic functions of the EMT in the Rehab Sector/Group.

7. List the conditions that usually require the establishment of a Rehab Sector/Group.

8. Describe factors that should be considered when siting the Rehab Sector/Group.

9. Describe the major divisions of the Rehab Sector/Group and explain what goes on in each of them.

10. Describe some common guidelines that mandate when firefighters must enter the Rehab Sector/Group.

11. Describe some common measures for assuring accountability in the Rehab Sector/Group.

12. List common vital sign findings that mandate a firefighter enter the Medical Evaluation/Treatment area.

13. List signs of potentially life-threatening emergencies that EMTs should be alert to when monitoring firefighters in the Rehab Sector/Group.

14. Explain the importance of remaining alert for unusual patterns of illnesses, injuries, or complaints when monitoring patients in the Rehab Sector/Group.

15. Explain the types of liquids that are desirable and the type that should be avoided when providing rehydration in the Rehab Sector/Group.

RESOURCES TO LEARN MORE

Emergency Incident Rehabilitation, FEMA—U.S. Fire Administration. FA-114 July 1992. USFA Publications, P.O. Box 70274, Washington, DC 20024 Provides a sample EIR SOP.

BASICS OF ESTABLISHING A REHAB SECTOR/GROUP

Situations requiring establishment of a Rehab/Sector Group
- Large, multi-jurisdiction incidents
- All multiple-alarm fires
- Hazardous materials incidents
- All incidents of long duration (greater than one hour)
- Extremes of weather conditions

Considerations for Rehab Sector/Group site selection:
- Outside and upwind of the operational hazard area or "hot zone"
- Allows prompt re-entry into emergency operations after rehabilitation
- Protected from environmental extremes
- Large enough for all who may need rehabilitation
- Free of vehicle exhaust
- Not immediately accessible to the media
- Provides access for SCBA replenishment/refill
- Close to a potential ambulance staging area
- Available supply of running and drinkable water
- Out of view of fatality recovery operations

Layout of the Rehab/Sector Group
- Single entry/exit point
- Accountability log-in/log-out point
- Space for gear storage
- Space for SCBA support
- Vital sign determination point
- Rest and Refreshment Area
  —Hydration
- Medical Evaluation/Treatment Area
  —Hydration
  —Access to ambulance staging area and transport

Common Criteria for Entry to the Rehab Sector/Group
- Crew member at physical or emotional limits
- Upon exhaustion of two SCBA cylinders
- Time limit after which Rehab is mandatory

Common Criteria for Entry into the Medical Evaluation/Treatment Area
- Heart rate faster than 120 beats per minute
- Blood pressure greater than 200 systolic or 110 diastolic or less than 90 systolic
- Any injuries

Common Criteria Mandating Continued Stay in Rehab After 20 Minutes
- Heart rate faster than 100 beats per minute
- Blood pressure greater than 160 systolic or 90 diastolic or less than 100 systolic
- Any injuries

EMS Special Operations

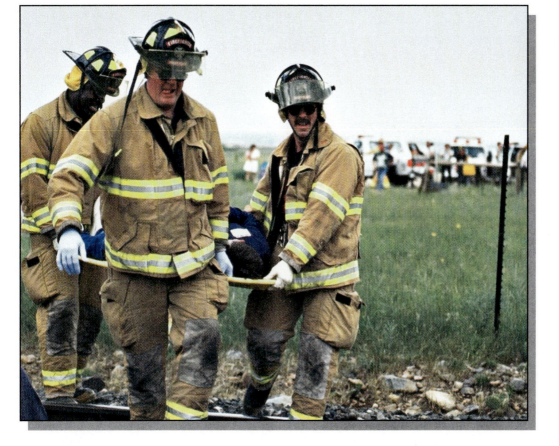

*F*irefighter-EMTs are dispatched to many situations that at first
appear to be routine medical calls. On arrival, however, the EMTs
find the situations to be anything but routine. They may
suddenly face a variety of dangers that the dispatcher who sent them out
knew nothing about. They might need to provide care to a patient who
has fallen down an icy slope or has been trapped in the cave-in of a
ditch. The EMTs might discover that the motor vehicle crash that they've
been dispatched to involves a tanker truck hauling deadly chlorine gas.
They might find at the scene a number of patients far greater than they
can handle. ▶

Situations such as these require personnel with special training and resources to ensure the safety of patients and fire and emergency crews involved in them. As a firefighter, you already have training that prepares you to handle some hazardous situations. At other times, your role will be to recognize the dangers or complications at a scene and to summon the appropriate personnel to rescue the patient or to stabilize the scene so that proper assessment and care can be provided.

OBJECTIVES

At the completion of this chapter, the EMT-Basic student should be able to meet the following objectives:

Knowledge and Understanding

1. Explain the EMT-Basic's role during a call involving hazardous materials. (pp. 733–742)

2. Describe what the EMT-Basic should do if there is reason to believe that there is a hazard at the scene. (pp. 732, 733–738)

3. Describe the actions that an EMT-Basic should take to ensure bystander safety. (p. 734)

4. State the role that the EMT-Basic should perform until appropriately trained personnel arrive at the scene of a hazardous materials situation. (pp. 733–738)

5. Break down the steps to approaching a hazardous situation. (pp. 733–742)

6. Discuss the various environmental hazards that affect EMS. (pp. 718–729)

7. Describe the criteria for a multiple-casualty situation. (p. 742)

8. Evaluate the role of the EMT-Basic in the multiple-casualty situation. (pp. 743–747)

9. Summarize the components of basic triage. (pp. 747–750)

10. Define the role of the EMT-Basic in a disaster operation. (pp. 743–752)

11. Describe the basic concepts of incident management. (pp. 742–743)

12. Explain the methods for preventing contamination of self, equipment, and facilities. (pp. 739–740)

13. Review the local mass casualty incident plan. (p. 742)

Skills

1. Given a scenario of a mass casualty incident, perform triage.

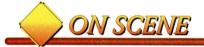

ON SCENE

DISPATCH: *STATION 24 AND COUNTY AMBULANCE 1, MEDIC 1. RESPOND FOR A REPORTED CAR THROUGH THE ICE AT WESTDALE POND AT CRAVITT'S PARK. TIME IS 2217.*

It's a cold December night. You respond as the EMT-trained officer on Rescue 24. En route to the call, you are advised that state troopers on scene are confirming a car through the ice at the deep pond. They say that two of the car's occupants have swum to safety, but there is a third person still beneath the ice.

Upon hearing the troopers' report, you radio the dispatcher requesting the immediate dispatch of the county's dive team as well as a mutual-aid hovercraft from the Goshen Fire Department. Knowing that there are at least three potential patients, you request that an additional paramedic ambulance be sent to the scene.

Upon arrival, you see a state trooper attending to two teenagers in the back of her patrol car. You notify dispatch that you have arrived and are establishing "Westdale Pond Command." You have the driver park your rescue vehicle off the road, near where tire tracks in the snow indicate that a car left the road and crashed through the ice.

You assign the two EMTs on your unit to care for the two shivering patients in the trooper's car. Your driver deploys your unit's floodlights so that they illuminate the pond. They reveal a large hole in the ice at the edge of the pond, but no vehicle. Meanwhile, one EMT reports to you that the two patients in the trooper's car are suffering from apparent generalized hypothermia. He also tells you that the patients say the person still under the ice is an 18-year-old male who was highly intoxicated.

Based on what you've learned so far, you radio in a report: "FireCom from Westdale Pond Command."

"Go ahead Westdale Pond Command."

"Dispatcher, at this time we have two teenagers out of the water suffering from generalized hypothermia. Advise County Ambulance 1

that they will be assigned to those two patients, who are in the state police car just south of Rescue 24."

"Copy that, Westdale Pond Command. ETA for the dive team is 4 minutes."

"Westdale Pond Command copies."

The dive team arrives minutes later, its members already in their dry suits and SCUBA equipment. They are in the water quickly and in a few minutes have recovered the missing patient, who is in cardiac arrest. Medic 1, the paramedic ambulance, has meanwhile arrived. The paramedic intubates the patient on scene. The patient is then packaged and loaded onto Medic 1 for transport. Two of the Rescue 24 crew members accompany the patient to assist with chest compressions and ventilations.

The cardiac arrest patient is pronounced dead at the hospital 2 hours later. The two other teenagers are discharged from the hospital the next day.

It's in the nature of firefighters and EMTs to respond in a crisis like the one described above in the attempt to save lives. People drawn to these occupations are action oriented. They want to do something rather than stand by and watch people whose lives are in danger. Action undertaken without adequate preparation and planning, however, can result in serious injury or death for the patient, for the would-be rescuers, and for those who try to rescue the rescuers. This lesson is driven home in countless newspaper stories:

◆ Would-be rescuers in California fall through the ice and die during a rescue attempt.

◆ An EMT who is first to arrive at a rescue operation in Ithaca, NY, falls on steep snow and slides out of control down an snow slope, falls into cold water, and drowns.

◆ A Pennsylvania paramedic and two firefighters are overcome by methane gas while trying to

rescue an infant who had fallen into an old well housing that is used as a depository for lawn clippings and leaves. The infant survives, but the three rescuers die.

Research data confirm the risks of taking hasty action in hazardous situations. One National Institute of Occupational Safety and Health (NIOSH) study found that approximately 60 percent of the fatalities that were reported in confined space emergencies were of first responders or would-be rescuers.

The true scope of danger to EMS workers may never be known because there is no national clearinghouse to track injuries to emergency responders. However, one thing is clear: rescue workers must have both an awareness and an understanding of the environments that they encounter in order to prevent tragedy and bring about successful rescue operations.

RESCUE SITUATION HAZARDS

This chapter describes common rescue situations firefighter-EMTs might encounter. It lists the hazards of those situations and suggests steps that can be followed to assure rescuer and patient safety.

Water-Related Hazards

Water sports are among the most popular recreational pastimes in this country. Children are naturally drawn to water, from mud puddles to ponds to swift-flowing streams. Adults play on water in more sophisticated and costly toys, from high-powered racing boats to jet skis to kayaks.

Because people are attracted to water in such large numbers, emergencies involving the water are common, even in arid parts of the country. Most water rescues are carried out without the involvement of public safety personnel. For example, people around a swimming pool pull a struggling swimmer out or other boaters rescue a person whose sailboat has capsized.

Some water emergencies, however, require that rescuers have special training and, often, special equipment. The most common of these situations involve rivers and fast-moving water. In these situations, the risks of victim entrapment and danger to rescuers are at their highest.

Failure to Use Personal Flotation Devices

Failure to wear personal flotation devices (PFDs) is a major reason for the large number of deaths of people engaging in water sports. PFDs assist wearers in several ways: they provide flotation; they help conserve body heat; they provide protection for the chest. Merely having a PFD in a boat or near at hand is not good enough. PFDs must be worn properly to be effective (Figure 28-1).

PFDs are not only for those engaged in water sports. Fire and EMS personnel called to water emergencies should wear them also. Body armor, turnout gear, or EMS clothing may be appropriate personal protective equipment for some activities, but the right PPE around water is a PFD!

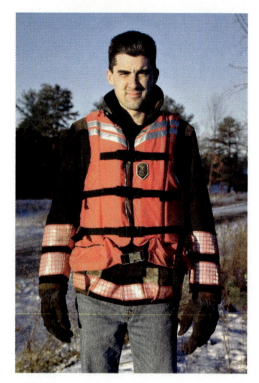

Figure 28-1 A personal flotation device (PFD) is mandatory equipment for any water-related rescue.

Water Temperature

Another factor that contributes to drowning deaths is water temperature. A person submerged in water colder than 98°F (37°C) will begin to lose body heat. The colder the water, the faster the heat loss. In water colder than 92°F (33°C), the body cannot maintain its normal core temperature and will start to become hypothermic. Immersion in water causes a loss of heat 25 times faster than exposure to still air. In fact, immersion for 15 to 20 minutes in 35°F (2°C) water is likely to result in death from hypothermia.

Even on seemingly warm days, water temperatures can be low enough to cause the swift onset of hypothermia. Remember this when dealing with river or swift-water emergencies. In the northern United States and Canada, melting snow as spring days grow warmer makes rivers rise and produces some of the best recreational white-water conditions. In southern and western areas, downpours from thunderstorms can create white-water conditions in dry river beds and storm water retention areas. Even though air temperatures are warm in these cases, the water is usually cold enough to cause an unprepared person to become hypothermic quickly.

People suffering from hypothermia rapidly lose the ability to help themselves. As the body's core temperature drops, motor skills and judgment deteriorate. Hypothermic patients are often unable to follow rescuers' instructions or to grab rescue devices thrown to them. This means that rescuers may have to use procedures that involve going to the victim.

Use of PFDs can be especially critical in cold water situations. PFDs provide flotation and keep people on the surface of the water. They also cover the victim's thorax, providing some insulation from the cold and allowing the victim to conserve energy.

Alcohol Consumption

Drinking and driving have long been publicized as a deadly combination. Unfortunately, drinking in combination with boating, swimming, diving, or any water sport can also be deadly. Alcohol consumption alters judgment, motor skills, and reaction time while increasing heat loss. Be alert to the possibility of alcohol involvement whenever you are called to a water emergency.

The Force of Moving Water

Many people are drawn to moving water for recreation. Moving water, however, poses special hazards, and even innocent-looking conditions can be deadly. Trained and experienced boaters learn how to read moving water, understand its hazards, and manage them. It's the less experienced and uninformed who are most often at risk in moving water incidents. This is true for both those engaging in sports and would-be rescuers. If you are not trained for moving water rescues, request assistance from units with such training.

Unless you have had experience as a white water boater, it can be difficult to understand the force that moving water can exert. That force is a factor of the water's depth, width, and velocity. For example, imagine a 4-foot (1.2 m) deep river that is 200 feet (60 m) with a current moving at a speed of 20 feet (6 m) per second. That river will move roughly 16,000 cubic feet (489 m³) of water

per second. A person trapped against an object in that river would have a force equivalent to roughly 550 pounds (249 kg) pressing against his body or 270 pounds (122 kg) if just his legs were trapped.

The force alone makes moving water dangerous. Other river features can further increase the risks.

Strainers or River Obstructions Strainers are partial obstructions to a river's flow. A strainer allows water to pass through but catches people or other objects (Figure 28-2). Some of the most common strainers are trees and tree branches in the river. If a swimmer or boater is pulled into a strainer, the force of the water can hold him there until he becomes hypothermic, tires, and drowns.

Fixed obstructions, such as bridge abutments, also pose problems in moving water. A boat or person can easily become trapped against such objects. Once trapped, the force of the moving water can make escape difficult.

Holes/Hydraulics Not all water on fast-moving rivers flows downstream! When water flows over a large uniform object in the current, a recirculating current, known as a **hydraulic** or "hole," is formed (Figure 28-3). Holes are often difficult to see from upstream, and escaping from large ones can be difficult. Boaters often play in hydraulics, surfing their standing waves. However, a person who is tossed out of his boat or enters a hydraulic unsuspectingly and without understanding what the current is doing can become trapped in the hydraulic's backwash until he eventually tires and drowns.

Low Head Dams Most people think that the danger associated with dams comes from their height. Yet low head dams, which have been called the perfect "drowning machines," are among the most dangerous river features (Figure 28-4). The dams appear harmless because they are only a few feet high. The dams, which are common on rivers in the eastern United States, were usually built to help control river flow and to raise water levels for locks or small hydroelectric sites. They are made of concrete and have vertical abutments on each side. Often, they span the river's entire width.

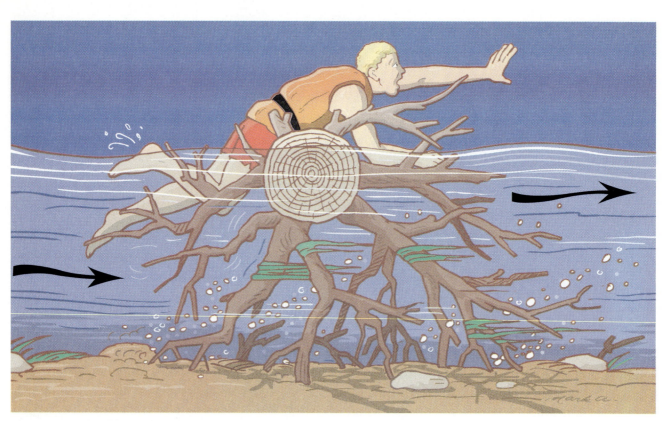

Figure 28-2 Strainers are objects that allow water to flow through them but that will trap other objects—and people.

Low head dams produce dangerous recirculating currents. These currents are like those in a hole, only larger and more uniform across the river. The dams are very difficult to see from upstream, and boaters who approach too closely can easily be swept over them and caught in the current. Boaters or fishermen on the downstream side may also approach too closely, capsize, and

Figure 28-3 When water flows over a large uniform object, it can create a hydraulic or hole with a recirculating current that moves against the river's flow and can trap people.

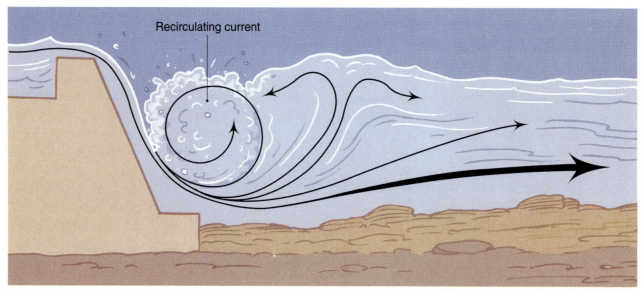
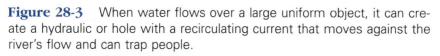

Recirculating current

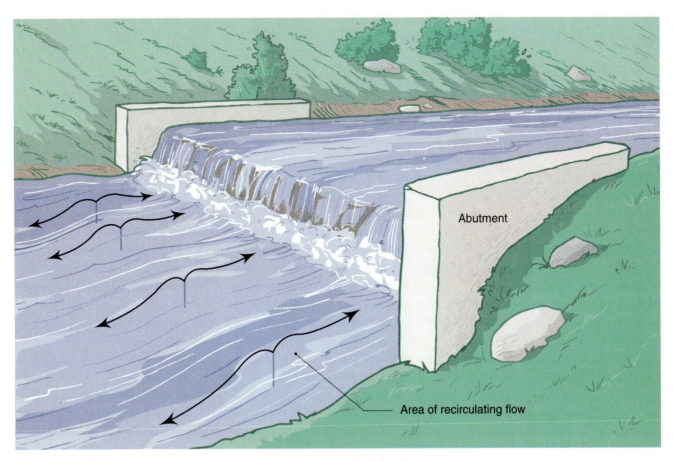

Figure 28-4   Their width, their recirculating currents, and their sheer abutments make low-head dams into treacherous river obstacles.

be caught by the upstream current. Once trapped in the recirculating flow, a person is pushed to the bottom, pulled to the surface, and pushed to the bottom again and again. Often, the force of the flow is so great that a PFD will not keep a person afloat; in fact, PFDs are usually ripped off by the current.

Sometimes, the only chance to get out of the recirculating flow is to swim out at the bottom, if one doesn't get caught in debris on the river bottom. Even if a person manages to work his way to the side of the dam, he may remain trapped by the vertical concrete abutments. Some dams are so wide that shore-based rescue attempts are very difficult.

Extremity entrapment   Attempts to stand up in any fast-moving water can be dangerous. This is especially true when the water is above a person's knees. When trying to stand, a person can easily trap a leg between rocks or other obstructions (Figure 28-5). This typically happens with an inexperienced boater, rafter, or tuber who falls out of his craft. His natural—but incorrect—reaction is to stand up. Instead, the proper thing to do is to get on one's back with the feet pointed downstream and to maneuver with a modified backstroke. When a person's extremity becomes caught, it must be extricated in exactly the same direction that it went in.

Rescue from Moving Water

The basic steps to follow for all water (and ice) rescues are *reach, throw, row,* and *go!*

◆ *Reach.* If the patient is close to shore, be sure you have firm, solid footing. You should be belayed or secured by a line so you cannot be pulled into the water. Reach out to the patient with an oar, a branch, a fishing pole, a towel, or some other object that won't break or pull apart. When he has grasped it, pull him to shore.

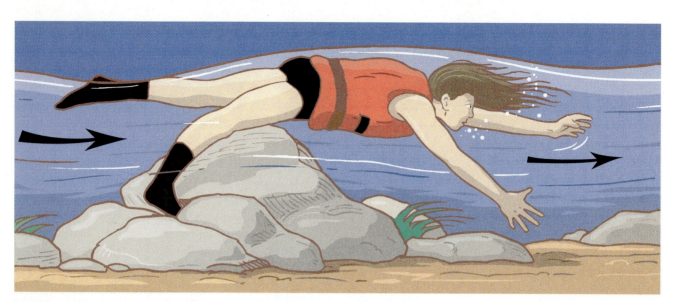

Figure 28-5 If a person's extremity becomes trapped in rocks or another underwater obstruction, a fast-moving current can complicate rescue attempts.

◆ *Throw.* While you remain on shore, throw the patient something and pull him back to shore with it. Emergency vehicles, especially those in jurisdictions with large bodies of water, should have a throw bag containing 100 feet (30 m) of polypropylene rope. The rope should be attached to an object that floats and is heavy enough to throw (Figure 28-6). Throw the object and rope to the patient and, when he grasps it, pull him to shore.

◆ *Row.* If the patient is unresponsive or out of throwing range, row to him in a boat if one is available.

Figure 28-6 Practice with the throw bag so you will be ready to use it in water or ice rescues.

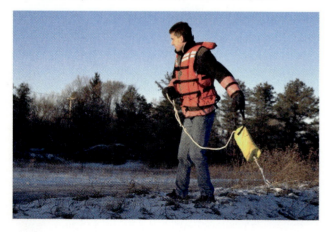

◆ *Go.* If the patient is unresponsive, out of throwing range, and a boat is not available, someone will have to go to him by wading or swimming.

Reach and throw are the two low-risk, shore-based steps that nearly any first responder can apply. *If you can't easily carry out a rescue using simple shore-based techniques, it's time to call for a team specializing in water rescue.*

Once a patient is safely on shore, he may need resuscitation. You can review the emergency care procedures to follow in cases of drownings and near drownings in Chapter 16, "Environmental Emergencies."

There are some things you can do to be better prepared for emergencies involving water rescue. They include the following:

◆ *Know your area.* Spend some time learning the hazards in your area. Where have rescues occurred in the past and why? What has been learned from those rescues? Study potential rescue sites to assess what the difficulty of rescue would be at different water levels.

◆ *Learn about the specialized rescue resources in your area.* What are the capabilities of the different water rescue units in the area? Where are they based? What basic procedures do

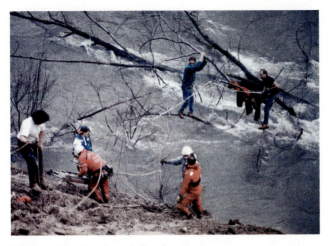

Figure 28-7 Specialized water rescue teams are familiar with techniques that will ensure the safest, most efficient operations.

COMPANY OFFICER'S NOTES

The most important thing you can do during a water rescue is to keep your crew members out of the water! The "go" of reach, throw, row, and go is a last resort after other methods have failed. When rescuers swim to retrieve patients, the results too often include injury or death for patients or rescuers. Unless you are part of a trained team or have special skills, stay out of the water and see that your crew does the same!

Whenever your crew is working near the water, be sure all members wear PFDs! In most cases, turnout gear and boots are not proper PPE for working around the water. While they do provide good insulation, they make swimming difficult and can cause a rescuer to sink.

they employ? Most teams have tremendous insight into local hazards and the techniques needed to rescue people from them (Figure 28-7).

◆ *Carry a PFD and throw bag and learn how to use them.* A PFD is mandatory equipment whenever you are working around the water or ice and especially when you are involved in a rescue. If you accidentally fall in, a PFD could save your life. A water rescue throw bag is an inexpensive tool that can enable you to reach a victim without entering the water. However, you must practice with it to use it effectively!

◆ *Don't enter the water!* Just because you can swim or have some previous water-safety training does not mean you can effect a rescue in moving water. Even specialized teams only attempt swimming rescues as their last resort.

Ice Rescue

People are drawn to water even when it is frozen. Skating, ice-fishing, snowmobiling, and just walking on frozen rivers, ponds, and lakes are all popular winter activities.

Judging the thickness and overall safety of ice is very tricky, however. The old adage "1 inch—keep off, 2 inches—one may, 3 inches—small groups, 4 inches—OK" is not really a very accu-

rate way to gauge safety. Many factors can affect the thickness of the ice over even a small area. For example, underwater springs or outlets can cause turbulence that produces thinner ice in one spot. Decaying plant matter at the bottom of a pond can also alter thickness.

Remember that a person submerged in near-freezing water does not have much time to live. Water near 32°F (0°C) can cause death quickly. Some factors such as clothing with a high insulation value can increase survival time. The longer a person is in the water, however, the lower the core body temperature will drop, lessening the chances of survival.

Whenever you as a first-responding firefighter-EMT encounter a victim who has fallen through ice, immediately call for a specialty rescue team. Then don a PFD and make reasonable attempts to reach or throw something to the victim from shore. If the attempt is successful, you can cancel the request for the specialty team. If it is not, valuable time will not have been wasted before the team is called. In addition to making reasonable rescue attempts from shore, you should prevent well-intentioned bystanders from going out onto the ice in their own rescue attempts. Such attempts will only complicate the rescue situation and may lead to the loss of more lives.

Special Reach and Throw Considerations

The reach, throw, row, go model used for water rescue is also used for ice rescue, but there are some additional things to keep in mind with patients who have fallen through ice.

The rope throw bag is the basic tool for heaving a line to a victim who has gone through the ice. Be aware, however, that as the victim becomes more hypothermic, his motor skills and mental capacities deteriorate. As time passes, he may not be able to grab or hold onto the line that you throw to him.

Another problem with the throw bag is its relatively limited range. It's hard to have much accuracy heaving a bag beyond about 75 feet (23 m). Often, victims who have gone through the ice are farther than that from shore.

Another reaching technique you might use involves an inflated fire hose. By using modified end caps and the air from a SCBA tank, you can quickly inflate a length of fire hose and push it out to the victim. The range this technique offers, however, is also limited.

Special Rowing Considerations

The "row" of reach, throw, row, and go refers to rescue attempts that use a boat as a rescue platform. Using a boat for ice rescues can be very challenging. When ice is thin, you can deploy a conventional boat and row or pole it, breaking through the ice as you head for the patient. Alternatively, you might use a small inflatable craft tethered with ropes fore and aft and pulled from shore. Perhaps the ultimate craft for ice rescue are airboats or hovercrafts. Either craft can be maneuvered over ice, water, or dry land. With skilled operators at the controls, they are able to make rescues when other shore or "live bait" rescues would be nearly impossible.

Going to a Patient Over Ice

Because of the effects of hypothermia on victims, rescuers must have a "go" technique at their disposal. When victims are too incapacitated to hang on to a line or other object, rescuers must go to them. Rescue personnel usually wear "dry" neo-prene ice rescue or exposure suits and are tethered to shore. The rescuer crawls, shuffles, or swims out to grab the victim and pull him to safety using the tether line. This type of rescue should only be attempted by personnel with special training.

Resuscitation

While cold water can be deadly, it can also help save the lives of people immersed in it. This is because of something called the *mammalian diving reflex*. This is how it works: When the face of a human, or any mammal, is plunged into cold water (less than 68°F, or 20°C), the heart rate rapidly decreases, breathing is inhibited, and blood vessels throughout the body constrict. Blood is redistributed from less vital organs to the heart and the brain, which are essential to sustaining life. The colder the water, the more oxygen is diverted to the heart and brain.

The mammalian diving reflex can significantly delay death. Some patients have been resuscitated after 45 minutes under water. The effects of the reflex are most pronounced in children.

As a guideline, start resuscitation on any pulseless, nonbreathing patient who has been submerged in cold water. Transport immediately to the closest medical facility where the patient can be rewarmed. Remember, in these situations a patient is never dead until he is warm and dead.

Confined Spaces and Hazardous Atmospheres

Breathing is normally an automatic process to which we give no thought. We assume that the air we are breathing is safe. At times when the air has a foul odor, irritates our respiratory systems, or is filled with smoke, we can easily perceive a potential danger. At those times, we can remove ourselves from the scene or don appropriate protective equipment.

Unfortunately, it is not always that easy to determine whether air is safe to breathe. This is especially true with air in **confined spaces.** Confined spaces are defined as places with limited access and egress that are not designed for human occupancy (Figure 28-8). In such places, oxygen levels can fall below the levels needed to

Recognizing Confined Spaces

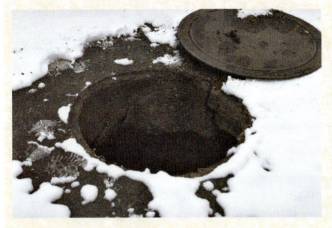

Figure 28-8A Manholes provide access to underground utility vaults.

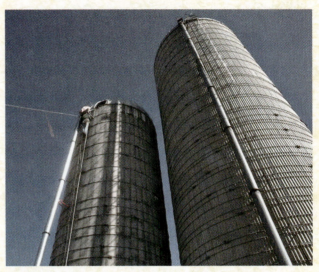

Figure 28-8B Silos.

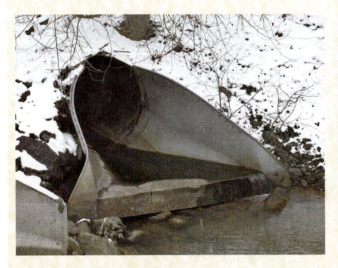

Figure 28-8C A culvert.

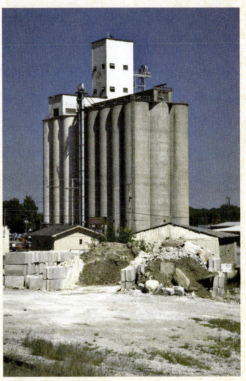

Figure 28-8D A grain elevator.

support life. Toxic or explosive gases can also collect in these places, posing serious dangers to those who enter. Some examples of confined spaces include the following:

- **Storage tanks and vessels** These containers can be designed for over-the-road use or for stationary sites such as oil refineries. They can hold compressed gases or different types of liquids, ranging from water to fuel to chemicals used in manufacturing.

- **Silos** Agricultural silos are perhaps the most common, but silos are also used to hold various types of solids that can flow (Figure 28-8B). Some silos are specifically designed to be oxygen limiting to cause fermentation. These oxygen-limiting silos traditionally have blue exteriors.

- **Storage bins** Grain bins or elevators that hold different types of solids often load at the top and dispense the material at the bottom (Figure 28-8D). The atmosphere in such a structure may be oxygen deficient. The material stored in the structure may also pose a threat of engulfing and suffocating or crushing anyone who falls into it or is trapped under it during an accidental release.

- **Underground vaults** These structures include utility vaults for water or sewer lines, electrical power, or telephone communications. They are usually accessed through manholes (Figure 28-8A). In addition to containing potentially deadly atmospheres, they may also pose threats from electrocution, drowning, hypothermia, and other hazards.

- **Wells, culverts, cisterns** The atmospheres in these structures may be oxygen deficient (Figure 28-8C). These structures also pose additional risks of drowning or entrapment.

Confined Space Hazards

The dangers associated with confined spaces can be subtle and difficult to detect. Too often, rescuers called to aid a patient who has collapsed in a confined space enter the space without properly sizing up the scene. If they fail to take proper precautions, these rescuers can become patients themselves. This can lead to additional casualties as other rescuers attempt to reach the downed rescuers. Be alert to the variety of hazards that you may encounter in confined spaces. These include the following:

Unsafe Oxygen Levels An oxygen-deficient atmosphere is perhaps the greatest hazard in a confined space and among the most common. Such an atmosphere is easily created. For example, as lawn clippings thrown into a cistern decay, they use and displace oxygen, causing an oxygen deficiency. The normal oxygen level in the air we breathe is about 21 percent. When the oxygen level drops below 16 percent, it poses a significant threat to life. The only reliable way to assess the atmosphere in a confined space is to monitor it using an atmospheric gas meter. Use the meter's probe to assess the atmosphere at the top, middle, and bottom of a confined space.

Oxygen levels can also be too high. If the meter reveals an oxygen level of 21 percent or higher, the possibility of rapid combustion poses a serious hazard in the space.

Other Gases Other gases that collect in confined spaces may be toxic or explosive. Monitor the atmosphere of the confined space with a meter before entering. Among the potentially dangerous gases most likely to be encountered are the following:

- Hydrogen sulfide (H_2S)
- Carbon dioxide (CO_2)
- Carbon monoxide (CO)
- Methane (CH_4)

Engulfment Another potential hazard in a confined space is that of engulfment by grain or any other dry material that will flow. Materials stored in grain elevators or other structures sometimes form seemingly solid crusts on their surfaces. The material can feel solid enough to walk on. However, these structures are emptied from the bottom. This can create voids, or empty spaces, in the material above. The crusted surface material can collapse under a person's weight like a snow bridge over a glacial crevasse. The person will then plunge down into the material and be engulfed and suffocated by it.

Machinery Grain elevators and other storage structures often contain various types of machinery to move the materials stored in them. Such machinery might include conveyors, augers, screws, pumps, and other mechanical devices that can entrap a person who is inside the structure. This machinery is usually powered by electricity, which means that the potential for electrocution is also present at such scenes. Motors and other mechanical devices can also "store" power, causing an unsuspecting person to become trapped or injured.

Basic Safety Procedures

OSHA has taken an aggressive approach to protect workers from the hazards of confined spaces. It has drawn up extensive regulations dealing with entry into confined spaces. The regulations require that sites where confined space entry may be necessary go through a permitting process before people are allowed to enter the spaces. The regulations also detail safety measures that should be taken to prevent emergencies. The OSHA regulations require that the following be done before entry into a confined space:

- The atmosphere be monitored for oxygen, carbon monoxide, hydrogen sulfide, and methane
- The space be properly ventilated
- Electrical systems be locked out and tagged out
- Stored energy be dissipated
- Pipes be disconnected or "blanked" out
- People entering the space use appropriate respiratory protection
- Fall-arresting and retrieval devices be used to extricate a person who cannot help himself

Many of the confined space emergencies you respond to will not be at permitted sites. This means that little may have been done to control dangers at the site. When you do respond to a permitted site, it will likely be for an emergency in which workers already on the scene have been unable to recover victims. This means that the rescue is a difficult one that poses significant risks. It can't be stressed too strongly that confined space rescues are complicated, dangerous affairs. Unless you are trained to function as part of a specialized rescue team and have proper equipment available, consider such sites as unsafe to enter.

If you are called to the scene of a confined space emergency, proceed as follows:

1. **Size up the scene and determine the nature of the emergency.**

   —Obtain a copy of the permit for the site and assess the type of work being done.

   —Determine how many patients are inside the space.

   —Determine what hazards the space poses without actually entering the space.

2. **Call for a specialized rescue team.**

3. **Establish a perimeter and do not allow anyone except rescue team members to pass beyond it and enter the space.**

4. **Assist workers at the site with extrication using any remote retrieval device they may be working with.**

5. **Take any reasonable actions to effect the rescue without adding to the risk of an explosion and without entering the space.**

COMPANY OFFICER'S NOTES

As a company officer, you must take the lead in quickly identifying the potential for oxygen-deficient or otherwise hazardous environments at a confined space emergency. Be sure to keep members of your crew from entering the space. Based on your scene size-up, begin to determine if the call is likely to be a rescue or a body recovery situation.

Trench Collapses

Another hazard you may face is a trench collapse at a construction site. Most collapses occur in trenches that are less than 6 feet (1.8 m) wide and 12 feet (3.6 m) deep. Trenches collapse for a variety of reasons. Sometimes dirt excavated from the trench is piled too close to its edge. There may be ground vibrations or water seepage that weaken trench walls. Sometimes trenches intersect and a common wall will give way.

When a trench does collapse, workers inside them may be completely or partially buried. Soil is heavy. A person whose chest is buried by 2 feet (0.6 m) of soil in a trench collapse may be trapped by a weight ranging from 700 to 1,000 pounds (318 to 454 kg). Being buried alive can thus rapidly lead to asphyxia for a victim whose chest is buried. Rapid rescue is necessary, but people who jump into a trench to attempt a rescue without carefully sizing up the scene risk being entrapped by a secondary collapse.

Once again, OSHA has acted aggressively to protect workers by setting certain requirements for trenches. These requirements have decreased, but not eliminated, trench collapses. One key requirement is that any excavation deeper than 5 feet (1.5 m) must use shoring or a protective device called a trench box to prevent trench cave-ins. The use of trench boxes is now common at construction sites around the country. You should be aware, however, that some contractors do not use the protective devices in hopes of cutting time and costs on the job. Also, many "do-it-your-selfers" who dig trenches on home construction projects may not be aware of OSHA regulations and safe procedures (Figure 28-9).

When you arrive at the scene of a trench collapse, remember that an immediate, aggressive rescue attempt may not be the best way to deal with the situation. Safe rescue requires careful

Figure 28-9 If trenches do not comply with OSHA regulations, the possibility of collapse is increased.

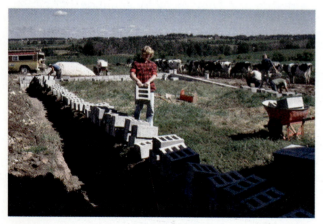

planning and a methodical approach. Avoid rescue attempts unless the trench is less than waist deep. Proceed following these steps:

1. **Secure the scene, and establish a perimeter around the site.**
2. **Do not allow anyone to enter the trench.**
3. **Call for a specialized trench rescue team.**

Rough Terrain Evacuations

Outdoor sports have become increasingly popular in recent years. These sports—hiking, rock climbing, mountain biking, and cross-country skiing—draw ever larger numbers of people into rugged terrain. Inevitably, this means more accidents in places where patients are hard to reach and from which their removal is difficult. As a firefighter-EMT, you must know how to perform litter evacuations over rough terrain without causing additional injury to patients. You must also know how to assess terrain and recognize when to call in a specialized rescue team.

Litter Carries

Carrying a patient on a litter over flat ground is a strenuous task under ideal conditions. As terrain becomes rougher, the litter carry becomes more demanding. Remember also that long litter carries are not confined to the wilderness. Long carries are common in suburban and rural areas. Even there, they are strenuous undertakings requiring many rescuers.

For a 1-mile (1.6 k) litter carry, 18 to 20 people should be available to assure sufficient manpower. Even with this many bearers, the carry could take up to an hour depending upon the terrain. A team of six litter bearers, as close to the same height as possible, should start the carry. After carrying the litter a short distance, the bearers change positions. After another short distance, the bearers change sides. As the carry continues, fresh bearers are rotated into the team, giving the original bearers a chance to rest.

Some devices are available that can ease the difficulty of a litter carry. For example, bearers can run webbing straps over the litter rails, across their shoulders and into their free hands. This will help distribute the weight across the bearers' backs.

Another helpful device is the litter wheel. It attaches to the bottom of a Stokes litter frame and takes most of the weight of the litter. The bearers then keep the litter balanced and control its forward motion. The wheel, however, works best over flatter terrain.

Carrying a litter looks easy but is deceptively difficult. Performing practice exercises is the best way of understanding just how difficult it is. Once you have carried a litter over different types of terrain, you will be better prepared to assess the various resources that may be necessary in emergency situations.

Low-Angle Rescue

As the angle of the terrain increases, it becomes more difficult for bearers to carry a litter, even with a litter wheel. In these situations, rescuers are forced to try to hold a heavy litter level while scrambling up hillsides. As slopes grow steeper, the risk of bearers falling and dropping the patient increases.

In these cases, bearers must perform what is known as a **low-angle rescue.** This procedure requires the use of ropes, hardware, and safety systems (Figure 28-10). In a low-angle rescue, a rope is secured at the top and bottom of the slope across which the litter is to be carried. The litter is then attached to the rope. The bearers hold the litter and walk with it up or down the slope. Low-angle rescue techniques should be considered under the following conditions:

◆ Slopes are as much as 40°.

Figure 28-10 A low-angle rescue operation.

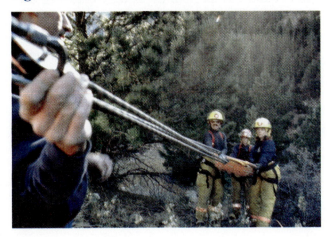

◆ The bearers do not need to use their hands to balance on or move up or down the slope.

◆ A fall is not likely to result in serious injury or death.

One of the most common low-angle rescue situations involves a car that has gone off the road and over the side of a steep bank in hilly or mountainous terrain. Responders who frequently deal with such situations develop their low-angle rescue skills and do not need to call for specialized teams.

High-Angle Rescue

Conditions more extreme than those described above call for **high-angle rescue** techniques. These conditions include the following:

◆ Slopes are greater than 40°.

◆ The bearers must use their hands to balance on or move up or down the slope.

◆ A fall is likely to result in serious injury or death.

◆ The patient is beyond the reach of firefighters working from aerial apparatus.

◆ Rappelling is required to reach a patient.

Generally, it is obvious when terrain requires high-angle rescue techniques—a cliff, a gorge, the side of a building. Rescue situations where slopes are only slightly greater than 40° might be treated as low angle if the terrain is smooth enough, but it is probably safer to use high-angle techniques on them. When your scene size-up reveals high-angle rescue conditions, call for a specialized team to carry out the rescue.

Helicopters in Rescue Operations

Chapter 25, "Emergency Vehicle Operations," discussed the basics of using helicopters to transport patients. The helicopter also has great potential in rescue operations. Its abilities to hover, to land in tight places, and to carry people and equipment make it a logical rescue platform. While the benefits of using a helicopter in a rescue operation may be great, so is the potential for disaster. Wind and weather conditions can make the handling of a helicopter difficult. The fact that helicopters can land in tight spaces means their rotors can pose a danger for ground rescue personnel. The use of helicopters in rescue efforts must be carefully planned and coordinated. In addition, a contingency plan must be ready in case the helicopter does not arrive or cannot carry out its intended mission. Before calling for a helicopter in a rescue situation, think carefully. Consider what the helicopter can and cannot do. Some of the helicopter's limitations and abilities are summarized below.

Visual Limitations

Aircraft can take off, fly to, and land at another airport in conditions of poor visibility by using instruments. In rescue situations, however, helicopters require good visibility. Helicopter crews must be able to make and maintain visual contact with ground personnel and to watch for hazards. If they are unable to do these things, both the rescue mission and the safety of helicopter and ground crews are in jeopardy. Usually, helicopters cannot be used in rescue operations when visibility falls below established minimum standards. While the standards can vary, the following are generally accepted minimums:

◆ Day—500-foot (150 m) cloud ceiling and 1 mile (1.6 k) of visibility

◆ Night—1,000-foot (300 m) cloud ceiling and 3 miles (4.8 k) of visibility

Even though minimum standards are provided for night operations, those operations are much more dangerous than daylight missions. Be sure that the benefits of conducting a night operation outweigh the potential risks.

Altitude and Air Temperature

Altitude plays a role in a helicopter's performance in rescue operations. The helicopter's ability to hover is what makes it especially useful as a rescue craft. As altitude increases, air density decreases. This means that the helicopter requires more power to hover. The more power the helicopter uses to hover, the less load it can carry. At some point, depending on the aircraft, the mission load requirements, and the elevation of the emergency scene, it may not be possible to accomplish the mission.

Air temperature also affects helicopter performance. The warmer the temperature, the less dense the air becomes. As with an increase in altitude, the helicopter must use more power to hover as the air grows warmer.

Helicopter Handling Considerations

Piloting a rotor craft is a far more complex job than piloting a fixed wing craft. The pilot must coordinate three main control systems simultaneously. At the same time, he must factor in the effects of altitude, temperature, the weight of load, and the distance from the ground on his craft's performance.

Take-offs, landings, and hovering maneuvers are especially difficult. It is at these times that the risk of a crash is greatest. Consider, for example, that when the craft is hovering to attempt a rescue or to deliver an external load the pilot cannot actually see the target, which is below the helicopter. He must rely on the crew chief to watch the target and to guide the pilot into the right position with spoken directions.

During these maneuvers, the pilot needs to see a reference point on the ground that he can use to position the aircraft. At night or in low light conditions, finding and holding such a reference point can be very difficult. The situation becomes even more complicated in windy or turbulent conditions.

Space and Load

The size of the helicopter and its engines directly affect what it can accomplish during a rescue mission. Some aircraft can carry a whole squad of people and still provide hoisting capability. Others are small and cannot carry much more than a pilot, a patient, and one crew member.

Helicopters are also very weight sensitive. Fuel load, equipment, number of crew members, and number of patients must be considered when a rescue operation is being planned. Prior to certain missions, a helicopter may have to be emptied to allow for pick-up of a patient. On other missions, a heavily weighted craft may be able to land in a tight spot but then be unable to take off from it without first off-loading some gear or crew members.

Every aircraft is different and has different flying and carrying characteristics. Learn what the rescue aircraft in your local jurisdiction can do *before* you need them.

Special Tactics

When a helicopter's mission is to land, pick up a patient, and transport him to a hospital, firefighter-EMTs need do nothing more than select a safe landing zone, mark it, and secure the area. One of the main reasons for using a helicopter, however, is its ability to insert rescuers and extract victims *without* landing. The helicopter allows rescue personnel to rappel from the craft to the ground. It can hoist victims or loads off the ground. It can also transport those loads as they dangle from cables beneath the aircraft.

Federal Aviation Administration (FAA) regulations control the use of special tactics. In general, hoisting of patients or personnel, rappelling from a craft, and flying with external loads are violations, unless undertaken by public aircraft during an emergency operation to save life. Under this rule, most hospital-based "medevac" helicopters could not perform the same functions as public aircraft in emergencies. Keep this restriction in mind if you are thinking of calling for a specialized helicopter rescue operation.

Special tactics are high-risk operations. Rescuers and victims being hoisted or carried during them are considered "external loads." If the craft becomes destabilized during flight or another emergency occurs, external loads are expendable cargo! The pilot or crew chief can jettison the load with the push of a button. They are within their rights to do so if the ship and its crew are in jeopardy. Because the risk level is potentially so high, you should be sure that use of special tactics is absolutely necessary before you request a rescue operation involving them.

Hoisting Some helicopters are equipped with mechanical hoists to insert and extract people from the ground. They are most commonly found on military and some public safety aircraft. There are a variety of devices used to attach a person to the cable and transport him to the helicopter. Hoisting operations require hover time. The hover time may vary depending on the speed of the hoist and the amount of cable payed out. Hoisting operations are also limited by the safe working load of the cable and by the number of duty cycles (raise/lower) of the system.

If you will be working around helicopters with hoisting capabilities, obtain some training with your area's air rescue service. Its members will familiarize you with both general safety procedures and those specific to the aircraft they use. For example, one procedure that applies to all helicopters that use hoist cables is grounding. When a cable is payed out from the ship, it builds up a charge of static electricity. As the cable is lowered, allowing it to touch the ground will ground it and dissipate the charge before anyone handles it. If this is not done, the first person to touch the cable will become the ground and get an electrical shock. This is an example of one of many safety issues associated with hoist operation.

Helicopter Short-Haul Technique The short-haul technique was developed by mountain rescue teams in Europe and Canada. It allows patients and rescue personnel to fly beneath helicopters as external loads. (The procedure has been called the "dope on a rope" technique.) It is a high-risk operation, one that should only be undertaken by specialized rescue teams.

The technique can be used by light-duty helicopters without hoisting capabilities. It allows these aircraft to both insert and extract rescuers and victims from an emergency scene where landing is not possible. Generally, a weighted rope (with a back up) is attached to the cargo hook or belly band of a helicopter. A rescuer wearing a flight helmet with communications capability and a harness is clipped onto the other end of the rope. The helicopter ascends, and the rescuer dangles beneath the ship as he is flown to the target area and gently lowered into position. To extract a patient, the ship flies into position and hovers. The ground team, meanwhile, clips the litter or a victim wearing a harness onto the line. The helicopter then ascends, flying the patient back to a staging area.

HAZARDOUS MATERIALS

The U.S. Department of Transportation (DOT) defines a hazardous material as "any substance which may pose an unreasonable risk to health and safety of operating or emergency personnel, the public, and/or the environment if not properly controlled during handling, storage, manufacture, processing, packaging, use, disposal, or transportation." Hazardous materials are all around us, as bleaches and cleansers under the kitchen sink, as anti-freezes and windshield washing solutions in the garage, and as fertilizers and pesticides in the garden shed.

Hazardous materials include chemicals and waste products. They can be solids, liquids, and gases. They can burn, poison, or corrode. More than 50 billion tons of them are manufactured in the United States. Some 4 billion tons are shipped within the United States.

Despite the dangers, we usually live in relative safety with the hazardous materials around us.

Federal, state, and local governments regulate nearly every aspect of their manufacturing, distribution, transportation, and use. These regulations aim to preserve the benefits derived from the use of the hazardous materials while limiting their dangers.

Unfortunately, the regulations too often fail to achieve their aims. Accidents still happen, and hazardous materials can be spilled or released because of equipment failure, vehicle accidents, environmental conditions, and human error. Also, many people ignore regulations, hoping to save money by scrimping on safeguards during transport or ignoring guidelines for disposal of hazardous materials. The consequences of accidental or intentional violation of regulations can be devastating and reach far beyond the immediate scene of the incident.

Sometimes it will be immediately obvious that an incident involves hazardous materials. There may be a fire at a chemical plant or a rollover of a tanker truck with "CORROSIVE" labels on it. You will naturally be suspicious of incidents at factories, along railroad lines, and on roads and highways. Be alert, though, for the possible presence of hazardous materials in rural and agricultural areas. Be prepared for the possibility of hazardous materials even on a call to a home. A malfunctioning heater/furnace may have filled the house with carbon monoxide, or someone attempting to make a more powerful cleaning solution may have mixed bleach and ammonia and instead produced chlorine gas.

Special training is required to deal with hazardous materials. If you discover or suspect the presence of hazardous materials at a scene, move back from the scene or do not enter it. Assess the situation, call dispatch, and request a hazardous materials (hazmat) team.

Training for Hazardous Materials Emergencies

Two federal agencies, OSHA and the Environmental Protection Agency (EPA), have developed regulations for dealing with hazardous materials emergencies. The regulations set out the knowledge, skills, and training required of rescuers in these situations. They are found in the OSHA publication "29 CFR 1910.120—Hazardous Waste Operations and Emergency Response Standard (1989)."

According to the standard, employers must provide training for "all employees who participate, or are expected to participate, in emergency response to hazardous substance accidents." The regulations describe four levels of training.

◆ *First Responder Awareness* This level is for those who are likely to witness or discover a hazardous materials emergency. These responders are trained to recognize a hazmat problem, to know the proper organization to deal with the problem, to know how to contact that organization, and to make the call for assistance. These responders then take no further action. No minimum number of training hours is required.

◆ *First Responder Operations* This level is for those who initially respond to a hazmat release for the purpose of protecting people, property, and the environment. They stay a safe distance from the material while trying to keep the emergency from spreading by limiting any further exposures to the material. A minimum of 8 hours of training is required.

◆ *Hazardous Materials Technician* This level is for responders who actually plug, patch, or stop the release of a hazardous substance. A minimum of 24 hours of training is required.

◆ *Hazardous Materials Specialist* These responders have advanced knowledge and skills. They provide command and support activities at the site of a hazardous materials incident. A minimum of 24 hours of training beyond Technician level is required.

The training levels outlined by OSHA have a fire service focus. To supplement them, the National Fire Protection Association has published NFPA 473, *Standard for Competencies for EMS Personnel Responding to Hazardous Materials Incidents*. This publication deals with competencies for EMS personnel at hazmat incidents.

The Role of EMTs at Hazmat Incidents

As a firefighter EMT, you stand a good chance of discovering a hazmat incident. You may be dis-patched to a reported traffic accident, poisoning, or "unknown" problem. Only when you arrive at the scene and size it up do you discover that hazardous materials are involved. The decisions you make and actions you take at that point lay the crucial groundwork for the handling of the incident. Be sure you know what your responsibilities are at a hazmat incident and carry them out fully.

Recognizing a Hazmat Incident

Some hazmat incidents are obvious even to untrained observers. Others offer only subtle signs. You must learn to recognize incidents at both extremes and all those that fall between. Start with the obvious. Think "hazmat" whenever you respond to the type of scene in which hazmat incidents are most common. These include incidents involving the following:

◆ Highway accidents involving common carriers.

◆ Trucking terminals

◆ Chemical plants or facilities where chemicals are used

◆ Delivery trucks

◆ Agricultural and garden centers

◆ Railway corridors

◆ Laboratories

Every community has sites where chemicals are used or hazardous materials are stored. Become familiar with the locations of those sites in your community. Spend time learning about your departments' and other public safety agencies' plans for dealing with hazmat incidents in your community.

Remember when dealing with a hazmat incident that you must ignore your natural impulse to rush to aid patients. Doing so can leave you injured or dead. Never assume that the scene is safe!

Take a command position upwind and uphill of the site. Stay a safe distance from the suspected hazardous material. Size up the scene before taking any action. Once you have confirmed that the scene is a hazmat incident, only personnel trained to the level of Hazardous Materials Technician and who are properly equipped should enter the immediate site.

Establishing Control of the Scene

Your priorities at the scene of a hazmat incident are your safety, the safety of your crew, and then the safety of the patient(s) and of the public. If yours is the first unit on scene, establish a "danger zone" and a "safe zone." Keep everyone out of the danger zone and try to convince onlookers to leave the area. Stay in the safe zone until trained hazmat personnel arrive.

To ensure that expert help does arrive, call for it. Request appropriately trained hazmat crews, but don't forget other resources that might be needed. Special rescue units might be needed to remove victims. Police units could help in keeping civilians from entering the scene. Public utilities crews can assist with requests involving electricity, gas, or water. Also request any additional EMS resources you think may be needed.

Implement your department's Incident Management System. Establish command and hold it until relieved by someone higher in the chain of command.

While waiting for hazmat crews to arrive, keep the situation from becoming worse. Evacuate people from the area around the incident, if necessary. Move bystanders as far back from the incident as possible. Do not risk your personal safety, or allow others on your crew to risk theirs, by making rescue attempts.

Prepare for the arrival of additional resources by setting up control zones (Figure 28-11):

◆ **The hot (red) zone**—This is the area of contamination or danger at the center of the incident. Isolate it. Allow no one to enter it without proper PPE. Hold any patients who escape from it in the next zone, the warm zone, for decontamination and/or treatment.

◆ **The warm (yellow) zone**—This is the area immediately adjacent to the hot zone. You should set up a decontamination corridor in the warm zone. That is where decontamination procedures for patients and rescue personnel leaving the hot zone should be performed.

◆ **The cold (green) zone**—This is the next zone after the warm zone. It is the staging ground for rescuers and their equipment. You and your crew should be in this zone.

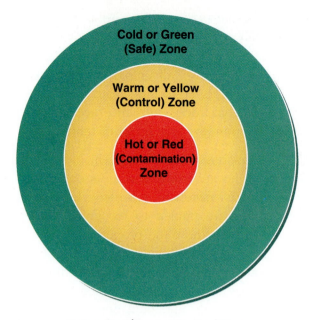

Hot or Red (Contamination) Zone
- Contamination is actually present.
- Personnel must wear appropriate protective gear.
- Number of rescuers limited to those absolutely necessary.
- Bystanders never allowed.

Warm or Yellow (Control) Zone
- Area surrounding the contamination zone.
- Vital to preventing spread of contamination.
- Personnel must wear appropriate protective gear.
- Life-saving emergency care and decontamination are performed.

Cold or Green (Safe) Zone
- Normal triage, stabilization, and treatment are performed.
- Rescuers must shed contaminated gear before entering the cold zone.

Figure 28-11 Zones at a hazmat incident.

Identifying the Substance

Once you have established control of the scene, attempt to identify the hazardous material involved in the incident (Figure 28-12). Doing this will help you determine the severity of the incident. If you know what the hazardous material is, you can better estimate the risks to rescuers, patients, the general public, and the environment. At this stage, you will also try to find out the following:

◆ What can you hear, see, and/or smell?

◆ What are the properties of the substance and the dangers posed by it?

◆ Is there any imminent danger of contamination spreading?

◆ How many victims are involved?

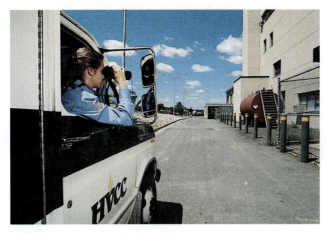

Figure 28-12 Use binoculars when inspecting the scene of a suspected hazmat incident for signs, labels, and placards.

◆ Is there any danger that the victims will contaminate other people—referred to as **secondary contamination**—upon leaving the scene?

Remember that you must try to identify the substance and answer these questions without getting too close to the scene. You can get the needed information in several ways.

◆ *Use binoculars to scan the scene for signs, labels, or placards warning of hazardous substances.* These indicators may be attached to railroad cars, trucks, or storage facilities such as tanks (Figure 28-13). The most common systems that use placards and labels include the following:

Figure 28-13 Vehicles carrying hazardous materials are required to display placards indicating the nature of their cargoes.

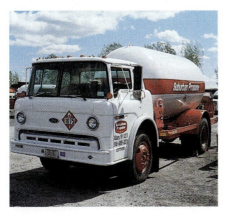

—*The National Fire Protection Association (NFPA) 704 System.* The NFPA 704 system is used at fixed storage facilities. It involves a diamond-shaped symbol divided into four smaller diamonds of different colors (Figure 28-14). The system uses both color and number coding. The color shows the type of hazard the material presents—fire (red), health (blue), or reactivity (yellow). The number shows how great a hazard the material presents on a scale of 0 to 4, with 0 being the lowest. In the smaller white diamond, other specific hazards are identified with abbreviations. Note that this system gives you basic information about the dangers of a substance but does not identify specific substances.

—*U.S. Department of Transportation labels and placards.* U.S. DOT regulations require that packages, storage containers, and vehicles carrying hazardous materials display warning labels or placards (Figure 28-15). The colors,

Figure 28-14 Key to the National Fire Protection Association (NFPA) 704 hazardous materials classification.

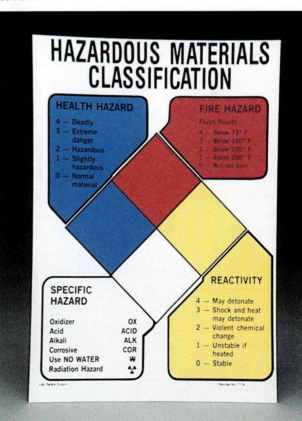

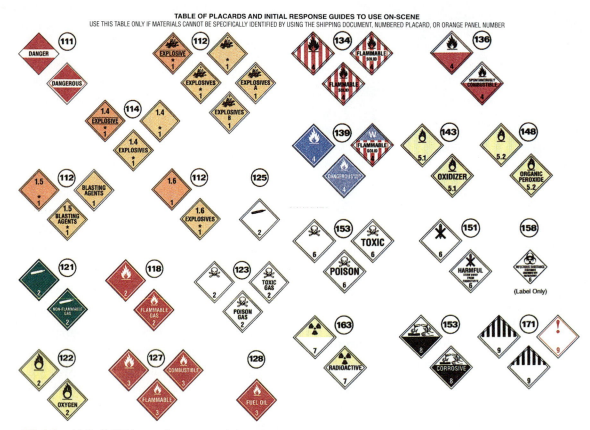

Figure 28-15   U.S. DOT hazardous materials placards.

legends, and code numbers on the labels and placards show the type of hazard the material presents—such as flammable, poison, explosive, radioactivity. Older placards are usually orange and display a United Nations (UN) or North American (NA) identification number. That number can help you determine the identity of the hazardous material.

◆ *Interview drivers, workers, or others leaving the hot zone.* Pay careful attention to their answers. Vehicle operators usually know the type of material they are hauling. Workers in factories know what types of chemicals their plant uses, their properties, and where they are stored. Some of these people may also be carrying or know where to get other types of information about the hazardous materials including the following:

—*Shipping documents.* Trucks, trains, boats, and aircraft should carry shipping papers describing the material being carried. If you can safely obtain these papers, do so. Unfor-

tunately, information on such papers is often incomplete or inaccurate.

—*Material Safety Data Sheets.* Employers at sites where hazardous materials are used are required to keep copies of these sheets and make them available to workers. The sheets usually list the names and characteristics of the materials, what types of health, fire, and reactivity dangers the materials pose, any special equipment or techniques required for safe handling of the materials, and suggested emergency first-aid treatment (Figure 28-16).

With the information that you gather using the methods above, you can find out more about the material and the actions you should take in dealing with it. Remember that it is difficult to take effective action in a hazmat incident unless the substance is identified! Other sources of more detailed information include the following:

◆ *North American Emergency Response Guidebook* (RSPA P 5800.7) This book, jointly

THE Clorox Company
7200 Johnson Drive
Pleasanton, California 94566
Tel. (415) 847-6100

Material Safety
Data Sheets

Health	2+
Flammability	0
Reactivity	1
Personal Protection	B

I – CHEMICAL IDENTIFICATION

Name	regular Clorox Bleach	CAS No.	N/A
Description	clear, light yellow liquid with chlorine odor	RTECs No.	N/A

Other Designations	Manufacturer	Emergency Procedure
EPA Reg. No. 5813-1 Sodium hypochlorite solution Liquid chlorine bleach Clorox Liquid Bleach	The Clorox Company 1221 Broadway Oakland, CA 94612	• Notify your supervisor • Call your local poison control center OR • Rocky Mountain Poison Center (303)573-1014

II – HEALTH HAZARD DATA

• Causes severe but temporary eye injury. May irritate skin. May cause nausea and vomiting if ingested. Exposure to vapor or mist may irritate nose, throat and lungs. The following medical conditions may be aggravated by exposure to high concentrations of vapor or mist: heart conditions or chronic respiratory problems such as asthma, chronic bronchitis or obstructive lung disease. Under normal consumer use conditions the likelihood of any adverse health effects are low. FIRST AID: EYE CONTACT: Immediately flush eyes with plenty of water. If irritation persists, see a doctor. SKIN CONTACT: Remove contaminated clothing. Wash area with water. INGESTION: Drink a glassful of water and call a physician. INHALATION: If breathing problems develop remove to fresh air.

III – HAZARDOUS INGREDIENTS

Ingredients	Concentration	Worker Exposure Limit
Sodium hypochlorite CAS# 7681-52-9	5.25%	not established

None of the ingredients in this product are on the IARC, NTP or OSHA carcinogen list. Occasional clinical reports suggest a low potential for sensitization upon exaggerated exposure to sodium hypochlorite if skin damage (e.g., irritation) occurs during exposure. Routine clinical tests conducted on intact skin with Clorox Liquid Bleach found no sensitization in the test subjects.

IV – SPECIAL PROTECTION INFORMATION

Hygienic Practices: Wear safety glasses. With repeated or prolonged use, wear gloves.

Engineering Controls: Use general ventilation to minimize exposure to vapor or mist.

Work Practices: Avoid eye and skin contact and inhalation of vapor or mist.

V – SPECIAL PRECAUTIONS

Keep out of reach of children. Do not get in eyes or on skin. Wash thoroughly with soap and water after handling. Do not mix with other household chemicals such as toilet bowl cleaners, rust removers, vinegar, acid or ammonia containing products. Store in a cool, dry place. Do not reuse empty container; rinse container and put in trash container.

VI – SPILL OR LEAK PROCEDURES

Small quantities of less than 5 gallons may be flushed down drain. For larger quantities wipe up with an absorbent material or mop and dispose of in accordance with local, state and federal regulations. Dilute with water to minimize oxidizing effect on spilled surface.

VII – REACTIVITY DATA

Stable under normal use and storage conditions. Strong oxidizing agent. Reacts with other household chemicals such as toilet bowl cleaners, rust removers, vinegar, acids or ammonia containing products to produce hazardous gases, such as chlorine and other chlorinated species. Prolonged contact with metal may cause pitting or discoloration.

VIII – FIRE AND EXPLOSION DATA

Not flammable or explosive. In a fire, cool containers to prevent rupture and release of sodium chlorate.

IX – PHYSICAL DATA

Boiling point....................................212°F/100°C (decomposes)
Specific Gravity (H$_2$O = 1)............1.085
Solubility in Water..........................complete
pH...11.4

Figure 28-16   A Material Safety Data Sheet.

published by the U.S. Department of Transportation, Transport Canada, and the Secretariat of Communications and Transportation of Mexico, should be on board every emergency vehicle (Figure 28-17). It contains a table of commonly used DOT placards and labels and lists more than a thousand chemicals. These chemicals are cross-referenced to a guide that briefly describes what actions should be taken in emergencies.

◆ *The Chemical Transportation Emergency Center (CHEMTREC).* This organization was established by the Chemical Manufacturer's Association. It maintains a 24-hour, toll-free telephone service to provide information about hazardous materials. CHEMTREC describes the properties of the chemicals involved in an incident and explains how to handle the emergency. CHEMTREC will even contact shippers or manufacturers of chemicals for more detailed information and field assistance. In the United States and Canada, the toll-free CHEMTREC number is 800-424-9300. For collect calls and calls from other

points of origin, the number is 703-527-3887. CHEMTREC can also refer you to the proper state and federal authorities for incidents involving radioactive materials.

◆ *CHEMTEL, Inc.* This is an emergency response communications center. In the United States and Canada, it can be reached, toll-free, 24 hours a day at 800-255-3924. For collect calls and calls from other points of origin, the number is 813-979-0626. CHEMTEL can also refer you to the proper state and federal authorities for incidents involving radioactive materials.

◆ *Your regional poison control center.* These centers are too frequently overlooked during hazmat incidents. Their reference and medical resources can provide essential guidance in the decontamination and treatment of patients affected by hazardous materials.

When you contact any of the organizations described above, be prepared to provide the following information:

◆ Your name and call-back number (and FAX number, if applicable)

◆ The nature and location of the problem

◆ The identification numbers of materials involved (if they can be obtained safely)

◆ The names of the carrier, shipper, manufacturer, consignee, and point of origin

◆ The container type and size

◆ Whether the container is in a fixed location or on a transport vehicle

◆ The estimated quantity of material transported and released

◆ Local conditions (weather, proximity to schools or housing, etc.)

◆ Number of injuries and/or exposures

◆ Emergency services that have been notified

Keep your line of communication to the organization open at all times.

Any information gathered both from on-scene witnesses and from resource centers such as CHEMTREC should be immediately communicated to the officer in charge of the responding hazmat team.

Figure 28-17 Always have the latest copy of the *North American Emergency Response Guidebook* aboard your vehicle.

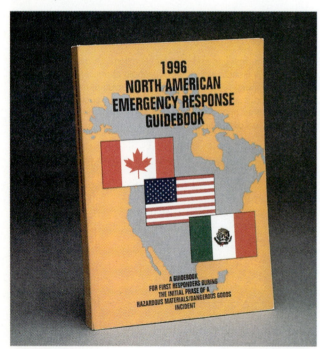

Establishing the Medical Treatment Sector

Rescue personnel and equipment must stage in the cold zone. As a firefighter providing emergency medical services at an incident, you will have two chief responsibilities: to monitor and rehabilitate hazmat team members and to take care of the injured.

Rehabilitation Operations To safely enter the hot zone, hazmat team members must wear chemical-protective clothing and breathing apparatus that impede heat loss and can increase risk of developing heat-related illnesses. Team members must be carefully monitored before, during and after emergency operations. This is done to make sure that their conditions do not deteriorate to the point where their safety or the integrity of the operation is endangered. Monitoring is carried out in the Rehab Sector. How to establish that sector and the procedures to follow in it were discussed in Chapter 27, "Emergency Incident Rehabilitation." You may wish to review that material at this time.

Decontamination Considerations As an EMT, you must work with the Incident Commander and hazmat team members to determine the most appropriate course of action to take with patients. The decision on whether to stay at the scene and decontaminate or to begin evacuation must be made after careful consultation with CHEMTREC, the regional poison control center, and other reference sources.

The hazmat team will set up a decontamination (decon) corridor in the warm zone. In it, they will provide field decon for both team members and any patients rescued (Figure 28-18). They should establish the decon corridor before sending any team members into the hot zone.

EMS providers have the responsibility of setting up the medical treatment area in the cold zone to receive decontaminated patients. Unless EMS providers are trained to the level of Hazmat Technician and function as part of the hazmat team, they must remain in the cold zone.

The field decon process is designed to remove most of the hazardous material and deliver a "clean" patient to EMS personnel for care and transportation. However, there may still be some chance of secondary contamination from patients to EMS personnel. It is important that EMS personnel work closely with the decon officer and consult with medical direction on both treatment and appropriate protection during transportation. Keep the following points in mind when you must treat and transport hazmat patients:

- *Field-decontaminated patients are not completely "clean."* Chemicals that pose a risk of secondary contamination to rescuers may settle in hard-to-clean areas of the body. These areas typically include the scalp/hair, groin, buttocks, arm pits, and between the fingers and toes.

- *Personal protective equipment or clothing is necessary to prevent secondary contamination of rescuers.* Standard PPE for EMS providers at a hazmat incident includes Tyvek coveralls and booties. A double layer of gloves may be necessary. Nitrile or neoprene gloves are often used because they are more resistant to chemicals than standard latex gloves. Check with the decon officer to determine if your equipment is appropriate or if the hazmat team might have some better items available for you to use.

- *Vehicles must be protected from contamination.* During the decon process, patients are thoroughly washed. When EMS providers receive patients, they are often dripping wet. Because the field decon process doesn't clean patients completely, some of the water dripping off a patient could contaminate an emergency vehicle. To prevent this, contain the water runoff. You can do this by placing the patient in a disposable decontamination pool or by covering the inside of the emergency vehicle with plastic sheeting.

- *Consider any equipment that is used to be disposable.* It may not be possible to decontaminate equipment used to move or treat a patient. You may have to dispose of spine boards, splints, blood-pressure cuffs, stethoscopes, and other gear.

9-Station Decontamination Procedure

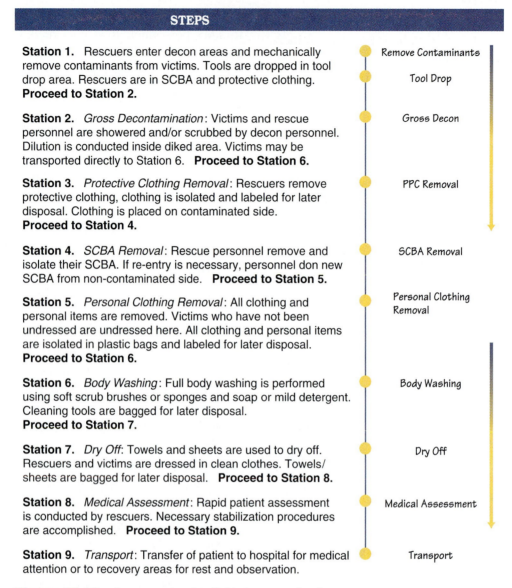

STEPS
Station 1. Rescuers enter decon areas and mechanically remove contaminants from victims. Tools are dropped in tool drop area. Rescuers are in SCBA and protective clothing. **Proceed to Station 2.**
Station 2. *Gross Decontamination*: Victims and rescue personnel are showered and/or scrubbed by decon personnel. Dilution is conducted inside diked area. Victims may be transported directly to Station 6. **Proceed to Station 6.**
Station 3. *Protective Clothing Removal*: Rescuers remove protective clothing, clothing is isolated and labeled for later disposal. Clothing is placed on contaminated side. **Proceed to Station 4.**
Station 4. *SCBA Removal*: Rescue personnel remove and isolate their SCBA. If re-entry is necessary, personnel don new SCBA from non-contaminated side. **Proceed to Station 5.**
Station 5. *Personal Clothing Removal*: All clothing and personal items are removed. Victims who have not been undressed are undressed here. All clothing and personal items are isolated in plastic bags and labeled for later disposal. **Proceed to Station 6.**
Station 6. *Body Washing*: Full body washing is performed using soft scrub brushes or sponges and soap or mild detergent. Cleaning tools are bagged for later disposal. **Proceed to Station 7.**
Station 7. *Dry Off*: Towels and sheets are used to dry off. Rescuers and victims are dressed in clean clothes. Towels/sheets are bagged for later disposal. **Proceed to Station 8.**
Station 8. *Medical Assessment*: Rapid patient assessment is conducted by rescuers. Necessary stabilization procedures are accomplished. **Proceed to Station 9.**
Station 9. *Transport*: Transfer of patient to hospital for medical attention or to recovery areas for rest and observation.

Station labels: Remove Contaminants, Tool Drop, Gross Decon, PPC Removal, SCBA Removal, Personal Clothing Removal, Body Washing, Dry Off, Medical Assessment, Transport

Figure 28-18 An example of a field decontamination process.

◆ *Decontaminate any equipment that is not disposed of before stowing it or using it again.* Be aware that much equipment may be out of service as the operation goes on.

Care of Injured and Contaminated Patients When providing care at a hazmat incident, you are likely to encounter four types of patients:

◆ Uninjured and not contaminated

◆ Injured but not contaminated

◆ Uninjured but contaminated

◆ Injured and contaminated

You should treat anyone who is not contaminated, whether injured or not, as you would a regular patient. However, patients who are contaminated, whether injured or not, pose the risk of secondary contamination. Normal hazmat procedures call for EMS personnel to treat patients only after they have received field decon from the hazmat team. Unfortunately, field decon may not be possible because of poor weather, because no one is available to perform the decon process, or because the patient is assessed as high priority and needs immediate care and transport. At other times, people fleeing the hot zone may bring a seriously injured and contaminated patient to you.

When you must treat a contaminated patient, identification of the hazardous material is crucial. Follow the treatment instructions given in the *North American Emergency Response Guidebook* or by the regional poison control center.

If you are confronted with priority patients who may cause secondary contamination before the arrival of a hazmat team, do the following:

1. **Take precautions appropriate to the substance as listed in the** *North American Emergency Response Guidebook.* This usually means isolation from the substance. Use PPE similar to that you would use for splash protection from bloodborne pathogens.

2. **Follow the first aid measures listed in the** *North American Emergency Response Guidebook.*

3. **Be sure to manage the patient's critical needs as you would those of any other patient.** Don't forget to manage the ABCs.

4. **If the treatment calls for irrigation with water, remember that water only dilutes most substances.** It does not neutralize them. Use large amounts of water and try to contain the runoff.

5. **To decontaminate a patient with water, cut the patient's clothing off and irrigate with large amounts of water.** If possible, use tepid or warm water to prevent hypothermia. If there are open wounds, try to avoid flushing contaminants directly into them. Pay particular attention to irrigating hard-to-clean areas such as dense body hair, the ear canals, the navel, the fingers and fingernails, the crotch, the arm pits, and so on. Try to use as much disposable equipment as possible. Discard it later.

6. **After treating the patient, decontaminate yourself.** You may need to dispose of some of your clothing as well.

Remember that the severity of any poisoning depends on the substance, route of entry, dosage, and duration of contact. Providing the immediate first-aid measures listed in the *North American Emergency Response Guidebook* may decrease the severity of poisoning and save lives. Whenever possible, the entire decontamination process should be carried out by qualified personnel from the hazmat team before you treat a patient. *When you do treat a contaminated patient, the benefits for the patient must outweigh the risks of contamination to you and your crew.*

Patient Assessment—Hazardous Materials Injuries

Be sure to wear appropriate PPE and SCBA, if necessary. Follow normal patient assessment procedures to determine injuries. Do not forget to conduct patient and bystander interviews. Do not let hazmat conditions and injuries distract you from the possibility that the patient may have other medical conditions or injuries.

◆ Emergency Care—Hazardous Materials Injuries

1. **If patients are not already in the cold zone, they must be moved to it from the hot zone.** In this situation, emergency moves may be necessary before assessment and care can begin.

2. **Provide basic life support.** For positive pressure ventilations and CPR, use oxygen from a flow-restricted, oxygen-powered ventilation device or bag-valve mask and oxygen reservoir so that you do not have to remove your own protective gear.

3. **Administer high concentration oxygen to any patient having difficulty breathing.**

4. **Immediately flush with water the skin, clothing, and eyes of anyone who has come into contact with the hazardous material.** Retain the runoff water.

5. **Remove clothing, shoes, and jewelry from all persons who have come into contact with the hazardous material.** Place those items in a sealed, labeled container. Continue flushing the patient's skin with water for no less than 20 minutes. Continue to retain runoff.

6. **Remove your protective gear only when recommended by local guidelines and in the manner described by them.**

7. **Transport the patient as soon as possible, providing care for shock, administering oxygen, and taking all steps necessary to maintain normal body temperature.**

MULTIPLE-CASUALTY INCIDENTS

A multiple-casualty incident (MCI)—or multiple-casualty situation (MCS) as it is termed in some areas—is an event that places great demands on the personnel and resources of an EMS system. Different jurisdictions define MCIs in different ways. Some systems define an MCI as any incident involving three or more patients. Other jurisdictions set the level for an MCI at five, seven, or more patients. The most common MCI is an automobile crash with three or more patients. You will likely respond to many incidents with three to fifteen potential patients. Incidents with large-scale casualties are rare and apt to be "once in a career" events.

The demands of an MCI usually go beyond what a single emergency unit can handle. In fact, the resources of multiple agencies—fire, EMS, and police—are often required to handle an MCI. With many people and different agencies involved in an incident, a clear plan for handling the situation is needed. Otherwise, confusion is likely to result. Personnel may fail to perform important tasks, or crews may not be where they are needed most at the proper times.

Coordination of personnel is the key to safe and efficient functioning at MCIs. To ensure this coordination, every jurisdiction should have a disaster plan. This is a pre-defined set of instructions that tells a community's various emergency responders what to do in different types of emergencies. No plan can predefine responses for all conditions that might arise. Nevertheless, every good disaster plan should be:

◆ *Flexible* The plan must be adaptable to a wide variety of incidents. It should be expandable to cover MCIs involving three patients to those involving fifteen or more.

◆ *Written to address the events conceivable for a particular location* This means that a plan for

a town in Kansas should address tornadoes, not hurricanes.

◆ *Well-publicized* Personnel in all responding agencies should know about the plan and how it operates.

◆ *Realistic* The plan should be based on the actual resources available.

◆ *Rehearsed* Agencies covered by the plan should practice using it.

Most well-trained emergency responders can handle small-scale MCIs pretty well. In theory, larger-scale incidents are managed using the same principles. However, the scope of the larger incidents can overwhelm responders. To handle these incidents, the jurisdiction must have a good plan and emergency personnel must know it and practice it.

The Incident Management System

There are many systems for organizing responses to large-scale emergency incidents. Historically, there have been two predominant systems used in the fire service, the FIRESCOPE/National Fire Academy Incident Command System (ICS) and the Phoenix Fire Ground Command (FGC) System. In recent years, these two systems have been merged into a common system called the National Fire Service Incident Management System (IMS). IFSTA has officially adopted the IMS system for use in all of its materials. This system is adaptable to all types of emergency incidents. In addition, it is mandated by law for the management of some types of incidents, such as those involving hazardous materials.

The system provides procedures for controlling personnel, facilities, equipment, and communications. It is designed for flexibility, from small-scale to large-scale incidents. Following the IMS structure can ensure good communications and coordination among different agencies who respond to an incident. IMS has five major functional areas. They are:

◆ *Command,* which is responsible for direction and oversight of all incident activities

◆ *Operations,* which is responsible for carrying out the goals of the mission as set by Command

♦ *Planning,* which is responsible for gathering and evaluating information about the incident, including the status of resources

♦ *Logistics,* which is responsible for providing facilities, services, and materials to support response at an incident

♦ *Finance/Administration,* which is responsible for costs and financial aspects of an incident

Not all of these components will be required at every incident. For example, Finance will only be of concern at really large-scale, long-term incidents. The most commonly used components at MCIs are Command and Operations.

Command

Command must be established at all incidents. Command is the person who assumes responsibility for management of an incident. This individual stays in command unless that role is transferred to another person or until the incident is brought to a conclusion.

IMS operates on the assumption that a manageable span of control is three to seven people or units, with five being the optimum number. As an incident escalates and becomes more complex, the number of people involved grows and becomes too great for one person to control. At this point, Command names Sector (also called Division or Group) Officers to help. These Sector Officers oversee specific functions at an incident, such as transportation or rehab. Command retains overall responsibility for directing the incident. If the incident expands still further, it may be necessary to implement a Medical Branch to supervise the various sectors.

There are two basic methods of Command—singular and unified. In singular command, one agency controls all resources and operations at an incident. As you know, EMS is often managed by a fire department. Singular command is often used at fire and rescue incidents.

There are incidents, however, that will involve fire, police, additional EMS providers, and other agencies. With such incidents, unified command is more appropriate. In unified command, several agencies work independently but cooperatively, rather than one agency assuming overall control.

Unified command is a highly effective means of incident management (Figure 28-19). It recognizes that large-scale incidents are complex and that the right agency must take the lead at the right time with the cooperation and support of the other agencies.

Command Functions

Initially, the most senior member of the first service to arrive at the scene of an incident assumes Command. He performs that role until someone of higher rank arrives on the scene. In a unified command structure, senior officers of the responding agencies would assume command cooperatively.

Command should be positioned at a location that is close enough to the scene to allow observation but also secure enough that management and communications will not be interrupted by a forced move. In a unified command, the various agencies establish one field command post and stay there. The Command post in the field is often identified by two traffic cones placed on the roof of an emergency vehicle, a flag, or some other device.

With Command assumed and a post established, the next priorities are scene size-up/triage and organization/delegation. First, Command and crew at an MCI do an initial scene size-up, start the triage process, and call for back-up. While waiting for help, initial triage is completed and Command gets ready for arriving resources.

Scene Size-Up

Traditionally, firefighters at MCIs have carried out fire suppression, rescue, and extrication duties. As a firefighter-EMT, you will probably be assigned to a role involving patient assessment and treatment.

If your unit is the first on the scene of an MCI, you will be performing the scene size-up. Remember that at this stage your job is to get an overall picture of the incident. Even though many patients may be in obvious distress and screaming for help, perform the scene size-up and triage before turning to any detailed assessment and treatment of individual patients. Only by doing this will you assure the rapid arrival of adequate resources to help the largest number of patients. When performing the scene size-up at an MCI, do the following:

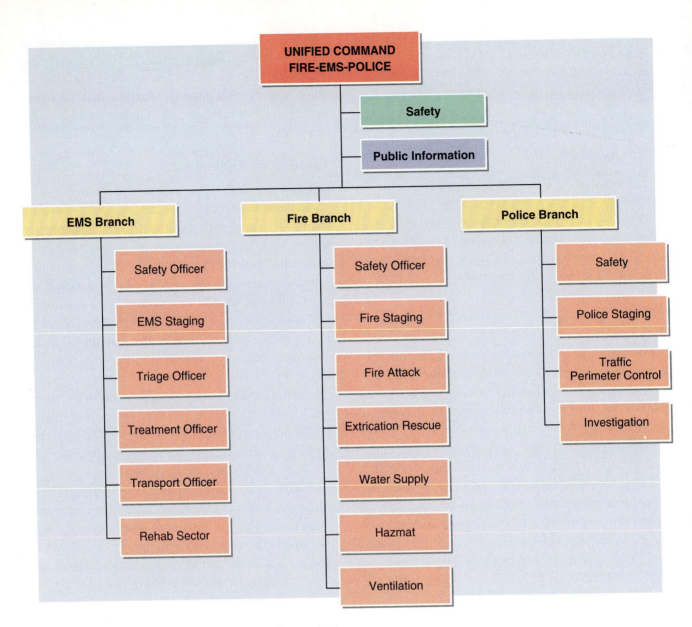

Figure 28-19   A typical unified command organization.

1. **Arrive at the scene and establish Command.** Put on proper identification.

2. **Do a quick walk through the scene** (or observe it from a safe distance if it's a hazmat incident). You may assign the remainder of your crew to perform this task and report back to you. Assess the scene for the following information:

   ◆ Number of patients (including "walking wounded")

   ◆ Scene hazards

   ◆ Apparent patient priorities

   ◆ Need for extrication

   ◆ Number of ambulances needed

   ◆ Other factors affecting the scene and resources needed to address them

   ◆ Areas to stage resources

3. **Radio in an initial scene report with your request for additional resources.**

Communications

Once the scene size-up has been done, an initial scene report should be made to the communications center. This report should be short and to the point. It must also make clear the severity of the situation and the need for additional resources. When making the report, Command should give itself a unique name to distinguish itself in from other units that may be using the same communications system. Command's location should also be a part of the initial report. One example of an initial report is this:

Firecom, this is Engine 62. We are on the scene of a two-car MVC with severe entrapment of four Priority 1 patients. Dispatch a rescue company and three paramedic ambulances. I will be establishing Central Avenue Command. Police are needed at the scene to assist with traffic and crowd control as soon as possible.

If the jurisdiction's disaster plan is to be put into effect, make sure that all responding units are informed of this. They must follow the same organizational chart for the incident that Command is using to assure that rescue efforts are coordinated. Command must tell responding units as early as possible what equipment to bring, how to access the scene, where to stage, and what they should do on arrival.

As help begins to arrive, control of on-scene communication is important. Use as much face-to-face communication as possible, especially between Command and Sector Officers and between Sector Officers and subordinates. This will help to reduce radio channel crowding. Command may have to designate a radio aide if radio communications take up too much time.

Basically, the flow of communications on the scene should correspond to the organizational chart being used for the incident. Accordingly, the only unit talking to the communications center and requesting resources is Command. The only ones who report to Command are the Sector Officers. Other personnel report only to their assigned Sector Officers.

Organization

Getting organized early and aggressively is very important. If you are serving as initial Command at an incident, you must have a plan to deploy resources when they arrive. You must have decided what Sector Officers will be needed and where resources will be placed.

A common mistake is to underestimate the resources needed. Somehow new patients not found during size-up have a way of appearing. Think big! Order big! Put resources in the staging area if they are not needed right away. In urban/suburban incidents, back-up can be fast and overwhelming. Think about supply and staging areas early or you will risk being overrun.

Another of the responsibilities of Command is to prevent "freelancing." Freelancing is uncoordinated or undirected activity at the emergency scene. Given the opportunity, most responders will arrive on the scene and begin setting their own priorities. Command can prevent this problem. When it is established early in the incident, people and crews can be assigned to tasks as they arrive.

Some tools are available to help in the organization of Command. For example, many agencies list the main points of their disaster plans on a "tactical worksheet' that can be used in the field (Figure 28-20). Such worksheets are useful aids for remembering all the steps that must be carried out during an incident.

EMS Sector Functions

In smaller MCIs, Command may be able to manage all aspects of the incident. As incidents grow in scale, they come to involve more information, resources, and personnel than a single person can effectively manage. In larger incidents, Command should designate Sector Officers to manage different aspects of the emergency operation. The number of sectors will vary depending upon the size and complexity of the incident (Figures 28-21 to 28-23). In MCIs, some of the common EMS sectors, in addition to Command, are the following:

◆ *Staging*—This sector, set up a safe distance from the emergency, holds, monitors, and inventories ambulances and emergency vehicles and their crews and releases them to other sectors as needed.

◆ *Supply*—This sector monitors, inventories, and distributes patient care equipment.

◆ *Extrication*—This sector oversees and directs rescue teams who are responsible for freeing patients from wreckage.

COLONIE EMS — Incident Tactical Worksheet

Location _____
Med. Command _____

— Establish underlined command with fire & police
— Place 2 cones on command vehicle
— Put bib on
— Designate triage office
— Advise inbound units where to stage
— Advise crews to stay with units until given instructions
— Advise units to switch to EMS Admin., 265 or 715

LEVEL 1 (3-10 Patients)

— Declare MCI
— EMS All Call
— Request # of Units Needed
— Cover Town/Sr. Medic Act 615
— Roll Call Hospitals
— Transport Officer?

(2-5 Amb. Needed)

LEVEL 2 (11-25 Patients)

— Declare MCI
— EMS All Call
— Request # of Units Needed
— Cover Town/Sr. Medic Act 615
— Roll Call Hospitals
— Get Mutual Aid Units
— Designate Treatment Officer
— Designate Transport Officer
— Designate Staging Officer
— REMO MD to Scene
— Consider Rehab & CISD

(6-13 Amb. Needed)

LEVEL 3 (over 25 Patients)

— Declare MCI
— EMS All Call
— Request # of Units Needed
— Cover Town/Sr. Medic Act 615
— Roll Call Hospitals
— Get Mutual Aid Units
— Designate Treatment Officer
— Designate Transport Officer
— Designate Staging Officer
— REMO MD to Scene
— Request Bus to Scene

(over 13 Amb. Needed)

FIRE

— Assess # of Units Needed
— EMS All Call Req. 619
— Designate Triage
— Set up Rehab at Air Bank
— Use 619 as ALS Unit

RESCUE

— Establish Perimeter
— Request Speciality Units
— Triage Officer Handles Inner Circle

HAZ-MAT

— Req. # of Units Needed
— EMS All Call
— Est. Command in Cold Zone
— Designate Triage
— Identify Agent
— Research Decontamination
— Research Med.
— Medical Baseline Assessment of Team
— Don Protective Barriers
— Assist With Decontamination
— Rehabilitate

HOSPITAL ROLL CALL

HOSPITAL ROLL CALL	AMCH	St. PETERS	MEMORIAL	VA	ELLIS	St. CLARE'S	LEONARD	St. MARY'S	SAMARITAN
CAN TAKE									
# PATIENTS SENT									

OF PATIENTS BY PRIORITY

1 (Red)	2 (Yellow)	3 (Green)	0 (Black)	TOTALS

UNITS RESPONDING

620	621	622
630	631	632
640	641	642
650	651	652
610	611	605
TSU-1	TSU-2	
619		
Guild.		
CPHM		
Albany		
Mohawk		
Empire		

UNITS IN STAGING

620	621	622
630	631	632
640	641	642
650	651	652
610	611	605
TSU-1	TSU-2	
619		
Guild.		
CPHM		
Albany		
Mohawk		
Empire		

Figure 28-20 An example of an incident tactical worksheet.

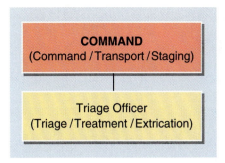

Figure 28-21 An organization for a smaller incident.

- *Triage*—This sector is responsible for sorting patients to determine the order in which they will receive medical care or transportation to definitive care.
- *Treatment*—This sector provides field care for patients. Triage also continues in this sector.
- *Transportation*—This sector is responsible for moving patients from treatment sectors to hospitals. The Transportation Sector Officer must communicate often with Command and with Sector Officers in staging, triage, and treatment to assure the smooth movement of patients out of the emergency scene. The Transportation Officer must know the priorities, identities, and destinations of all patients leaving the scene. The Transportation Officer may assign a Medical Communications Officer to communicate with the receiving hospital(s). This officer will continually monitor resource availability at the receiving hospitals to assure optimum patient care.
- *Rehab*—This sector is responsible for monitoring the health and well-being of rescue workers and providing them with rest, food, and rehydration as needed.

Individuals and agencies on the scene will be assigned roles in one or more sectors. Most systems use brightly colored reflective vests that can be worn over protective clothing to make each Incident Sector Officer easy to identify (Figure 28-24). Emergency personnel arriving at the scene after Command has been established would be expected to report to a Sector Officer for assignment to specific duties. Once assigned a task, an emergency worker should complete it, then report back to the Sector Officer.

Triage Sector

At an MCI, once EMS Command has been established, the next task is to quickly assess all the patients and assign each a priority for receiving emergency care or transportation to definitive care. This process is called **triage,** which comes from a French word meaning "to sort." The most knowledgeable EMS provider becomes the Triage Officer. The Triage Officer calls for additional help if needed, assigns available personnel and equipment to patients, and remains at the scene to assign and coordinate personnel, supplies, and equipment.

Initial Triage When faced with more than one patient, your goal must be to afford the greatest number of people the greatest chance of survival. To accomplish this, you must provide care to patients according to the seriousness of their illnesses or injuries. While you provide care, you must keep in mind that spending a lot of time trying to save one life may prevent a number of other patients from receiving needed treatment.

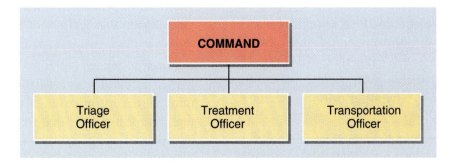

Figure 28-22 An organization for a medium-sized incident.

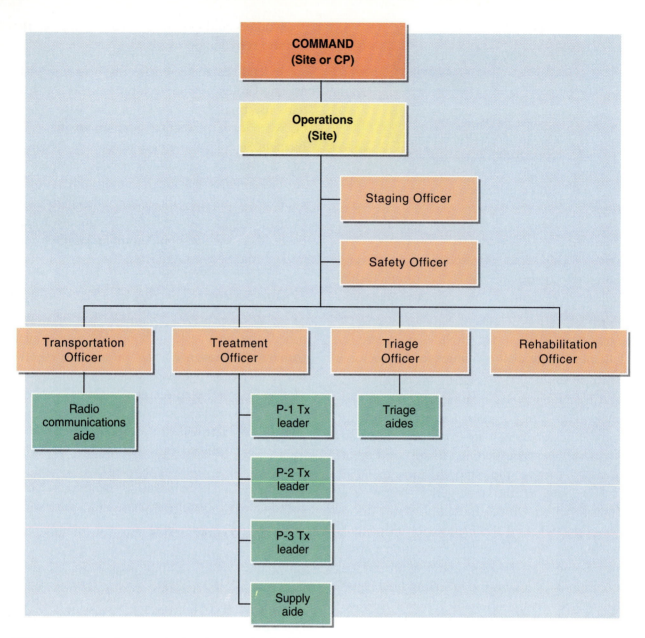

Figure 28-23 An organization for a major incident.

In performing triage on a group of patients, it is necessary to quickly assess them and assign them to one of the four following categories:

◆ *Priority 1: Treatable Life-Threatening Illnesses or Injuries*—Airway and breathing difficulties; uncontrolled or severe bleeding; decreased mental status; patients with severe medical problems; shock (hypoperfusion); severe burns.

◆ *Priority 2: Serious But Not Life-Threatening Illnesses or Injuries*—Burns without airway problems; major or multiple bone or joint injuries;

back injuries with or without spinal cord damage.

◆ *Priority 3: "Walking Wounded"*—Minor musculoskeletal injuries; minor soft tissue injuries.

◆ *Priority 4 (sometimes called Priority 0): Dead or Fatally Injured.* Patients with exposed brain matter, in cardiac arrest (no pulse for over 20 minutes except in cases of cold-water drowning, severe hypothermia, or lightning injuries); decapitated; with severed trunks; incinerated. Patients in arrest must be considered Priority 4 when resources are limited. The time that

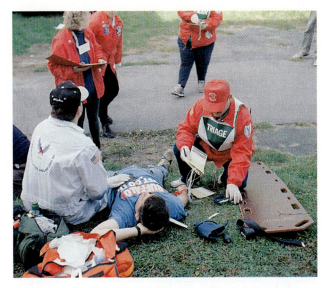

Figure 28-24 Using brightly colored reflective bibs will make personnel working in different sectors of the rescue operation readily identifiable.

must be devoted to rescue breathing or CPR for one person is not justified when there are many patients needing attention. Once ample resources are available, patients in arrest become Priority 1.

How triage is performed depends on the number of injuries, the immediate hazards to personnel and patients, and the location of backup resources. Your local operating procedures will supply guidance on the exact methods of triage to follow in a given situation. Some basic, standard triage procedures are described below.

If you are assigned to triage, begin the initial assessment. You can first request—using a bullhorn or loud voice—all patients who can walk to move to a particular area. This will identify Priority 3 "walking wounded" patients who have adequate airway and breathing. Then, quickly assess the remaining patients, checking for airway, breathing, and circulation. Do this as follows:

1. **If a patient's airway is not open, open it with a manual maneuver.** If the patient responds appropriately, move on to the next patient.
2. **If the patient is unresponsive, check for breathing and pulse. If there is no breathing or pulse, do not provide care for that person.** Move on to the next patient.

3. **If you feel a pulse, check for severe bleeding;** if there is severe bleeding, quickly apply a pressure dressing to the wound and move on to the next patient.

As long as there are other patients waiting to be triaged, the only initial treatment you should provide is airway management and control of severe bleeding. If there is an immediate danger to patients, begin moving them regardless of injuries. Your "walking wounded" patients may be able to assist in airway management and bleeding control procedures and in the movement of patients.

Patient Identification For triage procedures to work effectively, a system of identifying patients with the priorities assigned to them must be in place. Arriving EMS personnel must be able to look at patients and determine at a glance their treatment and transportation priorities or whether they have as yet been assessed.

Different jurisdictions use different systems for patient identification. One of the most common is the following color-coding method:

◆ Red = Priority 1
◆ Yellow = Priority 2
◆ Green = Priority 3
◆ Black (or gray) = Priority 4

Many systems use triage tags coded with these colors to identify patients (Figure 28-25). EMTs carrying out the initial assessment attach the tags to patients as they prioritize them. Often tags have space on them where basic medical information about a patient can be recorded.

Secondary Triage and Treatment As more personnel arrive at the incident scene, they should be directed to assist with the completion of initial triage. If triage has been completed, they can instead begin treatment.

Secondary triage generally begins at this point. In ideal triage systems, patients are gathered into a triage sector and, under the direction of the Triage Officer, are physically separated into treatment groups based on their priority levels as indicated on their triage tags.

An area to which patients are removed is referred to as a Treatment Sector. Each Treatment

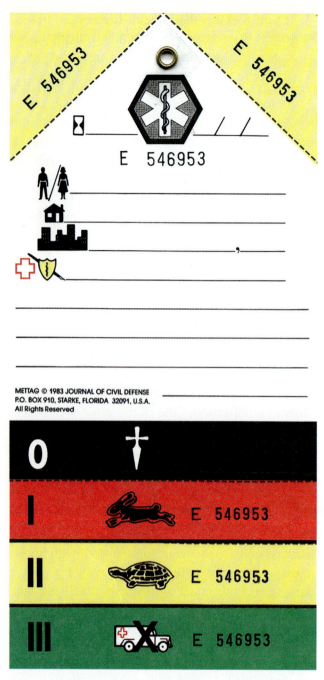
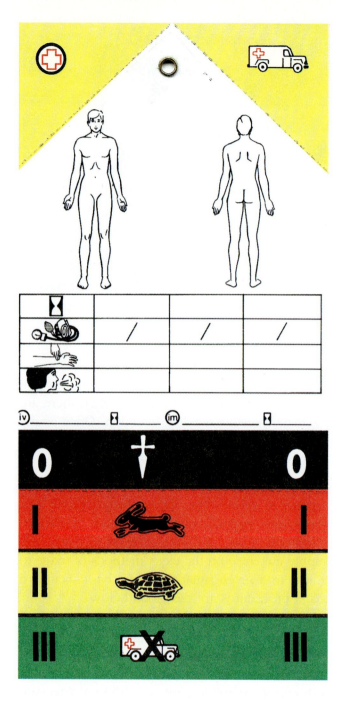

Figure 28-25 Front and back of a triage tag.

Sector should have its own Treatment Officer, an EMT responsible for overseeing the triage and treatment within that sector.

The Treatment Officer should again triage the patients in that sector to determine the order in which they will receive treatment. Patients' conditions may improve or deteriorate. If they do, it may be necessary to reassign a patient a higher or lower priority. The patient would then be moved to the appropriate Treatment Sector. Some sys-

tems use a different disaster tag during secondary triage on which more detailed information about the patient can be recorded (Figure 28-26).

The Treatment Sector EMTs will need supplies and equipment from ambulances such as bandages, blood pressure cuffs, and oxygen.

Transportation and Staging

Once patients have been properly prioritized and their treatment has begun, consideration must be

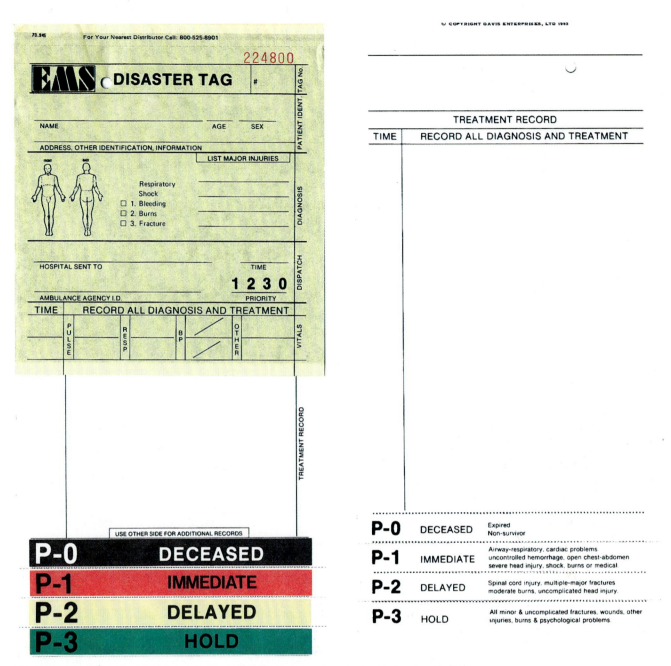

Figure 28-26 Front and back of an EMS disaster tag that can be used during both primary triage and secondary triage and treatment.

given to the order in which to transport the patients to a hospital. Again, this is done according to triage priority.

Ambulances for transport should be assembled in the Staging Sector. The Staging Officer is responsible for having vehicles and their operators ready to roll. No ambulance should proceed to a Treatment Sector without having been requested by the Transportation Officer and directed by the Staging Officer.

The Staging Officer should determine from each Treatment Sector the number and priority of patients in that sector. This information can then be used by the Transportation Officer to arrange that patients be taken from the scene to the hospital as efficiently as possible.

An ambulance should not transport any patient without the approval of the Transportation Officer. This is because the Transportation Officer is responsible for maintaining a list of patients and the hospitals to which they are transported. This information is relayed from the Transportation Officer (or the designated Medical Communications Officer) to each receiving hospital. In this way, the hospitals know what to expect and receive only those patients they are capable of handling. The EMTs on board the transporting ambulances must follow the Transportation Officer's directions. Failure to do so may result in patients being transported to the wrong facilities and delays in their treatment.

Once an ambulance has completed a run to a hospital, it will probably be directed to return to the staging area, perhaps bringing needed supplies. It should wait in the staging area for its next instructions from the Staging Officer.

Communicating with Hospitals

Receiving hospitals must be alerted about an MCI or disaster as soon as the scope of the incident is known. This allows them to call in additional personnel and otherwise prepare to receive the anticipated numbers of patients.

In an MCI, communications channels will be in heavy use. It is crucial that only the Transportation Officer, not individual EMTs, communicate with hospitals. This will help eliminate unnecessary radio traffic. It will also ensure that proper patient information is recorded at both ends of the ambulance ride.

In large-scale MCIs, individual patient reports are not necessary. Treating and transporting EMTs are usually different. Also, there are usually too many patients to permit EMTs to give good radio reports on each. In these circumstances, hospitals may only be provided with the most basic information—for example, that they are receiving a Priority 1 patient with respiratory problems.

Psychological Considerations

By their nature, MCIs are extremely stressful situations. This is true for both patients and rescuers involved in them. While they may outwardly show few signs of injury or emotional stress, people in MCIs face devastating circumstances with which they are normally unprepared to cope.

Proper early management of a psychologically stressed patient can support later treatment and help ensure a faster recovery. This management may require you to administer "psychological first aid." This may mean talking with a terrified parent, child, or witness. This does not mean that you should try to perform psychoanalysis. Nor should you lie to a patient in an attempt to calm him. Instead, present a caring, honest demeanor. Listen to the patient and show you are listening by acknowledging his fears and problems. This may be the only "psychological first aid" necessary.

Rescuers, too, face stress during MCIs. Those who become emotionally incapacitated should be treated as patients and removed to the Rehab Sector. They should be monitored there by an EMT or other clinically competent provider of care. These rescuers should not return to duty without first being evaluated by someone professionally trained to do so.

Critical incident stress debriefing (CISD) can be invaluable after an MCI or a disaster. You can review how CISD works in Chapter 2, "The Well-being of the EMT."

Chapter Review

SUMMARY

Firefighter-EMTs will face a variety of situations that may pose hazards to patients or EMS personnel. A basic guideline for dealing with these situations is "Think before you act." Rushing into an emergency that you're not trained or equipped to handle call spell disaster for you, your crew members, and your patients. If you face a complex rescue situation that you're not trained or equipped to handle, call for appropriate help and wait till it arrives and the situation is secure. Be familiar with hazardous situations likely to arise in your area. Also, be familiar with plans your jurisdiction has prepared for dealing with hazardous situations and large-scale emergencies, including MCIs.

REVIEWING KEY CONCEPTS

1. Describe some of the factors that can complicate water rescues.

2. List the different procedures for water rescue in the order in which they should be attempted.

3. List some common sites of confined space rescues and describe hazards commonly encountered in those spaces.

4. Describe steps to follow if you are called to the scene of a confined space rescue.

5. List the conditions that require use of low-angle rescue techniques. List conditions that require high-angle rescue techniques.

6. List the types of questions that must be answered before deciding that a helicopter rescue operation is justified.

7. List the four levels of training for people who expect to be involved in hazmat operations.

8. Describe the control zones that should be set up at a hazmat incident.

9. List resources for learning more about the material involved in a hazmat incident.

10. List the information you would be expected to provide when reporting a hazmat incident.

11. Describe procedures to follow when confronted with priority patients who may be contaminated at a hazmat incident.

12. Describe the steps of basic emergency care for patients with hazmat injuries.

13. Describe the major components and benefits of the Incident Management System.

14. Explain the purpose of triage.

15. List the basic priority categories of triage.

16. Explain how to perform an initial triage assessment.

RESOURCES TO LEARN MORE

Fire Service RESCUE, 6th Edition. Stillwater, OK: Fire Protection Publications, 1996.

Model Procedures Guide for Emergency Medical Incidents. Stillwater, OK: Fire Protection Publications, 1996.

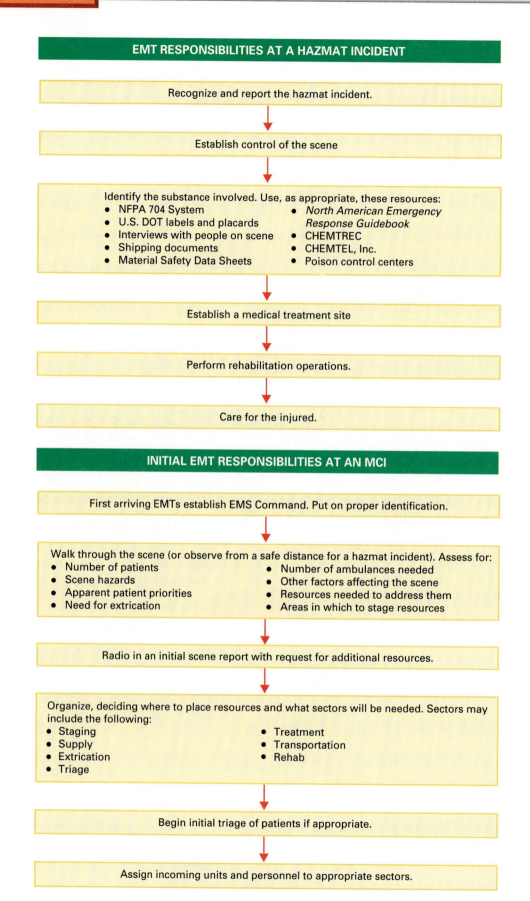

EMT RESPONSIBILITIES AT A HAZMAT INCIDENT

Recognize and report the hazmat incident.

Establish control of the scene

Identify the substance involved. Use, as appropriate, these resources:
- NFPA 704 System
- U.S. DOT labels and placards
- Interviews with people on scene
- Shipping documents
- Material Safety Data Sheets
- *North American Emergency Response Guidebook*
- CHEMTREC
- CHEMTEL, Inc.
- Poison control centers

Establish a medical treatment site

Perform rehabilitation operations.

Care for the injured.

INITIAL EMT RESPONSIBILITIES AT AN MCI

First arriving EMTs establish EMS Command. Put on proper identification.

Walk through the scene (or observe from a safe distance for a hazmat incident). Assess for:
- Number of patients
- Scene hazards
- Apparent patient priorities
- Need for extrication
- Number of ambulances needed
- Other factors affecting the scene
- Resources needed to address them
- Areas in which to stage resources

Radio in an initial scene report with request for additional resources.

Organize, deciding where to place resources and what sectors will be needed. Sectors may include the following:
- Staging
- Supply
- Extrication
- Triage
- Treatment
- Transportation
- Rehab

Begin initial triage of patients if appropriate.

Assign incoming units and personnel to appropriate sectors.

ADVANCED AIRWAY (ELECTIVE)

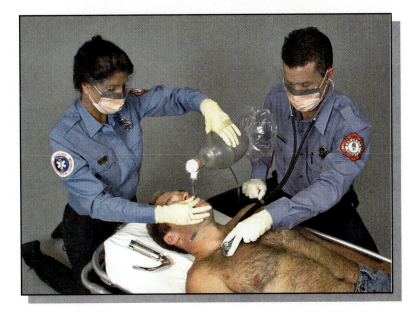

*I*n the final chapter of this textbook, you will learn about advanced airway management. The skills described in the chapter are optional for EMT-Basics under the 1994 DOT National Standard Curriculum. As has been the case with other skills you have learned up to this point, the descriptions and step-by-step procedures detailed in the chapter can in no way replace formal and repeated training in the techniques if you are authorized to use any of them by your department's medical direction. Rather, the chapter provides a broad overview of various advanced airway management devices and techniques that are currently available.

Advanced Airway Management

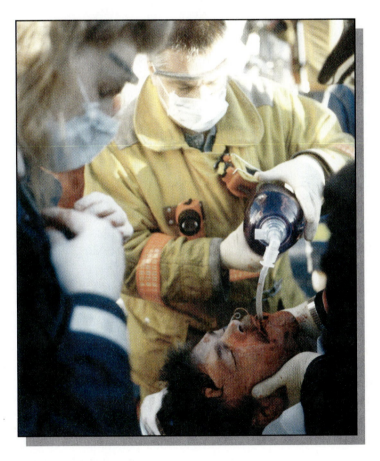

*N*o skill is more crucial for the EMT to master than the ability to assure that a patient has an adequate airway. Assuring an open airway is actually dependent on two separate skills. The first is the ability to assess and recognize airway and breathing problems. The second is the ability to maintain an open airway by using both manual techniques and airway adjuncts. Assuring an adequate airway is the first assessment and treatment priority in both basic and advanced life support. Control of a patient's airway is so crucial that advanced airway skills are now included as an elective in the EMT-

▶

Basic curriculum. The potential benefit of enabling EMTs to provide advanced airway skills cannot be overstated. EMTs are often the first care providers on the scene, and rapid and definitive control of the airway is essential to patient survival.

OBJECTIVES

At the completion of this chapter, the EMT student should be able to meet the following objectives:

Knowledge and Understanding

1. Identify and describe the airway anatomy in the infant, child, and adult. (pp. 760–763)

2. Differentiate between the airway anatomy in the infant, child, and adult. (pp. 760–763, 777)

3. Explain the pathophysiology of airway compromise. (pp. 762–763)

4. Describe the proper use of airway adjuncts. (p. 763)

5. Review the use of oxygen therapy in airway management. (p. 763)

6. Describe the indications, contraindications, and technique for insertion of nasogastric tubes. (p. 781)

7. Describe how to perform Sellick's maneuver (cricoid pressure). (pp. 774–775)

8. Describe the indications for advanced airway management. (pp. 769–770, 777–778)

9. List the equipment required for orotracheal intubation. (pp. 764–769)

10. Describe the proper use of the curved blade for orotracheal intubation. (p. 765)

11. Describe the proper use of the straight blade for orotracheal intubation. (pp. 765, 778)

12. State the reasons for and proper use of the stylet in orotracheal intubation. (pp. 768–769)

13. Describe the methods of choosing the appropriate size endotracheal tube in an adult patient. (pp. 767–768)

14. State the formula for sizing an infant or child endotracheal tube. (p. 778)

15. List complications associated with advanced airway management. (pp. 764, 777, 779)

16. Define the various alternative methods for sizing the infant and child endotracheal tube. (pp. 768–769)

17. Describe the skill of orotracheal intubation in the adult patient. (pp. 770–776)

18. Describe the skill of orotracheal intubation in the infant and child patient. (pp. 777–781)

19. Describe the skill of confirming endotracheal tube placement in the adult, infant, and child patient. (pp. 775–776, 780)

20. State the consequences of and the need to recognize unintentional esophageal intubation. (pp. 764, 775–776)

21. Describe the skill of securing the endotracheal tube in the adult, infant, and child patient. (pp. 769, 776, 780)

22. Recognize and respect the feelings of the patient and family during advanced airway procedures. (p. 763)

23. Explain the value of performing advanced airway procedures. (pp. 757–758, 763–764)

24. Defend the need for the EMT-Basic to perform advanced airway procedures. (pp. 763–764)

25. Explain the rationale for the use of a stylet. (pp. 768–769)

26. Explain the rationale for having a suction unit immediately available during intubation attempts. (p. 769)

27. Explain the rationale for confirming breath sounds. (pp. 775–776)

28. Explain the rationale for securing the endotracheal tube. (pp. 769, 776)

Skills

1. Demonstrate how to perform Sellick's maneuver (cricoid pressure).

2. Demonstrate the skill of orotracheal intubation in the adult patient.

3. Demonstrate the skill of orotracheal intubation in the infant and child patient.

4. Demonstrate the skill of confirming endotracheal tube placement in the adult patient.

5. Demonstrate the skill of securing the endotracheal tube in the adult patient.

6. Demonstrate the skill of securing the endotracheal tube in the infant and child patient.

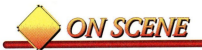

DISPATCH: *STATION 21, RESPOND TO THE SCENE OF AN MVC WITH INJURY. KIRKWOOD HIGHWAY AND HARMONY ROAD. TIME OUT IS 1221.*

On your arrival, you note that the state troopers have safely diverted traffic away from the crash scene and that an engine company is already on the scene. Only one car was involved in the crash, and it has sustained extensive damage. The vehicle is upright and stable, and there is no apparent fuel leak. As one trooper directs your ambulance into the scene, she informs you that there is a single victim, who was ejected from the car.

Approaching the vehicle, you and your partner find an unconscious male in his twenties, face down in the road. You note that he is lying in a pool of blood and hear gurgling respirations. While your partner maintains cervical stabilization, you and two first responders from the engine company log roll the patient onto his back. You see that the patient has sustained multiple facial lacerations and that there is a lot of blood in his airway. You begin to suction the patient's mouth with a large-bore, rigid-tip suction catheter and note that, even with aggressive suctioning, the patient has no gag reflex. You then insert an oropharyngeal airway, which the patient tolerates. The patient continues to bleed from the mouth, so you assign one of the first responders to suction the airway intermittently while you complete your initial assessment. The patient is breathing at only 6 breaths per minute, so you begin ventilations with a bag-valve mask. Assessment of the circulation reveals strong radial pulses and no apparent major external blood loss. The patient remains completely unresponsive to any stimuli.

You confer with your EMT partner and decide that you will go to the ambulance to prepare for orotracheal intubation while your partner continues to ventilate the patient. She and the first responders then secure the patient to a long spine board. Meanwhile, in the ambulance you select an 8.0 mm endotracheal tube and a curved laryngoscope blade and assure that both are functioning properly. Moments later, the patient is loaded into the ambulance. You see that he is now fully immobilized, with a cervical collar in place. One firefighter continues to ventilate the patient as you turn on the on-board suction and tuck the rigid-tip catheter between the spine board and the stretcher to the right of the patient's head. You assign one of the first responders to manually stabilize the patient's head while your partner opens the cervical collar and applies pressure to the cricoid cartilage. Using the laryngoscope, you then guide the endotracheal tube into the trachea. After quickly inflating the tube's cuff, you remove the mask from the BVM and begin to ventilate directly through the endotracheal tube. You listen for breath sounds and determine that the tube is properly placed. You secure the tube with tape and begin transport to the hospital. Your on-scene time was 11 minutes.

En route to the hospital, you complete your rapid trauma assessment and continue to reassess the patient. You again auscultate for the presence and equality of breath sounds and confirm that the tube is still properly placed. The patient begins to respond to pain by the time you arrive at the hospital.

Airway control is the highest priority in managing any critically ill or injured patient. Without an adequate airway, such a patient will die no matter what other care you provide. Advanced airway management can only be effective and successful, however, when you have mastered the basic airway techniques discussed in Chapter 6.

RESPIRATORY ANATOMY AND PHYSIOLOGY

The anatomy and physiology of the respiratory system have already been discussed in Chapters 5 and 6. There are, however, specific aspects of these subjects that the EMT who performs advanced airway skills must understand in greater depth to use the skills most effectively.

Anatomy

Air initially enters the respiratory tract through the nose and the mouth. Air that enters through the nose then passes through the *nasopharynx*. Air that enters the airway through the mouth passes through the *oropharynx* (Figure 29-1). The *hypopharynx* is the area directly above the openings of both the *trachea* (windpipe) and the *esophagus*. The *epiglottis* is a leaf-like structure that acts as a covering to the opening of the trachea. The epiglottis protects the airway by covering the entrance to the trachea when food or liquids are swallowed. Anterior to the epiglottis is a groove-like structure called the *vallecula*. The epiglottis allows air to pass into the opening of the trachea and through the larynx, or voice box. The larynx contains the two vocal cords.

Several rigid pieces of cartilage support the larynx and trachea. The *thyroid cartilage* is a shield-shaped structure that is anterior to, or in front of, the larynx. Multiple horseshoe-shaped cartilages that open posteriorly give support to the trachea. The *cricoid cartilage* is unique among them. Located at the lower portion of the larynx, it is the only tracheal cartilage to completely surround the windpipe.

Once air has passed through the larynx, it proceeds through the trachea. At the level of the

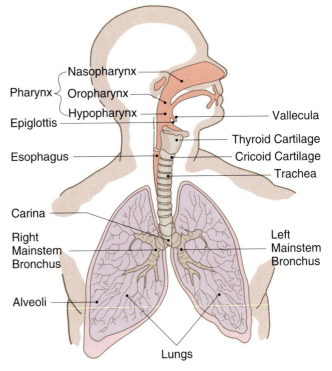

Figure 29-1 The airway, standard anatomical position.

carina, the trachea bifurcates, or splits, into the two mainstem *bronchi*. The right mainstem bronchus splits off the carina at less of an angle than the left mainstem bronchus. Because of the angle of the right mainstem bronchus, objects such as aspirated food that pass all the way down the trachea tend to lodge in it rather than in the left mainstem bronchus. The mainstem bronchi subsequently divide into smaller air passages down to level of the *alveoli*, where gas exchange takes place.

When trying to study and memorize the anatomy of the upper airway, remember that in the majority of cases in which you manage a critical airway problem the patient will be lying flat or supine. For this reason, it is important to visualize airway anatomy with the patient in both standard anatomical position and in the supine position (Figure 29-2).

Physiology

The most important aspect of respiratory physiology for the EMT who uses advanced airway skills to understand is what can cause the respiratory system to fail so severely that an advanced airway is necessary. In a properly functioning respiratory

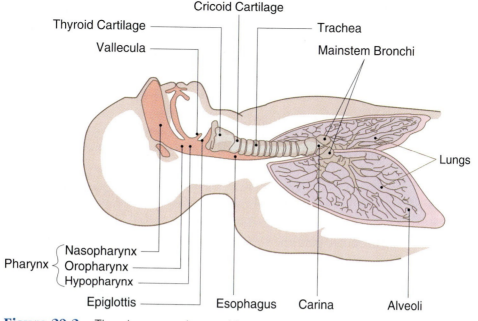

Thyroid Cartilage

Cricoid Cartilage

Vallecula

Trachea

Mainstem Bronchi

Lungs

Pharynx { Nasopharynx
Oropharynx
Hypopharynx }

Epiglottis

Esophagus

Carina

Alveoli

Figure 29-2 The airway, supine position.

system, many factors combine to produce adequate breathing. These factors include the following:

◆ A functioning brain stem, which is where the brain's centers of respiratory control are located

◆ An open airway

◆ An intact chest wall

◆ The ability of gas exchange to take place at the alveolar level

Injuries or illnesses affecting any of these components can result in inadequate breathing and respiratory failure. For example, a massive head injury could cause both brain stem injury and obstruction of the airway by blood and broken teeth. Similarly, a patient with massive pulmonary edema from congestive heart failure can go into respiratory failure because edema (or fluid) prevents adequate gas exchange at the level of the alveoli.

Assessing the adequacy of a patient's breathing is an essential skill for making decisions about what basic and advanced airway management to provide. A patient's respiratory status can range from normal, unlabored breathing to complete cessation of breathing, or respiratory arrest. Recognizing either adequate breathing or respiratory arrest is rarely challenging for the EMT. Recogniz-

ing the more subtle signs and symptoms of inadequate breathing is a more difficult, yet essential skill for the EMT.

In general, when assessing the adequacy of breathing you should carefully observe the *rate, rhythm, quality,* and *depth* of the patient's respirations. The normal rate of breathing varies with the age of the patient (Table 29-1). An adequately breathing patient will normally breath in a regular, rather than an irregular rhythm. The quality of a patient's breathing is assessed by listening for breath sounds and observing chest expansion and effort of breathing. The adequately breathing patient will have breath sounds that are equal and present bilaterally. In addition, the patient's chest will expand fully and equally, and the patient will

Table 29-1

Normal Rates of Breathing

Adult	12–20 breaths per minute
Child	15–30 breaths per minute
Infant	25–40 breaths per minute
Newborn/neonatal	Up to 50 breaths per minute

not use accessory muscles in the chest or neck during inspiration. Finally, the depth of breathing *(tidal volume)* will normally be sufficient not only to expand the lungs but also to assure adequate delivery of oxygen and removal of carbon dioxide at the level of the alveoli.

When a patient is in respiratory distress because of inadequate breathing, one or more of the following variations in rate, rhythm, quality, and depth of breathing may be noted:

◆ *Rate*—will be outside the normal range, either too fast or too slow

◆ *Rhythm*—will display an irregular pattern

◆ *Quality:*

   ◆ Breath sounds—will be diminished, unequal, or absent

   ◆ Chest expansion—will be unequal or inadequate

   ◆ Effort of breathing—will display increased effort and use of accessory muscles in the neck or chest, leaving the patient unable to speak in full sentences

◆ *Depth*—shallow

In addition, you may also note the following signs and symptoms in the patient with inadequate breathing:

◆ Cyanosis (bluish-gray color) in the lips, nail beds, and finger tips

◆ Cool and clammy skin

◆ Agonal breathing (gasping breaths just prior to respiratory arrest)

Pediatric Airway and Anatomy

The pediatric airway is not simply a miniature version of an adult airway. Infants and children possess some unique anatomic and physiologic features as compared to their grown-up counterparts. Not surprisingly, these younger patients may also have some signs and symptoms of respiratory failure different from those found with adults. These unique features of airway anatomy and physiology in infants and children compared with adults include the following: (Figure 29-3):

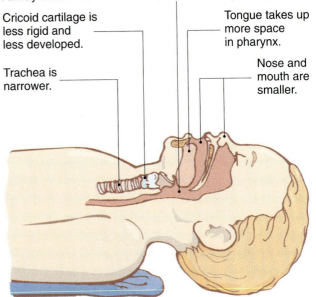

Airway structures are smaller and more easily obstructed.

Cricoid cartilage is less rigid and less developed.

Trachea is narrower.

Tongue takes up more space in pharynx.

Nose and mouth are smaller.

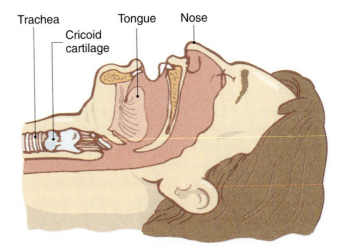

Trachea   Tongue   Nose

Cricoid cartilage

Figure 29-3   Adult and child airways compared.

◆ All structures in the mouth and nose are smaller in infants and children and can be more easily obstructed.

◆ The tongues of infants and children are proportionately larger, occupying more of the mouth and pharynx.

◆ The trachea of an infant or a child is softer and more flexible that that of an adult. This means that the airway can be easily closed off if the neck is extended too far forward or backward.

◆ The trachea is narrower, allowing the airway to become more easily obstructed if swelling occurs.

- The narrowest area in the infant or child airway is at the level of the cricoid cartilage.
- Because the chest wall is softer, the diaphragm is relied on heavily for the work of breathing.

Although infants and children may show inadequate breathing with the signs and symptoms mentioned above, they also frequently present with other signs or symptoms of respiratory distress. These include:

- A slower than normal heart rate
- Weak or absent peripheral pulses
- Retractions between and below the ribs, above the clavicles, and at the sternal notch
- Nasal flaring, in which the nostrils "flare" open with exhalation and clamp down with inhalation
- So-called "seesaw" breathing, in which the chest and abdomen move in opposite directions during breathing

PEDIATRIC NOTE

Recognition of respiratory distress and inadequate breathing is especially crucial in infants and children because respiratory failure is the leading cause of cardiac arrest in this age group.

MANAGEMENT OF THE AIRWAY

This chapter is about advanced airway management. However, the primary management of any airway is with basic airway techniques such as opening and suctioning the airway, administering supplemental oxygen, and using oro- and nasopharyngeal airways. The importance of mastering these skills cannot be overstated. You should review these skills from Chapter 6 before learning the techniques of advanced airway management.

Suctioning the Airway

The goal of airway management is keeping the airway open and free of obstructions. If the airway is obstructed with secretions, blood, or foreign materials, the airway will have to be suctioned. Suction equipment should always be within easy reach when managing any critically ill patient. If the patient is being managed outside the ambulance, either an electrical or hand-operated device should be brought to the patient's side. If the patient is in the ambulance, the on-board suction system should be set up and ready for immediate use. Fumbling around to get a suction unit working when the patient's airway is filled with vomitus or blood delays treatment and can harm the patient.

As you will see, a working rigid-tip suction catheter is an essential piece of equipment. The technique for using it was described in Chapter 6. You will potentially use this rigid-tip catheter to suction a patient's mouth and pharynx before and during an orotracheal intubation.

Orotracheal Intubation

Orotracheal intubation is the insertion of a specialized tube into a patient's mouth, through the vocal cords, and into the upper trachea. Orotracheal intubation is the most effective technique for controlling a patient's airway. This is because inserting the tube, called an **endotracheal tube,** allows direct ventilation of the lungs through the trachea, bypassing the entire upper airway. The endotracheal tube is placed through the vocal cords with *direct visualization* of the tube passing through the vocal cords. A **laryngoscope** is an illuminating instrument that is inserted into the pharynx and allows you to visualize the pharynx and larynx.

The advantages of orotracheal intubation of the apneic (nonbreathing) patient include the following:

- Complete control of the airway
- Minimized risk of aspiration
- Better oxygen delivery
- A means of deeper suctioning of the airway

◆ Provision of a route for the administration of certain drugs by advanced EMTs and paramedics, especially during cardiac arrests

Complications

Although orotracheal intubation can be a life-saving procedure, it has many potential complications. Orotracheal intubation is considered an "invasive" technique because it requires placement of equipment inside the body. Whenever you perform an invasive procedure, you must be aware of the potential complications and be prepared to recognize and treat them should they arise. These concerns are never more critical than in orotracheal intubation. Misplacement of the endotracheal tube into the esophagus in the apneic patient will rapidly lead to the patient's death if it is not immediately detected. Specific complications of orotracheal intubation include the following:

◆ *Slowing of the heart rate* Stimulating the airway with the laryngoscope and the endotracheal tube can lead to a slowing of the heart rate. This complication is especially common in infants and children. The patient's heart rate should be monitored throughout the intubation.

◆ *Soft tissue trauma to the teeth, lips, tongue, gums and airway structures*

◆ *Hypoxia* Prolonged attempts at intubation may lead to inadequate oxygenation of a patient. This condition of oxygen starvation is called **hypoxia**. To prevent hypoxia, a patient should be **hyperventilated** with high concentration oxygen (ventilations at about double the normal rate, or about 24 ventilations per minute) before intubation is attempted. Also, attempts to insert the tube should be limited to 30 seconds from the time ventilations cease until the patient is ventilated through the endotracheal tube.

◆ *Vomiting* Because stimulation of the airway may cause the patient to gag and vomit, you should always have a functioning rigid-tip suction catheter within reach when performing endotracheal intubation.

◆ *Right mainstem intubation* If the endotracheal tube is advanced too far during insertion, it is likely to go down the steep right mainstem bronchus. Mainstem intubation means that only one lung will be ventilated, leading to the development of hypoxia.

◆ *Esophageal intubation* This is the most serious complication. Unrecognized placement of the tube into the esophagus rather than the trachea prevents any ventilation of the lungs. It will rapidly lead to the patient's death.

◆ *Accidental extubation* Even if the endotracheal tube is properly placed at first, the tube can become dislodged when the patient is moved or when the patient himself moves upon regaining consciousness. Proper securing of the tube is essential. Be sure to reassess chest wall movement and breath sounds after every major move of an intubated patient such as from the floor to the stretcher.

Equipment

You must be thoroughly familiar with the following types of equipment in order to perform an endotracheal intubation.

Personal Protective Equipment Because of the high risk of splattering of sputum or blood during orotracheal intubation, body substance isolation (BSI) precautions must be taken. This means that gloves, a mask, and goggles or other protective eyewear are essential equipment during intubation. These items are mandatory because your face will be in the direct line of secretions, blood, and vomitus coming from the patient's mouth as you attempt to visualize the airway. In some intubation situations where there is excessive bleeding or vomiting, a gown or other impervious garment may also be required.

The Laryngoscope In addition to personal protective gear, orotracheal intubation requires specialized equipment. The **laryngoscope** is made up of two components—a handle that contains the batteries and a blade that is inserted into the airway and illuminates the airway (Figure 29-4). In most laryngoscopes, the handle and the blades are two separate pieces that must be assembled with each use (Figure 29-5). In these devices, the blade is placed parallel to the handle

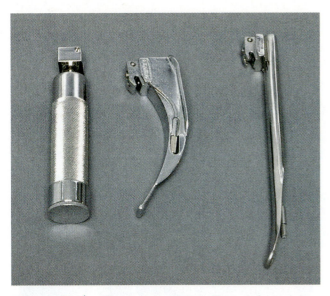

Figure 29-4 The laryngoscope. From left to right, the handle, the curved blade, and the straight blade.

There are two general types of laryngoscope blades: straight and curved. Both types come in assorted sizes ranging from the smallest size, 0, to the largest size, 4. The size of the blade used depends on the size of the patient. Most adult patients can be intubated using a size 2 or 3 straight blade or a size 3 curved blade. (Pediatric blade sizes will be discussed later in this chapter.) Whether to use a straight or curved blade is an individual choice. Straight blades, however, are preferred for pediatric orotracheal intubation.

Each blade type permits visualization of the vocal cords by taking advantage of different anatomical mechanisms. The tip of the straight blade is placed under the epiglottis to lift the epiglottis upwards, bringing the glottic opening and the vocal cords into view (Figure 29-8). The tip of the curved blade is inserted into the vallecula so that lifting the laryngoscope handle upward brings the glottic opening and the vocal cords into view (Figure 29-9).

The Endotracheal Tube The endotracheal tube (ET tube) is a single lumen—or channel—tube through which air and supplemental oxygen are delivered (Figure 29-10). At the proximal end of the tube (which remains outside the patient) is a standard 15 millimeter adapter for connection to the bag valve. At the distal end of the tube is a **cuff** designed to be inflated after the tube is placed to prevent leakage of air and fluid around the tip of tube. The cuff holds approximately 10 cc of air and should be inflated only enough to make a good seal around the tube. The cuff of the tube is filled by using a 10 cc syringe at the inflation valve. Just below the inflation valve is the **pilot balloon,** which fills with air when the cuff is inflated. Inflation of the balloon verifies that there is air in the cuff, which is out of sight once it is inserted. If the pilot balloon does not hold air, then assume that the cuff at the end of the tube has also failed. Endotracheal tubes used with infants and children less than 8 years old do not have cuffs. (See Orotracheal Intubation of Infants and Children later in this chapter.) Many endotracheal tubes have a small hole, known as a Murphy eye, on the left side of the tube at the distal end opposite the bevel. This feature lessens the

and the notch at the base of the blade is attached to the bar on the handle. The blade is then lifted to a 90°-angle with the handle and, as the blade locks into place, the light at the tip of the blade illuminates. Always check the bulb at the end of the blade to assure that it gives off a bright, white light and that the bulb is tightly secured to the blade. "White, bright, and tight" is an easy way to remember the proper condition of the instrument.

Some laryngoscopes are disposable, single-use units to eliminate the need for cleaning (Figure 29-6). Also, if you use a fiber-optic laryngoscope, you will not have to assure the bulb on the blade is secure, because the light source in located within the handle (Figure 29-7).

No matter what type of laryngoscope you use, you must check the device daily to assure that it is working properly. Spare batteries and bulbs should always be stored with the laryngoscope.

Laryngoscope Blades Laryngoscope blades are specifically designed for the anatomy of the airway. They provide optimal illumination of the vocal cords to enable insertion of the endotracheal tube through the cords. Most commercially available blades are designed with the light on the right side of the blade. This means that the scope's handle must be held in the left hand to best illuminate the airway.

Assembling the Laryngoscope

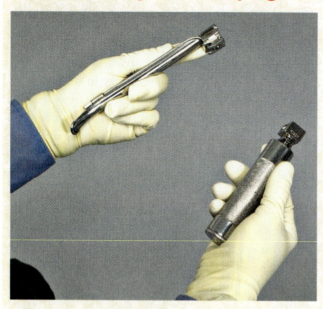

Figure 29-5A Hold the blade parallel to the laryngoscope handle.

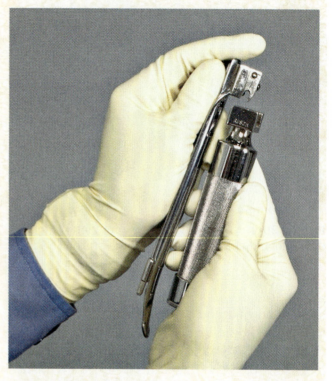

Figure 29-5B Attach the notch on the blade to the bar on the handle.

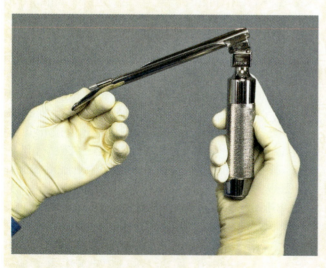

Figure 29-5C Lift the blade up so that it is at a 90°-angle to the handle.

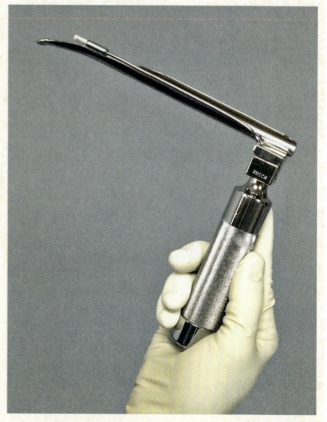

Figure 29-5D When the blade is properly positioned, it will lock into place at the 90°-angle to the handle and the light at its tip will illuminate.

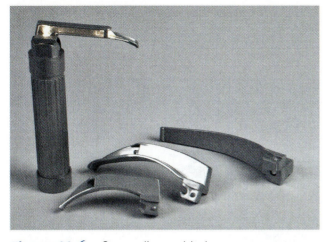

Figure 29-6 Some disposable laryngoscopes are pre-assembled with handle and blade as a fixed unit.

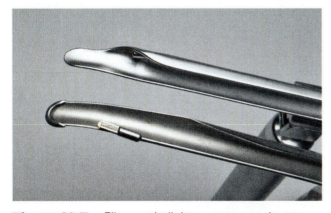

Figure 29-7 Fiber-optic light source on a laryngoscope blade (top) as compared to a conventional light bulb on a laryngoscope blade (bottom).

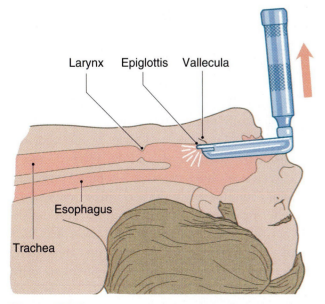

Figure 29-8 The straight laryngoscope blade lifts the epiglottis.

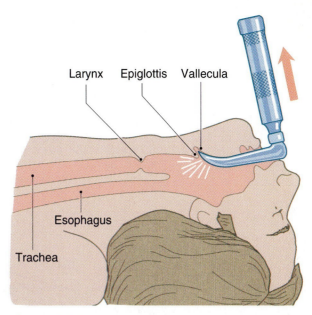

Figure 29-9 The curved laryngoscope blade lifts the vallecula.

chances of tube obstruction by providing an additional opening at the end of the tube.

Endotracheal tubes come in various diameters from 2.0 millimeters (used on premature infants) to 10.0 millimeters (used on very large adults). The diameter measured is the distance from one internal wall of the tube to the other, called the internal diameter or "i.d." No matter what the internal diameter of the tube is, a standard 15 millimeter adapter is affixed to the end of the tube to allow attachment to a BVM or other device.

When determining the proper size endotracheal tube to use in an adult patient, the rule of thumb is—in an emergency, use a 7.5 mm tube. For more precise sizing, it is generally accepted that an adult male should receive either an 8.0 or an 8.5 mm tube. An adult female should receive from a 7.0 to an 8.0 mm tube. The sizing of pediatric endotracheal tubes will be discussed later in this chapter.

The adult endotracheal tube has a standard length of 33 centimeters. The side of the tube is marked in centimeters starting from the distal tip. The most important of these marks is the one at 22 centimeters because, when the endotracheal tube is properly placed, the 22 centimeter mark will usually be at the patient's teeth. This position assures that the tip of the tube is in the trachea

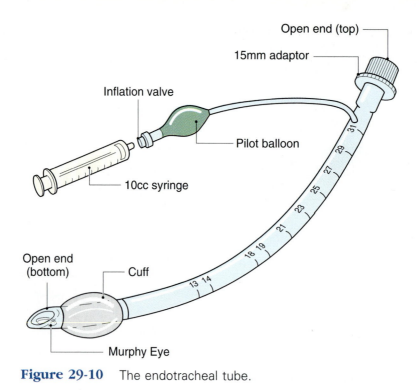

Inflation valve

10cc syringe

Open end
(bottom)

Cuff

Murphy Eye

Open end (top)

15mm adaptor

Pilot balloon

Figure 29-10   The endotracheal tube.

above the carina. (As you will learn, assuring proper placement of the tube is a critical skill, and checking the length marking is only a small part of this procedure.) It may be helpful to envision the depth of tube placement by reviewing the following anatomic distances in the average adult:

◆ 15 centimeters from the teeth to the vocal cords

◆ 20 centimeters from the teeth to the sternal notch

◆ 25 centimeters from the teeth to the carina

As you can see, there is very little room for error when placing the endotracheal tube, since only a few centimeters can mean the difference between proper placement of the tube just above the carina and misplacement beyond the carina and into the right mainstem bronchus.

Accessories   There are several other accessories to the endotracheal tube with which you must be familiar. These include the stylet; lubricant; the 10 cc syringe; devices for assuring proper tube placement; devices for securing the tube once it is properly placed; and a suction device.

◆ **Stylet and Lubricant**   Because the endotracheal tube is made of relatively flexible plastic, it is generally recommended that a **stylet,** a long, thin, bendable metal probe, be inserted into the tube before intubation (Figure 29-11). The stylet helps stiffen the tube and provides it with a shape that will ease its insertion through the vocal cords. The stylet should be lubricated with a water-soluble lubricant such as K-Y® jelly, Surgilube®, or Lubrifax® before insertion into the endotracheal tube. This will allow a smooth withdrawal of the stylet after the tube is successfully placed.

Once the lubricated stylet is inserted, the endotracheal tube should be shaped into a curved or "hockey stick" configuration. To avoid trauma to the airway, *do not* insert the stylet past the tip of the tube. Because stylets are longer than endotracheal tubes, it is easy to inadvertently allow the tip to extend beyond the end of the tube. Such an error could puncture the trachea. To avoid this complication, the tip of the stylet should not be inserted beyond the proximal end of the

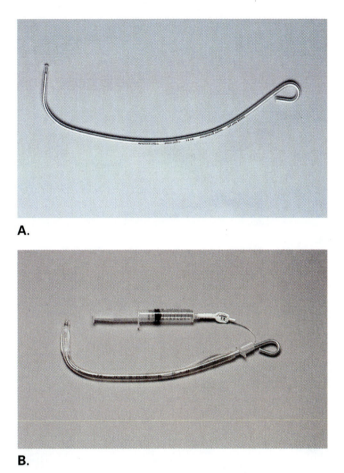

A.

B.

Figure 29-11 **A.** The stylet. **B.** The stylet in place in the endotracheal tube.

Murphy eye and the stylet's excess length should be bent over the 15 mm adapter.

During orotracheal intubation, excessive oral secretions often obstruct the view of the vocal cords. For this reason, always have an operational wide-bore suction device within easy reach during intubation attempts. The suction device should be turned on and placed by your right hand (since your left hand will be holding the laryngoscope).

Paradoxically, a patient's airway can sometimes be very dry. This can make insertion of the endotracheal tube difficult because of friction between the end of the tube and the patient's pharynx and glottis. To help ease this difficulty, apply water-soluble lubricant to the outside of the distal portion of the tube. In general, you can use half a packet of lubricant on the stylet and the other half of the packet on the outside of the tube.

◆ **Syringe** Another piece of essential equipment for use with the endotracheal tube is a 10 cc syringe. As noted above, use the syringe to inflate the cuff through the inflation valve. The syringe should also be used to test that the cuff is intact and holds air before inserting the tube. Once the integrity of the cuff has been assured, the air should be withdrawn, but the syringe should remain attached to the tube so that it is at hand when it is time to reinflate the cuff after the patient is intubated. Following final inflation of the cuff, the 10 cc syringe should be detached from the inflation valve to prevent leakage of air out of the cuff and back into the syringe.

◆ **Tube-securing Device** One of the final steps in orotracheal intubation is securing the tube to the patient so that it does not move or become dislodged. This is especially important in the prehospital setting where the tube can be easily dislodged during patient movement. Before securing the endotracheal tube, insert an oral airway or similar device such as a bite block in case the patient becomes responsive and gnaws at the tube. There are a number of methods for securing endotracheal tubes. These range from cloth tape (Figure 29-12) to commercially available devices (Figure 29-13). The medical director usually prescribes the manner of securing tubes in an EMS system. Whatever system is used to secure the tube, you must make sure the tube is firmly secured in place and able to withstand the tugs and pulls that are routine during moves of critically ill patients.

Indications for Endotracheal Intubation

When properly performed, orotracheal intubation is clearly a life-saving technique. It is essential, however, that you know under what conditions a patient needs to be intubated. The following is a listing of indications for when to perform orotracheal intubation:

◆ Inability to ventilate the apneic patient

◆ To protect the airway of a patient without a gag reflex or cough

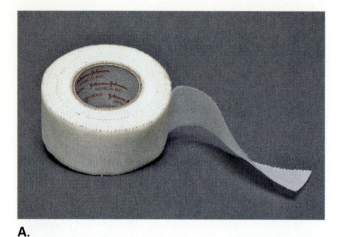

A.

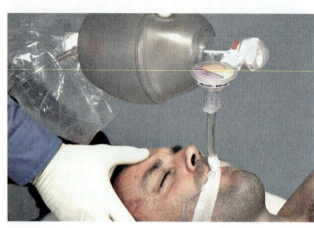

B.

Figure 29-12 **A.** Cloth tape for securing an ET tube. **B.** The tube secured using cloth tape.

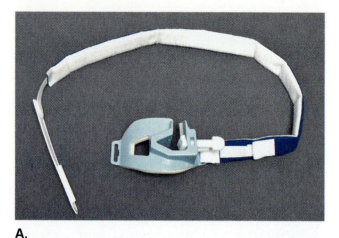

A.

B.

Figure 29-13 **A.** A commercially produced device for securing an ET tube. **B.** The tube secured using the device.

◆ To protect the airway of a patient unresponsive to any painful stimuli

◆ Respiratory or cardiac arrest

Technique of Intubation—Adult Patients

Orotracheal intubation is the most complicated and difficult procedure the EMT is expected to perform. Incorrectly performed, the EMT's actions can easily result in the patient's death. Because many EMTs will only rarely perform orotracheal intubation, it is essential that you not only learn and practice the technique extensively during your training but also continue to practice the technique on a regular basis once you are a certified EMT.

The following is a step-by-step guide to orotracheal intubation of the adult patient (Figure 29-14):

1. **Assure body substance isolation precautions.** These should include gloves, goggles or other protective eyewear, and a mask.

2. **Assure that adequate ventilation with a bag-valve mask and high concentration oxygen is being provided.**

3. **Hyperventilate the patient with high concentration oxygen at a rate of 24 breaths per minute prior to any intubation attempts.**

4. **Assemble, prepare, and test all equipment** including the following:

◆ *A suction unit with a large bore rigid tip.* It should be functional and positioned within easy reach of the intubator's right hand in case it is needed.

◆ *The cuff on the endotracheal tube.* It should be tested and then deflated with the 10 cc syringe left attached to the inflation valve.

(*text continues, page 774*)

Orotracheal Intubation

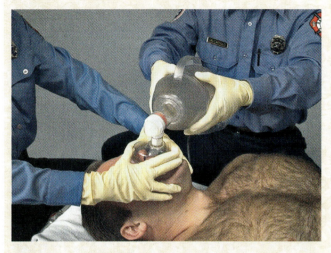

Figure 29-14A Hyperventilate the patient.

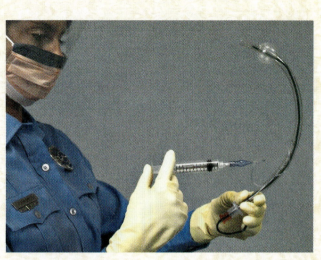

Figure 29-14B Assemble, prepare, and test the equipment.

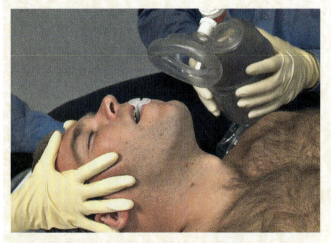

Figure 29-14C Position the patient's head.

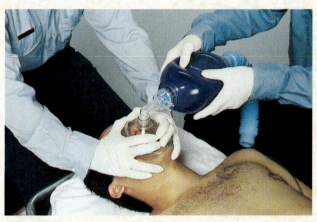

Figure 29-14D Make sure the airway is aligned. If you suspect trauma, keep the patient's head and neck in a neutral position.

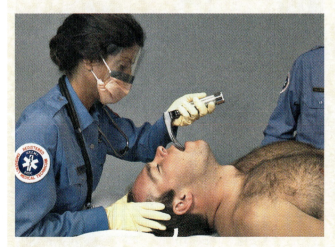

Figure 29-14E Prepare to insert the laryngoscope blade.

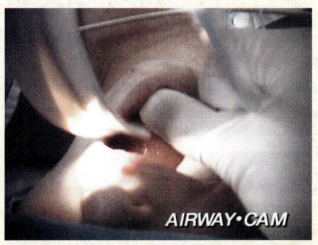

Figure 29-14F Open the mouth using a scissors technique.

(continued)

Orotracheal Intubation (continued)

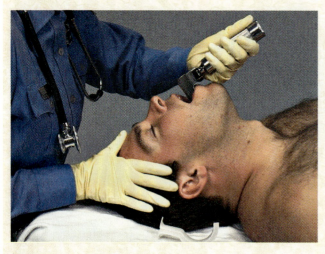

Figure 29-14G Insert the blade.

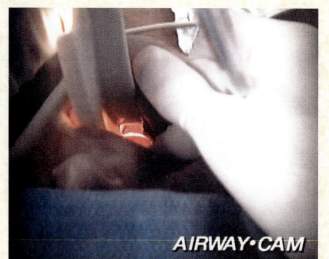

Figure 29-14H Insert the blade into its proper location, with a straight blade lifting the epiglottis and a curved blade (as shown) fitting into the vallecula.

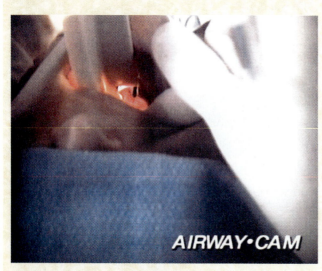

Figure 29-14I Visualize the glottic opening.

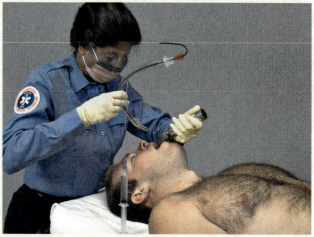

Figure 29-14J Insert the endotracheal tube.

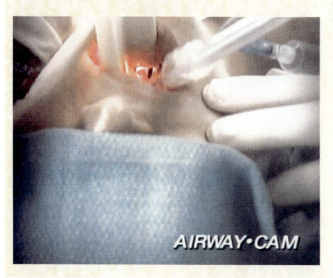

Figure 29-14K View of the tube going down the right side of the mouth toward the glottic opening.

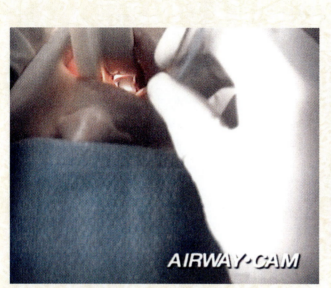

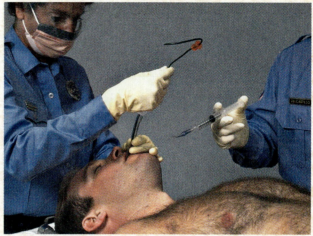

Figure 29-14L Pass the tube through the vocal cords.

Figure 29-14M Remove the laryngoscope and stylet. Inflate the cuff with 5 to 10 cc of air.

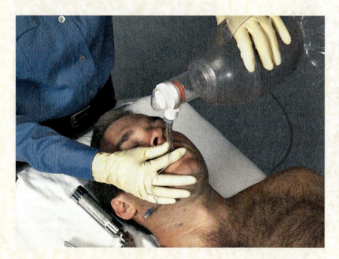

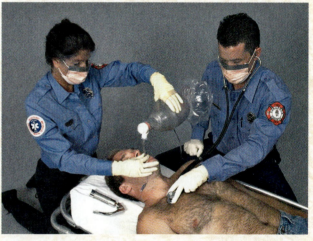

Figure 29-14N Attach the bag-valve unit or other ventilation device to the tube.

Figure 29-14O Auscultate over lungs and epigastrium to assure correct tube placement.

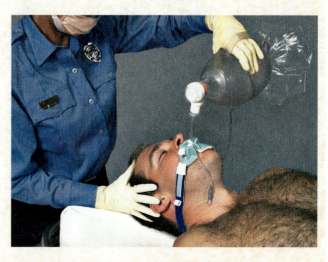

Figure 29-14P If correct placement is confirmed, secure the tube in place.

- ♦ *The laryngoscope.* Assemble it and assure that the bulb is firmly secured and that the light is bright and constant.

- ♦ *The stylet.* Lubricate the stylet and insert it into the tube and form the tube into a curved or "hockey stick" shape.

- ♦ *The device that will be used to secure the tube after successful intubation.*

5. **Position yourself at the patient's head.**

6. **Position the patient's head to assure good visualization of the vocal cords. Remove the oral airway.**

   - ♦ If trauma is not suspected, tilt the head, lift the chin, and attempt visualization of the vocal cords. If the cords cannot be seen, raise the patient's shoulders with a towel approximately 1 inch (25 mm) and attempt visualization again.

   - ♦ If trauma is suspected, the patient will have to be intubated with the head and neck in a neutral position while a second rescuer maintains in-line stabilization of the neck and head.

7. **Hold the laryngoscope in your left hand and insert the laryngoscope into the right corner of the patient's mouth.**

8. **Use a sweeping motion to lift the tongue upward and to the left, out of the way, to enable visualization of the glottis.**

9. **Insert the blade into the proper anatomical location:**

   - ♦ Curved blade fits into the vallecula.

   - ♦ Straight blade lifts the epiglottis.

10. **Lift the laryngoscope up and away from the patient; avoid using the teeth as a fulcrum.**

11. **Applying cricoid pressure (Sellick's maneuver) during intubation attempts may be beneficial.** Sellick's maneuver is performed by a second rescuer who uses his index finger and thumb to exert direct pressure on the patient's cricoid cartilage (Figure 29-15). Because the cricoid cartilage is the only cartilage in the neck that completely encircles the trachea, direct pressure helps to compress the esophagus, which is posterior to

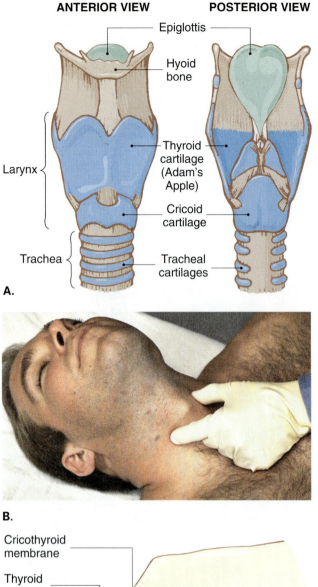

A.

B.

C.

Figure 29-15 **A.** The cricoid cartilage completely encircles the trachea. **B.** and **C.** In Sellick's maneuver, pressure is placed on the cricoid cartilage, compressing the esophagus, which reduces regurgitation and helps bring the vocal cords into view.

the trachea. This reduces the risk of vomitus entering the upper airway. In addition, the pressure often brings the vocal cords into better view. Cricoid pressure should be maintained until the patient is intubated.

12. **Visualize the glottic opening and vocal cords.** *Once the cords come into view do not loose site of them!*

13. **With the right hand, carefully insert the endotracheal tube through the vocal cords.** The tube should be inserted just deep enough so that the cuff is past the cords. Verify that the 22 cm mark on the tube is at the level of the patient's gums and teeth.

14. **Remove the laryngoscope.** Fold the blade down to extinguish the lamp.

15. **Remove the stylet.**

16. **Inflate the cuff with 5 to 10 cc of air and remove the syringe.**

17. **Continue to hold onto the endotracheal tube.** *Never let go of the endotracheal tube until it is secured in place.*

18. **Have a partner attach the bag valve to the endotracheal tube and deliver artificial ventilations.**

19. **Confirm tube placement.** The single most accurate way of assuring proper tube placement is visualizing the endotracheal tube as it passes through the vocal cords. All the following methods are for verification of tube placement.

◆ Observe the patient's chest rise and fall with each ventilation.

◆ Auscultate for the presence of breath sounds as follows:

a. Begin over the epigastrium. No breath sounds should be heard here during ventilations.

b. Listen over the left apex (top of the left lung area). Compare those breath sounds with those heard over the right apex. Breath sounds heard should be equal on both sides.

c. Listen over the left base (bottom of the left lung area). Compare those breath

sounds with those heard over the right base. Breath sounds heard should be equal on both sides.

◆ Observe the patient for signs of deterioration after tube placement. For example, if the patient develops cyanosis after intubation, it is a sign of hypoxia and probable incorrect tube placement.

◆ If local protocols permit, use other objective measures such as pulse oximetry, end tidal carbon dioxide detectors, or tube aspirators to confirm tube placement.

20. **An incorrect tube placement must be detected and corrected without delay.**

◆ If breath sounds are diminished or absent on the left but present on the right, it is likely the tube has intubated the right mainstem bronchus. If this occurs:

a. Deflate the cuff and *gently* withdraw the tube while artificially ventilating and while auscultating over the left apex of the chest.

b. Take care not to completely remove the endotracheal tube.

c. When the breath sounds become equal at both the left and right apex, reinflate the cuff and follow the directions below for securing the tube.

◆ If breath sounds are present only in the epigastrium, the esophagus has been intubated. Because esophageal intubation is a potentially fatal occurrence

a. Immediately deflate the cuff and withdraw the tube.

b. Hyperventilate the patient for at least 2 to 3 minutes before making a second attempt at intubation.

Warning! *The EMT should make only two attempts at orotracheal intubation. If both attempts fail, insert an oral airway and continue to ventilate the patient with high concentration oxygen via bag-valve mask, aggressively suctioning the airway as needed.* (Your local protocols may allow you to make additional attempts at intubation if the first two are unsuccessful.)

21. **If breath sounds are heard bilaterally and no sounds are heard over the epigastrium, secure the endotracheal tube using tape or the system approved by your medical director.** An oral airway may be inserted as a bite block to protect the endotracheal tube. Note the depth of the tube at the teeth both before and after securing it to assure the tube has not been dislodged during the procedure.

22. **Be sure to assess and reassess the breath sounds following every major move with the patient.**

    Warning! *It cannot be over-emphasized that the likely result of inadvertent esophageal intubation will be your patient's death.* Because of the magnitude of this complication, if at any time—despite your efforts to properly assess tube placement—you are in doubt of proper tube placement, immediately withdraw the tube and manage the airway with a bag-valve mask and basic airway adjuncts.

Although direct visualization of the endotracheal tube passing through the vocal cords is the most reliable way of assuring proper tube placement, many EMS systems require prehospital providers to use an additional "objective" device to confirm proper tube placement. Therefore, in addition to requiring you to listen for equal breath sounds in the chest and for a silent epigastrium, your system may direct that you use one of these devices. The most commonly used are the *syringe* or *bulb esophageal intubation detector devices* and the *end tidal carbon dioxide detectors.*

The syringe-style device (Figure 29-16) works on the premise that it is possible to withdraw air under pressure from the rigid trachea, but not from the collapsible esophagus. The device is attached to the 15 mm adapter of the endotracheal tube after the patient has been intubated and the cuff of the tube has been inflated. The plunger of the syringe is then pulled back. If air enters the syringe easily, the endotracheal tube is in the trachea. If there is resistance to pulling back the plunger, then it is presumed that the ET tube is in the esophagus, which has collapsed as air was withdrawn. With the bulb device (Figure 29-17), the device is attached to the tube and its

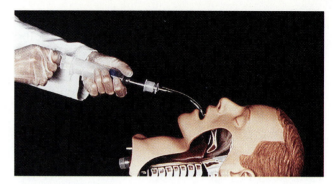

Figure 29-16   An esophageal intubation detector—syringe aspiration style.

bulb is squeezed. If the bulb refills easily, it indicates proper tube placement. If the bulb does not refill, the tube is incorrectly placed. If resistance to syringe aspiration is encountered or the bulb does not refill, withdraw the endotracheal tube immediately and hyperventilate the patient via BVM before making a second and final attempt at intubation.

End tidal carbon dioxide ($ETCO_2$) detectors measure the carbon dioxide in the exhalation portion of ventilations. These devices work on the premise that during exhalation CO_2 should be detected. If the tube is improperly placed, no CO_2 will be detected. The two types of $ETCO_2$ detectors in use are the colormetric and the digital (Figure 29-18). Colormetric detectors are single-use, disposable devices. They are attached between the endotracheal tube and the bag-valve device after intubation. They have a small window that displays color changes during ventilations. If the color in the window changes from purple to yellow during ventilations, then the tube is properly placed in the trachea. If the color remains purple during ventilations, then the tube is in the esophagus and must be withdrawn immediately. Colormetric devices can be difficult to use in low-light conditions. Also, in some cases of prolonged cardiac arrest, the amount of end tidal carbon dioxide given off by the patient may be too low for the device to detect.

Although more expensive than the colormetric models, digital $ETCO_2$ detectors are used by some EMS systems. These devices permit more precise measurement of end tidal carbon dioxide levels.

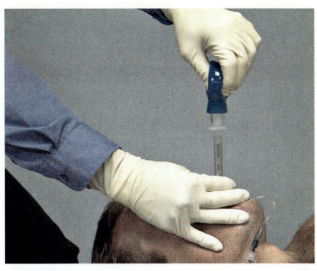

A.

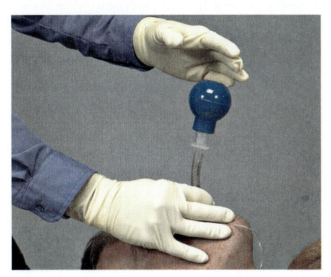

B.

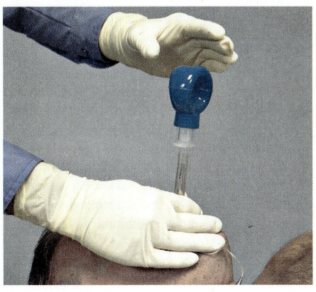

C.

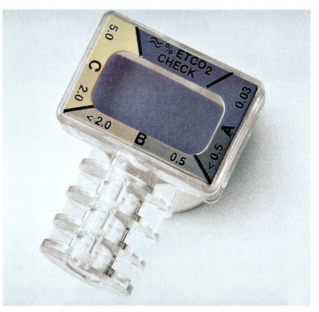

A.

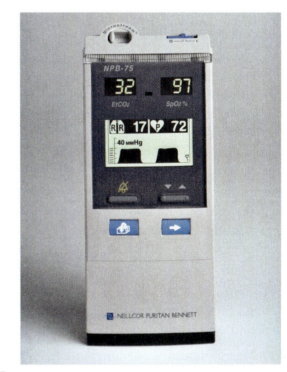

B.

Figure 29-18 **A.** A colormetric end tidal carbon dioxide detector. **B.** A digital end tidal carbon dioxide detector.

Figure 29-17 An esophageal intubation detector—bulb style. **A.** The device is attached to endotracheal tube and its bulb is squeezed. **B.** If the bulb refills easily upon release, it indicates correct tube placement. **C.** If the bulb does not refill, the tube is improperly placed.

Orotracheal Intubation of Infants and Children

Although the goal of orotracheal intubation is the same in both adult and pediatric patients, intubation of infants and children requires special training. This is because of various considerations of anatomy, physiology, and sizing. Special features of the anatomy and physiology of the pediatric airway have been discussed earlier in this chapter. These features relate to orotracheal intubation in infants and children in the following ways:

◆ In infants and children, it is often difficult to create a single clear visual plane from the mouth through the pharynx and into the glottis for orotracheal intubation because of such factors as the relatively large size of the tongue of the infant and child. To create such a plane, a straight larynoscope blade is usually preferred in infants and children.

◆ Because of size differences among infants and children coupled with the fact that the narrowest portion of the airway is at the level of the cricoid ring, the proper sizing of the endotracheal tube and the use of an *uncuffed* ET tube in children younger than 8 years of age are crucial.

◆ Because infants and children tend to develop hypoxia and bradycardia (slowed heart rate) easily during intubation attempts, pediatric intubations require careful monitoring coupled with swift and accurate technique.

The indications for orotracheal intubation of infants and children are similar to those for adult patients and include the following:

◆ Prolonged artificial ventilation is required

◆ Adequate artificial ventilation cannot be achieved by other means

◆ Ventilation of the clearly apneic patient

◆ Ventilation of the cardiac arrest patient

◆ Control of the airway in an unresponsive patient without a cough or gag reflex

The laryngoscope blades and the endotracheal tubes necessary for the orotracheal intubation of infants and children must be carefully sized to the patient. In general the straight blade, usually a size 1, is preferred in infants and small children because it provides for greater displacement of the tongue and better visualization of the glottis. As in adults, the blade lifts the epiglottis, bringing the vocal cords into view. In older children, the curved blade is often preferred because the blade's broad base displaces the tongue better, allowing better visualization of the vocal cords once the blade is placed into the vallecula and lifted.

Assorted sizes of endotracheal tubes should always be stocked in the pediatric airway kit. As previously mentioned, proper sizing of the tube is essential in children. Ideally a chart should be kept in the airway kit to assist the EMT in determining what size tube is generally used for a patient of a specific age. Alternatively, a Broselow™ tape can be used to estimate tube size based on the patient's height (Figure 29-19).

There is also a simple formula for estimating proper tube size. It is

$$\frac{\text{(Patient's age in years} + 16)}{4} = \text{Tube size}$$

You can also estimate correct tube size by using the diameter of the *patient's* little finger or the diameter of the nasal opening.

Infants are often the pediatric patients who require orotracheal intubation. Therefore, it is helpful to simply memorize that newborns and small infants generally require a 3.0 to a 3.5 tube and that a 4.0 tube can be used for older infants up to the age of 1 year.

No matter what system you use in determining tube size, it is always prudent to have tubes one half-size larger and one half-size smaller on hand at the time of intubation, since the size of the glottic structures does vary in infants and children.

Endotracheal tubes come in both cuffed and uncuffed versions. Cuffed tubes are always used in adult patients. Among pediatric patients, cuffed tubes are reserved for children 8 years of age and older. For younger children and infants, uncuffed tubes are used because the narrowing of the airway at the level of the cricoid cartilage serves as a functional cuff, snugging the tube in the airway. Uncuffed tubes (Figure 29-20) should display a vocal cord marker to assure proper placement of the tube. This marker is designed so that the vocal cords are at the level of the break in the translu-

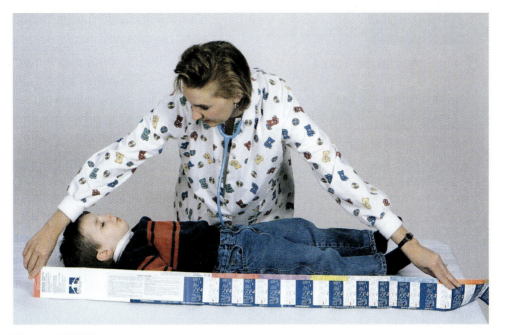

Figure 29-19   A Broselaw™ tape can be used to estimate tube size based on the pediatric patient's height.

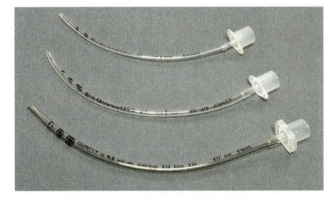

Figure 29-20   Three sizes of uncuffed pediatric endotracheal tubes.

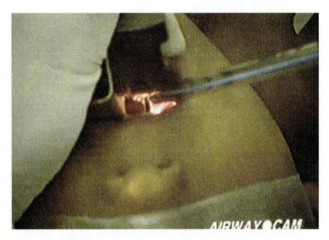

Figure 29-21   Insertion of an uncuffed endotracheal tube in a pediatric patient.

cent marker in the tube (Figure 29-21). If the child is old enough to get a cuffed tube, it should be inserted, like the adult tube, just deep enough so that the cuff material is distal to the cords.

Proper depth of tube can also be approximated by age (Table 29-2). However, direct visualization of the tube being placed at the proper depth is the best measure of tube depth.

The step by step procedure for orotracheal intubation of infants and children is very similar to the procedure outlined for adults (Figure 29-14). There are, however, some important differences that you must keep in mind when performing a pediatric intubation:

◆ The rate of hyperventilation both before and after intubation must be adjusted to the patient's age, with a faster rate for infants and children than for adults.

◆ The patient's heart rate must be continuously monitored during intubation attempts because both mechanical stimulation of the airway and hypoxia can slow the heart rate. If you note the heart rate slowing during intubation, immediately withdraw the blade and reventilate the infant or child with high concentration oxygen.

Table 29-2

Infant/Child Endotracheal Tubes

Age of Patient	Measurement of the Endotracheal Tube at the Teeth
6 months to 1 year	12 cm—teeth to mid-trachea
2 years	14 cm—teeth to mid-trachea
4–6 years	16 cm—teeth to mid-trachea
6–10 years	18 cm—teeth to mid-trachea
10–12 years	20 cm—teeth to mid-trachea

◆ The best way of positioning the patient's head during intubation is to gently tilt the head forward and lift the chin into the "sniffing position" (Figure 29-22).

◆ Very little force is needed to intubate the infant or child. Gentle finesse is the rule, not the exception.

◆ Sellick's maneuver can be helpful when intubating pediatric patients; however, the landmarks for performing it may be difficult to locate in infants and children. In addition, applying too much pressure to the relatively soft cartilage may collapse it, causing tracheal obstruction.

◆ When using a straight blade, realize that the epiglottis in infants and children is not as stiff

Figure 29-22 Place the pediatric patient's head in the "sniffing" position for intubation.

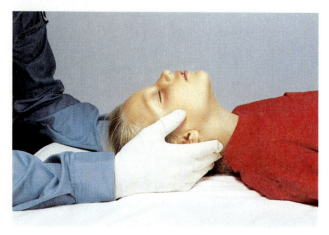

as in adults and may partially obscure a clear view of the vocal cords.

◆ Since distances in the infant and child are small, be certain to hold onto the tube until you are assured it is well secured. As with adults, reassess tube placement every time you move the patient.

◆ In infants and children, the best indicator of tube placement is symmetrical rise and fall of the chest during ventilation.

◆ Breath sounds in infants and children can often be misleading because the chest is small and sounds are easily transmitted from one area to another.

◆ Your EMS system may require the use of an aspiration device or an end tidal carbon dioxide detector at this point in the procedure.

◆ Observe the patient for increase in heart rate and improving color after intubation. An infant or child who becomes dusky in color and whose heart rate slows after intubation has probably been improperly intubated.

◆ Once tube placement is confirmed, the patient should be secured to an appropriate device to prevent any head movement from dislodging the tube.

◆ If the tube is properly placed but there is inadequate chest expansion, seek out the cause among the following:

—The tube is too small and there is an air leak around the tube at the glottic opening. This is detected by auscultating over the neck and mouth. Replace the first tube with a larger one after hyperventilating the patient.

—The pop-off valve on the bag-valve device has not been deactivated.

—There is a leak in the bag-valve device.

—The EMT is delivering an inadequate volume of air/oxygen with BVM ventilations.

—The tube is blocked with secretions. This can be treated initially with endotracheal suctioning (see below in this chapter). If suctioning fails, the tube should be removed.

Infants and children are at risk for the same complications of orotracheal intubation as adult patients. Inadvertent esophageal intubation is even more rapidly fatal in infants and children than in adults. In addition, excess pressure from over-inflation of the lungs can result in collapse of a lung, which can further compromise your ability to ventilate the patient.

Nasogastric Intubation of Infants and Children

An additional procedure the EMT must master along with pediatric orotracheal intubation is the placement of a **nasogastric tube** (NG tube). A nasogastric tube is inserted through the nose into an infant's or child's stomach. The NG tube is most commonly used in advanced airway management to decompress the stomach and proximal bowel of air. In infants and children, air frequently fills the stomach and proximal bowel after overly aggressive artificial ventilation or as a result of air swallowing. The NG tube provides a route for escape of this excess air. The NG tube can also be used to drain the stomach of blood or other substances. In the hospital setting, NG tubes can also be used to give medication and/or nutrition.

The indications for insertion of the NG tube in pediatric patients are as follow:

◆ Inability to ventilate the patient adequately because of distention of the stomach

◆ The unresponsive patient with gastric distention

Many experts believe that the NG tube should be inserted only after the airway has been secured with an endotracheal tube; this will prevent improper insertion of the NG tube into the trachea rather than the esophagus. Other complications of NG intubation include trauma to the nose, slowing of the heart rate, the triggering of vomiting, and—in very rare cases—passage of the NG tube into the cranium through a basilar skull fracture. *Because of the risk of cranial intubation with the NG tube, the presence of major facial trauma or head trauma is considered a contraindication for use of the NG tube.* In such cases, insertion of the tube through the mouth (orogastric technique) is preferred.

The equipment required for nasogastric tube insertion includes the following:

◆ Nasogastric tubes of various sizes:
  —Newborn/infant: 8.0 French
  —Toddler/preschool: 10.0 French
  —School age: 12 French
  —Adolescent: 14–16 French
◆ 20 cc syringe
◆ Water-soluble lubricant
◆ Emesis basin
◆ Tape
◆ Stethoscope
◆ Suction unit with connecting tubing

The procedure for insertion of the nasogastric tube illustrated in Figure 29-23 is as follows:

1. **Prepare and assemble all equipment.**
2. **Assure that the patient is well oxygenated prior to the procedure.**
3. **Measure the tube from the tip of the nose around the ear to below the xiphoid process.** (If the tube will be inserted by the orogastric technique, measure from the lips to below the xiphoid process.) This length will determine the depth to which the tube will be inserted.
4. **Lubricate the end of the tube.**
5. **Pass the tube gently downward along the nasal floor.**
6. **Confirm that the tube is in the stomach by:**
   ◆ Aspirating stomach contents
   ◆ Auscultating a rush of air over the epigastrium while injecting 10–20 cc of air into the tube
7. **Aspirate gastric contents by placing the tube to suction.**
8. **Secure the tube in place with tape.**

Orotracheal and Endotracheal Suctioning

You have already learned how to suction a patient's mouth and pharynx with a rigid-tip catheter. As part of your training in advanced air-

Nasogastric Intubation

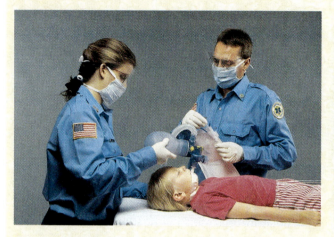

Figure 29-23A Oxygenate and continue to ventilate the patient.

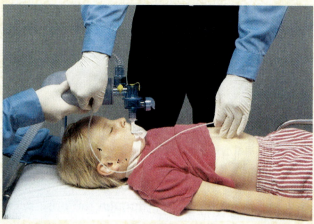

Figure 29-23B Measure the tube from the tip of the nose, over the ear, to the tip of the xiphoid process.

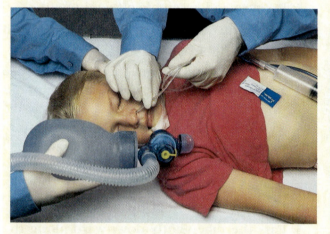

Figure 29-23C Pass the lubricated tube gently downward along the nasal floor to the stomach.

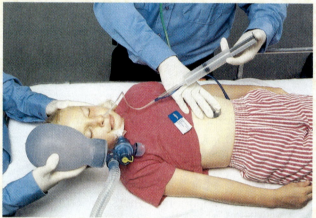

Figure 29-23D Auscultate over the epigastrium to confirm correct placement. Listen for bubbling while injecting 10 to 20 cc of air into the tube.

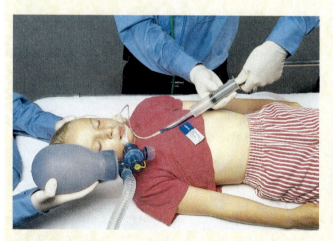

Figure 29-23E Use suction to aspirate stomach contents.

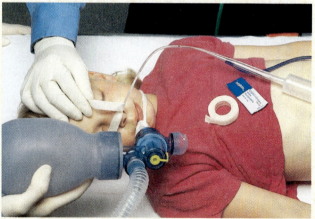

Figure 29-23F Secure the tube in place.

way management, you may learn the techniques of orotracheal and endotracheal suctioning. With these techniques, a flexible soft suction catheter is used to suction the trachea, usually down to the level of the carina in the artificially ventilated patient. These techniques are sometimes referred to as "deep suctioning."

In general, deep suctioning is best accomplished after an endotracheal tube has already been placed into the airway. Placing the suction catheter through the endotracheal tube (endotracheal suctioning) directly into the trachea below the vocal cords assures more effective suctioning. This is because it is usually difficult to blindly direct a soft suction catheter through the mouth (orotracheal suctioning) into the trachea. Such orally passed suction catheters frequently enter the esophagus rather than the trachea.

The indications for orotracheal and endotracheal suctioning are as follows:

◆ *Obvious secretions in the airway.* These may be detected either by moist bubbling sounds heard during ventilation with the bag-valve mask or by visible secretions seen inside the endotracheal tube after the patient has been intubated.

◆ *Poor compliance with bag-valve-mask ventilation.* Resistance to ventilation may be caused by secretions below the level of the larynx in the trachea.

The technique for endotracheal suctioning is shown in Figure 29-24. Specific steps in the procedure include the following:

1. **Hyperventilate the patient with high concentration oxygen before attempting to suction.**

2. **Check that all equipment is operating correctly.**

3. **Use sterile technique.** Don sterile gloves. Remove the catheter from its container without allowing it to touch anything until it is inserted into the endotracheal tube.

4. **Observe body substance isolation precautions.** Be certain to have eye protection and a mask in place, as splattering during deep suctioning is common.

5. **Approximate the desired length of the catheter to be inserted by measuring from the lips to the ear to the nipple line.** This will approximate the level of the carina.

6. **Advance the catheter to the desired location.**

7. **Apply suction and withdraw the catheter in a twisting motion.**

8. **Resume ventilations.**

9. **Attempts at deep suctioning should not exceed 15 seconds to prevent hypoxia.**

Deep suctioning can have complications. Most of the serious ones relate to the fact that the ventilated patient is deprived of oxygen during suctioning. Hyperventilation prior to suctioning, careful technique, and limiting suctioning to 15 seconds can help prevent the following complications of deep suctioning:

◆ Cardiac arrhythmias (especially slow heart rates)

◆ Hypoxia

◆ Coughing

◆ Damage to the lining (mucosa) of the airway

◆ Spasm of the bronchioles (bronchospasm) if catheter extends past the carina

◆ Spasm of the vocal cords (laryngospasm) during orotracheal suctioning

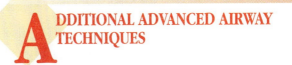

ADDITIONAL ADVANCED AIRWAY TECHNIQUES

There is a variety of advanced airway techniques that go beyond the standard EMT-Basic curriculum. Medical directors in some systems may elect to allow EMTs to use some of these techniques.

Automatic Transport Ventilators

Automatic transport ventilators (ATVs) have been used extensively in Europe for a number of years. The devices are rapidly gaining popularity in the United States as recent studies have demonstrated them to be superior in some ways to manual ventilation with the bag-valve mask.

Endotracheal Suctioning

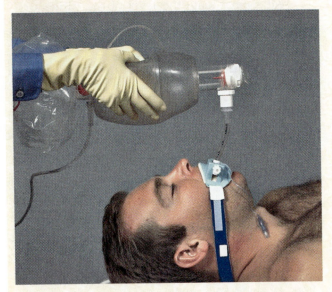

Figure 29-24A Hyperventilate the patient.

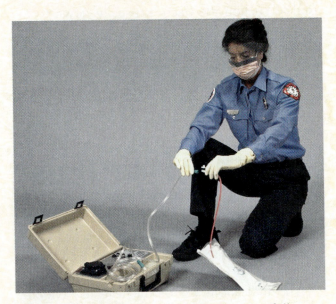

Figure 29-24B Check all equipment carefully.

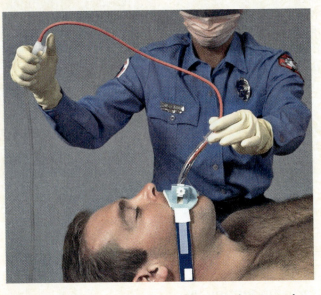

Figure 29-24C Insert the catheter without applying suction.

ATVs are compact devices with controls that set both the rate of ventilation and the tidal volume (Figure 29-25). Tidal volumes are determined by the patient's weight. A number of different ATV models are commercially available. The American Heart Association recommends that ATVs should meet certain minimum standards. The ATVs should

◆ Have the ability to deliver 100% oxygen

◆ Be able to provide at least two rates of ventilation: 10 breaths per minute for adults and 20 breaths per minute for children

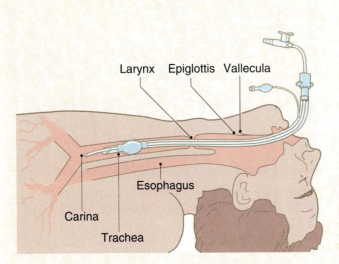

Larynx Epiglottis Vallecula

Esophagus

Carina

Trachea

Figure 29-24D The catheter may be advanced as far as the carina.

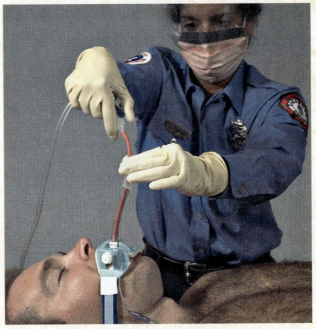

Figure 29-24E Apply suction. Withdraw the catheter with a twisting motion.

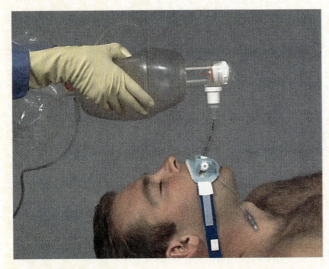

Figure 29-24F Resume ventilations. Suctioning should interrupt ventilations for no more than 15 seconds.

◆ Be lightweight (2 to 5 kg) and rugged

◆ Be equipped with an audible alarm to alert the user to problems in ventilation

◆ Have a standard 15 mm/22 mm coupling to connect with a mask or endotracheal tube

Although some units are marketed for pediatric use with controls for lower tidal volumes, the device is not suitable for children less than 5 years of age.

ATVs do require some additional training for safe use. The decision to use ATVs in an EMS sys-

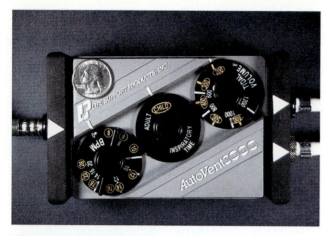

Figure 29-25 An automatic transport ventilator. (The coin shows the size of the device.)

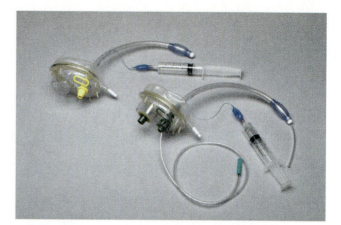

Figure 29-26 An esophageal obturator airway (EOA) (top) and an esophageal gastric tube airway (EGTA).

tem and the establishment of ATV protocols should be done by the medical director.

Esophageal and Multilumen Airways

In some EMS systems, medical direction may elect to allow EMTs to use esophageal airways such as the esophageal obturator airway and the esophageal gastric tube airway, multilumen airways such as the Combitube® and PtL®, and—most recently—the laryngeal mask airway. These devices do not provide the definitive airway control of an endotracheal tube. However, when properly used, they provide superior ventilation of the apneic patient as compared with a simple oral airway. Indeed, in some studies, ventilation with some of these devices has proven as effective as endotracheal tube ventilation.

If your EMS system uses one of these alternative devices, you must obtain additional training. What follows is an overview of the use of each of the devices. Remember that no matter what device is used to secure the patient's airway, it is likely that airway secretions, blood, and/or vomitus may be propelled toward the EMT. Gloves, a mask, and eye protection should be worn during any advanced airway procedure.

The EOA and EGTA

For over 20 years, the esophageal obturator airway (EOA) and its close cousin the esophageal gastric tube airway (EGTA) have been available as alternative methods of intubating patients. (Figure 29-26). Both devices are designed for insertion into the

patient's esophagus rather than the trachea. Once the device is seated in the esophagus, a cuff at the distal end of the tube is inflated, thereby blocking (or obturating) the esophagus. With the esophagus sealed, the ventilations delivered through the mask are delivered into the trachea and then the lungs. Both of these devices are passed "blindly" into the pharynx, eliminating the need to use a laryngoscope. The EGTA differs from the EOA in that the EGTA permits a gastric tube to be passed through it to decompress the stomach contents.

◆ *Insertion of the EOA/EGTA Airways*

The procedure for placing the EOA/EGTA is as follows (Figure 29-27):

1. **Hyperventilate the patient with high concentration oxygen via a BVM device.**

2. **Have suction ready.**

3. **Test the distal balloon with 35 cc of air.**

4. **Attach the mask to the tube.** Assure that it is properly seated by hearing the "click."

5. **Place the patient's head in a neutral or slightly flexed position if no spinal injury is suspected.**

6. **With one hand, lift the jaw anteriorly by placing a gloved thumb into the patient's mouth.**

7. **With the other hand, insert the airway tube until the mask is seated against the mouth and nose.**

8. **Give two ventilations to the mask and observe the chest rise.** If the chest does not rise, or if only one side of the chest rises, remove the airway, reventilate the patient, and reinsert the airway.

9. **If the chest does rise, inflate the cuff with 35 cc of air and detach the inflation syringe.**

10. **Ascultate over both sides of the chest for air movement. Also auscultate over the epigastrium, which should be silent.** If breath sounds are absent on one side of the chest or are present over the epigastrium, deflate the balloon, remove the device, and reventilate the patient.

11. **Once the device is properly placed, maintain a proper mask seal at all times.**

12. **If the patient regains consciousness, he will not be able to tolerate the EOA/EGTA. Turn the patient on his side, deflate the cuff, and withdraw the tube while suctioning.**

Insertion of an EOA/EGTA is contraindicated with the following patients:

◆ Children less than 16 years of age

◆ Patients under 5 feet (1.5 m) tall

◆ Those who have ingested caustic substances such as lye

◆ Those with a gag reflex

◆ Those with known esophageal diseases such as esophageal varices

Reported complications of EOA/EGTA use have included esophageal rupture and endotracheal rather than esophageal placement of the tube. The most common reason the device fails to provide adequate ventilation is lack of a proper mask seal. To avoid this, once the device is properly placed, the mask should be held in place with two hands by one rescuer and ventilations provided by a second rescuer.

The Esophageal Tracheal Combitube® Airway

The esophageal tracheal combitube (or Combitube®) airway has two separate ports for ventilations (Figure 29-28). Like the EOA/EGTA, the device is passed blindly into the pharynx. The Combitube®, however, allows for proper ventilation whether the tube is placed in the esophagus or in the trachea (Figure 29-29). If the tube is placed in the esophagus, then the esophagus is sealed off by a balloon. The pharynx and lungs are then ventilated in a manner much like an EOA. If the tube is placed into the trachea, then the trachea is directly ventilated in a manner similar to an endotracheal tube. Because the device is directly ventilated through a standard 15 mm adapter, the problem of mask seal encountered with the EOA/EGTA is eliminated.

The multilumen device requires the EMT to assess whether the distal tube is placed in the esophagus or the trachea in order to determine which port to ventilate. Because the device is more complicated than either an EOA/EGTA or a standard endotracheal tube, thorough initial training and on-going practice are essential.

Because the tubes of the Combitube® airway may be placed into the esophagus, the same contraindications as for the EOA/EGTA apply. These contraindications include:

◆ Children less than 16 years of age

◆ Patients under 5 feet (1.5 m) tall

◆ Those who have ingested caustic substances such as lye

◆ Those with a gag reflex

◆ Those with known esophageal diseases such as esophageal varices

◆ *Insertion of the Combitube® Airway*

Below are the steps to be followed when inserting the Combitube®:

1. **Hyperventilate the patient with high concentration oxygen via BVM device.**

2. **Have suction ready.**

3. **Insert the device blindly, watching for the two black rings on the Combitube® that are used for measuring the depth of insertion.** These rings should be positioned between the teeth or the bony cavities where the teeth have their roots.

Inserting the Esophageal Obturator Airway

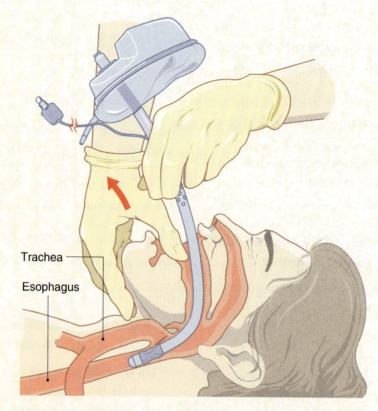

Figure 29-27A Insert the EOA completely assembled. Flex the patient's head forward while grasping the jaw and tongue. Lift up and forward.

Trachea

Esophagus

4. **Use the large syringe to inflate the pharyngeal cuff of the airway with 100 cc of air.** Once it is properly inflated, the device will seat itself in the posterior pharynx behind the hard palate.

5. **Use the smaller syringe to fill the distal cuff with 10 cc to 15 cc of air.**

6. **Usually the tube will have been placed in the esophagus. On this assumption, ventilate through the esophageal connector.** It is the external tube that is the longer of the two and is marked #1. You must listen for the presence of breath sounds in the lungs and the absence of sounds from the epigastrium in

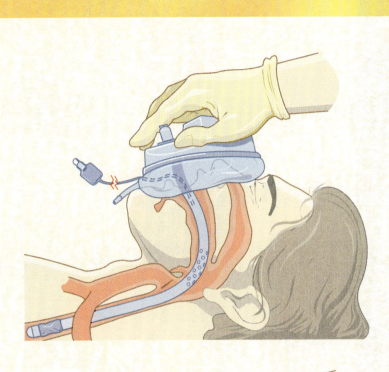

Figure 29-27B Advance the tube until the mask fits snugly over the patient's nose and mouth.

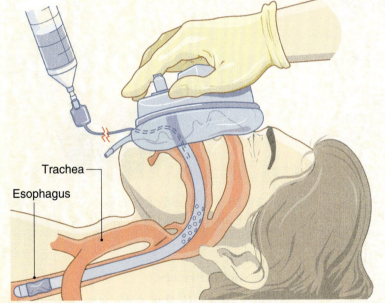

Trachea

Esophagus

Figure 29-27C Inflate the distal cuff. Check positioning of the device. Watch and auscultate for bilateral expansion of the chest and bilateral breath sounds. If the chest does not rise on both sides and breath sounds are not heard, withdraw the tube, hyperventilate, then attempt reinsertion.

order to be sure that the tube is, in fact, properly placed.

7. **If there is an absence of lung sounds and presence of sounds in the epigastrium, the tube has been placed in the trachea. In this case, attach the BVM and ventilate through the shorter tracheal connector, which is marked #2.** Listen again to be sure of proper placement of the tube.

The biggest advantage of the Combitube® is that rapid intubation is possible regardless of the position of the patient, which is helpful with trauma patients requiring limited cervical spine movement. As with the EOA/EGTA, if the patient

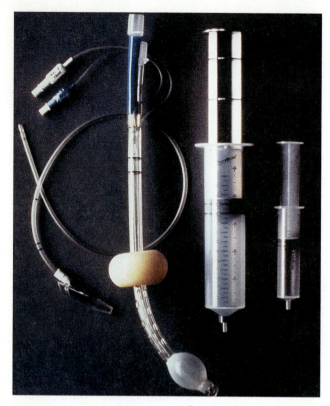

Figure 29-28 A Combitube® airway.

becomes conscious, you must remove the Combitube®. Remember that extubation is likely to be followed by vomiting. Have suction equipment ready. Follow the same guidelines as for removal of other airway devices.

The Pharyngo-Tracheal Lumen Airway (PtL®)

The PtL® is a multilumen airway somewhat similar to the Combitube®. The PtL® is no longer manufactured, but because some departments may still use it it will be briefly described here.

The PtL® is inserted in a slightly different manner than the Combitube®. The PtL® also has a semi-rigid stylet in its clear (endotracheal) tube that allows for better shaping of that tube. As with a standard endotracheal tube, this stylet must be removed if the PtL® is placed in the trachea.

◆ Insertion of the PtL®

Below are the steps to follow when inserting the PtL®:

1. **Hyperventilate the patient with high concentration oxygen via BVM device.**

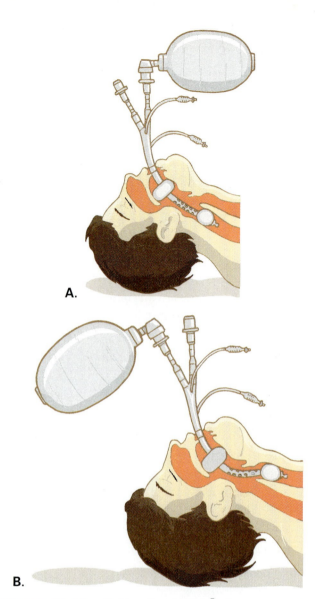

A.

B.

Figure 29-29 **A.** The Combitube® airway placed in the esophagus. **B.** The Combitube® airway placed in the trachea.

2. **Have suction ready.**
3. **Assure that all the cuffs are tested and then fully deflated.**
4. **Open the airway.** In a patient with potential spinal trauma, have a partner stabilize the head in a neutral in-line position while you pass the airway with minimal cervical manipulation. Use a thumb-in-mouth jaw-lift or tongue-lift method to open the airway. If you have ruled out spinal trauma, hyperextend the patient's head with one hand, insert your thumb deep into the patient's mouth, grasp the tongue and lower jaw between your

thumb and index finger and lift straight forward.

5. **Hold the PtL® in your free hand so that it curves in the same direction as the natural curvature of the pharynx. Then insert the tip of the airway into the patient's mouth and advance it carefully behind the tongue until the teeth strap contacts the lips and teeth.** (Positioning the airway in this manner with the teeth strap against the lips and teeth is proper for an average-sized adult. If the patient is very small, it may be necessary to withdraw the airway so that the teeth strap is as much as 1 inch from the teeth. When the patient is very large, it may be necessary to insert the airway beyond the normal depth so that the teeth strap is actually inside the patient's mouth, past the teeth.)

6. **When the tube is at the proper depth, flip the neck strap over the patient's head and tighten it with the hook-and-tape closures located on both sides of the strap.**

7. **Inflate the small cuff that seals either the esophagus or the trachea and the large cuff that seals the oropharynx, first making sure that the white cap is in place over the deflation port located under the inflation valve.** To inflate both cuffs simultaneously, deliver a sustained ventilation into the inflation valve. Failure to inflate the cuffs properly can be detected by the failure of the exterior pilot balloon to inflate or by feeling air escaping from the patient's mouth and nose. In this case, one of the cuffs, probably the large one, may be torn. Quickly remove the airway, ventilate the patient, then replace it with a new one. When you see by the pilot balloon that the two cuffs are inflated, deliver puffs of air to increase pressure in the cuffs and improve the seal.

8. **Determine the location of the PtL® by ventilating the short, green tube.** If the chest rises, the long tube is in the esophagus and air is, obviously, being diverted through the trachea into the lungs. In this case, deliver ventilations via BVM through the short, green tube.

9. **If the chest does not rise when the short, green tube is ventilated, the long, clear tube is probably in the trachea. In this case, remove the stylet and deliver ventilations through the clear tube.** Verify proper delivery of ventilations by listening to both lung fields (for sounds of air entering both lungs) and the epigastrium (where there should be *no* sounds of air entering the esophagus and stomach). Also verify chest rise with each breath.

10. **Continue ventilations through the airway until the patient regains consciousness or a protective airway gag reflex returns, or until the patient is transferred to the emergency department.**

Continually monitor the appearance of the pilot balloon during ventilation efforts. Loss of pressure in the balloon will signal a loss of pressure in the cuffs. If you suspect that a cuff is leaking, increase cuff pressure by blowing forcefully into the #1 inflation valve or replace the airway. Repositioning the PtL® to ensure that the teeth strap is snug against the patient's teeth is another way of reducing leakage.

Again, as with the EOA, EGTA or Combitube®, if the patient becomes conscious, you must remove the PtL®. Remember that extubation is likely to be followed by vomiting. Follow these guidelines for removing the PtL®.

◆ If there is no possibility of trauma, or if the patient is secured to a spine board, turn the patient onto his side.

◆ Remove the white cap from the deflation port to simultaneously deflate both cuffs.

◆ Carefully withdraw the airway and discard.

◆ Stay alert for vomiting.

The Laryngeal Mask Airway

The larygeal mask airway (LMA) has been in wide use in Europe for some time. It has recently been introduced into the United States. Although the device has largely been used in the operating room by anesthesiologists and nurse anesthetists, many feel the LMA may have prehospital value as well.

The LMA differs significantly in design from the other alternative advanced airway devices

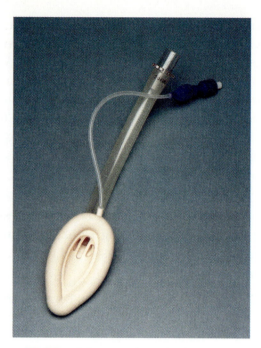

Figure 29-30   A laryngeal mask airway.

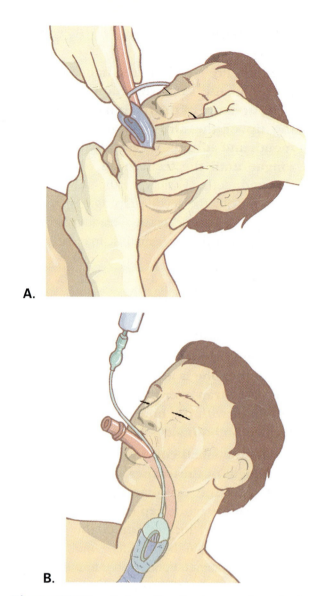

A.

B.

Figure 29-31   **A.** Inserting the laryngeal mask airway. **B.** The airway properly in place.

already described (Figure 29-30). The device is inserted neither into the trachea nor the esophagus, but rather into the hypopharynx. The device consists of an elliptical cuff on the distal portion of the tube. The LMA's inflatable cuff is designed to rest in the hypopharynx around the opening to the larynx. When inflated, it provides a tight seal around the opening to the larynx. Unlike other alternative advanced airway devices, the LMA comes in several different sizes, allowing its use in children as well as adults.

◆ *Insertion of the Laryngeal Mask Airway*

When properly used, the LMA can provide excellent control of the airway and assure adequate ventilation of the patient. The LMA is inserted using the following steps (Figure 29-31):

1. **Hyperventilate the patient with high concentration oxygen via the BVM device.**

2. **Have suction ready.**

3. **Assure that the cuff is tested and then fully deflated.**

4. **Lubricate the posterior surface of the cuff with a water-soluble lubricant.**

5. **Place the patient's head in the "sniffing position" with the neck slightly flexed and the head extended.**

6. **Have a second rescuer open the mouth by depressing the chin.**

7. **Hold the LMA like a pen and introduce the device with the opening of the cuff facing anteriorly so that the black line on the tube aligns with the nasal septum.**

8. **Advance the device with steady, gentle pressure past the hard and soft palates. Be careful not to allow the tube to rotate.**

9. **Advance the LMA into the hypopharynx until resistance is met.** At this point the tube

should be properly placed. Verify that the black line still aligns with the nasal septum.

10. **Inflate the cuff with the proper volume of air.** The tube will appear to rise 1 or 2 cm out of the mouth upon inflation of the cuff.

11. **Confirm proper placement in the breathing patient by listening for breath sounds through the proximal opening of the tube.** In the apenic patient, ventilate through the LMA and listen for presence of breath sounds over the lungs and absence of sounds over the epigastrium.

12. **Insert an oral airway or bite block into the mouth to protect the tube.**

13. **Once you have assured that the LMA is properly placed, secure the device in place.**

Complications associated with use of the LMA include the following:

◆ Gagging and vomiting during insertion of the airway in the semiconscious patient.

◆ Airway obstruction due to improper placement of the device. This can be caused by rotation of the tube or folding of the cuff material in the hypopharynx.

◆ Air leak around the cuff as detected by the escape of air through the mouth during breathing or ventilations.

Chapter Review

SUMMARY

There is no more important skill in the provision of emergency care than learning to open, maintain, and control a patient's airway. Endotracheal intubation is the "gold standard" of airway control and is taught as an optional skill to EMTs. If your EMS system allows you to perform endotracheal intubation or use another alternative advanced airway device, it is essential that you practice the procedure on a regular basis since its successful use may be truly life-saving for the patient with inadequate or absent respirations.

REVIEWING KEY CONCEPTS

1. Identify factors to observe when determining adequacy of breathing.

2. List the advantages of orotracheal intubation in the apneic patient.

3. Identify the possible complications associated with orotracheal intubation.

4. Contrast the uses of the straight and curved laryngoscope blades in intubation.

5. Describe the parts of an endotracheal tube and explain their various purposes.

6. List the indications for performing orotracheal intubation in adult patients.

7. Describe the purpose of Sellick's maneuver and explain how to perform it.

8. Explain various methods used to assess proper placement of the endotracheal tube.

9. Describe various ways of estimating endotracheal tube size for a pediatric patient.

10. Explain the reason for using uncuffed endotracheal tubes with pediatric patients.

11. Explain the purposes of nasogastric intubation and list the indications for performing the procedure.

12. Describe the method of measuring the nasogastric tube in the infant and child.

13. List the indications for orotracheal suctioning.

14. List possible complications of orotracheal suctioning.

RESOURCES TO LEARN MORE

Book

Roberts, J. R. and Hedges, J. R. *Clincal Procedures in Emergency Medicine, 3rd Editon.* Philadelphia: W. B. Saunders, 1997.

Video

Levitan, R. M. Airway•Cam Video Series. Airway•Cam Technology, PO Box 337, Wayne, PA 19087.

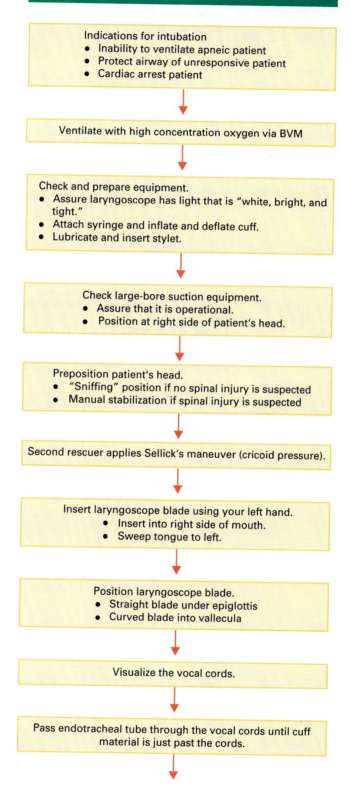

ADULT ENDOTRACHEAL INTUBATION

Indications for intubation
- Inability to ventilate apneic patient
- Protect airway of unresponsive patient
- Cardiac arrest patient

Ventilate with high concentration oxygen via BVM

Check and prepare equipment.
- Assure laryngoscope has light that is "white, bright, and tight."
- Attach syringe and inflate and deflate cuff.
- Lubricate and insert stylet.

Check large-bore suction equipment.
- Assure that it is operational.
- Position at right side of patient's head.

Preposition patient's head.
- "Sniffing" position if no spinal injury is suspected
- Manual stabilization if spinal injury is suspected

Second rescuer applies Sellick's maneuver (cricoid pressure).

Insert laryngoscope blade using your left hand.
- Insert into right side of mouth.
- Sweep tongue to left.

Position laryngoscope blade.
- Straight blade under epiglottis
- Curved blade into vallecula

Visualize the vocal cords.

Pass endotracheal tube through the vocal cords until cuff material is just past the cords.

(continued)

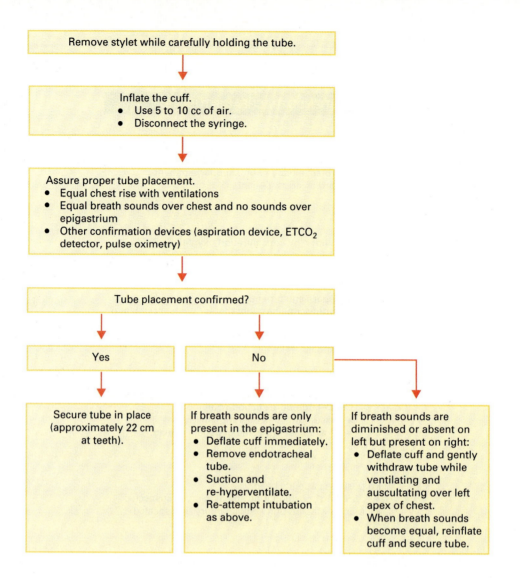

Remove stylet while carefully holding the tube.

Inflate the cuff.
- Use 5 to 10 cc of air.
- Disconnect the syringe.

Assure proper tube placement.
- Equal chest rise with ventilations
- Equal breath sounds over chest and no sounds over epigastrium
- Other confirmation devices (aspiration device, ETCO$_2$ detector, pulse oximetry)

Tube placement confirmed?

Yes

No

Secure tube in place (approximately 22 cm at teeth).

If breath sounds are only present in the epigastrium:
- Deflate cuff immediately.
- Remove endotracheal tube.
- Suction and re-hyperventilate.
- Re-attempt intubation as above.

If breath sounds are diminished or absent on left but present on right:
- Deflate cuff and gently withdraw tube while ventilating and auscultating over left apex of chest.
- When breath sounds become equal, reinflate cuff and secure tube.

ALS-Assist Skills

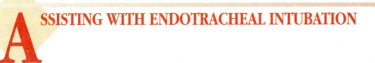

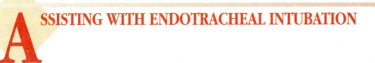

APPENDIX

A

Local protocol may require you to assist more highly trained EMS personnel in the administration of advanced life support (ALS) procedures. There are several new skills you can learn to enhance your capability as a "team player" on such calls. Your instructor will discuss the skills that are authorized by your medical director. However, the most common are:

◆ Assisting in the endotracheal intubation of a patient
◆ Applying ECG/defibrillator electrodes
◆ Using a pulse oximeter
◆ Assisting in intravenous (IV) fluid therapy

Note: The following information is intended as a summary of ALS-assist skills. More detailed information and additional in-service training may be required. Consult with your instructor on local protocols.

ASSISTING WITH ENDOTRACHEAL INTUBATION

Among the highest priorities of patient care is to assure a patient airway and to prevent aspiration. The "gold standard" for airway care is the endotracheal tube. Other airway devices, such as the EOA, EGTA, and Combitube®, are at best secondary. This is because the endotracheal tube is directly inserted into the trachea, forming an open pathway for air, oxygen, or medications to be blown into the lungs. In addition, adult sizes have an inflatable cuff that seals off the trachea to prevent aspiration. (In an infant or young child, the narrow trachea creates a seal.)

Patients who typically need to have an endotracheal tube inserted are those in pulmonary or cardiopulmonary arrest, trauma patients in need of airway control or supplemental oxygen, and those in respiratory distress or failure due to overdose, fluid in the lungs, asthma, asphyxia, or allergic reaction.

In some areas, EMT-Basics will be trained to perform endotracheal intubation of a patient. The skill is taught as an elective in Chapter 29, "Advanced Airway Management." In other areas, only EMT-Intermediates or EMT-Paramedics will perform endotracheal intubation, but EMT-Basics may be asked to assist with the procedure. The skills of assisting with endotracheal intubation are presented below.

Preparing the Patient for Intubation

Before the paramedic inserts the endotracheal tube, you may be asked to give the patient an extra amount of oxygen. This can easily be accomplished by ventilating with a bag-valve-mask device once every 2 seconds. Then the paramedic will position the patient's head to align the mouth, pharynx, and trachea. The paramedic will remove the oral airway and pass the endotracheal tube through the mouth (sometimes through the nose) into the throat past the vocal cords and into the trachea. This procedure usually requires a laryngoscope to move the tongue and other obstructions out of the way.

In order to maneuver the tube past the vocal cords correctly, the paramedic will need to see them. You may be asked to gently press on the throat to push the vocal cords into the paramedic's view. You will do this by pressing your thumb and index finger just to either side of the medial throat over the cricoid cartilage, the ring-shaped cartilage just below the thyroid cartilage, or Adam's apple. This procedure is known as cricoid pressure, or Sellick's maneuver (Figure ALS-1).

Once the tube is properly placed, the cuff is inflated with air from a 10 cc syringe. While holding the tube, the paramedic assures proper tube placement by using an esophageal intubation detector device and then listens with a stethoscope for lung sounds on both sides and over the epigastrium (the area of the upper abdomen just under the xiphoid process). If the tube has been correctly placed, there will be sounds of air entering the lungs but no sounds of air in the epigastrium. Air sounds in the epigastrium indicate that the tube has been incorrectly placed in the esophagus instead of the trachea so that air is entering the stomach instead of the lungs. The tube posi-

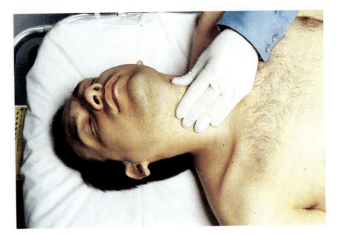

Figure ALS-1   In Sellick's maneuver, press your thumb and index finger on either side of the medial throat over the cricoid cartilage.

tion must be corrected immediately by removing the tube, re-oxygenating the patient, and repeating the process of intubation.

The correctly positioned tube is anchored in place with tape or a commercially made tube restraint. The entire procedure—including the last ventilation, passing the tube, and the next ventilation—should take less than 30 seconds.

Ventilating the Tubed Patient

When asked to ventilate a tubed patient, keep in mind that very little movement can displace the endotracheal tube. Look at the gradations on the side of the tube. In the typical adult male, for example, the 22 cm mark will be at the teeth when the tube is properly placed. If the tube moves, report this to the paramedic immediately.

Warning: *Be especially careful not to disturb the endotracheal tube.* If the tube is pushed in, it will most likely enter the right mainstem bronchus, preventing oxygen from entering the patient's left lung. If the tube is pulled out, it can easily slip into the esophagus and send all the ventilations directly to the stomach, denying the patient oxygen. This is a fatal complication if it goes unnoticed.

Hold the tube against the patient's teeth with two fingers of one hand (Figure ALS-2). Use the other hand to work the bag-valve-mask unit. A patient with an endotracheal tube offers less resistance to ventilations, so you may not need two hands to work the bag. If you are ventilating a

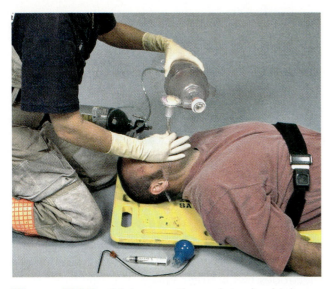

Figure ALS-2   Make sure the endotracheal tube does not move. Hold it with two fingers against the patient's teeth.

breathing patient, be sure to provide ventilations that are timed with the respiratory effort as much as possible so the patient can take full breaths. It is also possible to help the patient increase respiratory rate, if needed, by interposing extra ventilations. There are some cautions to remember.

◆ Pay close attention to what the ventilations feel like. Report any change in resistance. Increased resistance when ventilating with the bag-valve mask is one of the first signs of air escaping through a hole in the lungs and filling the space around the lungs, an extremely serious problem. A change in resistance can also indicate that the tube has slipped into the esophagus.

◆ With each defibrillation attempt, carefully remove the bag from the tube. If you do not, the weight of the unsupported bag may accidentally displace the tube.

◆ Watch for any change in the patient's mental status. A patient who becomes more alert may need to be restrained from pulling out the tube. In addition, an oral airway generally is used as a bite block (a device that prevents the patient from biting the endotracheal tube). If the patient's gag reflex returns along with increased consciousness, you may need to pull the bite block out a bit.

Finally, during a cardiac arrest in the absence of an IV line for administering medications, you may be asked to stop ventilating and remove the BVM. The paramedic may then inject a medication such as epinephrine down the tube. To increase the rate at which medication enters the blood stream through the respiratory system, you then may be asked to hyperventilate the patient for a few minutes (give ventilations at a faster-than-normal rate).

Assisting with a Trauma Intubation

Occasionally you will be asked to assist in the endotracheal intubation of a patient with a suspected cervical-spine injury. Since using the "sniffing position," which involves elevating the neck, risks worsening cervical spine injury, some modifications are necessary. Your role will change as well. You may be required to provide manual in-line stabilization during the whole procedure.

To accomplish this the paramedic will hold manual stabilization while you apply a cervical collar. In some EMS systems, the patient may be intubated without a cervical collar in place but with attention to manual stabilization during and after intubation. Since the paramedic must stay at the patient's head, it will be necessary for you to stabilize the head and neck from the patient's side (Figure ALS-3). Once you are in position, the paramedic will lean back and use the laryngo-

Figure ALS-3   To assist in the intubation of a patient with suspected cervical-spine injury, maintain manual stabilization throughout the procedure.

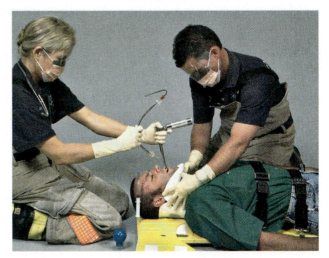

scope, which will bring the vocal cords into view. The patient can then be tubed.

After intubation, you will hold the tube against the teeth until placement is confirmed with both an esophageal intubation detector device and auscultation of both lungs and the epigastrium. Then the tube is anchored. At that time you can change your position to a more comfortable one. However, until the patient is immobilized on a long backboard, it will be necessary to assign another EMS worker to maintain manual stabilization while you ventilate the patient. Never assume that a collar provides adequate immobilization by itself. Manual stabilization must be used in addition to a collar until the head is taped in place on the backboard.

APPLYING ECG/DEFIBRILLATOR ELECTRODES

An electrocardiogram (ECG) provides data on the electrical activity of the heart. In the field, it is used to alert EMS personnel to life-threatening rhythm disturbances. Interpretation of an ECG has traditionally been a paramedic skill. However, to save time on calls you may be asked to assist. Make sure that you review the ECG equipment (Figure ALS-4). You should know how to turn on the monitor, how to record an ECG strip, how to change the battery, and how to change the roll of ECG paper. (These are the things that most often need to be done while the paramedic is involved with the patient.)

You also may be asked to carry out four steps in the process of applying the electrodes.

1. Turn on the ECG monitor
2. Plug in the monitoring cables or "leads."
3. Attach the monitoring cables to the electrodes.
4. Apply the electrodes to the patient's body.

Become familiar with the electrodes used by the paramedics with whom you work. There are two types: monitoring electrodes (with smaller pads) and combination monitoring/defibrillator electrodes (with larger pads). The one most commonly used by paramedics is the monitoring electrode.

If you are asked to apply monitoring electrodes to the patient's body, you will need three—each one giving a different "view" of the heart's electrical activity. First prepare the patient's skin. The best connection is on dry, bare skin, so it may be necessary to dry the area and shave excessive hair. Use a wash cloth to remove oil from the skin and consider using an antiperspirant on patients with very sweaty skin. Become familiar with the monitoring configuration (where to place the electrodes) used by ALS personnel in your system. The most common setup is placing

Figure ALS-5 The most common positioning of electrodes for an ECG is shown here. Become familiar with the monitoring configuration used by ALS personnel in your system.

Figure ALS-4 An ECG monitor/defibrillator.

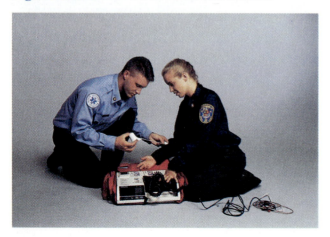

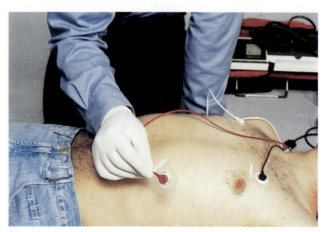

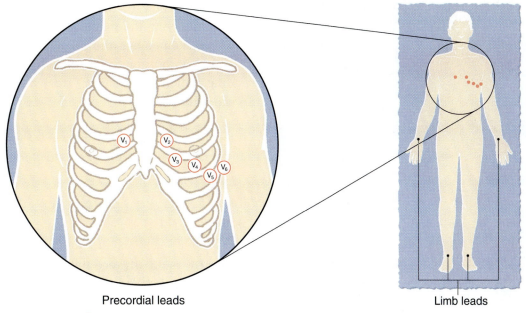

Precordial leads   Limb leads

Figure ALS-6   Placement of leads with a 12-lead ECG monitor.

the negative (white) electrode under the center of the right clavicle, the positive (red) electrode on the left lower chest, and the ground (black or green) electrode under the center of the left clavicle or the right lower chest (Figure ALS-5).

Some ALS systems have moved toward the routine use of a 12-lead ECG in the field. These machines usually provide a computerized interpretation of the patient's cardiogram that can easily be transmitted to the emergency department via cellular phone. A 12-lead ECG is used to assist in the diagnosis of an acute myocardial infarction (AMI). As the saying goes, in the case of an AMI "time is muscle." As the clock ticks, more and more heart muscle becomes dysfunctional and finally dies in the absence of oxygenated blood. With field diagnosis of AMI made possible by the 12-lead ECG, the time from AMI to the administration of "clotbuster" drugs, which break up the clots causing the AMI, can be reduced.

If 12-lead ECG monitors are used in your system, you may be asked to assist the paramedics in properly placing the leads. Application of the 12 leads is more complex than applying the 3 electrodes. Proper placement of the 12 leads is shown in Figure ALS-6. Ask the paramedics to review the lead placement with you.

USING A PULSE OXIMETER

A pulse oximeter is a photoelectric device that monitors the amount of oxygen circulating in the blood. It consists of a portable monitor and sensing probe (Figure ALS-7) that easily clips onto the patient's finger or earlobe. The oximeter screen displays a percentage measurement of oxygen saturation.

The oximeter should be used with all patients complaining of respiratory problems. It is useful in assessing the effectiveness of artificial respirations, oxygen therapy, bronchodilator therapy, and bag-valve-mask ventilations. It is important for you to note that

◆ Use of a pulse oximeter is helpful because it encourages you to be more aggressive about providing oxygen therapy and ventilations of a patient (in order to get the saturation reading up to 95%), especially a conscious patient in respiratory distress. The reverse situation is not true. That is, oxygen should not be withheld from a patient with signs and symptoms

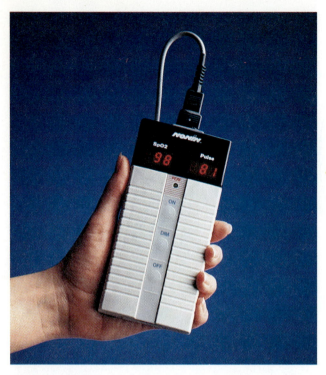

Figure ALS-7 A pulse oximeter is a photoelectric device that monitors the amount of oxygen circulating in the blood.

that indicate the need for oxygen, even if the reading is 95% or above.

◆ The oximeter is inaccurate with hypothermic patients (those whose body temperatures have been lowered by exposure to cold) and patients in shock.

◆ The oximeter will produce falsely high readings in patients with carbon monoxide poisoning. This is because carbon monoxide binds with hemoglobin in the blood, producing the red color read by the device. Also note that chronic smokers normally have 10% to 15% more residual carbon monoxide in their blood than nonsmokers, so they may show higher-than-normal readings while still requiring oxygen.

◆ Excessive movement of the patient can cause inaccurate readings. So can nail polish, if the device is attached to a finger. Carry acetone wipes to quickly remove the nail polish from a patient's fingernail before attaching the oximeter.

◆ Monitor the oximeter reading every 5 minutes.

◆ The accuracy of the unit should be checked by following the manufacturer's recommendations. Remember, the oximeter is just another tool. Do not rely on it solely for indications of the patient's condition. Treat the patient, not the machine.

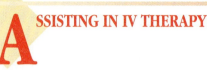

ASSISTING IN IV THERAPY

Setting Up an IV Fluid Administration Set

IV therapy is an advanced life support procedure. An intravenous (IV) line is inserted into a vein so that blood, fluids, or medications can be administered directly into the patient's circulation. A blood transfusion is almost always given at the hospital. An infusion of other fluids or medications can usually be done in the field.

The bag of fluid that feeds the IV is usually a clear plastic bag that collapses as it empties. The administration set is the clear plastic tubing that connects the fluid bag to the needle, or catheter. There are three important parts to this tubing.

◆ The drip chamber is near the fluid bag. There are two basic types: the mini drip and the macro drip. The mini drip is used when minimal flow of fluid is needed (with children, for example). Sixty small drops from the tiny metal barrel in the drip chamber equal one cubic centimeter (cc) or one milliliter (ml). The macro drip is used when a higher flow of fluid is needed (for a multi-trauma victim in shock, for example). There is no little barrel in the drip chamber of the macro drip, and only 10 to 15 large drops equal one cc or one ml.

◆ The flow regulator is located below the drip chamber. It is a device that can be pushed up or down to start, stop, or control the rate of flow.

◆ The drug or needle port is below the flow regulator. The paramedic can inject medication into this opening.

An extension set includes an extra length of tubing, which can make it easier to carry or disrobe the patient without accidentally pulling out the IV. Extension sets are sometimes not used with the macro drip set because lengthening tubing reduces the flow rate.

In most cases, a paramedic will insert the IV into the patient's vein. However, you may be enlisted to help set up the IV administration set. You will need to

1. Take out and inspect the fluid bag. The bags come in a protective wrapping to keep them clean. If you are setting up the IV, you must remove the wrapper, then inspect the bag to be sure it contains the fluid that has been ordered. Check the expiration date to make sure the fluid is usable, and look to see that the fluid is clear and free of particles. Squeeze the bag to check for leaks. Occasionally, the fluid comes in a bottle. If so, be sure it is free of cracks. If anything is wrong, report the problem and inspect another bag or bottle (Figure ALS-8).

2. Select the proper administration set. Uncoil the tubing, and do not let the ends touch the ground.

3. Connect the extension set to the administration set, if an extension set is to be used.

4. Make sure the flow regulator is closed. To do this, roll the stopcock away from the fluid bag.

5. Remove the protective covering from the port of the fluid bag and the protective covering from the spiked end of the tubing (Figure ALS-9). Insert the spiked end of the tubing

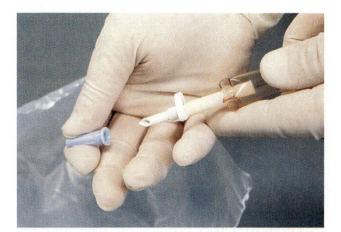

Figure ALS-9   Setting up the IV administration set includes removing the protective coverings from the port of the fluid bag and the spiked end of the tubing.

into the fluid bag with a quick twist. Do this carefully. Maintain sterility. If these parts touch the ground, they must not be used. Running germs or dirt directly into a patient's bloodstream can be extremely serious, even fatal.

6. Hold the fluid bag higher than the drip chamber. Squeeze the drip chamber a time or two to start the flow. Fill the chamber to the marker line (approximately one-third full).

7. Open the flow regulator and allow the fluid to flush all the air from the tubing. You may need to loosen the cap at the lower end to get the fluid to flow. Maintain the sterility of the tubing end and replace the cap when you are finished. Most sets can be flushed without removing the cap. Be sure that all air bubbles have been flushed from the tubing to avoid introducing a dangerous air embolism into the patient's vein.

8. Turn off the flow.

Make certain that the setup stays clean until the paramedic removes the needle and connects the IV tubing to the catheter inside the patient's vein. Occasionally, the paramedic will draw blood from the vein to obtain samples before inserting the IV. You may be asked to assist by placing the blood in sample tubes and labeling the tubes with the patient's name and any other information that your hospital requires. Remember that they are potential carriers of pathogens. Be sure to take BSI

Figure ALS-8   Inspect the IV bag to be sure it contains the solution that was ordered, for clarity, leaks, and to be sure it has not expired.

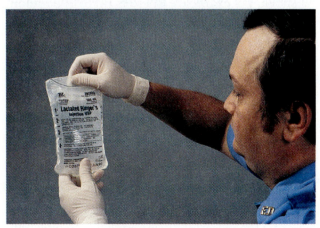

precautions. Carry the blood tubes to a safe place where they will not be in danger of breaking.

Do not be surprised if you are asked to hold up the arm for a few minutes during a cardiac arrest. During cardiac arrest, medications can be more effective if the patient's arm is temporarily raised after a drug is injected into the IV.

Maintaining an IV

An IV must continue to flow at the proper rate once it has been inserted into the patient's vein. However, a number of things may interrupt the flow. If you are charged with maintaining an IV, be sure to check for and correct the following problems.

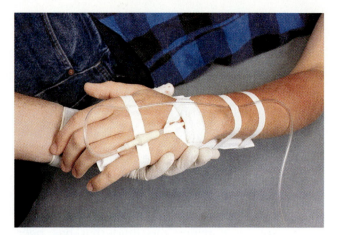

Figure ALS-10   Some IVs only flow when the IV site is in a certain position. Adjust or splint the body part as needed.

◆ Flow regulator may be closed.

◆ Clamp may be closed on the tubing.

◆ Tubing may kink.

◆ Tubing may get caught under the patient or the backboard.

◆ Constricting band used to raise the vein for insertion of the needle may have been mistakenly left on the patient's arm, perhaps covered by a sleeve.

◆ Tubing may have pulled out of the catheter.

The position of the IV or of the patient's arm also may need to be adjusted. Some IVs only flow when the patient's arm or IV site is in a certain position. Adjusting or even splinting the arm (Figure ALS-10) may be helpful as long as the splint is not too tight. Since the IV flow usually depends on gravity, be sure that the bag is held well above the IV site and the patient's heart.

Insufficient flow can cause blood to clot in the catheter. This can be prevented by adjusting the flow to an adequate "keep the vein open" or KVO rate. The KVO rate varies, but it is usually about 30 drops per minute for a micro drip and 10 drops per minute for a macro drip set. If the drip chamber is overfilled, clamp the tubing, in-

vert the drip chamber, and pump some fluid back into the bag.

An IV with a flow rate that is too fast is called a "runaway IV." It can rapidly overload the patient with fluid and cause serious problems, especially in an infant or child.

An infiltrated IV is one where the needle has either punctured the vein and exited the other side or has pulled out of the vein. In either case, the fluid is flowing into the surrounding tissues instead of into the vein. An unnoticed infiltrated IV can be very dangerous. Certain high concentration medications (such as 50% dextrose) can cause the death of the surrounding tissue. In addition to complaining of pain, the patient will show swelling at the site (noticeable in all but some obese patients). The person in charge of maintaining the IV must stop the flow and discontinue the IV according to local protocol. If you are not authorized to do this, report the problem immediately to the paramedic or medical direction.

If you learn how to help advanced life support personnel start an IV, run through an administration set, label blood tubes, and maintain an IV, valuable time can be saved at the scene and during transport.

Basic Cardiac Life Support Review

Before beginning your EMT-Basic course, you are required to have completed a course in cardiopulmonary resuscitation (CPR). The elements of CPR are reviewed here.

When a patient's breathing and heartbeat stop, *clinical death* occurs. This condition may be reversible through CPR and other treatments. However, when the brain cells die, *biological death* occurs. This usually happens within 10 minutes of clinical death, and it is not reversible. In fact, brain cells will begin to die after 4 to 6 minutes without fresh oxygen supplied from air breathed in and carried to the brain by circulating blood. *Cardiopulmonary resuscitation (CPR)* consists of the actions you take to revive a person—or at least temporarily prevent biological death—by keeping the person's heart and lungs working.

BEFORE BEGINNING RESUSCITATION: FIRST STEPS

Before you begin resuscitation (rescue breathing or CPR), you must take certain steps, including assessing the patient, activating EMS, positioning the patient, and assuring an open airway. These first steps are listed in Table BCLS-1.

Assessing the Patient

Patient assessment is crucial. Never initiate resuscitation without first establishing that the patient needs it. The required assessments are often categorized in two ways: (1) determining unresponsiveness, breathlessness and pulselessness; and (2) assessing the ABCs (airway, breathing, and pulse). As Table BCLS-1 shows, these categories overlap.

Determining Unresponsiveness

When you encounter a patient who has collapsed, your first action is to determine unresponsiveness. Tap or gently shake the patient (being careful not to move a patient with possible spinal injury) and shout, "Are you

Basic Life Support Sequence

ABCs	Assessment	Actions	Special Considerations
	Determine unresponsiveness. ("Are you OK?")	*If unresponsive:* Activate EMS. Position patient.	*For child/infant:* Activate EMS after 1 minute of resuscitation.
Airway	Airway open?	*If unresponsive, assume airway is or may become compromised.* Open the airway.	*If no trauma, use head-tilt, chin-lift. If trauma suspected, use jaw thrust.*
Breathing	Determine breathlessness. (Look, listen, feel.)	*If no breathing:* Provide 2 ventilations.	*If breathing is present:* Continue care as necessary. *If first ventilation is unsuccessful:* Reposition head and try again. *If ventilations are still unsuccessful:* Follow airway obstruction procedures.
Circulation	Determine pulselessness. (Carotid pulse)	*If no pulse:* Begin chest compressions (CPR).	*In an infant:* Feel for brachial pulse. *If pulse is present but breathing absent:* Continue rescue breathing.

okay?" The patient who is able to respond does not require resuscitation.

If the patient is unresponsive, immediately activate EMS (but if the patient is a child or an infant, activate EMS after 1 minute of resuscitation). Then position the patient and open the airway with the head-tilt, chin-lift or the jaw-thrust maneuver.

Determining Breathlessness

Determine breathlessness by the look-listen-feel method. Place your ear beside the patient's nose and mouth with your face turned toward the patient's chest. Look for chest rise and fall. Listen and feel for escape of air from the mouth or nose. The patient who is breathing adequately does not require resuscitation.

If the patient is not breathing, provide two ventilations (as explained later).

Determining Pulselessness

Determine pulselessness by feeling for the carotid artery in an adult or a child, by feeling for the brachial artery in an infant. (Pulse checks will be described in more detail under CPR, later.) The

patient who has a pulse does not require chest compressions.

If the patient has a pulse but is not breathing, provide rescue breathing (artificial ventilations). If the patient is pulseless, begin CPR (ventilations and chest compressions).

Assessing the ABCs

Assessments of the ABCs are included in the steps described above. Keep the ABCs in mind throughout every patient encounter, whether or not resuscitation is underway. If the answer to any of the ABC questions is *no,* take the appropriate steps to correct the situation.

◆ Is the patient's *airway* open?

◆ Is the patient *breathing?*

◆ Does the patient have *circulation* of blood (a pulse)?

Activating EMS

If you have assistance, the other person should call 9-1-1 or otherwise activate the EMS system as soon as a patient collapses or is discovered in collapse.

The quicker a defibrillator can reach the patient, the greater the patient's chances of survival.

If you are alone, and the patient is an adult, first determine unresponsiveness (as described earlier) and then activate EMS before returning to the patient to initiate the next steps. If the patient is a child or an infant, perform 1 minute of resuscitation before activating EMS.

The reason for the difference in timing of EMS activation is that cardiac arrest in an adult is likely to be the result of a disturbance of the heart's electrical activity that will require defibrillation; so getting defibrillation equipment to the patient takes precedence over starting CPR. Children and infants generally have healthy hearts, and cardiac arrest is likely to have resulted from respiratory arrest. In this situation, rescue breathing is more likely to be helpful than in an adult, and defibrillation will not help. So 1 minute of resuscitation before activating EMS is recommended for children and infants, but immediate activation of EMS is recommended for adults.

Positioning the Patient

As soon as you have determined unresponsiveness and activated EMS, make sure that the patient is lying supine (on his back) before attempting to open the airway and assess breathing and circulation. If you find the patient in some other position, help him to the floor or stretcher. If the patient is already lying on the floor, move him onto his back (Figure BCLS-1). If you suspect that the patient may have been injured, you or a helper must support the patient's neck and hold the head still and in line with his spine while you are moving, assessing, and caring for him.

Opening the Airway

Most airway problems are caused by the tongue. As the head tips forward, especially when the patient is lying on his back, the tongue may slide into the airway. When the patient is unconscious, the risk of airway problems is worsened because unconsciousness causes the tongue to lose muscle tone and muscles of the lower jaw (to which the tongue is attached) to relax.

Two procedures can help to correct the position of the tongue (Figure BCLS-2) and thus open

the airway. These procedures are the head-tilt, chin-lift maneuver and the jaw-thrust maneuver.

The Head-Tilt, Chin-Lift Maneuver

The head-tilt, chin-lift maneuver (Figure BCLS-3) provides for maximum opening of the airway. It is useful on all patients who need assistance in maintaining an airway or breathing. It is one of the best methods for correcting obstructions caused by the tongue. However, since it involves changing the position of the head, the head-tilt, chin-lift maneuver should be used only on a patient who you can be quite sure has not suffered a spinal injury.

Follow these steps to perform the head-tilt, chin-lift maneuver.

1. Once the patient is supine, place one hand on the forehead and the fingertips of the other hand under the bony area at the center of the patient's lower jaw.

2. Tilt the head by applying gentle pressure to the patient's forehead.

3. Use your fingertips to lift the chin and support the lower jaw. Move the jaw forward to a point where the lower teeth are almost touching the upper teeth. Do not compress the soft tissues under the lower jaw, which can press and close off the airway.

4. Do not allow the patient's mouth to close. To provide an adequate opening at the mouth, you may need to use the thumb of the hand supporting the chin to pull back the patient's lower lip. For your own safety (to prevent being bitten), do not insert your thumb into the patient's mouth.

The Jaw-Thrust Maneuver

The jaw-thrust maneuver (Figure BCLS-4) is most commonly used to open the airway of an unconscious patient or one with suspected head, neck, or spinal injuries.

Note: *The jaw-thrust maneuver is the only widely recommended procedure for use on patients with possible head, neck, or spinal injuries.*

Follow these steps to perform the jaw-thrust maneuver.

Positioning the Patient for Basic Life Support

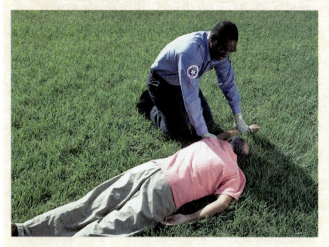

Figure BCLS-1A Straighten the legs and position the closer arm above the head.

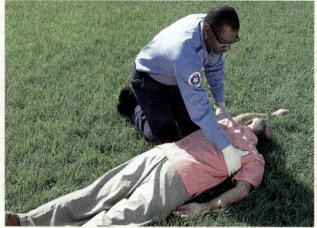

Figure BCLS-1B Cradle the head and neck. Grasp under the distant armpit.

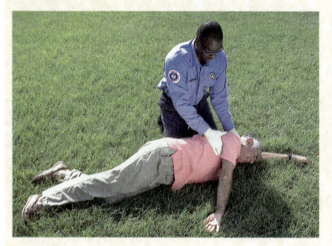

Figure BCLS-1C Move the patient as a unit onto his side.

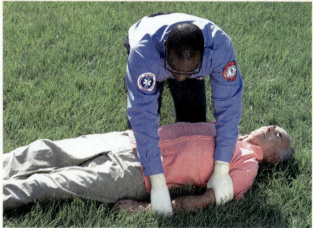

Figure BCLS-1D Move the patient onto his back and reposition the extended arm.

1. Carefully keep the patient's head, neck, and spine aligned, moving him as a unit, as you place him in the supine position.

2. Kneel at the top of the patient's head, resting your elbows on the same surface the patient is lying on.

3. Reach forward and gently place one hand on each side of the patient's lower jaw, at the angles of the jaw below the ears.

4. Stabilize the patient's head with your forearms.

5. Using your index fingers, push the angles of the patient's lower jaw forward.

6. You may need to retract the patient's lower lip with your thumb to keep the mouth open.

7. Do not tilt or rotate the patient's head. *Remember the purpose of the jaw-thrust maneuver is to open the airway with out moving the head or neck.*

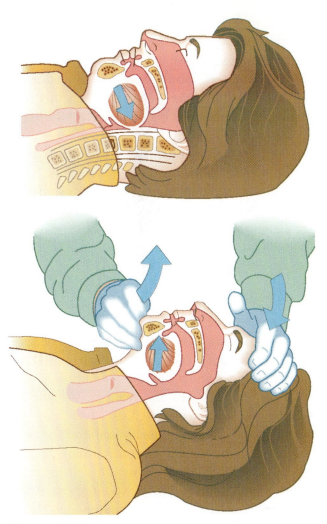

Figure BCLS-2   Procedures for opening the airway help reposition the tongue.

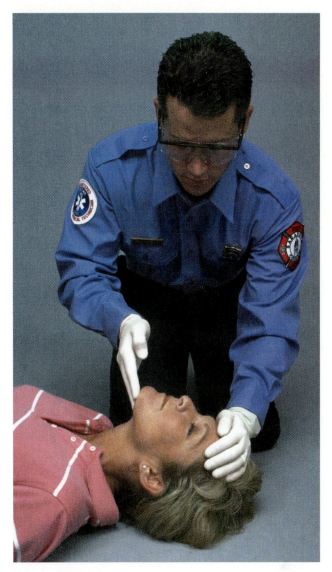

Figure BCLS-3   The head-tilt, chin-lift maneuver.

Initial Ventilations and Pulse Check

Deliver two slow breaths of sufficient volume to make the chest rise (Table BCLS-2). If the first breath is unsuccessful, reposition the patient's head before attempting the second breath. If the second ventilation is unsuccessful, assume that there is a foreign-body airway obstruction and perform airway clearance techniques (as described later).

If the initial ventilations are successful, you have confirmed an open airway and should feel for a pulse. If the patient has no pulse, begin chest compressions with ventilations (as described later under CPR). If the patient has a pulse but breathing is absent or inadequate, perform rescue breathing.

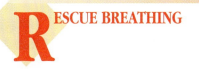

RESCUE BREATHING

Mouth-to-Mask Ventilation

Mouth-to-mask ventilation is performed using a pocket face mask. The pocket face mask is made of soft, collapsible material and can be carried in your pocket, jacket, or purse. The steps of mouth-to-mask ventilation are illustrated in Figure BCLS-5 on page 811 and summarized in Table BCLS-2.

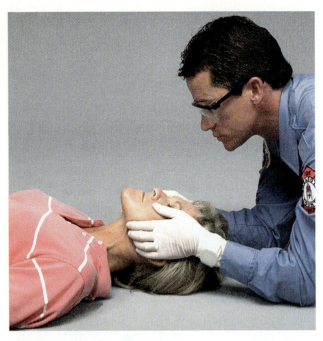

Figure BCLS-4   The jaw-thrust maneuver.

Gastric Distention

Rescue breathing can force some air into the patient's stomach, causing the stomach to become distended. This may indicate that the airway is blocked, that there is improper head position, or that the ventilations being provided are too large or too quick to be accommodated by the lungs or the trachea. This problem is seen more frequently in infants and children but can occur with any patient.

A slight bulge is of little worry, but major distention can cause two serious problems. First, the air-filled stomach reduces lung volume by forcing the diaphragm upward. Second, regurgitation (the passive expulsion of fluids and partially digested foods from the stomach into the throat) or vomiting (the forceful expulsion of the stomach's contents) are strong possibilities. This could lead to additional airway obstruction or aspiration of vomitus into the patient's lungs. When this happens, lung damage can occur and a lethal form of pneumonia may develop.

The best way to avoid gastric distention, or to avoid making it worse once it develops, is to position the patient's head properly, avoid too-forceful and too-quickly-delivered ventilations, and limit the volume of ventilations delivered. The volume delivered should be limited to the size breath that causes the chest to rise. This is why it is so important to watch the patient's chest rise as each ventilation is delivered and to feel for resistance to your breaths.

When gastric distention is present, be prepared for vomiting (Figure BCLS-6, page 812). If the patient does vomit, roll the entire patient onto his side. (Turning just the head may allow for aspiration of vomitus as well as aggravating any possible neck injury.) Manually stabilize the head and neck of the patient as you roll him. Be prepared to clear the patient's mouth and throat of vomitus with gauze and gloved fingers. Apply suction if you are trained and equipped to do so.

The Recovery Position

Patients who resume adequate breathing and pulse after rescue breathing or CPR, and who do not require immobilization for possible spinal injury, are placed in the recovery position (Figure BCLS-7, page 812). This position is also suitable for patients who are unconscious, but with ade-

Table BCLS-2

Rescue Breathing

	Adult	**Child**	**Infant**
Age	8 yrs and older	1 to 8 yrs	birth to 1 yr
Ventilation Duration	1½ to 2 sec	1 to 1½ sec	1 to 1½ sec
Ventilation Rate	10 to 12 breaths/min	20 breaths/min	20 breaths/min

Mouth-to-Mask Ventilation

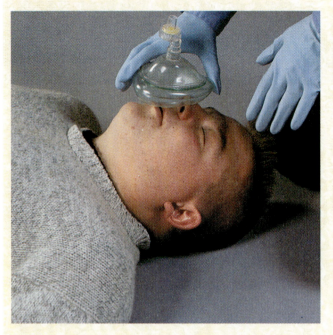

Figure BCLS-5A Position the patient and prepare to place the mask.

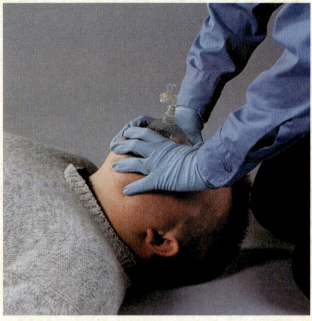

Figure BCLS-5B Seat the mask firmly on the patient's face.

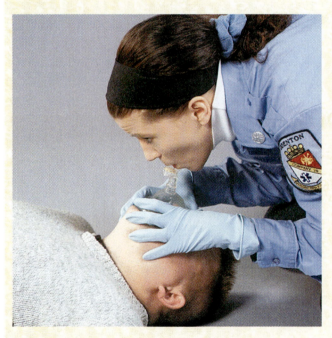

Figure BCLS-5C Open the patient's airway and watch the chest rise as you ventilate through the one-way valve.

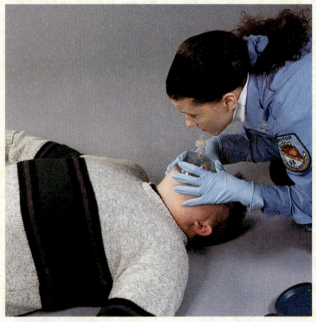

Figure BCLS-5D Watch the patient's chest fall during exhalation. Ventilate the adult patient 10 to 12 times a minute, a child or infant 20 times a minute. If the pocket mask has an oxygen inlet, provide supplemental oxygen.

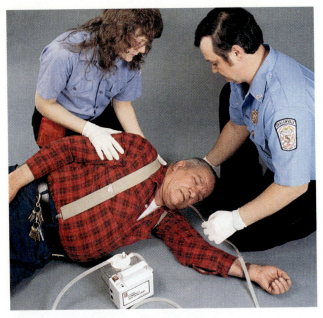

Figure BCLS-6   Be prepared for vomiting when attempting to relieve gastric distention.

quate pulse and respirations. The recovery position allows for drainage from the mouth and prevents the tongue from falling backward and causing an airway obstruction.

The patient should be rolled onto his side. This should be done moving the patient as a unit,

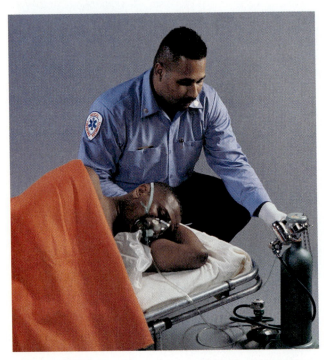

Figure BCLS-7   Place the breathing but unresponsive patient who has no head, neck, or spine injury in the recovery position (on his side) to protect the airway.

that is, not twisting the head, shoulders, or torso. The patient may be rolled onto either side; however it is preferable to have the patient facing you so that monitoring and suctioning may be more easily performed.

If the patient does not have respirations that are sufficient to support life, the recovery position must not be used. The patient should be placed supine and his ventilations assisted.

CPR

Checking the Pulse

Before beginning CPR, you must confirm that the patient is pulseless.

In an adult or child (not infant), check the carotid pulse (Figure BCLS-8). While stabilizing the patient's head and maintaining the proper head tilt, use your hand that is closest to the patient's neck to locate his "Adam's apple" (the prominent bulge in the front of the neck). Place the tips of your index and middle fingers directly over the midline of this structure. (Do not use your thumb. It has a pulse that you may feel instead of the patient's pulse.) Slide your fingertips to the side of the patient's neck closest to you. Keep the palm side of your fingertips against the patient's neck. (*Do not* slide your fingertips to the opposite side of the patient's neck, which may cause you to put pressure on the trachea and interfere with the patient's airway.) Feel for a groove between the Adam's apple and the muscles located along the side of the neck. Very little pressure needs to be applied to the neck to feel the carotid pulse.

In an infant, check for a brachial pulse (Figure BCLS-9).

If the patient is pulseless, begin CPR.

How CPR Works

CPR is a method of artificial breathing and circulation. When natural heart action and breathing have stopped, we must provide an artificial means to oxygenate the blood and keep it in circulation. This is accomplished by providing *chest compressions* and *ventilations*.

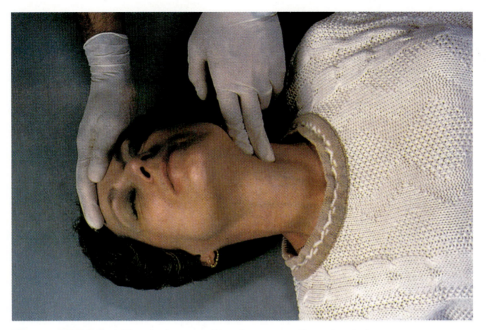

Figure BCLS-8 Check the carotid pulse to confirm circulation.

◆ To provide *chest compressions,* place the patient supine on a hard surface and compress the chest by applying downward pressure with your hands. This action causes an increase of pressure inside the chest and possible actual compression of the heart itself, one or both of which force the blood out of the heart and into circulation. When pressure is released, the heart refills with blood. The next compression sends this fresh blood into circulation and the cycle continues.

◆ To provide *ventilations,* use mouth-to-mask, mouth-to-mouth, mouth-to-nose, or mouth-to-

Figure BCLS-9 For infants, determine circulation by feeling for a brachial pulse.

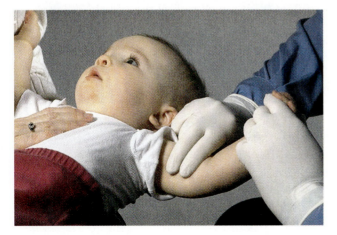

stoma methods. *It is highly recommended that CPR be performed using a pocket face mask or other barrier device as protection against infectious diseases.*

Both compressions and ventilations are necessary in CPR. Compressions without ventilations would circulate blood without enough oxygen in it to sustain brain or heart function. Ventilations without compressions would force oxygen into the lungs without circulating the blood to pick up the oxygen and deliver it to the body.

Remember: *Do not initiate CPR on any patient who has a pulse.*

How to Do CPR

CPR can be done by one or by two rescuers. All of the information under "Providing Chest Compressions," and "Providing Ventilations" applies to both one-rescuer and two-rescuer CPR. Specific information about each type of CPR then follows under "One-Rescuer CPR" and "Two-Rescuer CPR." Figures BCLS-10, 11, 12, 13, and 14 can help you follow and review these procedures as they are described below. These procedures are for an adult patient. Procedures for infants and children will be described later.

Locating the CPR Compression Site

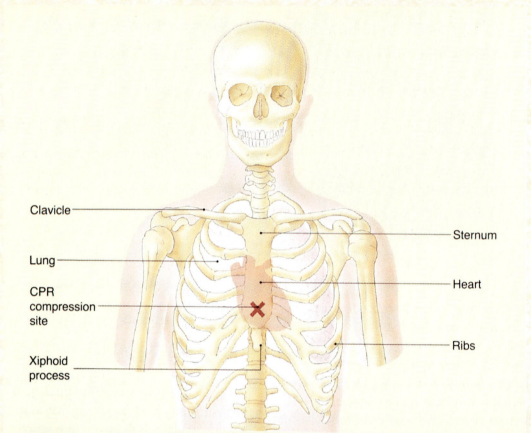

Clavicle

Lung

CPR compression site

Xiphoid process

Sternum

Heart

Ribs

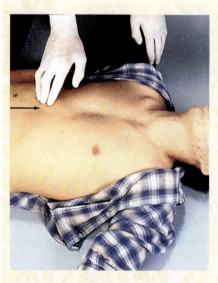

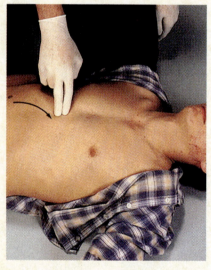

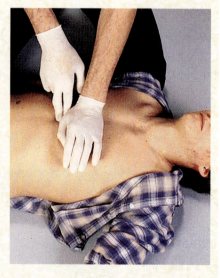

Figure BCLS-10A Use the index and middle fingers of the hand that is closer to the patient's feet to locate the lower border of the rib cage.

Figure BCLS-10B Move your fingers along the rib cage to the point where the ribs meet the sternum, the substernal notch. Keep your middle finger at the notch and your index finger resting on the lower tip of the sternum.

Figure BCLS-10C Move your hand to the midline. Place its thumb side against the index finger of the lower hand.

Providing Chest Compressions

After your hands are properly positioned on the CPR compression site (see Figure BCLS-20):

1. Straighten your arms and lock your elbows. You must not bend the elbows when delivering or releasing compressions.

2. Make certain that your shoulders are directly over your hands (directly over the patient's sternum). This will allow you to deliver compressions straight down onto the site. Keep both of your knees on the ground or floor.

3. Deliver compressions *straight down,* with enough force to depress the sternum of a typical adult 1½ to 2 inches.

   Note: Monitoring the depth of your compressions is one way to determine if they are adequate—the *only* way, if you are working alone. Another method for determining whether your compressions are adequate is to have someone else feel for a carotid pulse while you perform compressions. When CPR compressions are being performed properly, they should produce a carotid pulse. Never try to feel for a carotid pulse during compressions if you are by yourself; rather, perform compressions at 1½ to 2 inches until help arrives.

4. Fully release pressure on the patient's sternum, but *do not* bend your elbows and do not lift your hands from the sternum, which can cause you to lose correct positioning of your hands. Your movement should be from your hips, the hips acting as a fulcrum. Compressions should be delivered in a rhythmic, not a "jabbing," fashion. *The amount of time you spend compressing should be the same as the time for the release.* This is known as the 50:50 rule: 50% compression, 50% release.

Providing Ventilations

Ventilations are given between sets of compressions. The mouth-to-mask techniques described earlier for rescue breathing, and shown in Figure BCLS-5, are used.

One-Rescuer CPR

Figure BCLS-11 shows the techniques of one-rescuer CPR for the adult patient.

Compressions and Ventilations: Rates and Ratios

Table BCLS-3 on page 818 describes compression rates and ratios for adults, children, and infants.

Checking for Pulse and Breathing

CPR should be carried out for approximately *one minute,* or *four cycles* of 15 compressions and 2 ventilations. At this point you should check for a carotid pulse (3 to 5 seconds). At the same time look, listen, and feel for breathing. If there is no pulse, return to CPR. If there is a pulse but no breathing, perform rescue breathing. If there are both pulse and breathing, move the patient into the recovery position and continue to monitor carefully, taking care to check every few minutes for a carotid pulse.

CPR should not be delayed for more than a few seconds for a pulse-and-breathing check. If CPR is continued after the first check, break to check for a carotid pulse and the return of spontaneous breathing every few minutes thereafter. After breaking for the pulse-and-breathing check, resume CPR, beginning with chest compressions rather than ventilations.

Two-Rescuer CPR

Figure BCLS-12 on page 819 shows the technique of two-rescuer CPR for the adult patient.

How to Join CPR in Progress

If CPR has been started by someone who is trained to perform CPR but is not part of the EMS system and you join this person to perform CPR:

1. Identify yourself as someone who knows CPR and ask to help.

2. Ensure that EMS has been activated.

3. Allow the first rescuer to complete a cycle of 15 compressions and 2 ventilations.

One-Rescuer CPR (Adult)

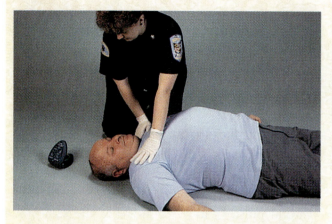

Figure BCLS-11A Establish unresponsiveness and position patient. (If you are working alone, call for help *as soon as* you establish unresponsiveness.

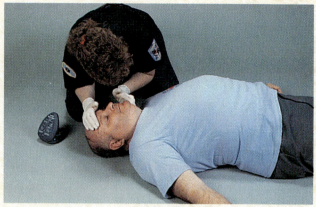

Figure BCLS-11B Open the airway.

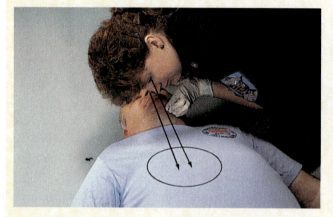

Figure BCLS-11C Look, listen, and feel for breath (3 to 5 seconds).

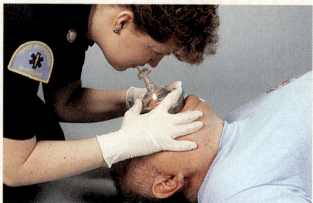

Figure BCLS-11D Ventilate twice (1½ to 2 sec/ventilation). If the first breath is unsuccessful, reposition the patient's head before attempting the second breath. Clear airway if necessary.

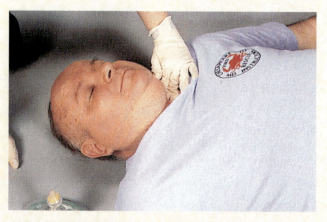

Figure BCLS-11E Determine that the patient is pulseless (5 to 10 seconds).

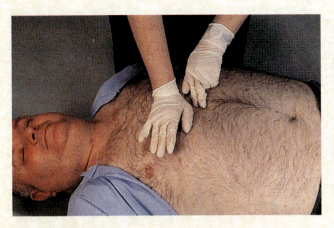

Figure BCLS-11F Locate compression site.

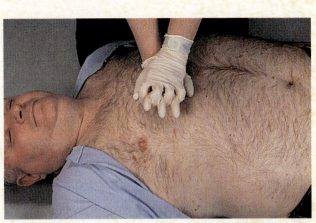

Figure BCLS-11G Position hands.

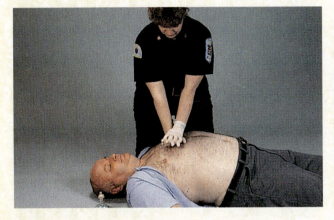

Figure BCLS-11H Begin compressions. (Compression at depth of 1½ to 2 inches or 35 to 50 mm, delivered at a rate of 80 to 100/minute.)

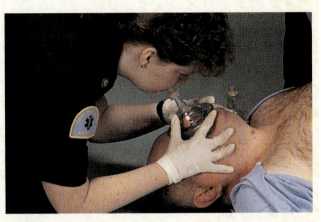

Figure BCLS-11I Ventilate twice. (Provide 2 ventilations every 15 compressions.)

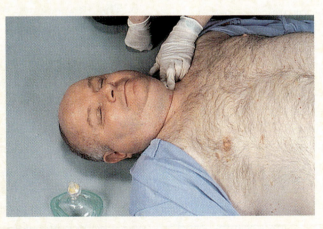

Figure BCLS-11J Recheck pulse and breathing after 4 cycles, then recheck every few minutes.

CPR for Adults, Children, and Infants

	Adult	Child	Infant
Age	8 yrs and older	1 to 8 yrs	birth to 1 yr
Compression Depth	1½ to 2 inches (35 to 50 mm)	1 to 1½ inches (25 to 35 mm)	½ to 1 inch (12 to 25 mm) [newborn—½ to 1¾ inch (12 to 18 mm)]
Compression Rate	80 to 100/min	100/min	at least 100/min (newborn—120/min)
Each Ventilation	1½ to 2 seconds	1 to 1½ = seconds	1 to 1½ seconds
Pulse Check Location	carotid artery (throat)	carotid artery (throat)	brachial artery (upper arm)
One-Rescuer CPR Compressions to Ventilations Ratio	15:2	5:1	5:1 (newborn—3:1)
Two-Rescuer CPR Compressions to Ventilations Ratio	5:1	5:1	5:1 (newborn—3:1)
When working alone: Call 9-1-1 or emergency dispatcher	After establishing unresponsiveness—before beginning resuscitation	After establishing unresponsiveness and 1 minute of resuscitation	After establishing unresponsiveness and 1 minute of resuscitation

4. Check for a pulse. If there is no pulse, start one-rescuer CPR. If you tire before EMS arrives, let the other rescuer perform CPR. Alternate until EMS arrives.

If you wish to join another member of the EMS System who has initiated CPR, you should

1. Identify yourself and your training and state that you are ready to perform two-rescuer CPR.

2. While the first rescuer is providing compressions, spend 5 seconds checking for a carotid pulse produced by each compression. This is to determine if the compressions being delivered are effective. Inform the first rescuer if there is or is not a pulse being produced. (If the first rescuer cannot deliver effective compressions, you will have to take over for him when CPR is resumed.)

3. You should say, "Stop compressions" and check for spontaneous pulse and breathing. This should take only a few seconds.

4. If there is no pulse, you should state, "No pulse. Continue CPR."

5. The switch from one-rescuer to two-rescuer CPR should take place after the first rescuer has completed a cycle of 15 compressions and 2 ventilations.

6. The first rescuer resumes compressions, and the second rescuer provides a ventilation during a brief pause after every fifth compression. If desired, the second rescuer can start compressions and allow the first rescuer to provide the ventilations.

How to Change Positions

When two rescuers are performing CPR, one of the rescuers may wish to change positions (Figure BCLS-13, page 821). Often the compressor is the one who becomes fatigued, but the ventilator also may request a change. The most important factor in the change is that it be done in as little time as

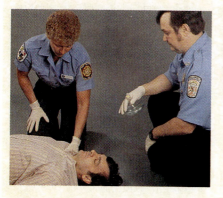

Figure BCLS-12A Determine unresponsiveness. Position patient.

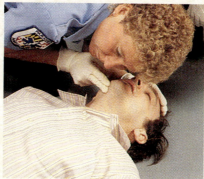

Figure BCLS-12B Open the airway and look, listen, and feel for breath (3 to 5 seconds).

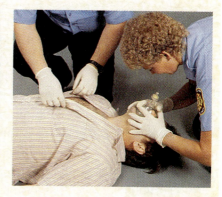

Figure BCLS-12C Ventilate twice (1½ to 2 sec/ventilation). If the first breath is unsuccessful, reposition the patient's head before attempting the second breath. Clear airway if necessary.

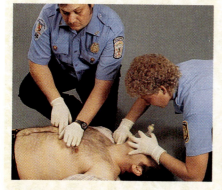

Figure BCLS-12D Determine pulselessness. Locate CPR compression site.

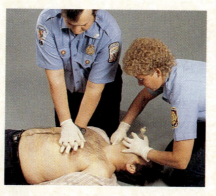

Figure BCLS-12E Say "no pulse." Begin compressions.

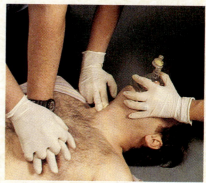

Figure BCLS-12F Check compression effectiveness. Deliver 5 compressions in 3 to 4 seconds (80 to 100/minute).

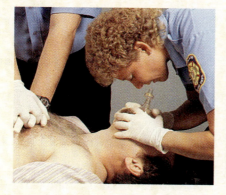

Figure BCLS-12G Stop compressions for ventilation. Ventilate once (1½ to 2 sec/ventilation). Continue with 1 ventilation every 5 compressions.

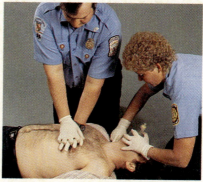

Figure BCLS-12H After a few minutes, reassess breathing and pulse. No pulse—say "Continue CPR." Pulse—say "Stop CPR."

possible. The compressor controls the change and will signal the pending change at the beginning of a series of compressions as follows: "CHANGE. One and two and three and four and five, BREATHE." The ventilator will provide one full breath, and the two rescuers will quickly change positions.

The rescuer who was previously providing compressions is now the ventilator. This rescuer opens the airway immediately upon reaching the patient's head and checks for a carotid pulse and respirations. These checks should take no more than 3 to 5 seconds. If a change takes place every 2 minutes or less, a check of pulse and breathing does not need to be done on every change.

For a review of CPR for the adult patient, see the summary in Figure BCLS-14, page 822.

CPR Techniques for Children and Infants

The techniques of CPR for children and infants are essentially the same as those used for adults. However, some procedures and rates differ when the patient is a child or an infant. (If younger than 1 year of age, the patient is considered to be an infant. Between 1 and 8 years of age, the patient is considered to be a child. Over the age of 8 years, adult procedures apply to the patient. Keep in mind that the size of the patient can also be an important factor. A very small 9-year-old may have to be treated as a child.)

The techniques of CPR for an infant are shown in Figure BCLS-16, page 824. For a child, CPR is conducted as for an adult, the chief difference in procedure being the hand position—using the heel of one hand—for chest compressions (Figure BCLS-15, page 823). To compare adult, child, and infant CPR, also review Table BCLS-3.

Positioning the Patient

When CPR must be performed, adults, children, and infants are placed on their backs on a hard surface. For an infant, the hard surface can be the rescuer's hand or forearm.

Opening the Airway

For an infant or a child, use the head-tilt, chin-lift or the jaw-thrust, but apply only a slight tilt for an infant. Too great a tilt may close off the infant's airway; however, make certain that the opening is adequate (note chest rise during ventilation). Always be sure to support an infant's head.

Establishing a Pulse

Take these steps to establish a pulse in an infant or a child.

◆ Infant—For infants, you should use the brachial pulse.

◆ Child—Determine circulation in the same manner as for an adult.

Special Considerations in CPR

How to Know if CPR Is Effective

To determine if CPR is effective

◆ *If possible have someone else feel for a carotid pulse* during compressions and watch to see the patient's chest rise during ventilations.

◆ *Listen for exhalation of air,* either naturally or during compressions, as additional verification that air has entered the lungs.

In addition to the above, any of the following indications of effective CPR may be noticed:

◆ Pupils constrict.

◆ Skin color improves.

◆ Heartbeat returns spontaneously.

◆ Spontaneous, gasping respirations are made.

◆ Arms and legs move.

◆ Swallowing is attempted.

◆ Consciousness returns.

Interrupting CPR

Once you begin CPR, you may interrupt the process for no more than a few seconds to check for pulse and breathing or to reposition yourself and the patient. The first recommended pulse and

(*text continues, page 823*)

Changing Positions

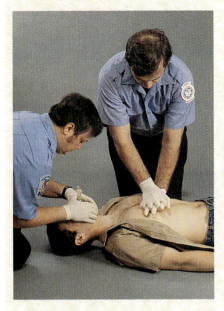

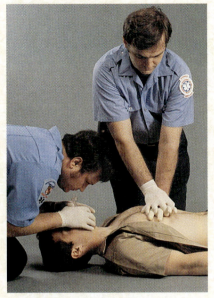

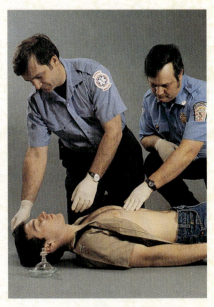

Figure BCLS-13A When fatigued, the compressor calls for the switch. (Note that in this sequence, both rescuers are shown on same side of patient for purposes of clarity. Normally, rescuers should be positioned on opposite sides of the patient.)

Figure BCLS-13B Compressor completes fifth compression. Ventilator provides one ventilation.

Figure BCLS-13C Ventilator moves to chest and begins to locate compression site. Compressor moves to head.

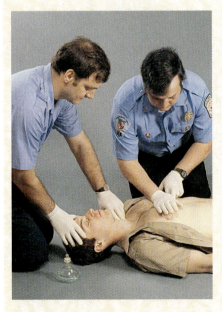

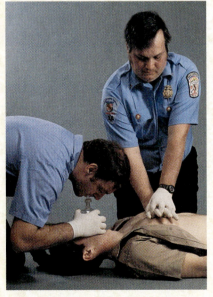

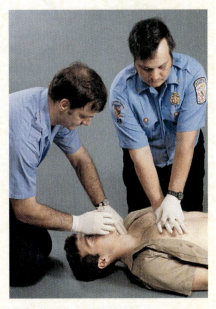

Figure BCLS-13D New compressor finds site. New ventilator checks carotid pulse.

Figure BCLS-13E New ventilator says, "No pulse." Both rescuers in new position, ready to continue CPR.

Figure BCLS-13F New compressor delivers 5 compressions (3 to 4 seconds) at a rate of 80 to 100/minute. New ventilator assesses effectiveness of compressions.

CPR Summary—Adt Patient

ONE RESCUER	FUNCTIONS	TWO RESCUERS
	• Establish unresponsiveness • If there's no response, call 911 • Position patient • Open airway • Look, listen, and feel (for 3-5 seconds)	
	• Deliver 2 breaths (1½–2 sec/ ventilation). If unsuccessful, reposition head and try again. Clear airway if necessary.	

	• Check carotid pulse. . .
	  (5-10 seconds)
	
	  If no pulse. . .
	• Begin chest compressions	

DELIVER COMPRESSIONS

ONE RESCUER			TWO RESCUERS
	1½–2 inches 80-100/min (15/9-11 sec)	1½–2 inches 80-100/min (5/3-4 sec)	

DELIVER VENTILATIONS
10-12 breaths/min

ONE RESCUER			TWO RESCUERS
	15:2	5:1 (Pause to allow ventilations)	
	• Do 4 cycles • Check pulse	• Ventilator checks effective-ness	

CONTINUE PERIODIC ASSESSMENT

Changing Positions

• Compressor—signal to change; provide 5 compressions • Ventilator—1 ventilation	New ventilator checks pulse If no pulse, instructs compressor to begin CPR	Continue CPR sequence

NOTE: Wear gloves and use either a pocket mask with one-way valve or bag valve mask

Figure BCLS-14

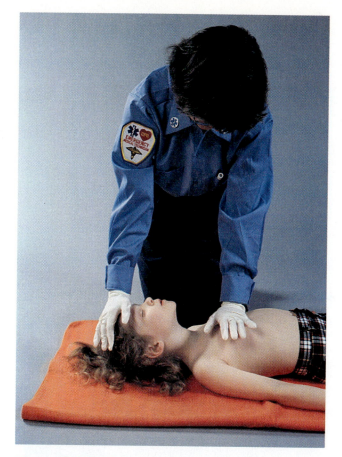

Figure BCLS-15 Performing chest compressions on a child.

even though unresponsive and perhaps not breathing—does have a pulse.

Usually, of course, you will perform CPR when the patient has no pulse. However, there are special circumstances in which CPR should not be initiated *even though the patient has no pulse.*

◆ Obvious mortal wounds—These include decapitation, incineration, a severed body, and injuries that are so extensive that CPR cannot be effectively performed (e.g., severe crush injuries to the head, neck, and chest).

◆ Rigor mortis—This is the stiffening of the body and its limbs that occurs after death, usually within 4 to 10 hours.

◆ Obvious decomposition.

◆ A line of lividity—Lividity is a red or purple skin discoloration that occurs when gravity causes the blood to sink to the lowest parts of the body and collect there. Lividity usually indicates that the patient has been dead for more than 15 minutes unless the patient has been exposed to cold temperatures. Using lividity as a sign requires special training.

◆ Stillbirth—CPR should not be initiated for a stillborn infant who has died hours prior to birth. This infant may be recognized by blisters on the skin, a very soft head, and a strong disagreeable odor. In all cases, if you are in doubt, seek a physician's advice.

breathing check is after the first minute of CPR. You should continue to check for these vital signs every few minutes.

In addition to these built-in interruptions, you may interrupt CPR to:

◆ Move a patient onto a stretcher.

◆ Move a patient down a flight of stairs or through a narrow doorway or hallway.

◆ Move a patient on or off the ambulance.

◆ Suction to clear vomitus or airway obstructions.

◆ Allow for defibrillation or advanced cardiac life support measures to be initiated.

When CPR is resumed, begin with chest compressions rather than with ventilations.

When Not to Begin or to Terminate CPR

As discussed earlier in this chapter, CPR should not be initiated *when you find that the patient—*

Once you have started CPR, you must continue to provide CPR until:

◆ Spontaneous circulation occurs . . . then provide rescue breathing as needed.

◆ Spontaneous circulation and breathing occur.

◆ Another trained rescuer can take over for you.

◆ You turn care of the patient over to a person with a higher level of training.

◆ You are too exhausted to continue.

◆ You receive a "no CPR" order from a physician or other authority per local protocols.

If you turn the patient over to another rescuer, this person must be trained in basic cardiac life support.

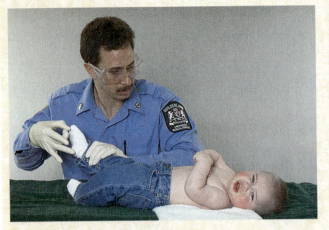

Figure BCLS-16A Establish unresponsiveness and position the patient. Send someone to call for help. If you are working alone, call for help after 1 minute of resuscitation. (Note that this sequence was photographed showing procedures with a real infant, who is awake. In practice, a baby requiring CPR would be unresponsive.)

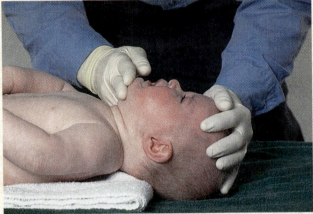

Figure BCLS-16B Open the airway with the head-tilt, chin-lift or jaw-thrust.

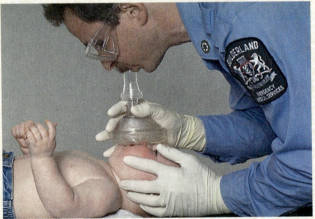

Figure BCLS-16D Give 2 slow breaths, taking 1 to 1½ seconds for each breath. Make sure the chest rises with each breath. If you cannot get a breath in, reposition the patient's head.

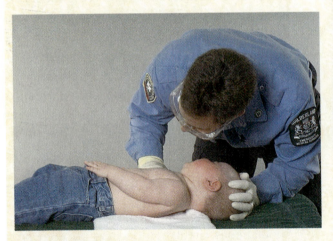

Figure BCLS-16C Look, listen, and feel for breathing (3 to 5 seconds).

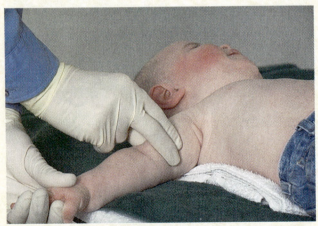

Figure BCLS-16E Check the brachial pulse.

A For a very small newborn, encircle chest with fingers and overlap thumbs on the sternum just below an imaginary line connecting the nipples.

B For an average-size newborn, encircle chest with fingers and place thumbs side by side on the sternum just below an imaginary line connecting the nipples.

C For an infant that is older or too large to encircle the chest, place middle and ring fingers on sternum one finger-width below imaginary line connecting nipples. Measure distance by first placing, then raising, index finger.

Figure BCLS-16F Position fingers for chest compressions according to the age and size of the infant.

(continued)

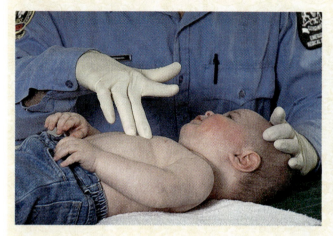

Figure BCLS-16G Begin compressing the chest at a rate of at least 100 per minute and at a depth of ½ to 1 inch (12 to 25 mm).

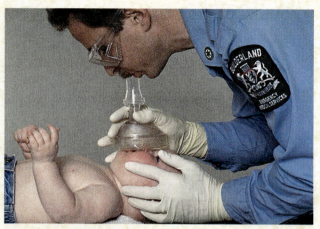

Figure BCLS-16H After every 5 compressions, give one slow breath.

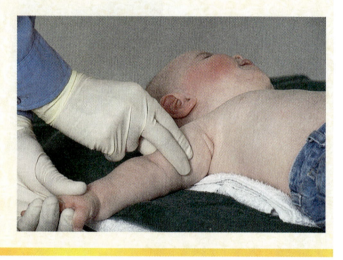

Figure BCLS-16I After about 1 minute, check the brachial pulse. If there is no pulse and you are working alone, active the EMS system. Resume cycles for 5 compressions to 1 ventilation, stopping every few minutes to check for a pulse.

CLEARING AIRWAY OBSTRUCTIONS

Not every airway problem is caused by the tongue (the situation in which you would use the head-tilt, chin-lift maneuver or the jaw-thrust maneuver, described earlier, to open the airway). The airway can also be blocked by foreign objects or materials. These can include pieces of food, ice, toys, or vomitus. This problem is often seen with children and with patients who have abused alcohol or other drugs. It also happens when an injured person's airway becomes blocked by blood or broken teeth or dentures or when a person chokes on food.

Airway obstructions are either partial or complete. Partial and complete obstructions have different characteristics that may be noted during assessment, and each type has a different procedure of care. It is important to understand the differences between partial and complete obstruction and the correct care for each.

Partial Airway Obstruction

A conscious patient trying to indicate an airway problem will usually point to his mouth or hold his neck. Many do this even when a partial obstruction does not prevent speech. Ask the patient if he is choking, or ask if he can speak or cough. If he can, then the obstruction is partial.

For the conscious patient with an apparent partial airway obstruction, have him cough. A strong and forceful cough indicates he is exchanging enough air. Continue to encourage the patient to cough in the hope that such action will dislodge and expel the foreign object. *Do not* interfere with the patient's efforts to clear the partial obstruction by means of forceful coughing.

In cases where the patient has an apparent partial airway obstruction but he cannot cough or has a very weak cough, or the patient is blue or gray or shows other signs of poor air exchange, treat the patient as if there is a complete airway obstruction, as described below.

Complete Airway Obstruction

Be alert for signs of a complete airway obstruction in the conscious or unconscious patient.

◆ *The conscious patient* with a complete airway obstruction will try to speak but will not be able to. He will also not be able to breathe or cough. Usually, he will display the distress signal for choking by clutching the neck between thumb and fingers.

◆ *The unconscious patient* with a complete airway obstruction will be in respiratory arrest. When ventilation attempts are unsuccessful it becomes apparent that there is an obstruction.

Procedures for Clearing the Airway

When you have determined that the airway is obstructed, you must take appropriate measures to clear it.

1. *Open the airway.* Since so many obstructions are caused by the tongue, you must first try to open the airway by using a head-tilt, chin-lift or a jaw-thrust maneuver.

2. *If the patient is unconscious and not breathing, attempt to provide ventilations (rescue breathing).* If the first ventilation is unsuccessful, readjust head position and attempt another ventilation. If still unsuccessful, then assume

that there is foreign matter in the airway that must be cleared. *If the patient is conscious and indicating that he is choking, do not attempt artificial ventilations, but instead move right to step 3.*

3. *Remove any foreign object.* If the patient is choking or, for the unconscious patient (if you have already opened the airway and unsuccessfully tried ventilation), two techniques are recommended for removal of a foreign object.

◆ Manual thrusts (abdominal or chest thrusts)
◆ Finger sweeps

On any given patient you may have to use both manual thrusts and finger sweeps.

Abdominal Thrusts The use of abdominal thrusts (the Heimlich maneuver) to clear a foreign body from the airway of an adult or child (not infant) patient is shown in Figure BCLS-17 and described below.

For the conscious adult or child (not infant) who is standing or sitting:

1. Make a fist and place the thumb side of this fist against the midline of the patient's abdomen between waist and rib cage. Avoid touching the chest, especially the area immediately below the sternum.

2. Grasp your properly positioned fist with your other hand and apply pressure inward and up toward the patient's head in a smooth, quick movement. Deliver five rapid thrusts..

For the unconscious adult or child (not infant) or for a conscious patient who cannot sit or stand, or if you are too short to reach around the patient to deliver thrusts:

1. Place the patient in a supine position.

2. Kneel and straddle the patient at the level of the thighs, facing his chest.

3. Place the heel of your hand on the midline of his abdomen, slightly above the navel and well below the sternum.

4. Now place your free hand over the positioned hand, shoulders directly over the patient's abdomen. Be sure that you are positioned

Clearing the Airway—Adult

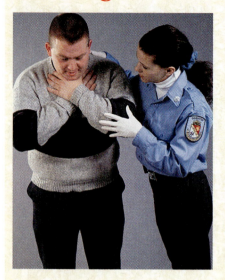

Figure BCLS-17A Recognize and assess for choking.

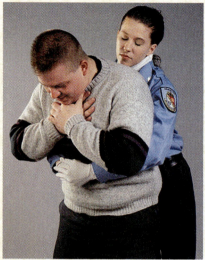

Figure BCLS-17B Position yourself to perform the Heimlich maneuver.

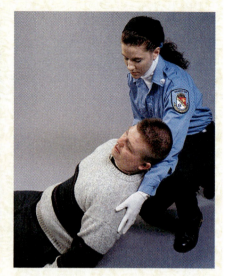

Figure BCLS-17C If the patient becomes weak or unconscious, assist him to the floor. If you are working alone, active the EMS system.

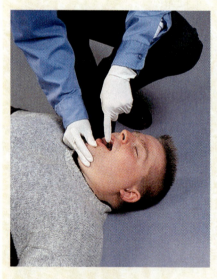

Figure BCLS-17D Do a tongue-jaw lift and a finger sweep.

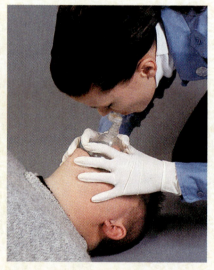

Figure BCLS-17E Attempt to ventilate. If this fails, reposition head and try again. If you are not successful . . .

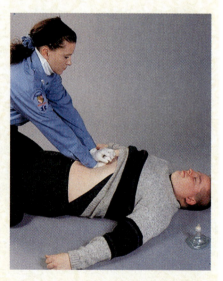

Figure BCLS-17F Perform the Heimlich maneuver. Repeat steps D through F if necessary.

over the midline so that thrusts will be delivered straight up, not off to one side.

5. Deliver five rapid thrusts by pressing your hands inward and upward toward the patient's diaphragm.

If the obstruction is not relieved after a series of five thrusts, reassess your position and the patient's airway (if the patient is unconscious, also attempt finger sweeps to attempt to remove the obstruction). Attempt to ventilate the patient and, if unsuccessful, repeat the series of thrusts. Repeat the sequence until the ostruction is relieved.

Chest Thrusts Chest thrusts are used in place of abdominal thrusts when the patient is in the late stages of pregnancy, or when the patient is too obese for abdominal thrusts to be effective. The use of chest thrusts to relieve an airway obstruction is shown in Figures BCLS-18 and 19 and described below.

For the conscious adult who is standing or sitting:

1. Position yourself behind the patient and slide your arms under his armpits, so that you encircle his chest.

2. Form a fist with one hand and place the thumb side of this fist on the midline of the sternum about two to three finger widths above the xiphoid process. This places your fist on the lower half of the sternum but not in contact with the edge of the rib cage.

3. Grasp the fist with your other hand and deliver five chest thrusts directly backward toward the spine.

For the unconscious adult:

1. Place the patient in a supine position.

2. Perform five chest thrusts as for CPR.

(*text continues, page 832*)

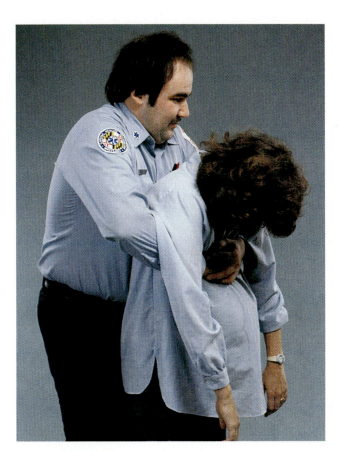

Figure BCLS-18 The chest thrust applied to a pregnant patient.

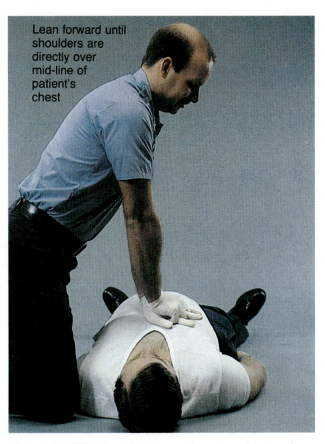

Figure BCLS-19 The chest thrust can be used when the patient is lying on his back.

Airway Clearance Sequence

	Adult	**Child**	**Infant**
Age	**8 yrs and older**	**1 to 8 yrs**	**birth to 1 yr**
Conscious	Ask: "Are you choking?" Heimlich maneuver until obstruction is relieved or patient loses consciousness	Ask: "Are you choking?" Heimlich maneuver until obstruction is relieved or patient loses consciousness	Observe signs of choking (small objects or food, wheezing, agitation, blue color, not breathing). Series of: 5 back blows 5 chest thrusts
Loses Consciousness During Procedure	Assist patient to floor. Establish unresponsiveness (ask, "Are you OK?"). If alone, call for help, then . . . Open airway. Perform finger sweeps. Attempt to ventilate. If unsuccessful, reposition head and attempt to ventilate again. If unsuccessful, perform Heimlich maneuver. (Repeat as needed.)	Assist patient to floor. Establish unresponsiveness (ask, "Are you OK?"). Open airway. Remove visible objects (NO blind sweeps). Attempt to ventilate. If unsuccessful, reposition head and attempt to ventilate again. If unsuccessful, perform Heimlich maneuver. (Repeat as needed.) After 1 minute, call for help if alone.	Establish unresponsiveness (tap or speak loudly). Open airway. Remove visible objects (NO blind sweeps). Attempt to ventilate. If unsuccessful, reposition head, and attempt to ventilate again. If unsuccessful, perform back blows and chest thrusts. (Repeat as needed.) After 1 minute, call for help if alone.
Unconscious When Found	Establish. If alone, call for help, then . . . Open airway. Perform finger sweeps. Attempt to ventilate. If unsuccessful, reposition head and attempt to ventilate again. If unsuccessful, perform Heimlich maneuver. (Repeat as needed.)	Establish unresponsiveness. Open airway. Attempt to ventilate. If unsuccessful, reposition head and attempt to ventilate again. If unsuccessful, Heimlich maneuver. Remove visible objects (NO blind sweeps). (Repeat as needed.) After 1 minute, call for help if alone.	Establish unresponsiveness. Open airway. Attempt to ventilate. If unsuccessful, reposition head and attempt to ventilate again. If unsuccessful, back blows and chest thrusts. Remove visible objects (NO blind sweeps). (Repeat as needed.) After 1 minute, call for help if alone.

Clearing the Airway—Infant

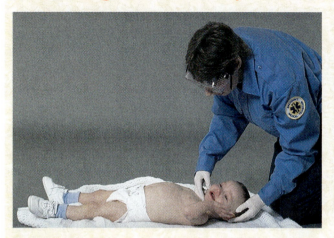

Figure BCLS-20A Recognize and assess for choking. Look for breathing difficulty, ineffective cough, and lack of a strong cry.

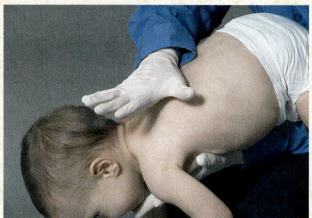

Figure BCLS-20B Give up to 5 back blows and . . .

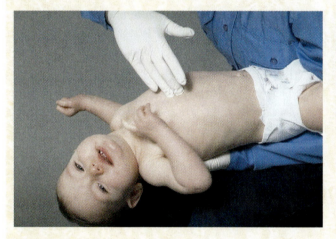

Figure BCLS-20C 5 chest thrusts.

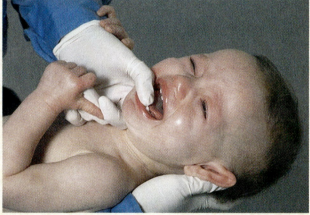

Figure BCLS-20D If the infant becomes unresponsive, perform a tongue-jaw lift and look for a foreign body. If you see one, use a finger sweep to remove it. (Never do blind finger sweeps in an infant or child.) Attempt to ventilate. If this fails, reposition the head and try again. If you are not successful, repeat the sequence shown above. If you are working alone, after 1 minute activate the EMS system and continue airway clearance and ventilation efforts. Transport as quickly as possible.

If the obstruction is not relieved after a series of five thrusts, reassess your position and the patient's airway (if the patient is unconscious, also attempt finger sweeps to attempt to remove the obstruction). Attempt to ventilate the patient and, if unsuccessful, repeat the series of thrusts. Repeat the sequence until the obstruction is relieved.

Airway Clearance Sequences Table BCLS-4 lists sequences of procedures to use in the event of a complete airway obstruction or a partial airway obstruction with poor air exchange. Note that, as discussed earlier, you should activate the EMS system as soon as unresponsiveness is determined, before carrying out the remainder of the airway clearance procedures.

Airway clearance procedures are considered to have been effective if any of the following happens.

◆ The patient re-establishes good air exchange or spontaneous breathing.
◆ The foreign object is expelled from the mouth.
◆ The foreign object is expelled into the mouth where it can be removed by the rescuer.
◆ The unconscious patient regains consciousness.

◆ The patient's skin color improves.

If a person has only a partial airway obstruction and is still able to speak and cough forcefully, do not interfere with his attempts to expel the foreign body. Carefully watch him, however, so that you can immediately provide help if this partial obstruction becomes a complete one.

Procedures for a Child or an Infant

The procedure for clearing a foreign body from the airway of a child is very similar to that used for an adult. The airway clearance procedure for an infant uses a combination of back blows and chest compressions as shown in Figure BCLS-20.

For both a child and an infant, two major differences from adult procedures are:

◆ If the child or infant becomes unconscious, send someone else to activate the EMS system. If no one else is available, wait until you have either relieved the obstruction or you have attempted the airway obstruction sequence for 1 minute.
◆ Do not perform blind finger sweeps. Instead, look in the mouth and perform a finger sweep only if you see a foreign body.

National Registry EMT-B Practical Examinations

The National Registry of Emergency Medical Technicians is an organization founded in 1970, one of whose goals is to establish nationwide professional standards for EMTs. Many state EMS systems use examinations developed by the National Registry to establish certification of EMTs.

The National Registry has prepared a certification examination correlated to the 1994 U.S. DOT Emergency Medical Technician-Basic: National Standard Curriculum. The examination includes both a written portion and a practical portion that consists of a series of performance-based skill stations.

To assist students in preparing for the skill stations that are part of the EMT-Basic examination, as well as to establish guidelines for those evaluating students' performance at the skill stations, the National Registry has developed a series of skill sheets. Each skill sheet contains a set of directions, the skill criteria, and the critical criteria that result in immediate failure of the station.

In studying for the National Registry examination, these skill sheets should be used in conjunction with the material presented in the textbook and not as the sole means of learning the skills. The skill sheets will aid you in organizing the steps necessary to perform each skill and in identifying the criteria that will be used to evaluate your perfor-mance. You can use these sheets to evaluate your own performance when practicing these skills and preparing for your practical skills evaluation.

Note: Three skill sheets regarding advanced airway management are included. The use of these skills will vary based on your medical director, training program, and local protocol.

ORGANIZATION OF THE NATIONAL REGISTRY EXAMINATION

The practical examination consists of six stations, five mandatory stations and one random basic skill station, consisting of both skill-based and scenario-based testing. The random skill station is conducted so the candidate is totally unaware of the skill to be tested until he or she arrives at the test site.

The candidate will be tested individually in each station and will be expected to direct the actions of assistant EMTs who may be present in the station. The candidate should pass or fail the examination solely on his or her actions and decisions.

On the next page is a list of the stations and their established time limits. The maximum time is determined by the number and difficulty of tasks to be completed.

Station 1:	Patient Assessment/Management—Trauma	10 min
Station 2:	Patient Assessment/Management—Medical	10 min
Station 3:	Cardiac Arrest Management/AED	15 min
Station 4:	Bag-Valve-Mask—Apneic Patient	10 min
Station 5:	Spinal Immobilization Station:	
	Spinal Immobilization—Supine Patient	10 min
	Spinal Immobilization—Seated Patient	10 min
Station 6:	Random Basic Skill Verification:	
	Long Bone Injury	5 min
	Joint Injury	5 min
	Traction Splint	10 min
	Bleeding Control/Shock Management	10 min
	Upper Airway Adjuncts and Suction	5 min
	Mouth-to-Mask with Supplemental Oxygen	5 min
	Supplemental Oxygen Administration	5 min

Instructions to the Candidate: Patient Assessment/Management—Trauma

This station is designed to test your ability to perform a patient assessment of a victim of multi-system trauma and voice-treat all conditions and injuries discovered. You must conduct your assessment as you would in the field, including communicating with your patient. You may remove the patient's clothing down to shorts or swimsuit if you feel it is necessary. As you conduct your assessment, you should state everything you are assessing. Clinical information not obtainable by visual or physical inspection, for example blood pressure, will be given to you after you demonstrate how you would normally gain that information. You may assume that you have two EMTs working with you and that they are correctly carrying out the verbal treatments you indicate. You have (10) ten minutes to complete this skill station. Do you have any questions?

Instructions to the Candidate: Patient Assessment/Management—Medical

This station is designed to test your ability to perform a patient assessment of a victim with a chief complaint of a medical nature and voice-treat all conditions and injuries discovered. You must conduct your assessment as you would in the field, including communicating with your patient. As you conduct your assessment, you

should state everything you are assessing. Clinical information not obtainable by visual or physical inspection, for example, blood pressure, will be given to you after you demonstrate how you would normally gain that information. You may assume that you have two EMTs working with you and that they are correctly carrying out the verbal treatments you indicate. You have (10) ten minutes to complete this skill station. Do you have any questions?

Instructions to the Candidate: Cardiac Arrest Management

This station is designed to test your ability to manage a pre-hospital cardiac arrest by integrating CPR skills, defibrillation, airway adjuncts, and patient/scene management skills. There will be an EMT assistant in this station. The EMT assistant will only do as you instruct him. As you arrive on the scene you will encounter a patient in cardiac arrest. A first responder will be present performing single rescuer CPR. You must immediately establish control of the scene and begin resuscitation of the patient with an automated external defibrillator. At the appropriate time, you must control the airway and ventilate the victim using adjunctive equipment. You may not delegate this action to the EMT assistant. You may use any of the supplies available in this room. You have (15) fifteen minutes to complete this skill station. Do you have any questions?

Instructions to the Candidate: Airway, Oxygen, Ventilation Skills Bag-Valve-Mask Apneic Patient with Pulse

This station is designed to test your ability to ventilate a patient using a bag-valve mask. As you enter the station you will find an apneic patient with a palpable central pulse. There are no bystanders and artificial ventilation has not been initiated. The only patient intervention required is airway management and ventilatory support using a bag-valve mask. You must initially ventilate the patient for a minimum of 30 seconds. You will be evaluated on the appropriateness of ventilator volumes. I will inform you that a second rescuer has arrived and will instruct you that you must control the airway and the mask seal while the second rescuer provides ventilation. You may use only the equipment available in this room. Do you have any questions?

Instructions to the Candidate: Spinal Immobilization—Supine Patient

This station is designed to test your ability to provide spinal immobilization on a patient using a long spine immobilization device. You arrive on the scene with an EMT assistant. The assistant EMT has completed the scene size-up as well as the initial and focused assessments. As you begin the station there are no airway, breathing, or circulatory problems. You are required to treat the specific, isolated problem of an unstable spine using a long spine immobilization device. When moving the patient to the device, you should use the help of the assistant EMT and the evaluator. The assistant EMT should control the head and cervical spine of the patient while you and the evaluator move the patient to the immobilization device. You are responsible for the direction and subsequent action of the EMT assistant. You may use any equipment available in this room. You have (10) ten minutes to complete this procedure. Do you have any questions?

Instructions to the Candidate: Spinal Immobilization Skills—Seated Patient

This station is designed to test your ability to provide spinal immobilization on a patient using a half spine immobilization device. You arrive on the scene with an EMT assistant. The assistant EMT has completed the scene size-up, initial and focused assessments. As you begin the station, there are no airway, breathing, or circulatory problems. You are required to treat the specific, isolated problem of an unstable spine using a half spine immobilization device. Continued assessment of airway, breathing, and central circulation is not necessary. You are responsible for the direction and subsequent actions of the EMT assistant.

Transferring the patient to the long spine board should be accomplished verbally. You may use any equipment available in this room. You have (10) ten minutes to complete this procedure. Do you have any questions?

Instructions to the Candidate: Immobilization Skills—Long Bone

This station is designed to test your ability to properly immobilize a closed, non-angulated long bone injury. You are required to treat only the specific, isolated injury. The scene size-up and initial assessment have been completed and during the focused assessment a closed, non-angulated injury of the _____ (radius, ulna, tibia, fibula) was detected. Ongoing assessment of the patient's airway, breathing, and central circulation is not necessary. You may use any equipment available in this room. You have (5) five minutes to complete this procedure. Do you have any questions?

Instructions to the Candidate: Immobilization Skills—Joint Injury

This station is designed to test your ability to properly immobilize a non-complicated shoulder injury. You are required to treat only the specific, isolated injury. The scene size-up and initial assessment have been accomplished on the victim and during the focused assessment a shoulder injury was detected. Ongoing assessment of the patient's airway, breathing, and central circulation is not necessary. You may use any equipment available in this room. You have (5) five minutes to complete this procedure. Do you have any questions?

Instructions to the Candidate: Immobilization Skills—Traction Splinting

This station is designed to test your ability to properly immobilize a mid-shaft femur injury with a traction splint. You will have an EMT assistant to help you in the application of the device by applying manual traction when directed to do so. You are required to treat only the specific, isolated injury. The scene size-up and initial assessment have been accomplished on the victim and during the focused assessment a mid-shaft femur deformity was detected. Ongoing assessment of the patient's airway, breathing, and central circulation is not necessary. You may use any equipment available in this room. You have (10) ten minutes to complete this procedure. Do you have any questions?

Instructions to the Candidate: Bleeding Control/Shock Management

This station is designed to test your ability to control hemorrhage. This is a scenario-based testing station. As you progress through the scenario, you will be offered various signs and symptoms appropriate for the patient's condition. You will be required to manage the patient based on these signs and symptoms. A scenario will be read aloud to you and you will be given an opportunity to ask clarifying questions about the scenario; however, you will not receive answers to any questions about the actual steps of the procedures to be performed. You may use any of the supplies and equipment available in this room. You have (10) ten minutes to complete this skill station. Do you have any questions?

Instructions to the Candidate: Airway, Oxygen, Ventilation Skills—Upper Airway Adjuncts and Suction

This station is designed to test your ability to properly measure, insert, and remove an oropharyngeal and a nasopharyngeal airway as well as suction a patient's upper airway. This is an isolated skills test comprised of three separate skills. You may use any equipment available in this room. Do you have any questions?

Instructions to the Candidate: Airway, Oxygen, Ventilation Skills—Mouth-to-Mask with Supplemental Oxygen

This station is designed to test your ability to ventilate a patient with supplemental oxygen using a mouth-to-mask technique. This is an isolated skills test. You may assume that mouth-to-mouth ventilation is in progress and that the patient has a central pulse. The only patient management required is ventilator support using a mouth-to-mask technique with supplemental oxygen. You must ventilate the patient for at least 30 seconds. You will be evaluated on the appropriateness of ventilatory volumes. You may use any equipment available in this room. Do you have any questions?

Instructions to the Candidate: Airway, Oxygen, Ventilation Skills, Supplemental Oxygen Administration

This station is designed to test your ability to correctly assemble the equipment needed to administer supplemental oxygen in the pre-hospital setting. This is an isolated skills test. You will be required to assemble an oxygen tank and regulator and administer oxygen to a patient using a nonrebreather mask. At this point you will be instructed to discontinue oxygen administration by the nonrebreather mask because the patient cannot tolerate the mask and start oxygen administration using a nasal cannula. Once you have initiated oxygen administration using a nasal cannula, you will be instructed to discontinue oxygen administration completely. You may use only the equipment available in this room. Do you have any questions?

PATIENT ASSESSMENT/MANAGEMENT—MEDICAL

Start Time: _____
Stop Time: _____ Date: _____
Candidate's Name: _____
Evaluator's Name: _____

	Points Possible	Points Awarded
Takes, or verbalizes, body substance isolation precautions	1	
SCENE SIZE-UP		
Determines the scene is safe	1	
Determines the mechanism of injury/nature of illness	1	
Determines the number of patients	1	
Requests additional help if necessary	1	
Considers stabilization of spine	1	
INITIAL ASSESSMENT		
Verbalizes general impression of patient	1	
Determines responsiveness/level of consciousness	1	
Determines chief complaint/apparent life threats	1	
Assesses airway and breathing — Assessment	1	
Initiates appropriate oxygen therapy	1	
Assures adequate ventilation	1	
Assesses circulation — Assesses/controls major bleeding	1	
Assesses pulse	1	
Assesses skin (color, temperature, and condition)	1	
Identifies priority patients/makes transport decision	1	

FOCUSED HISTORY AND PHYSICAL EXAM/RAPID ASSESSMENT

Signs and symptoms (Assesses history of present illness)

Respiratory	Cardiac	Altered Mental Status	Allergic Reaction	Poisoning/Overdose	Environmental Emergency	Obstetrics	Behavioral
•Onset?	•Onset?	•Description of the episode	•History of allergies?	•Substance?	•Source?	•Are you pregnant?	•How do you feel?
•Provokes?	•Provokes?	•Onset?	•What were you exposed to?	•When did you ingest/become exposed?	•Environment?	•How long have you been pregnant?	•Determine suicidal tendencies
•Quality?	•Quality?	•Duration?	•How were you exposed?	•How much did you ingest?	•Duration?	•Pain or contractions?	•Is the patient a threat to self or others?
•Radiates?	•Radiates?	•Associated symptoms?	•Effects?	•Over what time period?	•Loss of consciousness?	•Bleeding or discharge?	•Is there a medical problem?
•Severity?	•Severity?	•Evidence of trauma?	•Progression?	•Interventions?	•Effects—General or local?	•Do you feel the need to push?	•Interventions?
•Time?	•Time?	•Interventions?	•Interventions?	•Estimated weight?		•Last menstrual period?	
•Interventions?	•Interventions?	•Seizures?					
		•Fever?					

	Points Possible	Points Awarded
Allergies	1	
Medications	1	
Past pertinent history	1	
Last oral intake	1	
Events leading to present illness (rule out trauma)	1	
Performs focused physical examination (assesses affected body part/system or, if indicated, completes rapid assessment)	1	
Vitals (obtains baseline vital signs)	1	
Interventions (obtains medical direction or verbalizes standing order for medication interventions and verbalizes proper additional intervention/treatment)	1	
Transport (re-evaluates transport decision)	1	
Verbalizes the consideration for completing a detailed physical examination	1	
ONGOING ASSESSMENT (verbalized)		
Repeats initial assessment	1	
Repeats vital signs	1	
Repeats focused assessment regarding patient complaint or injuries	1	
	Total: 30	

Critical Criteria

___ Did not take, or verbalize, body substance isolation precautions when necessary
___ Did not determine scene safety
___ Did not obtain medical direction or verbalize standing orders for medication interventions
___ Did not provide high concentration of oxygen
___ Did not find or manage problems associated with airway, breathing, hemorrhage or shock (hypoperfusion)
___ Did not differentiate patient's need for transportation versus continued assessment at the scene
___ Did detailed or focused history/physical examination before assessing airway, breathing and circulation
___ Did not ask questions about the present illness
___ Administered a dangerous or inappropriate intervention

PATIENT ASSESSMENT/MANAGEMENT—TRAUMA

Start Time: _____
Stop Time: _____ Date: _____
Candidate's Name: _____
Evaluator's Name: _____

	Points Possible	Points Awarded
Takes, or verbalizes, body substance isolation precautions	1	
SCENE SIZE-UP		
Determines the scene is safe	1	
Determines the mechanism of injury	1	
Determines the number of patients	1	
Requests additional help if necessary	1	
Considers stabilization of spine	1	
INITIAL ASSESSMENT		
Verbalizes general impression of patient	1	
Determines responsiveness/level of consciousness	1	
Determines chief complaint/apparent life threats	1	
Assesses airway and breathing — Assessment	1	
Initiates appropriate oxygen therapy	1	
Assures adequate ventilation	1	
Injury management	1	
Assesses circulation — Assesses/controls major bleeding	1	
Assesses pulse	1	
Assesses skin (color, temperature, and condition)	1	
Identifies priority patients/makes transport decision	1	
FOCUSED HISTORY AND PHYSICAL EXAM/RAPID TRAUMA ASSESSMENT		
Selects appropriate assessment (**focused or rapid assessment**)	1	
Obtains or directs assistant to obtain baseline vital signs	1	
Obtains S.A.M.P.L.E. history	1	
DETAILED PHYSICAL EXAMINATION		
Assesses the head — Inspects and palpates the scalp and ears	1	
Assesses the eyes	1	
Assesses the facial areas including oral and nasal areas	1	
Assesses the neck — Inspects and palpates the neck	1	
Assesses for JVD	1	
Assesses for tracheal deviation	1	
Assesses the chest — Inspects	1	
Palpates	1	
Auscultates	1	
Assesses the abdomen/pelvis — Assesses the abdomen	1	
Assesses the pelvis	1	
Verbalizes assessment of genitalia/perineum as needed	1	
Assesses the extremities — 1 point for each extremity	4	
includes inspection, palpation, and assessment of motor, sensory and circulatory function		
Assesses the posterior — Assesses thorax	1	
Assesses lumbar	1	
Manages secondary injuries and wounds appropriately		
1 point for appropriate management of secondary injury/wound	1	
Verbalizes re-assessment of the vital signs	1	
	Total: 40	

Critical Criteria

___ Did not take, or verbalize, body substance isolation precautions
___ Did not determine scene safety
___ Did not assess for spinal protection
___ Did not provide for spinal protection when indicated
___ Did not provide high concentration of oxygen
___ Did not find, or manage, problems associated with airway, breathing, hemorrhage or shock (hypoperfusion)
___ Did not differentiate patient's need for transportation versus continued assessment at the scene
___ Did other detailed physical examination before assessing airway, breathing, and circulation
___ Did not transport patient within (10) minute time limit

BAG-VALVE-MASK APNEIC PATIENT

Start Time: _____
Stop Time: _____ Date: _____
Candidate's Name: _____
Evaluator's Name: _____

	Points Possible
Takes, or verbalizes, body substance isolation precautions	1
Voices opening the airway	1
Voices inserting an airway adjunct	1
Selects appropriately sized mask	1
Creates a proper mask-to-face seal	1
Ventilates patient at no less than 800 ml volume *(The examiner must witness for at least 30 seconds)*	1
Connects reservoir and oxygen	1
Adjusts liter flow to 15 liters/minute or greater	1
The examiner indicates the arrival of second EMT. The second EMT is instructed to ventilate the patient while the candidate controls the mask and the airway.	
Voices re-opening the airway	1
Creates a proper mask-to-face seal	1
Instructs assistant to resume ventilation at proper volume per breath *(The examiner must witness for at least 30 seconds)*	1
Total:	11

Critical Criteria

___ Did not take, or verbalize, body substance isolation precautions
___ Did not immediately ventilate the patient
___ Interrupted ventilations for more than 20 seconds
___ Did not provide high concentration of oxygen
___ Did not provide, or direct assistant to provide, proper volume/breath *(more than two (2) ventilations per minute are below 800 ml)*
___ Did not allow adequate exhalation

CARDIAC ARREST MANAGEMENT/AED

Start Time: _____ Date: _____
Stop Time: _____
Candidate's Name: _____
Evaluator's Name: _____

	Points Possible	Points Awarded
ASSESSMENT		
Takes, or verbalizes, body substance isolation precautions	1	
Briefly questions the rescuer about arrest events	1	
Directs rescuer to stop CPR	1	
Verifies absence of spontaneous pulse **(skill station examiner states "no pulse")**	1	
Directs resumption of CPR	1	
Turns on defibrillator power	1	
Attaches automated defibrillator to the patient	1	
Directs rescuer to stop CPR and ensures all individuals are clear of the patient	1	
Initiates analysis of the rhythm	1	
Delivers shock (up to three successive shocks)	1	
Verifies absence of spontaneous pulse **(skill station examiner states "no pulse")**	1	
TRANSITION		
Directs resumption of CPR	1	
Gathers additional information about arrest event	1	
Confirms effectiveness of CPR (ventilation and compressions)	1	
INTEGRATION		
Verbalizes or directs insertion of a simple airway adjunct (oral/nasal airway)	1	
Ventilates, or directs ventilation of, the patient	1	
Assures high concentration of oxygen is delivered to the patient	1	
Assures CPR continues without unnecessary/prolonged interruption	1	
Re-evaluates patient/CPR in approximately one minute	1	
Repeats defibrillator sequence	1	
TRANSPORTATION		
Verbalizes transportation of patient	1	
Total:	21	

Critical Criteria

___ Did not take, or verbalize, body substance isolation precautions
___ Did not evaluate the need for immediate use of the AED
___ Did not direct initiation/resumption of ventilation/compressions at appropriate times
___ Did not assure all individuals were clear of patient before delivering each shock
___ Did not operate the AED properly (inability to deliver shock)
___ Prevented the defibrillator from delivering indicated stacked shocks

SPINAL IMMOBILIZATION
SUPINE PATIENT

Start Time: _____

Stop Time: _____ Date: _____

Candidate's Name: _____

Evaluator's Name: _____

	Points Possible	Points Awarded
Takes, or verbalizes, body substance isolation precautions	1	
Directs assistant to place/maintain head in neutral in-line position	1	
Directs assistant to maintain manual immobilization of the head	1	
Re-assesses motor, sensory and circulatory function in each extremity	1	
Applies appropriately sized extrication collar	1	
Positions the immobilization device appropriately	1	
Directs movement of the patient onto the device without compromising the integrity of the spine	1	
Applies padding to voids between the torso and the board as necessary	1	
Immobilizes the patient's torso to the device	1	
Evaluates the pads behind the patient's head as necessary	1	
Immobilizes the patient's head to the device	1	
Secures the patient's legs to the device	1	
Secures the patient's arms to the device	1	
Reassesses motor, sensory and circulatory function in each extremity	1	
Total:	14	

Critical Criteria

____ Did not immediately direct, or take, manual immobilization of the head

____ Released, or ordered release of, manual immobilization before it was maintained mechanically

____ Patient manipulated, or moved excessively, causing potential spinal compromise

____ Patient moves excessively up, down, left or right on the patient's torso

____ Head immobilization allows for excessive movement

____ Upon completion of immobilization, head is not in the neutral position

____ Did not reassess motor, sensory, and circulatory function in each extremity after immobilization to the device

____ Immobilized head to the board before securing the torso

SPINAL IMMOBILIZATION
SEATED PATIENT

Start Time: _____

Stop Time: _____ Date: _____

Candidate's Name: _____

Evaluator's Name: _____

	Points Possible	Points Awarded
Takes, or verbalizes, body substance isolation precautions	1	
Directs assistant to place/maintain head in neutral in-line position	1	
Directs assistant to maintain manual immobilization of the head	1	
Reassesses motor, sensory and circulatory function in each extremity	1	
Applies appropriately sized extrication collar	1	
Positions the immobilization device behind the patient	1	
Secures the device to the patient's torso	1	
Evaluates torso fixation and adjusts as necessary	1	
Evaluates and pads behind the patient's head as necessary	1	
Secures the patient's head to the device	1	
Verbalizes moving the patient to a long board	1	
Reassesses motor, sensory and circulatory function in each extremity	1	
Total:	12	

Critical Criteria

____ Did not immediately direct, or take, manual immobilization of the head

____ Released, or ordered release of, manual immobilization before it was maintained mechanically

____ Patient manipulated, or moved excessively, causing potential spinal compromise

____ Device moved excessively up, down, left or right on patient's torso

____ Head immobilization allows for excessive movement

____ Torso fixation inhibits chest rise, resulting in respiratory compromise

____ Upon completion of immobilization, head is not in the neutral position

____ Did not reassess motor, sensory and circulatory function in each extremity after voicing immobilization to the long board

____ Immobilized head to the board before securing the torso

IMMOBILIZATION SKILLS
JOINT INJURY

Start Time: _____
Stop Time: _____ Date: _____
Candidate's Name: _____
Evaluator's Name: _____

	Points Possible	Points Awarded
Takes, or verbalizes, body substance isolation precautions	1	
Directs application of manual stabilization of the shoulder injury	1	
Assesses motor, sensory and circulatory function in the injured extremity	1	
Note: The examiner acknowledges "motor, sensory and circulatory function are present and normal."		
Selects the proper splinting material	1	
Immobilizes the site of the injury	1	
Immobilizes the bone above the injured joint	1	
Immobilizes the bone below the injured joint	1	
Reassesses motor, sensory and circulatory function in the injured extremity	1	
Note: The examiner acknowledges "motor, sensory and circulatory function are present and normal."		
Total:	8	

Critical Criteria

___ Did not support the joint so that the joint did not bear distal weight

___ Did not immobilize the bone above and below the injured site

___ Did not reassess motor, sensory and circulatory function in the injured extremity before and after splinting

---

IMMOBILIZATION SKILLS
LONG BONE INJURY

Start Time: _____
Stop Time: _____ Date: _____
Candidate's Name: _____
Evaluator's Name: _____

	Points Possible	Points Awarded
Takes, or verbalizes, body substance isolation precautions	1	
Directs application of manual stabilization of the injury	1	
Assesses motor, sensory and circulatory function in the injured extremity	1	
Note: The examiner acknowledges "motor, sensory and circulatory function are present and normal."		
Measures the splint	1	
Applies the splint	1	
Immobilizes the joint above the injury site	1	
Immobilizes the joint below the injury site	1	
Secures the entire injured extremity	1	
Immobilizes the hand/foot in the position of function	1	
Reassesses motor, sensory and circulatory function in the injured extremity	1	
Note: The examiner acknowledges "motor, sensory and circulatory function are present and normal."		
Total:	10	

Critical Criteria

___ Grossly moves the injured extremity

___ Did not immobilize the joint above and the joint below the injury site

___ Did not reassess motor, sensory and circulatory function in the injured extremity before and after splinting

IMMOBILIZATION SKILLS
TRACTION SPLINTING

Start Time: _____
Stop Time: _____ Date: _____
Candidate's Name: _____
Evaluator's Name: _____

	Points Possible	Points Awarded
Takes, or verbalizes, body substance isolation precautions	1	
Directs application of manual stabilization of the injured leg	1	
Directs the application of manual traction	1	
Assesses motor, sensory and circulatory function in the injured extremity	1	
Note: The examiner acknowledges "motor, sensory and circulatory function are present and normal"		
Prepares/adjusts splint to the proper length	1	
Positions the splint next to the injured leg	1	
Applies the proximal securing device (e.g., ischial strap)	1	
Applies the distal securing device (e.g., ankle hitch)	1	
Applies mechanical traction	1	
Positions/secures the support straps	1	
Re-evaluates the proximal/distal securing devices	1	
Reassesses motor, sensory and circulatory function in the injured extremity	1	
Note: The examiner acknowledges "motor, sensory and circulatory function are present and normal"		
Note: The examiner must ask the candidate how he/she would prepare the patient for transportation		
Verbalizes securing the torso to the long board to immobilize the hip	1	
Verbalizes securing the splint to the long board to prevent movement of the splint	1	
Total:	**14**	

Critical Criteria

____ Loss of traction at any point after it was applied
____ Did not reassess motor, sensory and circulatory function in the injured extremity before and after splinting
____ The foot was excessively rotated or extended after splint was applied
____ Did not secure the ischial strap before taking traction
____ Final immobilization failed to support the femur or prevent rotation of the injured leg
____ Secured the leg to the long board before applying mechanical traction

Note: If the Sagar splint or the Kendricks Traction Device is used without elevating the patient's leg, application of manual traction is not necessary. The candidate should be awarded one (1) point as if manual traction were applied.

Note: If the leg is elevated at all, manual traction must be applied before elevating the leg. The ankle hitch may be applied before elevating the leg and used to provide manual traction.

BLEEDING CONTROL/SHOCK MANAGEMENT

Start Time: _____
Stop Time: _____ Date: _____
Candidate's Name: _____
Evaluator's Name: _____

	Points Possible	Points Awarded
Takes, or verbalizes, body substance isolation precautions	1	
Applies direct pressure to the wound	1	
Elevates the extremity	1	
Note: The examiner must now inform the candidate that the wound continues to bleed.		
Applies an additional dressing to the wound	1	
Note: The examiner must now inform the candidate that the wound still continues to bleed. The second dressing does not control the bleeding.		
Locates and applies pressure to appropriate arterial pressure point	1	
Note: The examiner must now inform the candidate that the bleeding is controlled.		
Bandages the wound	1	
Note: The examiner must now inform the candidate that the patient is now showing signs and symptoms indicative of hypoperfusion.		
Properly positions the patient	1	
Applies high concentration oxygen	1	
Initiates steps to prevent heat loss from the patient	1	
Indicates the need for immediate transportation	1	
Total:	**10**	

Critical Criteria

____ Did not take, or verbalize, body substance isolation precautions
____ Did not apply high concentration of oxygen
____ Applied a tourniquet before attempting other methods of bleeding control
____ Did not control hemorrhage in a timely manner
____ Did not indicate a need for immediate transportation

AIRWAY, OXYGEN, AND VENTILATION SKILLS
UPPER AIRWAY ADJUNCTS AND SUCTION

OROPHARYNGEAL AIRWAY

Start Time: _____
Stop Time: _____
Candidate's Name: _____ Date: _____
Evaluator's Name: _____

	Points Possible	Points Awarded
Takes, or verbalizes, body substance isolation precautions	1	
Selects appropriately sized airway	1	
Measures airway	1	
Inserts airway without pushing the tongue posteriorly	1	
Note: The examiner must advise the candidate that the patient is gagging and becoming conscious.		
Removes the oropharyngeal airway	1	

SUCTION

	Points Possible	Points Awarded
NOTE: The examiner must advise the candidate to suction the patient's airway.		
Turns on/prepares suction device	1	
Assures presence of mechanical suction	1	
Inserts the suction tip without suction	1	
Applies suction to the oropharynx/nasopharynx	1	

NASOPHARYNGEAL AIRWAY

	Points Possible	Points Awarded
NOTE: The examiner must advise the candidate to insert a nasopharyngeal airway.		
Selects appropriately sized airway	1	
Measures airway	1	
Verbalizes lubrication of the nasal airway	1	
Fully inserts the airway with the bevel facing toward the septum	1	
Total:	13	

Critical Criteria

___ Did not take, or verbalize, body substance isolation precautions
___ Did not obtain a patent airway with the oropharyngeal airway
___ Did not obtain a patent airway with the nasopharyngeal airway
___ Did not demonstrate an acceptable suction technique
___ Inserted any adjunct in a manner dangerous to the patient

MOUTH TO MASK WITH SUPPLEMENTAL OXYGEN

Start Time: _____
Stop Time: _____
Candidate's Name: _____ Date: _____
Evaluator's Name: _____

	Points Possible	Points Awarded
Takes, or verbalizes, body substance isolation precautions	1	
Connects one-way valve to mask	1	
Opens patient's airway or confirms patient's airway is open (manually or with adjunct)	1	
Establishes and maintains a proper mask to face seal	1	
Ventilates the patient at the proper volume and rate (800–1200 ml per breath/10–20 breaths per minute)	1	
Connects mask to high concentration of oxygen	1	
Adjusts flow rate to at least 15 liters per minute	1	
Continues ventilation of the patient at the proper volume and rate (800–1200 ml per breath/10–20 breaths per minute)	1	
Note: The examiner must witness ventilations for at least 30 seconds		
Total:	8	

Critical Criteria

___ Did not take, or verbalize, body substance isolation precautions
___ Did not adjust liter flow to at least 15 liters per minute
___ Did not provide proper volume per breath
    (more than 2 ventilations per minute were below 800 ml)
___ Did not ventilate the patient at a rate of 10–20 breaths per minute
___ Did not allow for complete exhalation

OXYGEN ADMINISTRATION

Start Time: _____ Date: _____
Stop Time: _____
Candidate's Name: _____
Evaluator's Name: _____

	Points Possible	Points Awarded
Takes, or verbalizes, body substance isolation precautions	1	
Assembles the regulator to the tank	1	
Opens the tank	1	
Checks for leaks	1	
Checks tank pressure	1	
Attaches non-rebreather mask to oxygen	1	
Prefills reservoir	1	
Adjusts liter flow to 12 liters per minute or greater	1	
Applies and adjusts the mask to the patient's face	1	
Note: The examiner must advise the candidate that the patient is not tolerating the nonre-breather mask. The medical director has ordered you to apply a nasal cannula to the patient.		
Attaches nasal cannula to oxygen	1	
Adjusts liter flow to six (6) liters per minute or less	1	
Applies nasal cannula to the patient	1	
Note: The examiner must advise the candidate to discontinue oxygen therapy		
Removes the nasal cannula from the patient	1	
Shuts off the regulator	1	
Relieves the pressure within the regulator	1	
Total:	15	

Critical Criteria

_____ Did not take, or verbalize, body substance isolation precautions
_____ Did not assemble the tank and regulator without leaks
_____ Did not prefill the reservoir bag
_____ Did not adjust the device to the correct liter flow for the non-rebreather mask
       (12 liters per minute or greater)
_____ Did not adjust the device to the correct liter flow for the nasal cannula (6 liters per minute or less)

VENTILATORY MANAGEMENT
ENDOTRACHEAL INTUBATION

Start Time: _____ Date: _____
Stop Time: _____
Candidate's Name: _____
Evaluator's Name: _____

*Note: If a candidate elects to initially ventilate the patient with a BVM attached to a reservoir and oxygen, full credit must be awarded for steps denoted by "***" provided the first ventilation is delivered within the initial 30 seconds*

	Points Possible	Points Awarded
Takes or verbalizes body substance isolation precautions	1	
Opens the airway manually	1	
Elevates the patient's tongue and inserts a simple airway adjunct (oropharyngeal/nasopharyngeal airway)	1	
Note: The examiner must now inform the candidate "no gag reflex is present and the patient accepts the airway adjunct."		
**Ventilates the patient immediately using a BVM device unattached to oxygen	1	
**Hyperventilates the patient with room air	1	
Note: The examiner must now inform the candidate that ventilation is being properly performed without difficulty		
Attaches the oxygen reservoir to the BVM	1	
Attaches the BVM to high flow oxygen (15 liters per minute)	1	
Ventilates the patient at the proper volume and rate (800-1200 ml/breath and 10-20 breaths/minute)	1	
Note: After 30 seconds, the examiner must auscultate the patient's chest and inform the candidate that breath sounds are present and equal bilaterally and medical direction has ordered endotracheal intubation. The examiner must now take over ventilation of the patient.		
Directs assistant to hyper-oxygenate the patient	1	
Identifies/selects the proper equipment for endotracheal intubation	1	
Checks equipment — Checks for cuff leaks	1	
Checks laryngoscope operation and bulb tightness	1	
Note: The examiner must remove the OPA and move out of the way when the candidate is prepared to intubate the patient.		
Positions the patient's head properly	1	
Inserts the laryngoscope blade into the patient's mouth while displacing the patient's tongue laterally	1	
Elevates the patient's mandible with the laryngoscope	1	
Introduces the endotracheal tube and advances the tube to the proper depth	1	
Inflates the cuff to the proper pressure	1	
Disconnects the syringe from the cuff inlet port	1	
Directs assistant to ventilate the patient	1	
Confirms proper placement of the endotracheal tube by auscultation bilaterally and over the epigastrium	1	
Note: The examiner must ask, "If you had proper placement, what would you expect to hear?" (may be verbalized)		
Secures the endotracheal tube (may be verbalized)	1	
Total:	21	

Critical Criteria

_____ Did not take or verbalize body substance isolation precautions when necessary
_____ Did not initiate ventilation within 30 seconds after applying gloves or interrupts ventilations for greater than 30 seconds at any time
_____ Did not voice or provide high oxygen concentrations (15 liter/minute or greater)
_____ Did not ventilate the patient at a rate of at least 10 breaths per minute
_____ Did not provide adequate volume per breath (maximum of 2 errors per minute permissible)
_____ Did not hyper-oxygenate the patient prior to intubation
_____ Did not successfully intubate the patient within 3 attempts
_____ Used the patient's teeth as a fulcrum
_____ Did not assure proper tube placement by auscultation bilaterally over each lung **and** over the epigastrium
_____ The stylette (if used) extended beyond the end of the endotracheal tube
_____ Inserted any adjunct in a manner that was dangerous to the patient
_____ Did not immediately disconnect the syringe from the inlet port after inflating the cuff

VENTILATORY MANAGEMENT
ESOPHAGEAL OBTURATOR AIRWAY INSERTION FOLLOWING AN UNSUCCESSFUL ENDOTRACHEAL INTUBATION ATTEMPT

Start Time: _____
Stop Time: _____ Date: _____
Candidate's Name: _____
Evaluator's Name: _____

	Points Possible	Points Awarded
Continues body substance isolation precautions	1	
Confirms the patient is being ventilated high percentage oxygen	1	
Directs the assistant to hyper-oxygenate the patient	1	
Identifies/selects the proper equipment for insertion of EOA	1	
Assembles the EOA	1	
Tests the cuff for leaks	1	
Inflates the mask	1	
Lubricates the tube *(may be verbalized)*	1	
Note: The examiner should remove the OPA and move out of the way when the candidate is prepared to insert the device		
Positions the head properly with the neck in the neutral or slightly flexed position	1	
Grasps and elevates the patient's tongue and mandible	1	
Inserts the tube in the same direction as the curvature of the pharynx	1	
Advances the tube until the mask is sealed against the patient's face	1	
Ventilates the patient while maintaining a tight mask-to-face seal	1	
Directs confirmation of placement of EOA by observing for chest rise and auscultation over the epigastrium and bilaterally over each lung	1	
Note: The examiner must acknowledge adequate chest rise, bilateral breath sounds and absent sounds over the epigastrium		
Inflates the cuff to the proper pressure	1	
Disconnects the syringe from the inlet port	1	
Continues ventilation of the patient	1	
	Total: 17	

Critical Criteria
____ Did not take or verbalize body substance isolation precautions
____ Did not initiate ventilations within 30 seconds
____ Interrupted ventilations for more than 30 seconds at a time
____ Did not direct hyper-oxygenation of the patient prior to placement of the EOA
____ Did not successfully place the EOA within 3 attempts
____ Did not ventilate at a rate of at least 10 breaths per minute
____ Did not provide adequate volume per breath (maximum 2 errors/minute permissible)
____ Did not assure proper tube placement by auscultation bilaterally and over the epigastrium
____ Did not remove the syringe after inflating the cuff
____ Did not successfully ventilate the patient
____ Do not provide high flow oxygen (15 liters per minute or greater)
____ Inserted any adjunct in a manner that was dangerous to the patient

---

VENTILATORY MANAGEMENT
DUAL LUMEN DEVICE INSERTION FOLLOWING AN UNSUCCESSFUL ENDOTRACHEAL INTUBATION ATTEMPT

Start Time: _____
Stop Time: _____ Date: _____
Candidate's Name: _____
Evaluator's Name: _____

	Points Possible	Points Awarded
Continues body substance isolation precautions	1	
Confirms the patient is being properly ventilated with high percentage oxygen	1	
Directs the assistant to hyper-oxygenate the patient	1	
Checks/prepares the airway device	1	
Lubricates the distal tip of the device *(may be verbalized)*	1	
Note: The examiner should remove the OPA and move out of the way when the candidate is prepared to insert the device		
Positions the patient's head properly	1	
Performs a tongue-jaw lift	1	
☐ USES COMBITUBE ☐ USES THE PTL		
Inserts device in the mid-line and to the depth so that the printed ring is at the level of the teeth / Inserts the device in the mid-line until the bite block flange is at the level of the teeth	1	
Inflates the pharyngeal cuff with the proper volume and removes the syringe / Secures the strap	1	
Inflates the distal cuff with the proper volume and removes the syringe / Blows into tube #1 to adequately inflate both cuffs	1	
Attaches/directs attachment of BVM to the first (esophageal placement) lumen and ventilates	1	
Confirms placement and ventilation through the correct lumen by observing chest rise, and auscultation over the epigastrium and bilaterally over each lung	1	
Note: The examiner states, "You do not see rise and fall of the chest and hear sounds only over the epigastrium."		
Attaches/directs attachment of BVM to the second (endotracheal placement) lumen and ventilates	1	
Confirms placement and ventilation through the correct lumen by observing chest rise, and auscultation over the epigastrium and bilaterally over each lung	1	
Note: The examiner states, "You see rise and fall of the chest, there are no sounds over the epigastrium and breath sounds are equal over each lung."		
Secures device or confirms that the device remains properly secured	1	
	Total: 15	

Critical Criteria
____ Did not take or verbalize body substance isolation precautions
____ Did not initiate ventilations within 30 seconds
____ Interrupted ventilations for more than 30 seconds at any time
____ Did not hyper-oxygenate the patient prior to placement of the dual lumen airway device
____ Did not provide adequate volume per breath (maximum 2 errors/minute permissible)
____ Did not ventilate the patient at a rate of at least 10 breaths per minute
____ Did not insert the dual lumen airway device at a proper depth or at the proper place within 3 attempts
____ Did not inflate both cuffs properly
____ **Combitube** — Did not remove the syringe immediately following the inflation of each cuff
____ **PTL** — Did not secure the strap prior to cuff inflation
____ Did not conform, by observing chest rise and auscultation over the epigastrium and bilaterally over each lung, that the proper lumen of the device was being used to ventilate the patient
____ Inserted any adjunct in a manner that was dangerous to the patient

Glossary

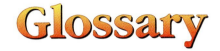

abandonment leaving a patient after care has been initiated and before the patient has been transferred to someone with equal or greater medical training.

abdominal quadrants four divisions of the abdomen used to pinpoint the location of a pain or injury: the right upper quadrant, the left upper quadrant, the right lower quadrant, and the left lower quadrant.

abortion spontaneous (miscarriage) or induced termination of pregnancy.

abrasion (ab-RAY-zhun) a scratch or scrape.

abruptio placentae (ab-RUPT-si-o plah-SENT-ta) a condition in which the placenta separates from the uterine wall; a cause of prebirth bleeding. Also called *placental abruption*.

absorbed poisons poisons that are taken into the body through unbroken skin.

acetabulum (AS-uh-TAB-yuh-lum) the pelvic socket into which the ball at the proximal end of the femur fits to form the hip joint.

acromioclavicular (ah-KRO-me-o-klav-IK-yuh-ler) **joint** the joint where the acromion and the clavicle meet.

acromion (ah-KRO-me-on) **process** the highest portion of the shoulder.

activated charcoal a powder, usually pre-mixed with water, that will adsorb some poisons and help prevent them from being absorbed by the body.

active rewarming application of an external heat source to rewarm the body of a hypothermic patient. See also *central rewarming*.

acute myocardial infarction (ah-KUTE MY-o-KARD-e-ul in-FARK-shun) **(AMI)** the condition in which a portion of the myocardium dies as a result of oxygen starvation; a heart attack.

afterbirth the placenta, membranes of the amniotic sac, part of the umbilical cord, and some tissues from the lining of the uterus that are delivered after the birth of the baby.

air embolism gas bubble in the bloodstream. The plural is *air emboli*. The more accurate term is *arterial gas embolism (AGE)*.

airway the passageway by which air enters or leaves the body. The structures of the airway are the nose, mouth, pharynx, larynx, trachea, bronchi, and lungs.

allergen something that causes an allergic reaction.

allergic reaction an exaggerated immune response.

alveoli (al-VE-o-li) the microscopic sacs of the lungs where gas exchange with the bloodstream takes place.

amniotic (am-ne-OT-ik) **sac** the "bag of waters" that surrounds the developing fetus.

amputation (am-pyu-TAY-shun) the surgical removal or traumatic severing of a body part, usually an extremity.

anaphylaxis (an-ah-fi-LAK-sis) a severe or life-threatening allergic reaction in which the blood vessels dilate, causing a drop in blood pressure, and the tissues lining the respiratory system swell, interfering with the airway. Also called *anaphylactic shock*.

anatomical position the standard reference position for the body in the study of anatomy. The body is standing erect, facing the observer. The arms are down at the sides and the palms of the hands face forward.

anatomy the study of body structure.

aneurysm (AN-u-rizm) the dilation, or ballooning, of a weakened section of the wall of an artery.

angina pectoris (AN-ji-nah [or an-JI-nah] PEK-to-ris) pain in the chest, occurring when blood supply to the heart is reduced and a portion of the heart muscle is not receiving enough oxygen.

anterior the front of the body or body part. Opposite of *posterior*.

antidote a substance that will neutralize a poison or its effects.

aorta (ay-OR-tah) the largest artery in the body. It transports blood from the left ventricle to begin systemic circulation.

apnea (ap-ne-ah) absence of breathing.

arrhythmia (ah-RITH-me-ah) a disturbance in heart rate and rhythm.

arteriole (ar-TE-re-ol) the smallest kind of artery.

arteriosclerosis (ar-TE-re-o-skle-RO-sis) a condition in which artery walls become hard and stiff due to calcium deposits.

artery any blood vessel carrying blood away from the heart.

artificial ventilation forcing air or oxygen into the lungs when a patient has stopped breathing or has inadequate breathing.

asystole (ay-SIS-to-le) when the heart has ceased generating electrical impulses.

atherosclerosis (ATH-er-o-skle-RO-sis) a buildup of fatty deposits on the inner walls of arteries.

atria (AY-tree-ah) the two upper chambers of the heart. There is a right atrium (which receives unoxygenated blood returning from the body) and a left atrium (which receives oxygenated blood returning from the lungs).

auscultation (os-skul-TAY-shun) listening. A stethoscope is used to auscultate for characteristic body sounds.

auto-injector a syringe pre-loaded with medication that has a spring-loaded device that pushes the needle through the skin when the tip of the device is pressed firmly against the body.

automaticity (AW-to-muh-TISS-it-e) the ability of the heart to generate and conduct electrical impulses on its own.

autonomic (AW-to-NOM-ik) **nervous system** the division of the peripheral nervous system that controls involuntary motor functions.

AVPU a memory aid for *alert, verbal response, painful response, unresponsive* as a classification of a patient's level of responsiveness. See also *mental status.*

avulsion (ah-VUL-shun) the tearing away or tearing off of a piece or flap of skin or other soft tissue. This term also may be used for an eye pulled from its socket or a tooth dislodged from its socket.

bag-valve mask (BVM) a hand-held device with a face mask and self-refilling bag that can be squeezed to provide artificial ventilations to a patient. Can deliver air from the atmosphere or oxygen from a supplemental oxygen supply system.

bandage any material used to hold a dressing in place.

base station a two-way radio at a fixed site such as a hospital or dispatch center.

behavior the manner in which a person acts.

behavioral emergency when a patient's behavior is not typical for the situation; when the patient's behavior is unacceptable or intolerable to the patient, his family, or the community, or when the patient may harm himself or others.

bilateral on both sides.

blood pressure the force of blood against the walls of the blood vessels. Usually arterial blood pressure (the pressure in an artery) is measured. See also *diastolic blood pressure; systolic blood pressure.*

blunt-force trauma injury caused by a blow that does not penetrate through the skin or other body tissues.

body mechanics the proper use of the body to facilitate lifting and moving and prevent injury.

body substance isolation (BSI) a form of infection control based on the presumption that all body fluids are infectious. BSI calls for always using appropriate barriers to infection at the emergency scene, such as gloves, masks, gowns, and protective eyewear.

bones hard but flexible living structures that provide support for the body and protection to vital organs.

brachial (BRAY-ke-al) **artery** artery of the upper arm.

brachial pulse the pulse felt in the upper arm; the pulse checked during infant CPR.

bradycardia (BRAY-duh-KAR-de-uh) a slow heart rate; any pulse rate below 60 beats per minute.

breech presentation when the baby appears buttocks or both legs first during birth.

bronchi (BRONG-ki) the two large sets of branches that come off the trachea and enter the lungs. There are right and left bronchi. The singular is *bronchus.*

bronchoconstriction constriction, or blockage, of the bronchi that lead from the trachea to the lungs.

calcaneus (kal-KAY-ne-us) the heel bone.

capillary (KAP-i-lair-e) a thin-walled, microscopic blood vessel where oxygen/carbon dioxide and nutrient/waste exchange with the body's cells takes place.

cardiac compromise a blanket term for any heart problem.

cardiac conduction system a system of specialized muscle tissues that conduct electrical impulses that stimulate the heart to beat.

cardiac muscle specialized involuntary muscle found only in the heart.

cardiogenic shock shock, or lack of perfusion, brought on not by blood loss but by inadequate pumping action of the heart. It is often the result of a heart attack or congestive heart failure.

cardiovascular system the heart and the blood vessels; the circulatory system.

carina (kah-RI-nah) the fork at the lower end of the trachea where the two mainstem bronchi branch.

carotid (kah-ROT-id) **arteries** the large neck arteries, one on each side of the neck, that carry blood from the heart to the head.

carotid (kah-ROT-id) **pulse** the pulse felt along the large carotid artery on either side of the neck.

carpals (KAR-pulz) the wrist bones.

cartilage tough tissue that covers the joint ends of bones and helps to form certain body parts such as the ear.

cellular phone a phone that transmits through the air instead of over wires so that the phone can be transported and used over a wide area.

central nervous system (CNS) the brain and spinal cord.

central pulses the carotid and femoral pulses, which can be felt in the central part of the body.

central rewarming application of heat to the lateral chest, neck, armpits, and groin of a hypothermic patient.

cephalic (se-FAL-ik) **presentation** when the baby appears head first during birth. This is the normal presentation.

cerebrospinal (suh-RE-bro-SPI-nal) **fluid (CSF)** the fluid that surrounds the brain and spinal cord.

cerebrovascular (suh-RE-bro VAS-ku-ler) **accident (CVA)** see *stroke.*

cervix (SUR-viks) the neck of the uterus at the entrance to the birth canal.

chief complaint in emergency medicine, the reason EMS was called, usually in the patient's own words.

circulatory system see *cardiovascular system.*

clavicle (KLAV-i-kul) the collarbone.

closed extremity injury an injury to an extremity with no associated opening in the skin.

closed wound an internal injury with no open pathway from the outside.

cold zone area where the command post and support functions that are necessary to control a hazardous material incident are located.

colostomy (ko-LOS-to-me) like an ileostomy, a surgical opening in the wall of the abdomen with a bag in place to collect excretions from the digestive system.

compensated shock when the patient is developing shock but the body is still able to maintain perfusion. See *decompensated shock; shock.*

concussion mild closed head injury without detectable damage to the brain. Complete recovery is usually expected.

conduction the direct transfer of heat from one material to another through direct contact.

confidentiality the obligation not to reveal information obtained about a patient except to other health care professionals involved in the patient's care, or under subpoena, or in a court of law, or when the patient has signed a release of confidentiality.

congestive heart failure (CHF) the failure of the heart to pump efficiently, leading to excessive blood or fluids in the lungs, the body, or both.

consent permission from the patient for care or other action by the EMT. See also *expressed consent; implied consent.*

constrict (kon-STRIKT) get smaller.

contamination the introduction of dangerous chemicals, disease, or infectious materials. See also *decontamination.*

contraindications (KON-truh-in-duh-KAY-shunz) specific signs or circumstances under which it is not appropriate and may be harmful to administer a particular drug to a patient.

contusion (kun-TU-zhun) a bruise; in brain injuries, a bruised brain is caused when the force of a blow to the head is great enough to rupture blood vessels.

convection carrying away of heat by currents of air or water or other gases or liquids.

coronary (KOR-o-nar-e) **arteries** blood vessels that supply the muscle of the heart (myocardium).

coronary artery disease (CAD) diseases that affect the arteries of the heart.

cranium (KRAY-ne-um) the bony structure making up the forehead, top, back, and upper sides of the skull.

crepitation (krep-uh-TAY-shun) the grating sound or feeling of broken bones rubbing together; also called *crepitus.*

cricoid (KRIK-oid) **cartilage** the ring-shaped structure that circles the trachea at the lower edge of the larynx.

cricoid pressure pressure applied to the cricoid cartilage to suppress vomiting and bring the vocal cords into view. Also called *Sellick's maneuver.*

critical incident stress debriefing (CISD) a process in which teams of professional and peer counselors provide emotional and psychological support to EMS personnel who are or have been involved in a critical (highly stressful) incident.

crowning when part of the baby is visible through the vaginal opening.

crush injury an injury caused when force is transmitted from the body's exterior to its internal structures. Bones can be broken, muscles, nerves, and tissues damaged, and internal organs ruptured, causing internal bleeding.

cyanosis (SIGH-uh-NO-sis) a blue or gray color resulting from lack of oxygen in the body (see *hypoxia*).

danger zone the area around the wreckage of a vehicle collision or other accident within which special safety precautions should be taken.

DCAP-BTLS A memory aid to remember deformities, contusions, abrasions, punctures/penetrations, burns, tenderness, lacerations, and swelling—signs and symptoms of injury found by inspection or palpation during patient assessment.

decompensated shock occurs when the body can no longer compensate for low blood volume or lack of perfusion. Late signs such as decreasing blood pressure become evident. See *compensated shock; shock.*

decompression sickness a condition resulting from nitrogen trapped in the body's tissues caused by coming up too quickly from a deep, prolonged dive. A symptom of decompression sickness is "the bends," or deep pain in the muscles and joints.

decontamination the removal or cleansing of dangerous chemicals and other dangerous or infectious materials. See also *contamination.*

delirium tremens (duh-LEER-e-um TREM-uns) **(DTs)** a severe reaction that can be part of alcohol withdrawal, characterized by sweating, trembling, anxiety, and hallucinations. Severe alcohol withdrawal with the DTs can lead to death if untreated.

dermis (DER-mis) the inner (second) layer of skin found beneath the epidermis. It is rich in blood vessels and nerves.

designated agent an EMT or other person authorized by a Medical Director to give medications and provide emergency care. The transfer of such authorization to a designated agent is an extension of the Medical Director's license to practice medicine.

detailed physical exam an assessment of the head, neck, chest, abdomen, pelvis, extremities, and posterior of the body to detect signs and symptoms of injury. The examination of the head includes detailed examination of the face, ears, eyes, nose, and mouth. It may be done en route to the hospital after earlier on-scene assessments and interventions are completed.

diabetes mellitus (di-ah-BEE-tez MEL-i-tus) also called "sugar diabetes" or just "diabetes," the condition brought about by decreased insulin production. The person with this condition is a diabetic.

diaphragm (DI-uh-fram) the muscular structure that divides the chest cavity from the abdominal cavity. A major muscle of respiration.

diastolic (di-as-TOL-ik) **blood pressure** the pressure remaining in the arteries when the heart is relaxed and refilling.

dilate (DI-late) get larger.

dilution (di-LU-shun) thinning down or weakening by mixing with something else. Ingested poisons are sometimes diluted by drinking water or milk.

direct carry a method of transferring a patient from bed to stretcher in which two or more rescuers curl the patient to their chests, then reverse the process to lower the patient to the stretcher.

direct ground lift a method of lifting and carrying a patient from ground level to a stretcher in which two or more rescuers kneel, curl the patient to their chests, stand, then reverse the process to lower the patient to the stretcher.

disaster plan a predefined set of instructions that tells a community's various emergency responders what to do in specific emergencies.

dislocation the disruption or "coming apart" of a joint.

distal farther away from the torso. Opposite of *proximal*.

distention (dis-TEN-shun) a condition of being stretched, inflated, or larger than normal.

do not resuscitate (DNR) order a legal document, usually signed by the patient and his physician, which states that the patient has a terminal illness and does not wish to prolong life through resuscitative efforts.

dorsal referring to the back of the body or the back of the hand or foot. A synonym for *posterior*.

dorsalis pedis (dor-sal-is PEED-is) **artery** artery supplying the foot, lateral to the large tendon of the big toe.

draw sheet method a method of transferring a patient from bed to stretcher by grasping and pulling the loosened bottom sheet of the bed.

dressing any material (preferably sterile) used to cover a wound that will help control bleeding and help prevent additional contamination.

drowning death caused by changes in the lungs resulting from immersion in water. See also *near-drowning*.

duty to act an obligation to provide care to a patient.

dyspnea (DISP-ne-ah) shortness of breath; labored or difficult breathing.

eclampsia (e-KLAMP-se-ah) a severe complication of pregnancy that produces seizures and coma.

ectopic (ek-TOP-ik) **pregnancy** when implantation of the fertilized egg is not in the body of the uterus, occurring instead in the oviduct, cervix, or abdominopelvic cavity.

edema (eh-DEEM-uh) swelling resulting from a buildup of fluid in the tissues.

embolism (EM-bo-lizm) a thrombus, or clot of blood and plaque, that has broken loose from the wall of an artery.

Emergency Incident Rehabilitation (EIR) method of assessing and treating personnel during emergency operations to prevent or provide early care for heat- and stress-related emergencies.

EMS Command the senior EMS person on the scene who establishes an EMS command post and oversees the medical aspects of a multiple-casualty incident.

endotracheal (EN-do-TRAY-ke-ul) **tube** a tube designed to be inserted into the trachea. Oxygen, medication, or a suction catheter can be directed into the trachea through an endotracheal tube.

epidermis (ep-i-DER-mis) the outer layer of skin.

epiglottis (EP-i-GLOT-is) a leaf-shaped structure that prevents food and foreign matter from entering the trachea.

epilepsy (EP-uh-lep-see) a medical condition that sometimes causes seizures.

epinephrine (EP-uh-NEF-rin) a hormone produced by the body. As a medication, it dilates respiratory passages and is used to relieve severe allergic reactions.

esophagus (eh-SOF-uh-gus) the tube that leads from the pharynx to the stomach.

evaporation the change from liquid to gas. When the body perspires or gets wet, evaporation of the perspiration or other liquid into the air has a cooling effect on the body.

evisceration (e-VIS-er-AY-shun) an intestine or other internal organ protruding through a wound in the abdomen.

exhalation (EX-huh-LAY-shun) a passive process in which the intercostal (rib) muscles and the diaphragm relax, causing the chest cavity to decrease in size and causing air to flow out of the lungs. Also called *expiration*.

expiration (EK-spuh-RAY-shun) See *exhalation*.

expressed consent consent given by adults who are of legal age and mentally competent to make a rational decision in regard to their medical well-being. See also *consent; implied consent*.

extremities (ex-TREM-i-teez) the portions of the skeleton that include the clavicles, scapulae, arms, wrists, and hands (upper extremities) and the pelvis, thighs, legs, ankles, and feet (lower extremities).

extremity lift a method of lifting and carrying a patient in which one rescuer slips hands under the patient's armpits and grasps the wrists, while another rescuer grasps the patient's knees.

femoral (FEM-or-al) **artery** the major artery supplying the thigh and leg.

femur (FEE-mer) the large bone of the thigh.

fetus (FE-tus) the baby as it develops in the womb.

fibula (FIB-yuh-luh) the lateral and smaller bone of the lower leg.

flow-restricted, oxygen-powered ventilation device (FROPVD) a device that uses oxygen under pressure to deliver artificial ventilations. Has automatic flow restriction to prevent over-delivery of oxygen to the patient.

flowmeter a valve that indicates the flow of oxygen in liters per minute.

focused history and physical exam the step of patient assessment that follows the initial assessment and includes the patient history, physical exam, and vital signs.

Fowler's position a sitting position.

fracture (FRAK-cher) any break in a bone.

full thickness burn a burn in which all the layers of the skin are damaged. There are usually areas that are charred black or areas that are dry and white. Also called a *third degree burn*.

gag reflex vomiting or retching that results when something is placed in the back of the pharynx. This is tied to the swallow reflex.

glottic opening the opening to the trachea.

glucose (GLU-kos) a form of sugar, the body's basic source of energy.

golden hour the optimum limit of one hour between time of injury and surgery at the hospital.

Good Samaritan laws a series of laws, varying in each state, designed to provide limited legal protection for citizens and some health care personnel when they are administering emergency care.

hallucinogens (huh-LOO-sin-uh-jens) mind-affecting or mind-altering drugs that act on the central nervous system to produce excitement and distortion of perceptions.

hazardous material according to the U.S. Department of Transportation, "any substance or material in a form which poses an unreasonable risk to health, safety, and property when transported in commerce."

hazardous materials incident the release of a harmful substance into the environment.

head-tilt, chin-lift maneuver a means of correcting blockage of the airway by the tongue by tilting the head back and lifting the chin. Used when no trauma, or injury, is suspected. See also *jaw-thrust maneuver*.

hematoma (hem-ah-TO-mah) a swelling caused by the collection of blood under the skin or in damaged tissues as a result of an injured or broken blood vessel; in a head injury, a collection of blood within the skull or brain.

hemorrhage (HEM-o-rej) bleeding, especially severe bleeding.

hemorrhagic (HEM-or-AJ-ik) **shock** shock resulting from blood loss.

hives red, itchy, possibly raised blotches on the skin that often result from allergic reactions.

hot zone area immediately surrounding a hazardous materials incident which extends far enough to prevent adverse effects from the released hazardous material to personnel outside the zone.

humerus (HYU-mer-us) the bone of the upper arm, between the shoulder and the elbow.

humidifier a device that is connected to the flowmeter in order to add moisture to the dry oxygen coming from an oxygen cylinder.

hyperglycemia (HI-per-gli-SEE-me-ah) high blood sugar.

hyperthermia (HI-per-THURM-e-ah) an increase in body temperature above normal.

hyperventilate (HI-per-VEN-ti-late) to provide ventilations at a higher rate than normal.

hypoglycemia (HI-po-gli-SEE-me-ah) low blood sugar.

hypoperfusion (HI-po-per-FEW-zhun) inadequate perfusion of the cells and tissues of the body caused by insufficient flow of blood through the capillaries. Also called *shock*. See also *perfusion*.

hypopharynx (HI-po-FAIR-inks) the area directly above the openings of both the trachea and the esophagus.

hypothermia (HI-po-THURM-e-ah) a generalized cooling that reduces body temperature below normal.

hypovolemic (HI-po-vo-LE-mik) **shock** shock resulting from blood or fluid loss.

hypoxia (hi-POK-se-uh) an insufficiency of oxygen in the body's tissues.

ileostomy (il-e-OS-to-me) See *colostomy*.

ilium (IL-e-um) the superior and widest portion of the pelvis.

implied consent the consent it is presumed a patient or patient's parent or guardian would give if they could, for example an unconscious patient or a parent who cannot be contacted when care is needed. See also *consent; expressed consent*.

Incident Command the person or persons who assume overall direction of a large-scale incident.

Incident Command System (ICS) see *Incident Management System*

Incident Management System (IMS) a system used for the management of a multiple-casualty incident, involving assumption of responsibility for command and designation and coordination of such elements as triage, treatment, transport, and staging.

index of suspicion awareness, often based on the mechanism of injury, that a patient may have suffered injuries.

indications specific signs or circumstances under which it is appropriate to administer a drug to a patient.

induced abortion expulsion of a fetus as a result of deliberate actions taken to stop the pregnancy.

inferior away from the head; usually compared with another structure that is closer to the head (e.g., the lips are inferior to the nose). Opposite of *superior*.

ingested poisons poisons that are swallowed.

inhalation (IN-huh-LAY-shun) an active process in which the intercostal (rib) muscles and the diaphragm contract, expanding the size of the chest cavity and causing air to flow into the lungs. Also called *inspiration*.

inhaled poisons poisons that are breathed in.

inhaler a spray device with a mouthpiece that contains an aerosol form of a medication that a patient can spray into his airway.

initial assessment the first element in assessment of a patient; steps taken for the purpose of discovering and dealing with any life-threatening problems. The six parts of initial assessment are: forming a general impression, assessing mental status, assessing airway, assessing breathing, assessing circulation, and determining the priority of the patient for treatment and transport to the hospital.

injected poisons poisons that are inserted through the skin, for example by needle, snake fangs, or insect stinger.

inspiration (IN-spuh-RAY-shun) See *inhalation*.

insulin (IN-suh-lin) a hormone produced by the pancreas or taken as a medication by many diabetics.

interventions actions taken to correct a patient's problems.

intubation (IN-tu-BAY-shun) insertion of a tube. See also *endotracheal tube; nasogastric tube; orotracheal intubation*.

involuntary muscle muscle that responds automatically to brain signals but cannot be consciously controlled.

irreversible shock when the body has lost the battle to maintain perfusion to vital organs. Cell and tissue damage occur, especially to the liver and kidneys. Even if adequate vital signs return, the patient may die days later due to organ failure.

ischium (ISH-e-um) the lower, posterior portions of the pelvis.

jaw-thrust maneuver a means of correcting blockage of the airway by moving the jaw forward without tilting the head or neck. Used when trauma, or injury, is suspected to open the airway without causing further injury to the spinal cord in the neck. See also *head-tilt, chin-lift maneuver.*

joints places where bones articulate, or meet.

jugular (JUG-yuh-ler) **vein distention (JVD)** bulging of the neck veins.

labor the stages of the delivery of a baby that begin with the contractions of the uterus and end with the expulsion of the placenta.

laceration (las-er-AY-shun) a cut.

laryngoscope (lair-ING-uh-skope) an illuminating instrument that is inserted into the pharynx to permit visualization of the pharynx and larynx.

larynx (LAIR-inks) the voicebox.

lateral to the side, away from the midline of the body.

lateral recumbent (re-KUM-bunt) **position** lying on the side. See *recovery position.*

liability being held legally responsible.

ligaments connective tissues that connect bone to bone.

limb presentation when an infant's limb protrudes from the vagina before the appearance of any other body part.

local cooling cooling or freezing of particular (local) parts of the body.

lungs the organs where exchange of atmospheric oxygen and waste carbon dioxide take place.

mainstem bronchi See *bronchi.*

malar (MAY-lar) the cheek bone, also called the *zygomatic bone.*

malleolus (mal-E-o-lus) protrusion on the side of the ankle. The *lateral malleolus,* at the lower end of the fibula, is seen on the outer ankle; the *medial malleolus,* at the lower end of the tibia, is seen on the inner ankle.

mandible (MAN-di-bl) the lower jaw bone.

manual traction the process of applying tension to straighten and realign a fractured limb before splinting. Also called *tension.*

manubrium (man-OO-bre-um) the superior portion of the sternum.

maxillae (mak-SIL-e) the two fused bones forming the upper jaw.

mechanism of injury a force or forces that may have caused injury.

meconium staining amniotic fluid that is greenish or brownish-yellow rather than clear as a result of fetal defecation; an indication of possible maternal or fetal distress during labor.

medial toward the midline of the body.

medical direction oversight of the patient care aspects of an EMS system by the Medical Director. *Off-line medical direction* consists of standing orders and protocols issued by the Medical Director that allow EMTs to give certain medications or perform certain procedures without speaking to the Medical Director or another physician. *On-line medical direction* consists of orders from the on-duty physician given directly to an EMT in the field by radio or telephone.

Medical Director a physician who assumes the ultimate responsibility for the patient care aspects of the EMS system.

mental status level of responsiveness. See also *AVPU.*

metacarpals (MET-uh-KAR-pulz) the hand bones.

metatarsals (MET-uh-TAR-sulz) the foot bones.

mid-axillary (mid-AX-uh-lair-e) **line** a line drawn vertically from the middle of the armpit to the ankle.

mid-clavicular (mid-clah-VIK-yuh-ler) **line** a vertical line through the center of each clavicle.

midline an imaginary line drawn down the center of the body, dividing it into right and left halves.

miscarriage see *spontaneous abortion.*

mobile radio a two-way radio that is used or affixed in a vehicle.

multiple birth when more than one baby is born during a single delivery.

multiple-casualty incident (MCI) any medical or trauma incident involving multiple patients.

muscles tissues or fibers that cause movement of body parts and organs.

musculoskeletal (MUS-kyu-lo-SKEL-e-tal) **system** the system of bones and skeletal muscles that support and protect the body and permit movement.

narcotics a class of drugs that affect the nervous system and change many normal body activities. Their legal use is for the relief of pain. Illicit use is to produce an intense state of relaxation.

nasal (NAY-zul) **bones** the bones that form the upper third, or bridge, of the nose.

nasal cannula (NAY-zul KAN-yuh-luh) a device that delivers low concentrations of oxygen through two prongs that rest in the patient's nostrils.

nasogastric (NAY-zo-GAS-trik) **tube (NG tube)** a tube designed to be passed through the nose, nasopharynx, and esophagus. It is used to relieve distention of the stomach in an infant or child patient.

nasopharyngeal (NAY-zo-fah-RIN-jul) **airway** a flexible breathing tube inserted through the patient's nose into the pharynx to help maintain an open airway.

nasopharynx (NAY-zo-FAIR-inks) the area directly posterior to the nose.

nature of illness what is medically wrong with a patient.

near-drowning the condition of having begun to drown, but still able to be resuscitated.

negligence a finding of failure to act properly in a situation in which there was a duty to act, needed care as would reasonably be expected of the EMT was not provided, and harm was caused to the patient as a result.

nervous system the system of brain, spinal cord, and nerves that govern sensation, movement, and thought. See also *central nervous system; peripheral nervous system; autonomic nervous system.*

neurogenic shock hypoperfusion due to nerve paralysis (sometimes caused by spinal cord injuries) resulting in the dilation of blood vessels that increases the volume of the circulatory system beyond the point where it can be filled.

9-1-1 system a system for telephone access to report emergencies. A dispatcher takes the information, and alerts EMS or the fire or police departments as needed. *Enhanced 9-1-1* has the additional capability of automatically identifying the caller's phone number and location.

nitroglycerin a medication that dilates the blood vessels.

nonrebreather mask a face mask and reservoir bag device that delivers high concentrations of oxygen. The patient's exhaled air escapes through a valve and is not rebreathed.

occlusion (uh-KLU-zhun) blockage, as of an artery by fatty deposits.

occlusive dressing any dressing that forms an airtight seal.

ongoing assessment a procedure for detecting changes in a patient's condition. It involves four steps: repeating the initial assessment, repeating and recording vital signs, repeating the focused history and physical exam, and checking interventions.

open extremity injury an extremity injury in which the skin has been broken or torn through from the inside by an injured bone or from the outside by something that has caused a penetrating wound with associated injury to the bone.

open wound an injury in which the skin is interrupted, exposing the tissue beneath.

OPQRST a memory device for the questions asked to get a description of the present illness: Onset, Provokes, Quality, Radiation, Severity, Time.

oral glucose (GLU-kos) a form of glucose (a kind of sugar) given by mouth to treat an awake patient (who is able to swallow) with an altered mental status and a history of diabetes.

orbits the bony structures around the eyes; the eye sockets.

organ donor a person who has completed a legal document that allows for donation of organs and tissues in the event of death.

oropharyngeal (OR-o-fah-RIN-jul) **airway** a curved device inserted through the patient's mouth into the pharynx to help maintain an open airway.

oropharynx (OR-o-FAIR-inks) the area directly posterior to the mouth.

orotracheal (OR-o-TRAY-ke-ul) **intubation** placement of an endotracheal tube through the mouth and into the trachea. See also *endotracheal tube*.

oxygen a gas commonly found in the atmosphere. Pure oxygen is used as a drug to treat any patient whose medical or traumatic condition may cause them to be hypoxic, or low in oxygen.

oxygen cylinder a cylinder filled with oxygen under pressure.

palmar referring to the palm of the hand.

palpation touching or feeling. A pulse or blood pressure may be palpated with the fingertips.

paradoxical (pair-uh-DOCK-si-kal) **motion** movement of a part of the chest in the opposite direction to the rest of the chest during respiration.

partial thickness burn a burn in which the epidermis (outer layer of skin) is burned through and the dermis (second layer) is damaged. Burns of this type cause reddening, blistering, and a mottled appearance. Also called a *second degree burn*.

passive rewarming covering a hypothermic patient and taking other steps to prevent further heat loss and help the body rewarm itself.

patella (pah-TEL-uh) the kneecap.

pathogens the organisms that cause infection, such as viruses and bacteria.

pedal edema accumulation of fluid in the feet or ankles.

penetrating trauma injury caused by an object that passes through the skin or other body tissues.

perfusion the supply of oxygen to and removal of wastes from the cells and tissues of the body as a result of the flow of blood through the capillaries.

perineum (per-i-NE-um) the surface area between the vagina and anus.

peripheral nervous system (PNS) the nerves that enter and leave the spinal cord and that travel between the brain and organs without passing through the spinal cord.

peripheral pulses the radial, brachial, posterior tibial, and dorsalis pedis pulses, which can be felt at peripheral (outlying) points of the body.

personal protective equipment (PPE) equipment such as eyewear, mask, gloves, gown, or turnout gear or helmet that protect the EMS worker from infection and/or from exposure to hazardous materials and the dangers of rescue operations.

phalanges (fuh-LAN-jiz) the toe bones and finger bones.

pharmacology (FARM-uh-KOL-uh-je) the study of drugs, their sources, characteristics, and effects.

pharynx (FAIR-inks) the area directly posterior to the mouth and nose. It is made up of the oropharynx and the nasopharynx.

physiology the study of body function.

placenta (plah-SEN-tah) the organ of pregnancy where exchange of oxygen, foods, and wastes occurs between a mother and fetus.

placenta previa (plah-SEN-tah PRE-vi-ah) a condition in which the placenta is formed in an abnormal location (low in the uterus and close to or over the cervical opening) that will not allow for a normal delivery of the fetus; a cause of prebirth bleeding.

placental abruption (plah-SEN-tahl ab-RUP-shun) condition in which the placenta separates from the wall of the uterus, often causing life-threatening bleeding.

plane a flat surface formed when slicing through a solid object.

plantar referring to the sole of the foot.

plasma (PLAZ-mah) the fluid portion of the blood.

platelets components of the blood; membrane-enclosed fragments of specialized cells.

pocket face mask a device, usually with a one-way valve, to aid in artificial ventilation. A rescuer breathes through the valve when the mask is placed over the patient's face. Also acts as a barrier to prevent contact with a patient's breath or body fluids. Can be used with supplemental oxygen when fitted with an oxygen inlet.

poison any substance that can harm the body by altering cell structure or functions.

portable radio a hand-held two-way radio.

positional asphyxia death of a person due to a body position that restricts breathing for a prolonged time.

positive pressure ventilation see *artificial ventilation.*

posterior the back of the body or body part. Opposite of *anterior.*

posterior tibial (TIB-ee-ul) **artery** artery supplying the foot, behind the medial ankle.

power grip gripping with as much hand surface as possible in contact with object being lifted, all fingers bent at the same angle, hands at least 10 inches apart.

power lift also called the *squat lift position.* It is a lift from a squatting position with weight to be lifted close to the body, feet apart and flat on the ground, body weight on or just behind balls of feet, back locked in. The upper body is raised before the hips.

preeclampsia (pre-e-KLAMP-se-ah) a complication of pregnancy where the woman retains large amounts of fluid and has hypertension (high blood pressure). She may also experience seizures and/or coma during birth, which is very dangerous to the infant.

premature infant any newborn weighing less than 5½ pounds or born before the 37th week of pregnancy.

pressure dressing a bulky dressing held in position with a tightly wrapped bandage to apply pressure to help control bleeding.

pressure point a site where a main artery lies near the surface of the body and directly over a bone. Pressure on such a point can stop distal bleeding.

pressure regulator a device connected to an oxygen cylinder to reduce cylinder pressure to a safe pressure for delivery of oxygen to a patient.

priapism (PRY-ah-pizm) persistent erection of the penis that may result from spinal injury and some medical problems.

prolapsed umbilical cord when the umbilical cord presents first and is squeezed between the vaginal wall and the baby's head.

prone lying face down.

protocols lists of steps, such as assessment and interventions, to be taken in different situations. Protocols are developed by the Medical Director of an EMS system.

proximal closer to the torso. Opposite of *distal.*

pubis (PYOO-bis) the medial anterior portion of the pelvis.

pulmonary (PUL-mo-nar-e) **arteries** the vessels that carry blood from the right ventricle of the heart to the lungs.

pulmonary edema accumulation of fluid in the lungs.

pulmonary veins the vessels that carry oxygenated blood from the lungs to the left atrium of the heart.

pulse the rhythmic beats felt as the heart pumps blood through the arteries.

pulse quality the rhythm (regular or irregular) and force (strong or weak) of the pulse.

pulse rate the number of pulse beats per minute.

pulseless electrical activity (PEA) a condition in which the heart's electrical rhythm remains relatively normal, yet the mechanical pumping activity fails to follow the electrical activity, causing cardiac arrest.

puncture wound an open wound that tears through the skin and destroys underlying tissues. A *penetrating puncture wound* can be shallow or deep. A *perforating puncture wound* has both an entrance and an exit wound.

pupil the black center of the eye.

quality improvement a process of continuous self-review with the purpose of identifying and correcting aspects of the system that require improvement.

radial artery artery of the lower arm. It is felt when taking the pulse at the wrist.

radial pulse the pulse felt at the wrist.

radiation sending out energy, such as heat, in waves into space.

radius (RAY-de-us) the lateral bone of the forearm.

rapid trauma assessment a rapid assessment of the head, neck, chest, abdomen, pelvis, extremities, and posterior of the body to detect signs and symptoms of injury.

reactivity (re-ak-TIV-uh-te) in the pupils of the eyes, reacting to light by changing size.

recovery position lying on the side. Also called *lateral recumbent position.*

red blood cells components of the blood. They carry oxygen to and carbon dioxide away from the cells.

repeater a device that picks up signals from lower-power radio units such as mobile and portable radios and retransmits them at a higher power. It allows low-power radio signals to be transmitted over longer distances.

respiration (RES-pir-AY-shun) breathing.

respiratory arrest when breathing completely stops.

respiratory failure the reduction of breathing to the point where oxygen intake is not sufficient to support life.

respiratory quality the normal or abnormal (shallow, labored, or noisy) character of breathing.

respiratory rate the number of breaths taken in one minute.

respiratory rhythm the regular or irregular spacing of breaths.

respiratory (RES-pir-uh-tor-e) **system** the system of nose, mouth, throat, lungs, and muscles that brings oxygen into the body and expels carbon dioxide.

rule of nines a method for estimating the extent of a burn. For an adult, each of the following areas represents 9% of the body surface: the head and neck, each upper extremity, the chest, the abdomen, the upper back, the lower back and buttocks, the front of each lower extremity, and the back of each lower extremity. The remaining 1% is assigned to the genital region. For an infant or child the percentages are modified so that 18% is assigned to the head, 14% to each lower extremity.

rule of palm a method for estimating the extent of a burn. The palm of the patient's hand, which equals about 1% of the body's surface area, is compared with the patient's burn to estimate its size.

SAMPLE history the present and past medical history of a patient, so called because the elements of the history begin with the letters of the word *sample:* signs/symptoms, allergies, medications, pertinent past history, last oral intake, events leading to the injury or illness.

scapula (SKAP-yuh-luh) the shoulder blade.

scene size-up steps taken by an ambulance crew when approaching the scene of an emergency call: checking scene safety, taking body substance isolation precautions, noting the mechanism of injury or nature of the patient's illness, determining the number of patients, and deciding what, if any, additional resources to call for.

scope of practice a set of regulations and ethical considerations that define the scope, or extent and limits, of the EMT's job.

seizure (SEE-zher) a sudden change in sensation, behavior, or movement. The most severe form of seizure produces violent muscle contractions called convulsions.

Sellick's maneuver see *cricoid pressure.*

shock See *hypoperfusion.* See also *cardiogenic shock; compensated shock; decompensated shock; irreversible shock; hemorrhagic shock; hypovolemic shock; neurogenic shock.*

shock position see *Trendelenburg position.*

side effect any action of a drug other than the desired action.

sign an indication of a patient's condition that is objective, or can be observed by another person; an indication that can be seen, heard, smelled, or felt by the EMT or others.

sphygmomanometer (SFIG-mo-mah-NOM-uh-ter) the cuff and gauge used to measure blood pressure.

spinous (SPI-nus) **process** the bony bump on a vertebra.

spontaneous abortion when the fetus and placenta deliver before the 28th week of pregnancy; commonly called a *miscarriage.*

sprain the stretching and tearing of ligaments.

staging officer the person responsible for overseeing and keeping track of ambulances and ambulance personnel at a multiple-casualty incident. The staging officer will direct ambulances to treatment areas at the request of the transportation officer.

staging sector the area where ambulances are parked and other resources are held until needed.

standing orders a policy or protocol that is issued by a Medical Director that authorizes EMTs and others to perform particular skills in certain situations.

status epilepticus (STAY-tus or STAT-us ep-i-LEP-ti-kus) a prolonged seizure or when a person suffers two or more convulsive seizures without regaining full consciousness.

sternum (STER-num) the breastbone.

stillborn born dead.

stoma (STO-mah) a permanent surgical opening in the neck through which the patient breathes. See also *tracheostomy.*

strain muscle injury resulting from over-stretching or over-exertion of the muscle.

stroke a condition of altered function caused when an artery in the brain is blocked or ruptured, disrupting the supply of oxygenated blood or causing bleeding into the brain. Also called a *cerebrovascular accident (CVA).*

stylet (STI-let) a long, thin, flexible metal probe.

subcutaneous (SUB-ku-TAY-ne-us) **layers** the layers of fat and soft tissues found below the dermis.

sucking chest wound an open chest wound through which air is "sucked" into the chest cavity.

suctioning (SUK-shun-ing) use of a vacuum device to remove blood, vomitus, and other secretions or foreign materials from the airway.

sudden death a cardiac arrest that occurs within two hours of the onset of symptoms. The patient may have no prior symptoms of coronary artery disease.

superficial burn a burn that involves only the epidermis, the outer layer of the skin. It is characterized by reddening of the skin and perhaps some swelling. An example is a sunburn. Also called a first degree burn.

superior toward the head (e.g., the chest is superior to the abdomen). Opposite of *inferior.*

supine lying on the back.

supine hypotensive syndrome dizziness and a drop in blood pressure caused when the woman in advanced pregnancy is in a supine position and the weight of the uterus, infant, placenta, and amniotic fluid compress the inferior vena cava, reducing return of blood to the heart and cardiac output.

symptom an indication of a patient's condition that cannot be observed by another person but rather is subjective, or felt and reported by the patient.

systolic (sis-TOL-ik) **blood pressure** the pressure created when the heart contracts and forces blood out into the arteries.

tachycardia (TAK-uh-KAR-de-uh) a rapid heart rate; any pulse rate above 100 beats per minute.

tarsals (TAR-sulz) the ankle bones.

temporal (TEM-po-ral) **bone** bone that forms part of the side of the skull and floor of the cranial cavity. There are a right and a left temporal bone.

temporomandibular (TEM-po-ro-mand-DIB-yuh-lar) **joint** the movable joint formed between the mandible and the temporal bone, also called the TM joint.

tendons tissues that connect muscle to bone.

thorax (THOR-ax) the chest.

thrombus (THROM-bus) a clot formed of blood and plaque attached to the inner wall of an artery.

tibia (TIB-e-uh) the medial and larger bone of the lower leg.

tiered response system type of EMS system in which multiple units and, possibly, multiple agencies respond to emergency calls.

torso the trunk of the body; the body without the head and the extremities.

tourniquet (TURN-i-ket) a device used for bleeding control that constricts all blood flow to and from an extremity.

toxin a poisonous substance secreted by bacteria, plants, or animals.

trachea (TRAY-ke-uh) the "windpipe"; the structure that connects the pharynx to the lungs.

tracheostomy (TRAY-ke-OS-to-me) a surgical incision in the neck held open by a metal or plastic tube. See also *stoma.*

traction splint a special splint that applies constant pull along the length of a lower extremity to help stabilize the fractured bone and to reduce muscle spasms in limb. Traction splints are used primarily on femoral shaft fractures.

transiton of care passage of care of a patient from one EMS provider to another.

transportation officer the person responsible for managing transportation of patients to hospitals from the scene of a multiple-casualty incident.

treatment officer the person responsible for overseeing treatment of patients who have been triaged at a multiple-casualty incident.

treatment sector the area in which patients are treated at a multiple-casualty incident.

Trendelenburg (trend-EL-un-berg) **position** a position in which the patient's feet and legs are higher than the head. Also called *shock position*.

trending the changes in a patient's condition over time, such as slowing respirations or rising pulse rate, that may show improvement or deterioration, and that can be shown by documenting repeated assessments.

triage the process of quickly assessing patients in a multiple-casualty incident and assigning each a priority for receiving treatment according to the severity of their illness or injuries. From a French word meaning "to sort."

triage officer the person responsible for overseeing triage at a multiple-casualty incident.

triage sector the area in which secondary triage takes place at a multiple casualty incident.

triage tag color coded tag indicating the priority group to which a patient has been assigned.

ulna (UL-nah) the medial bone of the forearm.

umbilical (um-BIL-i-kal) **cord** the fetal structure containing the blood vessels that carry blood to and from the placenta.

universal dressing a bulky dressing.

uppers stimulants such as amphetamines that affect the central nervous system to excite the user.

uterus (U-ter-us) the muscular abdominal organ where the fetus develops; the womb.

vagina (vah-JI-nah) the birth canal.

vallecula (val-EK-yuh-luh) a groove-like structure anterior to the epiglottis.

vein any blood vessel returning blood to the heart.

venae cavae (VE-ne KA-ve) the superior vena cava and the inferior vena cava. These two major veins return blood from the body to the right atrium. (*Venae cavae* is plural, *vena cava* singular.)

venom a toxin (poison) produced by certain animals such as snakes, spiders, and some marine life forms.

ventilation the breathing in of air or oxygen or providing breaths artificially. See also *artificial ventilation*.

ventral referring to the front of the body. A synonym for *anterior*.

ventricles (VEN-tri-kulz) the two lower chambers of the heart. There is a right ventricle (which sends oxygen-poor blood to the lungs) and a left ventricle (which sends oxygen-rich blood to the body).

ventricular fibrillation (ven-TRIK-u-ler fib-ri-LAY-shun) **(VF)** a condition in which the heart's electrical impulses are disorganized, preventing the heart muscle from contracting normally.

ventricular tachycardia (ven-TRIK-u-ler tak-i-KAR-de-uh) **(V-Tach)** a condition in which the heartbeat is quite rapid; if rapid enough, ventricular tachycardia will not allow the heart's chambers to fill with enough blood between beats to produce blood flow sufficient to meet the body's needs.

venule (VEN-yul) the smallest kind of vein.

vertebrae (VER-te-bray) the 33 bones of the spinal column (singular *vertebra*).

vital signs outward signs of what is going on inside the body, including respiration; pulse; skin color, temperature, and condition (plus capillary refill in infants and children); pupils; and blood pressure.

vocal cords two thin folds of tissue within the larynx that vibrate as air passes between them, producing sounds.

volatile chemicals vaporizing compounds, such as cleaning fluid, that are breathed in by the abuser to produce a "high."

voluntary muscle muscle that can be consciously controlled.

warm zone area at a hazardous material incident where personnel and equipment decontamination and hot-zone support take place.

water chill chilling caused by conduction of heat from the body when the body or clothing is wet.

watt the unit of measurement of the output power of a radio.

white blood cells components of the blood. They produce substances that help the body fight infection.

wind chill chilling caused by convection of heat from the body in the presence of air currents.

withdrawal referring to alcohol or drug withdrawal in which the patient's body reacts severely when deprived of the abused substance.

xiphoid (ZI-foid) **process** the inferior portion of the sternum.

zygomatic (ZI-go-MAT-ik) **bones** the cheekbones.

Index

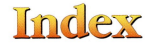

A

Abandonment, 55–58, 65
ABCs, 164, 307, 526, 527, 608–11, 628
  and pediatric patients, 608–11
Abdomen, assessment of, in unresponsive
    patient, 192
Abdominal injuries:
  in infants/children, 622
  open, 496–97
    emergency care, 498
Abdominal pain, in geriatric patients, 640
Abdominal thrusts, 827–28
Abnormal skin temperature and conditions,
    173
Abrasions, 463, 487
Absorption:
  poisoning by, 368
    assessment/emergency care, 373–75
Abuse:
  child abuse and neglect, 622–24
  defined, 622
  of geriatric patients, 639
  and stress, 23
Acceptance, as stage of dying, 22
Access, 686–92
  car doors, displacing, 690–91
  evolutions, 687–88
  front end of car, displacing, 692
  glass removal, 687
  initial and rapid trauma assessment,
    692–93
  roof of car, disposing of, 689
  simple vs. complex, 686–87
  tool staging, 687
  See also Extrication; Vehicle rescue
Accidental Death and Disability: The
    Neglected Disease of Modern Society, 5
Accidental extubation, 764
Accountability, in Rehab Sector/Group,
    707–8
Acetabulum, 75, 519
Acromion, 76, 520
Activated charcoal, 296
  and poisoning, 370–71
    administering, 371
Active suspensions, and vehicle rescue, 676
Acute confusion, in geriatric patients, 639
Adequate breathing:
  depth of, 101
  normal rates of, 101

quality of, 101
rhythm of, 101
signs of, 99
Adequate/inadequate artificial ventilation,
    305–6
Adequate/inadequate breathing, 304–6
Adhesive tape, 491
Administering oxygen, 130, 134
Advanced airway management, 757–96
  automatic transport ventilators (ATVs),
    783–86
  esophageal gastric tube airway (EGTA),
    786
    insertion of, 786–87
  esophageal obturator airway (EOA), 786
    insertion of, 786–87
  esophageal tracheal Combitube® airway,
    787–90, 797
    insertion of, 787–90
  laryngeal mask airway (LMA), 791–93
    insertion of, 792–93
  orotracheal intubation, 763–81
  pharyngo-tracheal lumen airway (PtL®),
    790–91
    insertion of, 790–91
  respiratory system, 760–63
    anatomy of, 760
    pediatric airway and anatomy, 762–63
    physiology of, 760–62
  on scene, 759–60
  suctioning the airway, 763
  See also Orotracheal intubation
Advanced cardiac life support (ACLS),
    332
Advance directives, 55
  and geriatric patients, 640
Advanced life support (ALS), 9, 143, 236,
    391, 705, 710
  assist skills, 797–804
    applying ECG/defibrillation electrodes,
      800–801
    endotracheal intubation, 797–800
    IV therapy, 802–4
    using a pulse oximeter, 801–2
AEDs, *See* Automated external defibrillators
    (AEDs)
AEMT-3, 9
Age:
  and burn severity, 506
  and heat-related emergencies, 395–96
  and hypothermia, 389–90

Aggressive patients, 449–50
Aging, anatomical/physiological changes
    with, 633–34
Agitated patients, communicating with,
    231
Agonal breathing, 762
Agonal respirations, 305
Airbags:
  injuries from, 156–59
  and vehicle rescue, 676–77
Airborne pathogens, protection from, 41–43
Aircraft safety programs, 666
Air embolus, 497
Air medical transport, 665–67
  ground safety procedures, 666
  landing zone, selecting, 665–66
  requesting, 665
  transition of care, 666
  value of, 665
  See also Helicopters in rescue operations
Air splints, 465, 491
Airway, 77
  clearing, 170
  defined, 98
Airway adjuncts, 112–18
  nasopharyngeal airways, 117–18
  oropharyngeal airways, 113–17
  rules for using, 113
Airway involvement, and burn severity,
    506
Airway management, 95–139
  airway adjuncts, 112–18
  artificial ventilation, 105–12
  goal of, 763
  head-tilt, chin-lift maneuver, 102–4
  importance of, 98
  and infants/children, 136–37
  jaw-thrust maneuver, 104–5
  opening the airway, 102–5
  oxygen therapy, 121–35
  respiration/breathing, 99–102
  on scene, 97–98
  suction/suction devices, 118–21
  See also Advanced airway management
Airway obstructions, 826–32
  complete obstructions, 827–29
    abdominal thrusts, 827–28
    airway clearance sequences, 828
    chest thrusts, 828
    clearing the airway, 827–30, 832
    in infants/children, 612–13, 828

Airway obstructions (*cont.*)
    partial obstructions, 612, 826–27
        with cyanosis/altered mental state,
            612–13
        in infants/children, 612
Airway skills, 601–5
    airway adjuncts, 604–5
    clearing complete airway obstructions,
        602–3
    opening the airway, 601
    suctioning, 602
Airway status, assessment of, 170–71
Allergens, defined, 365
Allergic reactions, 376–81
    anaphylactic shock, 376
    causes of, 376
    defined, 365
    emergency care, 378–81
        no signs/symptoms of severe reaction,
            381
        severe reaction/history of allergic
            reaction/prescribed auto-injector, 378
        severe reaction/without prescribed
            auto-injector, 378–81
    epinephrine auto-injector, 380
    patient assessment, 377–78
Allergies, and SAMPLE history, 178
ALS-assist skills, 797–804
Altered mental status, 168
    and brain injuries, 575
    and cerebrovascular accidents (CVAs),
        358–59
    and diabetes, 351–55
    emergencies, 347–62
    in geriatric patients, 636
    in infants/children, 615
    no history of diabetes:
        emergency care, 350–51
        patient assessment, 349–51
    and partial airway obstruction, 612–13
    on scene, 348–49
    and seizures, 356–58
Alupent®, 311
Alveoli, 77, 760
Alzheimer's disease, 636
Ambulances, 751
    portable ambulance stretcher, 277–79
    types of, 649–50
    typical ambulance equipment, 653–54
    wheeled ambulance stretcher, 276–77
American Heart Association, 108
American Red Cross, 705
Amniotic sac, 86–87, 414
    breaking of, 417
Amputations, 488, 500–501
    emergency care, 500–501
Anaphylactic shock, 376
Anatomical plane, 69
Anatomy, 67–93
    basic, 68–73
    body positioning, 72–73
    body regions, 71–72
    of body systems, 73–92
    surface/topographic, 68
    terms, 69–71
Anatomy/physiology of body systems, 73–92
Aneurysm, 192

Anger, as stage of dying, 22
Angina, 324
Ankle injuries, splinting, 535–36
Anterior, use of term, 69
Antibiotics, allergic reactions to, 376
Aorta, 84, 323
Arm injuries, splinting, 532, 539
Arrival at receiving facility, 662
Arterial bleeding, 462–63
Arteries, 84
Arterioles, 85
Artificial ventilation, 105–12
    adequate, 105
    bag-valve mask, 105, 107–12
    in children, 607–8
    flow restricted, oxygen-powered
        ventilation device (FROPVD), 105
    inadequate, 105–6
        mouth-to-mask ventilation, 105, 106–7
Artificial ventilation, 607–8
    adequate/inadequate, 305–6
    for infants/children, 607–8
Ascent-related barotrauma, 402
Aspirin, allergic reactions to, 376
Assault/battery, 59–60
Atria, 81, 322–23
Atrovent®, 311
Aura, 356
Auscultation, 184
Automated external defibrillators (AEDs), 9,
        14, 172, 324, 332, 333–44, 651
    advantages of, 334–35
    cardiac arrest patient assessment, 337–39
    and CPR, 336–37
    fully automated, 333, 343
    key ideas in, 339
    maintenance of, 343
    operator's shift checklist (illustration), 344
    post-resuscitation care, 339–42
    quality assurance, 343
    and recurring cardiac arrest, 342
    safety concerns, 335–36
    semi-automated, 333–34, 340–41
    single rescuer use of, 342
    training, 343
    when to use/when not to use, 335
Automated implantable cardioverter
        defibrillators (AICDs), 333
Automatic transport ventilators (ATVs),
        783–86
Automobile collisions, *See* Motor vehicle
        crashes
Autonomic nervous system, 88
Aviation crews, and transition of care, 259
AVPU scale, 169–70, 192
Avulsions, 488, 502
    emergency care, 502

B

Bag-valve mask (BVM), 105, 107–12
    assisting ventilations with, 110
    BVM-to-stoma ventilations, 110–11
    and CPR, 110
    in-line stabilization during ventilations,
        109

    mask seal, 108
    parts of, 107–8
    pop-off valves, replacing, 108
    two-rescuer BVM ventilation, 105, 108–10
Ball-and-socket joints, 76, 521
Bandages, 490–92
Bandaging, examples of, 491
Bargaining, as stage of dying, 22
Baseline vital signs, 144–45, 177, 180, 192
    in trauma patients, assessing, 201–4
Base station, 232
Basic cardiac life support (BCLS-1), 805–32
    See also Airway management; Airway
        obstruction; Cardiopulmonary
        resuscitation (CPR)
Basic life support (BLS), 9, 236
Basket stretcher, 281
Battery, 60
Battle's sign, 572
Behavior, defined, 445
Behavioral emergencies, 443–56
    behavioral changes, 445
    defined, 445
    documenting, 452–53
    emergency care, 447–48
    hostile/aggressive patients, 449–50
    medical-legal considerations, 453
    patient assessment, 447
    psychiatric emergencies, 446–47
    reasonable force and restraint, 450–52
    on scene, 444
    situational stress reactions, 446
    special considerations, 448–52
    suicide, 448–49
Bilateral, use of term, 70
Biological death, 805
Bipolar traction splint, applying, 540–42
Birth canal, 413
Bites/stings, 403–6
    insect bites, 403–4
    scorpion stings, 405
    snake bites, 405–6
        emergency care, 406
    spider bites, 404
Black outs, in geriatric patients, 636
Black widow spider, 404
Blanket drag, 270
Blast injuries, 160–61
    primary, 160
    secondary, 160
    tertiary, 160
Blasts, 469–70
Bleeding, 457–80
    arterial bleeding, 462–63
    body substance isolation (BSI), 462
    and broken bones/fractures, 521–23
    capillary bleeding, 463
    external bleeding, 462–69
    internal bleeding, 469–77
    and medication, 462
    on scene, 458–59
    severe, recognizing, 461–62
    venous bleeding, 463
    See also Circulatory system; External
        bleeding; Internal bleeding
Blood, 85–86, 461
Bloodborne pathogens, 45–46

Blood loss, body's responses to, 87
Blood pressure, 86, 183–85
  determining, 184–85
  in geriatric patients, 637
  normal ranges by age, 183–84
  sphygmomanometer, 184
Blood pressure cuff, *See*
  Sphygmomanometer
Blood vessels, 461
Bloody show, 417
"Blow-by" administration of oxygen, 606–7
Blunt trauma, 153–60
  mechanisms of injury (MOI), 153–60,
    469
  motor vehicle crashes, 153–59
  penetrating trauma, 159–60
  See also Motor vehicle crashes
Body, sternum, 75
Body language, in interpersonal
  communication, 229
Body mechanics, 264–68
  carrying techniques on stairs, 266
  log-rolling techniques, 267–68
  one-handed carrying techniques, 266
  and power lift/power grip, 264–65
  reaching/pulling techniques, 266–67
  special lifting/carrying considerations,
    265–68
Body positioning, 72–73
Body protection, and vehicle rescue, 678
Body regions, 71–72
Body substance isolation (BSI), 35–50, 142,
  147, 462, 471, 764
  and bleeding, 462
  defined, 38
Body surface area (BSA), 46, 503, 505–6
Body systems, 73–92
  circulatory system, 81–87
  defined, 73
  endocrine system, 88
  gastrointestinal (GI) system, 88
  genitourinary system, 88–89
  musculoskeletal system, 73–77
  nervous system, 87–88
  respiratory system, 77–81
  skin, 89–92
Brachial artery, 84
Bradycardia, 181, 326, 600
Brain injuries, 572–75
  and altered mental status, 575
Brand name, 289
Breach of duty, 59
Breast bone, 75
Breathing, 77–81, 99–102
  adequate/inadequate, 99
  depth of, 80–81, 762
  exhalation, 77–78
  inhalation, 77
  quality of, 80, 762
  rate of, 79–80, 761, 762
  respiratory failure:
    assessment of, 99–101
    emergency care, 101–2
  rhythm of, 80, 762
Breathing status assessment, 171–72
  responsive patient, 171
  unresponsive patient, 171–72

Breech presentation, 416, 430–31
Broken bones, 521–23
Broken utility pole:
  with wires down, 682
  with wires intact, 683
Bronchi, 77, 303, 760
Bronchiols, 303–4
Bronkometer®, 311
Bronkosol®, 311
Brown recluse spider, 404
Bulb esophageal intubation detector devices,
  776
Bullets, and penetrating injuries, 160
Bumpers, and vehicle rescue, 676
Burn centers, 13
Burnout, 24
Burns, 502–13
  and airway management, 135–36
  body surface area (BSA), 503, 505–6
  burn shock, 503
  chemical burns, 510–11
  circumferential, 507
  classification of, 503–6
  depth of, 503–5
  electrical burns, 511–13
  emergency care, 508–10
  full thickness burns, 504
  in geriatric patients, 503
  and hypothermia, 390
  in infants/children, 502, 510
  location of, 506
  mechanism of burn injury, 503
  partial thickness burns, 504–5
  patient assessment, 507–8
  and respiratory emergencies, 316
  rule of nines, 505–6
  severity of, 506–7, 510
  superficial thickness burns, 503–4
Burn severity, 506–7, 510
Burn shock, 503
BVM-to-stoma ventilations, 110–11
Bystander care, 258–59
Bystander safety, 152

C

Calcaneus, 76, 519, 533
Capillaries, 85, 461
Capillary bleeding, 463
Capillary refill, 470
  assessment of, 173
Cardiac arrest, 83, 328–32
  chain of survival, 328–32
  emergency care, 337–39
  and oxygen therapy, 121
  patient assessment, 337–39
  recurring, 342
Cardiac compromise, 324–28
  emergency care, 326–27
  nitroglycerin, 327–28
  patient assessment, 324–25
  signs/symptoms of, 325–26
Cardiac conduction system, 81–82
Cardiac emergencies, 319–46
  cardiac arrest, 328–32

cardiac compromise, 324–28
cardiovascular system,
  anatomy/physiology of, 322–24
defibrillation, 332–33
defibrillators, 333
  See also Cardiac arrest; Cardiac
    compromise; Defibrillation
Cardiac muscle, 77
Cardiac technician, 10
Cardiopulmonary resuscitation (CPR), 98,
  602, 805–26
  ABCs, determining, 806
  activating EMS, 806–7
  and automated external defibrillators
    (AEDs), 336–37
  and bag-valve mask (BVM), 110
  breathlessness, determining, 806
  changing positions, 818–20
  chest compressions, providing, 815
  determining effectiveness of, 820
  how it works, 812–13
  initial ventilations, 809
  interrupting, 820–23
  joining in progress, 815–19
  one-rescuer CPR, 815, 816–17
  opening the airway, 807–8
    head-tilt, chin-lift maneuver, 807
    jaw-thrust maneuver, 807–8
  patient assessment, 805–6
  positioning the patient, 807–8
  procedure for, 813–15
  pulse check, 809, 812
  pulselessness, determining, 806
  techniques for infants/children, 820,
    824–26
  two-rescuer CPR, 815, 819
  unresponsiveness, determining, 805–6
  ventilation, providing, 815
  when not to begin/terminate, 823
  See also Rescue breathing
Cardiovascular system:
  anatomy/physiology of, 322–24
  See also Circulatory system
Carina, 760
Carotid arteries, 84
Carpals, 76, 521
Carrying techniques on stairs, 266
Cells, 73
Cellular telephones, 233
Central intravenous lines, and pediatric
  patients, 626
Central lines, 626
Central nervous system, 87–88, 551–52
Cephalic presentation, 416
Cerebrovascular accidents (CVAs), 358–59
  and altered mental status, 358–59
  emergency care, 359
  and oxygen therapy, 121
  signs/symptoms of, 358–59
Certification, 10
Certified First Responder (CFR), 9
Cervical collars, 560–61
  applying, 563–64
  sizing, 562
Cervical vertebrae, 75, 550–51
Cervix, 413
  full dilation of, 417

Changing conditions, monitoring the scene
    for, 30
Charged fuel systems, and vehicle rescue,
    676
Charge nurse, 13
Chemical burns, 510–11
Chemical name, 289
Chemical Transportation Emergency Center
    (CHEMTREC), 738, 739
CHEMTEL, Inc., 738
Chest, assessment of, in unresponsive
    patient, 192
Chest injuries, in infants/children, 622
Chest pain, in geriatric patients, 639–40
Chest pains, and oxygen therapy, 121
Chest thrusts, 828
Chief complaint, 152
Child abuse and neglect, 622–24
    signs/symptoms of, 622–23
    suspected situations of, approaching,
        623–24
Childbirth, 417–29
    delivery procedures, 419–22
        delivering the baby, 420–22
        preparing the mother, 420
    EMT's role, 417
    equipment/supplies, 417–18
    evaluating the mother, 418–19
    keeping the baby warm, 427
    newborn assessment, 423–24
    newborn resuscitation, 424–25
    ongoing care of mother, 427–29
    placenta, delivering, 427–28
    post-delivery vaginal bleeding, controlling,
        428
    providing comfort to mother, 428–29
    transition of care, 419
    umbilical cord, cutting, 425–27
    See also Childbirth complications
Childbirth complications, 429–34
    breech presentation, 416, 430–31
    limb presentation, 431
    meconium, 433–34
    multiple births, 431–32
    premature birth, 432–33
    prolapsed umbilical cord, 429–30
Children, See Infants/children
Chronic obstructive pulmonary diseases
    (COPD), 293
Circulation, 391
Circulation status assessment, 172–73
    external bleeding, 172
    pulse, 172
    skin, 172–73
Circulatory system, 81–87
    anatomy/physiology of, 322–24
    bleeding, 461–71
    blood, 85–86, 461
    blood pressure, 86
    blood vessels, 461
    capillaries, 85, 461
    heart, 81–84, 322–23, 459–61
    hypoperfusion, 86–87
    perfusion, 86–87
    plasma, 85–86, 461
    platelets, 85, 461
    pulse, 86

red blood cells, 85, 461
vascular system, 84–85
veins, 85, 461
white blood cells, 85, 461
Circumferential burns, 507
Cisterns, 726
Civil law, 53
Civil wrong, 53
Classification of burns, 503–6
Clavicle, 76, 520
Cleaning/disinfection procedures, 43–45,
    663–65
Clinical death, 805
Closed musculoskeletal injuries, 525
Closed soft tissue injuries, 485–87
    assessment of, 486, 489–90
    contusions, 485
    crush injuries, 486
    emergency care, 486–87
    hematomas, 485–86
Clothes drag, 270
Coccyx vertebrae, 75, 551
Code of ethics, 53
Cold/cool environment, and hypothermia,
    389
Cold (green) zones, 734
Cold-related emergencies, 388–95
    generalized hypothermia, 389–90
        emergency care, 391–93
        patient assessment, 390–93
    local cold injuries, 393–95
        frostnip, 393–94
Collar bone (clavicle), 76, 520
Collection containers, suction units, 120
Combitube® airway, 787–90, 797
Commission, 59
Commonly encountered medications, 296–97
Common medical conditions, medications
    prescribed for, 298
Communications, 225–37
    after arrival at hospital/receiving facility,
        237
    communications systems, 232–34
    documentation, 237–50
    en route to hospital/receiving facility,
        237
    with geriatric patients, 231, 636
    interpersonal, 228–32
    with medical direction, 236–37
    and multiple-casualty incidents (MCI),
        744–45
    radio communications, 234–37
    on scene, 227–28
    and urgent moves, 269
    See also Communications systems;
        Documentation; Interpersonal
        communication; Radio
        communications
Communications systems, 8–9, 232–34
    base station, 232
    cellular telephones, 233
    components of, 232–34
    data terminals, 233–34
    digital radio equipment, 233
    mobile computer, 233–34
    mobile radios, 232
    portable radios, 232–33

repeaters, 233
system maintenance, 234
Company check-in/out sheet, 707
Company officer notes:
    access pathway, selection of, 687
    aircraft safety program, 666
    BSI, 41
    carbon monoxide (CO) poisoning, 374
    cardiac arrest in infants/children, 612
    cervical collar, 558
    child abuse, 623
    confined space emergencies, 727
    CPR, 336
    detailed physical examination, 210
    documentation, 246
    epinephrine auto-injector, 378
    extrication, 694
    forcible entry into residence, 637
    glove "balloons," 603
    Golden Hour, 524
    helicopter operations, 732
    helmet removal, 585
    HEPA respirators, 43
    hypothermia, 391
    immobilization, 558
    internal bleeding, 470
    legal issues, 246
    lifting and moving seminars, 661
    myocardial infarctions, 327
    near drowning, 618
    on-scene emergency childbirth, 423
        patient privacy during, 420
    oxygen delivery, 128
    poisoning, 368, 372, 374
    positional asphyxia, 452
    preassigned tasks, 660
    quality of care, 12
    radio communications, 234
    Rehab Sector/Group, 705
    resuscitation, 399
    seizures, 357
    smoke inhalation, 316
    stress in crew, 24
    traction splints, 533
    traffic laws and emergency vehicle
        operators, 656
    transition of care, 258
Complete airway obstructions, 612–13,
    827–29
Complete amputations, 488
Complex access, 686–87
Compression, and spinal injuries, 553
Conduction:
    heat loss by, 387
    and geriatric patients, 388
Cones, positioning, 680–81
Confidentiality, 60–61, 246
Confined spaces/hazardous atmospheres,
    724–27
    engulfment in, 726
    gases in, 726
    machinery hazards, 727
    safety procedures, 727
    silos, 726
    storage bins, 726
    storage tanks, 726
    underground vaults, 726

unsafe oxygen levels in, 726
  wells/culverts/cisterns, 726
Confused patients, communicating with, 231
Congestive heart failure, 192
Connective tissue, 76–77, 521
Consent, 54–55
  express, 54
  implied, 54–55
Continuous quality improvement (CQI), 12
Contusions, 485
Convection, heat loss by, 387, 702
Coral snake, 405
Coronary arteries, 84, 323
Corset-type, half-back immobilizer, 559
Coumadin®, 462, 638
Coverings for patient protection, 679
CPR:
  and automated external defibrillators
      (AEDs), 336–37
  See also Cardiopulmonary resuscitation
      (CPR)
Cradle carry, 271
Cranium, 551
Crepitus, 526
Cricoid cartilage, 77, 303, 760, 774
Crime scenes, and personal safety of EMT,
    149
Criminal law, 53
Critical care technician, 10
Critical incidents, 25
Critical incident stress debriefing (CISD),
    25–26, 33, 752
  defusing session, 26
  process, 33
Crush injuries, 486
Cuff, endotracheal tube, 765–68
Culverts, 726
CVAs, See Cerebrovascular accidents (CVAs)
Cyanosis, 99, 172, 470, 529, 531, 534, 612, 762
  and hypoxia, 124
  and partial airway obstruction, 612–13

D

Daily rescue vehicle checksheet, 652
Damaged pad-mounted transformer, and
    electrical hazards, 683
Damages, 59
Data terminals, 233–34
DCAP-BTLS, 201, 204, 210
Death of coworker, and stress, 23–24
Death and dying, 21–22
Decompression sickness (DCS), 402–3
Decontamination, 739–40
Defibrillation, 84, 328–33
  See also Cardiac emergencies
Defibrillator electrodes, applying, 800–801
Defibrillators, 333
  automated external defibrillators (AEDs),
      9, 14, 172, 324, 332, 333–44
  automated implantable cardioverter
      defibrillators (AICDs), 333
Defusing session, 26
Degloving injury, 488
Delivery procedures, childbirth, 419–22
Denial, as stage of dying, 21

Dental appliances, and airway management,
    136
Depression, as stage of dying, 22
Depth of burns, 503–5
Dermis, 90, 484
Descent-related barotrauma, 402
Designated officer (DO), 47–48
Detailed physical examination, 144
  and extrication, 695
  in responsive medical patient, 196–97
  in unresponsive medical patient, 194
Diabetes, 351–55
  and altered mental status, 351–55
  diabetes mellitus, 351
  emergency care, 335
  glucose, 351
  hyperglycemia, 352
  hypoglycemia, 352
  insulin, 351–52
  oral glucose, 296, 352–53
    administering, 355
  patient assessment, 352–53
  physiology of, 351–52
  Type I diabetics, 351–52
  Type II diabetics, 352
Diabetes mellitus, 351
Diaphoresis, 325
Diaphragm, 77, 304
Diastolic blood pressure, 86, 183
Diet, and stress, 24
Digital radio equipment, 233
Direct carry method, 272, 275, 276
Direct force, and musculoskeletal injuries,
    523–24
Direct ground lift, 272–73
Direct pressure, controlling bleeding by, 464
Disinfection, 43–45, 663
Dislocations, 524
Dispatch center, reaching, 8–9
Dispatch information, 146
Dispatch and response, 651–55
  Emergency Medial Dispatchers (EMDs), 651
  required dispatch information, 651–55
Distal, use of term, 70
Distal tarsal bones, 76
Distraction, and spinal injuries, 553
Disturbed patients, communicating with, 231
DNR orders, 55–56, 61, 641
Documentation, 237–50
  of behavioral emergencies, 452–53
  confidentiality of, 246
  falsification of, 248–49
  legal issues, 246–48
  patient refusal of treatment, 246–48
  prehospital care report, 239–46
  reasons for:
    administrative functions, 238–39
    educational/research functions, 239
    legal functions, 238
    medical functions, 238
  See also Communication; Prehospital care
      report
Do Not Resuscitate Order (DNR), 55–56, 61,
    641
Dorsal, use of term, 69–70
Dorsalis pedis artery, 85
Draw sheet method, 272, 274

Dressings, 490, 492
  pressure, 492
Drowning, 398, 399–400
  emergency care, 399–400
Drugs, and hypothermia, 390
Duty to act, 59
Dyspnea, 325
Dysrhythmias, 83, 182, 324, 326

E

Ears, external bleeding from, 468
Education, and injury prevention, 8
Effacement, 416
EGTA, See Esophageal gastric tube airway
    (EGTA)
EIR, See Emergency incident rehabilitation
    (EIR)
Elbow injuries, splinting, 535
Electrical burns, 511–13
Electrical hazards, 680–83
  broken utility pole:
    with wires down, 682
    with wires intact, 683
  damaged pad-mounted transformer, 683
Electrocardiogram (ECG), 83
  defibrillator electrodes, applying, 800–801
Electronic clipboard, 239
Elevation, controlling external bleeding
    using, 464–65
Emancipated minors, 60
Emergency care:
  abdominal open injuries, 496–97
  allergic reactions, 378–81
  amputations, 500–501
  avulsions, 502
  behavioral emergencies, 447–48
  breech presentation, 431
  burns, 508–10
  cardiac arrest, 337–39
  cardiac compromise, 326–27
  cerebrovascular accidents (CVAs), 359
  closed soft tissue injuries, 486–87
  diabetes, 335
  drowning, 399–400
  emotional aspects of, 21–26
  external bleeding, 464
  and fever, 616
  generalized hypothermia, 391–93
  hazardous materials, 741–42
  head injuries, 579
  heat-related emergencies, 397–98
  hypothermia, 391–93
  hypovolemic shock, 472–73
  impaled objects, 497
  insect bites/stings, 403–4
  internal bleeding, 471
  large open neck injury, 497–500
  limb presentation, 431
  local cold injuries, 394–95
  meconium, 434
  multiple births, 431–32
  musculoskeletal injuries, 526–27
  near-drowning, 399–400
  open chest injuries, 495–96
  open soft tissue injuries, 493–94

Emergency care (*cont.*)
  premature birth, 433
  prolapsed umbilical cord, 429–30
  respiratory distress, 309–10
  respiratory failure, 101–2
  SCUBA diving emergencies, 403
  seizures, 356–58
  sexual assault, 438
  snake bites, 406
  soft tissue injuries, 494–502
  spinal injuries, 565–69
  spontaneous abortion (miscarriage),
    434–35
  trauma in pregnancy, 436–37
  trauma to female external genitalia,
    437–38
  vaginal bleeding, 437
    late in pregnancy, 436
Emergency Care and Transportation of the
  Sick and Injured, 6
Emergency incident rehabilitation (EIR),
  699–713
  defined, 701
  heat exhaustion, 396–97, 703
  heat loss, mechanisms of, 702–3
  heat stroke, 397, 703
  Rehab Sector/Group, 701, 704–11
  on scene, 700–701
  stress-/heat-related emergencies, 701–4
    emergency care, 703–4
  See also Rehab Sector/Group
Emergency incident rehabilitation report,
  707
Emergency medical care, 3–17
  fire service and, 5–6
  on scene, 4–5
Emergency Medical Dispatchers (EMDs), 9,
  236, 258, 651
Emergency Medical Services (EMS) system, 5
Emergency Medical Service Systems Act, 6
Emergency Medical Technician-Basic
  (EMT), 3
  See also EMT
Emergency Medical Technician-Basic (EMT-
  B), 9
Emergency Medical Technician-Intermediate
  (EMT-I), 10
Emergency Medical Technician-Paramedic
  (EMT-P), 10
Emergency moves, 268–69, 270, 271
  one rescuer assists/carries, 271
  one-rescuer drags, 270
Emergency response employee (ERE), 47–48
Emergency scene, 658–61
  multiple-casualty incidents (MCIs), 658–60
  positioning units at, 658
  preparing patient for transport, 660
  reporting to dispatch, 658
  transition of care, 660–61
Emergency vehicle escorts, 657
Emergency vehicle operations, 647–69
  air medical transport, 665–67
  emergency response, 649–65
    at receiving facility, 662
    at the scene, 658–61
    dispatch and response, 651–55
    en route to receiving facility, 661

  en route to the scene, 655–58
  preparing for the call, 649–51
  returning to service, 662–65
  on scene, 648–49
  See also Dispatch and response;
    Emergency scene; Emergency
    vehicles; Receiving facilities;
    Returning to service
Emergency vehicles, 649–50
  ambulances, types of, 649–50
  equipment check, 650–51
  escorts, 657
  medium-duty truck chassis, 650
  parking, 656–57
  passing, 657
  preparing, 664–65
  right of way, 656
  sirens, 656
  speed, 656
  traffic signals, 656
  turning, 656
  typical ambulance equipment, 653–54
  vehicle check, 651
  vehicle inspection, 654
  warning lights, 656
EMS-initiated refusals (EMSIRs), 55
EMS sector functions:
  command sector, 743
  extrication sector, 745
  rehab sector, 747
  staging sector, 745, 750–52
  supply sector, 745
  transportation sector, 747, 750–52
  treatment sector, 747, 750
  triage sector, 745–50
EMS special operations, *See* Special
  operations
EMS system, 6–8
  elements of, 8–13
  health care professionals, 13–14
  standards, 6–8
EMT:
  personal safety, 26–31
  professionalism of, 14–15
  roles/responsibilities of, 14–15
  well-being of, 19–33
    on scene, 20–21
Endocrine system, 88
Endotracheal intubation:
  assisting with, 797–800
  preparing patient for, 798
  trauma intubation, 799–800
  ventilating the tubed patient, 798–99
Endotracheal suctioning, 781–83
Endotracheal tubes, 763, 765–68, 770
  cuffed/uncuffed, 778–79
  diameters of, 767
End tidal carbon dioxide ($ETCO_2$), 776–77
Engulfment, 726
En route to receiving facility, 661
En route to the scene, 655–58
  basic safety measures, 655–56
  emergency vehicle escorts, 657
  intersections, 657–58
  laws governing emergency vehicle
    operations, 656–57
  multiple-vehicle hazards, 657

En route to the station, 662–63
Environmental emergencies, 385–409
  bites/stings, 403–6
  cold-related emergencies, 388–95
  heat-related emergencies, 395–98
  on scene, 386–87
  temperature regulation, mechanisms of,
    387–88
  water-related emergencies, 398–403
  See also Bites/stings; Cold-related
    emergencies; Heat-related
    emergencies; Skin; Water-related
    emergencies
Environmental Protection Agency (EPA), 732
EOA, *See* Esophageal obturator airway
  (EOA)
Epidermis, 90, 484
Epiglottis, 77, 303, 760
Epinephrine, 294–95
Epinephrine auto-injector, 380
Equipment, cleaning/disinfecting, 43–45,
  663–65
Equipment check, 650–51
Escorts, emergency vehicles, 657
Esophageal gastric tube airway (EGTA), 786,
  797
  insertion of, 786–87
Esophageal intubation, 764
Esophageal obturator airway (EOA), 786,
  797
  insertion of, 786–87
Esophageal tracheal Combitube® airway,
  787–90
  insertion of, 787–90
Esophagus, 303, 760
Ethics, 53–54
Evaluation, 8, 11–12
Evaporation, heat loss by, 388
Eviscerations, 496–97
Exercise, and stress, 24
Exhalation, 77–78
Exposure control plan, 45–46
Express consent, 54
Expressed consent, 54
Extension, and spinal injuries, 553
External bleeding, 172, 462–69
  arterial, 462–63
  assessment for, 172
  capillary, 463
  controlling, 464–65
    by direct pressure, 464
    by elevation, 464–65
    devices used in, 465–68
    using pressure points, 465
  emergency care, 464
  from ears/eyes/nose, 468
  nosebleeds, 469
  pneumatic splints, 465
  rigid splints, 465
  tourniquets, 465–68
  venous, 463
External defibrillators, 333
External genitalia, trauma to, 437–38
Extremities, assessment of, in unresponsive
  patient, 192
Extremity injuries, in infants/children, 622
Extremity lift, 272, 274

Extrication, 671–96
  detailed physical examination, 695
  ongoing assessment, 695
  partial vs. full, 694–95
  rapid extrication:
    of child in safety seat, 580–81
    of high-priority patients, 576–77
    normal vs., 693–94
  terminating the rescue, 695
  transport, 695
  vehicle on its roof, 694–95
  vehicle on its side, 694
  vehicle on its wheels, 694
Extrication sector, 745
Eye contact, with patient, 229
Eye protection, 39–40
  and vehicle rescue, 678
Eyes, external bleeding from, 468

F

Facial bones, 74
Facial injuries, 569
  and airway management, 135–36
Facilities, 8, 12–13
Fallopian tubes, 413
Falls, 161
  from bikes, 619
  from height, 469
Female reproductive system, 413–14
Femoral artery, 85
Femur injuries, splinting, 533–34
Ferno (K.E.D.) Extrication Device, 566–67
Fetus, 414
Fever:
  in infants/children, 615–16
    emergency care, 616
Fibrillation, 328
  ventricular (VF/V-Fib), 83–84, 333
Fibula, 76
Fireman's carry, 271
Fireman's drag, 270
Fires, See Heat-related emergencies; Truck
    fires; Vehicle fires
FIRESCOPE/National Fire Academy Incident
    Command System (ICS), 742
Fire service, and emergency medical care,
    5– 6
First Responders, 8–9
Fixation splints, 465
Flares, positioning, 680–81
Flexible stretcher, 281–82
Flexion, and spinal injuries, 553
Flowmeters, 129–30
Flow restricted, oxygen-powered ventilation
    device (FROPVD), 105
Fluid replacement, 710–11
  and sports activity beverages, 711
Focused history and physical examination,
    143–44, 187–97
  approaches to, 188–89
  pediatric patients, 611
  and respiratory distress, 308
  responsive medical patient, 194–97
    assessing baseline vital signs, 196
    completing SAMPLE history, 195–96

detailed physical examination, 196– 97
    OPQRST, 195
    providing emergency care, 196
  on scene, 189, 194
  trauma patients:
    detailed physical examination, 197– 223
    reconsidering mechanism of injury,
        198–99
    on scene, 199–200
    significant mechanism of injury, 199–210
  unresponsive medical patient, 187–94
    baseline vital signs, 192
    detailed physical examination, 194
    obtaining SAMPLE history, 193–94
    positioning the patient, 192–93
    rapid physical examination, 189–92
Foods, allergic reactions to, 376
Foot drag, 270
Foot injuries, splinting, 533
Forearm injuries, splinting, 532, 539
Fowler's position, 73
Fractures, 521–23, 524
  in geriatric falls, 636
Frontal region, scalp, 74–75, 550
Front end of car, displacing, 692
Frostnip, 393–94
Fuel tanks, and vehicle rescue, 676
Full extrication, 694–95
Full thickness burns, 504
Fully automated AED, 333, 343

G

Gag reflex:
  and nasopharyngeal airway, 117
  and oropharyngeal airway, 113, 116, 604
Gaining access/extrication, 671–96
  access, 686–92
  extrication, 693–96
  vehicle rescue, 674–86
  See also Access; Extrication; Vehicle rescue
Gases in confined spaces, 726
Gastric distention, 810
Gastric feeding tubes, and pediatric patients,
    626–27
Gastrointestinal (GI) system, 88
Gastrostomy tubes, and pediatric patients,
    626–27
Gauze pads, 490
Gauze rolls, 491
General impression:
  forming, 165
  pediatric patients, 608–9
Generalized hypothermia, 389–90
  emergency care, 391–93
  patient assessment, 390–93
Generic name, 289
Genitourinary system, 88–89, 91
Geriatric patients, 503
  abuse of, 639
  alteration of mental status, 636, 639
  approaches to, 634–35
  black outs, 636
  blood pressure readings in, 637
  brain injuries, 575
  burns in, 503

communicating with, 231, 636
  and conductive heat loss, 388
  diabetes in, 355
  Do Not Resuscitate Order, 641
  heat-related emergencies in, 396
  and hypothermia, 389–90
  medical emergencies, 639–40
    abdominal pain, 640
    acute confusion, 639
    advanced directives, 640
    chest pain/shortness of breath, 639–40
    syncope, 639
  multiple diseases, presence of, 635
  multiple prescription medications, use of,
      635–36
  patient assessment, 635–40
  scene size-up, 635
  shock in, 637
  trauma emergencies, 636–39
    falls, 636–37
    head injuries, 638–39
    motor vehicle crashes, 637
Geriatrics, 631–44
  aging, anatomical/physiological changes
      with, 633–34
  on scene, 632–33
Glasgow Coma Scale, 575, 583
Glass removal, from vehicles, 687
Gloves, 38–39, 45
Glucose, 351
Golden hour, 524, 637
Good Samaritan laws, 59
Gowns, 41
Greater trochanter, 75
Gross negligence, 59
Ground gradient, 512, 682
Ground safety procedures, air medical
      transport, 666
Growth plates, 524
Gunshot wounds, 469
Gynecological emergencies, 437–38
  sexual assault, 438
  trauma to external genitalia, 437–38
  vaginal bleeding, 437
Gynecology, 411–41
  gynecological emergencies, 437–38
  See also Childbirth; Childbirth
      complications; Obstetrics/gynecology;
      Pregnancy emergencies

H

Hand injuries, splinting, 532–33, 539
Hand protection, and vehicle rescue, 678
Handwashing, 38
Hardened metals, and vehicle rescue, 676
Hazardous materials, 27, 732–42
  cold (green) zones, 734
  decontamination, 739–40
    nine-station decontamination procedure,
        740
  emergency care, 741–42
  establishing control of scene, 734
  hazmat incidents:
    EMT's role at, 733–42
    recognizing, 733

Hazardous materials (*cont.*)
  hazmat training, levels of, 27
  hot (red) zones, 734
  identifying the substance, 735–38
    by interviewing, 736
    using binoculars, 735
    using Chemical Transportation
      Emergency Center (CHEMTREC),
      738
    using CHEMTEL, Inc., 738
    using Material Safety Data Sheets,
      736–37
    using National Fire Protection
      Association (NFPA), 735
    using North American Emergency
      Response Guidebook, 736–38,
      741
    using regional poison control centers,
      738
    using shipping documents, 736
    using U.S. Department of Transportation
      labels/placards, 735–36
  medical treatment sector:
    care of injured/contaminated patients,
      740–41
    decontamination, 739–40
    establishing, 739–41
    rehabilitation operations, 739
  patient assessment, 741–42
  secondary contamination, 735
  training for emergencies, 732–33
  warm (yellow) zones, 734
Hazardous and toxic materials, and personal
  safety of EMT, 150
Hazmat encapsulating suits, 29
Hazmat training, levels of, 27
Head, 71
  assessment of, in unresponsive patient,
    190–91
  manual stabilization of, 168
Headgear, and vehicle rescues, 677–78
Head injuries, 569–79
  brain injuries, 572–75
  emergency care, 579
  facial injuries, 569
  in geriatric patients, 638–39
  Glasgow Coma Scale, 575, 583
  patient assessment, 575–79
  rapid extrication procedure:
    of child in safety seat, 580–81
    of high-priority patients, 576–77
  scalp injuries, 569
  scene size-up, 575
  skull injuries, 572
Head-on crashes, 154
Head-protection airbags, and vehicle rescue,
  677
Head/spine injuries, 547–91
  central nervous system, 87–88, 551–52
  helmet removal, 579–88
    alternative method, 588
  on scene, 548–50
  skull, 550
  spine, anatomy of, 550–51
  See also Head injuries; Spinal injuries
Head-tilt, chin-lift maneuver, 102–4
Head trauma, and hypothermia, 390

Health care professionals, 13–14
  nurses, 13
  physician assistants (PAs), 13
  physicians, 13
  public safety officers, 14
Health care proxies, 55
Hearing-impaired patients, communicating
  with, 231
Heart, 81–84, 322–23, 459–61
Heart attacks, 324
  and oxygen therapy, 121
Heat cramps, 396
Heat exhaustion, 396–97, 703
Heat loss, mechanisms of, 702–3
Heat-related airway injury:
  emergency care, 316
  signs/symptoms of, 316
Heat-related emergencies, 395–98, 701–4
  emergency care, 397–98
  in geriatric patients, 396
  heat cramps, 396
  heat exhaustion, 396–97
  heat stroke, 397
  risk factors, 395–96
Heat stroke, 397, 703
Heel bone (calcaneus), 76, 519, 533
Helicopters in rescue operations, 729–32
  altitude/air temperature, 730
  danger areas around helicopters, 667
  helicopter handling, 730
  hoisting, 731
  short-haul technique, 731
  space/load, 730
  special tactics, 731
  visual limitations, 730
  See also Air medical transport
Helmet removal, 579–88
  alternative method, 588
Helmets, and vehicle rescue, 677–78
Hematomas, 485–86
Hemorrhagic shock, 471
High-angle rescue, 729
High concentration oxygen, 134
High-efficiency particulate air (HEPA)
  respirator, 42–43, 147
High flow oxygen, 134
High-level disinfection, 663
Hinge joints, 76
Hip injuries, splinting, 534–35
HIV (human immunodeficiency virus), 47
Hoisting, by helicopter, 731
Home nebulizer, 311
Home ventilators, and pediatric patients, 626
Honesty, in interpersonal communication,
  230
Hormones, 88
Hostile/aggressive patients, 449–50
Hot (red) zones, 734
Human resources and training, 8, 9–10
Human skeleton, 520
Humerus, 76, 520
Humidifiers, 130
Hyperbaric centers, 13
Hyperglycemia, 352
Hypertension, 326
Hyperthermia, 387
Hyperventilation, 120, 764

Hypoglycemia, 352
Hypoperfusion, 86–87, 326, 376, 461
  and hypothermia, 390
  and oxygen therapy, 121
  See also Shock
Hypopharynx, 77, 303, 760
Hypotension, 326–27
Hypothermia, 387
  and burns, 390
  and drugs, 390
  emergency care, 391–93
  generalized, 389–90
  and geriatric patients, 389–90
  patient assessment:
    breathing, 391
    circulation, 391
    general impression, 390–91
    mental status, 391
Hypovolemic shock, 471–73
  emergency care, 472–73
Hypoxia, 124, 600, 764
  and cyanosis, 124
Hypoxic drive, 126, 310

I

Ice rescue, 400–402, 723–24
  going to a patient over ice, 724
  judging thickness/overall safety of ice, 723
  reach/throw considerations, 724
  resuscitation, 724
  rowing considerations, 724
  and specialty rescue team, 723
Identification of priority patients, 175–76
Iliac crest, 75, 519
Ilium, 75
Immersion in water, and hypothermia, 390
Immobilization, 557–69
  cervical collars, 560–61
    applying, 563–64
    sizing, 562
  corset-type, half-back immobilizer, 559
  devices, 559
  fiberglass long board, 559
  full-body spinal immobilization devices,
    559, 562–65
  with infants/children, 569, 578
  long spine board, 559, 568
    four rescuer log roll and, 570–71
    two rescuer log roll and, 572
  manual in-line stabilization, 558–60
    establishing, 560
  pediatric immobilization system, 620
  rapid extrication procedure:
    of child in safety seat, 580–81
    high-priority patients, 576–77
  short spinal immobilization devices, 559,
    560–62, 566–67
  standing takedown (three rescuers), 573
  standing takedown (two rescuers), 574
Impaled objects, 497
  emergency care, 497
  general patient care, 499–500
Impalements, 469
Implied consent, 54–55
Improvised splints, 528

Inadequate breathing, signs of, 99–101
Incident Command System (ICS), 30
Incident management system (IMS), 742–43
Incline drag, 270
Incorrect splinting, consequences of, 527
Indirect force, and musculoskeletal injuries, 524
Infants/children, 593–630
    abdominal injuries, 622
    advance directives, 627
    and airway management, 136–37
    airway management, 137
    airway obstruction, 611–12
        complete obstruction, 612–13
        partial obstruction, 612
        partial obstruction with cyanosis/altered mental state, 612–13
    altered mental status in, 615
    anatomy/physiology, 595–98
    bonds formed with EMS providers, 258
    burns in, 502, 510
    cardiopulmonary resuscitation (CPR) for, 820
    chest injuries, 622
    child abuse and neglect, 622–24
    common medical problems in, 611–18
    developmental considerations, 598
    diabetes in, 352
    EMT's response to, 628
    extremity injuries, 622
    eye damage, and oxygen therapy, 126
    family, 627–28
    fever in, 615–16
    heat-related emergencies in, 395
    and hypothermia, 389–90
    immobilization with, 569
    inadequate breathing in, 81
    initial assessment of, 173–74
    nasogastric intubation of, 781
    near-drowning of, 617–18
    organ systems of, 596
    orotracheal intubation of, 777–81
    pediatric airway and breathing management, 598–608
    pediatric emergency care, 595
    pediatric patient assessment, 608–11
    poisonings, 616
    psychological and social characteristics of, 599
    pulse oximetry, 126
    respiratory distress in, 763
    respiratory emergencies in, 311–15, 613–14
    respiratory system of, 79
    and rule of nines, 506
    on scene, 594–95
    seizures in, 614–15
    seriously ill/injured, 23
    shock, 616–17
    with slow pulse rate, 182
    with special needs, 624–27
        central intravenous lines, 626
        gastric feeding tubes/gastrostomy tubes, 626–27
        home ventilators, 626
        shunts, 627
        tracheostomy tubes, 625–26

    sudden infant death syndrome (SIDS), 618
    transition of care, 598
    trauma in, 618–22
        emergency care, 622
    See also Pediatric patient assessment
Infarction, 323
Infection control, 35–50
    airborne pathogens, protection from, 41–43
    basic safety precautions, 38
    cleaning/disinfection of equipment, 43–45
    handwashing, 38
    and the law, 45–48
    pathogens, 38
    personal health, monitoring, 43
    personal protective equipment (PPE), 38
    on scene, 36–37
Inferior, use of term, 70
Inferior vena cava, 85
Ingestion:
    poisoning by, 367
        assessment/emergency care, 369
Inhalation, 77
    poisoning by, 367, 373
        assessment/emergency care, 369–72
Inhaled bronchodilators, 293–94
Initial assessment, 143, 163–76
    ABCs, 164
    of airway status, 170–71
    of breathing status, 171–72
    of circulation status, 172–73
    general impression, forming, 165
    identification of priority patients, 175–76
    of infants/children, 173–74
    of mental status, 168
    pediatric patients, 608
    and respiratory distress, 307
    steps of, 164–65
Initial triage, 747–49
Injection:
    poisoning by, 367–68
        assessment/emergency care, 372–73
Injuries, and hypothermia, 390
Injury of coworker, and stress, 23–24
Injury prevention, 8
In-line stabilization during ventilations, 109
Insect bites/stings, 403–4
    allergic reactions to, 376
    emergency care, 403–4
    venom, 403
Insulin, 351–52
Intercostal muscles, 304
Intermediate-level disinfection, 663
Internal bleeding, 469–77
    emergency care, 471
    mechanisms of injury associated with, 469–70
    signs/symptoms associated with, 470
Internal defibrillators, 333
Interpersonal communication, 228–32
    with agitated/disturbed patients, 231
    body language, 229
    with confused/mentally disabled patients, 230–31
    eye contact, 229
    general guidelines, 229–32
    with geriatric patients, 231

    with hearing-impaired patients, 231
    honesty, 230
    introducing yourself to the patient, 229
    language, 230
    listening to the patient, 230
    with non-English-speaking patients, 232
    with pediatric patients, 231
    position, 229
    professional manner, 230
    speaking directly to the patient, 229–30
    tone of voice, 230
    with visually impaired patients, 232
Intersection collisions, factors contributing, 657
Intersections, and emergency vehicles, 657–58
Intravenous (IV) hydration, 711
Intravenous (IV) therapy, 802–4
    maintaining an IV, 804
    setting up fluid administration set, 802–4
Involuntary muscles, 77
Ischemia, 323, 324, 326
Ischium, 75, 519

J

Jaw-thrust maneuver, 104–5, 620
Joint injuries, splinting, 534–35, 544
Joints, 76, 521
Jugular vein distention (JVD), 191–92

K

Kubler-Ross, Elisabeth, 21–22
K-Y jelly, and endotracheal tube insertion, 768
Kyphosis, 639

L

Labor, 415–17
    stages of, 415–16
Labored breathing, 183
Labor pains, 416–17
Lacerations, 463, 487–88
Landing zone, for helicopter, 665–66
Language, in interpersonal communication, 230
Lap-belt complex injuries, 619
Large open neck injury:
    emergency care, 497–500
    patient care, 501
Laryngoscope, 763, 764–65, 766, 774
    assembling, 766
Laryngoscope blades, 45, 765, 778
Larynx, 77, 303
Last oral intake, and SAMPLE history, 179–80
Lateral, use of term, 70
Lateral bending, and spinal injuries, 553
Lateral malleolus, 76, 519
Laws, 53–54
Left, use of term, 71
Left lateral recumbent, 73
Liability, minimizing, 63–64

Licensing, 10
Lifting/moving patients, 261–84
  body mechanics, 264–68
  emergency moves, 268–69, 270, 271
  non-urgent moves, 269, 272–76
  packaging patients, defined, 263
  patient-carrying equipment, 276–82
  patient safety, 268–76
  planning for, 263–64
  positioning of patients, 282–83
  on scene, 262–63
  types of patient moves, 268–76
  urgent moves, 269
    See also Body mechanics; Patient-
      carrying equipment
Ligaments, 76, 521
Limb presentation, 431
Linear lacerations, 487
Listening to the patient, 230
Litter carries, 728–29
Living wills, 55
Local cold injuries, 393–95
  emergency care, 394–95
    early/superficial local cold injury, 394
    late/deep local cold injury, 394–95
  frostnip, 393–94
Location of burns, 506
Log-rolling techniques, 267–68
Long bone injuries, splinting, 532–44
Long spine boards, 280, 559, 568
  four rescuer log roll and, 570–71
  two rescuer log roll and, 572
Low-angle rescue, 729
Lower abdomen, assessment of, in
    unresponsive patient, 192
Lower extremities, 71, 75–76
  bones of, 521
Lower-leg injuries, splinting, 533
Low flow oxygen, 135
Lubrifax®, and endotracheal tube insertion,
    768
Lungs, 77

M

Machinery hazards, 727
Magnetic name tags, 707
Mammalian diving reflex, 724
Mandible, 74, 550
Mantoux, 42
Manual in-line stabilization, 558–60
  establishing, 560
Manubrium, sternum, 75
Masks, 40–41
Mask seal, 108
Material Safety Data Sheets, 736–37
Maxillae, 74, 550
MCI, *See* Multiple-casualty incidents (MCI)
Mechanisms of injury (MOI), 143, 153–60,
    469
  associated with internal bleeding, 469–70
  blast injuries, 160–61
  blunt trauma, 153–60, 469
  burns, 503
  falls, 161
  internal bleeding, 469–70

  musculoskeletal injuries, 523–24
  penetrating trauma, 469
  spinal injuries, 552–53, 554
  See also Blunt trauma
Meconium, 417, 433–34
  emergency care, 434
Medial, use of term, 70
Medial malleolus, 76, 519
Medical conditions:
  and burn severity, 506
  and heat-related emergencies, 396
  and hypothermia, 390
Medical control, *See* Medical direction
Medical direction, 8, 10–11
  communications with, 236–37
  off-line, 11
  on-line, 11
Medical identification device, 178
Medical/legal issues, 51–65
  advance directives, 55
  assault/battery, 59–60
  confidentiality, 60–61
  consent, 54–55
  laws and ethics, 53–54
  liability, minimizing, 63–64
  minors/special risk patients, 60
  negligence, 58–59
  potential organ donors, 61
  refusal of care/abandonment, 55–58, 65
  on scene, 52–53
  scope of practice, 54
  special reporting situations, 61–63
  suspected crime scenes, 63
Medical oversight, *See* Medical direction
Medical treatment sector:
  care of injured/contaminated patients,
      740–41
  decontamination, 739–40
  establishing, 739–41
  rehabilitation operations, 739
Medication, 289
  actions, 292
  administered by EMTs, 293–97
    epinephrine, 294–95
    inhaled bronchodilators, 293–94
    nitroglycerin, 293–94
  administration of, 292–93
  allergic reactions to, 376
  and bleeding, 462
  commonly encountered medications,
      296–97
  contraindications, 291
  dose, 291
  on EMS unit, 295–96
    activated charcoal, 296
    oral glucose, 296
    oxygen, 295–96
  forms of, 290
  and heat-related emergencies, 396
  and hypothermia, 390
  indications, 291
  prescription labeling, 290–91
  routes of administration, 290, 291
  and SAMPLE history, 178–79
  side effects, 292
  understanding, 291–92
Medication names, 289–90

Meditation, and stress, 24
Medium-duty truck chassis, 650
Mentally disabled patients, communicating
    with, 230–31
Mental status:
  assessment of, 168–70
  pediatric patients, 609
Metacarpals, 76, 521
Metaprel®, 311
Metatarsal bones, 76, 520
Metered dose inhaler (MDI), 293, 311
Mid-axillary line, 69
Mid-clavicular lines, 69
Midline, 69
Minors, as patients, 60
Miscarriage, 434–35
Mobile computer, 233–34
Mobile radios, 232
Motorcycle crashes, 469
Motor vehicle crashes, 153–59, 469
  ejections from vehicles, 156
  fatality in same vehicle, 156
  and geriatric patients, 637
  head-on crashes, 154
  rear-end collisions, 154
  rollover collisions, 156
  seatbelts and airbags, 156–59
  side-impact collisions, 155–56
Motor vehicle crash scenes, personal safety
    of EMT, 149
Mounted suction systems, 118
Mouth-to-mask ventilation, 105, 106–7, 809
Multi-drug resistant TB (MDR-TB), 42
Multiple births, 431–32
  emergency care, 431–32
Multiple-casualty incidents (MCI), 23,
    658–60, 742–52
  command functions, 743
  command sector, 743
  communications, 744–45
    with hospitals, 752
  EMS sector functions, 745–47
  extrication sector, 745
  incident management system (IMS),
      742–43
    command, 742
    functional areas, 742–43
  organization, 745
  and patient documentation, 250
  psychological considerations, 752
  rehab sector, 747
  scene size-up, 743–44
  staging sector, 745, 750–52
  supply sector, 745
  transportation sector, 747, 750–52
  treatment sector, 747, 750
  triage sector, 747–50
  See also Triage
Multiple diseases, in geriatric patients, 635
Multiple-vehicle hazards, 657
Murphy eye, 765–67
Muscle relaxants, allergic reactions to, 376
Muscles, 76–77, 521
  types of, 523
Musculoskeletal injuries, 517–46
  broken bones, 521–23
  and direct force, 523–24

dislocations, 524
emergency care, 526–27
fractures, 521–23, 524
and indirect force, 524
mechanisms of, 523–24
open/closed, 524–25
patient assessment, 526
on scene, 518–19
scene size-up, 526
and shock, 529
signs/symptoms of, 526
splinting, 527–44
sprains, 524
strains, 524
and twisting force, 524
types of, 524
See also Splinting
Musculoskeletal system, 73–77
anatomy/physiology of, 519–21
bones of, 73–77
connective tissue, 76–77
functions of, 73
joints, 76
muscles, 76–77
and trauma, 521–27
See also Musculoskeletal injuries
Mutual aid, requesting, 30
Myocardial infarction, 324

N

Nasal bones, 74, 550
Nasal cannula, 134–35
Nasal flaring, 81, 101, 609, 763
Nasogastric intubation, of infants/children,
781, 782
Nasogastric tube (NG tube), 781
Nasopharyngeal airways, 117–18
and gag reflex, 117
insertion of, 117–18
and nose bleeding, 605
in pediatric sizes, 604–5
Nasopharynx, 77, 303, 760
National Association of EMS Physicians,
45
National Fire Protection Association (NFPA),
733, 735
National Fire Service Incident Management
System (IMS), 742–43
National Highway Safety Act, 5
National Highway Traffic Safety
Administration (NHTSA), 6
National Institute of Occupational Safety and
Health (NIOSH), 42, 717
National Registry of Emergency Medical
Technicians (NREMT), 10
Natural hazards, and personal safety of EMT,
150
Nature of illness (NOI), 143, 152–53
Near-drowning, 398, 399–400
emergency care, 399–400
of infants/children, 617–18
Nebulizer, 293
Neck, 71
assessment of, in unresponsive patient,
191–92

Nec-Loc cervical collar, 561
Neglect:
defined, 622
and stress, 23
Negligence, 58–59
gross, 59
Neighboring jurisdictions, requesting
assistance from, 30
Nervous system, 87–88
autonomic, 88
central, 87–88
peripheral, 88
Newborn assessment, 423–24
Newborn resuscitation, 424–25
Newborns:
assessment of, 423–24
and radiation heat loss, 388
resuscitation of, 424–25
9-1-1 systems, 8–9
Nitroglycerin, 293–94, 327–28, 329
administration of, 330–31
automated external defibrillators (AEDs),
332
and cardiac compromise, 327–28
Noisy breathing, 81, 183
Nomex® jumpsuits, 677
Non-9-1-1 systems, 8–9
Non-English-speaking patients,
communication with, 232
Nonrebreather mask, 131–34
Non-urgent moves, 269, 272–76
direct carry method, 272, 275, 276
direct ground lift, 272–73
draw sheet method, 272, 274
extremity lift, 272, 274
Normal anatomic position, 69
Normal breathing, 183
Normal extrication, 693–94
*North American Emergency Response
Guidebook*, 28, 736–38, 741
Nosebleeds, 469
and nasopharyngeal airways, 605
Nurses, 13

O

Obstetrics/gynecology, 411–41
childbirth complications, 429–34
gynecological emergencies, 437–38
normal childbirth, 417–29
pregnancy:
anatomy/physiology of, 413–17
emergencies, 434–37
on scene, 412–13
Obstructions, and airway management, 136
Occipital region, scalp, 74–75, 550
Occupational Safety and Health
Administration (OSHA), 45
Occlusive dressings, 490
Occupation, and heat–related emergencies,
396
Occupational Safety and Health Agency
(OSHA), 732–33
Off-line medical direction, 11
Olecranon, 76, 520
Omission, 59

One-handed carrying techniques, 266
One rescuer assists/carries, 271
One-rescuer drags, 270
Ongoing assessment, 144–45
On-line medical direction, 11
Open chest injuries, emergency care, 495–96
Open crush injuries, 489
Open head injury, 575
Opening the airway, 102–5, 807–8
Open musculoskeletal injuries, 525
Open soft tissue injuries:
abdominal open injuries, 496–97
abrasions, 487
amputations, 488, 500–501
avulsions, 488, 502
emergency care, 493–94
impaled objects, 497
lacerations, 487–88
large neck injury, 497–500
penetrations/punctures, 489
OPQRST, 195, 325
Oral glucose, 296, 352–53
administering, 355
Oral rehydration, 704, 710–11
Orbits (eye sockets), 74, 550
Organs, 73
Oropharyngeal airways, 113–17, 118
and gag reflex, 113, 116
insertion of, 113–16
in pediatric sizes, 604–5
standard sizes of, 113
Oropharynx, 77, 303, 760
Orotracheal intubation, 763–81
advantages of, 763–64
complications, 764
depth of tub, approximating, 779
equipment, 764–69
accessories, 768–69
endotracheal tube, 763, 765–68, 770
laryngoscope, 763, 764–65, 766, 774
laryngoscope blades, 765, 778
personal protective equipment, 764
stylet/lubricant, 768–69, 774
syringe, 769
tube-securing device, 769
indications for, 769–70
of adult patients, 770–76
of infants/children, 777–81
as invasive technique, 764
orotracheal/endotracheal suctioning,
781–83
procedure, 771–73
Sellick's maneuver, 774–75, 780
tube size, estimating, 778
See also Nasogastric intubation
Orotracheal suctioning, 781–83
OSHA, 732–33
Overdose, 363
Oxygen, 295–96
for the heart, 323
Oxygen cylinders, 127–29
Oxygen delivery devices, 131
Oxygen delivery system, preparing, 132–33
Oxygen therapy, 121–35
administering oxygen, 130, 134
and cardiac arrest, 121
and cerebrovascular accidents (CVAs), 121

Oxygen therapy (*cont.*)
delivering oxygen to the breathing patient, 130–35
equipment, 127–35
flowmeters, 129–30
hazards of, 126–27
humidifiers, 130
hypoxia, 124
nasal cannula, 134–35
nonrebreather mask, 131–34
oxygen cylinders, 127–29
oxygen delivery devices, 131
oxygen delivery system, preparing, 132–33
pressure regulators, 129
pulse oximetry, 124–26
supplemental oxygen, importance of, 121–24

P

Pacemakers, 83
Pack strap carry, 271
Palliative care, 55
Palmar, use of term, 70
Palpation, 68, 184
Pantridge, Frank, 5
Parietal region, scalp, 74–75, 550
Parking, emergency vehicles, 656–57
Partial airway obstruction, 612
Partial airway obstructions, 612, 826–27
with cyanosis/altered mental state, 612–13
Partial amputations, 488
Partial extrication, 694–95
Partial thickness burns, 504–5
Past medical history, and SAMPLE history, 179
Patella, 75, 519
Pathogens, 38
Patient assessment, 141–223
allergic reactions, 377–78
behavioral emergencies, 447
burns, 507–8
cardiac arrest, 337–39
cardiac compromise, 324–25
components of, 142
detailed physical examination, 144
diabetes, 352–53
dispatch information, 146
focused history and physical examination, 143–44, 187–97
generalized hypothermia, 390–93
geriatric patients, 635–40
head injuries, 575–79
initial assessment, 143, 163–76
musculoskeletal injuries, 526
ongoing assessment, 144–45
poisoning, 368
priority patient, 143
respiratory distress, 307–8
SAMPLE history and vital signs, 176–87
scene assessment, 152–61
scene safety, 146–52
scene size–up, 142–43, 145–63
See also Detailed physical examination; Focused history and physical

examination; Initial assessment; SAMPLE history; Scene assessment; Scene safety; Scene size–up; Vital signs
Patient-carrying equipment, 276–82
basket stretcher, 281
flexible stretcher, 281–82
portable ambulance stretcher, 277–79
scoop stretcher, 280
spine boards, 280–81
stair chair, 279–80
wheeled ambulance stretcher, 276–77
Patient-initiated refusals (PIRs), 55
Patient narrative, 244–46
objective information in, 244
pertinent negatives in, 245
subjective information in, 244–45
Patient refusal checklist, 57
Patient refusal of treatment, 55–58, 246–48
Patient safety, 150–52
lifting/moving patients, 268–76
Pedestrian injuries, 469
Pediatric airway and breathing management, 598–608
airway skills, 601–5
airway adjuncts, 604–5
clearing complete airway obstructions, 602–3
opening the airway, 601
suctioning, 602
artificial ventilation, 607–8
supplemental oxygen therapy, 606–7
Pediatric Assessment Triangle, 611
Pediatric centers, 13
Pediatric considerations, and airway management, 136
Pediatric emergency care, 595
Pediatric immobilization system, 620
Pediatric notes, *See* Infants/children
Pediatric patient assessment, 608–11
ABCs, 608–11
focused history and physical examination, 611
general impression, 608–9
initial assessment, 608
mental status, 609
Pediatric patients:
communicating with, 231
EMT's response to, 628
Pediatrics, defined, 595
Pelvic injuries, splinting, 534–35
Pelvis, 75
assessment of, in unresponsive patient, 192
bones of, 519–21
Penetrating trauma, 159–60
mechanisms of injury, 469
Penetration, 489
and spinal injuries, 553
Penicillin, allergic reactions to, 376
Perfusion, 86–87, 459
Perineum, 414
Peripheral nervous system, 88, 551–52
PERRL, 186
Personal flotation devices (PFDs), failure to use, 718

Personal health, monitoring, 43
Personal protective equipment (PPE), 29–30, 38–41, 46, 147
eye protection, 39–40
gloves, 38–39
gowns, 41
masks, 40–41
when/which types to use, 41
Personal safety, 26–31, 147–50
crime scenes, 149
hazardous and toxic materials, 150
motor vehicle crash scenes, 149
natural hazards, 150
scene safety, 26–30
violence, 30–31
Pertinent negatives, 245
Phalanges (fingers), 76, 521
Phalanges (toes), 76, 520
Pharmacology, 287–300
essentials of, 289–93
medication, 289
administered by EMTs, 293–97
administration of, 292–93
forms of, 290
names, 289–90
understanding, 291–92
prescription labeling, 290–91
routes of administration, 290
on scene, 288–89
See also Medication
Pharyngo-tracheal lumen airway [PtL®], 790–91
insertion of, 790–91
Pharynx, 77, 303
Philadelphia cervical collar, 561
Phoenix Fire Department Rehabilitation SOP, 710
Phoenix Fire Ground Command (FGC) System, 742
Physical examination, 143–44
approaches to, 188–89
detailed, 144, 194
pediatric patients, 611
rapid, 189–92
trauma patients, with no significant mechanism of injury, 216–17
See also Rapid physical examination
Physician assistants (PAs), 13
Physicians, 13
Physiology, 67–93
Piggy back carry, 271
Pilot balloon, 765
Pin-index safety system, 129
Pit vipers, 405
Placards, warning of hazardous materials, 150–51
Placenta, 414
delivering, 427–28
Plantar, use of term, 70
Plants, allergic reactions to, 376
Plasma, 85–86, 461
Platelets, 85, 461
Pneumatic anti–shock garment (PASG), 465, 528
using, 476–77
Pneumatic splints, 465, 528

Pneumothorax, 495
Pocket face mask, 106
Poison, defined, 365
Poison control centers, 13, 738
Poisoning, 365–75
  and activated charcoal, 370
  by absorption, 368
  by ingestion, 367
    assessment/emergency care, 369
  by inhalation, 367
  by injection, 367–68
  and hypothermia, 390
  of infants/children, 616
  management techniques, 368–75
  patient assessment, 368
    techniques, 368–75
  routes of exposure, 367–68
Policies, EMS system, 8
Portable ambulance stretcher, 277–79
Portable radios, 232–33
Portable suction units, 118–19, 651
Position, in interpersonal communication,
    229
Positional asphyxia, 452
Position of function, 533
Positioning the patient, 192–93
Positioning of patients, in carrying device,
    282–83
Positioning units, at emergency scene, 658
Positive pressure ventilation, 105
Post-delivery vaginal bleeding, controlling,
    428
Posterior, use of term, 69
Posterior body, assessment of, in
    unresponsive patient, 192
Posterior tibial artery, 85
Postictal period, 614
Post-traumatic stress syndrome, 25
Potential organ donors, 61
Power grip, 265
Power lift, 264–65
Power lift/power grip, 264–65
PPD, 442
Pre-arrival instructions, 258
Pregnancy:
  amniotic sac, 86–87, 414
    breaking of, 417
  anatomy/physiology of, 413–17
  birth canal, 413
  bloody show, 417
  breech presentation, 416
  cephalic presentation, 416
  cervix, 413
  contractions, 417
  effacement, 416
  fallopian tubes, 413
  fetus, 414
  labor, 415–17
  labor pains, 416–17
  meconium staining, 417
  ovaries, 413
  physiologic changes during, 415
  placenta, 414
  presenting part, 416
  seizures during, 435
  supine hypotensive syndrome, 415

trauma in, 436–37
trimesters, 414
umbilical cord, 414
uterus, 414–16
  change in size of, 414
vagina, 413
vaginal bleeding late in, 435–36
See also Childbirth; Childbirth
    complications; Pregnancy
    emergencies
Pregnancy emergencies, 434–37
  seizures during pregnancy, 435
  spontaneous abortion (miscarriage),
    434–35
  trauma, 436–37
  vaginal bleeding late in pregnancy, 435–36
Prehospital care, 253–60
  on scene, 254–55
  tiered response systems, 255–56
  transition of care, 255
    procedures, 256–58
    special circumstances in, 258–59
Prehospital care report, 239–46
  administrative information, 243
  computerized report, 239
    electronic clipboard, 239
  correcting errors in, 248–49
  falsification of, 248–49
  formats, 239
  medical terminology in, 245
  minimum data set, 239–43
  multiple casualty incidents (MCIs), 250
  neatness of, 245
  patient data, 243–44
  patient narrative, 244–46
  radio codes in, 245
  special situations, 250–51
  standard abbreviations in, 245
  thoroughness of, 245–46
  written report, 239
Premature birth, 432–33
  emergency care, 433
Prescribed inhaler, 310–11, 312
  assisting with, 313
  with a spacer, assisting with, 314
Prescription labeling, 290–91
Presenting part, 416
Pressure dressings, 492
Pressure points, and external bleeding, 465
Pressure regulators, 129
Priapism, 557
Primary blast injuries, 160
Priority patients, identification of, 175–76
Privileged information, 61
Professionalism, 14–15
Professional manner, in interpersonal
    communication, 230
Prolapsed umbilical cord, 429–30
Prone position, 73
Protocols, 11
Proventil®, 311
Proximal, use of term, 70
Proximal tarsal bones, 76
Proximate cause, 59
Psychiatric emergencies, 446–47
Pubis, 75, 519

Public information and education, 8
Public safety officers, 14
Pulmonary artery, 84
Pulmonary tuberculosis (TB), 41–42
Pulmonary vein, 85
Pulse, 86, 172, 180–82
  quality of, 182
  slow, 81
Pulse oximeter, 124–26, 801–2
Punctures, 489
Pupils:
  abnormal findings in, 187
  assessment of, 186–87

Q

Quality, breathing, 305
Quality assessment (QA), 12
Quality assurance (QA), 12
  AEDs, 343
Quality of breathing, 80, 762
Quality improvement (QI), 11–12, 53

R

Raccoon eyes, 572
Radial artery, 85
Radiation heat loss, 387
  and newborns, 388
Radio communications, 9, 234–37
  after arrival at hospital/receiving facility,
    237
  communication/dispatch, 235–36
  en route to hospital/receiving facility,
    237
  general rules for, 234–35
  with medical direction, 236–37
Radius, 76, 520
Rapid extrication, 269
  of child in safety seat, 580–81
  of high-priority patients, 576–77
Rapid physical examination (unresponsive
    patient), 189–94
Rapid trauma assessment:
  by body region, 205
  performing, 201
  procedure, 206–9
Rate, breathing, 305
Rate of breathing, 79–80, 761, 762
Reaching/pulling techniques, 266–67
Realigning injured extremities, 531–32
Rear-end collisions, 154
Reasonable force and restraint, 450–52
Reassessment (ongoing assessment), 144
Receiving facility:
  arrival at, 662
  en route to, 661
Recovery position, 73
Recurring cardiac arrest, 342
Red bag, 43–44
Red blood cells, 85, 461
Refusal of care/abandonment, 55–58, 65
Regional poison control centers, 738
Regulations, EMS system, 8

Rehabilitation operations, 739
Rehab Sector/Group, 701, 704–11, 747
  accountability in, 707–8
  criteria for entering, 707
  design/location of, 705–7
  entry/triage, 708–9
  functions of, 704
  hydration/nourishment in, 710–11
  medical evaluation/treatment, 709–10
  staffing of, 704–5
Rehydration, 704, 710–11
Relaxation techniques, and stress, 24
Repeaters, 233
Reporting to dispatch, 658
Reproductive system, 91
Required dispatch information, 651–55
Rescue breathing, 809–12
  gastric distention, 810, 812
  mouth-to-mask ventilation, 809, 811
  recovery position, 810–11
Rescue plan, 30
Rescue situations, 29–30
  hazards, 718–23
Resource management, 8
Respiration, 77, 182–83
  See also Breathing
Respiratory arrest, 99
  and oxygen therapy, 121, 126
Respiratory depression, and oxygen therapy, 126
Respiratory distress, 306–10
  emergency care, 309–10
  focused history and physical examination, 308
  hypoxic drive, 310
  in infants/children, 763
  initial assessment, 307
  patient assessment in, 307–8
  scene size-up, 307
  signs/symptoms of, 308–9
Respiratory emergencies, 301–18
  adequate/inadequate artificial ventilation, 305–6
  adequate/inadequate breathing, 304–6
  and burns, 316
  home nebulizer, 311
  in infants/children, 311–15, 613–14
    early respiratory distress, 613–14
    respiratory arrest, 613
    severe respiratory distress/failure, 613–14
    upper airway obstruction vs. lower airway disease, 613
  prescribed inhaler, 310–11, 312
  respiratory distress, 306–10
  respiratory system, 303–4
  on scene, 302–3
  smoke inhalation, 315–16
Respiratory failure:
  assessment of, 99–101
  defined, 99
  emergency care, 101–2
Respiratory rate, 182
Respiratory system, 77–81, 760–63
  anatomy of, 77, 303–4, 760
  pediatric airway and anatomy, 762–63

physiology of, 77–81, 303–4, 760–62
Responsive patient:
  detailed physical examination of, 196–97
  and focused history and physical examination, 194–97
Retractions, 81
Returning to service, 662–65
  at the receiving facility, 662
  at the station, 663–65
  cleaning/disinfection procedures, 663–65
  en route to the station, 662–63
Rhythm, breathing, 305
Right, use of term, 71
Right lateral recumbent, 73
Right mainstem intubation, 764
Right of way, emergency vehicles, 656
Rigid splints, 465, 528, 532, 533
Road rash, 463
Roles/responsibilities, EMT, 14–15
Rollover collisions, 156
Roof of car, disposing of, 689
Rotation, and spinal injuries, 553
Rough terrain evacuations, 728–29
  high-angle rescue, 729
  litter carries, 728–29
  low-angle rescue, 729
Routes of administration, 290
Rule of nines, 505–6
Ryan White CARE Act, 47–48

S

Sacral vertebrae, 75, 550
SAMPLE history, 176–80
  allergies, 178
  elements of, 144
  events leading up to illness/injury, 180
  last oral intake, 179–80
  medications, 178–79
  obtaining, 193–94
  pertinent past medical history, 179
  responsive medical patient, 195–96
  signs and symptoms, 178
  trauma patients, with no significant mechanism of injury, 217
  for trauma patients, obtaining, 204–10
  unresponsive medical patient, 193–94
Scalp, regions of, 74–75, 550
Scalp injuries, 569
Scapula, 76, 520
Scene assessment, 152–61
  determining number of patients, 162–63
  mechanism of injury (MOI), 143, 153–61
  nature of illness (NOI), 143, 152–53
  See also Mechanism of injury (MOI)
Scene safety, 26–30, 146–52, 675–77
  assessing potential hazards, 146–47
  body substance isolation (BSI), 35–50, 142, 147
  bystander safety, 152
  danger zone, establishing, 148
  hazardous materials, 26–29
  listening for potential violence, 147
  patient safety, 150–52
  personal safety of EMT, 147–50

rescue situations, 29–30
scene size-up, 26, 142–43
and suicide/suicide attempts, 449
in vehicle rescues, 675–77
  See also Personal safety
Scene size-up, 26, 142–43, 145–63
  geriatric patients, 635
  and musculoskeletal injuries, 526
  and respiratory distress, 307
Schloendorf v. Society of the NY Hospital, 54
Scoop stretcher, 280
Scope of practice, 54
Scorpion stings, 405
SCUBA diving emergencies, 402–3
  ascent-related barotrauma, 402
  decompression sickness (DCS), 402–3
  descent-related barotrauma, 402
Seatbelts:
  injuries from, 156–59
  and vehicle rescue, 676
Secondary blast injuries, 160
Secondary contamination, 735
Secondary drowning syndrome, 617
Secondary triage, 749–50
Seesaw breathing, 81, 609, 763
Seizure medications, allergic reactions to, 376
Seizures, 356–58
  and altered mental status, 356–58
  during pregnancy, 435
    emergency care, 435
  emergency care, 356–58
  in infants/children, 614–15
    emergency care, 615
  patient assessment, 356
Self-adhering bandages, 491
Self-adhesive dressings, 490
Self-contained breathing apparatus (SCBA), 29, 150, 315, 683, 707
Sellick's maneuver, 774–75, 780
Semi-automated AEDs, 333–34, 340–41
Severe injuries, and stress, 23
Sexual assault, emergency care, 438
Shaken baby syndrome, 623
Shallow breathing, 183
Sharps container, 43–44
Shock, 86–87, 204, 326, 461
  anaphylactic shock, 376
  in geriatric patients, 637
  hemorrhagic shock, 471
  and hypothermia, 390
  hypovolemic shock, 471
  in infants/children, 616–17
  and musculoskeletal injuries, 529
  and oxygen therapy, 121–24
  patient assessment/care, 474–75
  pneumatic anti-shock garment, using, 476–77
  signs/symptoms of, 87
  See also Circulatory system; Hypoperfusion
Shock position, 73
Short-haul technique, helicopters, 731
Shortness of breath:
  in geriatric patients, 639–40
  and oxygen therapy, 121

Short spinal immobilization devices, 559, 560–62, 566–67
Short spine boards, 280–81
Shoulder blade (scapula), 76, 520
Shoulder drag, 270
Shoulder injuries, splinting, 535
Shunt failure, 627
Shunts:
    and pediatric patients, 627
    shunt failure, 627
Side-impact airbags, and vehicle rescue, 677
Side-impact collisions, 155–56
    and geriatric patients, 637
Signs, 178
Signs/symptoms:
    of cardiac compromise, 325–26
    of cerebrovascular accidents (CVAs), 358–59
    of child abuse and neglect, 622–23
    of internal bleeding, 470
    of musculoskeletal injuries, 526
    of respiratory distress, 308–9
Signs and symptoms, and SAMPLE history, 178
Silos, 726
Simple access, 686–87
Simple negligence, 58–59
Sirens, emergency vehicles, 656
Situational stress reactions, 446
Skeletal muscles, 76, 521
Skin, 89–92, 172–73
    assessment of, 172–73, 185–86
    capillary refill, 173
    color, 172
    dermis, 484
    epidermis, 484
    functions/structures, 484–85
    subcutaneous layers, 92, 484
    temperature/condition, 172–73
    See also Environmental emergencies
Skull, 550
Skull injuries, 572
Sling and swathe, 528, 532, 535
    applying, 537–38
Small volume nebulizers (SVNs), 311
Smoke inhalation, 315–16
    emergency care, 316
    signs/symptoms of, 316
Smooth muscles, 77
Snake bites, 405–6
    emergency care, 406
Soft tissue injuries, 481–516
    bandages, 490–92
    closed injuries, 485–87
        assessment of, 489–90
        contusions, 485
        crush injuries, 486
        hematomas, 485–86
    defined, 483
    dressings, 490, 492
    emergency care, 494–502
    open crush injuries, 489
    open injuries, 485, 493–94
        abdominal, 496–97
        abrasions, 487

amputations, 488, 500–501
avulsions, 488, 502
chest injuries, 495–96
general procedures for, 495
impaled objects, 497
lacerations, 487–88
large neck injury, 497–500
penetrations/punctures, 489
on scene, 483
skin, functions/structures, 484–85
Special facilities, 12–13
Special incident report, 62
Special lifting/carrying considerations, 265–68
Special operations, 715–55
    confined spaces/hazardous atmospheres, 724–27
    hazardous materials, 732–42
    helicopters in rescue operations, 729–32
    ice rescue, 723–24
    multiple-casualty incidents (MCI), 742–52
    rescue situation hazards, 718–23
    rough terrain evacuations, 728–29
    on scene, 716–17
    trench collapses, 727–28
    water-related hazards, 718–23
    See also Hazardous materials; Multiple-casualty incidents (MCI)
Special reporting situations, 61–63
Special risk patients, 60
Spectators, controlling, 680
Speed, emergency vehicles, 656
Sphygmomanometer, 84, 184
Spider bites, 404
Spinal column, 74–75, 550
Spinal cord, 551–52
Spinal injuries, 552–69
    emergency care, 565–69
    and head injuries, 620–21
    and hypothermia, 390
    and immobilization, 557–69
    mechanisms of injury, 552–53, 554
    patient assessment, 553–57
    See also Immobilization
Spine:
    anatomy of, 550–51
    manual stabilization of, 168
Spine boards, 280–81
Spine and head injury centers, 13
Splinting, 527–44
    ankle injuries, 535–36
    arm injuries, 532, 539
    bipolar traction splint, applying, 540–42
    elbow injuries, 535
    femur injuries, 533–34
    foot injuries, 533
    forearm injuries, 532, 539
    general guidelines for, 528–31
    hand injuries, 532–33, 539
    hip injuries, 534–35
    improvised splints, 528
    incorrect, consequences of, 527
    joint injuries, 534–35, 544
    long bone injuries, 532–44
    lower-leg injuries, 533
    pelvic injuries, 534–35

pneumatic anti–shock garments (PASGs), 528
pneumatic splints, 528
purpose of, 527
realigning injured extremities, 531–32
rigid splints, 528, 532, 533
shoulder injuries, 535
sling and swathe, 528, 532, 535
    applying, 537–38
step-down injuries, 535–36
thigh injuries, 533–34
traction splints, 528, 533–34, 540
unipolar traction splint, applying, 543
wrist injuries, 532–33, 539
Splints, types of, 527–28
Spontaneous abortion (miscarriage), 434–35
    emergency care, 434–35
Sports activity beverages, and fluid replacement, 711
Sprains, 524
Stab wounds, 469
Stages of labor, 415–16
Staging, 31, 146
Staging sector, 745, 750–52
Stair chair, 279–80
Stairs, carrying techniques on, 266
Standard disinfection, 663
Standards, EMS system, 6–8
Standing orders, 11
Standing takedown (three rescuers), 573
Standing takedown (two rescuers), 574
"Star of Life" symbol, 6
Status epilepticus, 356
Stellate lacerations, 487
Step chocks, 676
Step-down injuries, 535–36
Sterilization, 45, 663–64
Sternum, 75
Stifneck cervical collar, 561
Stoma, 111–12
Storage bins, 726
Storage tanks, 726
Strains, 524
Stress, 21–24
    burnout, 24
    family and friends' responses, 24–25
    as firefighting hazard, 24
    stressful situations, 21–24
    stress management, 24
        critical incident, 25–26
Stridor, 613
Strokes, See Cerebrovascular accidents (CVAs)
Stylet, 768–69, 774
Subcutaneous layer, 90
Subcutaneous layers, 484
Sucking chest wound, emergency care, 495–96
Suction catheters, 120–21
Suctioning the airway, 602, 763
Suctioning/suction devices, 118–21
    mounted suction systems, 118
    portable suction units, 118–19
    suctioning techniques, 120–21
    suction tips, 119
    tubing, 119

Sudden infant death syndrome (SIDS), 618
Suicide, 448–49
  scene safety, 449
Superficial thickness burns, 503–4
Superior, use of term, 70
Superior vena cava, 85
Supine hypotensive syndrome, 415
Supine patient transfer, 272
Supine position, 71
Supplemental oxygen, 606–7
  importance of, 121–24
  for infants/children, 606–7
Supply sector, 745
Surface anatomy, 68
Surgilube®, and endotracheal tube
  insertion, 768
Suspected crime scenes, 63
Symptoms, 178
Syncope, 326
  in geriatric patients, 639
Syringe esophageal intubation detector
  devices, 776
System maintenance, 234
Systolic blood pressure, 86, 183

T

Tachycardia, 181, 326
  ventricular (V-Tach), 333
Tarsal bones, 519
T-bone crashes, and geriatric patients, 637
Temperature regulation, mechanisms of,
  387–88
Temporal region, scalp, 74–75, 550
Tendons, 76, 521
Tension pneumothorax, 496
Tertiary blast injuries, 160
Thigh injuries, splinting, 533–34
Thoracic vertebrae, 75, 551
Thorax, 75
Thyroid cartilage, 760
Tibia, 75, 519
Tiered response systems, 255–56
Tone of voice, in interpersonal
  communication, 230
Tonsil sucker, 119
Tonsil-tip, 119
Tool staging, 687
Topographic anatomy, 68
Torso, 71
Tort, 53
Total quality management (TQM), 12
Touching a patient, 229
Tourniquets, 465–68
Toxic inhalation, signs/symptoms of, 315
Trachea, 77, 303, 600, 760
Tracheostomy tubes, 111–12
  and pediatric patients, 625–26
Traction splints, 528, 533–34, 540
Trade name, 289
Traffic hazards, 678–80
  positioning flares/cones, 680–81
Traffic signals, emergency vehicles, 656
Training, 8
Transition of care, 255, 381, 660–61
  air medical transport, 666

  and air medical transport, 666
  aviation crews, 259
  bystander care, 258–59
  childbirth, 419
  procedures, 256–58
  snakebites, 405
  special circumstances in, 258–59
Transportation, 8
Transportation sector, 747, 750–52
Trauma:
  in geriatric patients:
    falls, 636–37
    head injuries, 638–39
    motor vehicle crashes, 637
  in infants/children, 618–22
    bicycle-related injuries, 619
    burns, 619
    car vs. pedestrian injuries, 619
    head injuries, 619–22
    neck injuries, 619
    seat belt injuries, 618–19
  and musculoskeletal system, 521–27
  in pregnancy, 436–37
    emergency care, 436–37
  to female external genitalia, 437–38
Trauma centers, 13
Trauma intubation, assisting with, 799–800
Trauma patients:
  ALS support, requesting, 200
  baseline vital signs, assessing, 201–4
  detailed physical examination, 197–223
  mental status, reassessing, 201
  with no significant mechanism of injury,
    210–16
    detailed physical examination, 217–18
    focused physical examination, 216–17
    SAMPLE history, 217
    vital signs, 217
  ongoing assessment, 218–21
    in practice, 219–21
    steps of, 218
    trending of assessment components,
      218–19
    when to perform, 219
  rapid trauma assessment, performing, 201
  reconsidering mechanism of injury in,
    198–99
  SAMPLE history, obtaining, 204–10
  with significant mechanism of injury,
    199–210, 221
    detailed physical examination, 210
  spinal stabilization, continuing, 200
  transport decision, reconsidering, 200–201
Trauma systems, 8
Traumatic asphyxia, 486
Treatment guidelines, 11
Treatment sector, 747
Trench collapses, 727–28
Trendelenburg position, 73
Trending, 218–19
Triage, 708–9, 747–50
  initial, 747–49
  patient identification, 749
  secondary, 749–50
Triage nurse, 13
Triage sector, 747–50
Triangular bandages, 491

Trimesters, 414
Tripod position, 307
Truck fires, 684
Tuberculosis:
  guidelines, 46–47
  populations at high risk for, 42
Tubing, suction unit, 119
Turning, emergency vehicles, 656
Twisting force, and musculoskeletal injuries,
  524
Two-person bag–valve mask, 105
Two-rescuer BVM ventilation, 108–10
Type I diabetics, 351–52
Type II diabetics, 352

U

Ulna, 76, 520
Umbilical cord, 414
  cutting, 425–27
  prolapsed, 429–30
    emergency care, 429–30
Underground vaults, 726
Unipolar traction splint, applying, 543
Universal dressing, 490
Universal number, 8
Unresponsive patient:
  clearing airway of, 170
  detailed physical examination of, 194
Upper extremities, 71, 522
Urgent moves, 269
Urinary system, 91
U.S. Department of Transportation,
  labels/placards, 735–36
Uterus, 413, 414–16
  change in size of, during pregnancy, 414

V

Vacuum splints, 465
Vagina, 413
Vaginal bleeding, 437
  late in pregnancy, 435–36
    emergency care, 436
Vallecula, 760
Vascular system, 84–85
Vehicle check, 651
Vehicle fires, 683–84
  bumpers, 683
  in engine compartment, 683
  in passenger compartment, 683
  truck fire, 684
  under vehicle, 683–84
Vehicle inspection, 654
Vehicle rescue, 674–86
  body protection, 678
  electrical hazards, 680–83
    broken utility pole with wires down,
      682
    broken utility pole with wires intact,
      683
    damaged pad-mounted transformer, 683
  electrical system of vehicle, 684–85
  eye protection, 678

hand protection, 678
hazards:
    recognizing/managing, 675–85
    safeguarding patient from, 678
    safeguarding yourself from, 677–78
and headgear, 677–78
and helmets, 677–78
scene safety, 675–77
scene size-up, 674–75
spectators, controlling, 680
stabilizing the vehicle, 685–86
tools for, 674
traffic hazards, 678–80
    positioning flares/cones, 680–81
training for, 674
vehicle fires, 683–84
Veins, 85, 461
Velcro® name tags, 707
Venom, 403
Venous bleeding, 463
Ventilation, 105
   See also Artificial ventilation
Ventolin®, 311
Ventral, use of term, 69–70
Ventricles, 81, 322–23
Ventricular fibrillation (VF/V–Fib), 83–84,
    333
Ventricular tachycardia (V-Tach), 333
Ventricular (VF/V–Fib) fibrillation, 83–84, 333
Venules, 85
Vertebrae, 75, 550
Violence, 30–31
Visual imagery techniques, and stress, 24
Visually impaired patients, communicating
    with, 232

Vital signs, 180–87
    baseline, 144–45, 177, 180
    blood pressure, 183–85
    and cardiac compromise, 325–26
    pulse, 180–82
    pupils, 186–88
    respirations, 182–83
    skin, 185–86
    trauma patients, 217
Voice box, 77
Voluntary muscles, 76, 521, 551
Vomiting, and orotracheal intubation,
    764

W

Wafarin, 462
Warm (yellow) zones, 734
Warning lights, emergency vehicles, 656
Water containers, suction units, 120
Water-related emergencies, 398–403
    drowning, 398, 399–400
    emergency care, 399–400
    ice rescue, 400–402
    near-drowning, 398, 399–400
    SCUBA diving emergencies, 402–3
        ascent-related barotrauma, 402
        decompression sickness (DCS), 402–3
        descent-related barotrauma, 402
        emergency care, 403
Water-related hazards, 718–23
    alcohol consumption, 719
    extremity entrapment, 721
    moving water, force of, 719–21

    personal flotation devices, failure to use,
        718
    rescue from moving water, 721–23
    river features, 719–21
        holes/hydraulics, 719
        low head dams, 719–21
        strainers/river obstructions, 719
    water temperature, 718–19
Well-being, EMT, 19–33
Wells, 726
Wheeled ambulance stretcher, 276–77
    loading, 278
White blood cells, 85, 461
White Paper, The, 5
Wide-bore, rigid–tipped suction device, 105
Windpipe, 77
Work practice controls, establishing, 24
Work schedule, and stress, 24
Wrist, 76
Wrist injuries, splinting, 532–33, 539

X

Xiphoid process, 75

Y

Yankauer suction device, 105, 119

Z

Zygomatic bones, 74, 550